WG142 SIL V. 2

Volume 2

CARDIOVASCULAR PATHOLOGY

Second Edition

Volume 2

CARDIOVASCULAR PATHOLOGY

Second Edition

Edited by

Malcolm D. Silver, M.D., Ph.D.,
M.Sc., M.B.B.S.
Chair
Department of Pathology
University of Toronto Faculty of Medicine
Chief
Department of Pathology
The Toronto Hospital
Toronto, Ontario, Canada

CHURCHILL LIVINGSTONE
New York, Edinburgh, London, Melbourne, Tokyo

Library of Congress Cataloging-in-Publication Data

Cardiovascular pathology / edited by Malcolm D. Silver.—2nd ed.

    p.   cm.

  Includes bibliographical references and index.

  ISBN 0-443-08664-8

  1. Cardiovascular system—Diseases. I. Silver, Malcolm D.

  [DNLM: 1. Cardiovascular Diseases—pathology. WG 142 C264]

RC669.9.C37 1991b

DNLM/DLC

for Library of Congress   91-8294

                                                CIP

Second Edition © Churchill Livingstone Inc. 1991
First Edition © Churchill Livingstone Inc. 1983

Distributed in the United Kingdom by Churchill Livingstone, Robert Stevenson House, 1–3 Baxter's Place, Leith Walk, Edinburgh EH1 3AF, and by associated companies, branches, and representatives throughout the world.

Accurate indications, adverse reactions, and dosage schedules for drugs are provided in this book, but it is possible that they may change. The reader is urged to review the package information data of the manufacturers of the medications mentioned.

The Publishers have made every effort to trace the copyright holders for borrowed material. If they have inadvertently overlooked any, they will be pleased to make the necessary arrangements at the first opportunity.

Acquisitions Editor: *Beth Kaufman Barry*
Copy Editor: *Marian Ryan*
Production Designer: *Marci Jordan*
Production Supervisor: *Sharon Tuder*

Printed in the United States of America

First published in 1991   7 6 5 4 3 2 1

To my colleagues who have contributed to this book,
to all whose intellectual curiosity allowed
its contained knowledge to evolve,
and to my wife, children, and late parents

Contributors

James B. Atkinson, M.D., Ph.D.
Associate Professor, Department of Pathology, Vanderbilt University School of Medicine, Nashville, Tennessee

Giorgio Baroldi, M.D.
Chairman, Division of Cardiovascular Pathology, and Professor, Department of Pathology, University of Milan Medical School; Director, Department of Cardiology, Institute of Clinical Physiology CNR, Niguarda Hospital, Milan, Italy

Anton E. Becker, M.D.
Professor, Department of Pathology, University of Amsterdam Academic Medical Center, Amsterdam, The Netherlands

Margaret E. Billingham, M.D.
Professor, Department of Pathology, Stanford University School of Medicine; Director, Division of Cardiac Pathology, Department of Pathology, Stanford University Medical Center, Stanford, California

L. Maximilian Buja, M.D.
Professor and Chairman, Department of Pathology and Laboratory Medicine, University of Texas Medical School at Houston; Chief, Pathology Services, The Hermann Hospital and Lyndon Baines Johnson General Hospital; Director, Cardiovascular Pathology Research, St. Luke's Hospital-Texas Heart Institute, Houston, Texas

J. Butany, M.D.
Associate Professor, Department of Pathology, University of Toronto Faculty of Medicine; Staff Pathologist, Department of Pathology, The Toronto Hospital (Toronto General Division), Toronto, Ontario, Canada

David A. Chiasson, M.D.
Lecturer, Department of Pathology, University of Toronto Faculty of Medicine; Staff Pathologist, Department of Pathology, The Toronto Hospital (Toronto Western Division), Toronto, Ontario, Canada

J.A.G. Culham, M.D.
Professor, Department of Radiology, University of British Columbia Faculty of Medicine; Director, Cardiovascular and Interventional Radiology, British Columbia Children's Hospital, Vancouver, British Columbia, Canada

Giulia d'Amati, M.D.
Resident, Division of Anatomical Pathology, Department of Human Biopathology, University Lasapienza, Rome, Italy; Fellow, Division of Cardiovascular Pathology, The Toronto Hospital, Toronto, Ontario, Canada

B.N. Datta, M.D.
Professor, Department of Morbid Anatomy, Postgraduate Institute of Medical Education and Research, Chandigarh, India

Jesse E. Edwards, M.D.
Professor, Department of Pathology, University of Minnesota Medical School—Minneapolis, Minneapolis, Minnesota; Senior Consultant, Registry of Cardiovascular Disease, United Hospital, St. Paul, Minnesota

John J. Fenoglio, Jr., M.D.[*]
Associate Professor, Department of Pathology, Columbia University College of Physicians and Surgeons; Director, Department of Medical Pathology, Presbyterian Hospital, New York, New York

Victor J. Ferrans, M.D., Ph.D
Chief, Ultrastructure Section, Pathology Branch, National Heart, Lung and Blood Institute, National Institutes of Health, Bethesda, Maryland

Mervyn B. Forman, M.D.
Associate Professor, Department of Medicine, Vanderbilt University School of Medicine, Nashville, Tennessee

Robert M. Freedom, M.D.
Professor, Departments of Pediatrics and Pathology, University of Toronto Faculty of Medicine; Head, Division of Cardiology, Department of Pediatrics, The Hospital for Sick Children, Toronto, Ontario, Canada

Feroze N. Ghadially, M.D., Ph.D., D. Sc. (Lon.), M.B.B.S. (Bom.), M.B.B.S. (Lon.)
Professor Emeritus, Department of Pathology, University of Saskatchewan College of Medicine, Saskatoon, Saskatchewan; Adjunct Professor, Department of Pathology, University of Ottawa School of Medicine; Consultant, Division of Anatomical Pathology and Canadian Reference Centre for Cancer Pathology, Ottawa Civic Hospital, Ottawa, Ontario, Canada

[*]Deceased

Avrum I. Gotlieb, M.D.C.M.
Professor, Department of Pathology, University of Toronto Faculty of Medicine; Staff Pathologist, Department of Pathology, The Toronto Hospital (Toronto General Division), Toronto, Ontario, Canada

Michael G. Havenith, M.D.
Assistant Professor, Department of Pathology, University of Limburg School of Medicine; Staff Pathologist, Department of Pathology, University Hospital, Maastricht, Limburg, The Netherlands

H. Alexander Heggtveit, M.D.
Professor, Department of Pathology, McMaster University Faculty of Health Sciences; Staff Pathologist, Department of Pathology, Chedoke-McMaster Hospitals; Staff Pathologist, Department of Pathology, Hamilton General Hospital, Hamilton, Ontario, Canada

Reginald E.B. Hudson, M.D., Hon. D.Sc. (Emory), M.B.B.S.
Professor Emeritus, Department of Pathology, Institute of Cardiology, University of London; Honorary Consultant, Department of Pathology, National Heart Hospital, London, England

B. Lowell Langille, Ph.D.
Associate Professor, Department of Pathology, University of Toronto Faculty of Medicine; Staff Scientist, Department of Anatomic Pathology, The Toronto Hospital (Toronto General Division), Toronto, Ontario, Canada

J.T. Lie, M.D., M.S., M.B.B.S.
Professor, Department of Pathology, Mayo Medical School; Consultant, Departments of Pathology, Cardiovascular Diseases, and Internal Medicine, Mayo Clinic, Rochester, Minnesota

Hugh A. McAllister, Jr., M.D.
Clinical Professor, Department of Pathology, Baylor College of Medicine; Professor, Department of Pathology, University of Texas Medical School at Houston; Chief, Department of Pathology, St. Luke's Hospital-Texas Heart Institute, Houston, Texas

Eckhardt G.J. Olsen, M.D., M.B.B.S.
Consultant, Cardiovascular Division, Department of Histopathology, Royal Brompton and National Heart Hospital, London, England

Ariela Pomerance, M.D., M.B.B.S.
Consultant, Harefield and Mount Vernon Pathology Laboratories, Mount Vernon Hospital, Mount Vernon, Middlesex, England

E. René Rodríguez, M.D.
Assistant Professor, Department of Pathology, Rush Medical College of Rush University; Director, Cardiac Pathology Unit, Rush Heart Institute, Rush-Presbyterian-St. Luke's Medical Center, Chicago, Illinois

Alan G. Rose, M.D., M. Med. Path., M.B.B.S.
Professor and Chairman, Department of Pathology, University of Cape Town Medical School; Chairman, Department of Pathology, Groote Schuur Hospital, Cape Town, Republic of South Africa

Frederick J. Schoen, M.D., Ph.D.
Associate Professor, Department of Pathology, Harvard Medical School; Director, Division of Cardiac Pathology, Department of Pathology, Brigham and Women's Hospital, Boston, Massachusetts

Malcolm D. Silver, M.D., Ph.D., M.Sc., M.B.B.S.
Chair, Department of Pathology, University of Toronto Faculty of Medicine; Chief, Department of Pathology, The Toronto Hospital, Toronto, Ontario, Canada

Meredith M. Silver, M.Sc., M.B.B.S.
Associate Professor, Department of Pathology, University of Toronto Faculty of Medicine; Senior Staff Pathologist, Department of Pathology, The Hospital for Sick Children, Toronto, Ontario, Canada

C.J. Uys, M.D.
Professor Emeritus, Department of Pathology, University of Cape Town Medical School, Cape Town, Republic of South Africa

Harry V. Vinters, M.D.
Associate Professor, Department of Pathology, University of California, Los Angeles, UCLA School of Medicine; Member, Brain Research Institute, UCLA Center for Health Sciences, Los Angeles, California

Renu Virmani, M.D.
Clinical Professor, Department of Pathology, Vanderbilt University School of Medicine, Nashville, Tennessee; Clinical Professor, Department of Pathology, University of Maryland School of Medicine, Baltimore, Maryland; Clinical Professor, Department of Pathology, Georgetown University School of Medicine; Chairman, Armed Forces Institute of Pathology, Washington, D.C.

C.A. Wagenvoort, M.D.
Professor Emeritus, Department of Pathology, University of Amsterdam, Amsterdam; Honorary Consultant, Department of Pathology, Erasmus University, Rotterdam, The Netherlands

Noeke Wagenvoort
Professor, Department of Pathology, University of Amsterdam, Amsterdam, The Netherlands

Bruce F. Waller, M.D.
Professor, Department of Pathology, Indiana University School of Medicine; Member, Nasser, Smith, and Pinkerton Cardiology Group; Member, Heart Institute, St. Vincent's Hospital, Indianapolis, Indiana

Virginia M. Walley, M.D.
Clinical Assistant Professor, Department of Pathology, University of Ottawa Faculty of Medicine; Chief, Division of Anatomical Pathology, Ottawa Civic Hospital; Cardiac Pathologist, Department of Pathology, University of Ottawa Heart Institute, Ottawa, Ontario, Canada

James T. Willerson, M.D.
Edward Randall III Professor, and Chairman, Department of Internal Medicine, University of Texas Medical School at Houston; Chief, Medical Services, The Hermann Hospital and Lyndon Baines Johnson General Hospital; Director, Cardiology Research, St. Luke's Hospital-Texas Heart Institute, Houston, Texas

Gregory J. Wilson, M.D., M.Sc.
Associate Professor, Departments of Pathology, Surgery, and Physiology, University of Toronto Faculty of Medicine; Staff Pathologist, Department of Pathology, and Scientist, Research Institute, The Hospital for Sick Children, Toronto, Ontario, Canada

Preface to the Second Edition

This edition sees changes in authorship due to retirement and other considerations. In addition, I record, with great sadness, the death of John J. Fenoglio, Jr., in 1990.

The text has been revised, taking into consideration critiques of the first edition made by reviewers and many colleagues. New information and chapters have been added to deal with advances in clinical practice and, in particular, in therapeutic intervention. Also, new pathology is defined.

I am most grateful to my coauthors for their contributions to this edition. I thank interested colleagues who referred cases to me or to coauthors and so helped broaden our knowledge. The stimulus of discussion with clinical colleagues and students is invaluable in the practice of pathology.

The office staff of the Department of Pathology at the University of Toronto, particularly Julia Bella, gave me invaluable help. Again, Sophia Duda, librarian at the Banting Institute, has demonstrated that she deserves the epithet "national treasure." At Churchill Livingstone I am indebted to Beth Kaufman Barry, Marian Ryan, and Marci Jordan. My appreciation also goes to Julia Figures, who prepared the index. Finally, my thanks to Meredith Silver, for being herself.

Malcolm D. Silver

Preface to the First Edition

The idea for this book came from the continued success of the Core Curriculum Course in Acquired Heart Disease sponsored by the American College of Cardiology and arranged by Drs. Jesse E. Edwards and Maurice Lev and, lately, with the help of Dr. Saroja Bharati. Indeed, several authors of chapters have been participants in those courses.

The need for a comprehensive pathology text dealing with acquired cardiovascular disease in adults is self-evident. A discussion of congenital heart diseases, with the exception of those encountered in, or allowing survival to adulthood, has been omitted. This is a deliberate choice because congenital heart disease has its own excellent texts. Also, few individuals combine both pediatric and adult age groups in a cardiology, cardiovascular surgery, or pathology practice. In considering chapters that are included, the surgical correction or palliation of congenital heart lesions has allowed affected children to survive to adulthood and prompted a need to understand the morphological effects of such treatments. Also, new diagnostic methods (cardiac biopsies) are available and new methods of treatment have created a pathology of their own.

The book is designed to be useful to pathologists, cardiologists, and cardiovascular surgeons. It is also for clinicians, residents, and paramedical personnel who must maintain familiarity with the topics presented. For the pathologist, this book will be useful in both the surgical pathology and autopsy suites.

I wish to thank my co-authors for their contributions and my clinician colleagues in both Toronto and London, Ontario, for their enthusiasm and interest. Such enthusiasm makes the current practice of cardiology, cardiovascular surgery, and cardiovascular pathology as exciting as it is. My thanks too, to my colleagues in pathology who have allowed me to examine their interesting and often instructive cases.

It is a pleasure to acknowledge financial assistance, in the form of research grants, from the Ontario Heart Foundation. Grants from that body supported, in part, investigative studies that are reported in my chapters.

Ruth Asselin, Susan Budlovsky, Sophia Duda, and Maria Lorber at the University of Toronto and the staff of the photographic unit at Toronto General Hospital all greatly assisted me in the past and, at the University of Western Ontario, Dr. Hani Dick, Neil Falconer, Dr. Sally Ford, Hannah Koppenhoefer, and Sharon Wilton have had a similar role. I owe an especial debt to Sheila Collard for her excellent secretarial work and to my wife, Dr. Meredith M. Silver, for her ability to be, at the appropriate time, critic, inquisitor, helpmate, and goad.

I am grateful to the staff of Churchill Livingstone for their interest, cooperation, and helpfulness at all phases of the development of this book, especially Donna Balopole, Brooke Dramer, and William Schmitt.

Malcolm D. Silver

Contents

Volume 1

MYOCARDIAL DISEASES AND SUDDEN DEATH

PERICARDIAL DISEASES

Index

Volume 2

Infective Endocarditis

Malcolm D. Silver

Infective endocarditis is an inflammation of the endocardium induced by microorganisms. Morphologically, it presents with infected thrombotic vegetations. They are usually attached to the endocardium of a natural heart valve, with that valve often, although not invariably, showing evidence of an underlying congenital anomaly or acquired pathologic condition (Table 23–1). The infected vegetations may be large or small, and may or may not be associated with local destructive changes. Frequently, they are a source of either bland or infected emboli, which, with other pathologic sequelae, cause the systemic effects of the disease.

Much less frequently, infected vegetations are located on nonvalvular cardiac endocardium to produce *mural* endocarditis; least often, they are found on the intimal surface of the systemic or pulmonary arterial or venous system (*infective intimitis*). One notes, too, that infection occurs in thrombi attached to the surfaces of prostheses or patches (Fig. 23–1) inserted into the cardiovascular system for treatment (see Chs. 40 and 41) or, very rarely, in mural thrombi found in aneurysms or associated with myocardial infarction[71,95,99] (see Table 23–1).

Traditionally, clinicians classify the disease as *acute* or *subacute*, depending on its clinical course or infecting microorganism. Thus, acute endocarditis has a rapid and fulminant course whereas a subacute infection tends to be indolent, with inconspicuous or masked symptoms. Certain microorganisms, for example, *Staphylococcus aureus*, *Streptococcus pneumoniae*, *Neisseria meningitidis*, *Staphylococcus pyogenes*, and *Haemophilus influenzae* are often associated with an acute endocarditis; *Streptococcus viridans* or *Staphylococcus epidermidis* usually causes a subacute infection. This differentiation may have merit in defining the clinical course of the disease but it is not fundamental[76]: an acute endocarditis may be converted to a subacute phase by therapy, whereas subacute disease may suddenly threaten life when serious complications develop. Again, infections that usually produce a fulminant clinical course may, in some patients or circumstances, induce a subacute infective endocarditis and vice versa.

DISEASE INCIDENCE

It is uncertain whether, during the antibiotic era, the incidence of infective endocarditis has increased or decreased among adults in Western countries.[64,66,132,136] On the one hand the frequency of rheumatic valvular disease has diminished; antibiotics have been used widely to control infections, and chemoprophylaxis has been introduced for patients with congenital or acquired heart disease; on the other hand, medical and surgical practice have become much more aggressive so that invasive

Table 23–1. Cardiovascular Conditions and Infective Endocarditis

Conditions Frequently Associated with Infective Endocarditis/Intimitis	Conditions Infrequently Associated with Infective Endocarditis/Intimitis
Congenital Anomalies	Congenital Anomalies
Tetralogy of Fallot (especially if an anastomosis is created between systemic and pulmonary circulation)	Large ventricular septal defect Atrial septal defect
Ventricular septal defect (especially if small or associated with aortic regurgitation)	
Patent ductus arteriosus	
Coarctation of aorta	
Subvalvular membranous aortic stenosis	
Anomalies of heart valves (e.g., congenitally bicuspid aortic valve)	
Primum-type atrial septal defect	
Arteriovenous fistula	
Acquired Conditions	Acquired Conditions

Those causing valve incompetence, e.g.:
      Rheumatic valvular disease
      Mitral valve prolapse (irrespective of cause, but including Marfan syndrome and myxomatous degeneration)
      Calcification of mitral valve anomalies
	Those causing pure valve stenosis, especially mitral stenosis

Those causing combined valve stenosis and incompetence	
Hypertrophic cardiomyopathy	Mural thrombi in aneurysm or associated with myocardial infarcts
Prosthetic heart valves	Prosthetic arterial grafts/prostheses
Cardiac surgery	Pacemaker wires
Arteriovenous fistula	Bypass vein grafts

procedures are now used for investigation, patient monitoring, and therapy. In addition, cardiovascular surgery, hemodialysis, and immunosuppressive therapy have all become common, and, in some societies, use of narcotic drugs self-administered by the intravenous route has increased. Yet despite uncertainty about incidence infective endocarditis still occurs in Western countries and is still a medical problem, especially if it presents with minimal signs or symptoms.

There is no doubt, however, that treatment of the disease afforded by antibiotics has reduced mortality associated with it, especially that of the indolent form; that older patients are affected more frequently than in the past; that the disease often has a fulminant course; or that the types of microorganisms causing infective endocarditis have changed. For example, pneumococci and gonococci rarely cause it today while *Staphylococcus aureus* does so frequently.[64,132,136] Also, endocarditis caused by yeasts and fungi has increased in frequency, particularly associated with the use of heart-valve prostheses and long-term antibiotic therapy and with increased intravenous drug abuse. Furthermore, as rheumatic valvular disease is less often an

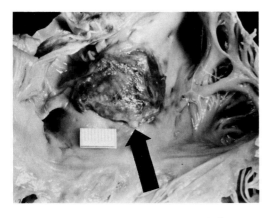

Fig. 23–1. Infective endocarditis (*Staphylococcus epidermidis*) confined to thrombus covering recently inserted pericardial patch occluding secundum-type atrial septal defect (arrow) in the right atrium of an 18-year-old male. The patient died of multiple pulmonary infarcts and abscesses. (Scale indicates 1 cm.)

underlying cause,[86] other forms of cardiac pathology have become associated with infective endocarditis more often, for example, prolapsed mitral valve[32,70,81] and hypertrophic cardiomyopathy.[124,128,132,133]

In contrast, Datta (see Ch. 33) and others[25] indicate that in Third World countries infective endocarditis is still commonly associated with rheumatic valvular disease, occurs in younger persons, is usually caused by *Streptococcus viridans* or *Staphylococcus aureus* and frequently has an indolent course. Nevertheless, in these countries too, the pattern of infective endocarditis is changing.[25,26,121]

In this chapter the pathogenesis of infective endocarditis will be presented, followed by a discussion of the pathology of the disease and its complications; its clinical manifestations and the microorganisms that cause it will be mentioned briefly; finally, infective endocarditis occurring under particular circumstances will be discussed. For greater detail on the disease occurring in infancy and childhood, the reader is referred to other sources.[52,58,62,77,89,92] A discussion of treatment is beyond the scope of this chapter.

PATHOGENESIS

In considering pathogenesis in this disease, explanations must be provided for:

1. The genesis of infected thrombotic vegetations found attached to heart valves and, if possible, the genesis of a variety of other but noninfected valvular vegetations and lesions.
2. The frequent association of infective endocarditis with certain congenital or acquired heart diseases.
3. The particular distribution of infective endocarditis, both in the heart and on heart valves.
4. The propensity of certain microorganisms to cause endocarditis frequently.

Genesis of Infected Vegetations

Current concepts regarding the pathogenesis of infective endocarditis are based on observations made on humans at autopsy and on experimental studies performed on animals.[3,41,50,90,125] These concepts are illustrated in Fig. 23–2.

A variety of noxious stimuli, of which blood turbulence may be a major one and trauma another, are thought to injure the endocardium or intima (see also Ch. 7). They initiate formation of sterile platelet-fibrin masses (nonbacterial thrombotic endocarditis), such as the mass that develops in a blood vessel as a hemostatic plug after vascular injury.[89]

Nonbacterial Thrombotic Endocarditis

In nonbacterial thrombotic endocarditis (NBTE), thrombotic vegetations that do not contain microorganisms develop on heart valves.[4,57,78–80] They are found in 1 to 2 percent of patients at autopsy (range 0.3 to 9.3 percent), are usually larger than the 1 to 2 mm diameter vegetations found in acute rheumatic fever (see Ch. 24), and are most fre-

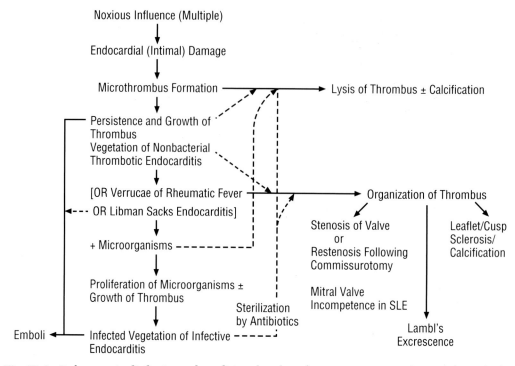

Fig. 23–2. Pathogenesis of infective endocarditis, other thrombotic vegetations, and some other valvular changes. Solid line arrows indicate progression of events to explain pathologic findings. Interrupted line arrows indicate possible progression of events. Verrucae of rheumatic fever are probably very rarely infected.

quently attached at the line of closure. They may be smooth-surfaced and firmly attached, or become quite bulky, nodular, and friable and spread over the adjacent surface of a cusp (Figs. 5–12, 23–3A). "Kissing" lesions affect adjacent sides of cusps and, in the aortic valve, individual lesions may be found attached to the nodulus Arantii at the midpoint of each cusp. The aortic valve is most often affected singly, followed in frequency by mitral and tricuspid valves. Multiple valve involvement is not infrequent. (NBTE is also discussed in Ch. 28.)

NBTE may occur at any age but most commonly affects patients from the fourth through eighth decades. It affects the sexes equally.

Histologically, vegetations consist of platelets admixed with fibrin and red blood cells, initially (Fig. 23–3B). The adjacent valve may show little damage or may contain fibrin material and a few leukocytes (mainly polymorphonuclear leukocytes [PMN]) and show destruction of connective tissue components. Subsequently, in healing, endothelium may grow across the surface of the vegetations and the thrombus may organize. They may also calcify.

Many examples of NBTE are found incidentally at autopsy and are throught to have developed during the terminal part of the patient's life. However, vegetations may be present for some time before death and act

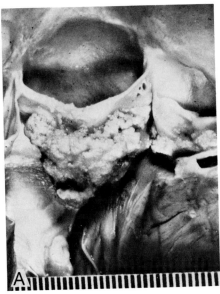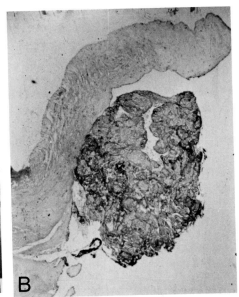

Fig. 23–3. Gross (scale marked in mm) (**A**) and microscopic (**B**) appearance of nonbacterial thrombotic endocarditis on an aortic valve cusp of a 68-year-old woman with metastatic adenocarcinoma of the pancreas. She had cerebral symptoms, thought to be caused by emboli, 7 days before she died. (H&E, × 4.) (Courtesy of M. M. Silver, M.D., Toronto.)

as a source of bland thromboemboli that cause clinical symptoms or signs[54] or kill the patient.[45,93] Lopez et al. put the incidence of visceral emboli in NBTE at approximately 42 percent.[79] Alternatively, the vegetations could become infected. A pathologist finding the lesions incidentally at autopsy must assume that they are infected until it is proven otherwise (see below).

Pathogenesis

The exact pathogenesis of NBTE is not known but it may be related to endothelial "injury" and loss. A percentage (50 percent) of cases develop in patients with hypercoagulable states or disseminated intravascular coagulation (DIC), suggesting a causal relationship.[4,67] The lesions are not seen infrequently in patients with terminal malignant disease, especially those with mucin-producing adenocarcinoma of the lung, pancreas, or colon,[111] and in association with other clinical conditions.[1,13] Occasionally, NBTE lesions in

patients with malignant disease contain tumor emboli.

The verrucae of acute rheumatic fever and the endocarditis of systemic lupus erythematosus (SLE) are examples of NBTE (see Ch. 30 and Fig. 30–26).

Considering the pathogenesis of thrombotic vegetations on valves in patients with SLE (Libman-Sacks endocarditis) and of valvular heart disease in general, the observations of the Fords and their colleagues are of interest.[47,48] The circulating lupus anticoagulant has been associated with an increased tendency to both venous and atrial thrombosis.[37,88] P. Ford and associates reported two cases of SLE with hemodynamically significant mitral valve dysfunction and associated lupus anticoagulant.[47] Both patients had their mitral valves replaced surgically, and both valves showed vegetations of Libman-Sacks type with calcification, fibrosis, and minimal commissural fusion. One valve was further occluded by a mass of thrombus attached to the subvalvular apparatus; it almost occluded the lumen. The second patient developed a thrombotic obstruction of a prosthetic valve 4 years after replacement. The authors indicated that phospholipid antibodies react in vitro with both platelets and endothelial cell surfaces and postulated that enhanced platelet aggregation or endothelial cell damage might promote coagulation in vivo.

In a subsequent study, S. Ford and colleagues looked for antiphospholipid antibodies in 48 consecutive patients undergoing prosthetic valve replacement.[48] Of the whole group, 15 (31%) had antibody levels > 2 SD above the mean for the control group and 11 (23%) had a level > 3 SD. There was an increased frequency of elevated antibody levels in patients with valves that were fibrocalcific and a significant association between antiphospholipid antibody and valve thrombosis. This striking association between valvular heart disease and the presence of elevated phospholipid antibodies in patients without SLE was strongest when viewed in relationship with the pathologic type of valve lesion rather than a morphologic designation in that 14 of 38 fibrocalcific valves were positive compared to 1 of 9 pliable valves. The authors are of the opinion that this finding tends to support the previous suggestion, both in patients with and without SLE, that the procoagulant effect of the phospholipid antibody promotes valve thrombosis, the organization of which results in fibrosis and calcification.

The authors indicate that these observations do not define whether the antibody alone can cause heart valve damage or whether a larger population with some predisposing heart valve lesion contains a subset of patients who have, by chance, acquired phospholipid antibodies that compound existing damage. Another possibility is that pre-existing heart valve lesions excite production of phospholipid antibodies by exposure of antigens in damaged endothelium, and endocardial basement-membrane that then may exert a prothrombotic effect.

This presence of a procoagulant state in a subset of patients with valvular heart disease is of interest, not only in terms of pathogenesis but also of thromboembolic complication before and after surgery.

NBTE vegetations on tricuspid and pulmonary valves are a common finding at autopsy in patients who had central venous lines or Swan-Ganz catheters. They, too, can be a source of emboli but, because they are small and enter the pulmonary system, rarely cause symptoms. The emboli can be demonstrated in histologic sections of the lung (see also Ch. 36).

Fate of NBTE Vegetations

The sterile thrombus on a valve may subsequently lyse or persist and increase in size and/or embolize, organize, calcify, or become infected.

Lysis. Possibly the injury-thrombus-lysis cycle is a continual one, occurring on heart valves and in the vascular system throughout a person's lifetime. Studies suggesting that minute thrombi are frequently found attached to the surface of human mitral valves support this concept.[56]

The vegetations of NBTE in its various clinical and morphologic forms and those of infective endocarditis sterilized by antibiotic therapy heal, in part, by lysis.

Organization and Calcification. The injury-thrombus-lysis cycle may be modified and the NBTE vegetation may organize. If these processes are repetitive, they could cause thickening of valvular tissue, stenosis of a damaged valve, or restenosis of a valve that had undergone previous surgical commissurotomy or repair (see above and Ch. 24). Also, Lambl's excrescences are probably produced by organization of such thrombi (see Ch. 5 and Figs. 5–43 and 5–44).

Organization may also occur as part of the healing mechanism in NBTE or cured infective endocarditis and lead to valve stenosis.[110] This process, by causing adhesions between NBTE vegetations of SLE found on the mitral valve and the adjacent mural endocardium, results in valvular incompetence in patients treated with steroids (see Chs. 25 and 30). A similar mechanism might cause adherence of valve tissue to endocardial friction lesion (see Ch. 5).

Infection of Thrombus

If microorganisms are present in the blood-stream, they may settle on the thrombi attached to the heart valves. If they do, the infected thrombi may still lyse and no infection results. However, if the microorganisms find a suitable milieu, they can grow and induce further thrombus formation to produce vegetations of infective endocarditis. This injury-thrombus-infection mechanism obviates a need to postulate that infective endocarditis is the result of a blood-borne infection carried into the valve substance through small blood vessels that exist in the base of normal cusps and are present in increased numbers in those thickened by pathologic processes. If that process occurs, it must be extremely rare.

Weinstein[132] agrees that the injury-thrombus-infection pathways is probably the mechanism in valvular infections that are clinically indolent. However, he implies that the presence of a sterile platelet-fibrin thrombus may not be necessary in the pathogenesis of clinically acute infective endocarditis. In the latter condition more than half the cases seem to develop on previously *normal* heart valves. The author postulates that, because microorganisms responsible for the acute infection are highly invasive, only a small number are required to establish an infection. Therefore, in Weinstein's opinion, a critical requirement is a bacteremia caused by an invasive organism and a sterile thrombus has little, if any, role in the pathogenesis of an acute infection. This seems reasonable if one believes that microorganisms attach to *abnormal* or *altered* endothelial cells. Whatever induces the abnormality would foster adherence by some microorganisms or promote thrombic formation, thereby facilitating adherence of other microorganisms to the resultant platelet-fibrin matrix. However, we know that platelets interact with particular matter (latex particles) in the bloodstream[53] and that, with the release of chemical factors from platelets, endothelial cell injury is likely.[91] Furthermore, it is known that heart valves respond rapidly to noxious stimuli.[5] Therefore, it may be unnecessary to postulate a different mechanism to explain the pathogenesis of acute infective endocarditis affecting normal heart valves. We return to this subject subsequently.

Associated Cardiovascular Diseases

Clinically, certain congenital and acquired heart conditions predispose the sufferer to infective endocarditis (see Table 23–1). In general, the infection occurs more frequently in hearts with valvular incompetence than in those with valvular stenosis.[35,51,106] Nevertheless, stenosed valves do become infected. Also, the risk is increased where a high-pressure jet of blood impinges on the endocardium or on the intima of a vessel. The reasons for these associations are now discussed.

Central to any concept of pathogenesis is a need to explain why:

1. Infective endocarditis is most often found affecting valves on the left side of the heart or at sites where a high-pressure jet of blood impinges on a chamber or vessel wall.
2. The disease is seen more often associated with valves that are incompetent than stenosed.
3. Both bland (NBTE) and infected vegetations occur characteristically on the atrial aspect of atrioventricular valves and on the ventricular aspect of semilunar valves, usually in relation to a valve's line of closure.

Again, hemodynamic factors seem to have an important role. In more than 1,000 autopsied cases reported in the literature Lepeschkin correlated the impact of pressure on heart valves with the frequency with which infective endocarditis affected them. Most frequently, the mitral valve was affected (86 percent of cases), followed in sequence by the aortic (55 percent), tricuspid (19.6 percent), and pulmonary (1.1 percent) valve. The author argued that mechanical stress was an important factor influencing the location of an infection because the average blood pressure on the mitral valve is 116 mgHg, and on the pulmonary valve 5 mmHg. Lepeschkin's study was done in 1952; many of the infected mitral valves reported in the literature and used in the study were likely damaged by rheumatic valvular disease. This indicates too that altered hemodynamics, associated with a heart valve damaged as a result of a congenital or an acquired condition, could increase the likelihood of endocardial damage and thus of infection, an association that is well-recognized in clinical practice.

Other experimental studies indicate that, if an infected fluid is forced at high pressure through a constriction, microorganisms settle out maximally and in a collarlike arrangement in the low-pressure "sink" immediately beyond the constriction.[110] Rodbard used this observation to explain the location of infected lesions on heart valves. His theory demands a minor degree of valvular incompetence so that, for instance, the atrial aspect of the mitral valve is a sink for the high-pressure left ventricle and the left ventricle a sink for the high-pressure aorta. In those circumstances microorganisms settle preferentially at sites where infected vegetations are found most commonly, that is, on the atrial aspect of atrioventricular-valves and on the ventricular aspect of semilunar valves in relation to a valve's line of closure. Rodbard used his observations to explain infected lesions found elsewhere in the vascular system—particularly, for example, on the downstream wall of the aorta in coarctation; "at the lips of the stenosis immediately distal to the coarctation," on the pulmonary artery wall immediately distal to the ostium of a patent ductus arteriosus, and on the right ventricular wall just beyond the ostium of a ventricular septal defect.[110] Also, in considering the localization of infected lesions associated with high pressure jets of blood it must be remembered that where the jet impacts, the endothelium/intima is damaged, increasing the risk of a subsequent infection at that site (see Fig. 23–2). The latter are called "satellite" lesions. Thus, MacCallum's patch in the left atrium may become infected in mitral regurgitation,[55,105] as may the ventricular surface of the anterior leaflet of the mitral valve in aortic regurgitation (see Ch. 27), the right ventricular wall or tricuspid valve leaflets opposite a ventricular septal defect (see Ch. 45), aortic valve cusps distal to a congenital subvalvular membranous stenosis (see Ch. 26), or the venous wall opposite an arteriovenous fistula. If there is a low-pressure jet of blood, as occurs in an atrial septal defect, associated infections are extremely rare. Presumably, the jet dissipates and does not impinge on the wall endocardium.

Microorganisms

Theoretically, any microorganism or bloodborne parasite (see Ch. 34) may induce infective endocarditis. Practically, certain microorganisms, and in particular gram-positive cocci, do so with a much greater frequency than others. For an infection to occur, an organism must:

1. Gain entry to the bloodstream.
2. Circumvent host defense mechanisms.
3. Adhere to a thrombus attached to a heart valve or, if Weinstein[132] is correct, to the valve itself.
4. Find a satisfactory milieu there in which to proliferate, while becoming covered by a fibrin-platelet thrombus to protect it against body defenses.

Entry of Microorganisms into Bloodstream

Usually microorganisms enter the bloodstream through lymphatics or by crossing a vessel wall.[40,77] The latter occurs directly or during injection of contaminated material explaining the frequency of infective endocarditis in those using intravenous drug administration in addiction. Rarely, infective endocarditis develops as a result of a foreign body penetrating the heart[84] following cardiac catheterization or other invasive procedure, or is introduced into the cardiovascular system during surgery. An infected mural thrombus formed as part of an infection may also act as a source of microorganisms.

In fact, spontaneously occurring transient bacteremias are likely a recurrent event in all human beings, the body having efficient defense mechanisms to control them and to prevent infection.[44] It is known that transient bacteremias occur in certain infections (e.g., pneumococcal pneumonia[10]) or following manipulative procedures done where microorganisms are normally found (e.g., tooth extraction[29]; sigmoidoscopy[73]; urinary tract manipulation[126]) and, clinically, that such events often precede the onset of infective endocarditis. In other cases a preexisting infection—e.g., in a decubitus ulcer, skin lesion following burns, or peritonitis—may be related microbiologically to that on a heart valve. Furthermore, certain invasive/therapeutic procedures increase the risk of infection. These include hemodialysis,[31] hyperalimentation (especially of candidal infections), and corticosteroid/or chemotherapy. Weinstein provides a lengthy list of procedures and conditions associated with infective endocarditis.[131] However, in some cases of infective endocarditis an obvious source of infecting organisms may not be apparent.

Circumvention of Host Defense Mechanisms

If, as is believed, both bacteremias and endocardial damage to heart valves are repeated and not rare events, one might ask why infective endocarditis does not occur more frequently? Obviously, the type of microorganism invading the bloodstream is im-

portant (see below) as is the dose. To survive in the bloodstream and cause an infection a microorganism must be able to deal with host defense mechanisms.[82] For example, determinants of pathogenecity among those causing infective endocarditis in experimental animals are (1) the microorganism's susceptibility to the cidal activity of serum complement; (2) its ability to circumvent immunoglobulin-mediated clearance; and (3) whether the microorganism triggers platelet aggregation—those that do are cleared from the blood more rapidly than those that do not.[125] (See subsequent discussion.)

Adherence of Microorganisms to a Heart Valve

The cell envelope of a microorganism is a complex structure, with its composition and organization differing from one species to another. These differences are reflected not only in an organism's Gram staining but also in its ability to adhere to cell surfaces and induce disease.[96] As Jann and Jann and the coauthors of the monograph that they edited indicate, bacterial adhesion is a surface phenomenon that, with very few exceptions, is carbohydrate specific and mediated by bacterial recognition proteins that are, according to the phenomenon studied, termed adhesive or hemagglutinin—the term "lectin" is sometimes used.[59] Adhesins may occur as structural subunits of fimbriae and form fimbriae that are mono- or multifunctional linear adhesion polymers. Other adhesins do not form recognizable structures and are tentatively called nonfimbrial. Adhesins may be components of bacterial cell walls; adhesion receptor specificities have been unraveled. The study of receptor distribution in tissue reveals implications about susceptibility to infection. The sequelae of adhesion may range from the action of toxins outside the target cell to their penetration into or through the tissues. However, besides the consequences of bacterial adhesion related to infection, the results may be colonization of a mucosal surface with bacteria that are normally harmless but that, in stress situations become virulent to produce nosocomial infections.

Other surface components of bacteria promote adhesion. Of these, the best characterized as promoting adhesion to NBTE vegetations is bacterial synthesis of dextran. More than 50 percent of endocarditis-associated strains are dextran-producing. Again, the binding in vitro of S. aureus, group A streptococci and viridans streptococci is augmented by the presence of fibronectin, a plasma glycoprotein that is a major surface constituent of mammalian cells.

Patients developing infective endocarditis caused by microorganisms regarded as normal flora may well have antibodies specific for these organisms present in their bloodstream before heart valve infection.[97] Such circulating antibodies, especially agglutinins, could encourage bacteria to settle on thrombotic vegetations, clumping them and allowing sufficient numbers to settle on the thrombus or a valve. However, Sande is of the opinion that prolonged exposure of the valve to microorganisms is more critical than the effects of antibodies in the development of infective endocarditis. Exactly how bacteria adhere to thrombi is not known. They may do so directly, because of cell wall constituents as indicated above, or indirectly because platelets may be aggregated by immune complexes[119] or because macrophages in the thrombus take up organisms.[40] Alternatively, the aggregated bacteria might themselves be surrounded by sticky platelets.

Proliferation and Incorporation into Vegetations

In their review of bacterial surface components and the pathogenesis of infectious disease, Peterson and Quie indicate that a successful defense against invading microorganisms involves an integrated function of humoral and cellular systems in the host; that the defense mechanisms are influenced by components of the microorganism's surface;

and that immunoglobulins and complement are important humoral elements of host defense with the bactericidal activity of serum depending on the activation of the entire complement sequence with the formation of the "membrane attack complex (C5b-C9)".[96]

Many gram-positive bacteria are resistant to the direct killing action of these serum factors, presumably because of the nature of their peptidoglycans, but many gram-negative bacteria are serum sensitive. This may explain, in part, why gram-positive organisms are more likely to be a cause of infective endocarditis than some gram-negative ones[40]; however, it is probable that other factors, which are also likely related to the composition of the bacterial coat and which independently or severally affect adhesion to cells, chemotaxis, opsinization, phagocytosis, and microbiocidal mechanisms within leukocytes, are also involved. Furthermore, the organism must find suitable substrates and an appropriate oxygen tension in the thrombus to permit growth.

The location of microorganisms within thrombi also offers protection from the host's defense mechanisms, especially PMN. Thus, success in causing this disease may be related to an organism's ability to stimulate endothelial cells to produce thromboplastin, their ability to activate prothrombin directly, or their ability to aggregate or bind platelets.[69] Monocytes that have ingested bacteria are also a source of procoagulant activity.

Eventually, the likelihood of an individual developing infective endocarditis is a result of an interplay among infecting microorganism, a thrombus on a heart valve or the heart valve itself, and the host's defense mechanisms. Much has been learned about factors involved but much also remains to be learned. A full understanding may, in the future, provide exact means of preventing the disease. Undoubtedly, subtle changes in these interactions involving either host, microorganisms, or both also explain why organisms that do not commonly cause infective endocarditis may do so occasionally.

PATHOLOGY

The pathology of infective endocarditis results from a variable combination of effects produced by microorganisms proliferating in the bloodstream, the physical bulk of infected vegetations, and local or systemic complications of the disease with the former affecting the valve and its environs and the latter the lungs, heart, or distal organs. Atkinson and Virmani[9] provide a review.

Complications produced by infective endocarditis develop most frequently during the active stage of the disease, but they, or the symptoms induced by them, may occur subsequently.

Morphology of Vegetations

Infective endocarditis is caused by microorganisms of varying virulence. Virulence also determines, to some extent, the morphology of vegetations and that of the adjacent heart valve, in that marked destructive lesions are often noted in fulminant infections whereas less-marked destruction plus a reparative response are features of indolent ones. Host factors too are important in determining outcome in that an organism usually associated with an indolent infection may, in some persons, assume a fulminant course and vice versa.

The vegetations of infective endocarditis are most commonly found attached to the atrial aspect of atrioventricular valves and to the ventricular aspect of semilunar valves. Usually, they are related to a valve's line of closure, but if large they may involve adjacent parts of a cusp or leaflet (Fig. 23–4) or contiguous structures—e.g., chordae tendineae or the sinus of Valsalva. Rarely valvular vegetations arise de novo at a site away from the line of closure, but, if so, a pathologic reason for their origin at that site is usually obvious.

Infected vegetations occur most frequently on valves on the left side of the heart. In patients with valves previously damaged by

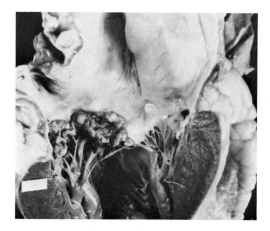

Fig. 23–4. Vegetations of infective endocarditis (*Candida albicans*) to left of picture affecting adjacent sides of anterior and posterior mitral valve leaflets producing "kissing lesions"—leaflets otherwise "normal." Patient, a 63-year-old man, had bilateral aortoiliac vascular grafts inserted and developed wound sepsis. Note large size of vegetations. (Scale indicates 1 cm.) (From Mambo et al.,[83] with permission.)

rheumatic disease, the mitral, aortic, tricuspid, and pulmonary valves are affected with decreasing frequency; an infection involving both the mitral and aortic valves is not uncommon. Nowadays ≃ 30% of infection occurs on previously normal valves.[9] When a valve is thought to be normal before an infection, the aortic valve seems involved more often than the others. However, tricuspid valve infections in drug addicts often develop on normal valves (see above discussion). Davies[33] has questioned whether such valves are indeed "normal" before the infection: in his words, "The recorded incidence of bacterial endocarditis on previously normal valves begs the question of what is normality for a valve." In general, single-valve infections are more frequent that those affecting several valves.

Vegetations vary in size, with fungal infections said to cause very large ones (Fig. 23–4). Small vegetations, or those remaining after embolization of superficial parts, may be overlooked by a pathologist, as they merely cause a focal irregularity or thickening of the line of closure. Vegetations may be gray-pink, soft, and friable, or gray, yellow-brown, and quite firm. They can have a smooth surface, but more often it is irregular or may be bosselated and appear somewhat granular. A vegetation may be single. If multiple, they may be contiguous on a single cusp or occur on different cusps in direct apposition—the so-called "kissing lesions" (Fig. 23–4). The involved cusp may have a "normal" anatomic configuration or show evidence of a congenital valvular anomaly or preexisting disease (see above).

Echocardiography can demonstrate lesions 2 to 3 mm or more in diameter.[38,120] Mügge and colleagues studied 105 patients with infective endocarditis by transthoracic and transesophageal echocardiography, correlating embolic events and in-hospital death to vegetation size.[90] A detailed comparison was made between anatomic and echocardiographic finding in a subgroup of 80 patients undergoing surgery or necropsy. The authors found that true valvular vegetations are reliably identified by echocardiography. The detection rate was better with transesophageal techniques (90 percent) than with transthoracic techniques (58 percent), especially when prosthetic valves were evaluated. However, an accurate echocardiographic differentiation between true vegetations and other endocarditis-induced valve destruction (ruptured leaflets or chordae) may be impossible. Patients with vegetations of diameters greater than 1 cm had a significantly higher incidence of embolic events than did those with vegetations of smaller diameter ($P < 0.01$). Particularly, in patients with mitral valve endocarditis, Mügge et al. were of the opinion that a vegetation larger than 1 cm in diameter was highly sensitive in identifying patients at risk for embolic events.[90] Vegetation size provided no indication of the degree of heart failure a patient had nor of the risk of death. No correlation was observed between vegetation size or location and the infecting microorganism.

Mural infections, whether in the heart or a blood vessel, present as thrombotic plaques of varying size with the variations in appearance noted above (Fig. 23–5).

A pathologist, finding such lesions at autopsy in a patient who had no clinical history to suggest an infection, is never certain whether the vegetations are infected or not. *Each should be regarded as infected until proven otherwise by microbiological and histologic examination.* Irrespective of whether a patient's history suggests an infection, such vegetations must be sampled. Swabbing them for microbiologic culture may yield a causative organism, but more constant results are likely if a fragment of the vegetation is forwarded for culture. Again, part of the vegetation must be removed to be smeared on a glass slide, or forwarded as a block for histologic examination and special stains to demonstrate microorganisms.

In such circumstances I always use both Gram and Gomori methenamine silver (GMS) stains. The combination is most useful because a GMS stain not only clearly defines fungal spores and hyphae but may also reveal cocci that have lost their staining characteristics to Gram stain, possibly as a result of an

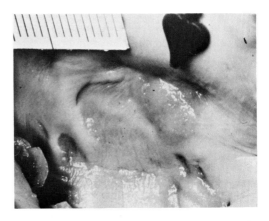

Fig. 23–5. Yellow-brown plaque of mural endocarditis (at tip of arrow) thickening endocardium and situated on the septal wall of the left atrium in a 29-year-old woman with leukemia and disseminated candidiasis. Mural endocarditis developed by spread of infection from intramyocardial abscess with formation of infected thrombotic vegetations over endocardium. (Scale indicates 1.4 cm.)

alteration in their surface coating or because they are dead. Other stains (e.g., Giemsa or Machiavello's) may also be used if particular infections (e.g., rickettsial) are suspected. If available, electron microscopy may also reveal microorganisms in thrombotic vegetations, particularly if an infection is caused by cell-wall deficient microorganisms that stain uncharacteristically with Gram's stain.[98] This procedure may help identification. The thrombotic vegetations of infective endocarditis can, with time, calcify, as may dead microorganisms. Care must be taken to distinguish between the irregularly sized granules of calcium occurring in thrombi and smaller, regularly sized calcified cocci.

Histologically and when freshly formed, vegetations consist of platelet and fibrin thrombi containing polymorphonuclear leukocytes and lesser numbers of other white blood cells. Later, the numbers of polymorphs may be more numerous at the edges of the thrombus and in the surrounding valve tissue. Colonies of bacteria or hyphae of an infecting organism may be demonstrated both at the edge of and within the thrombus. If the infection is indolent, the vegetation often shows a varying degree of organization and/or calcification (Fig. 23–6A). Chronic inflammatory cells and/or giant cells (Fig. 23–6B) also occur in the inflammatory infiltrate. Giant cells are a feature of vegetations in patients with endocarditis caused by *C. burnetti* (Q fever). Changes seen in adjacent cusp tissue are determined by preexisting lesions, are affected by the duration of the infective endocarditis, and may show changes caused by complications of the infection. Thus, a cusp may show tissue necrosis and a minimal acute inflammatory change, with edema and a polymorphonuclear leukocyte infiltrate in a virulent infection occurring on a previously normal cusp. Alternatively, evidence of both inflammation (acute, subacute, chronic, or, rarely, granulomatous) and repair and of preexisting pathology are likely in cusps infected by an organism of low virulence. Fistulae or sites of rupture may be seen.

Local Complications

Complications Caused by Vegetations

The physical bulk of vegetations can temporarily or permanently interfere with the normal function of a heart valve, especially of an

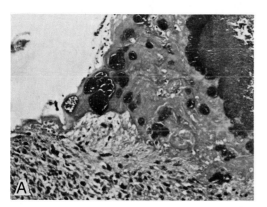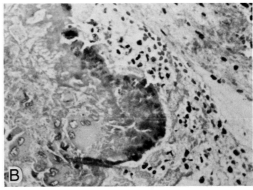

Fig. 23–6. Histology of vegetations in infective endocarditis. **(A)** Indolent infection showing clumps of coccal organisms (*Streptococcus viridans*) in thrombus to upper right of photograph. Note chronic inflammatory reaction in adjacent mitral valve leaflet. (H&E, × 40.) **(B)** Giant cell reaction in vegetation in enterococcal infection. (H&E, × 40.) Infections with *Coxiella burnetii* often produce such a giant cell response.

artificial one, causing *valvular stenosis or incompetence* and inducing transient or persistent heart murmurs and/or heart failure.[100]

Destructive Lesions

Functional disturbances also result from the local destructive effects of an infection. These usually induce valvular incompetence.

With tissue necrosis, the edge of a cusp may *ulcerate* (Fig. 23–7A), becoming ragged and irregular, or its body may be *perforated* (Fig. 23–7B). Sinus tracts may also be obvious. Such complications are not uncommon in virulent infections but also occur in indolent ones.

An infection may also weaken a cusp's fabric and lead to *aneurysm formation.* Aortic valve aneurysms are usually small (2 to 3 mm diameter) and bulge toward the left ventricle. Mitral valve aneurysms usually affect the anterior leaflet near its midpoint or base. They may be 3 to 4 mm in diameter and smooth-surfaced or have a larger orifice and a wind-sock-like appearance, with the sock being conical and several centimeters long (Figs. 23–8 and 23–9). Both types of mitral aneurysm

bulge toward the left atrium and can induce valve incompetence. An aneurysm may cause symptoms immediately or not until months or years after an infection has been successfully treated. Thus, the surgical pathologist may see these excised lesions. Occasionally, a leaflet perforation is found at the apex of such aneurysms (Fig. 23–8B).

By extending onto adjacent *chordae tendineae* or *papillary muscles* infective endocarditis may so weaken them that *rupture* results (Fig. 23–9). This is a rare event. A papillary muscle may also rupture following myocardial damage (see below). Chordal rupture and the much less common papillary muscle rupture are likely complications of virulent infections but also occur in indolent infections. In the latter instance and in my experience, rupture of chordae of the anterior mitral valve leaflet seems more common. The rupture may cause prolapse of the mitral valve. If the patient is successfully treated or has a subclinical or "missed" infection, the subsequent clinical presentation may suggest a prolapse due to myxomatous degeneration. Histologically, differentiation is usually not difficult if the valve is examined in surgical

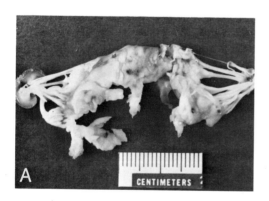 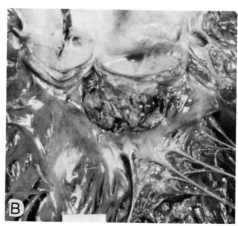

Fig. 23–7. (**A**) Surgically excised anterior mitral leaflet showing leaflet ulceration and destruction caused by Group A streptococcal endocarditis developed on a normal valve. (**B**) Acute *Staphylococcus aureus* infection on normal aortic valve cusp causing cusp perforation. (Scale indicates 1 cm.) The specimen is from a 23-year-old man who jabbed a skin pimple with a pin 5 days before presenting with acute, lethal aortic regurgitation.

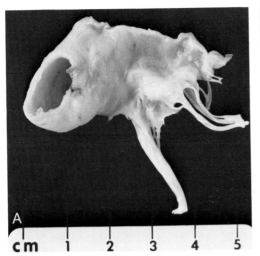 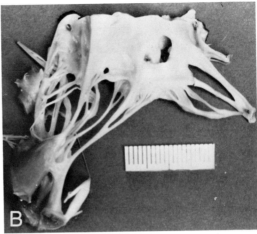

Fig. 23–8. **(A)** "Wind sock" type aneurysm of anterior leaflet of mitral valve excised surgically 1 month after an attack of infective endocarditis. The perforation at the apex of the aneurysm was increased in size during excision. (Specimen courtesy of A. Gotlieb, M.D., Toronto, Ontario.) **(B)** Ventricular ostium of a similar lesion from a second case. Mitral valve also excised surgically. (Scale indicates 2 cm.) (Specimen courtesy of N. Ranganathnan, M.D., Toronto.)

pathology or the autopsy suite. Myxomatous change is usually very marked where that condition is the cause of the prolapse and not obvious or focal where an infection has induced the prolapse. In addition, reparative changes in leaflet tissue may indicate a previous infection.

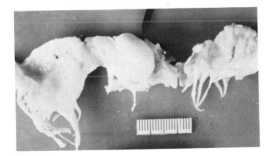

Fig. 23–9. Surgically excised mitral valve showing aneurysm (marker) of posterior leaflet following infective endocarditis. Adjacent chordae tendineae were also ruptured as a result of the infection. (Scale indicates 2 cm.) (From Russek,[113] with permission.)

Local Spread of Infection

Each of the destructive processes mentioned above, or others, may induce valve incompetence and set in motion a sequence of events that help *local spread* of an infection. For example, if an infected aortic valve is incompetent or becomes so during the infection, a regurgitant blood jet carrying microorganisms may impinge on the septal wall of the left ventricle or the ventricular aspect of the anterior mitral valve leaflet and induce *satellite infections* at these sites. The result may be a mural endocarditis, an acquired ventricular septal defect, or secondary endocarditis of the mitral valve (see also Ch. 25). In the latter instance infection starts on the ventricular aspect of the leaflet. However, subsequent complications of a satellite infection on the mitral valve may make it difficult to determine the original site of infection. In this manner too the posterior wall of the left atrium may develop a mural endocarditis when an infected mitral valve becomes incompetent. The previously mentioned *kissing lesions* on contiguous surfaces of cusps are another example of local spread.

Sinus of Valsalva Aneurysm

An aortic valve infection may spread locally to involve the sinus of Valsalva or the aortic intima. The former may induce a *sinus of Valsalva aneurysm* that bulges into surrounding tissue to produce a sinus, a fistula, or induce a bland or infected pericarditis.

Destruction of the sinus wall by infective endocarditis is not the only cause of these uncommon aneurysms, which are found mainly in middle-aged and elderly patients. Any process that weakens or destroys the sinus wall may cause a sinus of Valsalva aneurysm. Thus, they may be congenital or acquired (see Ch. 9).

The anatomic relationships of the aortic valve must be understood to appreciate the path of extension of these aneurysms and complications that may ensue (see also Ch. 27). Thus, a sinus of Valsalva aneurysm may extend distally along the aorta (Fig. 23–10A), laterally into adjacent heart tissue (Fig. 23–10B and C) or pericardium, or proximally toward the left ventricle (Fig. 23–10D).

If it extends distally it may rupture into the pericardium, the mediastinum, or the aortic lumen, inducing such complications as cardiac tamponade, sudden death, or a pseudoaneurysm. Alternatively, a sinus may be produced in the aortic wall, or a fistulous tract may develop that allows a paravalvular leak, which simulates aortic incompetence.[42]

The effect of a lateral extension of a sinus of Valsalva aneurysm depends on its site of origin. Edwards and Burchell arbitrarily divided each sinus into thirds (those related to the commissures and the middle third) and detailed the immediate anatomic relationships of each part[43] (Fig. 23–10B and C). Thus, lateral extension of an aneurysm may induce a sinus or fistula that is directed toward or reaches the epicardial surface, the right atrium (Fig. 23–11A), the right ventricle (inflow and outflow areas) (Fig. 23–11B), the

pulmonary artery, or the interatrial septum. A ventricular septal defect may be acquired by lateral extension toward the junction of right atrium and ventricle.

Lastly, a sinus of Valsalva aneurysm may extend proximally toward the left ventricle and produce a sinus that passes into ventricular muscle or a fistula that reaches right or left ventricular cavities. Because of the particular anatomic relationships, a sinus of Valsalva aneurysm extending from the posterior or left aortic cusp may destroy the conducting system and cause complete heart block, induce an acquired ventricular septal defect, or spread into the anterior leaflet of the mitral valve to cause a sinus or fistula directed toward the left atrium or left ventricle. The latter spread can produce a characteristic bulge or rupture at the base of the anterior leaflet on its atrial aspect. In this case the anterior leaflet may show no evidence of vegetation on its line of closure. Thus, a sinus of Valsalva aneurysm can cause a fistula that passes to any of the four heart chambers, to the aorta, or to the epicardium.

Annular or "Ring" Abscess

Infections on nontissue heart valve prostheses usually begin in the sewing-ring area. Such infections rapidly spread to the annular region and cause an infected sinus of Valsalva aneurysm or an *annular* or *ring abscess* (Figs. 23–11 and 23–12).[8,118] They are well-demonstrated by echocardiography. Most annular abscesses seen nowadays are associated with mechanical valve prostheses infected by virulent organisms and occur in the aortic area. However, tissue prosthetic valves may also develop annular abscesses, even though the infection in this instance is thought to commence on the valve cusps and to spread subsequently. These abscesses cause artificial heart valves to dehisce (see Fig. 23–12). Also, they burrow into surrounding tissue and, in the aortic area, their paths of spread and the sequelae they produce are like those induced by sinus of Valsalva aneurysms.

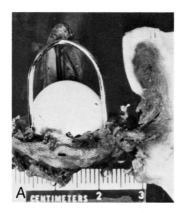

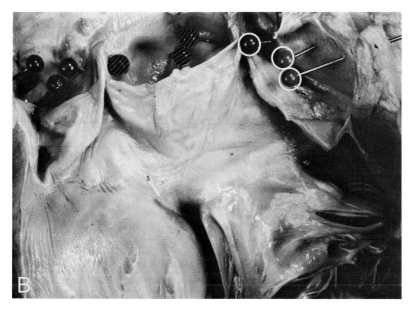

Fig. 23–10. Routes of spread of annular or ring abscesses following infective endocarditis on the aortic valve. (Note that aneurysms of Valsalva may extend by following comparable lateral or distal pathways.) **(A)** Infection (*Staphylococcus aureus*) spreading from Starr-Edwards prosthetic valve proximally in the aortic wall. This occurs rarely. It may induce a pericarditis, an external rupture, or lead to an aortico-left ventricular fistula and paravalvular leak that mimics aortic prosthesis/valve incompetence. **(B,C)** Lateral relationships of sinuses of Valsalva and the structures likely involved by spreading abscesses. Fig. B shows the outflow tract of the left ventricle. Note the close relationship between the anterior mitral valve leaflet and both posterior and left aortic valve cusps. This facilitates contiguous spread of infection from one to the other. Subsequent rupture sites may be at the base of the mitral leaflet and into the left atrium, or to atrial or ventricular aspects of the leaflet, distally. Sometimes multiple rupture sites are found. Pins have been placed through the sinuses in each of the thirds related to the commissures and at the middle third to define direction of likely spread. (*Figure continues.*)

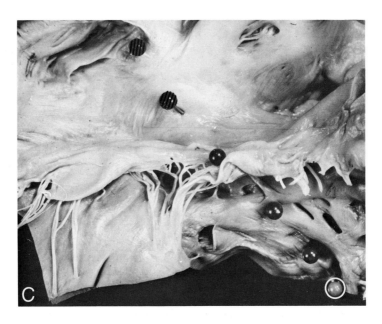

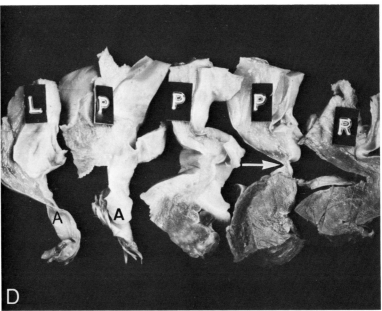

Fig. 23–10 (*Continued*). Fig. C shows that lateral spread of an infection from the left sinus (pins with white circles) may reach the pericardium and induce pericarditis or cardiac tamponade after rupture or cause fistulae between the sinus and the outflow tract of the right ventricle, the infundibulum, or pulmonary trunk (not shown). Abscesses from the posterior sinus (cross-hatched pins) pass into the right or left atria (not illustrated), while spread from the right sinus (black pins) forms fistulae passing into either the right atrium or ventricle. The latter may induce an acquired ventricular septal defect. Depending on the site of rupture the ventricular septal defect may pass into the right atrium, right ventricle, or both chambers. (**D**) Distal relationships of the aortic annulus and sinuses of Valsalva and structures likely involved if an infection spreads toward the heart apex. (L, left sinus; R, right sinus; P, posterior sinus.) Thus, an infection may spread into the left ventricular myocardium or the anterior mitral valve leaflet (Fig. A) or destroy the membranous interventricular septum (white arrow) and adjacent conducting systems, usually causing complete heart block. (Figs. **B, C,** and **D** from Russek,[113] with permission.)

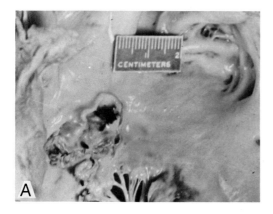
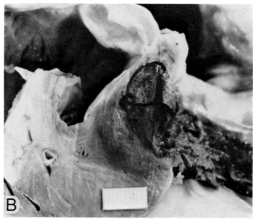

Fig. 23–11. (**A**) Fistula opening into right atrium at base of anterior mitral leaflet following spread of infection (*Staphylococcus pyogenes*) on aortic valve that induced an annular abscess in the right sinus of Valsalva. It subsequently spread laterally. (**B**) Annular abscess extending into outflow tract of right ventricle from enterococcal infection associated with aortic tissue valve prosthesis (removed for photograph). Before rupture, such lesions produce a reddish nodular elevation on the endocardial surface. They should be looked for in anatomic regions likely to be affected. (Scale indicates 1 cm.)

An annular abscess may also follow endocarditis on a natural heart valve.[18,118] They too are most commonly associated with aortic valve infections. The much less frequently occurring mitral annular abscess may spread proximally into the left atrial wall or interatrial septum, distally into the left ventricular muscle, or laterally to reach the epicardium. Most mitral annular abscesses that I have seen have spread laterally toward the epicardial surface (Fig. 23–13 & 23–18D). Such abscesses can compress a coronary artery[30] or induce an arteritis in the circumflex coronary artery, with the risk of a thrombotic occlusion and an acute myocardial infarction, a pericarditis (see Ch. 22), or a hemopericardium.

The sinuses or fistulous tracts produced by burrowing annular abscesses, irrespective of their origin, contain or are lined by thrombus. Arnett and Roberts[8] suggest that microorganisms are not demonstrated frequently in the thrombus, but this has not been my experience.

Annular abscesses rarely extend from tricuspid endocarditis. Again, an understanding of the anatomic relationships of the annulus is important in tracing their path. I have never seen an annular abscess associated with pulmonary valve endocarditis but do not doubt that they may occur.

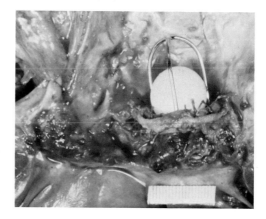

Fig. 23–12. Annular abscess developed in association with a *Candida* species infection on an aortic valve Starr-Edwards prosthesis and causing its dehiscence. (Scale indicates 2 cm.)

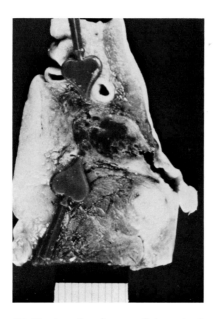

Fig. 23–13. Annular abscess of the mitral valve (defined by arrows) developed in association with annular calcification (white nodule in myocardium to right). Abscess spread laterally toward epicardium, where it produced a pericarditis. Cardiac tamponade could result if the abscess were to rupture. Note close anatomic relationship of circumflex coronary artery. In this situation it may be compressed or develop an arteritis. In the latter instance, thrombosis and a myocardial infarction would result. (Scale indicates 1 cm.)

Systemic Complications

In essence, systemic complications of infective endocarditis are caused by emboli from vegetations or by microorganisms proliferating in the bloodstream.

Embolization and Sequelae

Infected vegetations growing on heart valves are a source of emboli, particularly during the active phase of the disease and when they are friable. The emboli may be composed of bland thrombus or contain thrombus admixed with microorganisms. Rarely, fragments of damaged heart valve[18] or other cardiac tissue embolize.

Infection of right-sided valves induces emboli that pass into the pulmonary circulation and produce their sequelae in the lungs: those from left-sided heart valves pass into the systemic circulation with the brain (see also Ch. 28), heart, spleen, and kidney being common target organs. However, should an intracardiac shunt exist or develop as part of an infection, paradoxical emboli may occur or lung emboli may result from left-sided valve infections.

The effects of an embolus are related to its size and composition. Many are small and produce subclinical effects. Indeed, the extent of embolization found at autopsy in patients with infective endocarditis is usually more marked than is suggested by clinical manifestations. Other emboli cause minor or severe clinical manifestations that can be transient or permanent, and some (e.g., coronary or cerebral emboli) cause death. Recurrent embolic phenomena may be the first manifestation of infective endocarditis. In such circumstances, surgically recovered emboli must be examined with great care histologically, using Gram and GMS stains to demonstrate microorganisms. I cannot overemphasize this point, especially with regard to emboli recovered from patients bearing heart valve prostheses. By doing so, the surgical pathologist is, occasionally, the first to diagnose infective endocarditis.

Vascular occlusion produced by an embolus may be transient or permanent, and its effects may be aggravated by local vascular spasm. Pathologically the embolus may cause *ischemia* or *tissue infarction* or, if it occurs in a young person, its effects may lead to *organ atrophy*.

Infected emboli can induce localized infection where they impact. This may cause a *vasculitis* and lead to development of a *mycotic aneurysm* (Figs. 23–14 and 11–25) or, if the inflammation spreads into the tissue, formation of an *abscess* (Fig. 23–15). Generally, abscess formation is likely in virulent infections.

Mycotic aneurysms occur in cerebral, superior mesenteric (see Fig. 23–14), splenic,

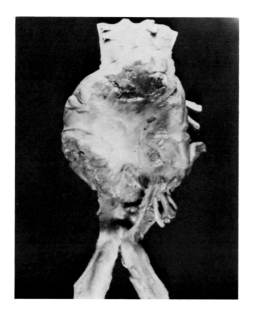

Fig. 23–14. Myotic aneurysm developed in the proximal part of the superior mesenteric artery in a 68-year-old woman. Its rupture caused the patient's death 3 months after mitral valve infective endocarditis had been successfully treated, medially.

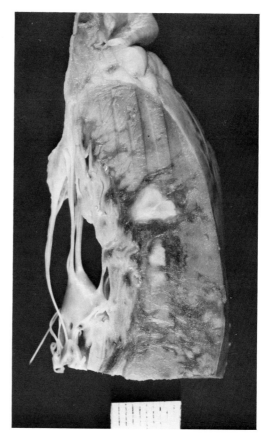

Fig. 23–15. Myocardial necrosis and abscesses developed in association with a *Staphylococcus aureus* endocarditis of the aortic valve. (Scale indicates 1 cm.) (From Russek,[113] with permission.)

coronary, and pulmonary vessels in particular, and may be multiple.[122] Most occur at vessel bifurcations, in the peripheral part of a vessel's distribution, and may not induce symptoms until long after the original infection has abated or is cured. Infective endocarditis is the most frequent precursor of these lesions[122] (see also Chs. 11 and 28). Durack and Beeson discuss the pathogenesis of mycotic aneurysms.[40]

Proliferation of Microorganisms in the Bloodstream

Microorganisms proliferating in the bloodstream cause a *bacteremia* (an important determinant in establishing a clinical diagnosis by blood culture), a *septicemia*, or stimulate *disseminated intravascular coagulation*. Because their proliferation also induces antibody formation (both a specific and nonspecific response),[97] immune-mediated disease can result (see below).

Complications Affecting Particular Organs

Heart

Most complications affecting the heart have been mentioned in this chapter, but further comment related to their particular effects on the pericardium (Ch. 22), myocardium (Ch. 19), and valves (Chs. 24–27) will be found in the chapters indicated.

Roberts illustrates that a pericarditis may follow extension of inflammation from (1) a ring abscess, (2) a mycotic aneurysm, (3) a septic arterial embolus, or (4) a myocardial abscess.[106]

It should be emphasized that infective endocarditis is a common cause of myocarditis found at autopsy (see Fig. 23–15) (see Ch. 19). Also, although heart failure in patients with infective endocarditis may be induced or aggravated by an accompanying myocarditis (particularly in aortic valve infections), the severity of congestive cardiac failure is, in the main, more closely related to the severity of associated valvular disease, especially that of valvular incompetence.

Small areas of myocardial necrosis and frank infarcts can be produced by coronary artery emboli with the complications expected in such circumstances. This may be another mechanism by which a ruptured papillary muscle develops in infective endocarditis.

Conducting system abnormalities, including complete heart block, may be directly related to destruction caused by myocarditic lesions, by the presence of a myocardial abscess, or by extension of an annular abscess.

Blood Vessels

Complications affecting small (Chs. 12 and 14) and large (Ch. 11) blood vessels in infective endocarditis are discussed in detail in the chapters indicated. Also, further information about mycotic aneurysms is found in Chapters 11 and 28.

Vascular complications are caused by several different mechanisms. A vasculitis may be caused by immunologic phenomena (likely in indolent infections), by the direct invasion of microorganisms into a vessel wall, or by their invasion following impaction of a septic embolus. Embolic occlusion of vasa vasorum could also cause a sterile infarction of a blood vessel wall.

Lungs

The characteristic lung findings in infective endocarditis are the result of bland or septic emboli producing pulmonary infarcts or abscesses. Indeed pulmonary symptoms are often the first clinical manifestations of right-sided endocarditis. Extension of the pulmonary lesions or reactions to them may affect the pleura or pericardium, inflaming them and inducing a serous effusion, an inflammatory exudate, or pus in the cavities. Bronchopleural fistulae and pulmonary mycotic aneurysms also occur.

Brain

Clinical manifestations of cerebral embolic phenomena in infective endocarditis[101,137] are most frequently caused by emboli impacting in the distribution of the middle cerebral arteries. The lesions produced may be microscopic or macroscopic, with symptoms that are transient. Embolic cerebral infarction is the most common neurologic complication of infective endocarditis, but cerebral abscesses also develop (see also Ch. 28). Embolic episodes affecting the spinal cord or peripheral nerves occur but are rare. Emboli to retinal arteries are found as a cause of sudden blindness.

Other cerebral manifestations may be due to mycotic aneurysms or result from their rupture or follow an acute septic or aseptic meningitis or meningocerebritis. Cerebral complications may be the initial presentation of infective endocarditis and can cause a patient's death.

Salgado et al. reported on a 12-year experience of neurologic complications occurring among 113 patients with native-valve endocarditis and 62 with infections on prosthetic valves.[114] The complications, which were defined as (1) cerebrovascular (stroke, transient ischemic attack, and mycotic aneurysm); (2) infectious (meningitis and abscess); and (3) nonspecific (encephalopathy, seizures, and headaches), occurred with the same frequency and distribution among the two groups. Cerebrovascular complications were the most common. *Staphylococcus aureus* endocarditis correlated statistically with the development of neurologic complications and death. The authors also concluded that mortality is not significantly increased by neurologic complication. In a follow-up study (median 2.2 years) the authors found that an episode of treated native endocarditis does not increase the natural history of stroke in valvular disease.

Kidney

Some renal complications are the direct result of bland or septic emboli, but immunologically induced glomerular disease also occurs.[72,94,135]

Embolic Complications

The incidence of renal infarctions at necropsy varies from series to series (38 to 91 percent), depending on the inclusion of microscopic lesions in the analysis. Tiny emboli can produce focal infarcts in glomeruli, but most focal glomerular lesions are thought to be the result of immune complex disease. It is unusual in infective endocarditis for renal infarcts to cause such severe renal damage that renal failure ensues. Septic emboli can induce abscess formation.

Immunologically Induced Glomerular Disease

Glomerular damage, caused by immunological mechanisms, may be the result of a direct action against glomerular basement membrane, or it can be produced by immune complexes. Current concepts favor the latter mechanism in the glomerulonephritis occurring in infective endocarditis. Bayer et al.[14] found circulating immunocomplexes in 28 of 29 patients with infective endocarditis. The lesions produced may be focal or diffuse.

Focal glomerulitis is segmental in the glomerulus (Fig. 23–16) and focal in that not all glomeruli are damaged. This form of the disease is seen particularly in indolent infections (antibody excess giving rise to large complexes). Usually, less than half the glomeruli visualized in histologic section are affected, but renal failure may ensue if the majority are damaged. Often, lesions are of varying age. Initially, an area of necrosis is seen accompanied by a polymorphonuclear leukocyte exudate, fibrin thrombi in adjacent capillaries, and swelling and proliferation of both endothelial and mesangial cells. Synechiae may form between the tuft and Bowman's capsule,

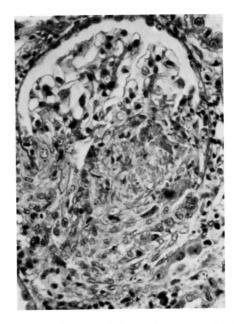

Fig. 23–16. Segmental glomerulonephritis developed in association with indolent *Streptococcus viridans* infection on a mitral valve affected by rheumatic valvular disease.

and occasionally crescents form. In the later stage scar develops. Electronmicroscopically, electron-dense deposits may or may not be demonstrable in the mesangium, within the basement membrane and subendothelial. It is likely that treatment with antibiotics has reduced the frequency of this complication.

The diffuse glomerulonephritis seen in infective endocarditis has the histology of an acute diffuse endocapillary glomerulonephritis of any cause. (It is caused by an antigen excess with small complexes.) Ultrastructurally, electron-dense deposits are usually observed between endothelial cells and glomerular basement membrane and within the mesangium. In cases of coagulase-positive staphylococcal endocarditis, the deposits may be confined to a subepithelial location. This form of glomerular disease may be encountered in fulminant infections. The diffuse lesions may cause renal failure, but even with extensive glomerular damage substantial recovery of renal function occurs with resolution.

Patterns of immunofluorescent staining are similar in both diffuse and focal glomerulonephritis. The most consistent finding is a diffuse, granular staining of C3 along capillary walls. In addition, immunoglobulin deposits, primarily IgG, are often present in the capillary walls, mesangium, or both. Fibrinogen is also demonstrable in crescents and areas of glomerular tuft necrosis. Specific antigens related to the infecting organism may also be located in the glomeruli.

Healed Lesions

The successful medical treatment of infective endocarditis means that a pathologist is seeing healed lesions in both the surgical pathology laboratory and autopsy suite much more frequently than in the past. Clinicians too must be able to diagnose the changes produced by such healed lesions in angiocardiographic or echocardiographic studies.

The healed form of any of the lesions mentioned above may be obvious,[108] but they are unlikely to be thought due to infective en-docarditis in the absence of a clear clinical history or unless valvular or paravalvular lesions are found. The clinician will recognize the latter through their effects. For the pathologist, the most obvious effects are healed ulcerations indenting the free margin of a cusp with associated cusp sclerosis, perforations with smooth, thick edges found in the body of a cusp (Fig. 23–17A), cusp aneurysms, or ruptured chordae tendineae. Other obvious effects, however, include healed sinuses or fistulae (Fig. 23–17B) caused by annular abscesses, large paravalvular defects found in association with artificial heart valves, or secondary changes induced in nearby tissue by such lesions.

CLINICAL MANIFESTATIONS

In areas where rheumatic valvular disease is prevalent, young persons (20 to 40 years) develop infective endocarditis; in such circumstances, men are affected much more

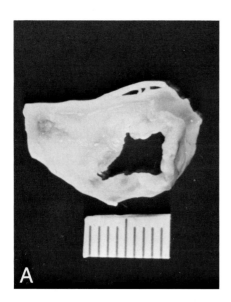
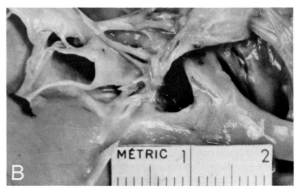

Fig. 23–17. (A) Healed endocarditis that caused a perforation in a surgically excised aortic valve cusp. Note thickened smooth edge of perforation. **(B)** Healed fistula found opening into the right ventricle at autopsy in a patient with an aortic Starr-Edwards aortic valve prosthesis and a history of infective endocarditis. Lesion was presumably caused by an annular abscess. (Courtesy of H. S. Asseltine, M.D., Windsor, Ontario.)

frequently than women. However, in Western countries the disease is seen with greater frequency in older persons (40 to 70 years) and, where it develops on heart valves that were thought to be previously normal, women have it as frequently as men. Carcinoma of the colon[68] and alcoholism, with or without associated liver cirrhosis,[21] are known factors that promote infective endocarditis.

Clinical manifestations caused by the disease mirror, to some extent, the virulence of an infecting organism. At one extreme they develop gradually, are of minor degree, and are so nonspecific that their cause is overlooked for a considerable period (clinical "subacute" endocarditis). At the other extreme manifestations evolve so rapidly and are of such a fulminant nature that their cause is not difficult to recognize (clinical "acute" endocarditis). A continuum exists between the two extremes. Refer to other sources[61,85,132] for a detailed description of the clinical manifestations of the disease. However, I present some principles that allow an appreciation of why they develop. In general, clinical findings in infective endocarditis are related to the effect of microorganisms proliferating in the bloodstream and to the local and systemic complications of the disease. It must be emphasized that a particular patient may not manifest all of them, nor does the mode of presentation of the disease necessarily follow any particular sequence.

Caused by Microorganisms Proliferating in the Bloodstream

Some clinical manifestations caused by microorganisms proliferating in the bloodstream are not specific; many represent the body's reaction to an infection. They include fingernail clubbing, purpuric and petechial hemorrhages, fever (which may be of low grade in indolent infections), anorexia, weight loss, and general lassitude. Patients may have splenomegaly.

Related laboratory findings include an elevation of the erythocyte sedimentation rate; anemia; a mild polymorphonuclear leukocytosis in indolent infections; a higher leukocyte count in fulminant ones, with the white cell count often showing a shift to the left; and proteinuria. When ancillary diagnostic methods are used, infected vegetations (if greater than 2 to 3 mm in diameter) and sinuses or fistulae induced by annular abscess can be diagnosed echocardiographically,[38,46,120,132] and the effects of localized cardiac complications recognized by changes in intracardiac pressures, oxygen tension, and both echocardiographic and angiographic findings.[12,132] Infective endocarditic lesions have been imaged with indium-III-labeled platelets.[103]

Other clinical manifestations are more closely related to a proliferation of microorganisms in the blood or to immunologic phenomena this induces. The latter include Osler's and Janeway's nodes, although there is some controversy as to whether these nodes are just due to immunologic phenomenon or are also caused by emboli. Roth's spots (probably the results of immune complex vasculitis in small peripheral vessels), renal failure, arthralgia, or arthritis. There may be an associated hypergammaglobulinemia and increased numbers of plasma cells present in the bone marrow. Circulating immune complexes can be present in the blood.[14] With a glomerulonephritis hematuria, proteinuria and casts may be found in the urine. The proliferation of microorganisms produces positive blood cultures (unless the patient has been treated previously with antibiotics or the infection is of very long standing) and may cause a disseminated intravascular coagulation.

Caused by Local or Systemic Complications

The patient may have a heart murmur initiated by the bulk of vegetations, caused by local complications of the endocarditis or as a result of heart failure. If valve destruction occurs, heart failure ensues and may be of gradual or sudden onset. Manifestations of a myocarditis, myocardial infarction, pericarditis, or cardiac arrhythmias, including varying degrees of heart block, may be observed.

The effects of embolic phenomena depend on whether an infection is present on right- or left-sided heart valves, on the size and nature of the embolus, and on the causative microorganism. Generally, embolic occlusion of a large blood vessel is uncommon in infections caused by bacteria but frequent where a fungal infection exists. Emboli from right-sided valvular infections induce "pneumonia" caused by single or multiple pulmonary infarcts or abscesses. The clinical manifestations produced by emboli arising from left-sided valvular infections depend on the site of impaction of the embolus in an organ and whether or not the embolus causes infarction or is infected and produces metastatic infections and their sequelae. Obviously, such manifestations may have a gradual or sudden onset.

MICROORGANISMS CAUSING INFECTIVE ENDOCARDITIS

As indicated above, any microorganism or blood-borne parasite may induce infective endocarditis. However, where the organism is identified streptococci and staphylococci induce most cases (90 to 95 percent) while *Candida* and *Aspergillus* species cause most fungal infections.[27,63,87,132]

Streptococci

Streptococcus viridans is the major cause of streptococcal endocarditis, especially in patients with heart valves damaged by rheumatic valvular disease. It usually induces an indolent infection. The next most frequent infecting organisms are enterococci; in such cases peripheral abscesses are a frequent complication. The remaining cases are caused by microerophilic and anaerobic streptococci, nonhemolytic streptococci, Group A β-hemolytic, and other streptococci. Enterococci and group A β-hemolytic streptococci may infect previously normal valves and induce a virulent infection.

Staphylococci

The frequency of staphylococcal infections has risen markedly in recent years; in some series these organisms are now as frequent a cause of infective endocarditis as streptococci. Staphylococcal infection is particularly common in patients who are drug addicts or who have artificial heart valves. Both coagulase-positive and coagulase-negative organisms can cause an infection. Coagulase-negative staphylococci often induce an indolent infection, whereas coagulase-positive organisms produce a fulminant one in which distal abscesses are a common complication. Overall, coagulase-positive organisms cause most cases of staphylococcal infective endocarditis.

Gram-Negative Organisms

Infection with gram-negative types of organism is much less common than that caused by gram-positive cocci. However, gram-negative endocarditis is not infrequent with intravenous narcotic abuse or in patients with diabetes mellitus.[27] Gram-negative infections may affect previously damaged heart valves, normal ones, especially in drug addicts, or occur as a nosocomial infection in patients with heart valve prostheses. *Pseudomonas aeruginosa* caused 59 percent of cases in one series of infective endocarditis among 110 intravenous drug abusers.[27] Pseudomonas usually produces an indolent infection whereas, on the other hand, an infection with *Serratia marcescens* is often fulminant.

Fungi

Fungal infections are most often indolent and present with the patient having repeated thromboembolic episodes occluding larger blood vessels. Fungal infections are common in patients with prosthetic heart valves or indwelling vascular catheters, those who are drug addicts, immunosuppressed, or who are receiving cytotoxic agents.[87,129] Candida is the most frequent infecting agent with Aspergillus and Histoplasma species[17] causing the bulk of the remaining cases.

Other Organisms

Lists of other microorganisms that cause infective endocarditis are provided by several authors.[63,87,132] Such lists have to be updated almost weekly as new causative organisms are recognized. Cell-wall deficient organisms and *Coxiella burnetii* may induce infective endocarditis. The latter is mentioned because of its long latent period and its clinical chronicity.[127,134] The importance of the pathologist collecting serum samples in cases of Q fever endocarditis, especially in culture-negative cases, cannot be overemphasized. This may provide the only means of diagnosis. "Mixed" infections and "superinfections" also occur. The latter occurs where a patient has been successfully treated with the appropriate antibiotic; symptoms disappear and then recur with a new organism being recovered from the bloodstream.

INFECTIVE ENDOCARDITIS IN PARTICULAR CIRCUMSTANCES

Affecting Left-Sided Heart Valves

From necropsy studies, Roberts[106] listed several findings applicable to infective endocarditis affecting left-sided heart valves.[20,108] They include the following:

1. Isolated left-sided endocarditis is about four times more common than either isolated right-sided infections or right- and left-sided endocarditis.
2. The initial clinical presentation usually suggests a systemic infection rather than cardiac disease.
3. A precordial murmur is almost always present, but the murmur does not necessarily indicate valvular damage.
4. A factor predisposing to infection is usually present.
5. The endocarditis involves previously anatomically and functionally normal valves in more than half the patients.
6. The aortic valve is now more frequently involved than the mitral.
7. Ring abscess is a common complication only when endocarditis involves the aortic valve. (I would agree with this statement but have found that annular abscesses occur not infrequently where infective endocarditis develops on a mitral valve showing calcification of the mitral annular ring—see later discussion.)
8. Pericarditis in patients with infective endocarditis is primarily a complication of aortic valve infection. (Again, I make an exception for infective endocarditis associated with calcification of the mitral valve annulus—see below.)
9. Among necropsy patients with isolated left-sided endocarditis, staphylococci rather than streptococci are now more frequently the infecting organism.
10. Associated acute meningitis and pneumonia is much less frequent in left-sided than in right-sided infective endocarditis.
11. Death in such infections is most commonly the result of abnormal cardiac function rather than of systemic infection or emboli.

Affecting Right-Sided Heart Valves

Again, Roberts[106] enumerated some findings applicable to right-sided heart valve endocarditis seen at necropsy.[107] They are:

1. The disease is considerably less frequent than left-sided endocarditis.
2. The clinical presentation primarily suggests an acute pneumonia rather than a cardiac disease.
3. A precordial murmur, particularly one of tricuspid or pulmonic valve origin, is often absent or of low intensity.
4. An obvious factor predisposing to infective endocarditis is usually identifiable—most frequently, opiate addiction, habitual alcoholism, an indwelling catheter, or chemotherapy for malignant neoplasms.
5. The infection is nearly always caused by a highly virulent organism.
6. The involved right-sided valve is nearly always anatomically and functionally normal before onset of the infection.
7. Of the right-sided valves, the tricuspid is involved in the majority of cases; it is distinctly uncommon for both the tricuspid and pulmonic valves to be involved.
8. About 50 percent of patients with active right-sided endocarditis at necropsy also have an active infection involving one or both left-sided valves. Furthermore, when both right- and left-sided endocarditis are present, "acute pneumonia" is nearly always the presenting feature, suggesting that the right-sided endocarditis preceded that on the left side.
9. Associated acute meningitis is fairly common.
10. Ring abscess is an infrequent complication.
11. Death is most commonly caused by "pulmonary insufficiency" secondary to repeated septic emboli from dislodged vegetative material.

Chan and colleagues confirm these observations in their review, pointing out that tricuspid valve infection accounts for 5 to 10 percent of all cases of endocarditis and that *Staphylococcus aureus* is the most common causative organism.[24] Polymicrobial infections of the tricuspid valve have become more prevalent, especially among drug addicts.

Among Drug Addicts

Drug addicts using the intravenous route of administration pay little attention to skin sterilization or to the source of fluids used to dissolve the drug to be administered; as a result, such persons are particularly prone to infections caused by staphylococci, streptococci gram-negative organisms (particularly Pseudomonas species), and Candida species.[23,102,123] (Their re-use and sharing of needles also increases their risk of contracting AIDS.) Many other organisms may induce endocarditis in addicts, but those listed cause the majority of cases.

Generally, the infection occurs in younger persons (teenager to 40 years old) and mainly in males. Usually it is fulminant, and symptoms develop rapidly. Mixed infections occur more frequently among this group than in nondrug abusers. Left-sided infections are the most common; infections involving valves on both sides of the heart are not uncommon. Often there is an underlying cardiac anomaly that predisposes the addict to the infection if left-sided valves are involved. If so, streptococci cause most infections. However, many cases, especially tricuspid valve infections, occur on "normal" valves.

Dressler and Roberts reported their necropsy study of 80 cases occurring in opium addicts.[39] Blacks were affected more often than whites in a ratio of $\simeq 7$ to 1 and males more often than females (ratio $\simeq 3$ to 1). The mean age at death was 34. Staphylococcal species caused the majority of cases (76 percent). Fifty-nine patients had active endocarditis, 11 healed endocarditis, and 10 both. The first episode of infective endocarditis involved a single right-sided valve in 30 percent of patients (tricuspid in 23 of 24); a single right- and left-sided valve in 16 percent; a single left-sided valve in 41 percent; both left-sided valves in 13 percent of the patients. The tricuspid valve was infected most often whether as an isolated infection or combined with infections or other valves (35 of 80 patients). Examination suggested that the infected valve had been normal in 81 percent of patients before infection. Dressler and Roberts noted that 53 percent of the patients died during the first episode of active endocarditis and that when active endocarditis was eradicated by antibiotics a recurrence commonly occurred at the sites of the previously healed infection. Valve-ring abscess occurred in 2.5 percent of infections appearing on the right side of the heart, in 9 percent of mitral valve infections, and in 55 percent of aortic valve infections.

On Prosthetic Valves

Although, overall, infectious endocarditis is not a common complication of prosthetic valves (less than 1 percent per year among patients with a prosthetic valve), it is a dreaded one.[2,7,16,75,131] Some infections become manifest soon after a valve is inserted and are a result of pre-existing contamination of the valve, contamination during surgery, particularly from a heart-lung machine, or from infection spreading from an adjacent locus (e.g., an infected wound site in the immediate postoperative period). Their frequency is diminishing. Alternatively, infective endocarditis associated with heart valve prostheses may develop at a later stage (generally classified as 2 months or more after insertion) and is the result of microorganisms entering the bloodstream as happens in infections in natural heart valves. This form of endocarditis is not decreasing in frequency.

Aortic and mitral valve prostheses are affected with about equal frequency, but infections on aortic valves produce clinical symptoms more often than those on the mitral valve. Also, aortic infections are likely to be more destructive.

The initial location of the infection may differ in tissue and nontissue valves. In tissue valves, the infection develops on the valve cusp, rather than on the sewing ring. This reduces the risk of a ready spread into annular tissue. However, annular abscesses occur frequently with both types of prostheses, indi-cating that in tissue valves the infection has either spread from the tissue cusp or, alternatively, started on the valve ring.

Staphylococci are a frequent cause of perioperative infections, whereas staphylococci (especially), streptococci, and fungi produce most of the late ones. The majority of microorganisms causing late-onset endocarditis are those likely to induce infection on a natural heart valve. It is possible that some cases of endocarditis caused by unusual organisms are the result of suprainfections induced by antibiotic treatment.[132]

The effects of such infections on the function of heart valve prostheses are discussed in Chapter 40.

In the Elderly

In the west, infective endocarditis is becoming more frequent among elderly patients.[6,104] It is a complication that must be suspected, especially among those who are hospitalized and who develop decubitus ulcers or another source of infection. Often the symptoms induced by the disease are atypical. Men are affected more frequently than women.

The causative organisms are those inducing infective endocarditis on natural heart valves (excluding infections in addicts), with streptococci and staphylococci causing most infections. Often there is an underlying valvular disease, but infection may develop on a normal valve.

Complicating Calcified Mitral Annulus

Calcification of the mitral valve annulus is a common finding at autopsy in elderly patients (see Ch. 5). Infective endocarditis may complicate this condition and in that setting affects elderly women particularly[22,53,130] (see Fig. 5–21; and Ch. 25).

Clinicopathologic correlations indicate that the disease should be suspected in elderly patients with a calcified mitral annulus (often

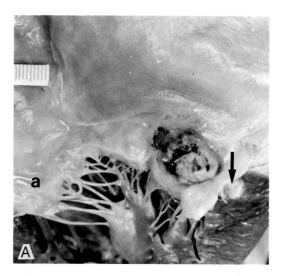

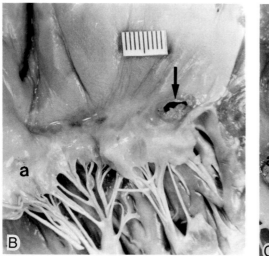
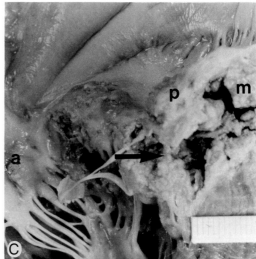

Fig. 23–18. Infective endocarditis associated with calcification of mitral valve annulus. (A) Infected vegetations at *base* of posterior mitral valve leaflet (characteristic location) related to calcium deposit in annulus (arrow). (a, anterior valve leaflet.) (B) Vegetations at base of leaflet with perforation, a common associated finding. (C) Large annular calcium mass (m) extending into adjacent base of left ventricle. *Note:* posterior leaflet stretched over calcium mass and tethered to it; this caused valve incompetence; absence of vegetation on atrial aspect of the leaflet and breakdown of tissue in calcium was due to pus formation and ulceration of abscess into ventricular cavity (arrow). Such events may give rise to systemic emboli of calcium and other debris. (p, posterior leaflet.) (Scales in Figs. A–C, each 1 cm) (*Figure continues.*)

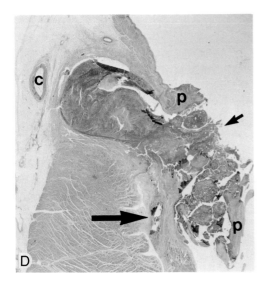
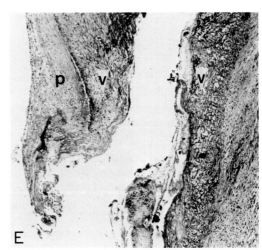

Fig. 23–18 (*Continued*). (**D**) Annular abscess extending into epicardial fat adjacent to circumflex coronary artery (c) from an infection associated with annular calcification. Posterior mitral leaflet has been perforated (small arrow). Section shows only a little of the calcification in the annular region (large arrow). (H&E, × 4.) (**E**) Infected vegetation (v) on both ventricular aspect of posterior mitral valve leaflet (p) and adjacent mural endocardium of left ventricle. (H&E, × 16.) (From Mambo,[83] with permission.)

better demonstrated by fluoroscopy or an overpenetrated chest radiograph than by a standard chest radiograph), especially if they are hospitalized. The patients may have a murmur of mitral insufficiency, fever, anemia, polymorphonuclear leukocytosis, and a positive blood culture regardless of evidence of peripheral embolism or of another disease that could cause the last four features.

Pertinent pathologic findings are the calcified mitral annulus (the aortic annulus may also be involved); the absence of other valvular disease; vegetations of infective endocarditis (staphylococci are the most frequent cause) found toward the *base* of the posterior leaflet rather than related to its line of closure and often associated with leaflet perforation, an annular abscess, and with or without a pericarditis (Figs. 23–13 and 23–18A–D).

The infection may develop on the atrial aspect of the leaflet elevated by the calcium mass or begin on the ventricular aspect, subsequently perforating it and producing vege-

tations on the atrial surface (Fig. 23–18C & E). In either case the infection readily spreads to the calcified tissue in the annulus (Fig. 23–18C & D). The resultant mitral ring abscess may induce a pericarditis or rupture into the left ventricle to produce distal tissue and/or calcium emboli.

Affecting Prolapsed Mitral Valve

Patients with myxomatous degeneration of the mitral valve (prolapsed mitral valve, floppy mitral valve) develop infective endocarditis (see Fig. 23–9).[32,70,81] Although endocarditis is a major complication of the condition, it is relatively infrequent.[60,70] Patients with mitral valve prolapse and a previously known systolic murmur have a higher risk.[32] The infection is presumed to develop in association with tiny thrombi, often found attached to the atrial aspect of the thickened prolapsed leaflet tissue. In some instances thrombus is also deposited in the angle between the base of a prolapsed posterior leaflet and the adjacent left atrial wall, and I have seen one case of infective endocarditis located at the latter site without any evidence of calcification in the underlying annulus. Incidentally, all these thrombi may be a possible source of emboli causing transient ischemic attacks in young people[11] (see Ch. 25 and Fig. 25–1 and Ch. 28). Microorganisms likely to cause the infection are those causing endocarditis in patients with other types of valvular disease. Streptococcal and staphylococcal infections cause most cases, but viridans streptococcal infections predominate.[60,70] However, the majority of cases in one series had staphylococcal infections.[28]

In Hypertrophic Cardiomyopathy and Membranous Subaortic Stenosis

Infective endocarditis has also been reported on the mitral valve associated with hypertrophic cardiomyopathy.[124,128,132,133] Its incidence is 5 to 9 percent.[133] The disease also develops on the aortic valve as a complication of membranous subaortic stenosis (see Ch. 26). Both situations reflect particular instances associated with hemodynamic "trauma" to the endocardium.

MURAL ENDOCARDITIS INTIMITIS

Mural endocarditis[19] is rare in the absence of a lesion such as a ventricular septal defect or cusp perforation that permits a jet of blood to impinge on the endocardial surface and promote the formation of satellite lesions. Most cases of mural endocarditis that I have seen occurred in debilitated patients, those who

were immunosuppressed, or those who were receiving chemotherapy as a result of a septicemic process occurring as part of an infection in an organ other than the heart (see Fig. 23–5). The causative organism was almost invariably a fungus (usually Candida), and the endocardial lesion resulted from the spread of the infection to involve the endocardium from an adjacent myocardial abscess. Mural endocarditis of this type is almost never diagnosed clinically, the cardiac signs and symptoms being lost in the general manifestation of the associated overwhelming infection.

Infections of the arterial or venous intima also occur. They are uncommon and may be difficult to diagnose unless they induce a mycotic aneurysm. Such lesions are usually associated with indwelling tubes, catheters, or shunts, but may develop at operative sites. I have seen infections involving the aortotomy wound in patients following the insertion of an aortic heart valve prosthesis. Most cases had an associated aortic prosthetic valve infection, but one was confined to the wound.

As indicated earlier, gram-negative organisms, particularly Salmonella species, may cause infection in mural thrombi found in aortic or cardiac aneurysms (see also Chs. 8 and 9).

REFERENCES

1. Allen AC, Sirota JH: The morphogenesis and significance of degenerative verrucal endocardiosis (terminal endocarditis), endocarditis simplex, nonbacterial thrombotic endocarditis. Am J Pathol 20:1025, 1944
2. Anderson DJ, Buckley BH, Hutchins GM: A clinicopathologic study of prosthetic valve endocarditis in 22 patients: Morphologic basis for diagnosis and therapy. Am Heart J 94:325, 1977
3. Angrist AA, Oka M: Pathogenesis of bacterial endocarditis. JAMA 183:249, 1963
4. Angrist A, Oka M, Nakao K: Vegetative endocarditis. Pathol Annu 2:155, 1967
5. Angrist AA, Oka M, Nakao K: Vegetative endocarditis. p. 91. In Sommers SC (ed): Car-

diovascular Pathology Decennial. Appleton-Century Crofts, East Norwalk, CT, 1975

6. Appelfeld MM, Hornick RB: Infective endocarditis in patients over age 60. Am Heart J 80:90, 1974

7. Arnett EN, Roberts WC: Prosthetic valve endocarditis. Clinicopathologic analysis of 22 necropsy patients with comparison of observations in 74 necropsy patients with active infective endocarditis involving natural left-sided cardiac valves. Am J Cardiol 38:281, 1976

8. Arnett EN, Roberts WC: Valve ring abscess in active infective endocarditis. Frequency, location and clues to clinical diagnosis from the study of 95 necropsy patients. Circulation 54:140, 1976

9. Atkinson JB, Virmani R: Infective endocarditis. Changing trends and general approach for examination. Hum Pathol 18:603, 1987

10. Austrian R, Gold J: Pneumococcal bacteremia with especial reference to bacteremic pneumoccal pneumonia. Ann Intern Med 60:759, 1964

11. Barnett HJM, Boughner DR, Taylor DW, et al: Further evidence relating mitral valve prolapse to cerebral ischemic events. N Engl J Med 302:139, 1980

12. Baron MG: Radiological and angiographic examination of the heart. p. 140. In Braunwald E (ed): Heart Disease. 3rd Ed. WB Saunders, Philadelphia, 1988

13. Barry WE, Scarpelli D: Nonbacterial thrombotic endocarditis: A clinicopathologic study. Arch Intern Med 109:151, 1962

14. Bayer AS, Theofilopoulos AN, Eisenberg R, et al: Circulating immune complexes in infective endocarditis. N Engl J Med 295:1500, 1976

15. Becker AE, Becker MJ, Martin FH, Edwards JE: Bland thrombosis and infection in relation to intracardiac catheter. Circulation 46:200, 1972

16. Ben Ismail M, Hannachi N, Abid F, et al: Prosthetic valve endocarditis. A survey. Br Heart J 58:72, 1987

17. Blair TP, Waugh RA, Pollack M, et al: Histoplasma capsulatum endocarditis. Am Heart J 99:783, 1980

18. Bloor CM: Endocarditis. p. 296. In: Cardiac Pathology. JB Lippincott, Philadelphia, 1978

19. Buchbinder NA, Roberts WC: Active infective endocarditis confined to mural endocardium. A study of 6 necropsy patients. Arch Pathol 93:435, 1972

20. Buchbinder NA, Roberts WC: Left-sided valvular active infective endocarditis. A study of forty-five necropsy patients. Am J Med 53:20, 1972

21. Buchbinder NA, Roberts WC: Alcoholism—an important but underemphasized factor predisposing to infective endocarditis. Arch Intern Med 132:689, 1973

22. Burnside JW, DeSanctis RW: Bacterial endocarditis on calcification of the mitral annulus fibrosus. Ann Intern Med 76:615, 1972

23. Cannon NJ, Cobbs CG: Infective endocarditis in drug addicts. p. 111. In Kaye D (ed): Infective Endocarditis. University Park Press, Baltimore, 1976

24. Chan P, Ogilby JD, Segal B: Tricuspid valve endocarditis. Am Heart J 117:1140, 1989

25. Cheng JJ, Ko YL, Chang SC, et al: Retrospective analysis of 97 patients with infective endocarditis seen over the past 8 years. Taiwan I Hsueh Hui Tsa Chih 88:213, 1989

26. Coard KCM, Prabhakar P, Bansal AS: Infective endocarditis at the University Hospital of the West Indies: A postmortem study. West Indian J Med J 38:217, 1989

27. Cohen PS, Maguire JH, Weinstein L: Infective endocarditis caused by gram-negative bacteria—a review of the literature 1947–1977. Prog Cardiovasc Dis 32:205, 1980

28. Corrigall D, Bolen J, Hancock EW, Popp RL: Mitral valve prolapse and infective endocarditis. Am J Med 63:215, 1977

29. Crawford JJ, Sconyers JR, Moriarty JD, et al: Bacteremia after tooth extractions studied with the aid of prereduced anerobically sterilized culture media. Appl Microbiol 27:927, 1974

30. Cripps T, Guvendik L: Coronary artery compression caused by abscess formation in infective endocarditis. Int J Cardiol 14:99, 1987

31. Cross AS, Steigbigel RT: Infective endocarditis and access site infection in patients on hemodialysis. Medicine 55:453, 1976

32. Danchin N, Vorriot P, Brianion S, et al: Mitral valve prolapse as a risk factor for infective endocarditis. Lancet 1:743, 1989

33. Davies MJ: Pathology of Cardiac Valves. Butterworths, London, 1980

34. Davis JM, Moss AJ, Schenk EA: Tricuspid candida endocarditis complicating a permanently implanted transvenous pacemaker. Am Heart J 77:818, 1969

35. Delahaye JP, Loire R, Milon H, et al: Infective endocarditis on stenotic aortic valves. Eur Heart J 9(Suppl E 43), 1988

36. Deppisch LM, Fayemi AO: Non bacterial thrombotic endocarditis. Clinicopathologic correlations. Am Heart J 92:723, 1976

37. Derkson RHWM, Kaker L: Lupus anticoagulant: Revival of an old phenomenon. Clin Exp Rheumatol 3:349, 1985

38. Dillon JC, Feigenbaum H, Konecke LL, et al: Echocardiographic manifestations of valvular vegetation. Am Heart J 86:698, 1973

39. Dressler FA, Roberts WC: Infective endocarditis in opiate addicts: Analysis of 80 cases studied at necropsy. Am J Cardiol 63:1240, 1989

40. Durack DT, Beeson PB: Protective role of complement in experimental endocarditis. Infect Immun 16:213, 1977

41. Durack DT, Beeson PB: Pathogenesis of infective endocarditis. p. 1. In Rahimtoola SH (ed): Infective Endocarditis. Grune & Stratton, New York, 1978

42. Edwards JE: Lesions causing or simulating aortic insufficiency. Cardiovasc Clin 5:127, 1973

43. Edwards JE, Burchell HB: The pathological anatomy of deficiencies between the aortic root and the heart, including aortic sinus aneurysm. Thorax 12:125, 1957

44. Everett ED, Hirschman JV: Transient bacteremia and endocarditis prophylaxis. A review. Medicine 56:61, 1977

45. Fayemi AO, Deppisch L: Coronary embolism and myocardial infarction associated with non bacterial thrombotic endocarditis. Am J Clin Pathol 68:393, 1977

46. Feigenbaum H: Echocardiography. p. 96. In Braunwald E (ed): Heart Disease. WB Saunders, Philadelphia, 1980

47. Ford PM, Ford SE, Lillicrap DP: Association of lupus anticoagulant with severe valvular heart disease in systemic lupus erythematosus. J Rheumatol 15:4, 1988

48. Ford S, Charette E, Knight J, et al: A possible role for antiphospholipid antibodies in acquired cardiac valve deformity. J Rheumatol (in press)

49. Ford S, Manley PN: Indwelling cardiac catheters. An autopsy study of associated endocardial lesions. Arch Pathol Lab Med 106:314, 1982

50. Freedman LR, Valone J, Jr: Experimental infective endocarditis. Prog Cardiovasc Dis 22:169, 1979

51. Gersony WM, Hayes CJ: Bacterial endocarditis in patients with pulmonary stenosis, aortic stenosis or ventricular septal defect. Circulation (suppl. 1)56:84, 1977

52. Geva T, Frand M: Infective endocarditis in children with congenital heart disease: The changing spectrum 1965–85. Eur Heart J 9:1244, 1988

53. Glynn MF, Movat HZ, Murphy EA, Mustard JF: Study of platelet adhesiveness and aggregation with latex particles. J Lab Clin Med 65:179, 1965

54. Goldstein RS, Zak FG: Skin lesions caused by embolism from heart valves with nonbacterial endocarditis. Arch Dermatol 93:585, 1966

55. Gonzales-Lavin L, Lise M, Ross D: The importance of the 'jet lesion' in bacterial endocarditis involving the left heart. J Thorac Cardiovasc Surg 59:185, 1970

56. Grant RT, Wood JE, Jr, Jones TD: Heart valve irregularities in relation to subacute bacterial endocarditis. Heart 14:247, 1928

57. Gross L, Friedberg CK: Nonbacterial thrombotic endocarditis: Classification and general description. Arch Intern Med 58:620, 1936

58. Hugo-Hamman CT, de Moor MM, Human DG: Infective endocarditis in South African children. J Trop Pediatr 35:154, 1989

59. Jann K, Jann B (eds): Bacterial adhesions. Curr Top Microbiol Immunol 151:1, 1990

60. Jeresaty RM: Mitral Valve Prolapse. Raven Press, New York, 1979

61. Johnson WD, Jr: The clinical syndrome. p. 87. In Kaye D (ed): Infective Endocarditis. University Park Press, Baltimore, 1976

62. Karl T, Wensley D, Stark J, et al: Infective endocarditis in children with congenital heart disease: Comparison of selected features and patients with surgical correction of palliation and those without. Br Heart J 58:57, 1987

63. Kaye D: Infecting microorganisms. p. 43. In Kaye D (ed): Infective Endocarditis. University Park Press, Baltimore, 1976

64. Kaye D: Changing patterns of infective endocarditis. Am J Med 78(6B):157, 1985

65. Keith JD: Bacterial endocarditis (infective endocarditis). p. 232. In Keith JD, Rowe RD, Vlad P (eds): Heart Disease in Infancy and Childhood. 3rd Ed. Macmillan, New York, 1978

66. Kerr A, Jr: Bacterial endocarditis—revisited. Mod Con Cardiovasc Dis 33:831, 1964

67. Kim HS, Suzuki M, Lie JT, Titus JL: Non bacterial thrombotic endocarditis (NBTE) and disseminated intravascular coagulation (DIC). Arch Pathol Lab Med 101:65, 1977

68. Klein RS, Catalano MT, Edberg SC, et al: *Streptococcus bovis* septicemia and carcinoma of the colon. Arch Intern Med 91:560, 1979

69. Kloster FE: Infective prosthetic valve endocarditis. p. 291. In Rahimtoola SH (ed): Infective Endocarditis. Grune & Stratton, Orlando, FL, 1978

70. Kolelar SL, Para MF: Mitral valve prolapse and infective endocarditis. p. 275. In Boudoulas H, Wooley CF (eds): Mitral Valve Prolapse and the Mitral Valve Prolapse Syndrome. Futura Publishing, Mt. Kisco, NY, 1988

71. Kortleve JW, Duren DR, Becker AG: Cardiac aneurysm complicated by salmonella abscess. A clinicopathological correlation in two patients. Am J Med 68:395, 1980

72. Krause JR, Levinson SP: Pathology of infective endocarditis. p. 55. In Kaye D (ed): Infective Endocarditis. University Park Press, Baltimore, 1976

73. LeFrock JL, Ellis CA, Turchik JB, Weinstein L: Transient bacteremia associated with sigmoidoscopy. N Engl J Med 289:467, 1973

74. Lepeschkin E: On the relation between the site of valvular involvement in endocarditis and the blood pressure resting on the valve. Am J Med Sci 224:318, 1952

75. Leport C, Vilde JL, Bricaire F, et al: Fifty cases of late prosthetic valve endocarditis: Improvement in prognosis over a 15 year period. Br Heart J 58:66, 1987

76. Lerner PI, Weinstein L: Infective endocarditis in the antibiotic era. N Engl J Med 274:199, 259, 323, 388, 1966

77. Levinson ME: Pathogenesis of infective endocarditis. p. 29. In Kaye D (ed): Infective Endocarditis. University Park Press, Baltimore, 1976

78. Loire R, Tabib A, Normand JC: L'endocardite thrombosante non bactérienne. Arch Mal Coeur 74:157, 1981

79. Lopez JA, Ross RS, Fishbein MC, Siegel RJ: Nonbacterial thrombotic endocarditis: A review. Am Heart J 113:773, 1987

80. MacDonald RA, Robbins SL: The significance of non-bacterial thrombotic endocarditis: An autopsy and clinical study of 78 cases. Ann Intern Med 46:255, 1957

81. MacMahon SW, Roberts JK, Kramer-Fox R, et al: Mitral valve prolapse and infective endocarditis. Am Heart J 113:1291, 1987

82. Maisch B: Autoreactive mechanisms in infective endocarditis. Springer Semin Immunopathol 11:439, 1989

83. Mambo N, Silver MD, Brunsdon DFV: Bacterial endocarditis of the mitral valve associated with annular calcification. Can Med Assoc J 119:323, 1978

84. Markowitz SM, Szentpetery S, Lower RR, Duma RJ: Endocarditis due to accidental penetrating foreign bodies. Am J Med 60:571, 1976

85. McAnulty JH, Rahimtoola SH, DeMots H, Griswold HR: Clinical features of infective endocarditis. p. 125. In Rahimtoola SH (ed): Infective Endocarditis. Grune & Stratton, Orlando, FL, 1978

86. McKinsey DS, Ratts TE, Bisno AL: Underlying cardiac lesions in adults with infective endocarditis: The changing perspective. Am J Med 82:681, 1987

87. McLeod R, Remington JS: Fungal endocarditis. p. 211. In Rahimtoola SH (ed): Infective Endocarditis. Grune & Stratton, Orlando, FL, 1978

88. Mueh JR, Herbst KD, Rapaport SI: Thrombosis in patients with the lupus anticoagulant. Ann Intern Med 92:156, 1980

89. Mustard JF, Packham MA: Normal and abnormal hemostasis. Br Med Bull 33:187, 1977

90. Mügge A, Daniel WG, Frank G, Lichtlen PR: Echocardiography in infective endocarditis: Reassessment of prognostic implications of vegetation size determined by the transthoracic and transesophageal approach. J Am Coll Cardiol 4:631, 1989

91. Nachman RL, Weksler B, Ferris B: Increased permeability produced by human platelet

granule cationic extract. J Clin Invest 49:247, 1970

92. O'Callaghan C, McDougall P: Infective endocarditis in neonates. Arch Dis Child 63:53, 1988

93. Olney BA, Schattenberg TT, Campbell JK, et al: The consequences of the inconsequential: Marantic (nonbacterial thrombotic) endocarditis. Am Heart J 98:513, 1979

94. Perez GO, Rothfield N, Williams RC: Immune complex nephritis in bacterial endocarditis. Arch Intern Med 136:334, 1976

95. Persuad V: Two unusual cases of mural endocarditis with a review of the literature. Am J Clin Pathol 53:832, 1970

96. Peterson PK, Quie PG: Bacterial surface components and the pathogenesis of infectious disease. Ann Rev Med 32:29, 1981

97. Phair JP, Clark J: Immunology of infective endocarditis. Prog Cardiovasc Dis 22:137, 1979

98. Piepkorn MW, Reichenbach DD: Infective endocarditis associated with cell wall-deficient bacteria. Hum Pathol 9:163, 1978

99. Pitlick S, Cohen L, Melamed R, Rosenfeld J: Mural endocarditis associated with recurrent false aneurysm of the left ventricle. Chest 71:227, 1977

100. Prasad TR, Valiathan MS, Venkitachalam CG, Kartha CC: Unusual manifestation of valvular vegetations. Thorac Cardiovasc Surgeon 36:170, 1988

101. Pruitt AA, Rubin RH, Karchmer AW, Duncan GW: Neurologic complications of bacterial endocarditis. Medicine 57:329, 1978

102. Reisberg BE: Infective endocarditis in the narcotic addict. Prog Cardiovasc Dis 22:193, 1979

103. Riba AL, Thakur ML, Gottschalk A, et al: Imaging experimental infective endocarditis with Indium-III-labeled blood cellular components. Circulation 59:336, 1979

104. Ries K: Endocarditis in the elderly. p. 143. In Kaye D (ed): Infective Endocarditis. University Park Press, Baltimore, 1976

105. Ringer M, Feen DJ, Drapkin MS: Mitral valve prolapse: Jet stream causing mural endocarditis. Am J Cardiol 45:383, 1980

106. Roberts WC: Characteristics and consequences of infective endocarditis (active or healed or both) learned from morphologic studies. p. 55. In Rahimtoola SH (ed): Infec-

tive Endocarditis. Grune & Stratton, Orlando, FL, 1978

107. Roberts WC, Buchbinder NA: Right-sided valvular infective endocarditis. A clinicopathologic study of twelve necropsy patients. Am J Med 53:7, 1972

108. Roberts WC, Buchbinder NA: Healed left-sided infective endocarditis. A clinicopathological study of 59 patients. Am J Cardiol 40:876, 1976

109. Roberts WC, Ewy GA, Clancy DL, Marcus FI: Valvular stenosis produced by active infective endocarditis. Circulation 36:449, 1967

110. Rodbard S: Blood velocity and endocarditis. Circulation 27:18, 1963

111. Rosen P, Armstrong D: Non bacterial thrombotic endocarditis in patients with malignant neoplastic diseases. Am J Med 54:23, 1973

112. Rosenthal A, Nadas AS: Infective endocarditis in infancy and childhood. p. 199. In Rahimtoola SH (ed): Infective Endocarditis. Grune & Stratton, Orlando, FL, 1978

113. Russek HI: Cardiovascular Problems. University Park Press, Baltimore, 1976

114. Salgado AV, Furlan AJ, Keys TF, et al: Neurological complications of endocarditis—a 12-year experience. Neurology 39:173, 1989

115. Sande MA: Experimental endocarditis. p. 11. In Kaye D (ed): Infective Endocarditis. University Park Press, Baltimore, 1976

116. Saner HE, Asinger RW, Homans DC, et al: Two-dimensional echocardiographic identification of complicated aortic root endocarditis. J Am Coll Cardiol 10:859, 1987

117. Schwartz IA, Pervez N: Bacterial endocarditis associated with a permanent transvenous cardiac pacemaker. JAMA 218:736, 1971

118. Sheldon WH, Golden A: Abscesses of the valve rings of the heart: A frequent but not well recognized complication of acute bacterial endocarditis. Circulation 4:1, 1951

119. Siqueira M, Nelson RA: Platelet agglutination by immune complexes and its possible role in hypersensitivity. J Immunol 86:516, 1961

120. Spangler RD, Johnson MC, Holmes J, Blount G: Echocardiographic demonstration of bacterial vegetations in active infective endocarditis. J Clin Ultrasound 1:126, 1973

121. Steiner I, Patel AK, Hutt MSR, Somers K: Pathology of infective endocarditis. Br Heart J 35:159, 1973

122. Stengel A, Wolferth CC: Mycotic (bacterial)

aneurysms of intravascular origin. Arch Intern Med 31:527, 1923

123. Stimmel B, Dack S: Infective endocarditis in narcotic addicts. p. 195. In Rahimtoola SH (ed): Infective Endocarditis. Grune & Stratton, Orlando, FL, 1978

124. Stulz P, Zimmerli W, Mihatsch J, Grädel E: Recurrent infective endocarditis in idiopathic hypertrophic subacute stenosis. Thorac Cardiovasc Surgeon 37:99, 1989

125. Sullam PM, Drake TA, Sande MA: Pathogenesis of endocarditis. Am J Med 78 (suppl 68):110, 1985

126. Sullivan NM, Sutter VL, Mims MM, et al: Clinical aspects of bacteremia after manipulation of the genitourinary tract. J Infect Dis 727:49, 1973

127. Turck WPG, Howitt G, Turnberg LA, et al: Chronic Q fever. Q J Med 45:193, 1976

128. Vecht RJ, Oakley CM: Infective endocarditis in three patients with hypertrophic obstructive cardiomyopathy. Br Med J 2:455, 1968

129. Walshe TJ, Hutchins GM, Bulkley BH, Mendelsohn G: Fungal infections of the heart: Analysis of 51 autopsy cases. Am J Cardiol 45:357, 1980

130. Watanakunakorn C: Staphylococcus aureus

131. Watanakunakorn C: Prosthetic valve infective endocarditis. Prog Cardiovasc Dis 22:181, 1979

132. Weinstein L: Infective endocarditis. p. 1093. In Braunwald E (ed): Heart Disease. 3rd E. WB Saunders, Philadelphia, 1988

133. Wigle ED, Sasson Z, Henderson MA, et al: Hypertrophic cardiomyopathy: The importance of the site and extent of hypertrophy. A review. Prog Cardiovasc Dis 28:1, 1985

134. Wilson HG, Neilson GH, Galea EG, et al: Q fever endocarditis in Queensland. Circulation 53:680, 1973

135. Wilson JW, Houghton DC, Bennett WM, Porter GA: The kidney and infective endocarditis. p. 179. In Rahimtoola SH (ed): Infective Endocarditis. Grune & Stratton, New York, 1978

136. Wilson LM: Etiology of bacterial endocarditis. Before and since the introduction of antibiotics. Ann Intern Med 58:946, 1963

137. Ziment I: Nervous system complications in bacterial endocarditis. Am J Med 47:593, 1969

endocarditis on the calcified mitral valve. Am J Med Sci 266:219, 1973

24

Blood Flow Obstruction Related to Tricuspid, Pulmonary, and Mitral Valves

Malcolm D. Silver

In so-called developed countries, a pathologist's experience with valvular heart disease is changing. This is a result, in part, of a diminution in the frequency of attacks of rheumatic fever in the community.[100] Also, valvular heart disease is treated surgically with growing success. Thus, the number of patients seen at autopsy in whom valvular heart diseases have followed their natural course has diminished, while the number who have had a heart valve prosthesis inserted, with or without associated complications, has increased. Nowadays, at centers where cardiovascular surgery is performed, diseased heart valves are seen more often in the surgical pathology laboratory than at the autopsy table. In contrast, the surgical treatment of valvular heart disease in underdeveloped countries, while changing practice in surgical pathology, has yet to make any impression on the huge reservoir of cases caused by rheumatic disease and likely to die of complications from their valvular disease.[55]

Datta, in Chapter 33, draws attention to differences in the frequency, clinical presentation, and morphology of valvular heart disease in the tropics as compared with Western countries. Pathologists must be aware of these differences, but, no matter where they practice, must examine with care any specimen of diseased heart valve encountered to define types of valvular disease that were not recognized in the past—either because they are new (e.g., methysergide-induced valvular disease) or because they were likely obscured, both clinically and pathologically, by the huge number of cases with rheumatic valvular disease that used to exist (e.g., prolapsed mitral valve).[138]

LEVELS OF OBSTRUCTION

In considering an obstruction to blood flow through the heart and relating it to valvular structures, an obstruction may occur at subvalvular, valvular, or supravalvular levels (Table 24–1). Most often, obstructions are at the valvular level.

933

Table 24–1.   Location, Frequency, and Mechanisms of Obstruction to Blood Flow Through the Heart.

Mechanisms of Obstruction/Frequency		*Level of Obstruction*
1. Congenital anomaly		
2. Leaflet/cusp stiffening		
3. Commissural fusion	Common	Valvular
4. Combination of 2 and 3		
5. Filling of valve lumen	Uncommon	
6. External compression of lumen		
Congenital anomaly or acquired lesion that encroaches upon lumen by		
1. Forming with lumen	Uncommon	
2. Originating from wall components	Common	Subvalvular or supravalvular
3. External compression	Uncommon	

MECHANISMS OF OBSTRUCTION

Natural valves become stenosed when, as a result of a congenital anomaly or acquired disease, their leaflets, or cusps stiffen, the adjacent side of cusps or leaflets are fused in the commissural regions (commissural fusion), or a combination of these processes occurs. Rarely, the orifice of a natural valve is stenosed by a mass filling its lumen or by external compression.

Subvalvular and supravalvular obstructions too may be congenital or acquired. They are usually the result of processes that encroach on the lumen of the inflow tract leading to valve or of the outflow tract leading from it. The obstruction may be caused by a mass forming within the lumen of the tract, by wall components impinging on the lumen, or by external compression of the tract wall (see Fig. 24–1).

Prosthetic heart valves are made either of tissue (tissue valves) or of metal, plastic, or other artificial components (nontissue or mechanical prostheses) (see Chs. 40 and 41). Tissue prostheses are narrowed by the same mechanisms that stenose a natural heart valve. Mechanical valves, for the most part, are stenosed by those mechanisms that induce supravalvular or subvalvular stenosis. All these mechanisms are listed in Table 24–2. Very

rarely, pathologic changes associated with a prosthetic valve will induce an obstruction proximal or distal to the prosthesis.

In this chapter, pathological processes producing obstruction to blood flow at subvalvular, valvular, and supravalvular levels will be discussed dealing with or related to tricuspid, pulmonary, and mitral valves in turn and obstructions encountered as one follows blood flow through the heart. As this book emphasizes conditions found in the adult, only congenital lesions that permit survival to adulthood are discussed.[36,97] Conditions causing stenosis of prosthetic heart valves are presented in Chapters 40 and 41.

OBSTRUCTION AT OR RELATED TO THE TRICUSPID VALVE

Supravalvular Obstruction

Supravalvular obstruction of the tricuspid valve is extremely uncommon.

Congenital Anomalies

Certain congenital anomalies that can persist to adulthood produce the so-called cor triatriatum dexter. When this anomaly is initially

Table 24–2.   Mechanism and Frequency of Obstruction to Blood Flow Through Prosthetic Heart Valves

Mechanism of Obstruction/Frequency		Prosthetic Valve Affected
Acquired lesions that cause:		
1. Leaflet stiffening		
2. Commissural fusion	Common	Tissue
3. Combination of 1 and 2		
4. Filling of lumen	Uncommon	
5. External compression		
Acquired lesions that		
1. Form within lumen	Common	
2. Encroach upon lumen		
3. Entrap occluder in lumen		Mechanical
4. Originate from lumen components	Uncommon	
5. Cause external compression and interfere with occluder excursion		

examined at autopsy, the right atrial chamber appears to be divided into two. This finding could give a false impression of a supraventricular stenosis in the right atrium. Hudson[54] illustrates an example of cor triatriatum dexter. It was found incidentally and at autopsy in a man of 78 and was caused by a greatly dilated coronary sinus receiving a left superior vena cava. Hudson[54] is of the opinion that other examples of an accessory septum that he cites as subdividing the right atrium to produce cor triatriatum dexter are examples of an anomalous development or regression of the right sinus venosus valve.

Several patterns of persistence exist.[27,36,38] The most common presents an abnormal membrane located to the right of the superior and inferior vena caval ostia and that of the coronary sinus. The second most common pattern has only the coronary sinus terminating to the right of the abnormal membrane.

Surgical correction of certain congenital anomalies can produce a small right atrial chamber that may behave as a supravalvular stenosis (see Ch. 45).

Acquired Lesions

An aneurysm of the septum primum[114]; a right atrial myxoma; other primary or secondary tumor masses that invade the right atrium or venae cavae (e.g., primary angio- or leiomyosarcoma or a renal carcinoma extending through the inferior vena cava); a large mural thrombus or an aneurysm of the sinus of Valsalva may all bulge into the right atrium and cause supravalvular tricuspid valve stenosis. Each is very rare. Some of these lesions might also cause valvular obstruction if they also project into the valve orifice.

Clinical Manifestations

Supravalvular stenosis induces clinical symptoms that mimic those of valvular stenosis (see below).

Valvular Obstruction

Congenital Anomalies

Perloff,[97] in discussing natural survival patterns in postpediatric congenital heart disease, lists Ebstein's anomaly of the tricuspid valve among the uncommon defects in which adult survival is expected and tricuspid atresia among the common defects in which survival is exceptional.

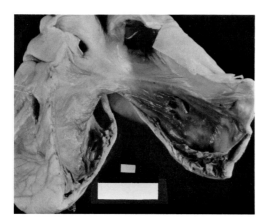

Fig. 24–1. Ebstein's anomaly of tricuspid valve in a 27-year-old woman with valvular patent foramen ovale and cerebral infarction. Note attachment of leaflets to right ventricular wall. (Small marker = 1 cm.) (Courtesy of M. Lipa, M.D., Toronto.)

Ebstein's Anomaly

Ebstein's anomaly[8,28,29,42,68,73,130,140] shows a displacement of fused or malformed tricuspid valvular tissue, usually the posterior and septal leaflets, into the right ventricular cavity so that the basal attachments of the leaflets adhere to the right ventricular cavity distal to the true annulus of the valve (Fig. 24–1). The valve tissue is often redundant, but the pathologic anatomy of the condition is variable. As a result of the anomaly, part of the right ventricle functions as part of the right atrium. The condition is commonly associated with a patent foramen ovale or fossa ovalis type of atrial septal defect but may occur as part of a complex congenital heart anomaly; abnormalities of left ventricular contraction and prolapsed mitral valves are also found in affected patients.[86,104,130] The abnormal tricuspid valve may be stenosed or incompetent but is usually neither.[30] The anomaly is best explained as an abnormality in the process of undermining of the right ventricular wall by which tricuspid valve leaflets and chordae are formed.[130]

Tricuspid Atresia

In tricuspid atresia (see also Ch. 45) no communication exists between the right atrium and ventricle, but the location of the valve may be marked by a dimple in the anterior wall of the right atrium. In this condition all right atrial blood must be shunted through an atrial septal defect to reach the left heart. Certain anatomic variants beyond the tricuspid valve affect longevity. They include the presence or absence of transposition of the great vessels, pulmonary stenosis, or a ventricular septal defect. If these conditions coexist, an affected patient's life expectancy is best when pulmonary stenosis permits an adequate but not excessive pulmonary blood flow and so prevents pulmonary vascular disease from developing. Thus, the very few patients with untreated tricuspid stenosis who survive to adulthood have coexisting pulmonary stenosis with a favorable regulation of pulmonary blood flow.[97]

Modern surgical procedures used to treat tricuspid atresia have affected its natural history so that patients are surviving longer even though few reach adult life (see Ch. 45).

Acquired Lesions

In the adult, acquired tricuspid valvular stenosis is seen much less frequently than mitral or aortic stenosis but is more common than pulmonary stenosis. Tricuspid stenosis may be an isolated lesion[87] but is usually associated with diseases affecting other valves—for example, rheumatic disease affecting mitral and aortic valves[79] (see Ch. 33) or in carcinoid heart disease also involving the pulmonary valve. Interestingly, the frequency of tricuspid stenosis seen in rheumatic valvular diseases in India (see Ch. 33) or Mexico[109] is much higher than is now encountered in Western countries.

Rheumatic Valvular Disease

Rheumatic valvular disease is the main cause of tricuspid stenosis.[25,52] It incites pathologic change mainly by causing commissural fusion (Fig. 24–2). The chordae of the tricuspid valve may thicken and shorten, but chordal fusion and, indeed, chordal changes in general (Fig. 24–4b) are not usually as severe as they are in rheumatic mitral stenosis. The commissural fusion is usually marked at the anteroseptal commissure (Fig. 24–4A) and, if all three commissures are affected, the shortened, thickened cusps, fused at their commissures, produce a diaphragm-like impediment to flow (Fig. 24–2C). The diaphragm funnels toward the right ventricle and has a fixed round, oval, or triangular orifice (Fig. 24–2C). Thus, in advanced rheumatic tricuspid stenosis, the valve is nearly always stenosed and incompetent. In contrast to mitral stenosis, secondary calcification of the stenosed tricuspid valve is relatively uncommon.[52]

Miscellaneous Causes

The leaflets of the tricuspid valve may also be thickened as a result of metabolic or enzymatic abnormalities; in Fabry's or Whipple's disease; or following methysergide therapy with resultant valvular stenosis (see also Ch. 31) Rightsided endocarditis is relatively uncommon, except among drug addicts who use the intravenous method of administration (see Ch. 23). Nevertheless, large, infected vegetations, filling the lumen, may cause transient valvular stenosis.

As indicated above, a right atrial myxoma or other intracavity tumor may, on rare occasions, induce symptoms of tricuspid stenosis. Secondary tumor invasion of the pericardium, usually from a primary tumor in the lung or the breast, can also cause obstruction by external compression of the valve.

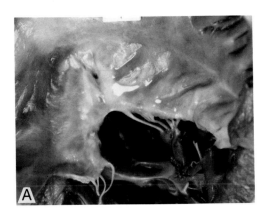

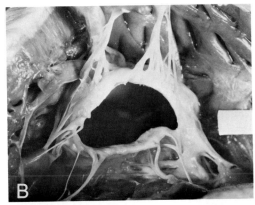

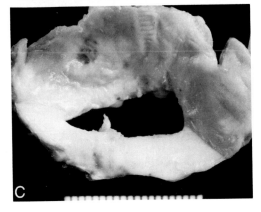

Fig. 24–2. Rheumatic disease affecting tricuspid valve and causing marked commissural fusion; chordal thickening and fusion is usually not severe. (A & C) Both valves viewed from atrial aspect; (B) valve viewed from ventricular aspect.) If commissural fusion is marked, a diaphragm-like orifice forms. (C) surgically excised tricuspid valve. (Scale in Figs. A and B = 1 cm; scale in Fig. C = 2 cm.)

Carcinoid heart disease, as a cause of tricuspid stenosis, is discussed in Chapter 31.

Pathologic Effects

Tricuspid valve stenosis causes a rise in right atrial pressure. This produces dilation of that chamber and a thickening of its wall due to hypertrophy. The right atrial endocardium may thicken and calcium plaques develop in it, but the latter change occurs far less commonly than it does in the enlarged left atrium associated with mitral stenosis. The raised intraluminal pressure causes dilatation of the ostia of veins draining into the right atrium, especially that of the coronary sinus, and congestion of liver and spleen; anasarca may develop.

Histologically, the liver shows severe congestion, which, if prolonged, will cause liver cell replacement and fibrosis (so-called cardiac cirrhosis).

Clinical Manifestations

As Braunwald indicates, the patient with tricuspid valve stenosis usually has a long history and is often female.[19] About 60 percent of patients have a history of attacks of rheumatic fever, and often, in this group, there is evidence of multivalvular disease. The low cardiac output associated with tricuspid stenosis causes progressive fatigue, edema, and anorexia. The patient may notice a fluttering in the neck veins caused by giant *a* waves in the jugular venous pulse. Often, they complain of discomfort due to hepatomegaly, abdominal swelling, or anasarca, which are all secondary to the elevated systemic venous pressure and out of proportion to the degree of dyspnea. Indeed, orthopnea and paroxsymal nocturnal dyspnea are both minimal and unusual whereas pulmonary edema and hemoptysis are rare, even if mitral stenosis coexists.

Evidence of multivalvular disease is often apparent at physical examination. The patient is wasted, has peripheral cyanosis, and neck vein distention with prominent V waves. There is a right ventricular lift and a holo-systolic murmur heard best at the left lower sternal border. A hepatic pulsation may be obvious and both anasarca and peripheral edema may be as well.

Electrocardiograms, (ECG) show full right atrial P waves and no right ventricular hypertrophy. Radiographs reveal marked cardiomegaly with a dilated right atrium and without an enlarged pulmonary artery segment. Two-dimensional echocardiography imaging shows diastolic doming of the valve leaflets with their thickening and restriction of excursion. Also, there is reduced separation of leaflet tips.

Treatment

Surgical treatment is preferred when the mean diastolic pressure gradient exceeds 5 mmHg and the valve orifice is less than 200 cm^2. It may involve balloon dilation, a commissurotomy, a plastic reconstruction, or valve excision and replacement with a prosthesis.

OBSTRUCTION AT OR RELATED TO THE PULMONARY VALVE

Subvalvular Obstruction

Congenital Anomalies

Isolated infundibular stenosis is a rare congenital anomaly.[33] Like subvalvular obstruction of the left ventricle, obstruction of the right ventricular outflow tract may be caused by: (1) a fibrous band, found at the junction of the main cavity of the right ventricle and the infundibulum and producing obstruction of the proximal infundibulum; or (2) muscle impinging on the lumen and narrowing it over a long or short segment.[31,74] An anomalous muscle bundle that forms a pyramidal mass between the septal wall, immediately adjacent to the septal leaflet of the tricuspid valve and the anterior wall of the right ventricle in the distal part of the inflow tract to the right ventricle, may also produce a right ventricular outflow tract obstruction.[35,41,77,108] The latter anomaly effectively produces a two-chambered outflow tract from the right ventricle. The anomalies described above almost invariably cause clinical problems in infancy or childhood but, in theory, minor forms could permit survival to adulthood.

In children, infundibular stenosis caused by myocardium impinging on the lumen may be associated with pulmonary valvular or supravalvular stenosis or occurs as part of the tetralogy of Fallot complex[97] (see Ch. 45) (Fig. 24–3).

However, the likelihood of finding these lesions at autopsy in adults in Western countries is diminishing as they are now usually corrected surgically in childhood. Rather, in adults surviving total correction of tetralogy of Fallot the endocardium at the infundibulectomy site is thickened and scarred and the muscle is locally thinned (Fig. 24–4). Sometimes, a pericardial or prosthetic patch has been inserted in the area and complications

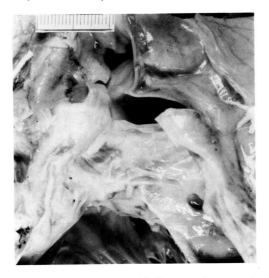

Fig. 24–4. Scarred infundibulum in right ventricle follow previous infundibulectomy during total correction of tetralogy of Fallot 2 years previously. Patient, a woman aged 36. (Scale indicates 2 cm.) (Courtesy of F. S. Sousa, M.D., Brampton, Ontario.)

of the ventriculotomy may be apparent. These may include recurrent stenosis (see Ch. 45). Jones et al.[58] described the ultrastructural changes in myocardium excised from the infundibulum in such cases.

In discussing other causes of right ventricular outflow tract obstruction, Freedom et al. (Ch. 45) list aneurysms of the membraneous septum.

Acquired Lesions

Marked hypertrophy of the interventricular septum can induce right ventricular outflow tract obstruction. Very rarely, hypertrophic cardiomyopathy causes a systolic movement of the anterior tricuspid valve leaflet and subpulmonic obstruction.

Clinical Features

Clinically, it may be difficult to distinguish valvular and subvalvular pulmonary stenosis because the symptoms caused by the latter mimic those due to the valvular disease. Nev-

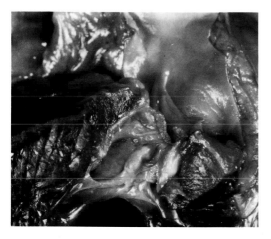

Fig. 24–3. Outflow tract of right ventricle illustrating infundibular stenosis in 23-year-old man with tetralogy of Fallot. The upper arch of a ventricular septal defect is seen in the lower part of the photograph. The patient had a pulmonary valve with three cusps.

ertheless, in subvalvular stenosis, post-stenotic dilation of the pulmonary artery is not a feature and angiographic and flow studies permit differentiation.

Valvular Obstruction

The majority (about 80 percent) of cases of right ventricular outflow tract obstruction occur at the valvular level.

Congenital Anomalies

Isolated pulmonary valvular stenosis is one of the common congenital cardiac defects in which adult survival is expected.[31,33,62,96,97] In fact, isolated pulmonary stenosis is more likely to be congenital than acquired.

Noonan Syndrome

Noonan and Ehmke[92] described a syndrome of pulmonary valve stenosis with other noncardiac anomalies that may affect both males and females. This syndrome, subsequently given the eponym Noonan syndrome, is better referred to as Turner's phenotype. This is in contrast to Turner's genotype in which an aortic coarctation is the most likely cardiovascular anomaly. Pulmonary stenosis is common in the phenotype syndrome, but other forms of congenital heart disease may occur.[83] The karyotype of affected persons is usually normal.

The pulmonary valve in Turner's phenotype syndrome or, indeed, in other congenital forms of pulmonary stenosis may be dome-shaped and have no commissures, or have either two or three cusps.[15] The dome-shaped valve is stenosed because of its frustrum shape, but, in those instances where three cusps exist, the stenosis is caused because the cusps are dysplastic and, as a result, greatly thickened, shortened, and rigid.[66] In such a dysplastic valve there is usually no associated commissural fusion, the valve annulus may be narrowed and the patient usually does not have a poststenotic dilation of the pulmonary

artery. Valve function in a patient with a dysplastic valve may be further impeded by fibrous masses present in the depths of the sinuses. Rarely, a stenosed pulmonary valve may calcify.[105]

Tetralogy of Fallot

Again pulmonary valvular stenosis may be a feature in tetralogy of Fallot.

LEOPARD Syndrome

Stenosis of the pulmonary valve may also occur as part of the LEOPARD syndrome (L = lentigenes, E = electrocardiographic conduction defects, O = ocular hypertelorism, P = pulmonic valve stenosis, A = abnormalities of genitalia, R = retardation of growth, and D = deafness, which is sensorineural), a rare, single gene determined complex of congenital malformations. Isolated stenosis of the pulmonary valve is the most common cardiac anomaly encountered in the syndrome, but it may be associated with aortic stenosis, endocardial fibroelastosis, or hypertrophic cardiomyopathy.[53,111]

Quadricuspid Valve

A quadricuspid pulmonary valve may become stenosed as a result of calcification and fibrosis.

Acquired Lesions

Rheumatic Disease

Rheumatic disease affecting the pulmonary valve and causing stenosis is uncommon and is almost invariably associated with rheumatic disease affecting other cardiac valves. Usually, there is slight commissural fusion; cusp thickening and the deformity is not severe.[112] However, Vela et al.[133] reported significant pulmonary valve lesions in patients from Mexico City and suggested that the pulmonary hypertension associated with the altitude of that city increases the stress on the valve, making it prone to damage.

Miscellaneous Causes

Carcinoid plaques may cause pulmonary stenosis by thickening the cusps (see Ch. 31). Cardiac tumors or aneurysms of the sinus of Valsalva can stenose the subvalvular or valvular area as may external pressure induced by calcification in the right atrioventricular groove, resulting from a tuberculous pericarditis.

Pathologic Effects

Pulmonary stenosis, whether congenital or acquired, causes dilation and hypertrophy of the right ventricle. If infundibular hypertrophy is marked, it may add to right ventricular outflow tract obstruction. Indeed, if right ventricular hypertension persists after an adequate valvulotomy, an infundibular resection may have to be done.[88] Endocardial fibroelastosis may develop in the right ventricle, particularly in the outflow tract; the jet of blood, forced through the stenosed valve, can produce an intimal jet lesion or cause poststenotic dilation of the pulmonary artery. Myocardial hypertrophy decreases the compliance of the right ventricle and impedes right atrial emptying. Patchy fibrosis of the right ventricle is a common finding at autopsy. If the intra-atrial pressure is increased markedly, it may cause a right to left shunt through a valvular, patent foramen ovale; with such a shunt, a patient's risk of developing a cerebral abscess is increased.

Clinical Manifestations

The majority of patients with mild pulmonary stenosis are asymptomatic.[32,62] Thus, the condition should be looked for as an incidental finding at autopsy. With severe valvular stenosis, dyspnea and fatigue can develop on exercise. Exertional syncope or lightheadedness are rare occurrences with severe stenosis, as is sudden death. Severe stenosis eventually induces tricuspid valve regurgitation with its associated symptoms and right heart failure.

A systolic murmur and thrill may be obvious in the pulmonary area. Echocardiography helps define both the pathology and the physiologic importance of pulmonary stenosis.

Treatment

Percutaneous balloon valvuloplasty appears to be both safe and effective treatment. Alternatively, valvulotomy may be used.

Supravalvular Obstruction

Congenital Anomalies

Supravalvular stenosis[33,37,54] occurs in the pulmonary trunk, in its main branches, or in the intrapulmonary arteries. Most often the trunk and/or its main branches are involved. Pulmonary arterial stenosis may be an isolated phenomenon but more often is associated with other congenital anomalies. The stenosis may be single or multiple, localized or segmental, or may be due to a generalized hypoplasia of the vessels (diffuse). Very rarely, a membranous ring is found in the pulmonary trunk immediately distal to the valve. Gay and colleagues[37] provided a useful classification of supravalvular pulmonary stenosis.

The cause of the condition is unknown. However, intrauterine infection with the rubella virus has been implicated in its pathogenesis.

Pathologic Effects

The physiologic abnormality is similar to that in valvular or isolated subvalvular pulmonary stenosis and is affected by the severity of obstruction. Because the majority of stenoses are centrally located, the pulmonary vessel proximal to the obstruction dilates and, because of an increased pressure in its lumen, causes a delayed closure of the pulmonary valve. The condition can be distinguished from other forms of right ventricular outflow tract obstruction by selective angiography and pressure measurements.

Most cases present with symptoms in infancy or childhood, but supravalvular stenosis may, in rare instances, be found as an isolated finding in adults. Possibly, some cases are missed at autopsy because of the usual techniques used to open the pulmonary arteries.

Treatment

Depending on the location of the stenosis and whether it is isolated, a graft or a patch graft may be used. Balloon angiography is also employed to treat the condition in children.

OBSTRUCTION AT OR RELATED TO THE MITRAL VALVE

Supravalvular Obstruction

Congenital Anomalies

Cor Triatriatum

This rare congenital anomaly usually presents in childhood: it may occur as an isolated abnormality or be associated with other congenital heart defects.[96] In children it usually causes severe venous obstruction. Rarely, the condition causes no symptoms until adulthood;[54,71,81,91] or it is found incidentally at autopsy.[75]

In cor triatriatum a membranous septum, containing variable numbers of myocardial fibers, divides the left atrium into two chambers. A dorsal, or obliquely inferior one, that receives the pulmonary veins and a ventral chamber that communicates with the left atrial appendage and through the mitral valve to the left ventricle.[131] Usually the mitral valve in cor triatriatum found in adults is normal, but mitral regurgitation may occur.[71] Van Praagh and Corsini[131] corrected the impression, easily gained from a gross specimen, that the chamber receiving the pulmonary veins is superior and the other inferior to the sep-

tum. The dividing septum usually stretches in an oblique plane and is in direct continuity with the septum primum. Niwayama[91] indicated that the foramen ovale may be opened or closed and could open into either chamber. However, Van Praagh and Corsini[131] were of the opinion that the foramen is always present in the ventral chamber and that communications between the dorsal chamber and right atrium are through abnormal communications between the common pulmonary vein chamber and the right wall of the sinus venosus.

In children the membrane may or may not be perforated. If perforated, the hole is usually single and small and located a short distance behind the posteromedial commissure of the normal appearing mitral valve.[131] The degree of obstruction caused by the membrane varies with the presence or absence of perforations and, in the former instance, with their size.[75,91] When the anomaly is found in adults, the perforation(s) is(are) usually large and may show calcification at their perimeter.

Histologically, the septum shows variable amounts of fibroelastic and myocardial tissue. Van Praagh and Corsini[131] indicated that the subdividing diaphragm in cor triatriatum is composed of the wall of the common pulmonary vein dorsally and that of the primitive left atrium ventrally. This viewpoint is supported by their finding that the composition of the diaphragm superiorly and ventrally is that of the left atrial free wall, whereas its composition inferiorly and dorsally is that of the common pulmonary vein.

In discussing theories of formation, Van Praagh and Corsini[131] favor the supposition that cor triatriatum results from entrapment of the left atrial ostium of the common pulmonary vein by tissue of the right wall of the sinus venosus from which the septum primum develops, leading to failure of incorporation of the common pulmonary vein to the left atrium during the fifth week of embryological development. Gharagozloo et al.[39] consider that the abnormal membrane is caused by the left superior vena cava impinging on the developing left atrium.

Other Anomalies

Anomalous fibromuscular bands, which may be found, although very rarely, in the left atrium of adults stretching from the intra-atrial septal wall to the base or free margin of the anterior or posterior mitral valve leaflet, must be mentioned at this point.[54,65,93] Hudson considered them a variant of cor triatriatum and one end of the spectrum of that anomaly. Knoblich and Ducey[65] suggested that the bands result from the septum primum not fusing with the septum secundum, with the dorsal part of the septum primum being drawn out by the developing mitral valve to produce the anomalous bands. Similar cords may pass through the mitral valve[93] or aortic orifice.[60]

Another form of congenital supravalvular stenosis exists in which the valve and its supporting structures are normal but the valve inlet is encroached on by a ridge of connective tissue at the base of the mitral valve.[118] This condition may occur as an isolated defect in adults. In children it frequently coexists with a parachute mitral valve or with the asplenia syndrome.[85] If the obstruction is caused by a supravalvular stenosing ring, the atrial appendage, unlike that in cor triatriatum, is located in the proximal chamber.

Acquired Lesions

I have seen several cases in which children have required insertion of several mitral valve prostheses. With each insertion the valve "annulus" has had to be advanced further proximally, to accommodate the new prosthesis. This decreases left atrial size and produces a level of stenosis above the original valve orifice.

Clinical Manifestations

Most cases of cor triatriatum present in childhood, but occasional patients are asymptomatic until the third decade. In adults the symptoms are similar to those of mitral stenosis.[53] The specific cause can be distinguished by echocardiography (especially in the 2D mode) or angiography.

Treatment

Surgical correction of cor triatriatum is undertaken if the patient develops symptoms of pulmonary hypertension.

Valvular Obstruction

Congenital Anomalies

Congenital fusion of mitral commissures or accessory mitral valve tissue are uncommon causes of mitral stenosis.[26] Most cases present in childhood,[20] but both Singh et al.[116] and Tank et al.[126] describe cases in teenagers. Possibly, minor forms of this congenital anomaly exist, causing mitral stenosis. They could be misinterpreted at autopsy as being due to rheumatic heart disease.

Acquired Lesions

Acquired mital stenosis is most often caused by repeated attacks of acute rheumatic fever (ARF).[94,106]

Epidemiology of Rheumatic Fever

In developed countries the frequency and severity of ARF has diminished, with fewer children being admitted to the hospital with the condition, or showing carditis, or dying of the acute attack.[9,67,100,124] Nevertheless, in North America, the disease still occurs in overcrowded areas of major cities, in areas where people on the lowest rung of the socioeconomic ladder live. Its incidence is high among blacks.[124]

Of note are reports of ARF affecting children in Utah[132] and other U.S. states and reports of it occurring among military recruits.[137] Whether this is due to a change in the virulence of the *Streptococcus* or has other explanations is uncertain.[10]

Acute rheumatic fever and its affects on the heart valves continue as major health problems in so-called third world countries, especially those located in the tropics[4,75,124] (see Ch. 33).

Climate, per se, has little effect on the prevalence of ARF; rather, in tropical countries, the populace often live in conditions promoting a rapid spread of pharyngeal streptococci of rheumatogenic potential. These include crowded living conditions, close person-to-person contact, and inadequate treatment or prevention of streptococcal infections. Furthermore, many people in these countries are undernourished. Correction of these problems in affluent societies has undoubtedly played a role in reducing the prevalence rate of ARF, but the behavior of rheumatogenic streptococci seems to have changed as well. Pharyngitis due to groups of streptococci is still common among populations in which rheumatic fever is now a rare disease. Changes in the virulence and serotypes of the Group A streptococci have been recorded.[9,123]

Rheumatic fever ordinarily occurs with greatest frequency and for the first time in children between 6 to 15 years old[11] It is uncommon before the age of 5 but may occur for the first time in adults. Recurrent attacks diminish with age, but a recurrence may present with unusual manifestation in an elderly patient. There is no sex difference in the attack rate, although certain valvular changes that develop as a result of repeated attacks may affect men (isolated aortic stenosis) or women (mitral stenosis) more frequently.

Pathogenesis of Rheumatic Fever

ARF develops in a susceptible person within 10 days to 6 weeks of a throat infection with β-hemolytic group A streptococci.[17,124,139] This is in contrast to acute glomerulonephritis, which is a result of a skin or throat infection with different strains of group A streptococci.[10,122,123,125] The susceptibility to ARF seems to run in families[117,142] but does not follow a Mendelian pattern of inheritance.[120,121] Nor is there a demonstrable relationship with human leukocyte antigen (HLA) genotypes. However, certain class II human histocompatibility antigens are en-

countered more frequently in patients with ARF than in controls. In particular, HLA-DR2 and DLA-DR4 phenotypes are encountered in a significantly higher frequency in black patients than in white patients.[101] Rheumatic subjects express a particular surface antigen on their B lymphocytes to a greater extent than do controls.[63] Whether these observations indicate genetic or acquired characteristics is not yet certain. In "closed" population—for example, navy recruits who were ill with frank exudative streptococcal pharyngitis caused by virulent Group A streptococci—ARF followed at a fairly predictable attack rate of approximately 3 percent regardless of the age, race, or ethnic group studied.[102] Other major variables that seem related to the attack rate are the magnitude of the immune response to antecedent streptococcal infection[110] and the duration the organism is carried during convalescence.

Between sore throat and initial or recurrent attack of ARF an immune response occurs. The evidence for this is based on clinical, epidemiologic, immunologic, and prophylactic evidence.[122–124] The streptococcal cell wall is a complex structure.[107] Its components enable the organism to successfully colonize and proliferate on the oropharyngeal mucosa. Stollerman[123] listed bacteriologic features of the strains of Group A streptococci related to ARF. Such organisms (1) are very rich in M protein and highly resistant to phagocytosis; (2) have very large hyaluronate capsules, as is evident from the huge mucoid colonies they form on blood agar; (3) are extremely virulent to mice when freshly isolated or may be made virulent by a few passages through mice; (4) are easily kept in the virulent phase by proper storage or culture and occasional mouse passage; (5) stimulate a good anti-M serum response against themselves in rabbits; and (6) lack the "sera opacity" factor.

A study of 15 families each having more than one sibling affected by rheumatic fever revealed a significant increased avidity of rheumatic fever-associated strains of streptococci to adhere to pharyngeal epithelial cells among rheumatic sibling when compared to normal sibling controls.[49] Components of the cell wall and extracellular products may have a direct toxic effect on heart muscle cells,[107] but, more importantly, they are capable of inducing immune reactions in a susceptible host. The reacting antigens (or antigen) are located in the cell wall and cytoplasmic membrane of the streptococcus and are closely related to the M protein, to the Group A polysaccharide of the cell wall, and to a glycoprotein and other proteins of the cytoplasm.[107,123]

It is postulated that large amounts of streptococcal antigens are absorbed by a hypersensitized host following a pharyngeal infection with virulent organisms and that a specific streptococcal product to which the host is allergic is bound to tissues affected by rheumatic fever. A subsequent humoral or cellular response (or both) is thought to damage the tissue, with the antibodies directed against the antigens cross-reacting with specific sites in the host. Human tissue components with an immunologic relationship to Group A streptococci have been identified in the myocardium (sarcolemma of cardiac muscle, subsarcolemmal sarcoplasm)[61,129]; heart valves[40]; skeletal muscle[146]; thymus; human glomerular basement membrane; skin; neuronal cytoplasm of human caudate and subthalamic nuclei; and human lymphocytes. Many monoclonal antibodies cross-react with M protein, the streptococcus virulence determinant, and host proteins such as myosin and tropomyosin.[24] Also, a specific pentapeptide of the M protein is immunologically cross-reactive with human cardiac myosin.[23] In their studies on diseased rheumatic valves recovered at surgery Gulizia et al.[48] reported that antistreptococcal monoclonal antibodies bind to valvular surface endothelium and immediate subendothelial structures such as elastin, microfibrils, and valvular interstitial cells. These findings may have pathologic significance. Furthermore, Yang and associates[145] demonstrated that Group A streptococcal antigens associated with the protoplast membrane induce cytotoxicity to guinea pig lymphocytes, with the lymphocytes specifically destroying allogenic myocardial cells grown in culture. These cellular mechanisms may also have a role. Studies on lymphocyte subsets in patients with acute rheumatic fever indicate a reduction of suppressor T cells with an absolute increase in helper T and B cells.[1,7] Nevertheless, although an infection with β-hemolytic Group A streptococci precedes the onset of ARF and the disease seems associated with immunologic reaction, the exact mechanisms are still unknown. One notes that this concept of pathogenesis is not universally accepted.[12,16]

Pathology of Rheumatic Fever

ARF produces proliferative and exudative inflammatory reactions in the connective tissue, particularly that of the heart, joints, and skin; Other organs may be affected, also. The disease is self-limiting, the signs presenting in most cases for less than 3 months, but attacks tend to recur.

Death in the Acute Phase   Relatively few of those affected with the disease die during the acute attack. If they do, the heart is usually enlarged and globular owing to dilation of all chambers and may show ventricular hypertrophy. A bland, fibrinous pericarditis may be observed, and occasionally a serous or serosanguinous pericardial effusion. Sometimes the myocardium shows remarkably little change—for example, myocardial edema with focal myocardial cell degeneration, despite florid clinical manifestations. Alternatively, a diffuse, nonspecific, mononuclear cell infiltrate consisting mainly of lymphocytes but with some histiocytes, plasma cells, polymorphonuclear leukocytes, and eosinophils with marked edema of the myocardium may be found (Fig. 24–5) with an associated nonspecific arteritis of small intramyocardial vessels (see Ch. 14). Occasionally, verrucae are present on the heart valves, but this is not a universal finding.

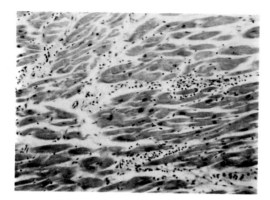

Fig. 24–5. Diffuse nonspecific myocarditis and edema in a 12-year-old girl dying acutely 3 weeks after onset of symptoms of acute rheumatic fever. (H&E, × 8.)

Death at Later Stages Patients dying later in the acute phase, whether during the first attack or subsequent ones, may manifest pathologic changes in the heart and other organs. These are discussed below.

Cardiac Lesions ARF produces a pancarditis. Lesions may involve endocardium, myocardium, pericardium, blood vessels, and the conducting system.

Endocardial Lesions. In the acute phase of rheumatic fever, *valvular* endocardial le-sions are found most commonly on the mitral valve and next in frequency on the aortic valve. They are not common on the tricuspid valve (probably because they are difficult to see) and are least frequent on the pulmonary valve.

Initially, they present as small, translucent beadlike vegetations 1 to 2 mm in diameter (verrucae) but subsequently they become gray-brown (Fig. 24–6A). They adhere firmly to the leaflet along the line of closure on the atrial aspect of atrioventricular valves and on the ventricular aspect of the cusps of semi-lunar valves. Usually verrucae are confined to the valvular endocardium but they may extend onto the chordae tendineae of atrio-ventricular valves and, in rare instances, be associated with chordal rupture.[56]

Histologically, the vegetations consist of platelets and fibrin and usually overlie a ne-crotic/inflammatory reaction in the adjacent valve (Fig. 24–6B). This, at varying stages, may be seen as an area of fibrinoid necrosis with mononuclear cells, fibroblasts, and oc-casional giant cells in the infiltrate around it. Alternatively, during healing, the inflamma-tory cells are arranged in a palisade fashion at right angles to the valve surface. The types of inflammatory cells present are comparable to those found in an Aschoff's nodule (see

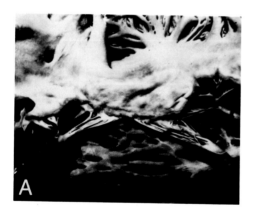
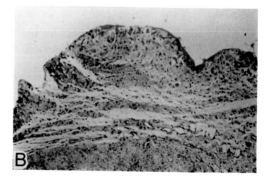

Fig. 24–6. Verrucae in acute rheumatic fever. In (A), verrucae have formed along the line of closure on the atrial aspect of the anterior mitral valve in a girl, aged 13. (B) shows the histologic equivalent with verruca composed of a ring thrombotic vegetation overlying a chronic inflammatory reaction in the adjacent leaflet. (H&E, × 20.)

below) and go through a life cycle like that of the nodule, but Aschoff's nodules, per se, are not commonly found in valves. The adjacent leaflet may be edematous, show a diffuse mononuclear cell infiltrate, and have small, thin-walled blood vessels invading it from its base.

It is presumed that verrucae develop as a result of damage to the connective tissue of the valve occurring as part of the immune reaction in acute rheumatic fever. This leads to ulceration of the surface endothelium with or without extrusion of damaged collagen and subsequent thrombus formation. The frequency of left-sided heart valve lesions is related to the pressure that these valves have to withstand; the location of verrucae, on the line of closure, is at a site most liable to trauma.

Aschoff's nodules (see below), are seen in the *mural* endocardium in ARF, particularly in the left atrium.[44,67] MacCallum[77] described a lesion in ARF with numerous Aschoff's nodules in the subendocardium related to a thickening of the overlying left atrial endocardium found proximal to the base of the posterior mitral valve leaflet. Nowadays, and in Western countries, this so-called MacCallum's patch is thought of as a jet lesion associated with the mitral regurgitation that often develops in ARF and, although the endocardial thickening is obvious, associated Aschoff's nodules are rarely seen.

A pathologist is likely to encounter *Aschoff's nodules* in the thickened endocardial connective tissue in approximately 40 percent of atrial appendages removed during cardiac surgery for mitral stenosis (Fig. 24–7). The nodules are uncommon in the atrial myocardium. Also, they are not often found if the atrial lumen contains an organized thrombus. The cellular components of the nodules are characteristic and are described below. Indeed, they must be identified carefully before a diagnosis is made because nonspecific granulomas are also found in the subendocardial tissue of approximately 20 percent of excised atrial appendages.

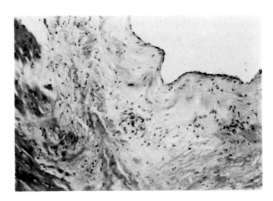

Fig. 24–7. Aschoff's nodules in endocardial tissue of surgically excised atrial appendage. (H&E, × 10.)

The presence of Aschoff's nodules in an appendage indicates that the patient has had ARF in the recent past but does not necessarily indicate a current acute attack. Hudson[54] observed Aschoff's nodules in 20 percent of papillary muscles attached to surgically excised mitral valves. Virmani and Roberts[134] found an incidence of only 2 percent.

In my practice, very few atrial appendages are now forwarded to surgical pathology from patients being treated for rheumatic valvular disease.

Myocardial Lesions. These lesions may be specific (Aschoff's nodule) or nonspecific. The nonspecific myocarditis found in the heart of those dead in the acute phase of rheumatic fever is described above. A giant cell myocarditis will be described subsequently.

Aschoff's nodules develop at many sites in the heart (for example, in the endocardium, pericardium, conducting system, etc.). They are, perhaps, most obvious in the myocardium. Indeed, the Aschoff's nodule in its granulomatous phase is the pathognomonic lesion of ARF in the myocardium.[5] However, this phase represents only one of several morphologic forms that a nodule may assume in its life cycle.

Microscopically, the nodules are round or oval focal lesions that vary in size. They are found in the interstitial tissue, often in close proximity to a small blood vessel, and usually in its adventitia (see Fig. 24–8A and B).

The frequency with which one finds Aschoff's nodules in the hearts of adult patients with rheumatic valvular disease varies. They are least common in patients dying of rheumatic valvular disease after the age of 30 but are not infrequent in younger patients.[127] They are most prevalent in the interventricular septum, posterior wall of the left ventricle, posterior papillary muscle of the left ventricle, pulmonary conus, and left atrium.[44]

The *earliest* lesions are not found in the heart until several weeks have elapsed from the onset of a clinical attack of ARF.[64] They are characterized by an area of swelling, edema, and subsequent fibrinoid necrosis of the connective tissue (Fig. 24–10A). Gammaglobulins may be demonstrated in the fibrinoid by immunofluorescence,[136] and lymphocytes, histiocytes, and plasma cells predominate in an infiltrate found at the perimeter of the fibrinoid necrosis. Gross and Ehrlich[44] described different forms of the nodule at this stage, depending on their morphologic structure.

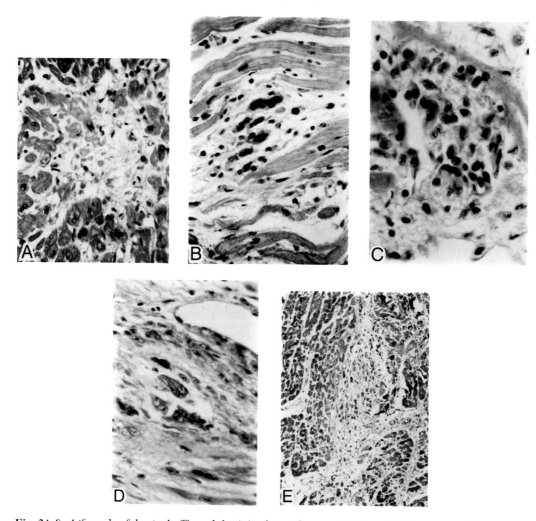

Fig. 24–8. Life cycle of the Aschoff's nodule. (A) Fibrinoid necrosis in interstitial tissue at earliest stage. (B–E) Granulomatous phase of nodule showing cellular components with (C) well-defined histiocytes and (D) giant cells. (E) Resolution of nodules with loss of inflammatory cells and replacement by scar. (H&E: Fig. A, × 32; Figs. B–D, × 64; Fig. E, × 4.)

A subsequent accumulation of cells produces the *granulomatous stage* of the Aschoff's nodule (Fig. 24–8B, C). This is found 1 month or more after an acute attack and is likely to remain in the tissue for 3 to 6 months or even longer and often persists long after clinical symptoms of an acute attack have subsided. A small area of fibrinoid necrosis may present at the center of the nodule in the early granulomatous phase. It becomes surrounded and eventually replaced by histiocytes, giant cells, plasma cells, lymphocytes, and fibroblasts arranged in roughly parallel rows. Histiocytes are large and have basophilic cytoplasm, an indistinct cellular outline, and hypertrophied nuclei. Often, the nuclei show a distinctive arrangement of their chromatin matter, giving the nucleus an "owls eye" or "caterpillar" appearance (Fig. 24–8C). These cells, also named Anitschow's myocytes, are derived from mesodermal cells and, in turn, give rise to giant cells (Aschoff cells) (Fig. 24–10D). When present, Aschoff cells are usually found toward the center of the nodule.

The life cycle of the Aschoff's nodules continue with a gradual diminution in their cellular content and transformation of those found into spindle-shaped cells with an associated growing accumulation of collagen at the site (Fig. 24–10E). Eventually the cellular lesion is replaced by an oval scar. Such scars broaden the interstitial connective tissue or, if a nodule was related to a small vessel, induce an onion-shaped scar centered on the vessel (see Ch. 14).

Patients with a myocarditis associated with clinically silent rheumatic fever may die suddenly.[59]

In very rare instances, a surgically excised atrial appendage shows a *giant cell myocarditis* (Fig. 24–9). The specimen may be yellow-brown, and the surgeon may comment on difficulties encountered in suturing the friable material of the stump of the appendage. A diffuse mononuclear cell infiltrate of histiocytes, lymphocytes, and plasma cells invades the muscle of the appendage, and giant cells are apparent in the reaction. Some giant cells seem derived from degenerating muscle cells,

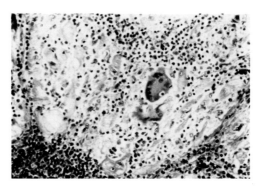

Fig. 24–9. Giant cell myocarditis in a surgically excised atrial appendage of a patient undergoing mital valve replacement for stenosis caused by rheumatic heart disease. (H&E, × 40.)

others from histiocytes. This association between rheumatic valvular disease and giant cell myocarditis may be a fortuitous one or represent an unusual tissue response by a particular patient.

Other Cardiac Lesions in Rheumatic Fever. An acute pericarditis is common in acute or recurrent attacks or ARF, and Aschoff's nodules are found in the tissue (see Ch. 22).

An acute vasculitis of coronary[47] (see Ch. 14 and Figs. 14–13A and B) and other arteries (see Ch. 11) in ARF has been recognized for many years.

Morphologic lesions of the conducting system are uncommon in acute rheumatic fever.[45]

Extracardiac lesions in acute rheumatic fever. Lesions may also occur in the joints,[64] skin and connective tissue, brain,[21,90] and vessels of the lung[135] in ARF.

Rheumatic Valvular Disease

A person who has had one attack of ARF is prone to others. Even following the first attack, 66 percent of the 1,000 patients studied by Jones and Bland[57] had some degree of rheumatic valvular disease, judged clinically, with the valvular disease worsening in 51 percent of this group at the end of a year. The minority, 34 percent, had no evidence of valvular disease following the first attack. Forty-four percent subsequently developed rheumatic heart disease during a 20-year observation.[11]

Explanations offered for the evolution of rheumatic valvular disease affecting any valve include damage wrought by the repeated attacks of ARF, with organization of resultant verrucae causing shortening and thickening of leaflets/cusps and chordae, and secondary damage caused by altered hemodynamics. This secondary damage is thought to induce minute thrombi on the valve surface with their subsequent organization and scarring of the valve.[2,78,128] (see Fig. 23–1).

A relationship between antiphospholipid antibodies and valvular heart disease has been demonstrated.[34] This may also have a role in the evolution of the valvular disease (see discussion in Ch. 23).

In the mitral valve and at an early stage, these changes cause obliteration of the clefts[103] of the posterior leaflet; as a result, the leaflet is shortened, puckered, and ap-

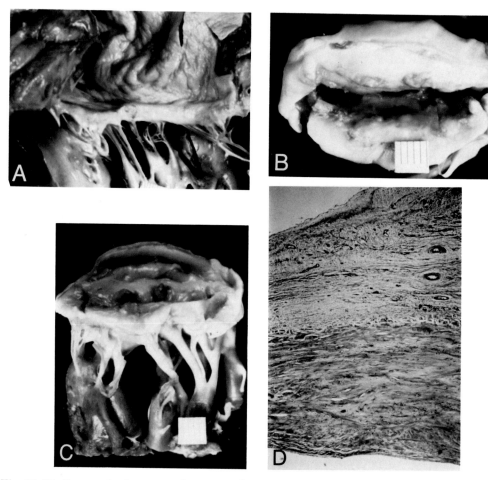

Fig. 24–10. Gross and microscopic changes produced by repeated attacks of rheumatic fever affecting mitral valve. (**A**) Effacement of scallops of posterior leaflets due to cleft fusion in 49-year-old man with mitral stenosis. (**B, C**) Atrial and ventricular aspects of stenosed mitral valve exercised surgically from a 27-year-old woman. Note: commissural and cleft fusion (*posterior leaflet at bottom of picture*); calcium nodules in leaflets Fig. B; and chordal changes in Fig. C. (**D**) Section of mitral leaflet showing sclerosis, vascularization, and nonspecific chronic inflammatory reaction. (Specimen in Figs. B and C courtesy of F. H. Oleniak, M.D., St. John's Hospital, Newfoundland.) (H&E, × 4.)

pears to have only one scallop instead of the usual three (Fig. 24–10A). Following this or concomitant with it, adjacent surfaces of both mitral valve leaflets fuse in the commissural area producing an ovoid, stenosed orifice with thin pliable leaflets (Fig. 24–10B). Alternatively, accompanying changes cause shortening, thickening, and fusion of leaflets and chordae tendineae; this may result in a funnel-shaped stenosis with stiff, rigid leaflets attached to the apices of the papillary muscles (Fig. 24–10C). A "buttonhole" stenosed valve forms when chordal shortening is less marked and a diaphragm with an oval or slitlike orifice results. Thus, the end result may be a valve stenosis, valve stenosis with insufficiency, or valve insufficiency alone[143,144] (see also Ch. 25). A subvalvular stenosis can result if chordal changes are severe. If mitral valvular stenosis is severe, the degree of turbulence that results can cause intravascular hemolysis and, over the years, renal hemosiderosis.

At this stage, after repeated attacks of rheumatic fever, valve leaflets are markedly thickened by fibroelastic connective tissue histologically (Fig. 24–12D). They show the presence of musculoelastic blood vessels, which initially were thin-walled capillaries during the acute phase.[46] These vessels extend well out into the substance of a leaflet toward its free margin, and a variable number of chronic inflammatory cells, mainly lymphocytes, may be present, particularly at the leaflet's base and surrounding the blood vessels. Dystrophic calcification appears in the stenosed leaflet and chordal tissue.

Intermediate stages are seen during periods of recurrent valvulitis, and if the disease is active, verrucae may be present on thickened leaflets. In countries with a high standard of living, 10 to 20 years may elapse between the attacks of ARF and evolution of a stenosed valve. However, in underdeveloped countries, probably as a result of the greater risk of repeated attacks of ARF, children or teenagers may present with clinical symptoms of severe valvular disease (see Ch. 33).

Surgically excised stenosed mitral valves or those examined at autopsy many years after the last attack of ARF usually do not show verrucae. Rather, thickening and fibrosis of the already damaged leaflets are obvious, and calcification of the tissues is prominent. The calcium may present as nodules within the thickened valve substance or as large yellow masses that ulcerate the endocardial surface, especially in the commissural areas. The ulcerated lesions can, in rare instances, be a source of calcium emboli[141] and have small thrombi associated with them. Lachman and Roberts[69] found that the amount of calcific deposits in surgically excised stenosed mitral valves correlated with the sex of a patient and with the mean diastolic pressure gradient across the valve but not with a patient's age, cardiac rhythm, or main pulmonary arterial or pulmonary arterial wedge pressure, or with previous mitral commissurotomy, presence of thrombus in the body of the left atrium, or presence of disease in one or more of the other cardiac valves. The authors reported that men tend to have heavier calcium deposits in stenosed mitral valves and at an earlier age than do women with the same hemodynamic lesions. These findings were made on adult patients in the United States, but Datta (see Ch. 33) indicates that calcification is seen less commonly in younger patients who develop severe stenosis rapidly. Lambl's excrescences or papillary tumors (see Ch. 5) are a frequent finding on such deformed valves in adults.

The process or valve stenosis is self-perpetuating, so a stenosed mitral valve may restenose after being subjected to a surgical commissurotomy in treatment.[3] The rate at which restenosis occurs depends in part on the adequacy of the commissurotomy and in part on the age of the patient. Clinically, estimates of the frequency of restenosis vary, but a restenosis can be diagnosed with certainty only on the basis of three satisfactory hemodynamic studies: a preoperative study; a second study following a satisfactory operation in which an increase in the size of the valvular orifice has been demonstrated; and third study after symptoms have reappeared when a reduction in size relative to the postoperative study is noted.[14] A study, using cross-sectional echocardiography to determine the size of the mitral valve orifice in 18 patients who had adequate commissurotomies, revealed no change in the mitral valve over a 10- to 14-year period in 13 patients and restenosis in 5 patients.[51] In younger persons restenosis may be due to further attacks of actue rheumatic fever, but restenosis in the adult occurs even in the absence of further attacks—probably by the organization of tiny thrombi found in relation to the commissurotomy[98] and related to damage caused by altered blood flow patterns through the valve. In other words, restenosis is caused by mechanisms comparable to those that produced the original stenosis. Nevertheless, other mechanisms that favor formation on a valve may be a factor[34] (see Ch. 23).

Pathologic Effects   In normal adults the area of the mitral valve orifice is 4 to 6 cm^2, a mild stenosis reduces this to 2 cm^2, and a critical stenosis to 1 cm^2.

Mitral stenosis raises the left atrial intraluminal pressure with resultant dilation and hypertrophy of the chamber wall (Fig. 24–11). Rarely, the enlarged atrium may compress surrounding structures. If the stenosis is prolonged, the hypertrophied atrial muscle eventually atrophies and is replaced by scar, a change likely a factor in promoting atrial fibrillation. The endocardium in the chamber thickens and egg-shell-like plaques of calcium may develop in it. These are visible on radiographs and are usually seen in the free atrial wall of patients with severe long-standing mitral stenosis and may, in some instances, derive from mural thrombi; they take years to develop.[50] Mural thrombi are found in the atrium, especially in patients with associated atrial fibrillation. They are either attached to the wall of the atrium (Fig. 24–11) or atrial appendage and are present in 25 percent of cases coming to autopsy. The thrombi are a frequent source of thromboemboli to the systemic circulation.[22,89] Huge left atrial mural thrombi or "ball" thrombi lying free in the lumen are not now seen very often at autopsy

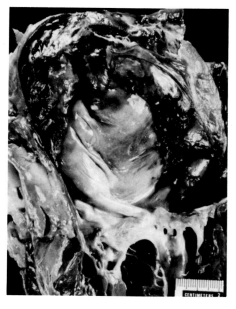

Fig. 24–11. Left atrial dilation and mural thrombus formation in a 47-year-old woman with severe mitral stenosis. Note marked chordal changes. They may induce a subvalvular stenosis.

in Western countries.[98] However, the surgeon may encounter such lesions and forward them for examination to the surgical pathologist. The raised left atrial pressure is transferred to the lungs, causing pulmonary hypertension (see Ch. 15) with resultant pulmonary congestion and intra-alveolar hemorrhage. Again, brown indurated lungs, the result of repeated intra-alveolar hemorrhage with subsequent fibrosis, are now not often seen in Western countries. Right ventricular hypertrophy is also a feature, and right ventricular failure may develop.

Clinical Features of Rheumatic Heart Disease

Acute Rheumatic Fever   The clinical signs and symptoms of ARF vary greatly.[123,124] They are determined by the organs affected and the severity of that affliction. Some, which occur simultaneously, in close succession, or singly, include arthritis, carditis, chorea, subcutaneous nodules, and erythema margination. They are *major* manifestations as diagnostic criteria. Others, such as fever, arthralgia, acute phase reactants in the blood, and a history of attacks of ARF, are not specific and are *minor* diagnostic criteria.

Arthritis. Roughly 75 percent of those with ARF develop an acute arthritis. Typically it affects large joints that are involved in succession, but any joint may be affected. The arthritis is usually self-limiting, lasting 2 to 3 weeks. Its presence is almost always associated with rising or peak titers of streptococcal antibodies.

Carditis. If the associated carditis causes minor symptoms or the patient does not have associated arthritis or chorea, the diagnosis may be missed. This provides an explanation for the roughly 50 percent of patients who have rheumatic valvular disease yet give no history of ARF. Alternatively and in a minority of patients, the carditis may cause death from acute heart failure. Heart murmurs, cardiomegaly due to dilation, and, less frequently overt signs of congestive heart failure or a pericarditis occur. Usually, there is a prolongation of atrioventricular conduction.

Extracardiac Manifestation. These manifestations may include subcutaneous nodules, erythema marginatum, chorea found in children or in women after puberty, and fever.

Laboratory Findings. These findings may reveal a persistent streptococcal throat infection, although this is uncommon; a leukocytosis or a normocytic, normochromic anemia; a raised erythrocyte sedimentation rate; and C reactive protein in the blood. Specific streptococcal antibodies, including antistreptolysin O and anti-DNAse B may be detectable in the first 3 weeks after onset of ARF. ECG patterns are nonspecific but may demonstrate a prolonged P–R interval or nonspecific ST–T changes.

Treatment. The patient is confined to bed during the acute phase of ARF. Usually, a course of penicillin is administered to control any persistent throat infection. Antirheumatic treatment consisting of salicylates or corticosteroids may be indicated to control toxic manifestations of the disease. The natural history of rheumatic heart disease has been radically changed by the use of antimicrobials in prophylaxis following an attack of ARF.

Rheumatic Valvular Disease ARF may induce univalvular disease, but more often it affects several valves. Here I concentrate on mitral stenosis, as effects on other valves are discussed in Chapters 25 through 27 and above.

Mitral stenosis. Mitral stenosis affects women more often than men.[14,70] Its principal symptom is dyspnea, caused by a reduced compliance in the lungs. As the valvular stenosis worsens, patients have orthopnea, are prone to episodes of pulmonary edema, and may develop right heart failure. Hemoptysis, thromboembolism, and infective endocarditis are complications. The markedly enlarged left atrium may compress surrounding anatomic structures.

Cardiac output is low. This may cause the so-called mitral facies with purplish-pink patches on the cheeks. The patient has a presystolic murmur; a loud, first heart sound, a long, but not loud, middiastolic murmur, and, usually, an opening snap. ECG examination is useful in patients with moderate or severe obstruction, recording changes attributable to atrial fibrillation and an enlarged left atrium. Radiographically, there is cardiomegaly with left atrial enlargement and possibly right ventricular hypertrophy; the left sternal heart border is straightened. M-mode echocardiography confirms the diagnosis in nearly all patients. Other sophisticated diagnostic tests provide complementary data.

As already indicated, the natural history of mitral stenosis varies in underdeveloped and developed countries (see Ch. 33).

A patient may be well-managed medically for many years. If symptoms become severe, a rapid downhill course ensues. Surgery is usually contemplated when valve stenosis is severe. Closed or open commissurotomy may be done or the valve excised and replaced by a prosthesis. The problem of valvular restenosis following commisurotomy has been discussed.

Nonrheumatic Causes

Nonrheumatic causes are extremely uncommon; most result from leaflet stiffening. Thus, mitral stenosis may develop in a patient with the carcinoid syndrome who has an intra-atrial communication or in one affected by a carcinoid tumor of the lung (see Ch. 31). Treatment with methysergide therapy may cause a deposition of fibrous tissue on this heart valve[6,84] (Fig. 24–12A-C) (see Ch. 34), whereas deposits of ceramide trihexoside in Fabry's disease[72] (Fig. 24–13) or mucopolysaccharide material in the Hurler-Scheie syndrome with or without associated dystrophic calcification may induce mitral stenosis (see Ch. 29). Also, mitral stenosis has been reported in patients with familial pseudoxanthoma elasticum in the valve; histologic sections show the irregular, coarse-fibered, abnormally fragmented elastic fibers seen in skin lesions (see Ch. 14). Whipple's disease can also induce mitral stenosis as part of the cardiac lesions seen in this disease.[80] The thickened mitral valves show a gross deformity resembling that seen in chronic rheumatic valvular disease. Characteristic PAS-positive macrophages and rod-shaped bacteria identical to those found in the mucosa of the small intestine of patients with Whipple's disease are seen in valvular lesions.

Large vegetations of infective endocarditis may induce mitral stenosis. The condition is also occasionally associated with calcification of the mitral annulus (see Ch. 5).

A left atrial myxoma or other tissue mass may also project into the valve lumen and produce the symptoms of mitral stenosis.

Subvalvular Obstruction

Although the chordae of the mitral valve and the left ventricular papillary muscles form integral parts of the mitral valve complex[115] and closure of the valves depends on their integrity, blood must flow through the chordae and past the papillary muscles in its passage into the left ventricle. Therefore, congenital or ac-

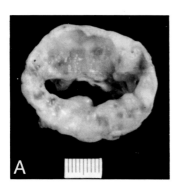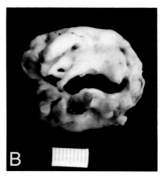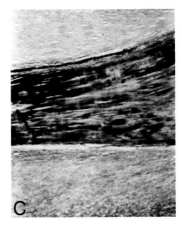

Fig. 24–12. Mitral stenosis attributed to methylsergide therapy in 46-year-old woman showing gross appearance of valve viewed from (**A**) atrial and (**B**) ventricular aspects. (Scale indicates 1 cm.) Note that gross appearance mimics that caused by mitral stenosis induced by rheumatic valvular disease. However, the histology is that of a proliferation of (**C**) fibromuscular tissue on valve components—coating a chorda tendineae (central dark area). (Masson trichrome—Verhoeff elastic, × 10.)

quired lesions of these structures may cause a subvalvular obstruction to blood flow.

Congenital Anomalies

Parachute Mitral Valves

In the condition known as parachute mitral valve, only one papillary muscle is present in the left ventricle, or two are very close together. All chordae tendineae passing to both mitral valve leaflets arise from the single head or the two, and, as a result, interchordal spaces are effectively narrowed, producing a subvalvular obstruction. In adults the condition may occur as an isolated phenomenon. In neonates or children, it is more often associated with other congenital cardiac anomalies.[113] In children, large papillary muscles may obstruct blood flow. Castenada et al.[18] reported a case with large papillary muscles associated with shortened chordae and mitral valve arcade. At autopsy, I have not recognized malpositioned or enlarged papillary muscles causing subvalvular mitral stenosis in adults. Others have made the diagnosis angiographically.[36]

Acquired Subvalvular Stenosis

Acquired subvalvular stenosis is most likely in rheumatic valvular disease, when chordal fusion is a major component of the valvular damage. The subvalvular stenosis is of importance when the valve disease is being treated by commissurotomy. The stenosis at both valvular and subvalvular levels must be alleviated if the patient is to benefit.

REFERENCES

1. Alarcon-Riquelme ME, Alarcon-Segovia D, Loredo-Abdala A, Alcocer-Varela J: T lymphocyte subsets, suppressor and contrasuppressor cell functions and production of interleukin-2 in the peripheral blood of rheumatic fever patients and their apparently healthy siblings. Clin Immunol Immunopathol 55:120, 1990

2. Angrist A, Oka M, Nakao K: Vegetative endocarditis. Pathol Anat 2:155, 1967

3. Arora R, Khalilullah M, Gupta, MP, Padmavati S: Mitral restenosis. Incidence and epidemiology. Indian Heart J 30:265, 1978

4. Aryanpur I, Nazarian I, Siassi B: Rheumatic heart disease in developing countries. p. 547. In Moss AJ, Adams FH, Emmanouilides GC (eds): Heart Disease in Infants, Children and Adolescents. 2nd ed. Williams & Wilkins, Baltimore, 1977

5. Aschoff L: The rheumatic nodules in the heart. Ann Rheum Dis 1:161, 1939

6. Bana DS, MacNeal PS, LeCompte PM, et al: Cardiac murmurs and endocardial fibrosis associated with methylsergide therapy. Am Heart J 88:640, 1974

7. Bhatia R, Narula J, Reddy KS, et al: Lymphocyte subsets in acute rheumatic fever and rheumatic valvular disease. Clin Cardiol 12:34, 1989

8. Becker AE, Becker MJ, Edwards JW: Pathologic spectrum of dysplasia of the tricuspid valve. Features in common with Ebstein's malformation. Arch Pathol 91:167, 1971

9. Bisno AL: The rise and fall of rheumatic fever. JAMA 254:538, 1985

10. Bisno AL: The resurgence of acute rheumatic fever in the United States. Ann Rev Med 41:319, 1990

11. Bland EF, Jones TD: Rheumatic fever and rheumatic heart disease. A twenty year report on 1000 patients followed since childhood. Circulation, 4:837, 1951

12. Boonpucknavig S, Udomsangpetch R, Pongpanich B: Immunologic studies on acute rheumatic fever and rheumatic heart disease. J Clin Lab Immunol 13:133, 1984

13. Borow KM, Braunwald E: Congenital heart disease in the adult. p. 976. In Braunwald E (ed): Heart Disease: A Textbook of Cardiovascular Medicine. 3rd ed. WB Saunders, Philadelphia, 1988

14. Braunwald E: Valvular heart disease. p. 1023. In Braunwald E (ed): Heart Diseases: A textbook of Cardiovascular Medicine. 3rd ed. WB Saunders, Philadelphia, 1988

15. Brock RC: The Anatomy of Congenital Pulmonic Stenosis. Paul B. Hoeber Inc., New York, 1957

16. Burch GE, Giles TD, Colcolough HL:

Pathogenesis of "rheumatic" heart disease: Critique and theory. Am Heart J 80:556, 1970

17. Cantanzaro FJ, Stetson CA, Morris AJ, et al: The role of streptococcus in the pathogenesis of rheumatic fever. Am J Med 17:749, 1954

18. Castenada AR, Anderson RC, Edwards JE: Congenital mitral stenosis resulting from anomalous arcade and obstruction papillary muscles. Am J Cardiol, 24:237, 1969

19. Coffman JD, Sommers SC: Familial pseudoxanthoma elasticum and valvular heart disease. Circulation 19:242, 1959

20. Collins-Nakai RL, Rosenthal A, Castenada AK, et al: Congential mitral stenosis. A review of 20 years experience. Circulation 56:1039, 1977

21. Costero I: Cerebral lesions responsible for death of patients with active rheumatic fever. Arch Neurol Psychiatr 62:48, 1949

22. Coulshed N, Epstein EJ, McKendrick CS, et al: Systemic embolism in mitral valve disease. Br Heart J 32:26, 1970

23. Cunningham MW, McCormack JM, Fenderson PG, et al: Human and murine antibodies cross-reactive with streptococcal M protein and myosin recognize the sequence GLN–LYS–SER–LYS–GLN in M protein. J Immunol 143:2677, 1989

24. Cunningham MW, McCormack JM, Talaber LR, et al: Human monoclonal antibodies reactive with antigens of the Group A streptococcus and human heart. J Immunol 141:2760, 1988

25. Datta BN, Nagrani B, Khattri HN, et al: Rheumatic heart disease at autopsy. An analysis of 260 cases in Chandigarh. Indian Heart, 30:39, 1978

26. Davachi F, Moller JH, Edwards JE: Diseases of the mitral valve in infancy: An anatomic analysis of 55 cases. Circulation 43:565, 1971

27. Doucette J, Knoblich R: Persistent right valve of the sinus venosus. So-called cor triatriatum dexter: Review of the literature and report of a case. Arch Pathol 75:105, 1963

28. Ebstein W: Uber einen sehr seltenen fall von Insufficienz der Valvula Tricuspidales bedintg durch eine engeborene hochgradige Missbildung der selben. Arch Anat Physiol 33:238, 1866

29. Edwards JE: Pathologic features of Ebstein's malformation of the tricuspid valve. Mayo Clin Proc 28:89, 1953

30. Edwards JE: Classification of congenital heart disease in the adult. Cardiovasc Clin 10/:11, 1979

31. Edwards JE, Carey LS, Neufeld HN, Lester RG: Congenital Heart Disease. WB Saunders, Philadelphia, 1965

32. Ellison RC, Freedom RM, Keane JF, et al: Indirect assessment of severity in pulmonary stenosis. Circulation 56 (Suppl. 1.):14, 1977

33. Emmanouilides GC: Obstructive lesions of the right ventricle and the pulmonary arterial tree. p. 226. In Moss AJ, Adams FH, Emmanouilides GC (eds): Heart Disease in Infants, Children and Adolescents. 2nd Ed. Williams Wilkins, Baltimore, 1977

34. Ford S, Charette E, Knight J, et al: A possible role for antiphospholipid antibodies in acquired cardiac deformity. J Rheumatol (in press)

35. Forster JW, Humphreys JO: Right ventricular anomalous muscle bundle: Clinical and laboratory presentations and natural history. Circulation 43:115, 1971

36. Freedom RM, Cullam JAG, Moes CAF: Angiography of congenital heart disease. Macmillan, New York, 1984

37. Gay BB, Jr, Franch RH, Shuford WH, Rogers JV, Jr: The roentgenologic features of single and multiple coarctations of the pulmonary artery and branches. Am J Roentgenol 90:599, 1963

38. Gerlis LM, Anderson RM: Cor triatriatum dexter with imperforate Ebstein's anomaly. Br Heart J 38:108, 1976

39. Gharagozloo F, Buckley BH, Hutchins GM: A proposed pathogenesis of cor triatriatum: Infringement of the left superior vena cava on the developing left atrium. Am Heart J 94:618, 1977

40. Goldstein I, Halpern B, Robert L: Immunologic relationship between streptococcus A polysaccharide and the structural glycoproteins of heart valves. Nature 213:44, 1967

41. Goor DA, Lillehei CW: Congenital Malformations of the Heart. Grune & Stratton, New York, 1975

42. Goosenhaven EJ, Stewart PA, Becker AE, et al: "Off-setting" of the septal tricuspid leaflet in normal hearts and in hearts with Ebstein's anomaly. Am J Cardiol 53:172, 1984

43. Gross L, Ehrlich JC: Studies on the myocardial Aschoff body. I. Descriptive classifi-

cation of lesions. Am J Pathol 10:467, 1934

44. Gross L, Ehrlich JC: Studies on the myo-cardial Aschoff body. II. Life cycle, sites of predilection and relation to clinical course of rheumatic fever. Am J Pathol 10:489, 1934

45. Gross L, Freid BM: Lesions in the A.V. con-duction system occurring in rheumatic fever. Am J Pathol 12:31, 1936

46. Gross L, Friedberg CK: Lesions of the cardiac valves in rheumatic fever. Am J Pathol 12:469, 855, 1936

47. Gross L, Kugel MA, Epstein EZ: Lesions of the coronary arteries and their branches in rheumatic fever. Am J Pathol 11:253, 1935

48. Gulizia JM, Cunningham MW, McManus BM: Evolving issues regarding the immu-nopathogenesis of rheumatic heart disease. Cor Notes. Society for Cardiovascular Pa-thology 5 (2):9, 1990

49. Hafez M, el-Battoty MF, Hawas S, et al: Ev-idence of inherited susceptibility of increased streptococcal adherance to pharyngeal cells of children with rheumatic fever. Br J Rheu-matol 28:304, 1989

50. Harthorne JW, Seltzer RA, Austen WG: Left atrial calcification. Review of literature and proposed management. Circulation 34:198, 1966

51. Heger JJ, Wann LS, Wyeman AE, et al: Long-term changes in mitral valve area after successful mitral commissurotomy. Circula-tion 59:443, 1979

52. Hollman A: The anatomic appearance in rheumatic tricuspid valve disease. Br Heart J 19:211, 1957

53. Hopkins BE, Taylor RR, Robinson JS: Fa-milial hypertrophic cardiomyopathy and len-tiginosis. Aust NZ J Med 5:359, 1975

54. Hudson REB: Cardiovascular Pathology. Vols. 1 & 3. Williams & Wilkins, Baltimore, 1965, 1970

55. Hutt MSR: Cardiac pathology in the tropics. p. 511. In Pomerance A, Davies MJ (eds): Pathology of the Heart. Blackwell Scientific Publications, Oxford, 1975

56. Hwang WS, Lam KL: Rupture of chordae tendineae during acute rheumatic carditis. Br Heart J 30:429, 1968

57. Jones TD, Bland EF: Rheumatic fever and heart disease: Completed ten-year observa-tion on 1000 patients. Trans Assoc Am Phy-sicians 57:267, 1942

58. Jones M, Ferrans VJ, Morrow AG, Roberts WC: Ultrastructure of crista supraventricu-laris muscle in patients with congenital heart disease associated with right ventricular out-flow tract obstruction. Circulation 51:39, 1975

59. Josselson A, Bagnall JW, Virmani R: Acute rheumatic carditis causing sudden death. Am J Forensic Pathol 5:151, 1984

60. Kamat PV, Ranganathan N, Yao J, Yu D: Con-genital intracardiac band. Arch Pathol Lab Med 101:81, 1977

61. Kaplan MH: The cross-reaction of group A streptococci with heart tissue and its relation to autoimmunity in rheumatic fever. Bull Rheum Dis 19:560, 1969

62. Kaplan S, Adolph RJ: Pulmonic valve stenosis in adults. Cardiovasc Clin 10(1):327, 1979

63. Khanna AK, Buskirk DR, Williams, RC, Jr, et al: Presence of a non-HLA B cell antigen in rheumatic fever patients and their families as defined by a monoclonal antibody. J Clin Invest 83:1710, 1989

64. Klinge F: Der Rheumatismus. J Bergman Munich, 1933

65. Knoblich R, Ducey EF: Anomalous fibro-muscular cord of the left atrium. Arch Pathol 73:86, 1962

66. Koretzky ED, Moeller JH, Korns ME, et al: Congenital pulmonary stenosis resulting from dysplasia of valve. Circulation 40:43, 1969

67. Krause RM: The influence of infection on the geography of heart disease. Circulation 60:972, 1979

68. Kumar AE, Fyler DC, Miettinen OS, Nadas AS: Ebstein's anomaly. Clinical profile and natural history. Am J Cardiol 28:84, 1974

69. Lachman AS, Roberts WC: Calcific deposits in stenotic mitral valves: Extent and relation to age, sex, degree of stenosis, cardiac rhythm, previous commissurotomy and left atrial body thrombus from study of 164 op-eratively-excised valves. Circulation 57:808, 1978

70. Lakier JB, Pocock WA: Mitral stenosis. p. 151. In Barlow JB (ed): Perspectives on the Mitral Valve. FA Davis, Philadelphia, 1987

71. Leavitt TW, Nixon JV: Cor triatriatum with mitral regurgitation in a 52-year old male. Cathet Cardiovasc Diag 5:75, 1979

72. Leder AA, Bosworth WC: Angiokeratoma corporis diffusum universale (Fabry's disease) with mitral stenosis. Am J Med 38:814, 1965

73. Lev M, Liberthson RR, Joseph RH, et al: The pathologic anatomy of Ebstein's disease. Arch Pathol 90:334, 1970

74. Lev M, Strauss S: Stenosis of the infundibulum. Arch Intern Med 70:53, 1942

75. Loeffler E: Unusual malformation of the left atrium: Pulmonary sinus. Arch Pathol 48:371, 1949

76. Lucas RV, Varco RL, Lillehei CW, et al: Anomalous muscle bundle of the right ventricle. Hemodynamic consequences and surgical considerations. Circulation 25:443, 1962

77. MacCallum WG: Rheumatic lesions of the left auricle of the heart. Bull Johns Hopkins Hosp 35:329, 1924

78. Magarey FR: Pathogenesis of mitral stenosis. Br Med J 1:856, 1951

79. Mahapatra RK, Agarwal JB, Wasir HS: Rheumatic tricuspid stenosis. Indian Heart J 30:138, 1978

80. McAllister HA, Jr, Fenoglio JJ, Jr: Cardiac involvement in Whipple's disease. Circulation 52:152, 1975

81. McGuire LB, Nolan TB, Reeve R, Dammann JR, Jr: Cor triatriatum as a problem of heart disease. Circulation 31:263, 1965

82. Mendelsohn G, Bulkley BH, Hutchins GM: Cardiovascular manifestations of pseudoxanthoma elasticum. Arch Pathol Lab Med 102:298, 1978

83. Mendez HM, Optiz JM: Noonan syndrome: The decline of rheumatic fever. A review. Am J Med Genet 21:493, 1985

84. Misch KA: Development of heart valve lesions during methylsergide therapy. Br Med J 2:365, 1974

85. Moller JH: Congenital causes of left ventricular inflow obstruction in the heart. IAP Monographs in Pathology 18:271. Williams & Wilkins, Baltimore, 1974

86. Monibi AA, Neches WH. Lenox CC, et al: Left ventricular abnormalities associated with Ebstein's malformation of the tricuspid valves. Circulation 57:303, 1978

87. Morgan JR, Forker AD, Coates JR, Myers WS: Isolated tricuspid stenosis. Circulation 44:729, 1971

88. Nadas AS: Pulmonic stenosis: Indication for surgery in children and adults. N Engl J Med 287:1196, 1972.

89. Neilson GH, Galea EC, Hossack KF: Thromboembolic complications of mitral valve disease. Aust NZ J Med 8:372, 1978

90. Neubuerger KT: The brain in rheumatic fever. Dis Nerv Syst 8:259, 1947

91. Niwayama G: Cor triatriatum. Am Heart J 59:291, 1960

92. Noonan JA, Ehmke DA: Associated noncardiac malformations in children with congenital heart disease. J Pediatr 63:468, 1963

93. Olsen EJG, Valentine JC: Anomalous bands in the heart. Br Heart J 34:210, 1972

94. Olsen LJ, Subramanian R, Ackermann DM, et al: Surgical pathology of the mitral valve. A study of 712 cases spanning 21 years. Mayo Clin Proc.

95. Padmavati S: Rheumatic fever and rheumatic heart disease in developing countries. Bull WHO 56:543, 1978

96. Perloff JK: The Clinical Recognition of Congenital Heart Disease. WB Saunders, Philadelphia, 1970

97. Perloff JK: Postpediatric congenital heart disease: Natural survival patterns. Cardiovasc Clin 10/1:27, 1979

98. Pomerance A: Cardiac involvement in rheumatic and "collagen" diseases. p. 279. In Pomerance A, Davies MJ, (eds): The Pathology of the Heart. Blackwell Scientific Publications, Oxford, 1975

99. Proceedings of the Third International Conference on Rheumatic Fever and Rheumatic Heart Disease. Rotarua, April 16–18, 1987. NZ Med J 101 Pt. 2:378, 1988

100. Quinn RW: Comprehensive review of morbidity and mortality trends for rheumatic fever, streptococcal disease and scarlet fever. Rev Infect Dis 11:928, 1989

101. Rajapaske CN, Halim K, Al-Orainey I, et al: A genetic marker for rheumatic heart disease. Br Heart J 58:659, 1987

102. Rammelkamp CH, Jr: Epidemiology of streptococcal infection. Harvey Lecture Series, 51:113, 1955–56

103. Ranganathan N, Lam JHC, Wigle ED, Silver MD: Morphology of the human mitral valve. II. The valve leaflets. Circulation 41:459, 1970

104. Roberts WC, Glancy GL, Seninger RP, et al: Prolapse of the mitral valve (floppy valve) associated with Ebstein's anomaly of the tricuspid valve. Am J Cardiol 38:377, 1976

105. Roberts WC, Mason DT, Morrow AG, Braunwald E: Calcific pulmonic stenosis. Circulation 37:973, 1968

106. Rose AG: Etiology of acquired valvular heart disease in adults. A survey of 18,123 autopsies and 100 consecutive valve-replacement operations. Arch Pathol Lab Med 110:385, 1986

107. Rotta J: Biological characteristics of Group A streptococcus and the pathogenesis of rheumatic fever. p. 3. In Shiokawa Y, Kawakita S (eds): Proceedings of the International Conference on Rheumatic Fever and Rheumatic Heart Disease. Japanese Circulation Society, Kyoto, 1979

108. Rowland TW, Rosenthal A, Castaneda AR: Double-chamber right ventricle: Experience in 17 cases. Am Heart J 89:455, 1975

109. Salinas-Madrigal L: Personal communication, 1980

110. Schwartz CJ, Korns ME, Edwards JE, Lillehei CW: Pathologic sequelae and complications of ventriculotomy. II. With particular reference to platelet thromboemboli in the small intramyocardial vessels. Arch Pathol 89:56, 1970

111. Seuanez H, Maine-Garzon F, Kolski R: Cardio-cutaneous syndrome (the "LEOPARD" Syndrome). Review of the literature and a new family. Clin Genet 9:266, 1976

112. Seymour J, Emanuel R, Pattinson N: Acquired pulmonary stenosis. Br Heart J. 30:776, 1968

113. Shone JF, Sellers RD, Anderson RC, et al: The developmental complex of "parachute mitral valve," supravalvular ring of left atrium, subaortic stenosis and coarctation of aorta. Am J Cardiol 11:714, 1963

114. Silver MD, Dorsey JS: Aneurysm of septum primum in adults. Arch Pathol Lab Med 102:62, 1978

115. Silverman ME, Hurst JW: The mitral complex. Am Heart J 76:399, 1968

116. Singh SP, Gotsman MS, Abrams LD, et al: Congenital mitral stenosis. Br Heart J 29:83, 1967

117. Spagnuolo M, Taranta A: Rheumatic fever in siblings. Similarity of its clinical manifestations. N Engl J Med 278:183, 1968

118. Srinivasan V, Lewin AN, Pieroni D, et al: Supravalvular stenosing ring of the left atrium. Case report and review of the literature. Bull Tex Heart Inst 7:149, 1980

119. Stetson, CA: The relation of antibody response to rheumatic fever. p. 208. In McCarthy M (ed): Streptococcal Infections. Columbia University Press, New York, 1954

120. Stevenson AC, Cheeseman EA: Heredity and rheumatic fever. A study of 462 families ascertained by an affected child and 51 families ascertained by an affected mother. Ann Eugen Lond 17:177, 1953

121. Stevenson AC, Cheeseman EA: Hereditary and rheumatic fever. Some later information about data collected in 1950–51. Ann Hum Genet 21:139, 1956

122. Stollerman GH: The relative rheumatogenecity of strains of Group A streptococci. Mod Concepts Cardiovasc Dis 44:35, 1975

123. Stollerman GH: Rheumatic Fever and Streptococcal Infection. Grune & Stratton, Orlando, FL, 1975

124. Stollerman GH: Rheumatic and hereditable connective tissue diseases of the cardiovascular system. p. 1706. In Braunwald E (ed): Heart Disease. A Textbook of Cardiovascular Medicine. 3rd Ed. WB Saunders, Philadelphia, 1988

125. Stollerman GH, Bisno AL: The relative rheumatogenecity of strains of Group A streptococci. p. 57. In Shiokawa Y, Kawakita S (eds): International Conference on Rheumatic Fever and Rheumatic Heart Disease. Japanese Circulation Society, Kyoto, 1979

126. Tank ES, Bernard WF, Gross RE: Surgical anatomy of congenital mitral stenosis. Circulation (Suppl. 11) 35, 36:246, 1967

127. Tedeschi CG, Wagner BM, Pani KC: Studies in rheumatic fever. I. The clinical significance of the Aschoff body based on morphologic observations. Arch Pathol 60:408, 1955

128. Tweedy PS: The pathogenesis of valvular thickening in rheumatic heart disease. Br Heart J 18:173, 1956

129. Van de Rijn I, Zabriskie JB, McCarthy M: Group A streptococcal antigens cross-reactive with myocardium. Purification of heart-reactive antibody and isolation and characterization of the streptococcal antigen. J Exp Med 146:579, 1977

130. Van Mierop LHS, Schiebler GL, Victorica BE: Anomalies of the tricuspid valve resulting in stenosis or incompetence. p. 262. In Moss AJ, Adams FH, Emmanouilides GC (eds): Heart Disease in Infants and Children. 2nd

Ed. Williams & Wilkins, Baltimore, 1977

131. Van Praagh R, Corsini I: Cor triatriatum: Pathologic anatomy and a consideration of morphogenesis based on 13 postmortem cases and a study of normal development of the pulmonary vein and atrial septum in 83 human embryos. Am Heart J 78:379, 1969

132. Veasey LG, Weidmeier SE, Orsmond GS, et al: Resurgence of acute rheumatic fever in the intermountain area of the United States. New Engl J Med 316:421, 1987

133. Vela JE, Contreras R, Sosa FR: Rheumatic pulmonary valve disease. Am J Cardiol 23:12, 1969

134. Virmani R, Roberts WC: Aschoff nodules in operatively excised atrial appendages and in papillary muscles. Frequency and clinical significance. Circulation 55:559, 1977

135. Von Glahn WC, Pappenheimer AM: Specific lesions of peripheral blood vessels in rheumatism. Am J Pathol 2:235, 1926

136. Wagner BM: Studies in rheumatic fever: III. Histochemical reactivity of the Aschoff body. Ann NY Acad Sci 86:992, 1960

137. Wallace MR, Garst PD, Papadimos TJ, Oldfield EC III: The return of acute rheumatic fever in young adults. JAMA 262:2557, 1989

138. Waller BF: Evaluation of operatively excised cardiac valves. Cardiovasc Clin 18:203, 1988

139. Wannamaker LW: The chain that links the heart to the throat. Circulation 48:9, 1973

140. Watson H: Natural history of Ebstein's anomaly of tricuspid valve in childhood and adolescence. An international cooperative study of 505 cases. Br Heart J 36:417, 1974

141. Wigle ED: Myocardial fibrosis and calcareous emboli in valvular heart disease. Br Heart J 19:539, 1957

142. Wilson MG, Schweitzer MD, Lubschez R: Familial epidemiology of rheumatic fever: Genetic and epidemiological studies. J Pediatr 22:468, 1943

143. Wood P: An appreciation of mitral stenosis. I. Clinical features. Br Med J 1:1051, 1954

144. Wood P: An appreciation of mitral stenosis. II. Investigations and results. Br Med J 1:1113, 1954

145. Yang LC, Soprey PR, Wittner MK, Fox EN: Cell mediated immune destruction of cardiac fibres in vitro. p. 36. In Shiokawa Y, Kawakita S (eds): International Conference on Rheumatic Fever and Rheumatic Heart Disease. Japanese Circulation Society, Kyoto, 1979

146. Zabriskie JB, Friemer EH: An immunological relationship between the group A streptococcus and mammalian muscle. J Exp Med 124:661, 1966

25

Pathology of Mitral Incompetence

Jesse E. Edwards

Mitral incompetence is caused by many etiologic factors and is based on malfunction of one or several components of the mitral apparatus. In most cases, a corresponding anatomic abnormality may be identified. It is therefore appropriate to summarize the anatomic features of the normal mitral valve (see Ch. 1 also).

The normal mitral valve is composed of two leaflets, each supported by a tensor apparatus in the form of chordae and papillary muscles (Fig. 25–1). One leaflet is anterior and the other posterior. The anterior leaflet, also called the medial or aortic leaflet, is longer from its free edge to its base than the posterior leaflet. It is of smaller dimension from side to side, however, than the posterior leaflet.

The anterior leaflet at its base is attached to the aortic-mitral intervalvular fibrosa, through which it makes fibrous continuity with the adjacent parts of the posterior (noncoronary) and left aortic cusps. The anterior leaflet participates along with the ventricular septum in forming the wall of the left ventricular outflow tract.

The posterior leaflet is related to the inferior wall of the left ventricle. It is composed of three separate elements, the so-called posteromedial, anterolateral, and middle scallops.

Bridging the two leaflets are the anterolateral and the posteromedial commissures, represented by continuity of valvular tissue. Supporting the leaflet tissue is the tensor apparatus, which has two parts corresponding to the commissures, the anterolateral and posteromedial papillary muscles and chordae. From the apical aspect of each muscle, chordae proceed upward and fan out to insert into the related parts of each of the leaflets. Therefore, each leaflet receives chordae from each papillary muscle, and each leaflet is supported by elements of each part of the tensor apparatus. As a given leaflet is supported by chordae from each of the sets of tensor apparatus, it is supported by opposing structures.

Each papillary muscle tends to show a longitudinal depression at its center, and from its apex a commissural cord proceeds upward to branch and insert into each leaflet.[55] The anterolateral papillary muscle tends to have one head, divided only by the aforementioned longitudinal depression. The posteromedial papillary muscle frequently shows multiple heads. The chordae insert into the ventricular aspect of the leaflets.

Anatomically, the basis for mitral incompetence may reside in the leaflets, at the commissures, in the tensor apparatus, or in the

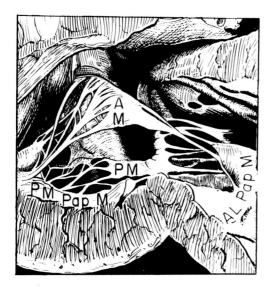

Fig. 25–1. Normal mitral valve viewed from the left ventricular aspect. AM, anterior mitral leaflet; PM, posterior mitral leaflet; PM pap M, posteromedial papillary muscle; AL pap M, anterolateral papillary muscle.

orifice of the valve.[47] The subject is broken down according to affections of the various components. When a given etiologic factor involves more than one component of the mitral apparatus, however, coverage of the changes caused by that etiologic factor is given under the most prevalent change.

COINVOLVEMENT OF LEAFLETS AND COMMISSURES

The classic basis for simultaneous involvement of leaflets and commissures is *rheumatic endocarditis.*

In the phase of acute rheumatic carditis, mitral insufficiency may occur. At this stage, the valvular changes are those of the acute process; major deformity of the valve does not occur. As the mitral incompetence of acute rheumatic carditis is classically transient, it is probable that the valvular malfunction depends on rheumatic myocarditis and resulting ventricular dilation. The so-called Mac-Cullum's patch that has been observed in the posterior wall of the left atrium is probably not a selective area of mural rheumatic endocarditis but a jet lesion secondary to the mitral incompetence.

Mitral incompetence resulting from the effects of chronic intrinsic valvular deformity takes on one of several appearances—namely, shortening of leaflets, fusion of one commissure, or fusion of both commissures.

When the primary cause of incompetence is shortening of leaflets, the latter resulting from recurrent inflammation with contracture, there may be no commissural fusion[45] (Fig. 25–2A). Insufficiency may then accentuate the degree of incompetence, so that "mitral insufficiency begets mitral insufficiency."[21] This situation comes about because the posterior wall of the enlarged left atrium is displaced posteriorly and inferiorly, pulling the posterior leaflet backward and inferiorly away from the anterior leaflet. At the same time, the free half of the leaflet, attached by chordae to the papillary muscles, is immobilized. This process may explain why some patients tolerate mitral regurgitation for years and then suddenly develop overwhelming mitral incompetence.

Commissural fusion may involve one or both commissures and be the dominant cause of incompetence of the valve. The fusion is primarily fibrous, but calcification is a common secondary effect. In contrast to the commissural fusion seen in mitral stenosis wherein the two leaflets are held in a closed position, in mitral incompetence the leaflets are held apart. The regurgitation occurs primarily at the site of fixation of the leaflets in the open position. Varying degrees of fibrous contracture of the leaflets may be observed, but the degrees of chordal shortening and interadhesion observed in mitral stenosis are usually absent.

It is more common for one commissure to be affected than two (Fig. 25–2B). The former

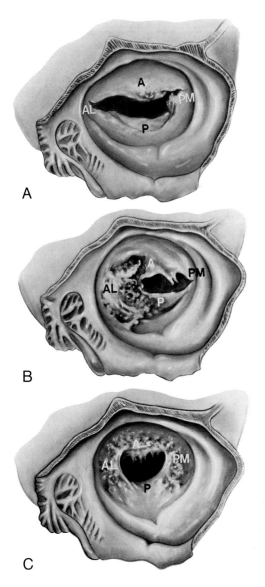

A

B

C

Fig. 25–2. Anatomic types of rheumatic mitral insufficiency. Each unopened mitral valve viewed from above. In each: A, anterior leaflet; P, posterior leaflet; AL, anterolateral commissure of mitral valve; PM, posteromedial commissure of mitral valve. (**A**) Intrinsically short leaflets. Commissures essentially unaffected. (**B**) Calcification and fusion of anterolateral commissure giving rise to the tear drop type of mitral insufficiency. (**C**) Calcification of the leaflets and commissures in continuity, yielding a wedding ring type of mitral insufficiency. Some restriction of the orifice is present, but incompetence is predominant.

type of deformity has been likened to a teardrop. Fusion of both commissures is often attended by calcification, not only of the commissural tissues but of all leaflet elements. The result is a totally fixed orifice, the so-called wedding ring deformity (Fig. 25–2C).

When commissural fusion occurs, some element of mitral stenosis is present, although its degree may be insignificant.

INVOLVEMENT OF LEAFLETS

While coinvolvement of the leaflets and commissures is usually the result of recurrent rheumatic endocarditis, there are several causes of mitral incompetence in which the leaflets are affected, while the commissures are normal.

Mitral incompetence caused by involvement of the leaflets varies anatomically. The leaflet tissue may be excessively lax, as in the myxomatous valve; it may be deficient, as in infective endocarditis and certain congenital states; or leaflet tissue, usually the posterior leaflet, may be immobilized as in left atrial enlargement, the hypereosinophilic syndrome, and in certain congenital states.

Prolapsed Leaflets

The myxomatous mitral valve, variously known as the floppy mitral valve, prolapsed mitral valve, and mid-late systolic click syndrome, may, under certain circumstances, be associated with mitral incompetence, although most subjects with this common condition do not exhibit incompetence of the valve.[27]

In fact, in clinical studies, including the use of echocardiography, the condition may be found in about 10 percent of apparently healthy young adults, with females more commonly affected than males.[7,35,37,40]

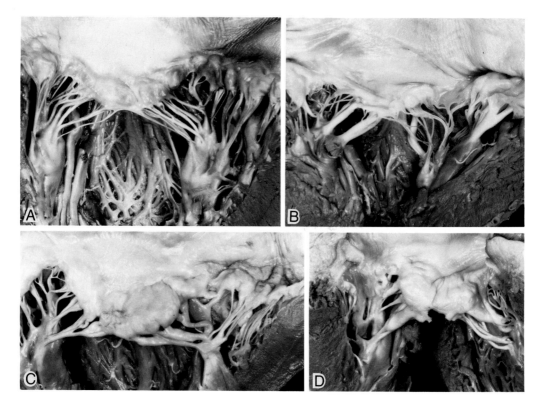

Fig. 25–3. Four examples of myxomatous alteration of the mitral valve. In each, the mitral valve has been opened in the classic fashion so that the anterior leaflet is in the center of the unit, while the posterior leaflet appears on each side of the illustration. (**A**) Interchordal hooding involving both the anterior, but principally elements of the posterior, mitral leaflet. (**B**) Prolapse of the posteromedial aspect of the anterior leaflet and the three scallops of the posterior leaflet. Stout chordae represent interchordal fusion. (**C**) Involvement of the posteromedial and middle scallops of the posterior leaflet (right) is dominant. The changes are associated with fibrous contracture. The posterior half of the anterior mitral leaflet is also affected, while the other half of this leaflet is relatively uninvolved. (**D**) The anterior leaflet shows major prolapse with secondary fibrosis of the leaflets and of subjacent chordae.

In systemic disorders of connective tissue, of which arachnodactyly (Marfan syndrome) is the most common, the myxomatous valve is commonly seen. The condition has also been noted in the Ehlers-Danlos syndrome[10] and in supravalvular aortic stenosis.[4] The question has been raised as to whether subjects with prolapse of the mitral valve are examples of Marfan syndrome in *forme fruste*.[52] Resolution of this question has not been reached, since the myxomatous mitral valve in subjects with Marfan syndrome is qualitatively like that in subjects without this con-

dition. In general, the changes are more marked in persons with Marfan syndrome than in non-Marfan subjects. A familial tendency for myxomatous mitral valve has been recognized in some non-Marfan subjects.[53,66]

The nature of the myxomatous mitral valve and its common presence in subjects with recognized systemic disorders of connective tissue indicate that the fundamental process is one of weakness of connective tissues of the body as a whole that is shared by the mitral valve.

Morphologically, the myxomatous mitral

valve is characterized by an excessive amount of myxomatous tissue in the spongiosa layer, the central part of the leaflet. As this material encroaches upon the supportive layer of the leaflet, the fibrosa, weakness and a lax state of the leaflets ensues.[24,49,60] Interchordal hooding or prolapse toward the left atrium results. While the anterior leaflet may be involved, elements of the posterior leaflet are more commonly affected.[51] When the posterior leaflet is involved, one or more of the three anatomic elements (scallops) of this leaflet may show the change. Fibrotic changes may occur (Fig. 25–3), while the intrinsic elements of the leaflet remain identifiable and the commissures are not fused. Grossly, this is an important distinction from rheumatic endocarditis. Histologically, the fibrotic changes are characterized by fibroelastic thickening of the contact surface layer, the atrialis, and padding by collagen on the ventricular surface of the leaflet[24,60] (Fig. 25–4).

Calcification of leaflet tissue may occur but does not, in general, constitute a major factor in the myxomatous valve. Calcified deposits in leaflet tissue, when present, tend to involve the basal aspect of the posterior leaflet. Grossly, such calcific deposits may be confused with annular calcification.

In the uncomplicated state, the chordae either appear normal or are elongated with some elements showing attenuation. Focal myxomatous changes may be noted histologically. Primary annular dilation has been noted in association with the myxomatous valve and claimed to be a basis for incompetence.[9] It has been recognized that dehiscence of valvular prostheses among subjects with the myxomatous valve is more common than when the mitral valve has been replaced for other conditions.[12,38,57] Such experiences suggest an intrinsic weakness of the connective tissue at the valvular annulus.

In most subjects with floppy mitral valve, the valve remains competent, although mitral insufficiency may occur with intact chordae. Among subjects with pure mitral insufficiency for which the valve was removed surgically,

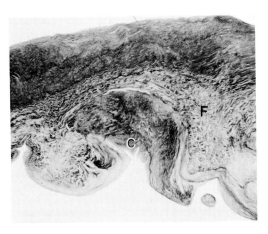

Fig. 25–4. Photomicrograph of mitral valve showing typical myxomatous change. The spongiosa is excessive and protrudes into the fibrosa (F), causing interruption in continuity of this layer. There is also fibrous thickening deposited on the ventricular aspect of the leaflet (C). The atrialis (upper) shows fibroelastic thickening. While changes are present, the basic structures of the valve are retained. (Elastic tissue stain, × 4.)

Hanson and associates[26] found myxomatous mitral valve, either with intact or ruptured chordae, to occur in 52 percent of cases studied.

The most common basis for significant mitral insufficiency in the myxomatous mitral valve is through rupture of chordae with a secondary flail state of the affected segment of the valvular apparatus.[57] Rupture of chordae may affect the anterior leaflet (Fig. 25–5), but the more common site for rupture of chordae is the posterior leaflet, where chordae to the middle scallop are most commonly involved[18,22,36] (Fig. 25–6). In this state, the regurgitant stream is directed toward the midportion of the atrial septum. At this site of impact, jet lesions occur. As this part of the atrial septum lies closely behind the aortic valve, the vibrations generated by the impact of the regurgitant stream may yield a murmur that from the points of view of time and location, may be misinterpreted as that of aortic stenosis.[1]

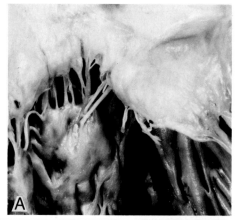

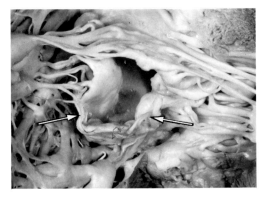

Fig. 25–6. Myxomatous alteration of mitral valve with rupture of chordae to the posterior leaflet. The unopened mitral valve viewed from below. The central part of the posterior leaflet (between arrows) shows fragments of ruptured chordae. The intact chordae are elongated and the leaflet tissue as seen through the orifice shows some prolapse and fibrous thickening as evidence of a pre-existing myxomatous state.

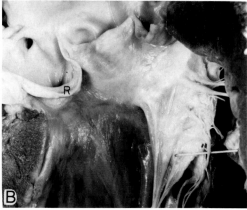

Fig. 25–5. Myxomatous alteration of mitral valve associated with rupture of chordae to anterior leaflet. **(A)** Anterolateral commissure of mitral valve and segment of each of the two leaflets. Chordae to the anterior leaflet have ruptured. **(B)** View of a portion of aortic valve and mitral valve from left ventricular aspect. Chordae inserting into the anterior leaflet have ruptured. The right aortic cusp (R) shows associated change represented by major prolapse of this cusp.

Another basis for mitral incompetence complicating the myxomatous mitral valve is through fusion of the left ventricular mural endocardium with chordae that insert into the posterior leaflet.[56] Such fusion, if extensive, causes effective shortening of chordae and may restrain motion of the posterior leaflet.

The process is first detectable as a series of linear fibrous thickenings of the left ventric-ular mural endocardium. These thickenings relate to the chordae and are interpreted as the result of friction by chordae upon the mural endocardium. In moderately advanced stages of the friction lesion, there is coalescence of the mural endocardial thickening (Fig. 25–7A). More advanced stages are uncommon and are characterized by extensive fusion of chordae to the thickened mural endocardium. Effective shortening of chordae results (Fig. 25–7B).

The mural lesion may show focal calcification; in one reported case, it was the site of primary mural infective endocarditis.[31]

With the mural fibrous lesions there may be concomitant fibrous deposits on the surfaces of chordae. Such deposits may lead to fusion of chordae (Fig. 25–8A). Uncommonly cartilagenous metaplasia may occur in chordae (Fig. 25–8B,C). Still another, yet relatively uncommon, complication of the myxomatous mitral valve is infective endocarditis.[13,41,46,49] Such a complication may be followed by mitral insufficiency if destructive changes occur[23] (Fig. 25–9).

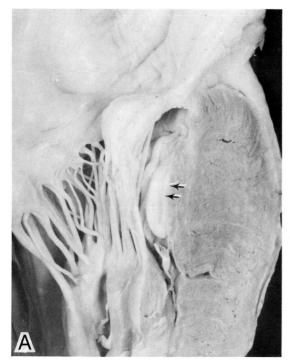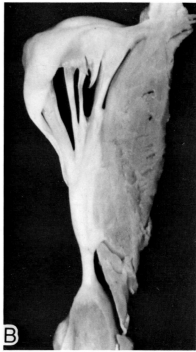

Fig. 25–7. Myxomatous mitral valve with mural friction lesions involving the endocardium of the left ventricle in relation to chordae attaching to the posterior mitral leaflet. (**A**) Beneath the chordae inserting into the prolapsing posterior mitral leaflet is fibrous thickening (arrows) of the mural endocardium of the left ventricle. (**B**) From a similar case. The chordae inserting into the posterior mitral leaflet have become adherent to the mural lesion of the left ventricular endocardium.

Other manifestations of the myxomatous mitral valve include premature ventricular contractions, ventricular fibrillation leading to sudden death, and transient ischemic attacks (TIAs). Usually, these manifestations are observed in subjects not having exhibited mitral incompetence.

Theories as to the cause of premature ventricular contractions and ventricular fibrillation include the following:

1. Friction of chordae upon the lining of the left ventricle.
2. Unusual degrees of tension on the chordae, perhaps with secondary vasospasm of supplying arteries.
3. Primary myocardial disease.[62] While peculiarities of left ventricular contraction have been noted in patients with myxo-

matous mitral valves, I have not observed any specific myocardial disease associated with classic examples of the valvular process.

It has been noted that transient neurologic manifestations occur among patients with the myxomatous valve, normal rhythm, and no infectious endocarditis; a reasonable cause is acute cerebral ischemia.[3] While pathologic substantiation is still wanting, it has been theorized that embolism arising from vegetative material forming on the contact surfaces of the mitral leaflets is the basis for the TIAs. This is a plausible explanation, as vegetations may indeed be deposited on the contact surfaces of the valves. In my experience, such vegetations are uncommon and are usually small; as a rule, their presence requires histologic

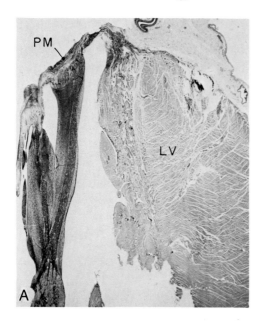

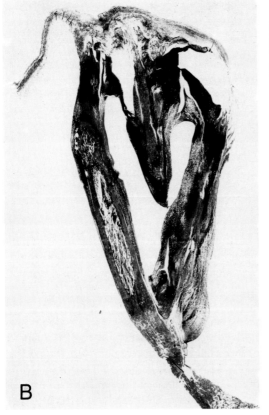

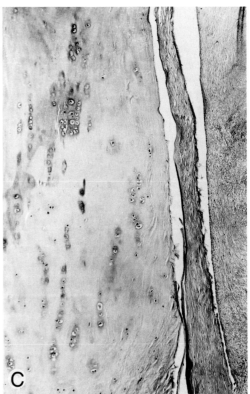

Fig. 25–8. Chordal changes in myxomatous mitral valve. (**A**) Low-power photomicrograph of posterior wall of left ventricle (LV) and posterior mitral leaflet (PM) with inserting chordae. Fibrous interadherence of chordae. (H&E, × 2.) (**B**) Low-power photomicrograph of chordae inserting into posterior mitral leaflet. Surface deposition of fibrous tissue and cartilagenous metaplasia. (Elastic tissue stain, × 2) (**C**) From case shown in Fig. B. Focus of cartilagenous metaplasia. (H&E × 42.)

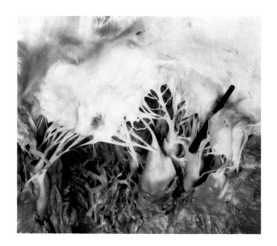

Fig. 25–9. Floppy mitral valve with infective endocarditis. The center of the anterior leaflet shows a vegetation, while a probe in the posterior leaflet is through a perforation.

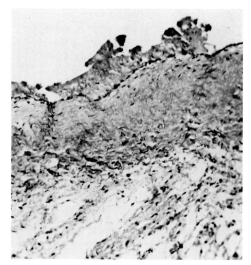

Fig. 25–10. Photomicrograph of atrial aspect of myxomatous mitral valve. Flat thrombotic vegetations are deposited on contact surface. (H&E, × 75.)

examination for identification (Fig. 25–10). A possible additional site for cerebral embolism is at the angle between the left atrium and the posterior mitral leaflet (Fig. 25–11). It has been observed that a linear thrombus may occur in this position representing the so-called angle lesion of the myxomatous mitral valve.[20] (See discussion in Ch. 28 also.)

Although myxomatous change in the mitral valve may appear as an isolated condition, it is common that when the condition is present, other valves and the great vessels may be simultaneously affected.[52,57] Either the aortic or the pulmonary valve, or both, may show varying degrees of myxomatous change. In the aortic valve, the process may lead to incompetence. In pathologic examination, the tricuspid valve commonly shows some degree of change, in association with a myxomatous mitral valve. In cases of pulmonary emphysema, the tricuspid valve is commonly affected and often to a greater degree than the mitral valve. This association is of particular interest. It suggests that a weakness of connective tissue is shared by both the lungs and the cardiac valves. In the lung, the process favors the development of emphysema. The resulting pulmonary and right ventricular hypertension challenge the tricuspid valve and brings out, strikingly in some cases, the phenomenon of prolapse of the tricuspid valve.

While the tricuspid valve may show isolated prolapse angiocardiographically and/or echocardiographically, usually prolapse of the tricuspid valve is associated with a similar process in the mitral valve.[28]

In the great vessels, cystic medial necrosis may occur; when present, it probably underlies the described difficulties of controlling the aortic perfusion site following replacement of the mitral valve.[39] The association of a myxomatous mitral valve and an atrial septal defect of the fossa ovalis (secundum) type is recognized.[33] This peculiar association may not relate to an inherent developmental association between the atrial septum and the mitral valve. Rather, the association may result from primary incompetence of the mitral valve with the atrial septal defect developing from an ordinary patent foramen ovale as a consequence of left atrial dilation.[63]

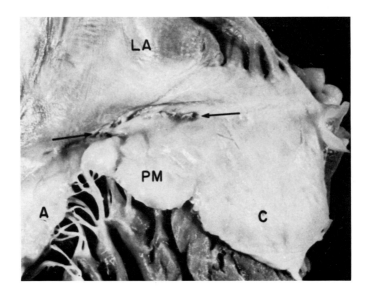

Fig. 25–11. Angle contact lesion in floppy mitral valve. Gross specimen shows a linear deposit of fibrin (between arrows) at the junction of the left atrium (LA) and the posteromedial scallop (PM) of the posterior leaflet. C, central scallop of posterior mitral leaflet; A, anterior leaflet. (From Edwards,[20] with permission.)

Deficiency of Leaflet Tissue

The most common basis for mitral incompetence caused by a deficiency of leaflet tissue is the destructive effect of infective endocarditis. The latter may cause mitral incompetence during the active phases of the disease. The effects of the destructive changes continue in spite of bacteriologic cure and appear as an example of chronic mitral insufficiency.

Destructive changes of infective endocarditis involving parts of the mitral apparatus and causing incompetence may result either from primary mitral endocarditis or from secondary involvement of the mitral valve in instances of primary aortic valvular infection.

Incompetence of the mitral valve from primary infection of this valve may result from interference with valvular closure by vegetations or from destruction of leaflet tissue, rupture of chordae, or a combination of the latter two conditions.

Another basis for mitral insufficiency resulting from primary infection of this valve is

through immobilization of the posterior leaflet. This comes about in the following way: in primary mitral infective endocarditis, infection may spread through the full thickness of the leaflet; vegetations may occur in the angle between the posterior mitral leaflet and the endocardium of the related inferior basal wall of the left ventricle (Fig. 25–12A). Healing of a vegetation in the latter position causes fibrous union between the left ventricular wall and the posterior mitral leaflet; the leaflet is thereby immobilized and cannot contribute to mitral valve closure[5] (Fig. 25–12B).

In a consideration of primary aortic valvular endocarditis being responsible for secondary mitral insufficiency, certain anatomic relationships between the two valves should be emphasized. Subjacent to the part of the aortic valve with which it is in fibrous continuity lies the anterior leaflet of the mitral valve. More inferiorly are the chordae of the mitral apparatus (Fig. 25–13A). Those chordae inserting into the anterior leaflet are more directly in line with a regurgitant stream beginning at

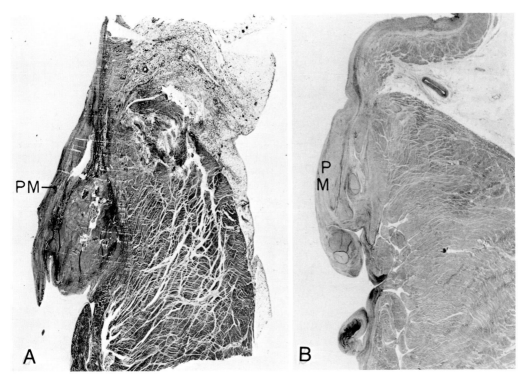

Fig. 25–12. Infective endocarditis causing adhesion of posterior mitral leaflet to mural endocardium of left ventricle. **(A)** Active infective endocarditis showing vegetation deposited between posterior mitral leaflet (PM) and left ventricular wall, setting the stage for the illustration shown in Fig. B. (Elastic tissue stain, × 2.3.) **(B)** Left atrium and left ventricle. Posterior mitral leaflet (PM) is adherent to mural endocardium of left ventricle as the result of healing of a vegetation in the angle between the leaflet and the ventricular wall. The process causes loss of valve function. (Elastic tissue stain, × 2.)

the aortic valve than are the chordae inserting into the posterior leaflet.

The anterior mitral leaflet is subject to secondary infection from aortic valvular endocarditis (Fig. 25–13) either by direct extension (Figs. 25–13A,B and 25–14) or from contamination by an infected regurgitant stream[19] (Fig. 25–13C,D). Gradual destruction may result in a mycotic aneurysm of the anterior leaflet, perforation of which leads to mitral regurgitation (Figs. 25–13C and 25–15). Infection of mitral chordae may result in rupture (Fig. 25–13). These chordae inserting into the anterior mitral leaflet are more subject to this complication than are those inserting into the posterior leaflet.

Congenital cleft of the anterior mitral leaflet may be included under the subject of deficiency of leaflet tissue. The most common state is that in which the cleft in the anterior mitral leaflet is part of the developmental complex variously known as the *persistent common atrioventricular canal* or *endocardial cushion defect*. The most common changes are a cleft in the anterior mitral leaflet and an atrial septal defect of the ostium primum type. An additional anomaly of this developmental syndrome observed in some cases includes a cleft in the septal leaflet of the tricuspid valve (the cleft mitral and tricuspid valves may together form the well-known common atrioventricular valve of the

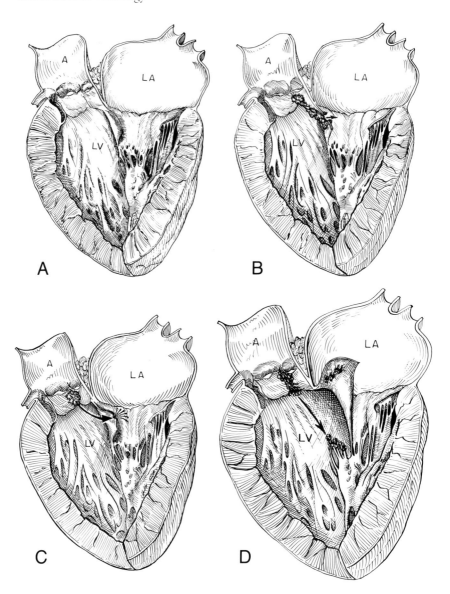

Fig. 25–13. Anatomic causes of mitral insufficiency complicating aortic valvular endocarditis. (**A**) Left atrium (LA), left ventricle (LV), and ascending aorta (A) in the normal. There is close relationship between the aortic valve and the anterior leaflet of the mitral valve. (**B**) Inflammation of the aortic valve involving the anterior leaflet of the mitral valve by direct extension of infection, with perforation (arrow) of anterior mitral leaflet. (**C**) Stream of aortic valvular regurgitation during active infection abuts on the ventricular surface of the anterior mitral leaflet, causing infection and perforation of that structure. (**D**) Regurgitation from aortic valve abuts on chordae of the mitral valve. The resultant infection allows for rupture of chordae and the appearance of a flail mitral leaflet.

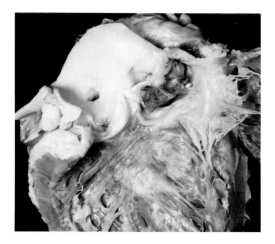

Fig. 25–14. Aortic valvular infective endocarditis extending directly onto the anterior mitral leaflet causing perforation (probe). Aortic valve shows a congenital bicuspid deformity.

endocardial cushion defect). A deficiency of the upper ventricular septum is also common, and superior to the deficient ventricular septum an interventricular communication may occur.

A particular point of interest is that chordae run between the edges of the cleft mitral valve, above, and the ventricular septum, below. If chordae insert into the ventricular septum some distance below the level of the mitral annulus and the cleft of the mitral valve is closed surgically, such chordae, if left intact, may lead to postoperative mitral regurgitation by preventing adequate excursion of a valve with a surgically obliterated cleft.[17]

Isolated cleft of the anterior mitral leaflet with intact atrial and ventricular septa may be viewed as a variant of the endocardial cushion defect (Fig. 25–16). In this uncommon con-

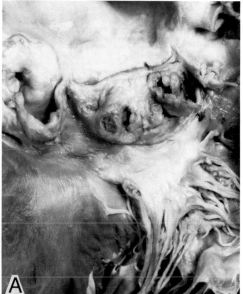
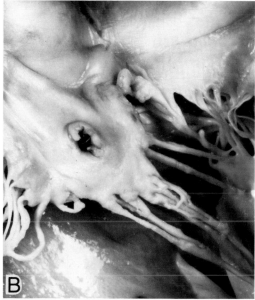

Fig. 25–15. Perforation of mitral leaflet secondary to aortic valvular endocarditis. (**A**) Primary bacterial endocarditis of aortic valve with numerous perforations in cusps of valve. The subjacent mitral valve shows a lesion representing a perforation. (**B**) Atrial aspect of mitral valve showing a perforation in the central portion of the anterior mitral leaflet. While the chordae are intact, they show nodular thickenings interpreted as secondary to infection of these structures by regurgitation of infected blood from the aortic valve.

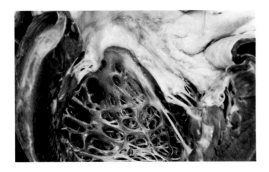

Fig. 25–16. Congenital cleft of anterior mitral leaflet from a child with major mitral insufficiency.

dition, significant mitral regurgitation is common.

Immobilization of Leaflet

The process of immobilization usually involves the posterior leaflet. Among acquired states causing this process are healed infective endocarditis, the hypereosinophilic syndrome, endomyocardial fibrosis, systemic lupus erythematosus, enlargement of the left atrium from mitral insufficiency, and, occasionally, calcification of the mitral ring. Certain congenital states may also be characterized by immobilization of leaflet tissue.

The process of adhesion of the posterior leaflet to the left ventricular wall in healing infective endocarditis has been mentioned earlier (see Fig. 25–12).

The hypereosinophilic syndrome is variously called Loeffler's fibroplastic endocarditis with eosinophilia, disseminated eosinophilic collagen disease, and eosinophilic leukemia. The condition, most commonly seen in men of the fifth decade, is frequently associated with loss of weight, evidence of cardiovascular disease, cutaneous rash, and eosinophilia. Total leukocyte counts, based on eosinophilia, may reach as high as 50,000 ml[3]. In this setting the syndrome is said to be present when other causes of eosinophilia, such as parasitic diseases and recognized allergic states, are excluded.

Many internal organs, including the liver, spleen, kidneys, and myocardium, may show interstitial eosinophilic infiltration. Controversy exists as to whether some or all cases are to be considered examples of eosinophilic leukemia. Support for a leukemic designation comes from those cases that show immature eosinophils and even blast cells in the peripheral blood and bone marrow. Negating this viewpoint are cases that do not show the types of hematologic abnormalities mentioned.

From a review of 14 personally observed cases and 57 acceptable cases in the literature, Chusid and associates[11] agree with the opinion of Roberts and associates[54] that the hypereosinophilic syndrome is a continuum of disease, ranging from apparent leukemia to a relatively mild disease characterized by a rash, although in all cases there is a strong tendency for cardiac disease.

The pathologic changes in the heart depend upon the stage of the disease. These were reviewed by Brockington and Olsen,[6] who describe the stages as follows:

1. Acute myocarditis, characterized by patchy necrosis and leukocytic infiltration with eosinophils present, although lymphocytes and plasma cells are dominant.
2. Mural thrombosis associated with endocardial leukocytic infiltration, including (but not dominantly) eosinophils. Patchy myocardial fibrosis is associated.
3. Endocardial thickening with blood vessels and leukocytes lying among collagenous fibers. This process is presumably derived from the organization of thrombus.
4. The healed stage, characterized by endocardial thickening with hyalin connective tissue within which are elastic fibers and blood vessels. Fingers of collagen extend from the thickened endocardium into the nearby myocardium. Leukocytic infiltration is either absent or minimal. Superimposed thrombus is common but not universal.

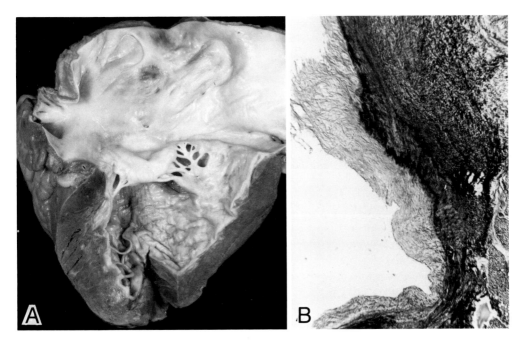

Fig. 25–17. Löeffler's endomyocardial fibrosis. (**A**) Left atrium and left ventricle. The posterior mitral leaflet is adherent to the fibrous, plaquelike lesion of the mural endocardium of the left ventricle. Immobility of the posterior leaflet results, allowing for mitral insufficiency and enlargement of the left atrium. (**B**) From the posterior wall of the left atrium, photomicrograph shows endocardial lesion interpreted as a jet lesion resulting from the mitral incompetence. (Elastic tissue stain, × 22.)

The process of thrombosis has two hemodynamic effects. That related to the posterior mitral leaflet becomes, by organization, adherent to the leaflet so as to immobilize it and cause mitral regurgitation[23,25] (Fig. 25–17). The other effect of the thrombus is that it may occupy luminal space and so restrict ventricular size.[25] Changes in the ventricles are usually more common and more extensive in the left ventricle than in the right. Apical involvement is characteristic, while the outflow tracts are usually unaffected.

The major cause of death in the hypereosinophilic syndrome is through cardiac involvement; the significant alterations of extracardiac organs relate more to complications of embolism and congestive heart failure than to infiltration by eosinophils.

The cardiac changes of the hypereosinophilic syndrome resemble the endomyocardial fibrosis described by Davies and Ball[15] as occurring in African natives; in fact, the two conditions may have similar etiologies.[54]

In lupus erythematosus[54] the valvular vegetations may involve the angle between the posterior mitral leaflet and left ventricular wall. This process usually does not cause mitral incompetence during active phases of the disease. With the use of steroid therapy, healing of valvular lesions tends to occur. In this area, organization of vegetations leads to a fibrous union of the posterior mitral leaflet with the left ventricular mural endocardium. Mitral incompetence results from immobilization of the posterior mitral leaflet[8] as in other etiologic states described.

Calcification of the mitral ring is characterized by a calcific deposit in the mitral annulus in relation to the posterior mitral leaflet. It is to be recognized that the term "ring" refers to the annulus and not to the shape of the calcification, the latter being semicircular.

The process appears to begin as a fatty alteration of the connective tissue involved. This is followed by calcification. Histologically, the process is similar to the changes in calcified aortic valves, being characterized by deposits of amorphous masses, some of which are calcified. Reactions in the form of non-specific inflammatory infiltration and foreign body giant cells are common.

The condition is a hallmark of the aged. In autopsy material, Pomerance[50] found an overall incidence of 8.5 percent in subjects over 50 years of age, with a sharp rise over 70 years. In females over 90 years of age, the incidence was about 43.5 percent, while in comparably aged males the incidence was 17 percent (see Ch. 5).

It is common for subjects with calcification of the mitral ring to manifest cardiac murmurs, although not all of these murmurs are to be charged to the process under discussion.

Uncommonly, mitral insufficiency is caused by calcification of the ring. The most likely mechanism by which this is brought about is by extension of the process from the ring to engage and immobilize the posterior mitral leaflet (Fig. 25–18). Simon and Liu[61] suggested that mitral regurgitation may result from interference with contraction of that myocardium related to the mitral orifice.

Other complications include ulceration through the leaflet with further complications of infective endocarditis and/or thrombosis with the potential for systemic arterial embolism.[50]

In *left atrial enlargement* associated with any type of mitral incompetence, except that in which both commissures are fused, a given degree of mitral insufficiency may, by its compounding effects, cause an accentuation of the degree of regurgitation, a phenomenon identified as "mitral insufficiency begets mitral insufficiency."[21]

This is brought about first by left atrial enlargement. As the wall of this chamber is continuous with the posterior mitral leaflet, the

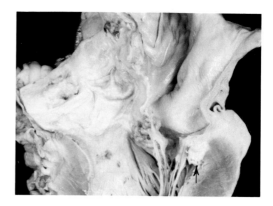

Fig. 25–18. Left atrium and portion of the mitral and the aortic valves in a case of calcification of the mitral ring. The lesion (point of arrow) lies at the junction of the left atrium, left ventricle, and posterior mitral leaflet. The latter is adherent to the internal aspect of the lesion. Associated changes in this case include calcification of the anterior leaflet and atherosclerosis of the aorta.

enlarged left atrium pulls the base of the posterior mitral leaflet backward and downward. The process may progress to the point at which the posterior mitral leaflet is strapped over the base of the left ventricular myocardial wall. Acting further to immobilize the posterior leaflet is the attachment of the free aspect of the leaflet through chordae with the subjacent papillary muscles (Fig. 25–19).

Of the various *congenital states* characterized by immobilization of leaflet tissue, the most common is *corrected transposition*.[16] In this condition, transposition of the great vessels and inversion of the ventricles and the atrioventricular valves occur. The left atrioventricular valve (anatomically inverted tricuspid valve) is subject to malformations, particularly that of the type known as Ebstein's malformation in normally oriented hearts. When associated with incompetence of the atrioventricular valve, the malformation on the left side gives a clinical and hemodynamic picture of mitral insufficiency. The principal basis for this appears to be a downward displacement with abnormal adhesion to the ventricular wall of the septal leaflet.

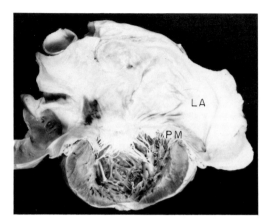

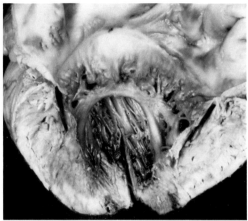

Fig. 25–19. Floppy mitral valve with intact chordae and extensive mitral insufficiency. The enlarged left atrium (LA) projects posteroinferiorly over the base of the left ventricle, pulling the posterior mitral leaflet (PM) over the left ventricular mass. Retention of the posterior mitral leaflet by chordae, along with the tensions of the enlarged left atrium, causes immobilization of the posterior mitral leaflet. The process illustrates the point that the effects of mitral insufficiency lead to more mitral insufficiency.

Anomalous mitral arcade is an uncommon primary anomaly that may cause mitral regurgitation, probably through restraint of both leaflets. The condition is characterized by an apparent underdevelopment of mitral valvular components. There are no clear-cut commissures, and the chordae lack differentiation into distinct strands. An arcade of fibrous tissue extends from one papillary muscle to the other as it runs along the inferior aspect of the anterior mitral leaflet[32] (Fig. 25–20).

Hurler syndrome is associated with an infiltration of valvular tissues and coronary arteries by the classical enlarged balloon cell (see Ch. 29). The gross picture is that of thickening with shortening and distortion of the leaflets of the valve. The basic alteration may be associated with mitral incompetence, principally through thickening and rigidity of leaflets.[30] In some cases, it may result from a myocardial infarction, incident to the coronary arterial lesions of this syndrome.

Fig. 25–20. Left atrium, left ventricle, and mitral valve showing anomalous mitral arcade. The mitral leaflets, commissures, and chordae are poorly developed. The arcade extends from the anterolateral to the posteromedial papillary muscle through the free extremity of the deformed mitral valve. (From Layman and Edwards,[32] with permission.)

TENSOR APPARATUS

Malfunction of the tensor apparatus as a basis for mitral incompetence may result from rupture of chordae or of a papillary muscle. In some instances the chordae may be intact but excessively long, as in the myxomatous mitral valve. Effective shortening of chordae as yet another complication of the myxomatous valve may underlie or contribute to mitral incompetence in some cases. The most common basis for mitral incompetence through malfunction of the tensor apparatus is myocardial infarction associated with nonruptured papillary muscles.

Rupture of Chordae Tendineae

There are two fundamental causes of rupture of chordae. One is a complication of the myxomatous mitral valve (Figs. 25–5 and 25–6). The other is infective endocarditis of the mi-

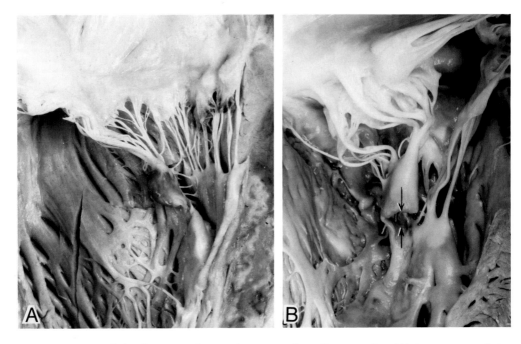

Fig. 25–21. Myocardial infarction with partial rupture of papillary muscles. (**A**) Acute myocardial infarction. There is partial rupture of one head of the posteromedial papillary muscle. (**B**) Healed myocardial infarction. One head of the posteromedial papillary muscle has ruptured, except for one retained strand of tissue (arrow on each side of rupture site).

tral valve, either primary or secondary to primary infection of the aortic valve. Rarely, chordae are ruptured as a result of cardiac trauma.

Rupture of a Papillary Muscle

Rupture of a papillary muscle may be a complication either of trauma or of acute myocardial infarction.

Isolated rupture of a papillary muscle on the basis of trauma is uncommon. When traumatic rupture of a papillary muscle occurs, it is usually attended by other major cardiac lesions, such as rupture of the ventricular septum and/or rupture of the free wall of one or both ventricles. The classic cause of rupture of a papillary muscle is acute myocardial infarction.

Among the ruptures that may complicate acute myocardial infarction, those involving either the free wall of the left ventricle or the ventricular septum are classically based on a transmural infarct. In contrast, rupture of a papillary muscle may complicate either transmural or subendocardial infarction.[65]

Rupture of part of a set of papillary muscles may be tolerated so as to leave a state of chronic mitral incompetence[34] (Fig. 25–21). When, as is more common, an entire set of muscles is involved, the resulting mitral insufficiency is overwhelming and leads to shock and early death (Fig. 25–22). Uncommonly, rupture of a papillary muscle may be followed by rupture of the free wall of the left ventricle with hemopericardium[65] (Fig. 25–23).

Classically, in cases of rupture of all or part of a set of papillary muscles, the underlying myocardial infarct occupies the lateral aspect of the left ventricle. Adjacent parts of the in-

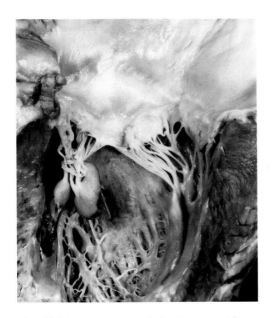

Fig. 25–22. Acute myocardial infarction with rupture of anterolateral papillary muscle.

ferior or anterior wall may be concomitantly affected. The posteromedial papillary muscle is more commonly involved than is the anterolateral one by a ratio of 4:1. Rupture usually occurs during the first week following onset of the infarction.

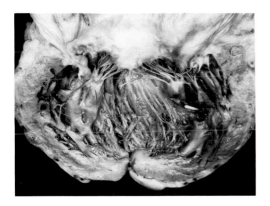

Fig. 25–23. Left atrium and left ventricle. Acute myocardial infarction with coexistent rupture of the posteromedial papillary muscle and of the free wall of the left ventricle. A probe lies in the tract of the rupture of the free wall of the left ventricle.

Myocardial Infarction with Intact Papillary Muscles

Mitral incompetence resulting from myocardial infarction is much more commonly associated with intact papillary muscles than with rupture of one of these structures. When the mitral insufficiency is associated with intact papillary muscles, it is rarely of massive intensity and acute (Fig. 25–24). Usually, it is a chronic process of varying degree that becomes recognized in the postinfarction period. This state is commonly called *papillary muscle dysfunction*. The pathologic counterparts of postinfarction mitral regurgitation vary (Fig. 25–25). The most common pattern is that of inferior or inferolateral healed subendocardial myocardial infarction with atrophy, through infarction, of the posteromedial papillary muscle.[2,59,64] Lateral or anterolateral myocardial infarction, with the single papillary muscle involved being the anterolateral one, is distinctly less common.

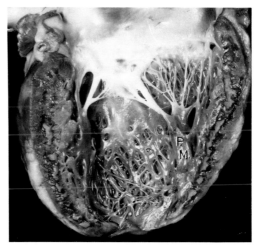

Fig. 25–24. Acute myocardial infarction associated with acute onset of massive mitral insufficiency. The pathologic process is that of extensive infarction involving the lateral wall of the left ventricle but without rupture of papillary muscles. PM, posteromedial papillary muscle.

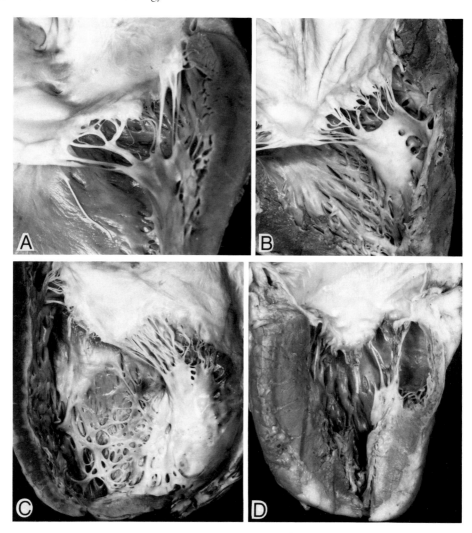

Fig. 25–25. Variations in gross appearance of the potential for mitral insufficiency in healed myocardial infarction with intact papillary muscles. (**A**) Atrophy and fibrosis of posteromedial papillary muscle, while little or no scarring appears in the free wall. (**B**) Coexistent subendocardial healed infarction of the free wall of the left ventricle and related posteromedial papillary muscle. (**C**) Healed extensive inferolateral myocardial infarction with involvement of posteromedial papillary muscle. (**D**) Transmural infarction of the inferior wall of the left ventricle, with scarring of the posteromedial papillary muscle.

Least common is healed myocardial infarction involving both papillary muscles. Usually there is concomitant extensive involvement of the free wall of the left ventricle. In this pattern of involvement, the infarction is extensive and the hemodynamic state is complicated by a congestive cardiac myopathy caused by the infarction and mitral regurgi-

tation. The mitral regurgitation, in turn, is to be viewed as resulting from two factors: (1) the state wherein a papillary muscle is involved as part of an infarction, and (2) the congestive cardiac myopathy of widespread loss of myocardial tissue. The usual basis for the myocardial infarction underlying mitral incompetence is coronary atherosclerosis, and the process is classically seen in adults. In infants or children, a similar picture may be observed as a complication of *anomalous origin of the left coronary artery* from the pulmonary trunk.[44]

Infarction of papillary muscles and related aspects of the left ventricular free wall may complicate *congenital aortic stenosis* and be a basis for mitral incompetence in the young.[43]

Effective Shortening of Chordae Tendineae

In considering the myxomatous mitral valve, it was pointed out that in some instances chordae related to the posterior mitral leaflet may rub upon the mural endocardium of the left ventricle. This process is followed by a fibrous reaction which, in turn, may cause chordae to adhere to the left ventricular wall. This causes effective shortening of the involved chordae. In extreme examples, the shortened chordae appear to unduly restrain motion of the posterior leaflet.

In late stages of *aortic valvular disease*, either stenosis but particularly regurgitation, mitral regurgitation may develop. The mechanism may be compounded of ventricular dilation and downward displacement of papillary muscles. The latter results from the enlargement of the left ventricle. As this occurs, the distance between the apices of the papillary muscles and the mitral orifice increases, thereby placing undue tension upon the chordae. This process, in turn, may restrict optimal positioning of the mitral leaflets and cause the orifice to be inadequately guarded.

ORIFICE OF THE MITRAL VALVE

For the purpose of this discussion, I will view the mitral valve orifice as part of the left ventricular cavity. Therefore, any condition that causes enlargement of the left ventricular cavity widens the mitral orifice. Mitral insufficiency may be a functional manifestation. The mechanism probably involves several factors, only one of which is the enlarged orifice that may make the mitral leaflets, even normal leaflets, relatively short. Another factor is inefficiency of the tensor apparatus, which is brought about by lateral deviation of the papillary muscles as the ventricle dilates. This displacement may disturb the lines of tension of the papillary muscles and chordae. The disturbance, in turn, may cause inefficient restraint of the leaflets, allowing them to prolapse.[21]

Among conditions that result in mitral incompetence by the mechanisms named are the various forms of chronic congestive cardiomyopathy[29] (Fig. 25–26); left ventricular failure for other reasons, including extensive myocardial infarction; and, in the young, so-called primary endocardial fibroelastosis[42] (Fig. 25–27). Systolic anterior motion of the anterior mitral leaflet is now a well-recognized phenomenon in hypertrophic obstructive cardiomyopathy.[58] The abnormal movement of this leaflet during the

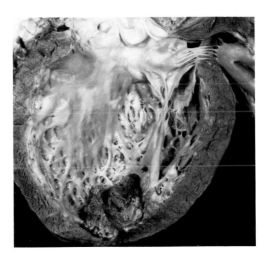

Fig. 25–26. Congestive cardiomyopathy. The left ventricle is dilated and shows focal endocardial fibroelastosis. A mural thrombus is present at the apex.

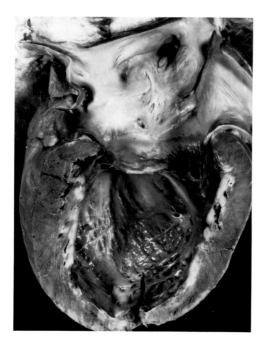

Fig. 25–27. Dilated type of endocardial fibroelastosis. The left ventricular cavity is enlarged, and its endocardium is thickened. The anterior leaflet of the mitral valve shows rolling of the free edge interpreted as secondary to the associated mitral insufficiency. As the left ventricle dilates, the two papillary muscles are moved away from each other. This process may account for the loss of efficiency of the mitral tensor apparatus.

period in which the mitral orifice should be closed accounts for the frequently present mitral incompetence in the type of cardiomyopathy named. Systolic anterior motion of the anterior mitral leaflet has also been observed in cases without hypertrophy of the ventricular septum.[14] (See Ch. 20 also.)

REFERENCES

1. Allen H, Harris A, Leatham A: Significance and prognosis of an isolated late systolic murmur: A 9- to 22-year follow-up. Br Heart J 36:525, 1974

2. Ballester M, Tasca R, Marin L, et al: Different mechanisms of mitral regurgitation in acute and chronic forms of coronary heart disease. Eur Heart J 4:557, 1983

3. Barnett HMJ: Embolism in mitral valve prolapse. Annu Rev Med 33:489, 1982

4. Becker AE, Becker MJ, Edwards JE: Mitral valvular abnormalities associated with supravalvular aortic stenosis. Observations in 3 cases. Am J Cardiol 29:90, 1972

5. Becker DL, Burchell HB, Edwards JE: Pathology of the pulmonary vascular tree. II. The occurrence in mitral insufficiency of occlusive pulmonary vascular lesions. Circulation 3:230, 1951

6. Brockington IF, Olsen EGJ: Löffler's endocarditis and Davies' endomyocardial fibrosis. Am Heart J 85:308, 1973

7. Brown OR, Kloster FE, DeMots H: Incidence of mitral valve prolapse in the asymptomatic normal. Circulation 51/52:77, 1975 (abst)

8. Bulkley BH, Roberts WC: Systemic lupus erythematosus as a cause of severe mitral regurgitation. New problem in an old disease. Am J Cardiol 35:305, 1975

9. Bulkley BH, Roberts WC: Dilatation of the mitral anulus. A rare cause of mitral regurgitation. Am J Med 59:457, 1975

10. Cabeen WR Jr, Reza MJ, Kovick RB, Stern MS: Mitral valve prolapse and conduction defects in Ehlers-Danlos syndrome. Arch Intern Med 137:1227, 1977

11. Chusid MJ, Dale DC, West BC, Wolff SM: The hypereosinophilic syndrome: Analysis of fourteen cases with review of the literature. Medicine (Baltimore) 54:1, 1975

12. Cooley DA, Gerami S, Hallman GL, et al: Mitral insufficiency due to myxomatous transformation: "Floppy valve syndrome." J Cardiovasc Surg 13:346, 1972

13. Corrigall D, Bolen J, Hancock E, Popp RL: Mitral valve prolapse and infective endocarditis. Am J Med 63:215, 1977

14. Crawford M, Groves B, Horwitz L: Mitral valve systolic anterior motion producing dynamic subaortic stenosis without asymmetric septal hypertrophy. Circulation 55/56:69, 1977 (abst)

15. Davies JNP, Ball JD: The pathology of endomyocardial fibrosis in Uganda. Br Heart J 17:337, 1955

16. Edwards JE: Differential diagnosis of mitral stenosis: A clincopathologic review of simulating conditions. Lab Invest 3:89, 1954

17. Edwards JE: The problem of mitral insufficiency caused by accessory chordae tendineae in persistent common atrioventricular canal. Mayo Clin Proc 35:299, 1960

18. Edwards JE: Mitral insufficiency resulting from "overshooting" of leaflets. Circulation 43:606, 1971

19. Edwards JE: Mitral insufficiency secondary to aortic valvular bacterial endocarditis. Circulation 46:623, 1972

20. Edwards JE: Floppy mitral valve syndrome. Cardiovasc Clin 18:249, 1987

21. Edwards JE, Burchell HB: Pathologic anatomy of mitral insufficiency. Mayo Clin Proc 33:497, 1958

22. Goodman D, Kimbiris D, Linhart JW: Chordae tendineae rupture complicating the systolic click-late systolic murmur syndrome. Am J Cardiol 33:681, 1974

23. Gottdiener JS, Maron BJ, Schooley RT, et al: Two-dimensional echocardiographic assessment of the idiopathic hypereosinophilic syndrome. Anatomic basis of mitral regurgitation and peripheral embolization. Circulation 67:572, 1983

24. Guthrie RB, Edwards JE: Pathology of the myxomatous mitral valve. Nature, secondary changes and complications. Minn Med 59:637, 1976

25. Hall SW Jr, Theologides A, From AHL, et al: Hypereosinophilic syndrome with biventricular involvement. Circulation 55:217, 1977

26. Hanson TP, Edwards BS, Edwards JE: Pathology of surgically excised mitral valves. One hundred consecutive cases. Arch Pathol Lab Med 109:823, 1985

27. Jeresaty RM: Mitral valve prolapse-click syndrome. Prog Cardiovasc Dis 15:623, 1973

28. Karayannis E, Stefadouros MA, Abdulla AM, Blackwell JC: Use of echocardiography in the diagnosis of prolapsed tricuspid valve. J Med Assoc Ga 67:205, 1978

29. Kaul U, Ramachandran P, Bhatia ML: Spontaneous conversion of long standing atrial fibrillation to sinus rhythm—an unusual preterminal phenomenon. Indian Heart J 35:241, 1983

30. Krovetz LJ, Schiebler GL: Cardiovascular

31. Kuhn D, Weber N: Mural bacterial endocarditis of a ventricular friction lesion. Arch Pathol 95:92, 1973

32. Layman TE, Edwards JE: Anomalous mitral arcade. A type of congenital mitral insufficiency. Circulation 35:389, 1967

33. Leachman RD, Cokkinos EV, Cooley DA: Association of ostium secundum atrial septal defects with mitral valve prolapse. Am J Cardiol 38:167, 1976

34. Lee KS, Johnson T, Karnegis JN, et al: Acute myocardial infarction with long-term survival following papillary muscular rupture. Am Heart J 79:258, 1970

35. Malcolm AD, Boughner DR, Kostuk WJ, Ahuja SP: Clinical features and investigative findings in presence of mitral leaflet prolapse. Study of 85 consecutive patients. Br Heart J 38:244, 1976

36. Marchand P, Barlow JB, du Plessis LA, Webster I: Mitral regurgitation with rupture of normal chordae tendineae. Br Heart J 28:746, 1966

37. Markiewicz W, Stoner J, London E, et al: Mitral valve prolapse in one hundred presumably healthy females. Circulation 51/52:77, 1975 (abst)

38. McKay R, Yacoub MH: Clinical and pathological findings in patients with "floppy" valves treated surgically. Circulation 47/48(suppl III):63, 1973

39. McKay R, Yacoub MH: Acute aortic dissection and medial degeneration in patients with "floppy" mitral valves. Thorax 31:49, 1976

40. McLaren MJ, Hawkins DM, Lachman AS, et al: Non-ejection systolic clicks and mitral systolic murmurs in Black schoolchildren of Soweto, Johannesburg. Br Heart J 38:718, 1976

41. Mills P, Rose J, Hollingsworth BA, et al: Long-term prognosis of mitral-valve prolapse. N Engl J Med 297:13, 1977

42. Moller JH, Lucas RV Jr, Adams P, et al: Endocardial fibroelastosis. A clinical and anatomic study of 47 patients with emphasis on its relationship to mitral insufficiency. Circulation 30:759, 1964

43. Moller JH, Nakib A, Edwards JE: Infarction of papillary muscles and mitral insufficiency

manifestations of the genetic mucopolysaccharidoses. Birth Defects 8:192, 1972 associated with congenital aortic stenosis. Circulation 34:87, 1966

44. Noren GR, Raghib G, Moller JH, et al: Anomalous origin of the left coronary artery from the pulmonary trunk with special reference to the occurrence of mitral insufficiency. Circulation 30:171, 1964

45. Olson LJ, Subramanian R, Ackermann DM, et al: Surgical pathology of the mitral valve: A study of 712 cases spanning 21 years. Mayo Clin Proc 62:22, 1987

46. Osmundson PJ, Callahan JA, Edwards JE: Mitral insufficiency from rupture of chordae tendineae simulating aortic stenosis. Mayo Clin Proc 33:235, 1958

47. Perloff JK, Roberts WC: The mitral apparatus. Functional anatomy of mitral regurgitation. Circulation 46:227, 1972

48. Pocock WA, Lakier JB, Hitchcock JF, Barlow JB: Mitral valve aneurysm after infective endocarditis in the billowing mitral leaflet syndrome. Am J Cardiol 40:130, 1977

49. Pomerance A: Ballooning deformity (mucoid degeneration) of atrioventricular valves. Br Heart J 31:343, 1969

50. Pomerance A: Pathological and clinical study of calcification of the mitral valve ring. Br J Clin Pathol 23:354, 1970

51. Ranganathan N, Silver MD, Robinson TI, et al: Angiographic-morphologic correlation in patients with severe mitral regurgitation due to prolapse of the posterior mitral valve leaflet. Circulation 48:514, 1973

52. Read RC, Thal AP, Wendt VE: Symptomatic valvular myxomatous transformation (the floppy valve syndrome). A possible forme fruste of the Marfan syndrome. Circulation 32:897, 1965

53. Rizzon P, Biasco G, Brindicci G, Mauro F: Familial syndrome of midsystolic click and late systolic murmur. Br Heart J 35:245, 1973

54. Roberts WC, Buja LM, Ferrans VJ: Loeffler's fibroplastic parietal endocarditis, eosinophilic leukemia, and Davie's endomyocardial fibrosis: The same disease at different stages? Pathol Microbiol (Basel) 35:90, 1970

55. Rusted IE, Scheifley CH, Edwards JE, Kirklin JW: Guides to the commissures in operations upon the mitral valve. Mayo Clin Proc 26:297, 1951

56. Salazar AE, Edwards JE: Friction lesions of ventricular endocardium. Relation to chordae tendineae of mitral valve. Arch Pathol 90:364, 1970

57. Salomon NW, Stinson EB, Griepp RB, Shumway NE: Surgical treatment of degenerative mitral regurgitation. Am J Cardiol 38:463, 1976

58. Shah PM, Gramiak R, Adelman AG, Wigle ED: Role of echocardiography in diagnostic and hemodynamic assessment of hypertrophic subaortic stenosis. Circulation 44:891, 1971

59. Shelburne JC, Rubinstein D, Gorlin R: A reappraisal of papillary muscle dysfunction: Correlative clinical and angiographic study. Am J Med 46:862, 1969

60. Shrivastava S, Guthrie RB, Edwards JE: Prolapse of the mitral valve. Mod Concepts Cardiovasc Dis 46:57, 1977

61. Simon MA, Liu SF: Calcification of the mitral valve annulus and its relation to functional valvular disturbance. Am Heart J 48:497, 1954

62. Swartz MH, Teichholz LE, Donoso, E: Mitral valve prolapse. A review of associated arrhythmias. Am J Med 62:377, 1977

63. Tandon R, Edwards JE: Atrial septal defect in infancy. Common association with other anomalies. Circulation 49:1005, 1974

64. Tsakiris AG, Rastelli GC, Amorim D de S, et al: Effect of experimental papillary muscle damage on mitral valve closure in intact anesthetized dogs. Mayo Clin Proc 45:275, 1970

65. Vlodaver Z, Edwards JE: Rupture of ventricular septum or papillary muscle complicating myocardial infarction. Circulation 55:815, 1977

66. Weiss AN, Mimbs JW, Ludbrook PA, Sobel BE: Echocardiographic detection of mitral valve prolapse. Exclusion of false positive diagnosis and determination of inheritance. Circulation 52:1091, 1975

26

Blood Flow Obstruction Related to the Aortic Valve

Malcolm D. Silver

Obstruction to blood flow in the vicinity of the aortic valve occurs at subvalvular, valvular, or supravalvular levels. The mechanisms of obstruction are those that cause stenosis at comparable locations related to other heart valves and are listed in Table 24–1. In the adult, aortic valvular stenoses are most frequent, subvalvular stenoses much less common, and supravalvular stenoses least common. Lesions causing stenosis may be congenital or acquired and, at the valvular level, a natural or an artificial heart valve may be stenosed; obviously, conditions that stenose a prosthetic valve are all acquired. In this chapter, obstruction at each level is considered in a sequence related to frequency, with emphasis given to acquired lesions. The congenital lesions discussed are those likely to cause problems in adults.

ANATOMY OF LEFT VENTRICULAR OUTFLOW TRACT, AORTIC VALVE, AND ASCENDING AORTA

To better appreciate the pathology of subvalvular, valvular, and supravalvular aortic stenoses, the reader must have a good understanding of the anatomy of these areas.

The outflow tract of the left ventricle extends from the apex of the left ventricle to the aortic valve.[135,136] Anteriorly, it is defined by the septal wall of the left ventricle with, at its distal end, the membranous interventricular septum. Posteriorly, its boundaries are formed by the anterior mitral valve leaflet, its associated chordae tendineae, and the anterior papillary muscle of the left ventricle with the "intervalvular septum,"[136] and, in its distal part, with the curtain formed by fusion of the anterior and posterior mitral leaflets.

Movement of the anterior mitral leaflet during the cardiac cycle alters the caliber of the distal outflow tract in the subaortic area. Thus, in ventricular diastole, when the mitral valve opens, the tract is narrowed as the anterior leaflet moves toward the ventricular septum. Conversely, during systole, that leaflet moves away from the septum to close the mitral valve orifice and, in doing so, enlarges the outflow tract as blood is discharged through it. Figures 1–9 and 1–20 illustrate the anatomy of the left ventricular outflow tract.

Chapter 1 provides a description of the left ventricle, the aortic valve apparatus, the sinuses of Valsalva, and the coronary artery ostia. Considering the aortic valve, Angelini and colleagues[2] studied 30 normal valves and 64 with two cusps; the authors prefer the term "leaflet" to "cusp." They found that the cusps

985

attached to the aortic wall in a crescentic or semilunar fashion. In doing so, the cusps crossed the ringlike junction of the aortic wall and ventricular mass, ascended to the commissures, and descended to the trough of each cusp. In this study neither gross nor histologic examination demonstrated any cordlike ring supporting the cusps' attachment at the ventriculoarterial junction. On the aortic aspect, the aortic wall was found to expand to form the sinuses of Valsalva, with each sinus supporting the corresponding cusp in a semilunar fashion. When viewed from the ventricular aspect, the sinuses were separated by triangles of fibrous tissue that were thinner than the aortic wall in the sinuses. The triangles extend to the apex of a commissure. Angelini and colleagues[2] indicated that the number of sinuses and cusps that a valve has at its formation can be determined by identifying these intercusp triangles, found between each adjacent sinus.

Aortic valve cusps in most normal hearts vary both in height and width.[100,133] Vollebergh and Becker[133] from their study indicate that most are approximately 2.5 cm wide along their free margin and 14 mm high at their midpoint. In my experience, if a cusp is tensed when measured at the autopsy table, it is 15 to 22 mm high at its midpoint.

Normal aortic valve cusps are slightly redundant (the cross-sectional area of the aortic root is less than the sum of the areas of the cusps) and overlap in their closed position. Visible semilunar ridges 2 to 3 mm from a cusp's free edge and rising to meet the corpus arantius located at the cusp's midpoint are found on its ventricular surface. The ridges indicate the line of valve closure. In addition, normal commissures have a circumferential amplitude of approximately 120°.[2]

Anatomically, the aortic valve has one cusp placed anteriorly and two posteriorly. For convenience they are named for their relationship to the coronary artery ostia. Thus, a normal valve is said to have right and left cusps and a noncoronary cusp.

Schoen, in Chapter 41, presents details of the structural-functional relationships of aortic valve cusps. Thubrickar et al.[128] have compared the mechanical properties of aortic valve cusps both in vivo and in vitro. Important to the subsequent discussion of the congenitally bicuspid valve is that adjacent sides of normally formed cusps curve toward each other at the commissural region with their free margins eventually running a short, roughly parallel course before they insert into the commissural mound on the aortic wall. Adjacent cusps are separated by a very small distance at the site of insertion and, normally, the commissural mound extends no more than one-sixth of the distance between the aortic wall and the center of the aortic lumen.[134]

Chapters 23 and 27 give details of the immediate anatomic relationships of the aortic valve ring and sinuses of Valsalva (see Fig. 23–10); the schematic diagrams in the paper by Sud and colleagues[123] allow direct visualization of these relationships. Chapter 8 presents the anatomy of the ascending aorta.

CLINICAL AND PATHOLOGIC EFFECTS OF OBSTRUCTIONS RELATED TO THE AORTIC VALVE

The general effects of subvalvular, valvular, and supravalvular aortic stenoses are mentioned here; specific changes, induced by particular levels of stenosis, will be presented when they are discussed.

Symptoms Caused by These Obstructions

Clinically, the symptoms produced by subvalvular obstruction are also those of aortic valvular stenosis and supravalvular stenosis.

They include fatigue on exertion, dyspnea, effort syncope or light-headedness, angina pectoris, left ventricular failure, and an increased liability to sudden death. Each level of obstruction induces slight differences in associated clinical/investigative findings that permit differentiation among them.[6,28] In these analyses Doppler echocardiography is a valuable adjunct.[83,86]

Sudden Death

As Kulbertus reported,[62] sudden death accounts for about one-third of the mortality among patients with valvular aortic stenosis who have not been treated surgically. It occurs most often in those with a history of heart failure, but it may kill asymptomatic persons. The mechanism is obscure. Complex ventricular arrhythmias are much more prevalent in those with aortic stenosis than in control subjects. However, the frequency of these arrhythmias is significantly more common only in patients with aortic stenosis and normal coronary arteries. Patients with aortic stenosis and coronary artery disease experience complex ventricular arrhythmias as prevalently as persons without aortic stenosis. In their study, Olshausen et al.[84] found that the severity of arrhythmias was strongly influenced by myocardial performance. Thus, severe arrhythmias in these patients are frequently a sign of impaired left ventricular function.

The risk of sudden death in valvular aortic stenosis is not entirely prevented by valve replacement. Gohlke-Bärwolf and colleagues[34] reported a similar incidence of arrhythmias among 234 patients with isolated aortic stenosis treated by valve replacement who were studied both pre- and postoperatively. They observed sudden death uncommonly in this group (0–3 percent/year), it being responsible for 18 percent of late deaths. Those with subvalvular or supravalvular aortic stenosis are also prone to sudden death.

General Pathologic Effects

Obstruction of Sudden Onset

In an adult the sudden onset of severe obstruction at any level related to the aortic valve is very rare. It may be seen, for example, if there is rapid growth of a malignant tumor on the septal wall, in acute cardiac tamponade, or in conditions of prosthetic valve thrombosis. In these eventualities the left ventricle dilates.

Obstruction of Gradual Onset

Coronary Blood Flow in Aortic Stenosis

Factors that maintain coronary blood flow in the normal heart are interfered with in a patient with aortic stenosis.[7] For example, coronary flow is impaired by an elevated left ventricular end-diastolic pressure and a shortened diastole. In addition, the hypertrophied left ventricular muscle mass and elevated systolic pressure increase myocardial oxygen requirements.[6] As a result, the myocardium is prone to ischemia during diastole, and that makes the patient with aortic stenosis liable to syncope, ventricular arrhythmias, and sudden death; to focal myocardial necrosis; and to myocardial fibrosis, particularly in the subendocardial zone.

Myocardial Changes

Because these obstructions are commonly self-perpetuating and worsen gradually, they produce concentric left ventricular hypertrophy. Often, the hypertrophied ventricle can sustain a large pressure gradient across an obstruction without any reduction in cardiac output or the production of symptoms. Thus, in the natural history of aortic stenosis, especially valvular stenosis, there may be a long latent period with gradually worsening stenosis before symptoms occur. However, when they do appear the patient's prognosis is usually poor, unless the obstruction is relieved.[6]

In other words, symptoms in a patient with aortic stenosis are almost invariably associated with severe obstruction, but severe obstruction is not necessarily associated with symptoms.[6] Indeed, some cases of sudden death occurring in elderly patients and seen at autopsy show such severe valvular stenosis that one wonders how the patient functioned. Yet, the history subsequently obtained from family or friends, yields no story of apparent clinical dysfunction.

At autopsy the heart weight in an adult with such an obstruction is usually in the 600 to 800 g range, but it may weigh up to 1 kg. The left ventricular wall is thickened concentrically, and both papillary muscles and trabeculae carneae are brawny. As a result, the left ventricular chamber may seem small. Also, the hypertrophied septal wall often bulges into and encroaches on the right ventricular cavity. If the left ventricle fails, its wall, while still thickened, may be less obviously so because of chamber dilation. In such cases left atrial dilation, pulmonary congestion with or without edema, and right heart dilation and/ or hypertrophy may be obvious.

Ventricular hypertrophy associated with aortic stenosis increases diastolic stiffness. As a result, a greater intracavitary pressure is required for ventricular filling. Some patients with aortic stenosis develop "chamber" stiffness caused by an increased muscle mass, others have both increased "chamber" and "muscle" stiffness. Both types of stiffness may regress if an obstruction is relieved, but not all patients lose muscle stiffness. This may relate to the persistence of fibrosis in the ventricular myocardium.[6]

Histologically, left ventricular myocardial fibers are hypertrophied, there is often an increased amount of interstitial fibrous tissue, and, because perfusion of the subendocardium is reduced in the pressure-loaded left ventricle, foci of myocardial necrosis or fibrosis replacing muscle fibers may be seen in this zone. Among a group of 32 patients with isolated aortic stenosis whose hearts did not demonstrate coronary atherosclerosis at postmortem angiography, Hutchins et al.[47] found contraction band necrosis or focal fibrous tissue replacement in the subendocardial myocardium of 9 percent of their hearts. Contraction band necrosis results when periods of no myocardial perfusion are followed by reflow. In 13 hearts, subendomyofiber vacuolization was demonstrated. This lesion, the authors believe, results from ischemia not accounted for by coronary atherosclerosis. Hutchins et al.[47] used these morphologic findings as evidence that both an episodic and a sustained reduction of blood flow occur in the left ventricular subendocardium in the presence of aortic stenosis.

During the early days of corrective surgery, patients with aortic valvular stenosis and marked left ventricular hypertrophy were prone to both usual and unusual morphologic forms of myocardial necrosis. The latter, including "stone heart" and "circumferential hemorrhagic necrosis" are discussed in Chapter 40. Better methods of myocardial preservation during surgery mean that all these lesions are now encountered much less commonly.

Ultrastructurally, left ventricular myocardial cells may show features of hypertrophy alone or of hypertrophy with degenerative changes, the latter including fibrosis, cellular atrophy, cellular or myofibrillary disorganization, Z-band abnormalities, myofibrillar lysis, myelin figures, proliferation of the sarcoplasmic reticulum, lipid accumulation, spherical microparticles associated with plasma membranes, intramitochondrial glycogen, thickened external laminae, intracytoplasmic junctions and cellular isolation with partial dissociation, and a complete loss of intracellular connections.[53,74,117] The latter degenerative changes are not specific for the myocardial hypertrophy associated with left ventricular outflow tract obstruction but also occur in other forms of heart disease.[53]

Hemolysis and Dystrophic Calcification

Hemolysis and dystrophic calcification are discussed subsequently.

VALVULAR AORTIC STENOSIS

Obstruction to the outflow of blood from the left ventricle is most often caused by changes affecting the natural aortic valve itself. The changes may be congenital or acquired and induce clinical manifestations at any age. However, they do so most often in middle or later adult life.

Natural History

As indicated above, and regardless of how it is induced, valvular aortic stenosis is a self-sustaining and slowly progressive condition.

Among 142 patients with mild stenosis (aortic valve opening >1.5 cm^2) irrespective of its cause, Horstkotte and Loogen[43] found that clinical progression within 10 years of initial diagnosis occurred in 12 percent. Twenty-five years after diagnosis, the severity of aortic stenosis was clinically unchanged in 38 percent, whereas 25 percent had developed moderate stenosis and 38 percent had had the valve replaced. Progression of moderate stenosis (aortic opening area decreased to 1.5 to 0.8 cm^2) was more rapid, the average interval between manifestations of moderate stenosis and surgery was 13.4 years. Thirty-five patients with hemodynamically severe stenosis (aortic valve area 0.8 to 0.4 cm^2) who had refused surgery had a poor prognosis overall. The symptoms of angina pectoris, syncope, and congestive heart failure were indications of severe stenosis and usually occurred in that order. The mean survival after onset of angina pectoris was 45 ± 13 months; 27 ± 15 months after syncope, and 4 ± 10 months after congestive heart failure. The mean survival in the group averaged 23 ± 5 months, and the 5-year probability of survival was 18 ± 7 percent. All of these patients died within 12 months of observation.

Jonasson and colleagues[52] followed 26 patients with valvular aortic stenosis an average of 9 years. The valve area was 0.7 to 1.9 (mean 1.2) cm^2 at the first study and 0.3 to 2.0 (mean 0.9) cm^2 at the last. The mean annual decrease in valve area was about 0.1 cm^2 in 10 patients and less in the others. The authors agree that the rate of progression of valvular aortic stenosis in adults is usually slow, but moderate stenosis may become severe within a few years.

Roberts et al.,[104] in a clinical pathologic study, reported a man and a woman who, within 15 years, each developed severe aortic stenosis as a result of calcification developing in previously normal valves that had three cusps.

The risk of sudden death occurring in patients with valvular aortic stenosis is discussed above.

Mechanisms of Aortic Stenosis: Calcific Aortic Stenosis

As indicated in Chapter 24, acquired valvular stenosis may be initiated (1) by cusp stiffening, no matter whether it is caused by sclerosis, by the deposition of material (particularly of calcium) in the cusp parenchyma, or by combinations of these changes; (2) by fusion of adjacent sides of the cusps near the commissural area, that is, "commissural fusion," or (3) by a combination of these changes. Significant aortic stenosis has been defined, clinically, as a peak systolic pressure gradient greater than 50 mmHg and/or an aortic valve area index of less than 0.7 cm^2/m^2 body surface area.[115]

Irrespective of the mechanism initiating aortic valvular stenosis, with time further cusp sclerosis and dystrophic calcification occur as secondary phenomena. They may be associated with commissural fusion, which can be a cause or sequence of aortic stenosis. The extent of the secondary changes vary from patient to patient and with the cause of calcific aortic stenosis. As in mitral stenosis (see Ch. 24), the altered hemodynamics and other changes associated with aortic stenosis likely induce local endothelial or tissue injury. An adaptive/reparative response, which may involve thrombus deposition and/or calcification, follows, with these processes aggravating the original stenosis.[121] Ford et al.[25a] provide some evidence for a role for antiphospholipid antibodies promoting thrombosis in valvular deformity. Increasing dystrophic calcification is probably the result of degenerative changes in collagen (see later discussion). The end-product is a calcified, stenosed aortic valve.

Differential Diagnosis of the Causes of Calcific Aortic Stenosis

Because the functional effects of calcific aortic stenosis are relatively constant, a clinician may be satisfied with that diagnosis. However, calcific aortic stenosis, like a granular contracted kidney, has several different causes. A pathologist, studying such a diseased aortic valve in surgical pathology or at autopsy, is obliged to establish the underlying cause of the changes. A correct diagnosis can be made in the majority (>95 percent) of cases.[16,93,101,122] It may be difficult when morphologic changes are severe and is fraught with pitfalls even if they are less advanced. Nevertheless, diagnosis must be attempted if the natural history of each form of calcific aortic stenosis is to be better appreciated, treatment improved, and preventive measures instituted.

In attempting a differential diagnosis at autopsy, keep the valve intact and open the aorta from above to the upper level of the sinus of Valsalva; then examine the valve in detail. Careful study of surgically excised valves will allow a differential diagnosis, but fragmentation during excision may interfere with this. Subramanian et al.,[122] who studied 374 valves excised surgically from patients with pure aortic stenosis, found 20 percent in one piece, 46 percent in two, 20 percent in three pieces, and 14 percent in four or more pieces. The

fact that 86 percent of the aortic valves had been excised in three or fewer pieces facilitated the authors' ability to evaluate commissures for acquired or congenital fusion and to classify the valves confidentially on gross inspection alone. Classification as to cause in the remainder was aided by the surgeon's description of the valve. Unlike the authors, I have less faith in either a clinician's or surgeon's ability to distinguish the exact morphology or cause of a case of calcific aortic stenosis.

I agree with Roberts and Morrow[109] that a careful gross examination of a surgically excised valve will likely allow the diagnosis of all pathologic features. Histologic examination merely confirms them. If an excised valve shows no other abnormality grossly (e.g., attached vegetations), I often block sections but forgo histologic examination. In doing so, I risk missing the diagnosis of amyloidosis. It must be kept in mind that amyloid is found histologically, in some calcified, stenosed, aortic valve cusps.[12]

Calcific Aortic Stenosis and a Patient's Age

In Chapter 33, Datta reports 100 examples of isolated aortic stenosis found in Indian patients. He notes that fibrous sclerosis was seen in those over 30 years of age and calcification in patients older than 40. Fibrous sclerosis may cause aortic stenosis in Western countries and especially affects congenitally abnormal valves in the young, but, overall, calcific aortic stenosis is much more common in the West, even in the young. Its pathogenesis varies with a patient's age.[20,93,101,110]

There is overlap as to the cause of valvular aortic stenosis in different age groups. In general, calcific aortic stenosis seen in children, teenagers, and young adults (20 to 30 years) will likely be due to a congenital anomaly—either a unicuspid aortic valve or one with no obvious commissure (acommissural valve).

Roberts et al.[108] reported a case of calcific

aortic stenosis in a 28-year-old patient with homozygous type 2 hyperlipidemia, suggesting that a few cases of calcific aortic stenosis in the 20 to 40 age group may have this cause (see later discussion). It must be emphasized that with this exception and despite being able to demonstrate some lipid associated with fibrosis and calcium histologically in stenosed aortic valve cusps, atherosclerosis, per se, is *not* a cause of calcific aortic stenosis.[58]

More frequently, in the 35 to 55 age group and especially in women, rheumatic valvular disease induces aortic stenosis. If so, the aortic lesion is almost always combined with mitral rheumatic valvular disease.[101] Acquired bicuspidization of the aortic valve with stenosis may result from rheumatic disease but is uncommon (see Ch. 33).

Congenitally bicuspid aortic valves usually induce calcific aortic stenosis in patients 40 to 70 years old and are said to be the most common cause of isolated aortic stenosis in men 50 to 60 years old.[16,100] Datta (Ch. 33) recorded 52 cases of congenitally bicuspid valve among 100 East Indian patients with aortic stenosis.

Degenerative calcific changes (Monckeberg's calcification) affecting all three cusps are the likely cause of calcific aortic stenosis after that age.

Davies,[16] in his series of 187 surgically excised stenosed aortic valves, noted that the mean age of patients with stenosis caused by rheumatic disease was 52 years, 62 years for those with bicuspid valves, and 69 years for those with degenerative calcification. Comparable mean ages in the study of Subramanian et al.[122] were 60, 59, and 72 years, while the mean age of patients with unicommissural valves was 48 years. Of interest, in this context, is the clinical report of Horskotte and Loogen.[43] They found that the age of onset of clinical symptoms of aortic stenosis was 39 ± 18 years in patients with rheumatic aortic stenosis, 48 ± 6 years in those with a stenosed bicuspid valve, and 66 ± 12 years in those with degenerative calcification.

Pathologic Effects and Complications

The general pathologic effects of valvular aortic stenosis are described above. Specific effects are discussed here.

Poststenotic Dilation of the Ascending Aorta

Poststenotic dilation of the ascending aorta is a common finding in patients with valvular aortic stenosis. It is caused by a high-pressure jet of blood leaving the stenosed valve and dissipating its energy in the ascending aorta. Turbulence and the frequency of vibration produced by that turbulence are considered important factors that induce aortic dilation.[98] If the jet is localized it may, in rare instances, produce a focal aneurysm in the ascending aorta rather than a generalized poststenotic dilation. If so, the aneurysm wall may be at risk during sternotomy at open heart surgery and catastrophic hemorrhage may result. Also, a plaque of intimal thickening can develop on the vessel wall at the site of jet impaction, providing a locus for infection. The intima of the dilated or aneurysmal ascending aorta may be wrinkled and the vessel may be thin-walled. Histologically, its media shows focal elastic tissue degeneration and an increased accumulation of glycosaminoglycans. These changes are not unlike those found in the media of older persons or those with systemic hypertension.[9,117] If they are severe, fibrosis may replace the foci of destroyed elastic tissue in the media. The histologic changes also make the dilated ascending aorta prone to intimal tears and dissecting aneurysms, with these complications occurring either spontaneously,[31,40] during,[5] or following surgery. Larson and Edwards[63] recorded a much greater frequency of aortic dissection and rupture among patients with congenitally unicuspid or bicuspid valves, than among those with stenosed aortic valves with three cusps.

Coronary Artery Luminal Diameter and Atherosclerosis

Morphologically, the luminal diameter of coronary arteries seems greater in patients with aortic stenosis and a hypertrophied left ventricle. In an angiographic study, Abdalali and colleagues[1] compared coronary luminal diameter in 32 patients with aortic stenosis with those of 24 control subjects without left ventricular hypertrophy and found significantly larger coronary arteries in the former group ($P < 0.01$). The increased coronary luminal diameter had a weak correlation to left ventricular wall thickness ($r = 0.32$) and mass ($r = 0.34$).

An association between an aberrant origin of the coronary arteries and valvular aortic stenosis is rare. Northcote et al.[81] report a left coronary artery arising from the right sinus of Valsalva in a 73-year-old man with a calcified stenosed aortic valve.

Hudson[44,45] stressed the healthy state of coronary arteries found at autopsy in cases of calcific aortic stenosis. However, widespread use of preoperative coronary angiography indicates that patients with aortic stenosis may have coexistent severe coronary atherosclerosis.[37,39,73] As a result of this finding, aortocoronary bypass surgery is often done when a stenosed valve is excised. However, the value of a "near-routine" insertion of aortocoronary bypass grafts in patients with combined aortic stenosis and coronary artery disease is controversial.[60,70]

Gastrointestinal Hemorrhage

An arteriovenous malformation (also known as angiodysplasia) is a common cause of recurrent gastrointestinal bleeding in elderly patients. Following correspondence in the *New England Journal of Medicine* more than 30 years ago, many papers have been published linking valvular aortic stenosis, angiodysplasia, and gastrointestinal hemorrhage.[59,69,113,118] The incidence of aortic stenosis in patients with angiodysplasia is reported in the 10 to 60 percent range. Surgical alleviation of a patient's aortic stenosis seems to cure the gastrointestinal hemorrhage.[69,113]

Gilinsky and Giles[33] report bleeding that first developed in a patient with gastric antral vascular ectasia ("watermelon stomach")[50] 1 year after aortic valve replacement. The patient was anticoagulated and had a prothrombin time of 14.7 seconds (control 12.3 seconds). The authors[33] note that this uncommon form of vascular ectasia has not previously been associated with aortic stenosis. They were uncertain whether the association thought to exist between angiodysplasias, gastrointestinal bleeding, and aortic stenosis also applied to the "watermelon stomach" variety.

Mehta and colleagues[78] challenge the association between aortic stenosis and gastrointestinal hemorrhage. In their opinion it was established mainly on case reports or retrospective analyses. They noted that in most previous studies the diagnosis of aortic stenosis had been based on clinical examination. The authors re-examined the situation in 29 men with gastrointestinal angiodysplasia recorded by endoscopy and used two-dimensional and Doppler echocardiography to define the presence or absence of aortic stenosis. Among the 29 patients, 22 had ejection systolic murmurs, 18 had echocardiographic evidence of aortic sclerosis, but none had aortic stenosis as assessed by Doppler echocardiography. Although acknowledging some limitations in their study Mehta et al.[78] concluded that it did support an association between the vascular dysplasia and aortic sclerosis but not aortic stenosis. They suggest the need for a prospective trial before there is complete acceptance of this proposed association.

Infective Endocarditis

Infective endocarditis may develop on stenosed aortic valves.[18,107] However, the risk of infection is low. The disease is much more prevalent in patients with aortic incompetence.[107]

Calcific Nodules on Aortic Valves

Calcific nodules on aortic valves are discussed later in the chapter.

Congenital Anomalies That Cause or Lead to Aortic Stenosis

The Acommissural and Unicommissural Aortic Valve

Acomissural and unicommissural aortic valves both are congenitally anomalous valves that are frustrum-shaped. The acommissural valve has a domed appearance (like a volcanic cone) when viewed from the aortic aspect and no commissural attachments to the sinus wall (Fig. 26–1). In the unicommissural valve the cusp's free margin is attached to the sinus wall at one spot, usually at the site of one of the

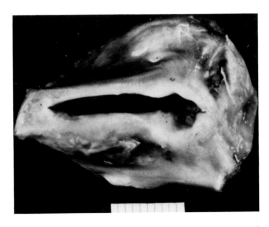

Fig. 26–2. Surgically excised congenital unicuspid aortic valve causing calcific aortic stenosis in a 22-year-old man. Note single commissure, orifice shape that suggests an exclamation mark, and raphes on right of photograph. (Scale indicates 1 cm.)

aortic commissures (anterior, posteromedial, or posterolateral). The free margin then extends toward the opposite sinus wall and, without forming any other commissures, returns to reattach to the sinus wall near the first attachment.[21] This gives the valve orifice an appearance resembling an exclamation mark (Fig. 26–2).[103]

Initial stenosis is likely to be greater with an acommissural valve, but both types cause a heart murmur, heard first in childhood. Usually, the symptoms produced by an acommissural valve cause death or require surgical intervention when cusp tissue is still supple and before it becomes calcified. However, if a lesion is palliated by a commissurotomy and the child reaches young adulthood, the tissue may calcify before the valve restenoses. If calcification develops in the so-treated acommissural valve or nontreated unicommissural valve, it may or may not be severe. In either anomaly, aborted commissures forming ridges of tissue (raphes) that pass from the sinus wall to the cusp may be seen in the depth of the sinus. In the adult, both forms of congenital anomaly are infrequent causes of calcific aortic stenosis, with unicommissural valves being somewhat more common than

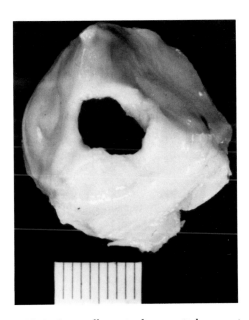

Fig. 26–1. Surgically excised congenital acommissural aortic valve from an 18-year-old woman with murmur of aortic stenosis since birth. Note the valve's domed-shaped, rounded orifice and ridges of aborted commissures. (Scale indicates 1 cm.)

acommissural ones. They formed 6 percent of cases studied by Subramanian et al.[122] Both unicuspid and bicuspid valves are more common in men than in women.

The Congenitally Bicuspid Aortic Valve

The bicuspid aortic valve (see also Ch. 27) also occurs with greater frequency in males than females (4 to 1). However, its true incidence is not known. This congenital anomaly, now considered the most frequent cause of isolated aortic stenosis in the 50- to 70-year old age group is, by conventional wisdom, thought to occur as an isolated phenomenon in approximately 2 percent of the population.[101] Practically, and for reasons to be discussed, its frequency may be greater or less than that. Certainly, that frequency is higher when the valvular anomaly is associated with certain congenital cardiovascular defects, for example, coarctation of the aorta.[125] Becker et al.[3] recorded the association in 46 of 100 infant cases. The bicuspid valve was the only accompanying congenital lesion in nine cases and was found together with other congenital anomalies in the remainder. On that point one may speculate that, in the future, diseased bicuspid aortic valves may be encountered more frequently clinically and at autopsy because the associated congenital heart anomalies are now corrected surgically, allowing the affected child to live and, possibly, to develop complications in the bicuspid valve. Therefore, this anomaly must be studied in detail to provide more succinct information about the natural history of the bicuspid valve.

An alternate viewpoint that could, on further study, reduce the number of "true" congenital bicuspid valves has been published.[2] In their review of the morphology of normal and bicuspid aortic valves and by defining a congenitally bicuspid valve as one having but two "interleaflet triangles," Angelini et al.[2] found only seven examples among 64 valves with two cusps. The authors accepted these seven as "true" bicuspid valves and suggest that the others started with three cusps (because they had three interleaflet triangles) and became bicuspid during intrauterine or postnatal life. Because these observations are new and need confirmation, subsequent discussion focuses on the morphologically bicuspid aortic valve in which the number of interleaflet triangles has not been defined.

Morphology

The cusps of a congenitally bicuspic aortic valve may be of equal size and have commissures opposite each other (180-degree circumferential amplitude between commissure). Such cusps may remain supple and function normally throughout a patient's life.

More often, however, the cusps are of unequal size. In this instance, the circumferential amplitude of the commissures is more than 180 degrees. This produces a larger "conjoint" cusp formed because commissural development did not occur or was aborted at one commissure. A bicuspid valve may have crescentic valve orifice (Fig. 26–3) or one shaped like the old sinuous logo of Northwest Airlines. Cusps of equal or unequal size are prone to complications.

The bicuspid valve may become incompetent through a number of mechanisms (see Ch. 27) or undergo cusp sclerosis and calcification and stenose with time. Fenoglio et al.,[23] from their study, estimated that approximately one-third of congenitally bicuspid valves cause no problems, one-third become incompetent and one-third stenose. Of the bicuspid valves I see in surgical pathology and at autopsy, stenosed ones are much more frequent than incompetent ones.

Theoretically, the commissures of a congenitally bicuspid aortic valve may be located anywhere around the circumference of the sinus part of the aorta. Practically, they may be located anteriorly and posteriorly, producing medial and lateral cusps (36 percent of the series of Angelini et al.[2]), or one is placed medially and one laterally with asso-

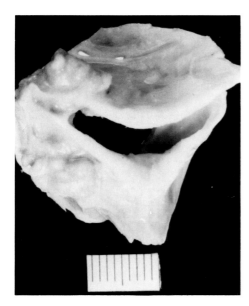

Fig. 26–3. Congenitally bicuspid valve causing calcific aortic stenosis in a 59-year-old man. Note similunar valve orifice and calcific masses in cusp substance. (Scale indicates 1 cm.)

ciated anterior and posterior cusps (64 percent of the series of Angelini et al.[2]). If the commissures are located anterioposteriorly, the right and left coronary arteries are likely to arise from each sinus; if commissures are located mediolaterally, both arteries arise from the anterior cusp.[101]

The height of a conjoint cusp is often least at its midregion, adjacent to a raphe, if one is present. If the cusp is supple, this deficiency in height may favor development of valve incompetence. Equally, this shortened zone may be stiffened either by attachment to the raphe or by secondary calcification in the raphe. Then, with some cusp redundancy or secondary changes of cusp eversion caused by valvular insufficiency, the valve assumes a gross appearance that I compare to an underwire brassiere that permits decolletage (Fig. 26–4A). Edwards discusses the incompetent bicuspid aortic valve in Chapter 27.

Unlike normal aortic valve cusps the larger conjoint cusp of a congenitally bicuspid aortic valve is often 3 to 3.5 cm wide. Indeed, its

large size, when seen in surgical pathology, may be a clue that one is dealing with this anomaly. Usually, the location of the aborted third commissure or raphe is obvious in the sinus of the conjoint cusp, but it is not always present. Davies found a raphe in 66 percent of the congenitally bicuspid valves he studied;[16] Subramanian et al. in 59 percent of their cases.[122]

The morphology of a raphe presents a spectrum of abnormal development. This is best appreciated if the raphe is thought to have height and length and to show a variable degree of differentiation at its upper or free margin. Thus, a raphe may extend a varying distance from the sinus wall toward the cusp (length), vary in its height related to the free edge of the cusp, and show partial separation of its free margin into cusp margins. Waller and colleagues[134] have emphasized these differences. Variations in the length and height of a raphe usually do not cause diagnostic difficulties for the clinician or pathologist because, in the majority of bicuspid valves, the upper margin of the raphe does not show any separation and presents a flattened if rounded surface that ends slightly short of the cusp's free margin.[85]

However, a raphe may reach the free margin of a conjoint cusp. Waller et al.,[134] who describe this condition as "pseudoacquired congenital bicuspid valve," observed it in 20 percent of the noncalcified bicuspid valves they studied. It is appreciated that such a high raphe, in a patient with calcific aortic stenosis, may provide diagnostic difficulties for both clinician and pathologist. Another diagnostic problem for pathologists arises when there is separation of the upper margin of a raphe into two cusp margins (Fig. 26-4A). The separation is usually partial and may be located near either the commissural ridge or a cusps' free margin. This finding has been called "bridging of cuspid tissue across insertion of a bicuspid ridge."[134] Complete separation along the length of the upper margin of a raphe is uncommon in my experience. Again, one has difficulty deciding if the fusion is congenital

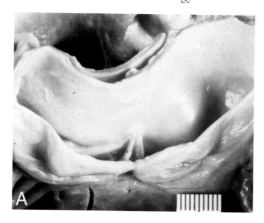
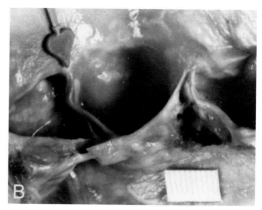

Fig. 26–4. (**A, B**) Partial separation of upper margin of raphe into cusp edges in two different congenitally bicuspid valves. Also note the variation in height of raphes. (Scale indicates 1 cm.)

or acquired. Distinction may be possible by examining the commissural region (see later discussion), but in a calcified valve this is often of no help. Nevertheless, I suspect that some congenitally bicuspid valves are regarded as acquired lesions and attributed to rheumatic valvular disease because they show these latter variations, which are not generally appreciated. If so, the frequency of congenitally bicuspid valves may be slightly higher than is currently thought.

Very rarely, and in another variant of maldevelopment seen with congenitally bicuspid valves, a strand of tissue that is rounded or oval in cross section and 1 mm in diameter or less, extends from the commissural mound to the free margin of the conjoint cusp in its midregion and at approximately that height (see Fig. 27–9). There is, in other words, a fenestration between this strand, the sinus side of the cusp, and the adjacent sinus wall, with this fenestration allowing free communication between adjacent parts of the conjoint cusp. The importance of the lesion is that the strand may rupture suddenly, allowing the conjoint cusp to prolapse and cause acute aortic incompetence (see Ch. 27). Roberts,[103] Waller and colleagues,[134] and Carter et al.[10] have described this lesion.

Histologically, Lewis and Grant[68] reported that a raphe consisted mainly of elastic tissue like the aortic media, whereas cusps fused as

a result of an inflammatory reaction consisted mainly of fibrous tissue. Other authors in the 1930s and 1940s confirmed these findings.[4,61] However, current opinion does not accept this histologic differentiation unequivocally because a raphe may or may not contain elastic tissue and because severe calcification may destroy the elastic tissue. Thus, in the adult, histologic section of commissural areas in calcific aortic stenosis may not help distinguish underlying pathology.

Calcification

With time, the uneven cusps of a congenitally bicuspid valve often develop dystrophic calcification, the process beginning in the raphe and then extending to the cusps themselves. It is demonstrable by echocardiography.[140] Aortic valves with three or four cusps may also calcify with increasing age,[89] either de novo or following rheumatic or other disease. The following comments apply to calcification occurring in them, too.

Schoen, in Chapter 41, discusses the mechanisms of calcification in bioprosthetic valves. He notes that the chemical composition and structural characteristics of such calcium deposits are very similar to those that occur in atherosclerotic plaques, in natural aortic valves, or on the membranes of mechanical blood pumps. As in a bioprosthetic valve cusp, the extent of calcification of natural heart valves varies from person to person.

The mechanism of calcification is obscure. A variation in cusp size, whether the valve is bicuspid or tricuspid and variation in hemodynamic forces experienced by the cusps may be important factors increasing "wear and tear" on cusp tissue.[19,123] Kim and colleagues,[58] studying aging changes in aortic valves in relation to dystrophic calcification, found that calcification appeared to result from cellular aging and death followed by petrification of cellular degeneration products. Presumably, calcification occurring in other conditions inducing calcific aortic stenosis also causes increased wear and tear in the tissue (see Ch. 5). In all instances the calcium is deposited initially in the zona fibrosa. With accumulation, the spongiosa is involved and the connective tissue surrounding the deposit becomes loosened and may show a chronic inflammatory cell reaction, that is, in rare instances, granulomatous. Lipid deposits are commonly related, but the calcific process is not thought to be atherosclerotic; Schoen[115] stresses this point. Bone and bone marrow metaplasia may develop in the calcium deposits.

A large calcium mass may ulcerate the surface of the cusp in which it develops (Fig. 26–5) or, through "kissing" trauma perforate an adjacent one, causing valve incompetence.[106] If such calcium masses are spontaneously excavated, they release calcium emboli into the bloodstream. Such emboli are uncommon but may cause strokes.[42,95,138] The subsequent formation and organization of bland thrombi related to such ulcers may raise suspicion of infective endocarditis on gross examination. Histologic examination with demonstration of microorganisms is required to prove that diagnosis. Calcium emboli may also be dislodged from calcified stenosed aortic valves during cardiac catheterization, balloon valvuloplasty,[15] or corrective surgery.

Calcification may also extend from the valve cusps into adjacent tissues. For example, a bar of calcium commonly extends 1 to 2 cm into the base of the anterior leaflet of the mitral

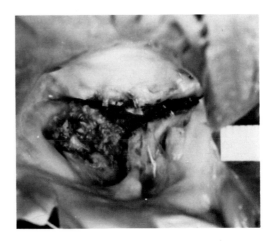

Fig. 26–5. Ventricular aspect of aortic valve with calcific stenosis following rheumatic valvular disease in a 55-year-old woman. Note ulcerated calcified mass on one of the cusps. (Scale indicates 6 mm.)

valve at its midpoint (Fig. 26–6). Michel et al.[78a] observed such calcium deposits in 32 percent of their 675 patients with aortic stenosis. In one it was so severe it caused mitral stenosis. Also, calcium can extend into the upper septal wall and damage or destroy conducting system tissue (either branches of the left bundle or the atrioventricular node itself), inducing arrhythmias or complete heart block. Mitral annular calcification is also associated with aortic stenosis.[78a]

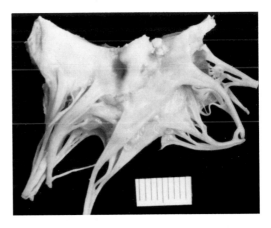

Fig. 26–6. Bar of calcium extending into anterior mitral valve leaflet in a 55-year-old woman with calcific aortic stenosis caused by rheumatic valvular disease. (Scale indicates 1 cm.)

Wong et al.[140] assert that general calcification is heaviest in congenital valves. One notes that renal dialysis[72] and Paget's disease are said to favor cusp calcification leading to aortic stenosis.

Thrombosis and Infection

The formation of bland thrombi on the cusps or on calcium masses and infective endocarditis are complications of the congenitally bicuspid valve. Both the thrombi and infected vegetations may be sources of emboli.

Hemolysis

If a valve is markedly stenosed, red cells are damaged in their passage through it, inducing hemolysis that is defined by renal hemosiderosis at autopsy.[99] See Chapter 40 for a discussion of the mechanism of hemolysis associated with artificial heart valves.

Dissecting Aneurysm

A dissecting aneurysm of the aorta is a complication that is found associated with the congenitally bicuspid aortic valve, whether or not the patient has an associated coarctation.[22]

Distribution of Coronary Arteries

The frequency of left coronary artery dominance is two to four times greater in the hearts of patients with congenitally bicuspid aortic valves.[49,51,66,116] Also, in such hearts, the left coronary ostium is twice as frequently located distal to the sinotubular junction, that is, in the proximal ascending aorta, than it is in normal hearts.[66]

Rheumatic Disease Causing Aortic Stenosis

Rheumatic valvular disease may affect a congenitally bicuspid aortic valve.[45,77] Much more often it damages a valve with three cusps. Isolated aortic rheumatic valvular disease occurs, being somewhat more common in tropical countries (see Ch. 33), but in the West isolated aortic stenosis attributable to this cause is uncommon. Rheumatic aortic stenosis is more often associated with mitral valvular disease.

The end result of repeated attacks of acute rheumatic fever directly, or of attacks associated with the passage of time, may be aortic valvular incompetence caused by sclerosis and shortening of the cusps (see Ch. 27), but, for this discussion, fusion of adjacent sides of the cusps in the commissural areas with or without cusp sclerosis is of greater importance. Commissural fusion is a major morphologic feature that helps distinguish this cause of aortic stenosis from others. Often it affects each commissural area equally, producing a triangular valve orifice (Fig. 26–7). In this circumstance and when viewed from the aortic aspect the orifice has the configuration of the filter of a "True" cigarette seen end-on. Rarely, fusion affects one commissure to a greater extent, inducing acquired bicuspidization. Damaged aortic cusps in rheumatic valvular disease thicken as a result of fibrosis but remain pliable for a long time. They and the commissural areas eventually calcify, aggravating the valvular stenosis. The calcification is, however, less marked than occurs in a stenosed bicuspid valve. In Western countries this process takes several decades to evolve. However, rheumatic aortic stenosis may progress much more rapidly in third-world countries. Then cusps are usually sclerosed and may not calcify (see Ch. 33).

If a valve is not heavily calcified it is possible to distinguish the margin of the two cusps joined by connective tissue if the commissural area is examined histologically. The cusps show sclerosis, collections of chronic inflammatory cells at their base, focal myxomatous change, and calcification and increased vascularization, the small vessels having thickened walls. All of these changes are nonspecific and nondiagnostic (see Ch. 24). In the West, Aschoff's nodules are rarely seen in such cusps.

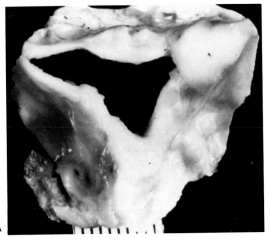 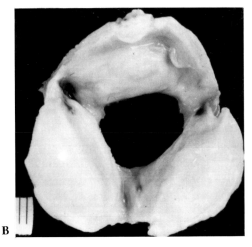

Fig. 26–7. (**A**) Aortic and (**B**) ventricular aspects of different surgically excised aortic valves with stenosis caused by rheumatic valvular disease. Note triangular orifice caused by commissural fusion. (Scale in Fig. A indicates 1 cm; in Fig. B, 3 mm.)

A discrepancy exists between the number of cases that have morphologic features of rheumatic heart disease and those who have a history of rheumatic fever. Less than one-half the cases give such a history. This raises the question of other nonrheumatic aortic diseases producing gross lesions indistinguishable from those caused by rheumatic valvular disease (see Ch. 24).

Degenerative Cusp Calcification Causing Aortic Stenosis (Mönckeberg's Calcification)

Pomerance discusses this topic in detail in Chapter 5. I reiterate that in this condition the dystrophic calcification affects valves with three cusps and that the nodular calcification is usually confined to the base and basal half of the cusps. It rarely affects the free margins (Fig. 26–8; see also Figs. 5–13 and 5–14). Also, commissural fusion is an unusual finding in this form of calcific aortic stenosis so that the valve orifice is triradiate. The condition is most common in patients over the age of 65 years and affects the sexes equally.

Rare Forms of Aortic Valvular Stenosis

Quadricuspid Aortic Valve

A quadricuspid valve is a congenital anomaly much less likely to affect an aortic valve than a pulmonary valve. Nevertheless, a quadricuspid aortic valve may become calcified[89] and stenosed.[46]

Aortic Stenosis Associated with Type II Hyperlipidemia

Young adults with aortic stenosis that is associated with type II hyperlipidemia develop marked lipid deposits in their aortic valve cusps. These, with associated dystrophic calcification, induce calcific aortic stenosis. The family history, associated clinical findings and marked deposits of atheromatous-like material in the cusps permit diagnosis.[57,108] The condition is uncommon. If the hyperlipidemia is controlled therapeutically, valvular stenosis may resolve (see also Ch. 29).

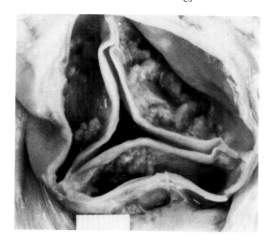

Fig. 26–8. Calcific aortic stenosis occurring in 77-year-old male and due to dystrophic calcification alone. Note triradiate valve orifice lack of commissural fusion and calcification confined to base of cusps. (Scale indicates 1 cm.)

Other Rare Causes of Aortic Valvular Stenosis

The large vegetations of active endocarditis[107] or of nonbacterial thrombotic endocarditis may cause a transient and acute aortic stenosis. Also, healed calcified vegetations of infective endocarditis induce aortic stenosis.[105]

Rheumatoid granulomata in the aortic annulus may encroach upon the valve lumen and cause aortic stenosis (see Ch. 30). Pritzker and colleagues[93a] reported aortic stenosis in two patients with systemic lupus erythematosus caused by massive thrombosis on the valves.

Patients with inborn errors of metabolism accumulate metabolic products in their hearts. The accumulations themselves or associated with calcium deposits may induce aortic stenosis by stiffening cusps. Figure 26–9 illustrates calcific aortic stenosis in a patient with Fabry's disease. The valvular disease also occurs in gout. Ochronosis may be complicated by aortic stenosis with or without commissural or cusp fusion. The relationship between ochronosis and the valvular lesions is uncertain[36,67] (see Ch. 29).

As indicated previously, renal dialysis and Paget's disease of bone are said to favor development of aortic stenosis.

Calcific Aortic Stenosis and the "Porcelain" Aorta

Coselli and Crawford[13] discuss replacement of a stenosed calcified aortic valve in elderly patients who have concomitant severe and extensive calcification of the ascending aorta, the so-called porcelain aorta. Calcification of the vessel is so extensive, in this rare situation, that the ascending aorta presents as a rigid tube with its tubular shape maintained by either a solid calcified plate or a lattice of calcification within the medial wall. If the aorta is clamped in the usual manner during valve replacement, cerebral embolism of aortic debris, aortic wall laceration, or aortic dissection may result from or at the point of cross clamping. The authors imply that the severe calcification is a complication of atherosclerotic disease in the ascending aorta. Such severe calcification also occurs in syphilis.

In contrast McLoughlin et al.[76] described clinical and radiologic findings in two young women who had extensive dystrophic calcification of the ascending aorta and aortic valve without dilation of the aorta. The cause of this

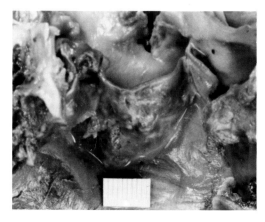

Fig. 26–9. Calcific aortic stenosis in a patient with Fabry's disease. (Scale indicates 1 cm.) (Specimen courtesy of G.W. Mackenzie, M.D. and F.W. Woods, M.D., Victoria, British Columbia.)

rare condition is not known. Further investigation in the patient who survived revealed other features, compatible with Singleton-Merten syndrome.[120] Theman and colleagues[127] studied the morphology in the cases who died. They found that a varying width of media throughout the aorta and extending into its proximal branches was devoid of nuclei (medionecrosis), although elastic lamellae were present. Plaques of calcium found in the acellular media were confined to the ascending aorta. Electron microscopically the calcium seemed to have an affinity for elastic tissue elements of all sizes. The mode of deposition appeared to be by "avenues" of the microfibrillar component. The cause of the medionecrosis was not established.

Rose and Forman[111] described another case in a 24-year-old woman who had, in addition, calcification of the mitral valve. The authors related the findings to an idiopathic aortitis.

The pathogenic relationship, if any, between these different cases is uncertain, as is the relationship between valvular and aortic lesions. What is certain is that in rare instances calcific aortic stenosis may be associated with severe calcification in the ascending aorta.

Aortic Stenosis Caused by Artificial Heart Valves

All artificial heart valves produce some degree of stenosis when inserted,[126] the transvalvular gradient being greater with some models and with smaller sizes. Stenosis may be aggravated with time if a prosthesis is inserted into a growing child. Prosthetic valves also become stenosed if thrombus, pannus, or infected vegetations encroach on their lumen. Indeed, a problem in many older models of mechanical valves is the gradual accumulation of pannus that encroaches on the in-flow orifice (see Ch. 40).

The cusps of all tissue valves presently in use calcify and stiffen as the period following insertion lengthens. This induces valvular stenosis (see Ch. 41).

SUBVALVULAR AORTIC STENOSIS

Theoretically, an excess or redundancy of any of the structures forming the boundaries of the outflow tract of the left ventricle or their congenital malposition may cause them to encroach on the tract and induce subvalvular obstruction.[20,21,27,29,64,71,119,131,141] In the young, fixed subaortic stenosis is commonly associated with other congenital cardiac anomalies. In the adult, an excess of "endocardium" or myocardium cause most cases.

Perloff[91] classifies subvalvular stenosis among the uncommon postpediatric congenital heart diseases in which adult survival is exceptional. In the adult, subvalvular aortic stenosis is far less common than valvular stenosis but is more frequent than supravalvular stenosis. A pathologist is likely to encounter cases of subvalvular stenosis in teenagers and young adults as a clinically unsuspected cause of sudden death (see Ch. 21) or to review fragments of tissue in surgical pathology excised to alleviate the obstruction. Rarely, adults with the condition are encountered at autopsy. Like subvalvular stenosis related to the pulmonary valve (see Ch. 24), isolated aortic subvalvular obstruction is most often membranous (fibrous) or muscular. Also, the lesion causing the obstruction may be discrete or affect a longer segment of the outflow tract.

Discrete Membranous Subvalvular Stenosis

Discrete membranous subvalvular stenosis (DMSS) accounts for 8 to 10 percent of all cases of congenital aortic stenosis and affects males twice as frequently as females. Several authors[38,54,91] have drawn attention to its rarity among older patients despite its relative frequency among children with congenital left ventricular outflow tract obstruction. The

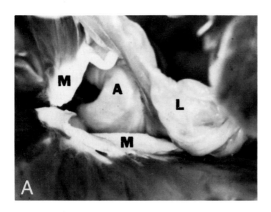
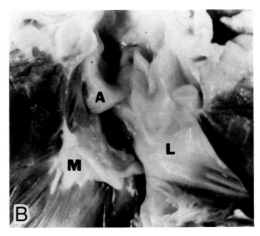

Fig. 26–10. Membranous subaortic stenosis found at autopsy following sudden death of a 16-year-old male at an ice hockey game. **(A)** View up outflow tract of left ventricle towards aortic valve (A) showing membrane (M) obstructing tract. **(B)** Opened outflow tract revealing membranous obstruction in more detail. In this instance the membrane did not extend across the anterior mitral valve leaflet (L) but note extension towards base of aortic cusp. Note that the distal ventricular aspect of the anterior mitral leaflet is normal in this condition. (Specimen courtesy of J. Ferris, M.D., Hamilton, Ontario.)

authors[54,91] could not account for this difference. They did not favor early death, either in or out of hospital, as the explanation. However, most cases I have seen at autopsy occurred suddenly, in athletic male teenagers. Possibly, such deaths are handled by coroners rather than by hospital pathologists. If so, this would favor early death as a cause of the apparent discrepancy observed clinically. Alternatively, the features of DMSS may change with age so that it overlaps with hypertrophic cardiomyopathy. Indeed, left ventricular obstructive lesions are found among 10 percent of relatives of patients with DMSS.[54]

Morphology

In DMSS[11,20,21,97,101–104,124,141] tough, gray-white fibroelastic tissue obstructs the outflow tract of the left ventricle in an area 1 to 2 cm proximal to the aortic valve cusps and in the plane of the annulus fibrosis of the mitral valve (Fig. 26–10). The tissue varies in width (2 to 4 mm) and is most obvious on the membranous intraventricular septum; it may form a discrete band, an accumulation of several bands, or, most commonly in the adult, a diffuse ridge. That on the septal wall sometimes extends toward the right aortic valve cusp (Fig. 26–10B). The membranous obstruction may be crescentic, extending across the anterior part of the left ventricular outflow tract with its ends inserting into the ventricular aspect of the base of the anterior mitral valve leaflet or, more commonly and in the adult, extend onto the base of the anterior mitral valve leaflet to form a distinct circumferential collar. These lesions can be missed if not thought of. One gains a better impression of the stenosis they cause by reconstructing the outflow tract, if it has been opened at autopsy and sighting along the tract toward the aortic valve. It is emphasized that the distal ventricular surface of the anterior mitral leaflet is usually normal in DMSS and not thickened as it is in hypertrophic cardiomyopathy accompanied by systolic anterior movement of the anterior leaflet. Also, in DMSS the outflow tract of the left ventricle does not appear narrowed, except at the site of the membrane.

Usually, the aortic annulus is of normal size and the aortic valve has three cusps. They may be normal, delicate, and competent. If the high-pressure jet of blood passing through the membranous subvalvular obstruction impinges on them, however, it often thickens them on their ventricular surface and they become distorted, leading to aortic incompetence. Again, these changes can be compared with those found in hypertrophic cardiomyopathy, where aortic valve cusps usually are normal (see Ch. 20). Damaged aortic cusps in DMSS are prone to infective endocarditis. Roberts[103] has indicated that, if aortic valve cusps are destroyed by infective endocarditis in a patient with DMSS, the heart is somewhat protected from the severe effects of the resultant valvular incompetence by the subaortic stenosis. Also, the aortic valve cusps may calcify, but this is not common.

In general, subvalvular obstructions do not cause poststenotic dilation of the aorta, but there may be dilation in the area between membrane and aortic valve cusps.

Histology

Ferrans and colleagues[25] described five distinct layers in surgically excised discrete subaortic fibrous rings examined histologically and ultrastructurally: an endothelial cell layer, a subendothelial layer rich in acid mucopolysaccharides, a fibroelastic layer, a layer of smooth muscle cells, and a central layer of densely packed collagenous tissue. The layers varied in width and in some specimens were discontinuous. The excised tissue was completely avascular. Thus, the rings had a structure comparable to that of endocardium of the outflow tract of the left ventricle and, in the authors'[25] opinion, represented a large fold of endocardium that projected into the lumen of the outflow tract. At present, it is uncertain if the fibrous tissue lining the endocardium in patients with tunnel-type subaortic stenosis has a similar structure. That found in the DMSS of the Newfoundland dog is different; it contains chondrocyte-like cells.[94] Studies

also indicate that the endocardial plaques in carcinoid disease have no elastic tissue in them.[24] Thus, endocardial plaques do not all have the same histologic structure.

Small intramyocardial vessels may show changes in DMSS.[79] They include intimal fibrous tissue proliferation, medial muscle hypertrophy and muscle cell disorganization. The changes are like those described in intramyocardial vessels in hypertrophic cardiomyopathy (see Ch. 20). They induce ischemic damage.

Pathogenesis

The cause of DMSS is not known. Theories range from a failure of resorption of the bulbus cordis[55] to malformation of the proximal extremity of the truncus septum where it joins the conus septum[129] or a malformation of the atrioventricular cushion surrounding the subaortic left ventricular outlet.[130] The condition occurs in animals and has been particularly studied in the Newfoundland dog.[94]

In that animal, a range of lesions, varying from a discrete membrane to a segmental stenosis may be found causing subvalvular stenosis. Pyle and colleagues[94] believe that the discrete lesions represent a persistence of embryonal tissue in the left ventricular outflow tract and that such tissue is capable of proliferating after birth. The process in dogs seems controlled by a specific polygenic system or a major gene with modifiers. The affected dog is prone to infective endocarditis on the aortic valve beyond the obstruction and shows changes in intramyocardial coronary arteries like those described in humans with DMSS.[79]

Many authors[8,38,56,97,141] have provided clinical/anatomic classifications of the lesions seen in discrete subaortic stenosis. The observations in Newfoundland dogs[94] taken with these classifications suggest a range of subvalvular stenotic lesions. DMSS may be at one end of the range, and "tunnel" subaortic stenosis, a much less common condition, at the other. In the latter condition the outflow tract of the left ventricle is markedly narrowed in an area extending 1 to 3 cm proximal to the aortic annulus. This long stenosed segment is associated with a marked thickening of the myocardium of the outflow tract and has on its luminal surface a thick layer of fibrous tissue that invariably extends onto the anterior leaflet of the mitral valve. The aortic valve cusps are thickened, and the valve annulus may be small. Histologically, the myocardium is hypertrophied, shows an orderly arrangement of muscle fibers, and may show focal scarring. Abnormalities of intramyocardial coronary arteries also occur in this condition.[75] Its separation as an entity is important because of the difficulties in medical and surgical management.

Treatment

Surgical treatment with or without a need to replace aortic or mitral valve is the usual mode of therapy. Restenosis may occur after surgery.[8]

Muscular Subaortic Stenosis

Morphology

Normally, the distal third of the septal wall, as it forms a boundary of the outflow tract of the left ventricle, appears either flat or bulges convexly and very slightly into the left ventricular cavity. The muscle bulge may be accentuated in the very young or the elderly to produce the so-called sigmoid septum[35] (see Chs. 1 and 20). The sigmoid septum is found in hearts of normal weight and does not usually cause muscular subaortic stenosis. However, in 4 of 22 hearts with this condition examined by Goor and colleagues,[35] friction lesions were found on adjacent sides of the anterior mitral valve and the septal endocardium, producing endocardial thickenings coincident in nature and location with those found in hypertrophic cardiomyopathy. Histologically, the myocardium of the sigmoid septum is normal and does not show the bizarre arrangement of fibers and fascicles seen in hypertrophic cardiomyopathy.

On gross examination, the left ventricular myocardium in muscular subaortic stenosis is usually hypertrophied; in hypertrophic cardiomyopathy that hypertrophy may be marked. Whatever the cause of the subaortic stenosis, the septal wall usually bulges asymmetrically and prominently into the ventricular outflow tract and narrows it. This change is found most frequently in its distal, subvalvular third, but sometimes occurs in the midventricular region or a "tunnel" outflow tract is obvious. Usually, the aortic annulus and valve cusps are normal and muscular subaortic stenosis does not induce poststenotic dilation of the aorta. If there is associated systolic anterior movement of the anterior mitral valve leaflet, mirror-image plaques of endocardial thickening may develop on the ventricular aspect of the leaflet, its associated chordae tendineae, and the apices of the anterior left ventricular papillary muscle posteriorly and on the septal wall anteriorly.

Histology

Histologically, in muscular subaortic stenosis, myocardial fibers may have the usual morphologic pattern of hypertrophied myocardium and may or may not show intracytoplasmic inclusions, depending on the cause of the obstruction. Panza and Maron[88] discuss the 10 percent of patients who have significant valvular aortic stenosis and show asymmetric thickening of the left ventricle, clinically. The authors emphasize that the ventricular septum and free left ventricular wall of such hearts rarely, if ever, have the histologic appearance of hypertrophic cardiomyopathy. In the latter condition the myofibers demonstrate a bizarre architectural arrangement. This and other conditions causing muscular subaortic stenosis are discussed in Chapter 20. Histology may also reveal other pathology causing the subvalvular "muscular" stenosis, for example, rhabdomyoma[17] or other cardiac tumor.

Etiology

Muscular subaortic stenosis may be congenital or acquired. If acquired, it may occur as part of a disease process involving the myocardium locally or diffusely (see also Ch. 29). Alternatively, muscular subaortic stenosis may be a functional response of the left ventricle (see previous discussion).

Treatment

Treatment of these conditions may be medial or surgical.

Heart Valve Prostheses and Subvalvular Aortic Stenosis

Subvalvular stenosis results if fresh or infected vegetations, or organized thrombus (pannus) extends across a valve's ostium from the sewing ring.

An angled or normally inserted mitral valve prosthesis can cause left ventricular outflow obstruction. This uncommon complication is more likely with a prosthesis of high profile but has also been reported with those of low profile.[14]

SUPRAVALVULAR AORTIC STENOSIS

Stenosis of the ascending aorta, or supravalvular aortic stenosis,[20,44,45,80,87,90,92,101] is the least common form of blood flow obstruction observed in relation to the aortic valve. A lesion may be congenital or acquired and either discrete and localized or diffuse and it affect a tubular segment of the ascending aorta.

Congenital Forms of Supravalvular Aortic Stenosis

Morphology

Three morphologic forms have been described in children with supravalvular aortic stenosis.[92] They are (1) an hourglass narrowing associated with severe thickening of the aortic media and often associated with superimposed fibromuscular intimal thickening, (2) a fibrous membrane that presents as a diaphragm, with a central or eccentric opening, stretching across the vessel lumen, usually in an aorta of normal size, and (3) a hypoplastic form of supravalvular stenosis characterized by a diffuse or tubular hypoplasia of the ascending aorta. These supravalvular obstructions are located at, or begin in, the ascending aorta immediately distal to the sinus of Valsalva. Presumably, the elastic tissue band described crossing the aortic lumen immediately distal to the aortic valve cusps in a stillborn boy[129] is part of the spectrum of supravalvular aortic stenosis.

In supravalvular aortic stenosis, the coronary arteries are subject to a systolic hypertension and are perfused, in the main, during systole.[80] As a result, they are often of large bore and tortuous, show intimal thickening, and are prone to premature atherosclerosis. Indeed, the severity of clinical disease in adults often correlates better with abnormalities of the coronary arteries than with the severity of the supravalvular obstruction, although both may be significant.[87] Usually the aortic valve has three cusps; these may become sclerosed and incompetent. Also, the free margin of an aortic valve cusp may adhere to the tissue producing the obstruction. In some instances when this occurs, the associated sinus and any coronary artery arising from it may be completely isolated from the aortic lumen. Isolation of the coronary artery increases the risk of ischemic heart disease. The aortic sinuses are usually not dilated in supravalvular aortic stenosis, nor is poststenotic dilation common. Indeed, the aorta beyond a localized obstruction may be relatively hypoplastic.

Histology

O'Connor and colleagues[82] described the histologic evidence from six patients aged $1\frac{1}{2}$ to 12 years. Three had Williams syndrome and two had familial supra-aortic stenosis. Four had an hourglass deformity, one a diffuse stenosis, and the sixth had a membranous deformity. Tissue was recovered from four at surgery and from two at autopsy.

Microscopically, disorganized medial elements with a fibrotic intima were found in five cases, the other had valvelike tissue only. Ultrastructurally, thick irregular elastic fibers, abundant swirling collagen, hypertrophied smooth muscle cells, and scant ground substance characterized the medial tissue changes.

The authors[82] suggest that hemodynamics during intrauterine development might predispose to the localization of the stenosis to the supravalvular region. The cause of the mural dysplasia is uncertain.

Pathogenesis

Supravalvular aortic stenosis may be inherited as an autosomal dominant with variable penetrance, or occur sporadically. They are more common in males than females (4:1).

Supravalvular aortic stenosis may be part of the so-called hypercalcemic[32,96] or Williams[139] syndrome. In newborn rabbits, the syndrome seems related to hypervitaminosis D in the pregnant doe[30]; in affected humans, it seems associated with an abnormal calcium metabolism.[26] It is of interest, although of uncertain significance, that Hutchins et al.[48] described hyperplasia of the parafollicular (C) cells in the thyroid of a 30-year-old man with an hourglass-type supravalvular aortic stenosis and the hypercalcemic syndrome. In Williams syndrome the affected person may have a characteristic facies, mental retardation, stenosis of peripheral and pulmonary arteries, an inguinal hernia, strabismus, and abnormalities of dental development. In some patients pulmonary valvular stenosis may be associated with stenosis of peripheral pulmonary arteries. Rarely, mitral valve prolapse and mitral insufficiency are complications.

Supravalvular aortic stenosis may also be part of the congenital rubella syndrome.[132]

Clinical Features

As with other forms of left ventricular outflow tract obstruction, usual presenting symptoms are angina pectoris, congestive heart failure, and a heart murmur; once developed, these symptoms usually indicate a poor prognosis. Sudden death also occurs.[31]

Children with severe hypoplasia of the aorta do not survive to adulthood. However, aortas of small bore (5 cm in circumference or less) are found, occasionally, in cases of sudden death in athletic teenagers.[65] In these cases, the coronary vessels are normal and the left ventricle may or may not be hypertrophied. Having seen four such cases, I am tempted to assume that the anatomic finding produces the equivalent of a supravalvular aortic stenosis and causes the sudden death. It may, but the association is not proven. Certainly, such small-bore aortas cause difficulties during the surgical correction of aortic valvular disease.

Congenital supraaortic stenosis is uncommon in adults.[87,90] In a group of 26 cases studied by Pansegrau et al.,[87] all were 16 years or older and each patient had an hourglass type of deformity. Most did not have evidence of the hypercalcemic syndrome, and only five had abnormal facies, mental retardation, or both. Of these five patients, three had the hypercalcemic syndrome, one Marfan syndrome, and one the congenital rubella syndrome. Nineteen patients had the sporadic form of the disease and two the familial form.

Acquired Supravalvular Aortic Stenosis

Acquired supravalvular aortic stenosis is an extremely rare condition. The only examples I have seen have been caused by cardiac surgery. Angulation of a heart valve prothesis or disproportion may induce symptoms of a supravalvular stenosis. Also, healing of an aortotomy wound may cause this problem,[101] as may kinking, stenosis, or obstruction of a vascular graft in the ascending aorta.

Patients with homozygous type II hyperlipoproteinemia develop severe atherosclerosis in the ascending aorta. This may cause a supravalvular stenosis.[137]

"Porcelain" Aorta

See previous discussion of "porcelain" aorta.

REFERENCES

1. Abdalali SA, Baliga G, Clayden AD, Smith DR: Coronary artery luminal diameter in aortic stenosis. Am J Cardiol 55:460, 1985
2. Angelini A, Ho SY, Anderson RH, et al: The morphology of the normal aortic valve as compared with the aortic valve having two leaflets. J Thorac Cardiovasc Surg 98:362, 1989
3. Becker AE, Becker MJ, Edwards JE: Anomalies associated with coarctation of the aorta: Particular reference to infancy. Circulation 41:1067, 1970
4. Bishop LF, Jr., Truber M: Bicuspid aortic valve: A differential study between inflammatory and congenital origin. J Tech Mech 15:111, 1936
5. Black LL, McComb J, Silver MD: Vascular injury following heart valve replacement. Ann Thorac Surg 16:19, 1973
6. Braunwald E: Valvular heart disease. p. 1023. In Braunwald E (ed): Heart Disease. 3rd Ed. WB Saunders, Philadelphia, 1988
7. Braunwald E, Sobel BE: Coronary blood flow and myocardial ischemia. p. 1191. In Braunwald E (ed): Heart Disease. 3rd Ed. WB Saunders, Philadelphia, 1988
8. Cabrera A, Galdeano JM, Zumalde J, et al: Fixed subaortic stenosis: The value of cross-sectional echocardiography in evaluating different anatomical patterns. J Cardiol 24:151, 1989
9. Carlson RG, Lillehei CW, Edwards JE: Cystic medial necrosis of the ascending aorta in relation to age and hypertension. Am J Cardiol 25:411, 1970
10. Carter JB, Sethi S, Lee GB, Edwards JE: Prolapse of semilunar cusps as causes of aortic insufficiency. Circulation 43:922, 1971
11. Chevers N: Observations on diseases of the orifice and valves of the aorta. Guys Hosp Rep 7:387, 1842
12. Cooper JH: Isolated dystrophic amyloidosis of heart valves. Hum Pathol 14:649, 1983
13. Coselli JS, Crawford ED: Aortic valve replacement in the patient with extensive calcification of the ascending aorta (porcelain aorta). J Thorac Cardiovasc Surg 91:184, 1986
14. Currie PJ, Seward JB, Lam JB, et al: Left ventricular outflow tract obstruction related to a valve prosthesis: Case caused by a low-profile mitral prosthesis. Mayo Clin Proc 60:184, 1985
15. Davidson CJ, Skeleton TN, Kisslo KB, et al: The risk of systemic embolization associated with percutaneous balloon valvuloplasty in adults. Ann Intern Med 108:557, 1988
16. Davies MJ: Pathology of cardiac valves. p. 18. In Crawford T (ed): Postgraduate Pathology Series, 1980
17. De Deominicis E, Frigiola A, Thieme G, et al: Subaortic stenosis by solitary rhabdomyoma. Chest 95:470, 19
18. Delahaye JJ, Loire R, Milon H, et al: Infective endocarditis in stenotic aortic valves. Eur J Cardiol 9(suppl E):43, 1988
19. Edwards JE: Editorial: The congenital bicuspid aortic bicuspid aortic valve. Circulation 23:485, 1961
20. Edwards JE: Pathology of left ventricular outflow obstruction. Circulation 31:586, 1965
21. Edwards JE, Carey LS, Neufeld HN, Lester RG: Congenital Heart Disease, Vol. 2, WB Saunders, Philadelphia, 1965, p. 723
22. Edwards WD, Leaf DS, Edwards JE: Dissecting aortic aneurysm associated with congenital bicuspid aortic valve. Circulation 57:1022, 1978

23. Fenoglio JJ, Jr, McAllister HA, Jr, DeCastro CM, et al: Congenital bicuspid aortic valve after age 20. Am J Cardiol 39:164, 1977

24. Ferrans VJ, Roberts WC: The carcinoid endocardial plaque: an ultrastructural study. Hum Pathol 7:387, 1976

25. Ferrans VJ, Muna WFT, Jones M, Roberts WC: (1978) Ultrastructure of the fibrous ring in patients with discrete subaortic stenosis. Lab Invest 39:30, 1978

25a. Ford S, Charrette F, Knight J, et al: A possible role for antiphospholipid antibodies in acquired cardiac valve deformity. J Rheumatol (in press)

26. Forbes GB, Bryson MF, Manning J, et al: Impaired calcium homostasis in the infantile hypercalcemic syndrome. Acta Paediat Scand 61:305, 1972

27. Freedom RM, Dische MR, Rowe RD: Pathologic anatomy of subaortic stenosis and atresia in the first year of life. Am J Cardiol 39:1035, 1977

28. Friedman WF: Congenital heart disease in infancy and childhood. p. 967. In Braunwald E (ed): Heart Disease. WB Saunders, Philadelphia, 1980

29. Friedman WF, Kirkpatrick SE: Congenital aortic stenosis. p. 178. In Moss AJ, Adams FH, Emmanouilides GC (eds): Heart Disease in Infants, Children and Adolescents. 2nd ed. Williams & Wilkins, Baltimore, 1977

30. Friedman WF, Roberts WC: Vitamin D and the supravalvular aortic stenosis syndrome. The transplacental effects of vitamin D on the aorta of the rabbit. Circulation 34:77, 1966

31. Fukada T, Tadavarthy SM, Edwards, JE: Dissecting aneurysm of aorta complicating aortic valvular stenosis. Circulation 53:169, 1976

32. Garcia RE, Friedman WF, Kaback MM, Rowe RD: Idiopathic hypercalcemia and supravalvular aortic stenosis. Documentation of a new syndrome. New Engl J Med 271:117, 1964

33. Gilinsky NH, Giles OA: Gastric antral vascular ectasia ("watermelon stomach"): First bleeding after aortic valve replacement J Clin Gastroenterology 9:612, 1987

34. Gohlke-Bärwolf CH, Peters K, Petersen J, et al: Influence of aortic valve replacement on sudden death in patients with pure aortic stenosis. Eur Heart J 9(suppl E):139, 1988

35. Goor DA, Lillehei CW, Edwards JE: The "sigmoid septum." Variation in the contour of the left ventricular outlet. Am J Roentgen 107:366, 1969

36. Gould L, Reddy CVR, DePalma D, et al: Cardiac manifestations of ochronosis. J Thorac Cardiovasc Surg 72:788, 1976

37. Graboys TB, Cohn PF: The prevalence of angina pectoris and abnormal coronary arteriograms in severe aortic valvular disease. Am Heart J 93:683, 1977

38. Greenspan AM, Morganroth J, Perloff JK: Discrete fibromembranous aortic stenosis in middle age. Natural history and case report. Cardiology 64:306, 1979

39. Hancock EW: Aortic stenosis, angina pectoris and coronary artery disease. Am Heart J 93:382, 1977

40. Heath D, Edwards JE, Smith LA: The rheologic significance of medial necrosis and dissecting aneurysm of the ascending aorta in association with calcific aortic stenosis. Mayo Clin Proc 33:228, 1958

41. Heyde EC: Gastrointestinal bleeding in aortic stenosis (letter to the editor). N Engl J Med 259:196, 1958

42. Holley KE, Bahn RC, McGoon DC, Mankin HT: Spontaneous calcific embolization associated with calcific aortic stenosis. Circulation 27:197, 1963

43. Horstkotte D, Loogen F: The natural history of aortic valve stenosis. Eur Heart J 9(suppl E):57, 1988

44. Hudson REB: Cardiovascular Pathology. Vol. 1. Edward Arnold (Publishers), London, 1965, p. 1037

45. Hudson REB: Cardiovascular Pathology, Vol. 3. Edward Arnold (Publishers), London, 1970, p. 581

46. Hurwitz LE, Roberts WC: Quadricuspid semilunar valve. Am J Cardiol 31:623, 1973

47. Hutchins GM, Kuhajda FP, Moore GM: Myocardial injury in patients with aortic stenosis. Am J Cardiovasc Pathol 1:31, 1986

48. Hutchins GM, Mirvis SE, Mendelsohn G, Bulkley BH: Supravalvular aortic stenosis with parafollicular cell (C-cell) hyperplasia. Am J Med 64:967, 1978

49. Hutchins GM, Nazarian IH, Bulkley BH: Association of left dominant coronary arterial system with congenital bicuspid aortic valve. Am J Cardiol 42:57, 1978

50. Jabari M, Cherry R, Zough ZO, et al: Gastric

antral vascular ectasia: the watermelon stomach. Gastroenterology 87:1165, 1984

51. Johnson AD, Detwiler JH, Higgins CB: Left coronary artery anatomy in patients with bicuspid aortic valves. Br Heart J 40:489, 1978

52. Jonasson R, Jonsson B, Nolander R, et al: Rate of progression or severity of valvular aortic stenosis. Acta Med Scand 213:51, 1983

53. Jones M, Ferrans VJ: Myocardial ultrastructure in children and adults with congenital heart disease. Cardiovasc Clin 10:501, 1979

54. Katz NM, Buckley MJ, Liberthson RR: Discrete membranous subaortic stenosis. Report of 31 patients, review of the literature and delineation of management. Circulation 56:1034, 1977

55. Keith A: Malformations of the heart. Lancet 2:359, 1909

56. Kelly DT, Wulfsberg E, Rowe RD: Discrete suboartic stenosis. Circulation 46:309, 1972

57. Khachadurian AK: The inheritance of essential familial hypercholesterolemia. Am J Med 37:402, 1964

58. Kim KM, Valigorsky JM, Mergner WJ, et al: Aging changes in the human aortic valve in relation to dystrophic calcification. Hum Pathol 7:47, 1976

59. King RM, Pluth JR, Giuliani ER: The association of unexplained gastrointestinal bleeding with calcific aortic stenosis. Ann Thorac Surg 44:514, 1987

60. Kirklin JW, Kouchoukos NT: Editorial: Aortic valve replacement without myocardial revascularization. Circulation 63:252, 1981

61. Koletsky S: Congenital bicuspid aortic valves. Arch Intern Med 67:129, 1941

62. Kulbertus HE: Ventricular arrhythmias, syncope and sudden death in aortic stenosis. Eur Heart J 9(suppl E):51, 1988

63. Larson EW, Edwards WD: Risk factors for aortic dissection: a necropsy study of 161 cases. Am J Cardiol 53:849, 1984

64. Lauer RM, DuShane JW, Edwards JE: Obstruction of left ventricular outlet in association with ventricular septal defect. Circulation 22:110, 1960

65. Laurie W: Aortic hypoplasia as a possible cause of sudden death. Med J Aust 2:710, 1968

66. Lerer PK, Edwards WD: Coronary arterial anatomy in bicuspid aortic valve. Necropsy study of 100 hearts. Br Heart J 45:142, 1981

67. Levine HD, Parisi AF, Holdsworth DE, Cohn LH: Aortic valve replacement for ochronosis of the aortic valve. Chest 74:466, 1978

68. Lewis T, Grant RT: Observations relating to subacute infective endocarditis. Heart 10:21, 1923

69. Love AW: The syndrome of calcific aortic stenosis and gastrointestinal bleeding: Resolution following aortic valve replacement. J Thorac Cardiovasc Surg 83:779, 1982

70. Lytle BW, Cosgrove DM, Goormastic M, Loop FD: Aortic valve replacement and coronary bypass grafting for patients with aortic stenosis and coronary artery disease: Early and late results. Eur Heart J 9(suppl. E):143, 1988

71. MacLean LD, Culligan JA, Kane DJ: Subaortic stenosis due to accessory tissue on the mitral valve. J Thorac Cardiovasc Surg 45:382, 1963

72. Maher ER, Curtis JR: Calcific aortic stenosis in chronic renal failure. Lancet 2:1007, 1985

73. Mandel AB, Gray IR: Significance of angina pectoris in aortic valve stenosis. Br Heart J 38:811, 1976

74. Maron BJ, Ferrans VJ, Roberts WC: Myocardial ultrastructure in patients with chronic aortic valve disease. Am J Cardiol 35:725, 1975

75. Maron BJ, Redwood DR, Roberts WC, et al: Tunnel subaortic stenosis. Left ventricular outflow tract obstruction produced by fibromuscular tubular narrowing. Circulation 54:404, 1976

76. McLoughlin MJ, Pasternac A, Morch J, Wigle ED: Idiopathic calcification of the ascending aorta and aortic valve in two young women. Br Heart J 36:96, 1974

77. McReynolds RA, Ali N, Cuadra M, Roberts WC: Combined acute rheumatic fever and congenitally bicuspid aortic valve. A hitherto unconfirmed combination. Chest 70:98, 1976

78. Mehta PM, Heinsimer JA, Bryg RJ, et al: Reassessment of the association between gastrointestinal arteriovenous malformation and aortic stenosis. Am J Med 86:275, 1989

78a. Michel PL, Vitoux B, Dermine P, et al: Mitral calcification in aortic stenosis. Europ Heart J 9(suppl E):77, 1988

79. Muna WFT, Ferrans VJ, Pierce JE, Roberts WC: Discrete subaortic stenosis in New-

foundland dogs: association of infective endocarditis. Am J Cardiol 41:746, 1978

80. Neufeld HN, Wagenvoort CA, Ongley PA, Edwards JE: Hypoplasia of the ascending aorta: an unusual form of supravalvular aortic stenosis with special reference to localized coronary arterial hypertension. Am J Cardiol 10:746, 1962

81. Northcote RJ, Sethia B, McGuiness JB: Aberrant origin of the left coronary artery with associated aortic stenosis. Thorax 40:152, 1985

82. O'Connor WN, Davis JB, Jr, Geisser R, et al: Supravalvular aortic stenosis: clinical and pathologic observations in six patients. Arch Pathol Lab Med 109:179, 1985

83. Ohlsson J, Liranne B: Non invasive assessment of valve area in patients with aortic stenosis. J Am Coll Cardiol 7:501, 1986

84. Olshausen KV, Schwarz F, Apfelbach J, et al: Determinants of the incidence and severity of ventricular arrhythmias in aortic valve disease. Am J Cardiol 51:1103, 1983

85. Osler W: The bicuspid condition of the aortic valves. Trans Assoc Am Physicians 2:185, 1886

86. Otto CM, Pearlman AS, Comess KA, et al: Determination of the stenotic aortic valve area in adults using Doppler echocardiography. J Am Coll Cardiol 7:509, 1986

87. Pansegrau DG, Kioshos JM, Durnin RE, Kroetz FW: Supravalvular aortic stenosis in adults. Am J Cardiol 31:635, 1973

88. Panza JA, Maron BJ: Valvular aortic stenosis and asymmetric septal hypertrophy: Diagnostic considerations and clinical and therapeutic implications. Eur Heart J 9(suppl E):71, 1988

89. Peretz DI, Changfoot GH, Gourlay RH: Four-cusped aortic valve with significant hemodynamic abnormality. Am J Cardiol 23:291, 1969

90. Perloff JK: The Clinical Recognition of Congenital Heart Disease. 2nd Ed. WB Saunders, Philadelphia, 1978, p. 81

91. Perloff JK: Postpediatric congenital heart disease: Natural survival patterns. Cardiovasc Clin 10/1:27, 1979

92. Peterson TA, Todd DB, Edwards JE: Supravalvular aortic stenosis. J Thorac Cardiovasc Surg 50:734, 1965

93. Pomerance A: Pathogenesis of aortic stenosis and its relation to age. Br Heart J 34:569, 1972

93a. Pritzker MR, Ernst JD, Caudill C, et al: Acquired aortic stenosis in systemic lupus erythematosis. Ann Intern Med 93:434, 1980

94. Pyle RL, Patterson DF, Chacko S: The genetics and pathology of discrete subaortic stenosis in the Newfoundland dog. Am Heart J 92:324, 1976

95. Rancurel G, Marcelle L, Vincent D, et al: Spontaneous calcific cerebral embolus from a calcific aortic stenosis in a middle cerebral artery infarct. Stroke 20:691, 1989

96. Rashkind WJ, Golinko R, Arcasoy M: Cardiac findings in idiopathic hypercalcemia of infancy. J Pediatr 58:464, 1961

97. Reis RL, Peterson LM, Mason DT, et al: Congenital fixed subvalvular aortic stenosis. An anatomical classification and correlations with operative results. Circulation 1(suppl 43):11, 1971

98. Roach MR: Hemodynamic factors in arterial stenosis and poststenotic dilatation. p. 439. In Stehbens WE (ed): Hemodynamics and the Blood Vessel Wall. Charles C Thomas, Springfield, Ill., 1979

99. Roberts WC: Renal hemosiderosis (blue kidney) in patients with valvular heart disease. Am J Pathol 48:409, 1966

100. Roberts WC: The congenitally bicuspid aortic valve. A study of 85 autopsy cases. Am J Cardiol 26:72, 1970

101. Roberts WC: Valvular, subvalvular and supravalvular aortic stenosis: Morphological features. Cardiovasc Clin 5/1:97, 1973

102. Roberts WC: Left ventricular outflow tract obstruction and aortic regurgitation. p. 110. In Edwards JE, Lev M, Abell MR (eds): The Heart. Williams & Wilkins, Baltimore, 1974

103. Roberts WC: Congenital cardiovascular abnormalities usually "silent" until adulthood: morphologic features of the floppy mitral valve, valvular aortic stenosis, discrete subvalvular aortic stenosis, hypertrophic cardiomyopathy, sinus of Valsalva aneurysm and the Marfan syndrome. Cardiovasc Clin 10/1: 407, 1979

104. Roberts WC, Arnett EA, Cabin HC, et al: Documented development of severe stenoses of previously confirmed normally functioning aortic valves. Am Heart J 104:306, 1982

105. Roberts WC, Buchbinder NA: Healed left-

sided infective endocarditis: A clinicopathologic study of 59 patients. Am J Cardiol 40:876, 1977

106. Roberts WC, McIntosh CL, Wallace RB: Aortic valve perforation with calcific aortic valve stenosis and without infective endocarditis or significant aortic vegetation. Am J Cardiol 59:476, 1987

107. Roberts WC, Ewy GA, Glancy DL, Marcus FI: Valvular stenosis produced by active infectious endocarditis. Circulation 36:449, 1967

108. Roberts, WC, Ferrans VJ, Levy RI, Fredrickson DS: Cardiovascular pathology in hyperlipoproteinemia: Anatomic observations in 42 necropsy patients with normal or abnormal lipoprotein patterns. Am J Cardiol 31:557, 1973

109. Roberts WC, Morrow AG: Cardiac valves and the surgical pathologist. Arch Pathol 82:309, 1966

110. Roberts WC, Perloff JK, Constantino T: Severe valvular aortic stenosis in patients over 65 years of age. A clinicopathologic study. Am J Cardiol 27:497, 1971

111. Rose AG, Forman R: Idiopathic aortitis with calcification of ascending aorta and aortic and mitral values. Br Heart J 38:650, 1976

112. Ross J, Jr, Braunwald E: Aortic stenosis. Circulation 5(suppl 37):61, 1968

113. Scheffer SM, Leatherman LL: Resolution of Heyde's syndrome of aortic stenosis and gastrointestinal bleeding after aortic valve replacement. Ann Thorac Surg 42:477, 1986

114. Schlatmann TJM, Becker AE: Histologic changes in the normal ageing aorta: implications for dissecting aortic aneurysm. Am J Cardiol 39:13, 1977

115. Schoen FJ: Interventional and Surgical Cardiovascular Pathology. Clinical Correlations and Basic Principles. WB Saunders, Philadelphia, 1989, p. 112

116. Scholz DG, Lynch JA, Willerscheidt AB, et al: Coronary arterial dominance associated with congenital bicuspid aortic valve. Arch Pathol Lab Med 104:417, 1980

117. Schwarz F, Flameng W, Schaper J, et al: Myocardial structure and function in patients with aortic valve disease and their relation to postoperative results. Am J Cardiol 41:661, 1978

118. Schwartz BM: Additional note on bleeding in aortic stenosis (letter to the editor). N Engl J Med 259:456, 1958

119. Sellers RD, Lillehei CW, Edwards JE: Subaortic stenosis caused by anomalies of the atrioventricular valves. J Thorac Cardiovasc Surg 48;289, 1964

120. Singleton EB, Merten DF: An unusual syndrome of widened medullary cavities of the metacarpals and phalanges, aortic calcification and abnormal dentition. Pediatr Radiol 1:2, 1973

121. Stein PD, Sabbah HN, Pitha JV: Continuing disease process of calcific aortic stenosis. Role of microthrombi and turbulent flow. Am J Cardiol 39:159, 1977

122. Subramanian R, Olsen LJ, Edwards WD: Surgical pathology of pure aortic stenosis: a study of 374 cases. Mayo Clin Proc 59:683, 1984

123. Sud A, Parker F, Magilligan DJ Jr: Anatomy of the aortic root. Ann Thorac Surg 38:76, 1984

124. Sung C-S, Price EC, Cooley DA: Discrete subaortic stenosis in adults. Am J Cardiol 42:283, 1978

125. Tawes RL, Berry CL, Aberdeen E: Congenital bicuspid aortic valves associated with coarctation of the aorta in children. Br Heart J 31:127, 1969

126. Taylor DEM, Whamond JS: Velocity profiles and impedance of prosthetic mitral valves. p. 261. In Kalmanson D (ed): The Mitral Valve. A Pluridisciplinary Approach. Publishing Sciences Group, Acton, Mass. 1976

127. Theman TE, Silver MD, Haust MD, et al: Morphological findings in idiopathic calcification of the ascending aorta afflicting a young woman. Histopathology 3:181, 1979

128. Thubrikar MJ, Aouad J, Nolan SP: Comparison of the in vivo and in vitro mechanical properties of aortic valve leaflets. J Thorac Cardiovasc Surg 92:29, 1986

129. Torres ET, Cavalcanti AR: Congenital elastic band of aortic valve. Am Heart J 45:630, 1953

130. Van Mierop LHS: Pathology and pathogenesis of the common cardiac malformations. Cardiovasc Clin 2:27, 1970

131. Van Praagh R, Corwin RD, Dahlquist EH, Jr, et al: Tetralogy of Fallot with severe left ventricular outflow tract obstruction due to anomalous attachment of the mitral valve to

the ventricular septum. Am J Cardiol 26:93, 1970

132. Varghese PJ, Izukawa T, Rowe RD: Supravalvular aortic stenosis as part of rubella syndrome, with discussion of pathogenesis. Br Heart J 31:59, 1969

133. Vollebergh FEMG, Becker AE: Minor congenital variations of cusp size in tricuspid aortic valve. Br Heart J 39:1006, 1977

134. Waller BF, Carter JB, William HJ, Jr, et al: Bicuspid aortic valve. Comparison of congenital and acquired types. Circulation 48:1140, 1973

135. Walmsley R: Anatomy of the left ventricular outflow tract. Br Heart J 41:263, 1979

136. Walmsley R, Watson H: Clinical Anatomy of the Heart. Churchill Livingstone, New York, 1978, p. 183

137. Wennevold A, Jacobsen JG: Acquired supravalvular aortic stenosis in familial hypercholesterolemia. A hemodynamic and angiocardiographic study. Am J Med 50:823, 1971

138. Wigle ED: Myocardial fibrosis and calcareous emboli in valvular heart disease. Br Heart J 19:539, 1957

139. Williams JCP, Barratt-Boyes BG, Lowe JB: Supravalvular aortic stenosis. Circulation 24:1311, 1961

140. Wong M, Tei C, Sadler N, et al: Echocardiographic observation of calcium in operatively excised stenotic aortic valves. Am J Cardiol 59:324, 1987

141. Wright GB, Keane JF, Nadas AS, et al: Fixed subaortic stenosis in the young: Medical and surgical course in 83 patients. Am J Cardiol 52:830, 1983

27

Pathology of Aortic Incompetence

Jesse E. Edwards

A review of the essential features of the normal aortic valve is appropriate before consideration of the pathologic processes underlying aortic valvular incompetence.

The aortic valve is equipped with three semilunar cusps, each attached to the aortic wall along its periphery. The superolateral edges of each cusp insert into the aortic wall independently of the neighboring cusp. This attachment occurs at a mound of tissue that also receives the edge of the neighboring cusp. The two edges form a commissure or hinge.[44] There are three commissures. The length of the upper free edge of each cusp is longer than the straight-line distance between its two lateral attachments. This extra length allows for free mobility of the cusps during the cardiac cycle (Fig. 27–1). During ventricular diastole, the extra length allows the center of each cusp to move to the center of the aortic orifice to effect valve closure. During ventricular systole, the extra length allows the free edge of the cusp to move to the wall of the aorta, thereby permitting the valve orifice to open widely.[8]

The space between a cusp and the aortic wall is called the aortic sinus (sinus of Valsalva). The names given to the sinuses correspond to those of the cusps. Two of the sinuses are located more or less anteriorly.

That toward the right and related to the origin of the right coronary artery is the right aortic sinus; that toward the left and related to the origin of the left coronary artery is termed the left aortic sinus. The third sinus, the posterior or noncoronary sinus, is located posteriorly.

The relationships to adjacent structures of the aortic sinuses vary. The posterior aortic sinus is related to the atrial septum. Proximal to it lies the membranous ventricular septum with the contained bundle of His. The right aortic sinus is related to the right ventricular infundibulum. The left aortic sinus is partly related to the atrial septum, posteriorly, and to the pulmonary trunk, anteriorly. The mid-portion of the left aortic sinus is related to the epicardium at the site of origin of the left coronary artery.

Approximately two-thirds of the circumference of the origin of the aorta is attached directly to the anterior or septal portions of the left ventricular wall. The remainder of the aorta, that related to the junction of the posterior and left sinuses, is attached primarily to the anterior leaflet of the mitral valve through the interposition of a thin fibrous sheet, the mitral-aortic intervalvular fibrosa.[14]

Incompetence of the aortic valve may result from intrinsic disease of the cusps or from primary diseases of the ascending aorta, the

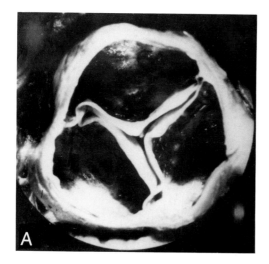 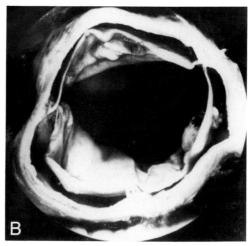

Fig. 27–1. Specimen of a normal aortic valve viewed from above and unopened. (**A**) Simulated state of valve closure. The three cusps are of a sufficient length to allow the center of each to approach the center of the aortic orifice. (**B**) The phase of ventricular systole wherein the aortic valve is open is simulated, showing how "the extra length" of the cusps allows each to approach the aortic wall to open the valve to a caliber approaching that of the aorta itself. (From Edwards,[9] with permission.)

latter having effects upon the aortic valve as to interfere with its competence.[10] There remain not a small number of cases in which there is uncertainty as to the basis for the valvular incompetence.[2] In some of these, there is myxomatous change of the aortic cusps, so-called mucoid degeneration as described by Allen and co-workers.[2] In other cases it is possible that changes occur in the ascending aorta that are more subtle than the classic examples of aortitis or extensive cystic medial necrosis, so-called annulo-aortic ectasia.[35] In addition, a large variety of shunts allow an abnormal escape of blood from the aorta. The effects of the latter process may yield hemodynamic disturbances, which, in some respects, may mimic aortic valvular insufficiency.[11]

INTRINSIC DISEASE OF AORTIC VALVE

Intrinsic diseases of the aortic valve leading to aortic incompetence are principally of rheumatic and inflammatory nature. Less common

changes are those associated with rheumatoid arthritis and lupus erythematosus. The principal congenital disease is the congenital bicuspid aortic valve.

Rheumatic Disease

Rheumatic diseases of the aortic valve may cause either pure aortic incompetence or aortic incompetence associated with some degree of stenosis (see Ch. 24).

In the study of aortic valves removed from 225 patients with pure aortic insufficiency, Olson and associates[28] applied the designation *postinflammatory* aortic insufficiency to 103 cases (46 percent). In three of these cases, the patients had ankylosing spondylitis, while in the remainder, Olson et al. considered the so-called postinflammatory state a result of rheumatic disease. Cases with infective endocarditis were considered in a separate category by these investigators.

Pure aortic incompetence of rheumatic origin results from recurrent active inflammation leading to fibrosis and contracture of the

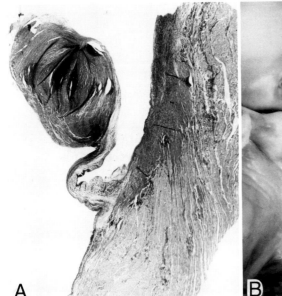

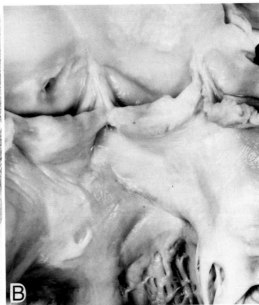

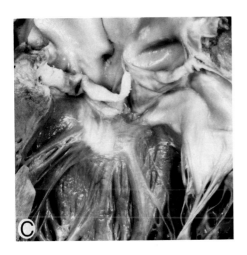

Fig. 27–2. Rheumatic incompetence of aortic valve. (**A**) Low power photomicrograph of root of aorta and aortic cusp. The distal portion of the cusp shows major thickening with fibrous contracture as a result of recurrent rheumatic endocarditis. (Elastic tissue stain, × 5.) (**B**) Portion of opened aortic valve showing fusion at one commissure. The principal feature is shortening of the cusps. The septal wall of the subaortic tract shows a semicircular regurgitant jet lesion from aortic incompetence. The shortening of the cusps is more or less equal. (**C**) Opened aortic valve and related structures. The right aortic cusp (center) shows shortening and retraction of a greater degree than is exhibited by the other two cusps. The white patch on the subjacent ventricular septum is interpreted as a regurgitant jet lesion.

cusps (Fig. 27–2A). Calcification is either absent or present in minor degree.[28] The cusps become shorter than normal (Fig. 27–2B). In some instances, the effect on cusps is unequal, so that one undergoes greater contracture than the other two (Fig. 27–2C). The result is a malalignment of cusps, leading to regurgitation of blood across the valve. The regurgitant stream may strike either the left ventricular lining or the anterior mitral leaflet,[21,42] leaving a tell-tale jet lesion (Fig. 27–2B).

In pure rheumatic aortic incompetence, commissural fusion is either absent or minimal (Fig. 27–3A). If contracture is coupled with fusion of two or three commmissures, the effect is a combination of aortic stenosis and incompetence (Fig. 27–3B,C).

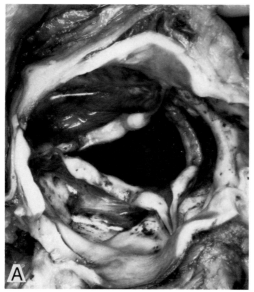

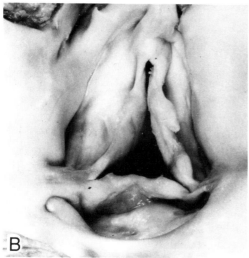

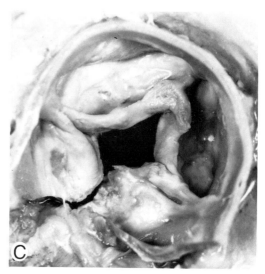

Fig. 27–3. Rheumatic aortic valvular disease. In each instance, the aortic valve is unopened and viewed from above. **(A)** Shortening of each cusp without commissural fusion. The condition is that of pure aortic incompetence. **(B)** Fusion of each of the three commissures restraining the valve from opening completely; the major effect appears to be a shortening of cusps yielding a triangular-shaped defect at the center of the orifice. **(C)** Fusion of each of the aortic commissures with fibrosis and calcification yielding a stenotic valve but, since the orifice is incompletely guarded, incompetence is associated. (Fig. A from Edwards,[9] with permission.)

Infective Endocarditis

Except for rheumatic disease, inflammation involving the aortic valve so as to make it incompetent is most commonly of the infectious type (see Ch. 23).

Infective endocarditis of the aortic valve may involve a tricuspid aortic valve, but not infrequently the valve is bicuspid, either congenitally (Fig. 27–4A) or as a result of acquired disease. While interposition of vegetations be-

tween the closing aspects of the cusps may cause aortic incompetence, the usual basis is destruction of cusp tissue (Fig. 27–4B). This is manifested either as one or several perforations or as destruction along the aortic attachment of a cusp with secondary prolapse. As the major conduction tissue is closely related to the aortic valve, the association of atrioventricular conduction disturbance is more common with an infectious cause of aortic incompetence than with other causes.

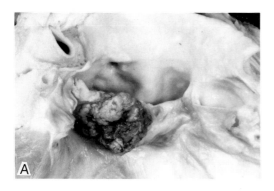

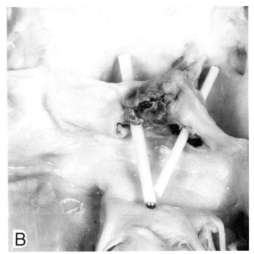

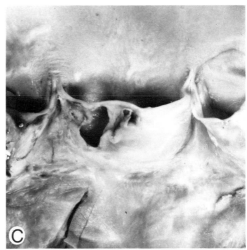

Fig. 27–4. Infective endocarditis. (**A**) Congenital bicuspid aortic valve with a large vegetation attached to the conjoined cusp. The vegetation may have interfered with adequate closure of the valve. (**B**) Each of two cusps of the aortic valve shows perforation (probes) as part of active bacterial endocarditis. (**C**) Perforations in an aortic cusp as a manifestation of bacteriologically healed bacterial endocarditis. (Fig. B from Edwards,[9] with permission.)

It is of particular significance that destructive changes complicating the active phase of infective endocarditis continue as a cause of aortic incompetence after bacteriologic cure (Fig. 27–4C). Infective aortic valvular endocarditis may cause secondary infection of the mitral apparatus resulting in mitral regurgitation.[7]

Myxomatous Valve

In recent years, aortic insufficiency ascribed to myxomatous change of the aortic valve has become increasingly prominent.[2,40] Tonne-

macher and associates[41] indicated their criteria for myxomatous aortic valve (so-called myxomatous degeneration or floppy aortic valve). Of the three histologic features identified, each was present for these investigators to use the diagnosis of myxomatous degeneration. These features are (1) discontinuity of the fibrosa, (2) widening of a zona spongiosa with acid mucopolysaccharides, and (3) more than 50 percent of the valve involved by excess acid mucopolysaccharide deposit (Fig. 27–5). Using these criteria, it was found that among 37 aortic valves surgically removed for pure aortic insufficiency, 12 (32 percent) qualified for this diagnosis.

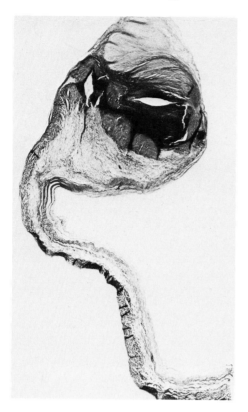

Fig. 27–5. Myxomatous aortic valve. Cusp is viewed vertically. Fibrosa is to the left. This shows focal interruption because of excess spongiosa. Knobby distal end is secondary to aortic regurgitation. (Elastic tissue stain, × 15.)

Similar findings were reported by Allen and associates.[2] In studying 55 aortic valves removed for isolated aortic insufficiency, these workers found that 13 (24 percent) had myxomatous change. Sudden death with isolated floppy aortic valve was described by Pounder.[30]

It is to be recognized that the myxomatous aortic valve, as defined, may be observed in Marfan syndrome. It may also be associated with floppy or prolapsed mitral valve. Also, an increase in acid mucopolysaccharides within cusps may complicate hypertension, traumatic disease, and infective endocarditis, among other conditions. Thus, the distinction between a primary or secondary process may not be easy to make.

Collagen Diseases

Aortic regurgitation may complicate lupus erythematosus.[27,36] Attenuation of valvular tissue with secondary perforation has been described.[3]

Among 225 patients with pure aortic insufficiency, Olson and associates[28] noted three subjects with ankylosing spondylitis and fibrosis of aortic valvular cusps.

In rheumatoid arthritis (see Ch. 30), granulomas of this condition may involve the pericardium, myocardium, cardiac skeleton, and valves, particularly the aortic and mitral. The rheumatoid granulomas may undergo fibrosis and calcification, leading to a loss of their specific histologic morphology (Fig. 27–6). When causing aortic incompetence, the condition usually involves the root

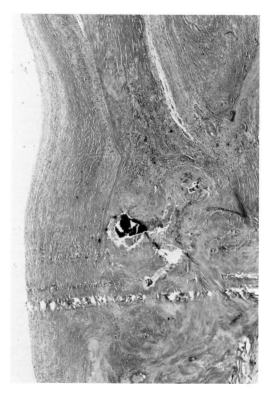

Fig. 27–6. Base of aortic valve showing fibrotic and calcified granuloma of rheumatoid valvulitis. (H&E; × 20.)

of the aorta and related cardiac skeleton and, to varying degree, the cusps as well.[19,33]

Trauma

A traumatic basis for aortic insufficiency is usually the result of laceration of the aorta (see Ch. 36). Only uncommonly will blunt external trauma cause a laceration of a cusp (Fig. 27–7). It has been reported that rupture of an aortic cusp complicated straining.[38] Violent coughing has also been claimed as a cause of tearing of cuspid tissue.[18] Valvuloplasty for the treatment of aortic stenosis may induce incompetence of the valve.[1]

Congenital Anomalies of or Related to the Aortic Valve

Two principal causes of intrinsic aortic incompetence are associated with congenital disease—namely, congenital bicuspid aortic valve (see Ch. 26) and ventricular septal defect. Fenestration of aortic cusps, while common, is a rare cause of aortic regurgitation.[39] In Olson's series,[28] noninfected congenital bicuspid valve accounted for 20 percent of cases

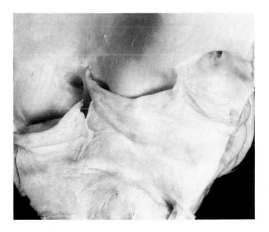

Fig. 27–7. Traumatic rupture of an aortic cusp. (From Carter et al.,[5] with permission.)

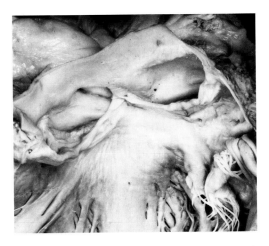

Fig. 27–8. Congenital bicuspid aortic valve with prolapse of conjoined cusp resulting in aortic incompetence. (From Eliot et al.,[11] with permission.)

of pure aortic insufficiency. In the series of Roberts and associates,[34] the comparable figure was 7 percent. The unusual tendency for the noninfected congenital bicuspid aortic valve to be incompetent was emphasized by Fenoglio and colleagues.[12]

The classic congenital bicuspid aortic valve shows anterior and posterior cusps. The anterior is the larger, and the two coronary arteries arise from its sinus. Classically, a low ridge, the so-called raphe, extends from the aortic wall onto the center of the aortic face of the wider cusp. Under usual circumstances, the cusps make adequate apposition so as to allow for valvular competence. Unusually, the larger cusp is sufficiently redundant to prolapse beyond the optimal position for closure of the valve, and incompetence results[8] (Fig. 27–8). Usually, a classic congenital bicuspid valve known to be incompetent during adult life had not been incompetent in earlier years.

In an uncommon type of congenital bicuspid valve, the raphe is represented by a thin strand of tissue running from near the free aspect of the larger cusp, on one hand, to the aortic wall, on the other. Rupture of this strand causes the larger cusp to lose support, so that it prolapses. This may account for the sudden appearance of major aortic re-

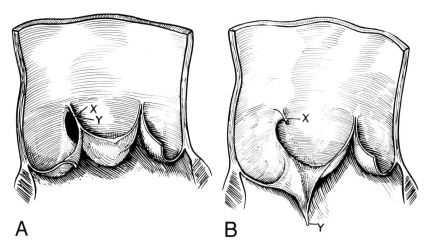

Fig. 27–9. Congenital bicuspid aortic valve in which the conjoined cusp is supported by a strand. (**A**) The natural state. Points X and Y are contiguous. (**B**) Spontaneous rupture of the strand allows points X and Y to move away from each other and be associated with prolapse of the related cusp. (From Carter et al.,[5] with permission.)

gurgitation[5,34] (Fig. 27–9). The congenital quadricuspid aortic valve may also be incompetent.[28]

In aortic incompetence associated with ventricular septal defect,[40,43] the defect is closely related to the aortic root and valve (see Ch. 45 also). Usually the defect is of supracristal type; less commonly, infracristal (Fig. 27–10A). The basis for aortic incompetence appears to be an inadequate attachment of the

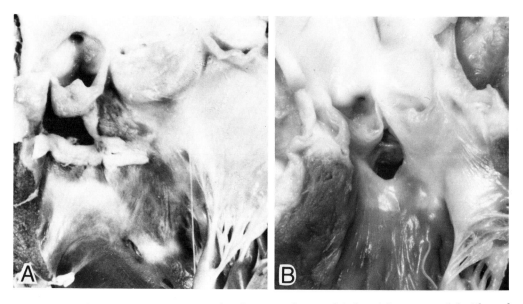

Fig. 27–10. Aortic incompetence associated with ventricular septal defect. (**A**) From an adult. The right aortic cusp is prolapsed in relation to a subjacent ventricular septal defect of the supracristal type. (**B**) From an infant. The right aortic cusp is prolapsed in relationship to a defect of the infracristal type. Aortic insufficiency had been demonstrated by angiography during the patient's life.

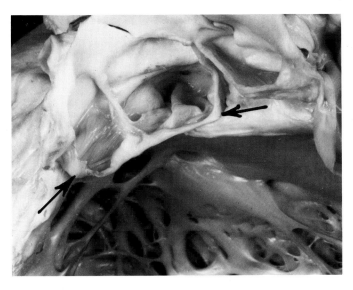

Fig. 27–11. Bicuspid aortic valve with prolapse associated with a subjacent ventricular septal defect. The conjoined cusp (between arrows) has prolapsed, obscuring the subjacent ventricular septal defect.

aortic root to the cardiac skeleton. As a result, that part of the aorta related to the defect moves away from its optimal position. The related cusp(s) (usually the right, less commonly the left) are carried laterally with the displaced aorta and "tip." The result is malalignment of the cusps and incompetence of the valve. As with the usual case of aortic incompetence complicating a congenitally bicuspid valve, the aortic incompetence is classically the result of progressive change and not commonly observed in the very young (Fig. 27–10B). Uncommonly, the prolapsed cusp may occlude the ventricular septal defect during ventricular diastole (Fig. 27–11).

Recently, using Doppler echocardiography, Sasson and associates[35] analyzed blood flow in 52 patients with hypertrophic cardiomyopathy. Each had been treated by transaortic ventriculomyectomy/myotomy and was studied a mean of 7.8 years after surgery. Twenty-eight patients had aortic regurgitation. Among a subgroup of 22 studied both pre- and postoperation, 8 developed new aortic regurgitation. Sasson et al. note that the regurgitation is usually trivial but may progress with time. By contrast, they found

only 1 patient who had aortic regurgitation among 34 others with this cardiomyopathy who did not have surgery. The cause of the aortic regurgitation is not certain. The Toronto group suggest that valve cusp injury during surgery or a loss of subvalvular support following surgery are possible morphologic explanations. A third possibility is altered velocity, direction, and/or dynamics of the turbulent jet of blood in the left ventricular outflow tract after surgery. Pathologists must help define the cause of this new observation.

Myxomatous alteration of the aortic cusps ("floppy aortic valve") is usually associated with extensive cystic medial necrosis of the aorta (Fig. 27–12). Nevertheless, myxomatous change may be an isolated process.[2,41]

PRIMARY DISEASE OF ASCENDING AORTA

While the aortic valve is intrinsically normal, aortic incompetence may result from primary disease of the ascending aorta.[9,10] Either one of two fundamental processes underlie this

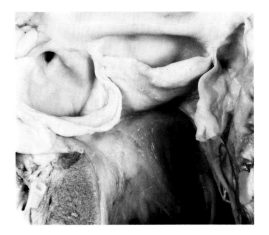

Fig. 27–12. Aortic valve in an instance of extensive cystic medial necrosis of aorta. The right aortic cusp (left side of illustration) shows marked prolapse. Mitral incompetence from ruptured chordae was also associated.

process, namely (1) ectasia of the aortic root, or (2) laceration of the ascending aorta.

Ectasia of the Aortic Root

Dilation or ectasia of the aortic root places tension on the individual cusps, causing them to bow and to lose their "extra length," thus making them relatively short for the orifice they guard. Commissural widening may accompany this change (Fig. 27–13). Ectasia of the aortic root may be associated with widening of more distal segments of the aorta such as the upper ascending aorta, the arch, or even the descending aorta.

The classic cause of this condition is aortitis, of which syphilitic aortitis[16] is the example par excellence. Aortic changes associated with

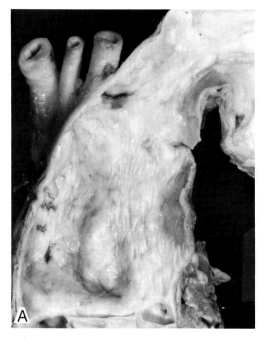

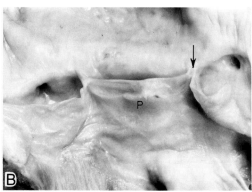

Fig. 27–13. Aortitis as a basis for aortic incompetence. (**A**) Interior of ascending aorta and a portion of the arch. A portion of the aortic valve lies in the lowermost portion of the illustration. The aorta is dilated and shows a characteristic wrinkled lining. Ostia of the branches of the arch are obscured. (**B**) Closeup of the aortic valve. There is commissural separation (beneath arrow) between left and posterior (P) aortic cusps. The posterior cusp also shows bowing incident to the aortic dilation.

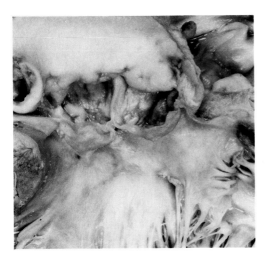

Fig. 27–14. Aortic valve and ascending aorta. The root of the aorta is markedly distorted on the basis of aortitis associated with multijoint rheumatoid arthritis. Aortic insufficiency was associated in the 12-year-old child from whom the specimen was obtained. (From Edwards,[9] with permission.)

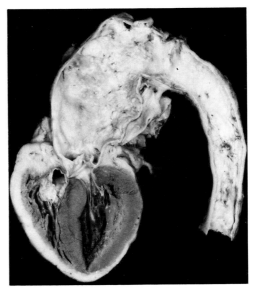

Fig. 27–15. Senile dilation of the aorta. The principal effects lie in the ascending aorta. (From Edwards,[9] with permission.)

rheumatoid spondylitis[22] yield a similar picture, as do various types of aortitis of unknown etiology.[17,23,24,32] In rheumatoid arthritis, the root of the aorta may be affected (Fig. 27–14), and inflammatory and fibrotic changes of the valve cusps may be associated.

It is commonly recognized that the thoracic aorta widens progressively with age (Fig. 27–15). In an occasional subject of advanced age, the process of aortic dilation affecting the root may be of such proportion as to be responsible for aortic incompetence. Associated hypertension possibly accentuates the process of aortic dilation leading to incompetence of the valve.[45]

Yet another cause of aortic incompetence is extensive cystic medial necrosis of the aorta,[36] either of the idiopathic type[46] or associated with Marfan syndrome,[4,13,29] even in the absence of laceration of the aorta (Fig. 27–16). In this condition, a contributing factor to aortic incompetence may be associated with intrinsic changes of the cusps that allow them to prolapse[31] or, rarely, to rupture.[15,26] In extensive cystic medial necrosis, the ascending aorta is the segment most affected. Minor changes may occur in the arch and less beyond.

Laceration of the Aorta

Laceration of the ascending aorta may complicate hypertension, extensive cystic medial necrosis, external blunt trauma (Fig. 27–17A,B) or, uncommonly, aortitis.

If the laceration occurs near a commissural attachment of two cusps, the secondary retraction of tissue causes prolapse of the cusps at the related commissure. The consequent cusp malalignment underlies the sudden appearance of valvular incompetence[9,10] (Fig. 27–17). The state is among those underlying acute aortic insufficiency.[6] If the patient survives, chronic aortic incompetence results (Fig. 27–17).

Laceration of the aorta may remain as such

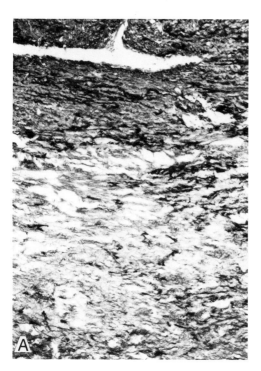

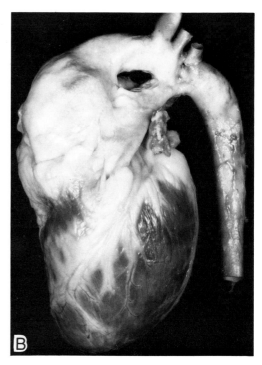

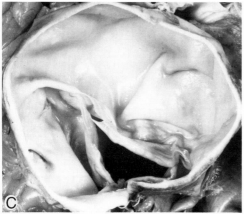

Fig. 27–16. Marfan syndrome associated with aortic cystic medial necrosis and aortic insufficiency. Specimens from three different cases. (**A**) Photomicrograph of ascending aorta showing interruptions of the media on the basis of extensive cystic medial necrosis. (Elastic tissue stain, × 100.) (**B**) Exterior of heart and aorta. There is characteristic pronounced dilation of the ascending aorta. (**C**) Interior of ascending aorta and aortic valve viewed from above. Marked dilation of aorta. The aortic cusps have been stretched and also show some features of prolapse. (Fig. B from Edwards,[9] with permission.)

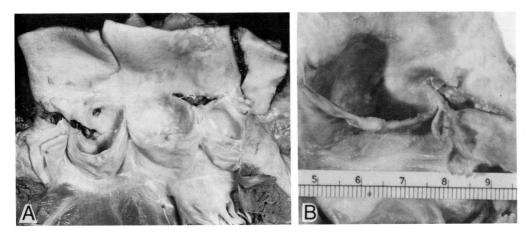

Fig. 27–17. Aortic insufficiency complicating laceration of the aorta. (**A**) Traumatic lacerations of the aorta showing prolapse of two of the commissures secondary to the lacerations. (**B**) A portion of the ascending aorta and aortic valve. There is an old laceration of the aorta above one of the commissures. The associated retraction of the aortic tissues caused prolapse of related cusps and incompetence of the valve. (Fig. A from Edwards,[9] with permission.)

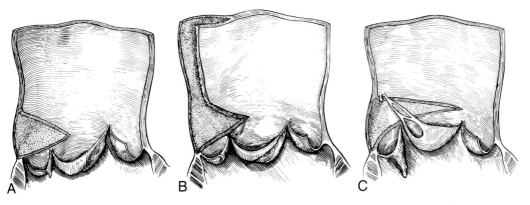

Fig. 27–18. Diagrammatic portrayal of consequences of laceration of the aorta in relationship to an aortic commissure. (**A**) Laceration without dissecting aneurysm. Retraction of the edges of the laceration allows for commissural prolapse and aortic incompetence. (**B**) The process shown in Fig. A with regard to the aortic valve is the same, with the additional feature of classic dissecting aneurysm. (**C**) Laceration of the aorta has been at a level just below the upper level of the commissure causing attenuation of one aortic cusp and rupture of the other. (From Edwards,[10] with permission.)

(Fig. 27–18A) or may become complicated by aortic dissection[20] (Fig. 27–18B). In any event, the effects on the aortic valve are principally those of prolapse incident to the underlying laceration.

In either event, if the aortic laceration lies below the upper aspect of a commissure, there is, additionally, the chance of tearing of related cusps by the process of retraction of the edges of the laceration[25] (Fig. 27–18).

REFERENCES

1. Alexopoulous D, Sherman W: Unusual hemodynamic presentation of acute aortic regurgitation following percutaneous balloon valvuloplasty. Am Heart J 116:1622, 1988

2. Allen WM, Matloff JM, Fishbein MC: Myxoid degeneration of the aortic valve and isolated severe aortic regurgitation. Am J Cardiol 55:439, 1985

3. Bernhard GC, Lange RL, Hensley GT: Aortic disease with valvular insufficiency as a principal manifestation of systemic lupus erythematosus. Ann Intern Med 71:81, 1969

4. Brown OR, DeMots H, Kloster FE, et al: Aortic root dilation and mitral valve prolapse in Marfan's syndrome. An echocardiography study. Circulation 52:651, 1975

5. Carter JB, Sethi S, Lee GB, Edwards JE: Prolapse of semilunar cusps as causes of aortic insufficiency. Circulation 43:922, 1971

6. Dervan J, Goldberg S: Acute aortic regurgitation: pathophysiology and management. Cardiovasc Clin 16:281, 1986

7. Dianzumba SB, Montello NJ, Joyner CR: Intermittent premature mitral valve closure in combined acute severe aortic and mitral regurgitation. South Med J 77:1449, 1984

8. Edwards JE: The congenital bicuspid aortic valve. Circulation 23:485, 1961

9. Edwards JE: Lesions causing or simulating aortic insufficiency. Cardiovasc Clin 5:128, 1973

10. Edwards JE: Pathology of acquired valvular disease of the heart. Semin Roentgenol 14:96, 1979

11. Eliot RS, Woodburn RL, Edwards JE: Conditions of the ascending aorta simulating aortic valvular incompetence. Am J Cardiol 14:679, 1964

12. Fenoglio JJ Jr, McAllister HA, DeCastro CM, et al: Congenital bicuspid aortic valve after age 20. Am J Cardiol 39:164, 1977

13. Glaser J, Whitman V, Liebman J: Aortic regurgitation in a young girl with severe form of Marfan syndrome. J Pediatr 83:685, 1973

14. Gross L, Kugel MA: Topographic anatomy and histology of the valves in the human heart. Am J Pathol 7:445, 1931

15. Hays FB, Boggan WH: Rupture of aortic valve cusp attachment due to cystic medionecrosis of the aorta. Ann Intern Med 43:1107, 1955

16. Heggtveit HA: Syphilitic aortitis. A clinicopathologic autopsy study of 100 cases, 1950 to 1960. Circulation 29:346, 1964

17. Heggtveit HA, Hennigar GR, Morrione TG: Panaortitis. Am J Pathol 42:151, 1963

18. Jaworsky C, Smith DW, Shindler D, Kostis J: Recurrent nontraumatic aortic tears resulting in valvular avulsion and aortic insufficiency. Clin Cardiol 8:173, 1985

19. Lebowitz WB: The heart in rheumatoid arthritis (rheumatoid disease): A clinical and pathological study of sixty-two cases. Ann Intern Med 58:102, 1963

20. Levy MJ, Siegal DL, Wang Y, Edwards JE: Rupture of aortic valve secondary to aneurysm of ascending aorta. Circulation 27:422, 1963

21. Louie EK, Mason TJ, Shah R, et al: Determinants of anterior mitral leaflet fluttering in pure aortic regurgitation from pulsed Doppler study of the early diastolic interaction between the regurgitant jet and mitral inflow. Am J Cardiol 61:1085, 1988

22. Malette WG, Eiseman B, Danielson GK, et al: Rheumatoid spondylitis and aortic insufficiency. An operable combination. J Thorac Cardiovasc Surg 57:471, 1969

23. McGuire J, Scott RC, Gall EA: Chronic aortitis of undetermined cause with severe and fatal aortic insufficiency. Am J Med Sci 235:394, 1958

24. Miehle W: Aortic insufficiency in non-syphilitic mesaortitis. Fortschr Med 104:735, 1986

25. Murray CA, Edwards JE: Spontaneous laceration of ascending aorta. Circulation 47:848, 1973

26. O'Brien KP, Hitchcock GC, Barratt-Boyes GB, Lowe JB: Spontaneous aortic cusp rupture associated with valvular myxomatous transformation. Circulation 37:273, 1968

27. Oh WMC, Taylor RT, Olsen EGJ: Aortic regurgitation in systemic lupus erythematosus requiring aortic valve replacement. Br Heart J 36:413, 1974

28. Olson LJ, Subramanian R, Edwards WD: Surgical pathology of pure aortic insufficiency: A study of 225 cases. Mayo Clin Proc 59:835, 1984

29. Phornphutkul CH, Rosenthal A, Nadas AS: Cardiac manifestations of Marfan syndrome in infancy and childhood. Circulation 47:587, 1973

30. Pounder DJ: Floppy aortic valve presenting as sudden death. Forensic Sci Int 25:123, 1984

31. Read RC, Thal AP, Wendt VE: Symptomatic valvular myxomatous transformations (the floppy valve syndrome). Circulation 32:897, 1965

32. Restrepo C, Tejeda C, Correa P: Nonsyphilitic aortitis. Arch Pathol 87:1, 1969

33. Roberts WC, Kehoe JA, Carpenter DF, Golden A: Cardiac valvular lesions in rheumatoid arthritis. Arch Intern Med 122:141, 1968

34. Roberts WC, Morrow AG, McIntosh CL, et al: Congenitally bicuspid aortic valve causing severe, pure aortic regurgitation without superimposed infective endocarditis: Analysis of 13 patients requiring aortic valve replacement. Am J Cardiol 47:206, 1981

35. Sasson Z, Prieur T, Skrobik Y, et al: Aortic regurgitation: A common complication after surgery for hypertrophic cardiomyopathy. J Am Coll Cardiol 13:63, 1989

36. Savunen T, Aho HJ: Annulo-aortic ectasia. Light and electron microscopic changes in aortic media. Virchows Arch [A] 407:279, 1985

37. Shulman HJ, Christian CL: Aortic insufficiency in systemic lupus erythematosus. Arthritis Rheum 12:138, 1969

38. Spurny OM, Hara M: Rupture of the aortic valve due to strain. Am J Cardiol 8:125, 1961

39. Symbas PN, Walter PF, Hurst JW, Schlant RC: Fenestration of aortic cusps causing aortic regurgitation. J Thorac Cardiovasc Dis 57:464, 1969

40. Tatsuno K, Konno S, Sakakibara S: Ventricular septal defect with aortic insufficiency. Am Heart J 85:13, 1973

41. Tonnemacher D, Reid C, Kawanishi D, et al: Frequency of myxomatous degeneration of the aortic valve as a cause of isolated aortic regurgitation severe enough to warrant aortic valve replacement. Am J Cardiol 60:1194, 1987

42. Trappe HJ, Daniel WG, Frank G, Lichtlen PR: Comparisons between diastolic fluttering and reverse doming of anterior mitral leaflet in aortic regurgitation. Am Heart J 114:1399, 1987

43. Van Praagh R, McNamara JJ: Anatomic types of ventricular septal defect with aortic insufficiency. Am Heart J 75:604, 1968

44. Waller BF, Carter JB, Williams HJ, et al: Bicuspid aortic valve. Comparison of congenital and acquired types. Circulation 48:1140, 1973

45. Waller BF, Zoltick JM, Rosen JH, et al: Severe aortic regurgitation from systemic hypertension (without aortic dissection) requiring aortic valve replacement: Analysis of four patients. Am J Cardiol 49:473, 1982

46. Weaver WF, Edwards JE, Brandenburg RO: Idiopathic dilation of the aorta with aortic valvular insufficiency: A possible forme fruste of Marfan's syndrome. Mayo Clin Proc 34:518, 1959

28

Interactions Between the Heart and Brain

Harry V. Vinters

This chapter summarizes the effects of lesions of the heart and great vessels on the brain and those of encephalic lesions on the heart. Discussion of the former topic is more extensive, simply because these interactions are more clearly understood, there is more abundant literature, and cerebral lesions resulting from cardiac abnormalities have been somewhat better documented in terms of pathology and pathogenetic mechanisms.

Throughout this discussion, several terms are used, meriting definition and explanation. The term *stroke* denotes a clinical syndrome characterized by a sudden, nonconvulsive, focal neurologic deficit.[2] Implicit in this definition is the understanding that a stroke need not necessarily be caused by vascular disease. The term *stroke* defines a clinical syndrome, not a pathologic entity; although it is sometimes used more loosely and is used extensively throughout this chapter. By convention, clinicians often use the term to describe a cerebral infarct: a frequently used synonym is *cerebrovascular accident* (CVA). Strokes are usually caused by cerebral infarcts or hemorrhages or by a combination of the two. When it becomes important to make this distinction, it is made in the text.

The bibliography to this chapter is not exhaustive, nor is it intended to be. Emphasis is placed on the current literature, especially clinicopathologic and clinical reviews. The American Heart Association journal *Stroke* is an excellent source of such reviews.

Illustrations consist mainly of relevant brain lesions. This is done because cardiac lesions are illustrated much more extensively throughout the text. For readers interested in pursuing the subjects of stroke and cerebrovascular disease in general, and the role that cardiac lesions play in the pathogenesis of stroke, several excellent books and monographs or chapters within larger texts have been published.[65,70,105,153] It is the goal of this chapter to interest the reader in further investigating the renaissance in the study of important interactions between heart and brain.

ATHEROSCLEROSIS OF CEREBRAL VERSUS SYSTEMIC AND CORONARY VESSELS

The pathogenesis of atherosclerosis is discussed at length in Chapter 7. Of particular interest to the neuropathologist is an understanding of the degree of atherosclerosis that might be expected in the cerebral vessels in the presence of severe systemic atherosclerotic disease. One of the best studies, that by Fisher and colleagues,[45] closely examined the extent and severity of atherosclerosis in carotid and vertebral arteries (both extra- and intracranial) at necropsy in nearly 180 patients. It was concluded that atherosclerosis of extracranial carotid arteries is usually less than that in the aorta but greater than that in vertebral and intracranial cerebral arteries. This finding was valid for both men and women, whether normotensive or hypertensive. Severe atherosclerosis, including occlusive atheromatous disease, was common in the great vessels of the neck, although not always symptomatic. When occlusive atherosclerotic disease was symptomatic, occlusion had usually occurred extracranially in the carotid arteries, when intracranially in arteries of the vertebrobasilar system. (This observation may have contributed to the popularity of surgical carotid endarterectomy.) Focal atherosclerosis was more likely in carotid than in vertebral arteries. Hypertension had, in general, aggravated cerebral atherosclerosis and, in particular, basilar atherosclerosis with resultant stenosis. The results of this study must be interpreted with the caveat that it was done during the 1960s, when aggressive antihypertensive therapy was not as prevalent as it is currently. Not surprisingly, Fisher et al.[45] found that atherosclerosis increased significantly for all patients after the age of 50 years, particularly in the aorta. A similar rapid increase in the severity of carotid atherosclerosis occurred after the age of 50 years, but with a slower rate of incline than the progression of atherosclerosis found in the aorta.

It must be remembered that coronary artery disease is a significant cause of death in patients with cerebrovascular disease, precisely because the two often coexist.[111] Symptomatic cerebrovascular disease usually begins later than coronary artery disease, at least in western populations, and intracranial vessels undergo atherosclerotic change approximately 10 years after their coronary counterparts. In addition, coronary and extracranial carotid atherosclerosis precede intracranial atherosclerosis, especially in white males. The role of some risk factors for vascular disease (e.g., hypercholesterolemia, cigarette smoking) is better defined for coronary atherosclerosis than for symptomatic atherosclerosis of cerebral vessels.

Among patients undergoing cerebrovascular surgical procedures (e.g., carotid endarterectomy), operative mortality is relatively high in those with symptomatic coronary artery disease. The most common cause of death for patients with a cerebral infarct or transient ischemic attack (TIA) is a myocardial infarct, rather than neurologic disease.[62] Stroke after coronary artery bypass grafting is said to occur in less than 5 percent of patients.[62] Occasionally, carotid artery reconstruction is performed before elective coronary artery bypass grafting in patients with symptomatic carotid disease reflected in the central nervous system (CNS). Simultaneous procedures on cervical and coronary artery vessels are infrequently warranted and inherently more risky.[62]

Furlan and Craciun[51] studied patients who had undergone coronary artery bypass grafting (CABG) and angiographically documented significant stenosis of the internal carotid artery (significant stenosis being defined as greater than 50 percent stenosis of the vascular lumen). Of 144 patients, 115 had bilateral internal carotid artery (ICA) lesions and combined surgical procedures with unilateral ICA endarterectomy. Another 29 (including 11 with bilateral carotid lesions) had CABG only. In the 115 with bilateral carotid disease and combined surgery, there were eight perioperative strokes (7 percent of patients), and three-fourths were on the same side as the endarterectomy. Furlan and Craciun[51] concluded that asymptomatic unilateral ICA stenosis of less than 90 percent severity did not increase stroke risk during open heart surgery for CABG.

EFFECTS OF CARDIAC LESIONS ON THE ADULT NERVOUS SYSTEM

This section deals with effects on the brain of specific groups of cardiac diseases (e.g., endocarditis, mitral valve prolapse, arrhythmias). There are several excellent reviews on the subject.[11,12,27,49,72] Furlan[49] defined five key areas of interest for investigators studying the interactions between heart and brain. The first, cardiovascular neurobiology or autonomic neurophysiology, is more broadly defined as "cerebral mechanisms of (autonomic) cardiovascular and respiratory control." The neurologic and neuropathologic consequences of open heart surgery are discussed in the section on sequelae of open heart surgery and cardiac arrest, as are complications of cardiopulmonary resuscitation, especially that of global brain ischemia. The interaction of risk factors for cerebrovascular and cardiovascular disease is discussed in the section on atherosclerosis of cerebral versus systemic and coronary vessels. The importance of cardioembolic causes of stroke will become manifest in the present section.

In general, emboli to the CNS produce hemorrhagic infarcts.[12,69,71,161] On clinical grounds, however, a patient who experiences a hemorrhagic infarct may have either an atheroembolic or a cardioembolic stroke; the two entities are not always easily distinguishable.

Cardiac lesions as causes of brain infarcts are especially important in young people.[72] Nevertheless, stroke is unusual in the young. In children and young adults, a probable cause for a cerebral infarct can be identified in approximately 70 to 90 percent of persons.[72] The relevant causes include arterial dissections of the cervical carotid or vertebral arteries (the cause of approximately 4 to 22 percent of brain infarcts in the young), a prothrombic state, and cardiogenic embolism (the cause of approximately one-third of strokes in this age group). The relative importance of cardiogenic embolism to the clinician investigating a stroke in a young person, however, is apparent; extensive studies of heart structure and function including two-dimensional echocardiography, wall-motion studies, and transesophageal echocardiography are required. The overall importance of cardioembolic stroke has also become clear in the detailed clinical data collected by several stroke registries.[20,47,108]

Figures vary from center to center, but one-fifth to one-sixth of ischemic strokes are secondary to cardiogenic embolism. The clinician must appreciate this, because many of these causes of stroke are preventable or treatable, provided appropriate modalities are used. Several clinical features may suggest a cardiogenic embolism to the brain.[11,27] They include an acute onset of a neurologic deficit, which is maximal from the onset, the presence of a potential cardiac source of embolism, the existence of multiple infarcts in several vessel territories of the CNS, and the presence of a hemorrhagic component (Fig. 28–1) to an infarct[100,101] as assessed by computed tomographic (CT) scans. Supportive evidence consists of the existence of little or no atherosclerosis in the great vessels demonstrated by cerebral angiography, as well as the occurrence of emboli to other end organs (e.g., kidneys and spleen), although the latter may be clinically silent, whereas cerebral lesions usually declare themselves by a neurologic deficit. Hemorrhagic infarcts may be caused by nonembolic sources, such as watershed phenomena secondary to hypotension, or venous thrombosis.

Cardiogenic emboli usually travel to the middle cerebral artery (MCA) bifurcation (Fig. 28–2) in the Sylvian fissure or to parietal or angular branches of the MCA.[11] When they pass to the vertebrobasilar system (approximately 10 percent), such emboli usually lodge in the basilar tip and may cause occipital ischemia, producing visual complaints. Anterior cerebral artery (ACA) territory emboli are

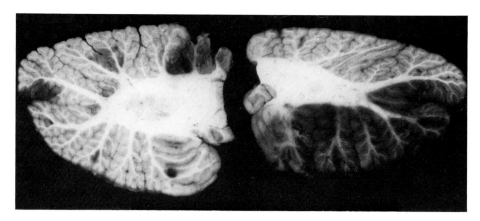

Fig. 28–1. Parasagittal sections of fixed cerebellar hemispheres. Patient had severe cardiomyopathy with biventricular mural thrombi (heart weight: 500 g). There was extensive endomyocardial fibrosis in both ventricles. Note large hemorrhagic infarcts secondary to emboli from the ventricular thrombi in both cerebellar hemispheres, but larger in the right cerebellar hemisphere. Infarct in the right cerebellar hemisphere is approximately in the distribution of the posterior inferior cerebellar artery.

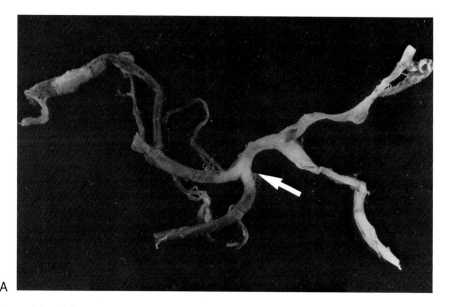

A

Fig. 28–2. (A) Middle cerebral artery dissected out of the Sylvian fissure from the fixed brain of a patient with endocarditis. Note the pale, Y-shaped embolus (arrow) lodged at the bifurcation of the right middle cerebral artery. (*Figure continues.*)

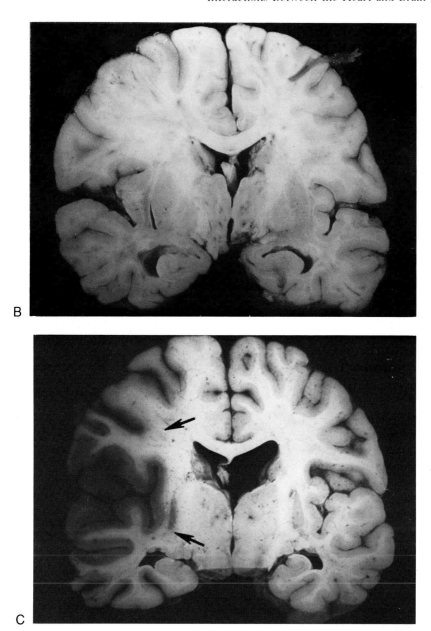

Fig. 28–2 (*Continued*) (**B**) Resultant right hemisphere infarct, with cerebral edema and right-to-left shift of midline structures. (**C**) Effects of a recent embolus that lodged in the left middle cerebral artery at a comparable location, in a 12-year-old boy with a complex history of congenital heart disease and multiple cardiac thrombi. The patient had a Fontan procedure performed 13 days before death and became hemiparetic 6 days later. Note the large area of dusky gray discoloration of the cortex (arrows) and relative loss of distinction in the cortex–white matter junction of the left cerebral hemisphere. The changes are essentially confined to the territory of the middle cerebral artery, with sparing of the anterior and posterior cerebral artery territories. Cerebral edema, which is usually maximal 2 to 4 days after an infarct, has subsided, so that the two hemispheres appear roughly symmetric in size and shape despite the large left cerebral infarct.

1034   Cardiovascular Pathology

much less common than MCA territory emboli. Table 28–1 presents the relative importance of different cardiac conditions as causes of embolic stroke. Each entity presented in Table 28–1 is discussed below.

When a cardioembolic stroke is suspected, one must remember that echocardiography, advanced though the technology may be, is not a foolproof method of demonstrating a cardiac source of emboli.[152] Two-dimensional echocardiography is said to have a limit of resolution of approximately 4 mm and is also a relatively poor investigational procedure with which to assess the presence of thrombi within the atrial appendage. It is incumbent, then, upon the pathologist investigating an unusual cerebral infarct (particularly of sudden onset and especially in a young patient) at necropsy to examine the heart and great vessels diligently for a source of emboli. Ventricular thrombi usually occur with large infarcts of the anterior myocardial wall and transmural myocardial infarcts, as well as infarcts that involve the cardiac septum.

DeBono and Warlow[35] emphasize the importance of seeking a source of emboli in patients with TIA or retinal ischemia who come to the attention of a neurologist. In more than 100 such patients who were investigated, approximately one-third had structural abnormalities of the heart, including mitral valve prolapse, aortic or mitral regurgitation, or aortic or mitral stenosis. Approximately one-third showed arrhythmias on appropriate 24-hour Holter cardiac monitoring, and approximately 15 percent showed evidence of ischemic cardiac disease. One-third of patients had a history or clinical evidence of hypertension. Only slightly more than one-third of patients who received cerebral angiograms had significant arterial lesions, and many had both cardiac and cervical carotid lesions. Of interest, even after extensive and relatively exhaustive investigation, was that one-fourth of patients had no evidence of cardiovascular disease. Nevertheless, the study demonstrates the etiologic diversity of cerebral or retinal ischemia in a large group of patients and the importance of considering a cardiac source of brain or retinal ischemia. The need for a detailed car-

diac investigation in patients who experience cerebral ischemia has been stressed by others.[19,146] The investigation assumes added importance if cerebral angiography shows the carotid and vertebral arteries to be free of disease.[146]

Endocarditis

Endocarditis may be caused by an infectious organism or it may occur without infection, such as nonbacterial thrombotic endocarditis (NBTE) (see Ch. 23). Although these two entities have important interrelationships themselves, they are considered separately.

Infective Endocarditis

Infective endocarditis (IE) may occur on a patient's native heart valve, or on a prosthetic valve.[11,27] Of patients with IE involving a native valve, 13 to 33 percent will experience emboli. By contrast, in patients with IE involving a prosthetic valve and who do not receive anticoagulant treatment emboli will develop more commonly (approximately 50 to 70 percent). Anticoagulant treatment significantly decreases this percentage to the range of 5 to 15 percent but increases the risk of serious intracerebral hemorrhage.[27] The pattern of IE has recently changed and continues to change in an era of evolving social mores and surgical practice. Patients who have open heart surgery for coronary, valvular, or congenital heart disease are at increased risk of IE, as are intravenous drug abusers.[7] Over the past 20 years, the age of patients in whom IE develops has increased, and up to one-third of those with IE appear to have no underlying cardiac disease or "silent" disease if it is present. IE is also more common in the immunocompromised host (Fig. 28–3). The infectious microorganisms that cause IE are discussed in Chapter 23. Peripheral emboli as complications of IE are clinically apparent in more than one-tenth of patients but are found significantly more often at postmortem examination.[7] Complications of infectious emboli shed by an infected cardiac valve (native or prosthetic) include abscesses, ischemia, infarcts, and mycotic aneurysm, although these are by no means mutually exclusive entities, in terms of pathogenesis.

Pruitt et al.[124] studied more than 200 patients with IE seen during the mid-1960s and early 1970s. Their age range was 3 months to 89 years, and more than one-third had clinically apparent neurologic complications. When the literature was reviewed, an estimated 25 percent of patients with IE were noted to develop neurologic complications, with a broad range from study to study. In general, neurologic complications are a poor prognostic feature in patients with IE. Many studied died as a direct complication of their neurologic difficulties. In 36 of the more than 200 patients, neurologic problems were the first sign of IE. The most common manifestation was that of cerebral embolism, although seizures, meningismus, subarachnoid hemorrhage, intracerebral hemorrhage, and even subdural hematomas occurred. CNS symptoms were especially likely when the infectious agent was *Staphylococcus aureus*, *Streptococcus pneumoniae*, anaerobic streptococci, or Enterobacteriaceae. Neurologic problems were much more frequent in patients with infection of the mitral than aortic valve.

The types of cerebral abnormality identified included infarcts in the MCA territory (34 of 218 patients), meningeal signs and symptoms (33), seizures (24), multiple microemboli (23), and microscopic evidence of brain abscess (8). Mycotic aneurysms were seen in four patients, whereas subarachnoid hemorrhage without an obvious mycotic aneurysm occurred in five, and watershed infarcts in three patients. A large brain abscess was identified in a single patient. Embolism, when present, was to the MCA and was often fatal. Large and small cerebral emboli were more common with mitral valve infection, and this did not appear to be related to associated atrial fibrillation. Of interest was that noncerebral peripheral emboli occurred with the same incidence when vegetations were on mitral or aortic valves. Almost 50 percent of patients with cardiogenic cerebral emboli experienced emboli to other viscera. Emboli that had occurred within 2 weeks of the onset of IE were

associated with endocarditis caused by virulent microorganisms (especially *S. aureus* and *Enterococcus*). Those that occurred later in the clinical course were more commonly secondary to IE caused by *Streptococcus*.

Cerebral embolism of infected material was also thought to be of pathogenetic importance in causing cerebral abscess or mycotic aneurysm when these lesions were found. Infectious or mycotic aneurysms (the former term is preferable) of peripheral vessels in the brains of IE patients occur much less commonly than does cerebral embolism. In older series, infectious aneurysms account for 2.5 to 6 percent of all intracerebral aneurysms identified at centers where vascular disease is studied in detail. Infectious microaneurysms (Fig. 28–4) frequently rupture, producing fatal intracerebral or subarachnoid hemorrhage. As expected, the aneurysms may be single or multiple. There is evidence that they may heal with antibiotic therapy.

In an older study, Roach and Drake[129] found infectious aneurysms in 4.6 percent of patients with IE. They most commonly involved branches of the MCA, less commonly the ACA and PCA. Various organisms were cultured. It is important to remember that, even in this day, a pathologist examining brain tissue from an intracerebral hematoma or the surrounding brain parenchyma (Fig. 28–4) should carefully examine the resected tissue rather than treating it simply as "clot." In this way, a clinician may be alerted to the presence of IE not previously suspected on clinical grounds.

Theories of the pathogenesis of infectious aneurysms center on two main mechanisms: (1) a septic embolus lodges within a vessel (Fig. 28–4), and microorganisms and inflammatory cells move into the vessel wall and weaken it; and (2) infectious material moves into vasa vasorum of cerebral vessels with resultant thrombosis and necrosis of the vessel wall and subsequent weakening, possibly leading to rupture.[109]

A recent study of IE with or without infectious aneurysms[134] found that, among patients with such aneurysms, more than one-half experienced subarachnoid hemorrhage without warning whereas just under 50 per-

Table 28–1.   Causes of Cardioembolic Stroke (Brain Infarcts)[a]

Clinical Condition	Location of Potential Emboli
Atrial fibrillation	Left atrium (e.g., appendage)
Ischemic heart disease	
Acute/recent	Left ventricle, endocardial surface
Chronic/old	Apical (e.g., left ventricle), ventricular aneurysm surface
Rheumatic heart disease (i.e., mitral stenosis/ regurgitation)	Auricle/dilated atrium; atrial endocardial "jet" lesions
Endocarditis	
Infective	Valve surface and attachment, mitral endocardium
Nonbacterial thrombotic emboli (NBTE)/ marantic	Valve surface
Prosthetic heart valve	Site of attachment and/or device surface
Mitral valve prolapse (MVP)—myxomatous degeneration	Atrial site of valve attachment, valve surface
Mitral annulus calcification	Attached to valve surface
Calcific aortic stenosis	Attached thrombi or calcified degenerate material
Congenital heart disease (including paradoxical embolism)	Miscellaneous
Cardiomyopathy	Atrium/ventricle—usually in muscular trabeculae
Cardiac tumors (usually atrial myxoma)	Usually attached to margin of septum secundum

[a] Entities are listed in approximately decreasing order of frequency.

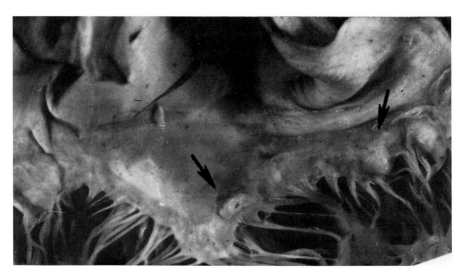

Fig. 28–3. Mitral valve from a 39-year-old patient with AIDS and disseminated Kaposi's sarcoma and cytomegalovirus (CMV) infection. Acute infective endocarditis was seen with vegetations involving tricuspid, mitral, and aortic valves. Histologically, the vegetations, including those seen on the mitral valve (arrows), showed predominantly gram-positive cocci but also gram-negative cocci and rods.

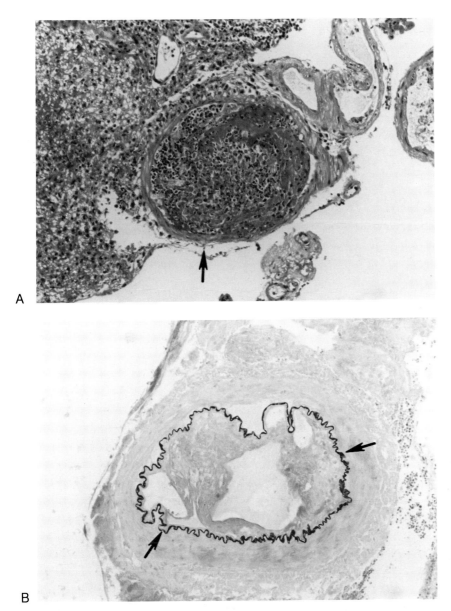

Fig. 28–4. Brain biopsy material from a young man with a long history of drug abuse and infective endocarditis. Resected material consisted of blood clot, brain tissue, and several blood vessels. (**A**) Small artery occluded by thrombus, within which inflammatory cells (including polymorphonuclear leukocytes) are prominent (arrow). Surrounding brain tissue shows vacuolization and scattered inflammatory cells. (H&E × 210.) (**B**) Another small artery that has undergone thrombosis and recanalization (Elastic van Gieson, × 210.) Elastica (arrows) is clearly visible. (*Figure continues.*)

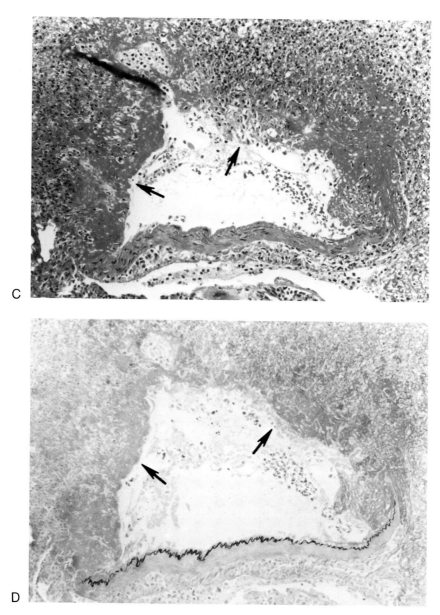

Fig. 28–4 *(Continued)*. **(C, D)** Parallel sections, showing intact lower portion of the artery, whereas superior portion (arrows) shows extensive fibrinoid necrosis, and surrounding acute and chronic inflammatory cells. This represents an infectious aneurysm and was the presumed site of intraparenchymal bleeding in this patient. (Fig. C: H&E, × 210; Fig. D: Elastic van Gieson, × 210.) *(Figure continues.)*

cent had some type of neurologic prodrome, suggesting focal signs and symptoms consistent with cerebral embolism. Overall, patients with IE showed no significant difference in the frequency of neurologic symptoms whether they harbored mycotic aneurysms. The risk of rupture of an infectious aneurysm after antibiotic therapy was extremely low.

Infectious or mycotic aneurysms have also been observed in children with various types

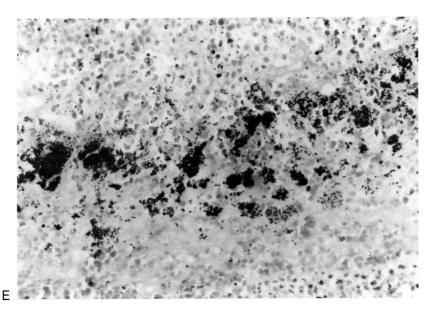

E

Fig. 28–4 (*Continued*). (**E**) Clusters of gram-positive cocci among the inflammatory cells within the brain parenchyma and the aneurysm wall. (Gram, × 530.)

of heart disease, including ventricular septal defect and rheumatic heart disease.[16] Neurologic signs and symptoms preceded evidence of IE or sepsis, just as they may in adults. Clinical presentations included intracerebral hemorrhage, seizures, and hemiparesis. When considering intracerebral hemorrhage in patients with IE,[74] it is apparent when all patients with IE and intracerebral hemorrhage are considered, that mycotic or infectious aneurysms are a relatively infrequent cause of hemorrhage.

A recent review of neurologic complications of endocarditis (involving 113 patients with native valve IE and 62 with prosthetic valve IE followed clinically for 12 years)[135] concluded that neurologic complications occur with comparable frequency in patients with native or prosthetic valve IE. *S. aureus* endocarditis increased the risk of neurologic complications and death, and mortality did not appear to be significantly higher in those who had experienced neurologic morbidity.

Brain abscess as a complication of IE occurs with a postmortem incidence of approximately 4 to 5 percent.[124] When abscesses are found, they are usually caused by highly virulent mi-

croorganisms, especially *S. aureus*. In the older literature (i.e., before computed tomography scans were in general use), abscesses were often not suspected during life. Scanning techniques now make the diagnosis of a mass lesion fairly straightforward, although even the best scans may fail to distinguish between abscess and tumor, and microabscesses may be found only at necropsy. As with mycotic or infectious aneurysms, abscesses probably originate from septic emboli. When cerebrospinal fluid (CSF) was examined in patients with IE and neurologic complaints,[124] approximately one-third of samples showed no significant abnormality, less than one-third yielded purulent CSF, significant numbers of patients (25 percent) showed a predominant lymphocytosis in the spinal fluid, and 13 percent showed evidence of hemorrhage.

Nonbacterial Thrombotic Endocarditis

Nonbacterial thrombotic endocarditis (NBTE) is a clinicopathologic entity of unknown etiology. Generally seen in patients who have a wasting disease such as cancer, it has also been described in patients with acquired immune deficiency syndrome (AIDS) and in a significant proportion of patients treated by bone marrow transplantation.[4,11,26,27,55,119,168]

Studies that emphasize the clinicopathologic aspects of neurologic complications of NBTE[18,96] conclude that NBTE can occur at any age, although its peak incidence is between the ages of 61 and 70 years. It occurs as often in males as in females. Vegetations (more accurately described as thrombi) were seen most commonly on the aortic valve and in decreasing frequency on mitral, tricuspid, and pulmonic valves, although significant numbers of patients have more than one valve involved.

In the series reported by Biller et al.,[18] malignant neoplasms were found at postmortem examination in almost one-half of NBTE patients, and some patients had more than one primary tumor. Brain emboli occurred in one-third of patients, whereas almost two-thirds had emboli to other organs. Coagulation abnormalities were present in approximately 20 percent of patients, and disseminated intravascular coagulation (DIC) was seen in 10 percent. Of underlying malignancies associated with NBTE, the largest number were adenocarcinomas (with the pancreas being the organ most commonly involved), whereas approximately 10 percent of cases had lymphoreticular or hematologic malignancies. All tumors were widespread at the time NBTE was discovered. Non-neoplastic disorders were also commonly associated with NBTE. These included cardiac disorders (18 percent of patients), hepatic or gastrointestinal disease (less than 10 percent), and pulmonary disorders (e.g., chronic obstructive pulmonary disease, in approximately 5 percent of patients). Other syndromes associated with NBTE included renal disease, vasculitis, drug overdose, and miscellaneous infections. The cause of NBTE could not be identified in approximately 7 percent of patients. Neurologic signs and symptoms were prominent in some patients but were not necessarily the most common clinical manifestation of NBTE. From a practical perspective, it is significant that NBTE is not the most common cause of a cerebral infarct in a patient with underlying malignancy.[63]

Other large clinicopathologic studies of NBTE[132] found that it occurs with a frequency of more than 7 percent in patients with bronchiolar carcinoma or adenocarcinoma of the lung and have confirmed the frequent association with carcinomas of pancreas and prostate. It has also been seen in children,[176] in whom it may also generate cerebral emboli. Many affected children had had a history of cardiac catheterization and were in multisystem failure. The diagnosis was frequently made only at postmortem examination. In general, children and young adults with NBTE have a broader spectrum of systemic disease than do older patients, including lymphoma, collagen vascular disease, and Goodpasture syndrome.

The pathologist examining the brain of a patient with cancer and multiple cerebral infarcts at autopsy must be aware of this possible cause of cerebral infarcts, since one group[27] estimated that brain emboli may occur in 30 percent of patients with NBTE. In addition, cerebral emboli may antedate the definitive diagnosis of an underlying cause of NBTE or an associated lesion, in the event that one is eventually found.

Mitral Valve Prolapse

Several excellent reviews have emphasized the clinical, pathologic, and etiologic aspects of mitral valve prolapse (MVP).[34,64,84,171,172] This enigmatic disease of the mitral valve is discussed in Chapter 25. Its overall incidence has been estimated at 3 to 4 percent in males and at more than 5 percent in females.[34] The severity of the lesion can be graded clinically with the most severe grades associated with infective endocarditis or dysfunction of the mitral valve. MVP may be a cause of sudden, unexplained death and arrhythmias develop in patients with MVP.[36] This is obviously of diagnostic and therapeutic importance in considering the etiology of a stroke syndrome that occurs in a patient with MVP.

The association of stroke with MVP appears well established.[21] Boughner and Barnett[21] re-emphasized the frequent finding of MVP in the adult population and highlighted the fact that the entity is discovered more commonly at autopsy than is suspected by clinical examination. Although an increased risk of stroke exists in patients with MVP, the cause is not always apparent and indeed may be multifactorial. Echocardiography, refined though it is, may not always reveal the lesion. In addition, the extent of mitral valve involvement is extremely variable from patient to patient and the extent of the valvular disease may influence the risk of stroke, at least of embolic stroke. The clinical difficulty is summarized by Boughner and Barnett[21] as follows: "It is increasingly difficult to argue that there is no relationship between the two [MVP and stroke]. The greatest difficulty is in anticipating [the patient] in whom the association will occur."

The association between MVP and stroke was suggested on clinical grounds during the late 1970s and early 1980s. Echocardiography demonstrated evidence of MVP in 40 percent of patients under the age of 45 years who experienced stroke or TIA, but in only 6.8 percent of age-matched control patients.[13] In 18 of 24 patients who had experienced a TIA or stroke, MVP was the only recognizable probable cause. Other studies by Barnett and his group[10,14] have established the association between MVP and amaurosis fugax, retinal artery occlusion, TIA, stroke, and seizure disorders. MVP with retinal or cerebral ischemic events is more likely to occur in women than in men, and the symptomatic age group is usually 35 to 55 years. MVP has often been unsuspected prior to a cerebral ischemic event, and some patients have an entirely un-

remarkable clinical history and physical examination. Cardiac rhythm disturbances associated with MVP have included premature ventricular contractions, atrial flutter and fibrillation, and bursts of ventricular tachyarrhythmia. Familial stroke syndromes related to MVP have also been described.

The pathogenesis of events leading to stroke in patients with MVP may include fissuring and thrombus formation on abnormal valves that show myxomatous degeneration, with resultant embolization. It is important to remember that only an embolus as small as 5 mm in diameter is required to obstruct the middle cerebral artery at its bifurcation in the Sylvian fissure (see Fig. 28–2). Infective endocarditis may complicate MVP, but is an infrequent occurrence (less than 10 percent of patients). With MVP, systemic emboli occur much less frequently than emboli to the brain. In some respects, the diagnosis of MVP as a cause of stroke is one of exclusion, and a clinician faced with a patient with stroke or TIA must exclude other causes of cerebral ischemia, even in the presence of MVP.

Some investigators have shown that patients with MVP at risk of stroke also have significant prolapse of the aortic valve.[9] The prolapse may be associated with significant diffuse thickening of the affected valves, either aortic or mitral, or both.

Despite the association of MVP and stroke, autopsy documentation of fatal stroke from an embolic source associated with MVP is relatively scarce.[142] In the small number of autopsy-confirmed cases of embolic stroke in patients with MVP, only a myxomatous mitral valve has been demonstrated whereas a cardiac thrombus was not seen grossly, although it may be detected microscopically.[142] The association of MVP and cerebral ischemic events is especially significant, however, in patients without other risk factors for stroke or cerebrovascular disease.[91] It must also be re-emphasized that stroke occurring in young adults with MVP is extremely rare (approximately 1 in 5,000 to 6,000 patients per year[27]). A large research effort aims to ascertain which subset of patients with MVP is at increased risk of cerebral or retinal ischemic events.[76]

Rice et al.[126] described a family with 27 members, 8 of whom were found to have MVP by echocardiography. Four within this family suffered a total of eight cerebral ischemic events by the age of 40 years, and MVP appeared to be the only risk factor for the stroke syndrome. MVP has also been suggested as one cause of infantile hemiplegia.[127]

Arrhythmias

Of cardiac arrhythmias, the one most commonly associated with an increased incidence of embolic stroke is atrial fibrillation. Those with chronic atrial fibrillation have a fivefold increase in stroke risk over patients without fibrillation, and those who have atrial fibrillation and rheumatic heart disease have almost a 20-fold increased risk of stroke.[27,67] Atrial fibrillation accounts for 12 to 15 percent of all ischemic strokes. It is estimated that more than one-third of strokes in elderly patients are associated with atrial fibrillation. Also, that one-third of persons with chronic atrial fibrillation will have a stroke at some point in their lives.[67] In addition, "silent" strokes are a frequent finding in patients with atrial fibrillation.

Atrial fibrillation may not itself be as significant a predictor of stroke as it is of underlying cardiac disease, which may produce emboli to the brain. However, this point is disputed. Subgroups of patients with atrial fibrillation at increased risk of stroke include those with congestive heart failure. Controversy exists as to the mechanism of atrial fibrillation-associated cerebral infarcts,[75] as well as the criteria used to make the clinical diagnosis.[73] Some studies[37] attempted to analyze subgroups with atrial fibrillation at high or low risk for emboli, with limited success. Anticoagulant prophylaxis in the treatment of patients with atrial fibrillation is also controversial, since treatment may lead to more serious sequelae than the arrhythmia itself.

Nevertheless, more than one-half of strokes associated with atrial fibrillation are secondary to cardiogenic emboli. In younger patients, atrial fibrillation without other cardiopulmonary disease carries a relatively low risk of emboli.[67] In other patients, such as those with atrial fibrillation related to thyrotoxicosis, emboli are most likely in older patients with cardiac dilation and congestive heart failure. Whereas the association of chronic atrial fibrillation with stroke is relatively well established, the association between intermittent atrial fibrillation and cardiogenic emboli is less clear. Patients without rheumatic heart disease but with atrial fibrillation who have sustained a clinically significant stroke show a significant risk of a later stroke, with a recurrence rate estimated at 15 to 20 percent in the first year alone. It has also been claimed that the greatest risk of cerebral thromboembolism is at the onset of sustained atrial fibrillation.[112] Recurrent embolic events are common and embolic infarcts related to atrial fibrillation tend to be large and clinically disabling.

A review of 150 patients with atrial fibrillation[145] revealed that approximately one-third had evidence of stroke or peripheral embolism. Most infarcts that occurred had no preceding TIA as a warning. Thromboemboli also occurred in persons in whom atrial fibrillation was unsuspected before the cerebral infarct. CT scan analysis of patients with chronic atrial fibrillation showed that a significant percentage (10 to 15 percent) had evidence of previous, clinically silent cerebral infarcts.[92] A Scandinavian study[122] estimated an even higher percentage of clinically "silent" encephalic lesions.

Patients with paroxysmal atrial fibrillation[120] may have cerebral emboli at the onset of the arrhythmia. After this syndrome evolved into chronic atrial fibrillation, the incidence of emboli increased significantly and many occurred during the first year of chronic atrial fibrillation. The same group[121] demonstrated that atrial fibrillation associated with thyrotoxicosis does not carry an increased risk of stroke above that for individuals of comparable age.

Although clinically of much less importance than atrial fibrillation, the sick sinus syndrome, a chronic disorder of sinoatrial function, is also associated with stroke. The mechanism may be that of decreased brain perfusion or thromboembolism.[11] Sick sinus syndrome is associated with myotonic dystrophy, other types of muscular dystrophy, and Friedreich's ataxia. Cardiac pacing in affected patients is not protective against strokes.[46] The cerebral ischemic symptoms experienced by many patients[44] are often vague and nonspecific and include syncope, possibly due to decreased cerebral perfusion. Such symptoms may also occur with paroxysmal tachycardia and atrioventricular disorders with complete heart block.[11]

Myocardial Infarct and Coronary Angioplasty

Persons who suffer a myocardial infarct are at increased risk of stroke because impaired cardiac function may limit the amount of blood that reaches the brain, or hypokinetic segments of the myocardial wall may provide a nidus where a thrombus can form, creating the potential for cardioembolic stroke (Fig. 28–5). Emboli may arise from thrombi that form soon after an acute myocardial infarct in regions of mural dyskinesia or akinetic segments or from thrombi formed at the site of a ventricular aneurysm that develops during organization and repair of infarcted myocardium. In general, stroke risk after a myocardial infarct varies directly with the size of the infarct as judged by elevation in serum creatine phosphokinase (CPK) levels. In one study,[159] when the CPK was greater than 1,160 IU/L, stroke incidence was approximately 24 times that when the peak CPK was less than 1,160. Many strokes occurred less than 10 days after the myocardial infarct, and virtually all developed less than 18 days after the infarct.

A pathologist examining, at autopsy, a person who suffered a myocardial infarct and ebral symptoms must be aware that cardiopulmonary resuscitation carries its own risks of neurologic injury. Bone marrow emboli, for instance, have been seen in the cerebral circulation after closed cardiac massage.[131] Also, other materials may enter the systemic circulation and find their way to the brain, including air, fat, and small amounts of pulmonary and bronchial epithelium.[165] Whenever bones are fractured, fat emboli may pass to the brain and produce a syndrome characterized by restlessness, confusion, stupor, and coma.[40,87] The pathologic correlate is the presence of petechial hemorrhages found predominantly within the cerebral white matter. The pathologist must have a high index of suspicion that such emboli will be present and must perform appropriate fat stains on frozen material before processing brain tissue.

In view of the increasing use of coronary angioplasty to treat patients with significant coronary artery disease, the pathologist must be aware that CNS complications may also arise, although they are decidedly rare.[54] Their frequency has been estimated at 0.2 percent; documented complications include hemispheric infarcts, a brainstem infarct, and a TIA. Emboli were thought to be the likely source of neurologic difficulties in three cases, including an air embolus in one patient. In two patients, the severely atherosclerotic aorta was traumatized during catheter insertion, presumably inducing the passage of atheroembolic material to the brain. Another patient suffered a hypotensive episode after an otherwise successful angioplasty procedure.

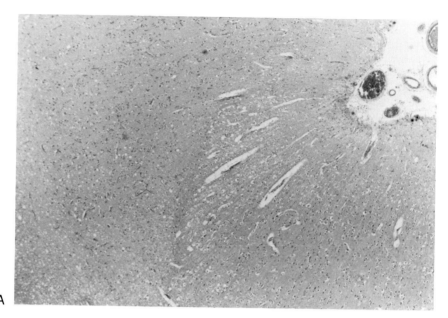

A

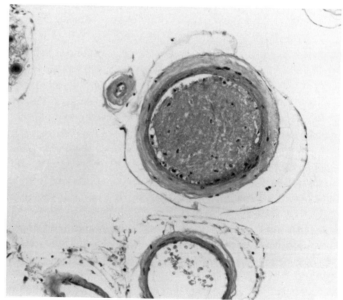

B

Fig. 28–5. Section of brain parenchyma (cortex and subcortical white matter, leptomeninges and meningeal blood vessels at upper right) from an 85-year-old woman with atherosclerotic coronary artery disease, an old anteroseptal infarct, and a significant history of cardiac arrhythmias requiring pacemaker insertion. Brain was grossly unremarkable, despite a history of dementia. (**A**) A recent infarct involving cortex and subcortical white matter, visualized as subtle vacuolization of the tissue. Eosinophilic neuronal change was also seen at higher magnification. (**B**) A leptomeningeal artery occluded by embolic material consisting of platelets and fibrin. (H&E; Fig. A: × 55; Fig. B: × 210.)

Complications of Catheterization and Artificial Cardiac Valves

Any reader of this text need not be reminded that atherosclerosis is a systemic disease and that atheromatous material within the vessel wall is brittle and relatively fragile, particularly in complicated atherosclerotic plaque. Atheromatous emboli are frequently seen at autopsy when persons over the age of 60 years are examined.[90] They were found in almost 1 percent of such patients examined postmortem, with sites of predilection including the kidneys, spleen, and brain. Obviously, not all lesions had been symptomatic, although it is again stressed that lesions in the brain are much more likely to be symptomatic than are those secondary to atheromatous emboli in other organs, particularly if the atheromatous emboli lodge within "eloquent" regions of the CNS.

Cardiac catheterization is not without hazard, although it is hoped that new technology and materials will minimize embolization of artificial materials to the brain.[39] In a study of children who had cardiac surgery or catheterization, "foreign" particles with a foreign body giant cell reaction were often found within distal organs, including the brain. Fiber emboli were detected in 8 percent of almost 200 patients during routine postmortem examination. All in whom fiber emboli were present had had angiograms and/or intracardiac surgical procedures or extracardiac procedures (e.g., pulmonary banding). One patient had fatal embolization of fiber material to the cerebral vessels, with extensive occlusion of the cerebral vasculature. The embolized materials included cotton and paper; particles were of variable size, but many had a width of approximately 2 μm and length of up to 40 μm. The authors showed that many fibers had been shed from drape material, gowns, caps, and masks.[39] The presumption is that such emboli would be preventable if

appropriate filtering techniques were used. In general, the importance of iatrogenic emboli to the brain cannot be overestimated.[57,167,170]

Cholesterol emboli, presumably originating in atheromatous plaques, have been documented in various organs after cardiac catheterization.[30] Other cerebral infarcts that follow cardiac catheterization[118] have been caused by one or more of several mechanisms, including dislodged atheromatous emboli, thrombus embolization from the catheter tip, in situ thrombosis or spasm of vessels, and hypotension.

A further complication, admittedly rare, of cardiac catheterization is that of cerebral hemorrhage after ergonovine administration.[123] The mechanism may be a transient increase in blood pressure caused by discomfort of the procedure and infusion of the drug, although the administration of a small dose of heparin at the beginning of the procedure may have been a contributory factor.

Prosthetic heart valves (Fig. 28–6) may produce emboli to the brain by one of several mechanisms. Such valves may be the nidus for infectious endocarditis (IE).[11,27] More importantly, they may be the site of thrombus formation, elements of which then embolize to the CNS. Also, components of a prosthetic heart valve may dislodge and travel to or obstruct the cerebral circulation.[147] A more extensive discussion of artificial cardiac valves and their complications is found in Chapters 39 and 40. It is important to remember that many patients with prosthetic valves are on anticoagulant therapy; a complication may be intracerebral hemorrhage or significant hemorrhagic transformation of an ischemic infarct. However, a group at the Mayo Clinic found that, at least in patients with IE related to prosthetic cardiac valves, anticoagulation did not significantly increase morbidity and mortality.[173] In fact, the incidence of major CNS complications increased, and mortality was significantly higher if anticoagulation was discontinued. It has been estimated that

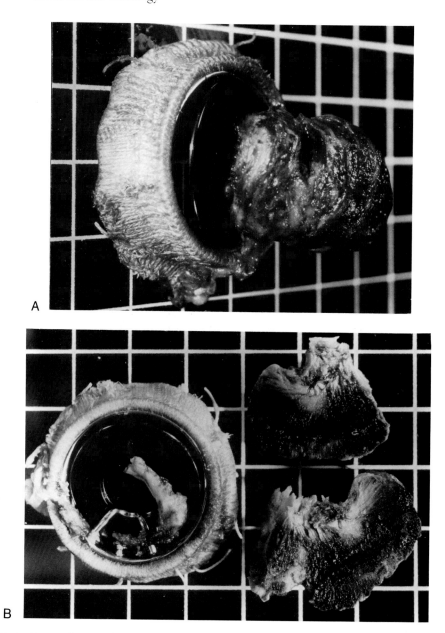

Fig. 28–6. Heart valve prosthesis (Björk-Shiley) showing extensive large adjacent thrombus. (**A**) Thrombus in situ. (**B**) Cross section. (Courtesy of Nir Kossovsky, M.D., Department of Pathology, UCLA Medical Center.)

the risk of embolization from prosthetic heart valves is 1 to 5 percent per year and is greater for the mitral than aortic valve.[11,27]

Cardiomyopathy

Cardiomyopathy is rarely associated with stroke or cerebrovascular symptoms.[27] However, intracardiac thrombi are relatively common in patients with dilated or restrictive cardiomyopathy (Fig. 28–7). Dilated, hypokinetic ventricular segments may also be present, and secondary atrial fibrillation may arise. The latter as an important risk factor of stroke is discussed above. Rarely, brain embolism may be the presenting feature of a cardiomyopathy.

Idiopathic hypertrophic cardiomyopathy (IHC) usually presents with cardiac symptoms or syncope.[52] In a series with follow-up of 150 patients, none presented with a stroke syndrome. All deaths in the follow-up period of (on average) more than 5 years were apparently attributable to cardiac causes, but approximately 7 percent of patients had cerebrovascular complications. A minority had stroke, whereas the remaining patients had TIAs only. The stroke risk was considered greater if a patient was in atrial fibrillation. Other groups[42] detected IHC in several patients in whom stroke was the presenting symptom. The strokes appeared to be embolic in origin. In two of the affected patients, echocardiography showed mitral valve vegetations with apparent infective endocarditis and intracardiac thrombus in a patient with a dilated form of cardiomyopathy that had developed from a hypertrophic form.

Clinically, intracardiac thrombi in persons with cardiomyopathy or other forms of cardiac disease are detectable by Indium-111 platelet scintigraphy.[94] Serial-echocardiography has shown that ventricular thrombi may disappear after a stroke.[38] Thus, a patient who has an embolic cerebral infarct at necropsy may have no remaining trace of an atrial or ventricular thrombus, even after a diligent search is made using histologic sections. Nevertheless, such a search is mandatory in these patients.

Recurrent cerebral embolism has also been clinically demonstrated in a young patient with cardiomyopathy probably secondary to amyloidosis,[128] and TIAs were attributed to a ventricular mural thrombus in a 58-year-old woman with adriamycin-induced cardiomyopathy.[140]

Mitral Annulus Calcification, Aortic Stenosis, and Rheumatic Heart Disease

Calcification of the mitral valve annulus (MAC) is a common clinical and autopsy finding in elderly patients (see Ch. 5). This age-related phenomenon occurs more frequently in hypertensive patients with diffuse atherosclerotic disease.[27] Patients at risk of this lesion may also have stroke related to atherosclerotic disease of the great vessels feeding the brain or intracranial vessels, making it difficult to assess the relative importance of MAC as a cause of cerebral infarcts. Nevertheless, studies in which large numbers of patients with MAC were followed[53] addressed the likely contribution of this cardiac lesion to the development of cerebral infarcts. The conclusions have been that MAC is probably better identified as a marker of generalized calcific atherosclerosis than as a source of cerebral emboli. MAC is also frequently complicated by infective endocarditis, atrioventricular block, and mitral regurgitation, and abnormalities of the conduction system of the heart are common.[48] Thus, while MAC is by no means a benign condition and is associated with other abnormalities that may give rise to embolic stroke, the association with specific stroke syndromes is not clear.

Embolic infarcts of the brain rarely complicate calcific aortic stenosis.[88] Indeed, calcific emboli within cerebral vessels have been

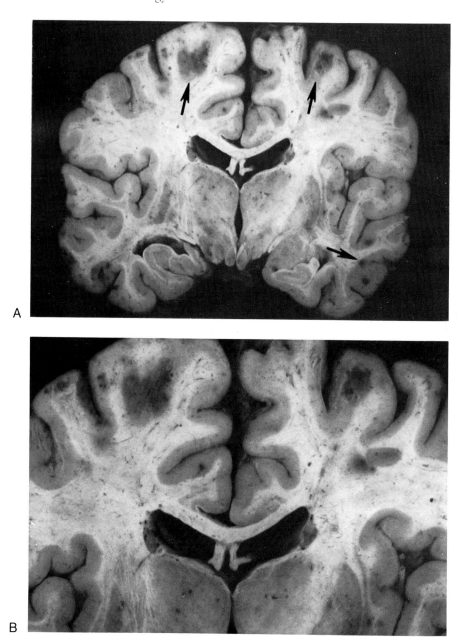

Fig. 28–7. Multiple embolic cerebral infarcts in a patient with Löffler's restrictive cardiomyopathy. At autopsy, biventricular mural thrombi were seen and there was extensive myocardial fibrosis within both ventricles. Coronal section of fixed brain at the level of the mammillary bodies (**A**) shows multiple recent infarcts, visualized as patchy areas of gray discoloration in multiple vessel territories of both cerebral hemispheres (arrows). (**B**) A magnified view of the larger cortical and subcortical infarcts.

confirmed at postmortem examination. Such emboli are more likely to occur in a patient who has had cardiac surgery or cardiac catheterization. Calcific emboli may also be seen in retinal arteries.[25]

It should not be forgotten that rheumatic heart disease may be a cause of significant morbidity and mortality.[27] Neurologic complications often result from thrombi on the atrial wall or within the atrial appendage. Mitral stenosis and atrial fibrillation also occur in affected persons, adding to the risk of cardiogenic emboli. A recent clinicopathologic conference[115] poignantly illustrated the clinical problem. A thrombus within the left ventricular apex was discovered in a patient who had clinical and pathologic criteria of rheumatic myocarditis, and massive cerebral infarcts had resulted from thromboembolism.

Cardiac Tumors

Neoplasms of the myocardium or endocardial surface are a rare cause of stroke (see also Ch. 35). Of tumors associated with neurologic dysfunction, the most common is atrial myxoma. In a retrospective analysis of 11 patients with pathologically documented atrial myxoma,[95] five had abnormalities on neurologic examination. The tumor was more common in females and much more common in the left atrium than in the right. All five patients who had neurologic abnormalities on examination showed CT scan evidence of bland cerebral infarcts. Neurologic symptoms were the presenting feature of the atrial myxoma in four patients, and echocardiography was frequently diagnostic. Gated magnetic resonance imaging (MRI) scans of the heart showed position and movement of the myxoma in two patients. In follow-up evaluation of the patients, which extended for 1 month to 7 years after tumor resection, 9 of 11 showed no recurrence of neurologic abnormalities.

This study[95] supports the reported incidence of neurologic complications in atrial myxoma, which is given as 25 to 45 percent.

Many neurologic complications are the result of cerebral emboli. Other complications of the tumor may include multiple fusiform aneurysms in peripheral branches of the cerebral vasculature, secondary to invasion of vessel walls by myxomatous tissue. These are thought to arise directly from emboli of myxomatous material. Of interest is that aneurysms caused by this mechanism may resolve after resection of the primary tumor. However, aneurysm formation and enlargement with resultant intracerebral hemorrhage may be delayed, manifesting several months after resection.[130] Mass effect may also result from the proliferation of myxomatous tissue in the brain.

Other large studies of atrial myxoma and associated neurologic complications[138] indicate the predominance of this tumor in females and emphasize that the tumor may occur at any age from the teens to the geriatric period. Rarely, tumors are bilateral. Transient or permanent ischemic events have been noted in all areas of the central neuraxis, including the spinal cord and retina. In most patients, cardiac and systemic complaints dominate the clinical picture, whereas neurologic abnormalities are of minor importance.

However, rare patients with atrial myxoma may present with CNS embolic disease and without a history of cardiac dysfunction.[160] In one, emboli of myxomatous material were actually visualized within retinal arterioles. Atrial myxoma may also present clinically as a peripheral vasculitis.[83] In one patient, myxomatous embolic material was seen in the blood vessels of a muscle biopsy. A pathologist must remember this unusual cause of peripheral embolic disease when examining biopsy tissues from patients with cryptic neurologic or systemic diseases.

Multiple strokes secondary to atrial myxoma have also been reported in individuals several months before they presented with cardiac symptoms related to their myxoma.[158] In one patient, multiple strokes in the vertebrobasilar distribution antedated detection

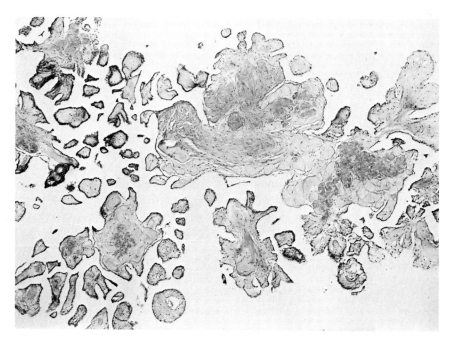

Fig. 28–8. Section of papillary fibroelastoma from a patient who experienced embolic stroke. In cross section, the neoplasm shows variably thickened avascular cores with overlying single layers of endothelial cells. (PAS, × 17.5.) (From Kasarskis et al.,[89] with permission.)

of the cardiac myxoma by 10 months. Myxomatous emboli to the spinal cord have also been described.[80]

A tumor much less frequently associated with stroke is the papillary fibroelastoma (Fig. 28–8). Kasarskis et al.[89] found this lesion in two patients with cardiogenic cerebral emboli and discovered six other similar patients in a review of the literature. Excision of the tumor appears to be curative. The tumor is composed of a variably thick avascular core covered by a single layer of endothelium-like cells (Fig. 28–8). Males are more commonly affected than females, but the number of cases described is small.

Miscellaneous

Some neurologic disorders are associated with cardiac or aortic disease, although not necessarily caused by the cardiac or aortic disease. There is a well-described association between coarctation of the aorta and berry aneurysms on the circle of Willis.[153] In addition, coincident rupture of a berry aneurysm and dissection of the aorta during sexual intercourse in a 34-year-old man have been reported.[102] The coincidence of clinical presentations was attributed in part to the rise in blood pressure observed during intercourse.

Embolic stroke has also been associated with aneurysm of the atrial septum.[41] This is an uncommon entity, and clinical examination and electrocardiography do not necessarily confirm the diagnosis. It can, however, be detected by two-dimensional echocardiography. Although an atrial septal aneurysm may coexist with a stroke syndrome, the causal relationship between the two is not well established in every case.

In a review of 36 patients with echocardiographic findings typical of atrial septal aneuryms,[15] more than one-fourth had significant cerebrovascular events. In one-half of 10 patients with strokes, a definite embolic origin related to the atrial septal aneurysm could be established. TIAs of probable embolic origin occurred in two patients, and one had a peripheral embolus. The cause of the embolic events was postulated as a thrombus associated with the septal aneurysm.

Some investigators stress that atrial septal aneurysm should be considered in those who have simultaneous emboli in both pulmonary and systemic circulations.[28] Cheng and Kisslo[28] emphasize that the only clinical entities that can produce such a syndrome are atrial septal aneurysm, biatrial myxoma, and paradoxic embolism.

CONGENITAL HEART DISEASE

Congenital heart disease predisposes to cerebral emboli by one or more of the following mechanisms: (1) right-to-left shunts, (2) an increased predisposition to endocarditis, and (3) associated arrhythmias, especially atrial fibrillation.[27] Stroke is quite rare in children and full-term infants but, when it occurs, a cardiac problem is very often the cause.[144] One must remember that many patients with congenital heart disease now have an excellent life expectancy, indicating that congenital heart disease may be anticipated as a significant and increasing cause of stroke in adults and even the elderly in the years to come (Fig. 28–9). Schoenberg et al.[144] have estimated the average annual incidence rate for strokes in children at approximately 2.5 cases/100,000; most of these are ischemic events. Of ischemic events, 26 percent are associated with preexisting heart disease and, overall, this is the commonest cause of ischemic stroke in this age group. Any discussion of congenital heart disease as a cause of stroke must be considered with the caveat that treatment modalities (both surgical and nonsurgical) for these disorders are changing and evolving, so that the

pattern of neuropathology seen in such patients is likely to change as well.

In a review of 29 patients with stroke complicating cyanotic congenital heart disease, Cottrill and Kaplan[33] found the commonest lesion to be cerebral venous thrombosis, including thrombosis of the dural sinuses. By contrast, only three arterial occlusions were identified. At particularly high risk of stroke were young cyanotic children whose hematologic indices showed hypochromic microcytic anemia. Strokes were especially common under the age of one year. Terplan[157] performed a detailed autopsy analysis on approximately 500 children with congenital heart disease, 17 percent of whom had experienced thromboembolic infarcts. Thromboemboli had occurred four to five times more commonly in surgical than in nonsurgical patients, and 18 thromboemboli were seen in direct association with catheterization, whereas 21 were seen after catheterization and surgical procedures. (A diligent search for thromboemboli by the examining pathologist is often required to find the responsible lesions.) The incidence of anoxic-ischemic necrosis of the cortex, either diffuse or focal, was also four times higher in the surgical group. Except in infants, venous thromboses were uncommon. The underlying cardiac disease in Terplan's series included shunting lesions in 172 patients, hypoplastic right heart syndrome in 125, hypoplastic left heart in 89, transposition of the great vessels in 86, and coarctation of the aorta in 26. The older literature[29] supports Terplan's finding that necrosis is much more common in the operative group than in persons who have not had surgery.

An eastern European study[23] of postmortem cerebral complications of congenital heart disease and cardiac surgery carried out on 45 patients showed that damage to white matter was more likely to occur in persons under the age of 3 months, whereas injury to gray matter was more likely in older persons. In this study, necrosis (when detected) was usually not a complication of microembolization. Figure

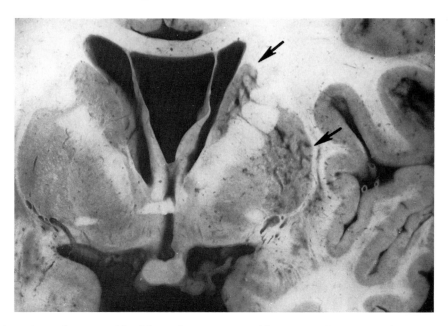

Fig. 28–9. Coronal section of fixed brain from a 22-year-old patient with Down syndrome in whom an atrioventricular canal defect, atrial septal defect, and ventricular septal defect were treated surgically. An organized and calcified thrombus was identified in the right atrium in the region of the atrial septal defect repair. Multifocal (probably embolic) brain infarcts, similar to those identified in the right basal ganglia (arrows), were identified throughout the brain. Infarcts showed severe calcification, as did the foci of myocardial necrosis seen on histologic sections.

28–10 illustrates severe necrotizing leukoencephalopathy observed in an infant who had an Ebstein's anomaly repaired surgically.

Cerebral abscess is still a feared complication of congenital heart disease, usually with superimposed infective endocarditis secondary to a right-to-left shunt.[137] Again, patterns of disease in this area are changing, but the older literature is of considerable interest.[61,68] During the 1950s, Newton[116] studied hematogenous brain abscesses in seven patients with cyanotic congenital heart disease. He stressed the difficulty of detecting a primary site of infection in patients with abscess. Abscesses occasionally followed surgical procedures (e.g., the Blalock-Taussig procedure). A study from the early 1960s[104] stressed that in children under the age of 2 years, cerebral infarct secondary to thrombosis was a more common cause of neurologic morbidity than was abscess. In considering all causes of cerebral abscess, admittedly an uncommon mass lesion when compared with brain neoplasms, congenital heart disease as a likely predisposing factor is less common than is infection of the middle ear and paranasal sinuses.[85,136]

Several cardiogenic causes of stroke in young adults have already been reviewed. When clinicians or pathologists are faced with young patients who have experienced a stroke, a cardiac source (especially of emboli) must be considered. Atherosclerotic and cardiac disease may be responsible for as many as 50 percent of ischemic strokes in persons under the age of 45 years.[114] As a result, clinicians frequently perform detailed cardiac imaging studies in young people with stroke.[107]

Previously unsuspected congenital heart disease is frequently detected in young patients studied using detailed cardiac imaging modalities.[99] Patent foramen ovale is signifi-

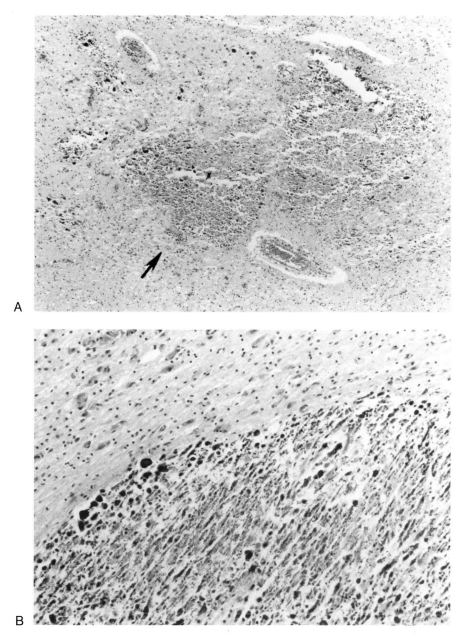

Fig. 28–10. Severe necrotizing leukoencephalopathy in a patient with congenital heart disease after surgical repair. The 2-month-old patient had Ebstein's anomaly, including pulmonary atresia and an atrial septal defect. A complicated clinical course followed the Blalock-Taussig procedure. Eventually, renal insufficiency and sepsis occurred, as did increasing lethargy and a seizure disorder. This patient died 2 months after the surgery. Numerous sections throughout the brain showed foci of necrosis and calcification within the white matter. (**A**) A focus at low magnification (arrow), with surrounding edema and astrocytic gliosis of the brain. (**B**) Higher magnification showing large foci of calcification, including linear calcified regions of necrotic axons, whereas the adjacent brain (upper left-hand corner) shows some intact neurons and astrocytic gliosis. (H&E; Fig. A: × 80; Fig. B: × 210.)

cantly more frequent in young stroke patients than in controls. Among young persons with significant cerebral infarcts, the prevalence of a patent foramen ovale was 21 percent in patients with an identifiable cause of stroke, and 40 percent in those with no identifiable cause but a significant risk factor for stroke (e.g., MVP or use of oral contraceptives). These results imply that paradoxic embolus through a patent foramen ovale may be responsible for a significant number of strokes. This conclusion is supported by the literature.[174] Other possible causes of paradoxic embolism include atrial septal defect.[86] Such emboli are usually not preceded by clinically apparent pulmonary emboli or deep venous thrombosis. Paradoxic emboli to the brain may follow a Valsalva maneuver and may be precipitated by placement of a Swan-Ganz catheter.[17] They have been associated with right atrial myxoma and with the use of oral contraceptives.[17]

SEQUELAE OF OPEN HEART SURGERY AND CARDIAC ARREST

Open heart surgery generally leads to neurologic morbidity and mortality because of hypoxic-ischemic episodes that occur during the surgical procedure and/or as a result of the release of variable amounts of embolic material into the cerebral circulation. Modern filtering techniques used in cardiopulmonary bypass have effectively eliminated many potential embolic materials (e.g., muscle, calcium, and silicone), but platelet-fibrin and atheromatous material may enter the brain from the extracorporeal circulation.[11]

Furlan and Breuer[50] found major cerebral infarcts in fewer than 2 percent of patients undergoing open heart surgery at an institution with a large volume of complex cardiothoracic surgical procedures. Of more than 30,000 patients who had cardiac catheterization, focal ischemic events were seen in approximately 0.1 percent.[50] When infarcts occurred, they were (not surprisingly) related to emboli associated with dysrhythmias, ventricular mural thrombi, brittle atherosclerotic aortas, microaggregate formation in the extracorporeal circulation, or to pre-existing cerebrovascular disease. Furlan and Breuer[50] believed that asymptomatic internal carotid artery stenosis did not significantly increase stroke risk. An encephalopathy, thought to be multifactorial in origin, occurs in approximately 12 percent of patients undergoing open heart surgery while more subtle neuropsychological abnormalities may be even more common. Induced hypotension to levels acceptable for routine cardiopulmonary bypass may be an underappreciated cause of brain ischemia in patients with microvascular brain disease and defective autoregulation. When postoperative coma is seen, it is usually secondary to hypoxic-ischemic events or frank cerebral infarcts, including watershed infarcts. Stroke incidence has decreased markedly in patients undergoing open heart surgery since the 1960s,[59] largely through the efforts of more advanced monitoring techniques and surgical methodologies, membrane oxygenators, and filtration techniques that decrease microaggregate formation in the circulation. However, benefits derived from these technical advances may have plateaued since the 1970s.

Furlan and Breuer[50] found a 5 percent rate of local brain or ocular infarcts among more than 400 patients undergoing CABG; 2 percent of patients were left with a major neurologic disability. These investigators were unable to correlate any specific pre- or postoperative variables with stroke risk. Even transient postoperative atrial fibrillation did not appear to increase stroke risk. Coma not attributable to metabolic factors was present in fewer than 1 percent of patients, but the specific cause often failed to be detected. An interesting suggestion was that some anesthetic agents affect the neuronal cytoplasmic cytoskeleton, and these effects may be manifested as an inhibition of axoplasmic flow, leading to neuronal dysfunction and resultant neurologic morbidity. Others have stressed the importance of embolization of cholesterol or atheromatous material in patients with significant atherosclerosis.[32]

Two detailed autopsy studies of neuropathologic sequelae of cardiac surgery[3,79] concluded that neuropathologic complications were greater in patients who had undergone open heart surgery or been on cardiac bypass than in those who had no surgical treatment or simply closed heart or peripheral vascular procedures. Of more than 200 patients studied in the open heart surgery group, more than 85 percent had significant neuropathologic changes, the most commonly encountered lesions being focal hemorrhages, neuronal necrosis, and emboli. The latter included fibrin-platelet aggregates, crystalline material (seen best with polarization microscopy), and neutral fat, all seen primarily within microvessels. Nonfat emboli were more common, the longer the perfusion time in patients on bypass, and were not encountered in patients in whom a Dacron wool filter had been placed in the arterial line during perfusion.[3]

In a companion study, the same group reported finding fat emboli in 80 percent of patients after open heart surgery and in almost 50 percent of nonoperated patients, whereas nonfat emboli were seen in almost one-third of patients following open heart surgery.[79]

Neurologic morbidity and mortality associated with cardiac valve prostheses has been discussed, but re-emphasis is warranted (Fig. 28–11). Thromboemboli may be associated with various valve prostheses.[43] Their incidence is said to be less than 2/100 patient-years for aortic valves made of biologic

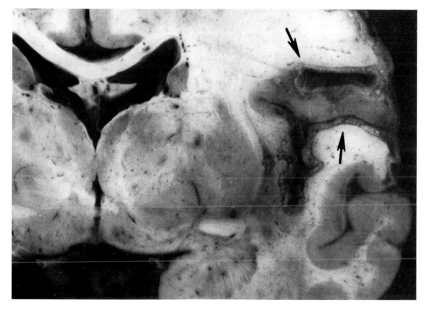

Fig. 28–11. A 15-year-old had aortic valve replacement because of infective endocarditis. Hemiparesis was observed soon after the patient awoke from anesthesia. The patient died six months later. Coronal section of the fixed brain at level of the anterior commissure shows an extensive cortical infarct (arrows) involving the insular cortex and inferior frontal and superior temporal cortex. Infarct almost certainly occurred intraoperatively or soon after the operative procedure. Note that the infarct does not have a large cystic component, although separation between the cortical ribbon and the subcortical white matter is obvious.

materials (patients not on anticoagulants) and for the best mechanical valves (patients on anticoagulants). For mitral valve prostheses, comparable figures are in the range of 4/100 patient-years. Morbidity and mortality may obviously be associated with hemorrhagic complications of anticoagulation. Particulate emboli from artificial cardiac valves may also be seen in the retinal circulation.[133] A detailed study of particulate microemboli in the circulation during open heart surgery[150] found that particles 13 to 80 μm in size could be detected in the patient's blood before and during bypass. During the first 10 minutes of cardiopulmonary bypass, the volume of particles in the arterial blood drawn from the oxygenator was greater than that in venous blood. However, the volume of particles in blood from the cardiotomy return line was markedly elevated and remained elevated throughout the surgical procedure. The particles had a size distribution approximating that of platelet aggregates that could be induced in vitro in the patient's blood. Dacron filters were effective in removing almost 90 percent of microemboli. Fatal cerebral microemboli, some calcified, have been seen in a small number of patients after aortic valve replacement.[98]

Atheroemboli to the brain may occur any time a severely atherosclerotic aorta or its branches are traumatized during a vascular surgical procedure, such as during or after correction of a stenotic aortic valve.[151] Patients who are examined many months or years after atheroemboli have occurred will show recanalized vessels in terminal or circumferential branches of the vertebrobasilar and carotid system. Fatal cerebral atheromatous embolization has been observed after cardiopulmonary bypass, secondary to ruptured atherosclerotic plaque in the ascending aorta at the site of aortotomy for cardiopulmonary bypass.[106]

A fatal cerebral embolic infarct with a thrombus in the MCA was observed after CABG, the apparent cause being thrombosis of the vein grafts with extension of thrombus into the aortic lumen.[22] Stroke in the form of a cerebral infarct has occurred in a patient with unsuspected fibromuscular dysplasia after surgery for aortic coarctation.[103] Patients with congenital heart disease who undergo the Blalock-Taussig procedure have a new vascular anatomy[97] that predisposes them to a subclavian steal syndrome. Vertebrobasilar ischemia may result.

Hypoxic-ischemic injury to the brain after cardiac arrest or during cardiac surgery is a dreaded complication, because the patient (although resuscitated from cardiac standstill) may be left in a persistent neurologic vegetative state for months or years. Clinical aspects of the prognosis and treatment of anoxic-ischemic encephalopathy after cardiac arrest have been discussed.[149] Usually, one of two neuropathologic findings is detected after such an arrest or a profound hypotensive episode, and it is difficult to predict which will be discovered in a given patient. Diffuse anoxic-ischemic encephalopathy may result, with ischemic neuronal cell change throughout the brain but is especially common in anoxia-sensitive structures (hippocampus, cerebellar Purkinje cells). With time, the ischemic neurons disappear and resultant astrocytic gliosis will occur. In severe cases, patchy laminar necrosis of the cortex may result.[24] The degree of anoxic damage to the brain depends on the severity and duration of the cardiac arrest. Discrete infarcts occurring in watershed territories of the cerebral circulation may also result (Fig. 28–12). These appear grossly as (usually) hemorrhagic infarcts, for example, between the MCA and ACA territories, or between any other two or three vascular territories of supply within the brain. Watershed infarcts have also been observed in the cerebellum and brain stem. Torvik[162] estimated that watershed infarcts represent 10 percent of all brain infarcts. The probable mechanisms are hypotension, microemboli consisting of platelet-fibrin or atheromatous material (Fig. 28–12), large vessel

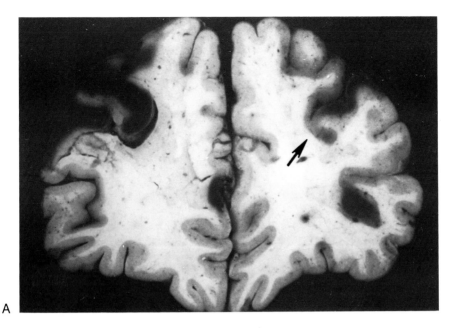

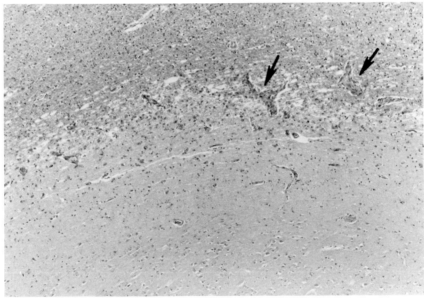

Fig. 28–12. A 58-year-old woman with hypertensive and arteriosclerotic cardiovascular disease had coronary artery bypass surgery performed during a prolonged and complicated surgical procedure that lasted 18 hours. Postoperatively, she was in a coma until death several days later. At autopsy, recent and healed myocardial infarcts were identified, as were organizing mural thrombi within the left ventricle cavity. Severe and complicated atherosclerotic disease was seen throughout the body. **(A)** Coronal section of frontal lobes, with multiple focally hemorrhagic infarcts in both cerebral hemispheres, seen as dusky gray discoloration of the cortex. At least one infarct (arrow) in the right cerebral hemisphere is in the watershed between the anterior cerebral and middle cerebral territories of vascular supply. The multiple cerebral infarcts almost certainly accounted for the patient's postoperative coma. **(B)** Interface between a region of cerebral infarct (lower portion of frame) and more normal brain tissue (upper portion). Note vascular endothelial hyperplasia (arrows) at the interface between the two, consistent with the infarct occurring several days previously. Atheroembolic material was seen within numerous leptomeningeal blood vessels. *(Figure continues.)*

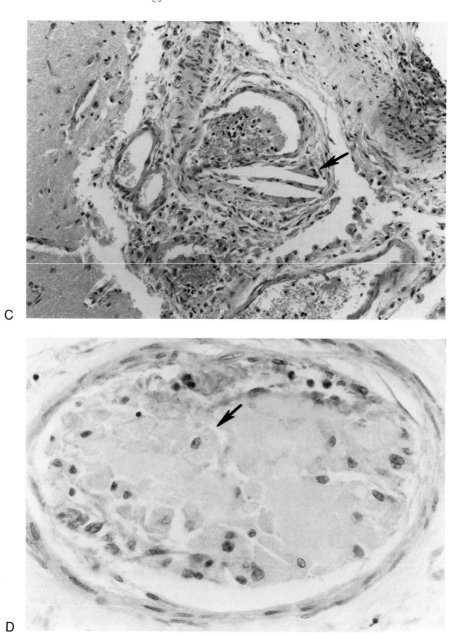

Fig. 28–12 (*Continued*). (**C**) Cholesterol clefts, with a foreign body giant cell adjacent to one (arrow). Some vessels had undergone recanalization. (**D**) Leptomeningeal vessel adjacent to the cerebellum, in which foamy histiocytes (presumably originating in a proximal atherosclerotic plaque) can be identified (arrow). Such findings are relatively common in individuals who experience watershed infarcts (see text). (H&E; Fig. B: × 80; Fig. C: × 210; Fig. D: × 530.)

occlusions in persons with severe atherosclerotic disease, or any combination of these three.[163]

More than 20 years ago, Adams et al. published a detailed clinicopathologic study of the effects of hypotension on the CNS in 11 patients who survived a cardiovascular event by 2 days to 23 months.[1] Large watershed lesions were seen in some patients, whereas smaller watershed infarcts associated with patchy neuronal loss were seen in others. A third group showed more subtle degrees of neuronal loss and astrocytic gliosis. Of interest was the fact that one anoxia-sensitive structure, the hippocampus, was normal in many patients. Large watershed infarcts were thought to result from a precipitate drop in blood pressure, whereas subtle neuronal loss and gliosis was more likely to be associated with a sustained diminution in blood pressure. Occasionally, unusual patterns of anoxic-ischemic change may be seen in patients who survive cardiac arrest or profound hypotension; for example, we have occasionally observed unusual necrotizing lesions in the white matter (especially in the corpus callosum) in such patients (Fig. 28–13). In humans, hypoxic-ischemic leukoencephalopathy, although much less common than hypoxic polioencephalopathy (i.e., resulting in cortical and/or hippocampal injury), has been associated with prolonged hypoxemia and periods of profound hypotension and metabolic imbalance (e.g., acidosis).[60]

ISCHEMIC LESIONS OF THE SPINAL CORD

The spinal cord may also be affected in patients who have a cardiopulmonary arrest or profound sustained hypotension. In some respects, the spinal cord is a microcosm of the brain, but with a lower blood flow (15 to 20 ml/min/100 g versus 50 in the brain).[139] Anoxic-ischemic events or infarcts in the spinal cord may result from cardiac emboli or sustained hypotension, for example, that seen after cardiac arrest, aortic rupture, and dissecting aneurysm of the aorta.[93,139] The latter entities are particularly important because any disruption of the aorta will also disrupt important radicular arterial feeding branches to the spinal cord parenchyma.[139] The watershed area within the spinal cord is generally thought to be the thoracic region. Aortic coarctation may also produce a relative steal of blood from the spinal cord.

Ischemic spinal cord injury has been seen after cardiac surgery in children.[125] This was especially common in aortic coarctation but was seen in other children who were operated upon for congenital heart disease. The risk of spinal cord ischemia, however, did not appear to be related to the length of time the aorta was cross-clamped or the number of collateral vessels divided.

Paraplegia has also been observed in patients given intra-aortic balloon pump counterpulsation.[148] Possible mechanisms include vascular occlusion secondary to positioning of the balloon, vasospasm, thromboemboli, hypotension, or arterial dissection.

Persons with severe atherosclerotic disease of the aorta are susceptible to the development of atheroembolic spinal cord infarcts, even if the atherosclerotic disease is otherwise asymptomatic. Central gray matter is more likely to show infarcts than is peripheral white matter, and atheromatous emboli including cholesterol clefts are frequently seen within affected and infarcted spinal cord tissue.[56,77,78,82,175]

The spinal cord shows a propensity to undergo anoxic-ischemic change. Again, this usually affects the central gray matter more than the white matter, in patients who experience cardiac arrest. This is especially likely in children and affects the thoracolumbar areas in particular, with resultant severe loss of anterior horn cells should the patient survive. Usually, patients also show diffuse anoxic-ischemic change throughout the brain.[8,58,169]

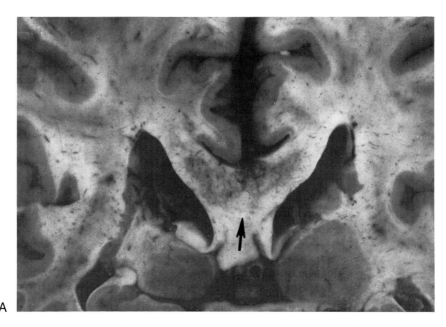

A

Fig. 28–13. Unusual anoxic-ischemic white matter lesions seen in a 69-year-old man following surgery. Patient had severe atherosclerotic aortic disease and had several peripheral vascular surgical procedures including aortobifemoral bypass grafting and aortorenal grafts. After his most recent surgery (aortorenal graft), done 1 month before death, the patient was paraplegic secondary to ischemic myelopathy (see text). He also showed encephalopathic features clinically. At autopsy, multiple necrotic lesions were seen throughout the cortex and the deep white matter. (**A**) Necrotic lesion (arrow) within the splenium of the corpus callosum. (*Figure continues.*)

NEUROPATHOLOGY OF CARDIAC TRANSPLANTATION

As cardiac transplantation becomes more widely used, neurologic complications are certain to be frequently observed (Table 28–2). The series published to date have been relatively small but informative. In 23 patients examined at postmortem after heart transplant,[110] 70 percent had neurologic complications, the most common cause being vascular disease. Of neurologic or neuropathologic complications, 60 percent were vascular in nature, and most were related to prolonged hypotension and failure of cerebral autoregulation. Vascular abnormalities included cerebral infarcts, anoxic-ischemic change or laminar necrosis, and, less commonly, hemorrhage (including small petechial hemorrhages). Infection, when present, was attributable to one or more of several organisms, including *Toxoplasma gondii*, *Candida albicans*, *Aspergillus*, and cytomegalovirus (CMV). In a study of 18 patients, Ang et al.[5] also found that approximately two-thirds of the lesions were vascular and when infarcts were present they frequently had an appearance that suggested that they antedated the heart transplantation. Hemorrhages were often caused by coagulopathy and sepsis. Infection, when present, was caused by the same types of organisms found by the Pittsburgh group.[110] Of interest is that neither group reported lymphomas or lymphoproliferative disorders affecting the brain in any patient.

Clinical and neuropathologic studies from the Stanford transplant group[81,143] previously

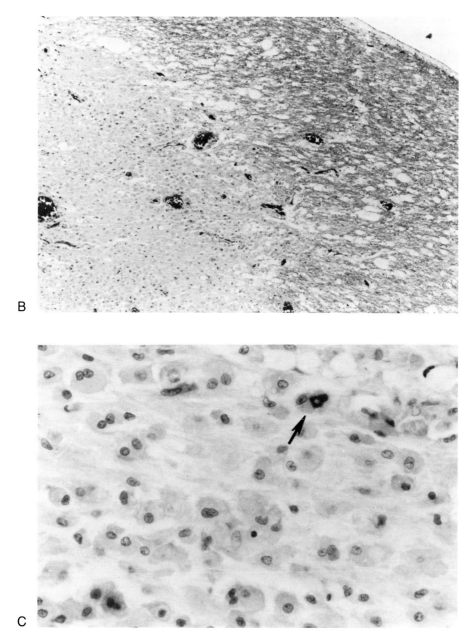

Fig. 28–13 (*Continued*). (**B**) Stained for myelin, the interface between relatively normal white matter (right of frame) and necrotic focus is shown at left. The necrotic focus shows diminished staining and numerous histiocytes. (**C**) Histiocytes at higher magnification. Note an unusual mitotic figure among the histiocytes (arrow). (H&E; Fig. B: × 80; Fig. C: × 530.)

Table 28–2. Neurologic/Neuropathologic
Complications of Cardiac and
Heart-Lung Transplantation

Vascular
    Anoxic-ischemic lesions, infarcts, laminar
      necrosis (i.e., secondary to hypotension,
      loss of microvascular autoregulation)
    Emboli (e.g., air, particulate, fat)
    Hemorrhages (e.g., with coagulopathy)
Infection
    Fungal
        Candida
        Aspergillus
        Mucormycosis
    Parasitic
        Toxoplasma gondii
    Viral
        Cytomegalovirus
        Other herpesviruses
Lymphoma
Metabolic encephalopathy

identified a range of pathologic findings similar to that seen in later studies. Clinical classification of the neurologic complications indicates that almost one-fifth are the result of operative morbidity (including anoxic brain changes after cardiac arrest, air emboli from chambers of the heart, particulate emboli, or inadequate brain perfusion), whereas more than one-third are related to opportunistic infection of the CNS by fungi or viruses. Less than 10 percent were attributed to cerebrovascular disorders and approximately 12 percent to metabolic encephalopathy. Autopsy study of selected patients[143] showed that CNS infections were as common as vascular lesions, and included infection by *Aspergillus*, *Candida*, *Mucormycosis*, and *Toxoplasma*. The Stanford group found cerebral lymphoma after heart transplant in rare patients.[143] Viral infections included those caused by CMV, herpes simplex virus (HSV), and herpes zoster virus (HZV). Vascular complications included an embolus to the MCA and multiple fat emboli. Hotson and Pedley[81] estimated (in 1976) that approximately one-fifth of patients who died after cardiac transplantation did so as a

result of neurologic complications, although this figure may now be different.

It is of interest to compare the patterns of neuropathology seen in patients after cardiac transplantation with those seen in patients who undergo a kidney or liver transplant or even in those who are immunosuppressed for other reasons (e.g., those with AIDS). For instance, progressive multifocal leukoencephalopathy related to papovavirus infection is an uncommon problem in cardiac transplant patients but is not infrequent in the other groups, such as patients with AIDS.[168] Also, cerebral lymphomas and other lymphoproliferative disorders appear more common in patients with AIDS or with iatrogenic immunosuppression after renal transplant.[141,168]

Heart-lung transplantation is a therapeutic modality not yet in widespread use. The neurologic and neuropathologic complications of this procedure have not been described in detail,[6,156] although preliminary reports[66] indicate that CNS infection, especially by fungal and bacterial agents, may frequently arise as a result.

EFFECTS OF NERVOUS SYSTEM LESIONS ON THE HEART

Although the emphasis in this chapter has been on neurologic and neuropathologic complications of cardiac, valvular, and related vascular lesions, we now turn to consideration of effects of CNS lesions on the heart. Indications that vascular lesions or other forms of mass lesion in the brain might cause functional or structural cardiac abnormalities began to emerge during the 1940s, when electrocardiographic (ECG) changes suggestive of subendocardial ischemia were found in some patients with subarachnoid hemorrhage.[117] Since that time, and especially during the past 10 to 15 years, the study of possible myocardial injury resulting from cerebral events (especially strokes) has yielded interesting data.

Cardiac lesions are usually seen after hemorrhagic stroke, especially massive subarachnoid hemorrhage. The resultant cardiac lesions include subendocardial hemorrhages (Fig. 28–14) and focal micronecrosis within the myocardium, also referred to as myocytolysis.[31,117] Subtle lymphocytic infiltrates may be seen in the myocardium. It was soon recognized that the types of cardiac lesion identified were similar to those seen in patients with pheochromocytoma or caused in animals by infusion of large amounts of catecholamines. A hypothesis was thus formulated that rapidly evolving or acute intracranial lesions stimulated the hypothalamus to produce a systemic or local release of catecholamines as a result of sympathetic excitation.[117] It was also apparent that cardiac myocytolysis was seen in patients who had many different types of intracranial lesion, but the observation has continued to be made most frequently in patients with subarachnoid hemorrhage. Myocardial abnormalities associated with lesions producing increased intracranial pressure are found in territories that differ from those associated with ischemia secondary to coronary artery disease or with agonal ischemic events and are seen in patients who survive an intracranial catastrophe by at least 6 to 8 hours.

Evidence of myocardial injury in patients with stroke has also come from the measurement of cardiac enzymes,[117] which rise after the ictus in a pattern that is different from that observed with myocardial infarct. Support for the previously described catecholamine hypothesis of myocardial injury has been obtained from measuring plasma norepinephrine and epinephrine levels in patients with subarachnoid hemorrhage. Levels of both catecholamines are increased above control levels. The enzyme dopamine β-hydroxylase, taken as a measure of sympathetic tone, is also elevated in many stroke patients, and especially those with subarachnoid hemorrhage. Another systemic manifestation of severe cerebral damage is that of neurogenic pulmonary edema. This may occur almost instantly (e.g., after a gunshot wound to the head), but is also seen with massive subarachnoid or intracerebral bleeding. The finding is also associated with ECG changes and myocytolysis. It is thought to represent a centrally mediated sympathetic effect resulting from a massive increase in pulmonary blood volume, possibly caused by sympathetic overactivity that occurs with hypothalamic injury.

Myers et al.[113] examined data on 100 stroke patients who were carefully observed in a stroke unit using 24-hour Holter rhythm monitors; serial cardiac enzymes and norepinephrine concentrations were measured. It was concluded that there were significantly more serious arrhythmias in stroke than in nonstroke patients, especially in older patients. Arrhythmias were more common in patients who had large cerebral hemispheric infarcts, as opposed to those who had brain stem strokes. The occurrence of arrhythmias appeared to be independent of the presence of coexistent cardiac disease. Fifteen stroke patients with abnormally elevated CPK values had higher mean plasma norepinephrine concentrations than did stroke patients with normal CPK levels. It was concluded that stroke may cause cardiac arrhythmias and myocardial cell damage, the latter related to increases in sympathetic tone resulting from the stroke.

Cardiac arrhythmias have also been documented in patients with massive subarachnoid hemorrhage related to berry aneurysms.[166] Approximately one-fifth of patients had such arrhythmias, especially within the first 2 days of a subarachnoid hemorrhage, and arrhythmias occurred in patients without underlying cardiac disease, hypoxia, or electrolyte imbalance. One group found a significant correlation between vasospasm affecting the left half of the brain and specific ECG abnormalities, including T-wave inversion and prolongation of the QT interval.[154]

Some clinical features and ECG abnormalities seen in patients after subarachnoid hemorrhage have been reproduced in a rabbit model.[164] Various cardiac arrhythmias, in-

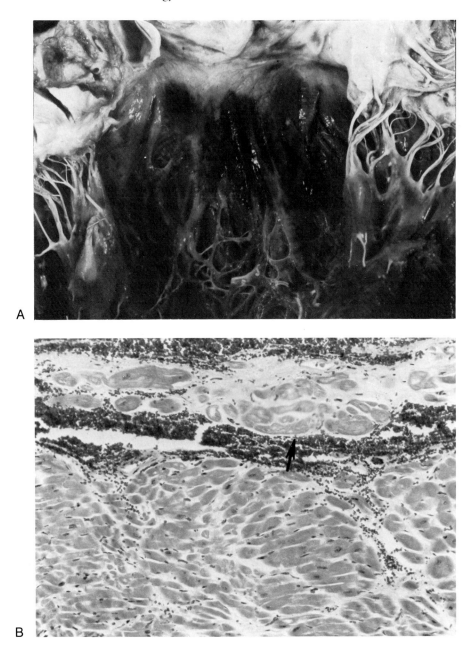

Fig. 28–14. Endocardial surface of left ventricle in a patient who had multiple cerebral hemorrhages related to deposits of metastatic melanoma. Hemorrhagic deposits were also present within the brain stem. **(A)** Extensive subendocardial hemorrhage. **(B)** Microscopic section of the endocardial surface (ventricular cavity at top) showing acute subendocardial hemorrhage. Some fibers adjacent to the hemorrhage show probable early ischemic change (arrow). (H&E, × 210.)

cluding premature atrial and ventricular contractions were seen when small volumes of prostaglandin $F_{2\alpha}$ ($PGF_{2\alpha}$) were injected into the basal cistern. Intracisternal lidocaine was effective in suppressing the arrhythmias. Stober et al.[155] found that, in patients with spontaneous intracerebral hemorrhage, there was a significant correlation between clinical manifestations of brain stem compression and cardiac arrhythmias, the latter including sinus arrythmia, multifocal PVCs, and ventricular tachycardia. Stober and co-workers believed that transtentorial herniation led to compression of the brain stem, which may have triggered changes within hypothalamic autonomic centers. However, these investigators emphasized the important point that cardiac arrhythmias represent only a single manifestation of a relatively complex cardiovascular reaction that occurs in anyone with stroke, but especially hemorrhagic stroke, as well as in patients with increased intracranial pressure from other causes.

ACKNOWLEDGMENTS

The assistance of Beverly Chandler, Laurel Reed, and Carol Appleton in preparation of tissues for microscopy and text illustrations is appreciated. Scott D. Brooks provided expert secretarial and editorial assistance in final preparation of the manuscript. Ongoing work in my laboratory was supported by grant NS 26312–01 from the National Institutes of Health and by a John Douglas French Foundation/Wilson Foundation Fellowship.

REFERENCES

1. Adams JH, Brierley JB, Connor RCR, Treip CS: The effects of systemic hypotension upon the human brain. Clinical and neuropathological observations in 11 cases. Brain 89:235, 1966

2. Adams RD, Victor M: Principles of Neurology. 2nd Ed. McGraw-Hill Book Co, New York, 1981

3. Aguilar MJ, Gerbode F, Hill JD: Neuropathologic complications of cardiac surgery. J Thorac Cardiovasc Surg 61:676, 1971

4. Anders KH, Guerra WF, Tomiyasu U, et al: The neuropathology of AIDS. UCLA experience and review. Am J Pathol 124:537, 1986

5. Ang LC, Gillett JMR, Kaufmann JCE: Neuropathology of cardiac transplant: A review of 18 cases. J Neuropathol Exp Neurol 46:402, 1987

6. Atkinson JB: The pathobiology of heart-lung transplantation. Hum Pathol 19:1367, 1988

7. Atkinson JB, Virmani R: Infective endocarditis: Changing trends and general approach for examination. Hum Pathol 18:603, 1987

8. Azzarelli B, Roessmann U: Diffuse "anoxic" myelopathy. Neurology (NY) 27:1049, 1977

9. Barletta GA, Gagliardi R, Benvenuti L, Fantini F: Cerebral ischemic attacks as a complication of aortic and mitral valve prolapse. Stroke 16:219, 1985

10. Barnett HJM: Embolism in mitral valve prolapse. Annu Rev Med 33:489, 1982

11. Barnett HJM: Heart in ischemic stroke—A changing emphasis. Neurol Clin 1:291, 1983

12. Barnett HJM: Cardiac causes of cerebral ischemia. p. 168. In Toole JF (ed): Cerebrovascular Disorders. 3rd Ed. Raven Press, New York, 1984

13. Barnett HJM, Boughner DR, Taylor DW, et al: Further evidence relating mitral-valve prolapse to cerebral ischemic events. N Engl J Med 302:139, 1980

14. Barnett HJM, Jones MW, Boughner DR, Kostuk WJ: Cerebral ischemic events associated with prolapsing mitral valve. Arch Neurol 33:777, 1976

15. Belkin RN, Hurwitz BJ, Kisslo J: Atrial septal aneurysm: Association with cerebrovascular and peripheral embolic events. Stroke 18:856, 1987

16. Bell WE, Butler C II: Cerebral mycotic aneurysms in children. Two case reports. Neurology (NY) 18:81, 1968

17. Biller J, Adams HP Jr, Johnson MR, et al: Paradoxical cerebral embolism: Eight cases. Neurology (NY) 36:1356, 1986

18. Biller J, Challa VR, Toole JF, Howard VJ: Nonbacterial thrombotic endocarditis. A neu-

rologic perspective of clinicopathologic correlations of 99 patients. Arch Neurol 39:95, 1982

19. Biller J, Johnson MR, Adams HP Jr, et al: Echocardiographic evaluation of young adults with nonhemorrhagic cerebral infarction. Stroke 17:608, 1986

20. Bogousslavsky J, Van Melle G, Regli F: The Lausanne Stroke Registry: Analysis of 1,000 consecutive patients with first stroke. Stroke 19:1083, 1988

21. Boughner DR, Barnett HJM: The enigma of the risk of stroke in mitral valve prolapse. Stroke 16:175, 1985

22. Bounds JV Jr, Sandok BA, Barnhorst DA: Fatal cerebral embolism following aorto-coronary bypass graft surgery. Stroke 7:611, 1976

23. Bozóky B, Bara D, Kertész E: Autopsy study of cerebral complications of congenital heart disease and cardiac surgery. J Neurol 231:153, 1984

24. Brierley JB, Graham DI: Hypoxia and vascular disorders of the central nervous system. p. 125. In Adams JH, Corsellis JAN, Duchen LW (eds): Greenfield's Neuropathology. 4th Ed. Edward Arnold, London, 1984

25. Brockmeier LB, Adolph RJ, Gustin BW, et al: Calcium emboli to the retinal artery in calcific aortic stenosis. Am Heart J 101:32, 1981

26. Cammarosano C, Lewis W: Cardiac lesions in acquired immune deficiency syndrome (AIDS). J Am Coll Cardiol 5:703, 1985

27. Cerebral Embolism Task Force: Cardiogenic brain embolism. Arch Neurol 43:71, 1986

28. Cheng TO, Kisslo J: Atrial septal aneurysm as a cause of cerebral embolism in young patients. Stroke 19:408, 1988

29. Cohen MM: The central nervous system in congenital heart disease. Neurology (NY) 10:452, 1960

30. Colt HG, Begg RJ, Saporito JJ, et al: Cholesterol emboli after cardiac catheterization. Eight cases and a review of the literature. Medicine (Baltimore) 67:389, 1988

31. Connor RCR: Heart damage associated with intracranial lesions. Br Med J 3:29, 1968

32. Coppeto JR, Furlan AJ, Breuer AC: Major embolic complications of open heart surgery and DDA. Stroke 16:899, 1985

33. Cottrill CM, Kaplan S: Cerebral vascular ac-

cidents in cyanotic congenital heart disease. Am J Dis Child 125:484, 1973

34. Davies MJ, Moore BP, Braimbridge MV: The floppy mitral valve. Study of incidence, pathology, and complications in surgical, necropsy, and forensic material. Br Heart J 40:468, 1978

35. DeBono DP, Warlow CP: Potential sources of emboli in patients with presumed transient cerebral or retinal ischaemia. Lancet 1:343, 1981

36. DeMaria AN, Amsterdam EA, Vismara LA, et al: Arrhythmias in the mitral valve prolapse syndrome. Prevalence, nature, and frequency. Ann Intern Med 84:656, 1976

37. Dewar HA, Weightman D: A study of embolism in mitral valve disease and atrial fibrillation. Br Heart J 49:133, 1983

38. DeWitt LD, Pessin MS, Pandian NG, et al: Benign disappearance of ventricular thrombus after embolic stroke. A case report. Stroke 19:393, 1988

39. Dimmick JE, Bove KE, McAdams AJ, Benzing G III: Fiber embolization—A hazard of cardiac surgery and catheterization. N Engl J Med 292:685, 1975

40. Dines DE, Burgher LW, Okazaki H: The clinical and pathologic correlation of fat embolism syndrome. Mayo Clin Proc 50:407, 1975

41. Di Pasquale G, Andreoli A, Grazi P, et al: Cardioembolic stroke from atrial septal aneurysm. Stroke 19:640, 1988

42. Di Pasquale G, Pinelli G, Andreoli A: Idiopathic hypertrophic subaortic stenosis and cerebral ischemia. Stroke 16:537, 1985

43. Edmunds LH Jr: Thromboembolic complications of current cardiac valvular prostheses. Ann Thorac Surg 34:96, 1982

44. Fairfax AJ, Lambert CD: Neurological aspects of sinoatrial heart block. J Neurol Neurosurg Psychiatry 39:576, 1976

45. Fisher CM, Gore I, Okabe N, White PD: Atherosclerosis of the carotid and vertebral arteries—Extracranial and intracranial. J Neuropathol Exp Neurol 24:455, 1965

46. Fisher M, Kase CS, Stelle B, Mills RM Jr: Ischemic stroke after cardiac pacemaker implantation in sick sinus syndrome. Stroke 19:712, 1988

47. Foulkes MA, Wolf PA, Price TR, et al: The

stroke data bank: Design, methods, and baseline characteristics. Stroke 19:547, 1988

48. Fulkerson PK, Beaver BM, Auseon JC, Graber HL: Calcification of the mitral annulus. Etiology, clinical associations, complications and therapy. Am J Med 66:967, 1979

49. Furlan AJ: Stroke: The heart of the matter. Stroke 17:583, 1986

50. Furlan AJ: Breuer AC: Central nervous system complications of open heart surgery. Stroke 15:912, 1984

51. Furlan AJ, Craciun AR: Risk of stroke during coronary artery bypass graft surgery in patients with internal carotid artery disease documented by angiography. Stroke 16:797, 1985

52. Furlan AJ, Craciun AR, Raju NR, Hart N: Cerebrovascular complications associated with idiopathic hypertrophic subaortic stenosis. Stroke 15:282, 1984

53. Furlan AJ, Craciun AR, Salcedo EE, Mellino M: Risk of stroke in patients with mitral annulus calcification. Stroke 15:801, 1984

54. Galbreath C, Salgado ED, Furlan AJ, Hollman J: Central nervous system complications of percutaneous transluminal coronary angioplasty. Stroke 17:616, 1986

55. Garcia I, Fainstein V, Rios A, et al: Nonbacterial thrombotic endocarditis in a male homosexual with Kaposi's sarcoma. Arch Intern Med 143:1243, 1983

56. Garland H, Greenberg J, Harriman DGF: Infarction of the spinal cord. Brain 89:645, 1966

57. Ghatak NR: Pathology of cerebral embolization caused by nonthrombotic agents. Hum Pathol 6:599, 1975

58. Gilles FH, Nag D: Vulnerability of human spinal cord in transient cardiac arrest. Neurology (NY) 21:833, 1971

59. Gilman S: Cerebral disorders after open-heart operations. N Engl J Med 272:489, 1965

60. Ginsberg MD, Hedley-Whyte ET, Richardson EP Jr: Hypoxic-ischemic leukoencephalopathy in man. Arch Neurol 33:5, 1976

61. Gluck R, Hall JW, Stevenson LD: Brain abscess associated with congenital heart disease. Pediatrics 9:192, 1952

62. Graor RA, Hetzer NR: Management of coexistent carotid artery and coronary artery disease. Stroke 19:1441, 1988

63. Graus F, Rogers LR, Posner JB: Cerebrovascular complications in patients with cancer. Medicine (Baltimore) 64:16, 1985

64. Gravanis MB, Campbell WG Jr: The syndrome of prolapse of the mitral valve. An etiologic and pathogenic enigma. Arch Pathol Lab Med 106:369, 1982

65. Hachinski V, Norris JW: The Acute Stroke. FA Davis, Philadelphia, 1985

66. Hall WA, Martinez AJ, Dummer JS, et al: Central nervous system infections in heart and heart-lung transplant recipients. Arch Neurol 46:173, 1989

67. Halperin JL, Hart RG: Atrial fibrillation and stroke: New ideas, persisting dilemmas. Stroke 19:937, 1988

68. Hanna R: Cerebral abscess and paradoxic embolism associated with congenital heart disease. Report of seven cases, with a review of the literature. Am J Dis Child 62:555, 1941

69. Harrison MJG: Thromboembolism. p. 171. In Harrison MJG, Dyken ML (eds): Cerebral Vascular Disease. Neurology. Vol. 3. Butterworths, London, 1983

70. Harrison MJG, Dyken ML (eds): Cerebral Vascular Disease. Neurology. Vol. 3. Butterworths, (Publishers) London, 1983

71. Hart RG, Easton JD: Hemorrhagic infarcts. Stroke 17:586, 1986

72. Hart RG, Freeman GL: Stroke in young people—The heart of the matter. West J Med 146:596, 1987

73. Hart RG, Britton M, Gustafsson C: Atrial fibrillation and the diagnosis of cardioembolic stroke. Stroke 16:1043, 1985

74. Hart RG, Kagan-Hallet K, Joerns SE: Mechanisms of intracranial hemorrhage in infective endocarditis. Stroke 18:1048, 1987

75. Hart RG, Sherman DG, Easton JD, et al: Atrial fibrillation and stroke. Stroke 15:387, 1984

76. Hart RG, Sherman DG, Wolf PA, Kannel WB: Mitral valve prolapse and embolic stroke. Stroke 16:334, 1985

77. Henson RA, Parsons M: Ischaemic lesions of the spinal cord: an illustrated review. Q J Med 36:205, 1967

78. Herrick MK, Mills PE Jr: Infarction of spinal cord. Two cases of selective gray matter involvement secondary to asymptomatic aortic disease. Arch Neurol 24:228, 1971

79. Hill JD, Aguilar MJ, Baranco A, et al: Neuropathological manifestations of cardiac surgery. Ann Thorac Surg 7:409, 1969

80. Hirose G, Kosoegawa H, Takado M, et al: Spinal cord ischemia and left atrial myxoma. Arch Neurol 36:439, 1979

81. Hotson JR, Pedley TA: The neurological complications of cardiac transplantation. Brain 99:673, 1976

82. Hughes JT, Brownell B: Spinal cord ischemia due to arteriosclerosis. Arch Neurol 15:189, 1966

83. Huston KA, Combs JJ Jr, Lie JT, Guiliani ER: Left atrial myxoma simulating peripheral vasculitis. Mayo Clin Proc 53:752, 1978

84. Jaffe AS, Geltman EM, Rodey GE, Uitto J: Mitral valve prolapse: A consistent manifestation of type IV Ehlers-Danlos syndrome. The pathogenetic role of the abnormal production of type III collagen. Circulation 64:121, 1981

85. Jefferson AA, Keogh AJ: Intracranial abscesses: A review of treated patients over 20 years. Q J Med 66:389, 1977

86. Jones HR Jr, Caplan LR, Come PC, et al: Cerebral emboli of paradoxical origin. Ann Neurol 13:314, 1983

87. Kamenar E, Burger PC: Cerebral fat embolism: A neuropathological study of a microembolic state. Stroke 11:477, 1980

88. Kapila A, Hart R: Calcific cerebral emboli and aortic stenosis: Detection of computed tomography. Stroke 17:619, 1986

89. Kasarskis EJ, O'Connor W, Earle G: Embolic stroke from cardiac papillary fibroelastomas. Stroke 19:1171, 1988

90. Kealy WF: Atheroembolism. J Clin Pathol 31:984, 1978

91. Kelley RE, Pina I, Lee S-C: Cerebral ischemia and mitral valve prolapse: Case-control study of associated factors. Stroke 19:443, 1988

92. Kempster PA, Gerraty RP, Gates PC: Asymptomatic cerebral infarction in patients with chronic atrial fibrillation. Stroke 19:955, 1988

93. Kepes JJ: Selective necrosis of spinal cord gray matter. A complication of dissecting aneurysm of the aorta. Acta Neuropathol (Berl) 4:293, 1965

94. Kessler C, Henningsen H, Reuther R, et al: Identification of intracardiac thrombi in stroke patients with Indium 111 platelet scintigraphy. Stroke 18:63, 1987

95. Knepper LE, Biller J, Adams HP Jr, Bruno A: Neurologic manifestations of atrial myxoma. A 12-year experience and review. Stroke 19:1435, 1988

96. Kooiker JC, MacLean JM, Sumi SM: Cerebral embolism, marantic endocarditis, and cancer. Arch Neurol 33:260, 1976

97. Kurlan R, Krall RL, Deweese JA: Vertebrobasilar ischemia after total repair of tetralogy of Fallot: Significance of subclavian steal created by Blalock-Taussig anastomosis. Stroke 15:359, 1984

98. Larmi TKI, Kärkölä P, Kairaluoma MI, et al: Calcium microemboli and microfilters in valve operations. Ann Thorac Surg 24:34, 1977

99. Lechat PH, Mas JL, Lascault G, et al: Prevalence of patent foramen ovale in patients with stroke. J Engl J Med 318:1148, 1988

100. Lodder J, Krijne-Kubat B, Broekman J: Cerebral hemorrhagic infarction at autopsy: Cardiac embolic cause and the relationship to the causes of death. Stroke 17:626, 1986

101. Lodder J, Krijne-Kubat B, van der Lugt PJM: Timing of autopsy-confirmed hemorrhagic infarction with reference to cardioembolic stroke. Stroke 19:1482, 1988

102. Lovas JGL, Silver MD: Coincident rupture of berry aneurysm and aortic dissection during sexual intercourse. Arch Pathol Lab Med 108:271, 1984

103. Malloy DS, Sangalang VE, Fraser GM: Cerebral infarction secondary to unsuspected intracranial fibromuscular dysplasia following bypass of aortic coarctation. Stroke 15:908, 1984

104. Matson DD, Salam M: Brain abscess in congenital heart disease. Pediatrics 27:772, 1961

105. McCormick WF: Vascular diseases. p. 35. In Schochet SS Jr (ed): The Clinical Neurosciences. Vol. 3: Neuropathology. Churchill Livingstone, New York, 1983

106. McKibbin DW, Bulkley BH, Green WR, et al: Fatal cerebral atheromatous embolization after cardiopulmonary bypass. J Thorac Cardiovasc Surg 71:741, 1976

107. Mohr JP: Cryptogenic stroke. N Engl J Med 318:1197, 1988

108. Mohr JP, Caplan LR, Melski JW, et al: The

Harvard Cooperative Stroke Registry: A prospective registry. Neurology (NY) 28:754, 1978

109. Molinari GF, Smith L, Goldstein MN, Satran R: Pathogenesis of cerebral mycotic aneurysms. Neurology (NY) 23:325, 1973

110. Montero CG, Martinez AJ: Neuropathology of heart transplantation: 23 cases. Neurology (NY) 36:1149, 1986

111. Moossy J: Cerebral atherosclerosis: Morphology and some relationships with coronary atherosclerosis. p. 253. In Zülch KJ, Kaufmann W, Hossmann K-A, Hossmann V (eds): Brain and Heart Infarct. Springer-Verlag, Berlin, 1977

112. Moss AJ: Atrial fibrillation and cerebral embolism. Arch Neurol 41:707, 1984

113. Myers MG, Norris JW, Hachinski VC, et al: Cardiac sequelae of acute stroke. Stroke 13:838, 1982

114. Nencini P, Inzitari D, Baruffi MC, et al: Incidence of stroke in young adults in Florence, Italy. Stroke 19:977, 1988

115. Nespeca MP, Townsend JJ: Multiple cerebral emboli in a young man. West J Med 146:589, 1987

116. Newton EJ: Haematogenous brain abscess in cyanotic congenital heart disease. Q J Med 25:201, 1956

117. Norris JW: Effects of cerebrovascular lesions on the heart. Neurol Clin 1:87, 1983

118. Oliva A, Scherokman B: Two cases of occipital infarction following cardiac catheterization. Stroke 19:773, 1988

119. Patchell RA, White CL III, Clark AW, et al: Nonbacterial thrombotic endocarditis in bone marrow transplant patients. Cancer 55:631, 1985

120. Petersen P, Godtfredsen J: Embolic complications in paroxysmal atrial fibrillation. Stroke 17:622, 1986

121. Petersen P, Hansen JM: Stroke in thyrotoxicosis with atrial fibrillation. Stroke 19:15, 1988

122. Petersen P, Madsen EB, Brun B, et al: Silent cerebral infarction in chronic atrial fibrillation. Stroke 18:1098, 1987

123. Piatt JH Jr: Massive intracerebral hemorrhage complicating cardiac catheterization with ergonovine administration. Stroke 15:904, 1984

124. Pruitt AA, Rubin RH, Karchmer AW, Duncan GW: Neurologic complications of bacterial endocarditis. Medicine (Baltimore) 57:329, 1978

125. Puntis JWL, Green SH: Ischaemic spinal cord injury after cardiac surgery. J Neurol Neurosurg Psychiatry 60:517, 1985

126. Rice GPA, Boughner DR, Stiller C, Ebers GC: Familial stroke syndrome associated with mitral valve prolapse. Ann Neurol 7:130, 1980

127. Rice GPA, Ebers GC, Bondar RL, Boughner DR: Mitral valve prolapse: A cause of stroke in children? Dev Med Child Neurol 23:352, 1981

128. Rice GPA, Ebers GC, Newland F, Wysocki GP: Recurrent cerebral embolism in cardiac amyloidosis. Neurology (NY) 31:904, 1981

129. Roach MR, Drake CG: Ruptured cerebral aneurysms caused by micro-organisms. N Engl J Med 273:240, 1965

130. Roeltgen DP, Weimer GR, Patterson LF: Delayed neurologic complications of left atrial myxoma. Neurology (NY) 31:8, 1981

131. Roessmann U, Zarchin LE: Cerebral bone marrow embolus after closed chest cardiac massage. Arch Neurol 36:58, 1979

132. Rosen P, Armstrong D: Nonbacterial thrombotic endocarditis in patients with malignant neoplastic diseases. Am J Med 54:23, 1973

133. Rush JA, Kearns TP, Danielson GK: Cloth-particle retinal emboli from artificial cardiac valves. Am J Ophthalmol 89:845, 1980

134. Salgado AV, Furlan AJ, Keys TF: Mycotic aneurysm, subarachnoid hemorrhage, and indications for cerebral angiography in infective endocarditis. Stroke 18:1057, 1987

135. Salgado AV, Furlan AJ, Keys TF, et al: Neurologic complications of endocarditis: A 12-year experience. Neurology (NY) 39:173, 1989

136. Samson DS, Clark K: A current review of brain abscess. Am J Med 54:201, 1973

137. Sancetta SM, Zimmerman HA: Congenital heart disease with septal defects in which paradoxical brain abscess causes death. A review of the literature and report of two cases. Circulation 1:593. 1950

138. Sandok BA, von Estorff I, Giuliani ER: CNS embolism due to atrial myxoma. Clinical features and diagnosis. Arch Neurol 37:485, 1980

139. Satran R: Spinal cord infarction. Stroke 19:529, 1988

140. Schachter S, Freeman R: Transient ischemic attack and adriamycin cardiomyopathy. Neurology (NY) 32:1380, 1982

141. Schneck SA, Penn I: De-novo brain tumours in renal-transplant recipients. Lancet 1:983, 1971

142. Schnee MA, Bucal AA: Fatal embolism in mitral valve prolapse. Chest 83:285, 1983

143. Schober R, Herman MM: Neuropathology of cardiac transplantation. Survey of 31 cases. Lancet 1:962, 1973

144. Schoenberg BS, Mellinger JF, Schoenberg DG: Cerebrovascular disease in infants and children: A study of incidence, clinical features, and survival. Neurology (NY) 28:763, 1978

145. Sherman DG, Goldman L, Whiting RB, et al: Thromboembolism in patients with atrial fibrillation. Arch Neurol 41:708, 1984

146. Shuaib A, Hachinski VC, Oczkowski WJ: Transient ischemic attacks and normal cerebral angiograms: A follow-up study. Stroke 19:1223, 1988

147. Silver MD: Late complications of prosthetic heart valves. Arch Pathol Lab Med 102:281, 1978

148. Singh BM, Fass AE, Pooley RW, Wallach R: Paraplegia associated with intraaortic balloon pump counterpulsation. Stroke 14:983, 1983

149. Snyder BD, Tabbaa MA: Assessment and treatment of neurological dysfunction after cardiac arrest. Stroke 19:269, 1988

150. Solis RT, Noon GP, Beall AC Jr, DeBakey ME: Particulate microembolism during cardiac operation. Ann Thorac Surg 17:332, 1974

151. Soloway HB, Aronson SM: Atheromatous emboli to central nervous system. Report of 16 cases. Arch Neurol 11:657, 1964

152. Starkey IR, Nishide M: Cardiac abnormalities in ischemic cerebrovascular disease. Stroke 15:1081, 1984

153. Stehbens WE: Pathology of the Cerebral Blood Vessels. CV Mosby, St. Louis, 1972

154. Stober T, Kunze K: Electrocardiographic alterations in subarachnoid haemorrhage. Correlations between spasm of the arteries of the left side on the brain and T inversion and QT prolongation. J Neurol 227:99, 1982

155. Stober T, Sen S, Anstätt T, Bette L: Correlation of cardiac arrhythmias with brainstem compression in patients with intracerebral hemorrhage. Stroke 19:688, 1988

156. Tazelaar HD, Yousem SA: The pathology of combined heart-lung transplantation: An autopsy study. Hum Pathol 19:1403, 1988

157. Terplan KL: Patterns of brain damage in infants and children with congenital heart disease. Am J Dis Child 125:175, 1973

158. Thompson J, Kapoor W, Wechsler LR: Multiple strokes due to atrial myxoma with a negative echocardiogram. Stroke 19:1570, 1988

159. Thompson PL, Robinson JS: Stroke after acute myocardial infarction: Relation to infarct size. Br Med J 2:457, 1978

160. Tipton BK, Robertson JT, Robertson JH: Embolism to the central nervous system from cardiac myxoma. Report of two cases. J Neurosurg 47:937, 1977

161. Toole JF: Cerebral embolism. p. 187. In Toole JF (ed): Cerebrovascular Disorders. 3rd Ed. Raven Press, New York, 1984

162. Torvik A: The pathogenesis of watershed infarcts in the brain. Stroke 15:221, 1984

163. Torvik A, Skullerud K: Watershed infarcts in the brain caused by microemboli. Clin Neuropathol 1:99, 1982

164. Uchida M, Saito K, Niitsu T, Okuda H: Model of electrocardiographic changes seen with subarachnoid hemorrhage in rabbits. Stroke 20:112, 1989

165. Vagn-Hansen PL: Complications following external cardiac massage, with special emphasis on cerebral embolism. Acta Pathol Microbiol Immunol Scand [A] 79:505, 1971

166. Vidal BE, Dergal EB, Cesarman E, et al: Cardiac arrhythmias associated with subarachnoid hemorrhage: Prospective study. Neurosurgery 5:675, 1979

167. Vinters HV: Iatrogenic cerebral emboli: Accidental and intentional. In Platt WR (ed): Pathology Update Series. Vol. 2. Continuing Professional Education Center, Princeton, NJ, 1985

168. Vinters HV, Anders KH: Neuropathology of AIDS. CRC Press, Boca Raton, FL, 1990

169. Vinters HV, Gilbert JJ: Hypoxic myelopathy. Can J Neurol Sci 6:380, 1979

170. Vinters HV, Kaufmann JCE, Drake CG: "Foreign" particles in encephalic vascular malformations. Arch Neurol 40:221 1983

171. Virmani R, Atkinson JB, Forman MB, Ro-

binowitz M: Mitral valve prolapse. Hum Pathol 18:596, 1987

172. Wigle ED, Gilbert BW, Boughner DR, et al: Mitral valve prolapse—A modern epidemic? Proc R Coll Phys Surgeons Can 10:286, 1977

173. Wilson WR, Geraci JE, Danielson GK, et al: Anti-coagulant therapy and central nervous system complications in patients with prosthetic valve endocarditis. Circulation 57:1004, 1978

174. Webster MWI, Smith HJ, Sharpe DN, et al: Patent foramen ovale in young stroke patients. Lancet 2:11, 1988

175. Wolman L, Bradshaw P: Spinal cord embolism. J Neurol Neurosurg Psychiatry 30:446, 1967

176. Young RSK, Zalneraitis EL: Marantic endocarditis in children and young adults: Clinical and pathological findings. Stroke 12:635, 1981

29

Metabolic and Familial Diseases

Victor J. Ferrans

This chapter describes pathologic cardiovascular findings associated with metabolic and familial diseases, including glycogen storage diseases, mucopolysaccharidoses, and other diseases of carbohydrate metabolism; diseases of amino acid and protein metabolism; diseases of lipid metabolism; diseases related to iron, copper, and calcium metabolism; diseases caused by a deficiency of minerals, vitamins, or other nutrients; and diseases affecting the neuromuscular system. Cardiac lesions produced by endocrine disorders are reviewed separately (see Ch. 31), as are familial syndromes of dilated and hypertrophic cardiomyopathy (see Ch. 20).

DISEASES OF CARBOHYDRATE METABOLISM

Glycogen Storage Diseases

The glycogen storage diseases are characterized by deficiencies in the activity of different enzymes of glycogen metabolism. They are transmitted as autosomal recessive traits and manifested by an accumulation of glycogen (which may be structurally normal or abnormal, depending on the nature of the enzymatic defect). The diagnosis of glycogen storage disease should not be based only on the demonstration of increased glycogen content (which is not always elevated), but must be confirmed by analysis of glycogen structure and by demonstration of the specific enzymatic defect, that is, in leukocytes or cultured skin fibroblasts. Evidence of cardiac involvement is found in type II (Pompe's disease), type III (Cori's disease), and type IV (Andersen's disease) glycogen storage diseases.

Type II Glycogen Storage Disease

The spectrum of type II glycogen storage disease (deficiency of a lysosomal α-1, 4-glucosidase or acid maltase) includes not only classic Pompe's disease or infantile form,[219] as described herein, but also two other, milder forms: a *juvenile form*[117,219] and an *adult form*,[3,117,225,232,410] both of which progress very slowly and show, predominantly, manifestations of skeletal muscle disease simulating muscular dystrophy. A few patients with features typical of Pompe's disease have normal levels of acid maltase[448]; the nature of the biochemical defect in these patients remains to be established.

In Pompe's disease the heart is grossly enlarged, with a weight up to 6.5 times normal.[111] The walls of all chambers are thickened, especially the left ventricular free wall and papillary muscles. In some patients, severe degrees of wall thickening are associated with small cardiac cavities and with obstruction to left[112,373,421] and/or right[45,223] ventricular outflow. Other patients, however, show cardiac dilation.[431] In one patient,[373] obstruction to left ventricular outflow was thought due to myocardial hypercontractility and to anterior systolic motion of the anterior mitral leaflet (without asymmetric septal hypertrophy). In another patient,[112] the obstruction was considered a result of narrowing of the left ventricular outflow tract, by a greatly hypertrophied posteromedial papillary muscle. In 13 patients, the left ventricular free wall was hypertrophied to a much greater extent than was the ventricular septum; no obstruction to left ventricular outflow was observed in any patient at rest, after isoproterenol infusion, or after ventricular premature contractions.[43]

Fibroelastotic thickening of the endocardium occurs in about 20 percent of patients with Pompe's disease.[103] On gross examination, the heart is rubbery in consistency and pale pink. In histologic preparations stained with hematoxylin and eosin (H&E), the central portions of the cardiac muscle cells show severe vacuolization, which imparts a lacework appearance to the tissue (Fig. 29–1). This is caused by massive glycogen deposits that displace myofibrils to the periphery of the cells. The deposits have histochemical characteristics of normal glycogen. Appreciable degrees of myofibrillar loss also occur and may be related to cardiac failure, which often is the cause of death. Glycogen deposits are also present in vascular smooth muscle and endothelium.[62,103,219,245] Most of the glycogen in tissues of patients with Pompe's disease is located within lysosomes. This is also the case in the heart (Fig. 29–1 and 29–2). Previously, it had been reported that much of the cardiac glycogen was free in the cytoplasm of myocytes.[45,52,128,159,233] However, my colleagues

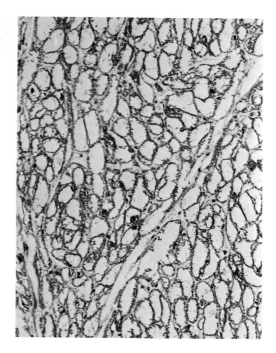

Fig. 29–1. Vacuolated appearance of muscle cells in histologic section of a heart from a child with type II glycogen storage disease. (H&E, × 300.)

and I believe this appearance results from extreme mechanical fragility of lysosomes. In well-preserved tissue, most glycogen deposits in cardiac myocytes in Pompe's disease are confined to lysosomes. These are greatly enlarged and distended by numerous particles of morphologically normal glycogen (β form). The conduction system of the heart is also involved by glycogen deposits in Pompe's disease. The short PR interval evident in the electrocardiogram (ECG) of many patients with Pompe's disease has been attributed to extreme enlargement of the conducting cells.[37] As expected, myocardial glycogen content is increased[52,500] up to 9 percent of wet tissue weight (normal, 0.77 percent[112]).

Cardiac involvement in juvenile and adult forms of type II glycogenosis is clinically minimal, although extensive deposits of a basophilic glycogen-like material have been found in the hearts of some older patients who, clinically, are thought to have type II glycogenosis.[15,225] Detailed cardiac anatomic

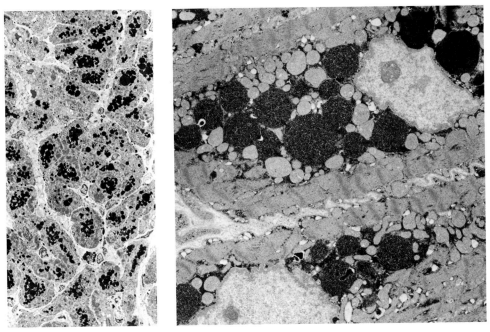

A   B

Fig. 29–2. (**A**) Myocardial biopsy from a child with type II glycogen storage disease. (Specimen was fixed with glutaraldehyde, postfixed with OsO_4, embedded in Epon, cut at a thickness of 0.5 μm, and stained with toluidine blue.) Glycogen-filled lysosomes appear as round structures. ($\times$ 700.) (**B**) Electron micrograph of the tissue seen in Fig. A, stained histochemically[53] to demonstrate periodate-reactive materials and show intralysosomal deposits of glycogen. ($\times$ 8,000.)

observations on adults with biochemically proven acid maltase deficiency reveal deposits of carbohydrate material that are histochemically and ultrastructurally similar to that observed in basophilic degeneration of the heart (see below).[330,469]

Type III Glycogen Storage Disease

Cardiac involvement in type III glycogen storage disease (deficiency of amylo-1, 6-glucosidase or debrancher enzyme) is common,[335] but usually considerably less severe than in type II.[51,288,327,468] Levine et al. found cardiomegaly in 5 of 22 patients, although none had clinical symptoms of cardiac dysfunction.[289] Cardiac morphologic findings have been described in only a few patients. One had markedly vacuolated myocytes distended with glycogen in the deeper layers of the heart

(cardiac glycogen content, 4.9 percent).[468] Other patients had massive cardiomegaly and died in infancy.[51,327] Glycogen deposits in type III glycogenosis are biochemically abnormal (short outer branches) but ultrastructurally normal and free in the cytoplasm. In a myocardial biopsy from a patient with type III glycogen storage disease (Fig. 29–3), we found intramitochondrial and intranuclear glycogen deposits in addition to large accumulations in the main cytoplasmic compartment (unpublished observations).

Type IV Glycogen Storage Disease

In type IV glycogen storage disease (deficiency of brancher enzyme or α-1,4-glucan: α-1,4-glucan 6-glucosyl transferase), clinical manifestations of heart disease and cardiomegaly are variable, but gross cardiac en-

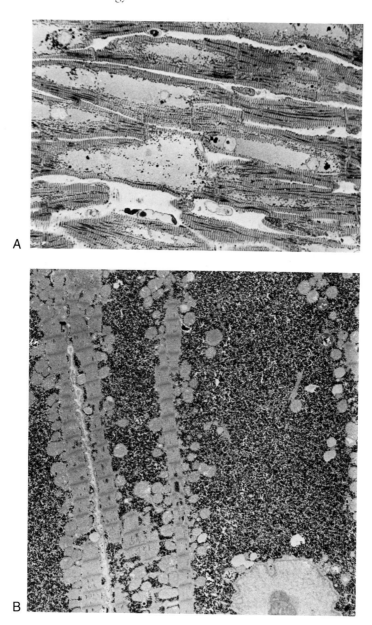

Fig. 29–3. (**A**) Phase contrast micrograph of semithin section, stained with toluidine blue, of myocardial biopsy specimen from a patient with type III glycogen storage disease, showing large, centrally located accumulations of glycogen in cytoplasm of cardiac myocytes. (× 500.) (**B**) Electron micrograph of tissue seen in Fig. A, showing accumulation of monoparticulate glycogen. (Thiery stain,[53] × 10,000.)

largement has been reported.[65,372,425] Extensive deposits of glycogen in cardiac muscle cells (Fig. 29–4) are a consistent finding.[65,239,371,411,425] Death from hepatic cirrhosis usually occurs in the first few years of life. Several patients with the clinical picture of type IV glycogenosis have survived beyond 10 years of age; it has been suggested that they have a juvenile form of the disease.[462] However, such cases are extremely

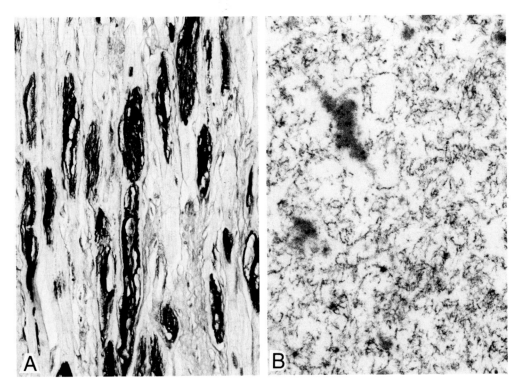

Fig. 29–4. Type IV glycogen storage disease. (**A**) Histologic section of myocardium showing large, darkly stained glycogen deposits occupying the central areas of muscle cells. (PAS, × 400.) (From Ishihara et al.,[239] with permission.) (**B**) Electron micrograph showing fibrillar structure of glycogen deposits in cytoplasm of hepatocyte in type IV glycogen storage disease. (Uranyl acetate and lead citrate, × 52,000.) (From Schochet et al.,[411] with permission.)

rare and, because of the variation in clinical and enzymatic findings,[192,462] it remains uncertain whether they represent a single disease entity. One patient with possible type IV glycogenosis also had aortic valvular stenosis and endocardial fibroelastosis.[65]

Glycogen deposits in type IV glycogenosis differ from those in other types of glycogen storage disease in that they are basophilic and relatively resistant to amylase digestion and are biochemically (long outer branches) and ultrastructurally abnormal.[130,239,371] These deposits consist of fibrils or plates, rather than granules, although glycogen granules also are present. The fibrils and plates are 5 to 6 nm thick and are free in the cytoplasm. They are not diagnostic of type IV glycogenosis, because they also occur in cardiac muscle cells

in Lafora type of myoclonic epilepsy (in which no biochemical defect has been detected) and in basophilic degeneration of the heart.[98] The stored materials in type IV glycogenosis also share some antigenetic similarities with the materials in these other disorders.[506]

Other Forms of Glycogen Storage Disease

Eishi et al.[113] described a patient in whom glycogen storage disease was limited to the heart, was manifested by cytoplasmic and intramitochondrial accumulation of glycogen in myocytes, and was caused by deficiency of phosphalase kinase. In another patient, glycogen storage disease involving myocardium was associated with deficiency of phosphofructokinase.[207]

Other Disorders of Cardiac Glycogen

Abnormalities of cardiac glycogen that occur in diseases other than the glycogen storage diseases include basophilic degeneration, intramitochondrial glycogen, and intranuclear glycogen.

Basophilic Degeneration

Basophilic degeneration is the name given to deposits, localized in the cytoplasm of cardiac muscle cells, of material that stains blue-gray with H&E and is periodic acid-Schiff (PAS)-positive.

Three types of material have been described.[130] The most common is characterized by fibrils that are similar to those of glycogen in type IV glycogen storage disease and can be digested, albeit slowly, by amylase (Fig. 29–5). This type of basophilic degeneration material is found in a small number of cardiac myocytes in the hearts of the majority of patients over 65 years of age (see Ch. 5).[384] The other two types are much less common: one consists of fibrils, the other of large masses of finely granular material in which dense inclusions are embedded.[130] The biochemical disorders responsible for these lesions have not been identified.

Intramitochondrial Glycogen

Intramitochondrial glycogen deposits occur in a small percentage of cardiac muscle cells in some patients with myocardial hypertrophy.[304] In experimental animals, the deposits develop as a delayed response to severe hy-

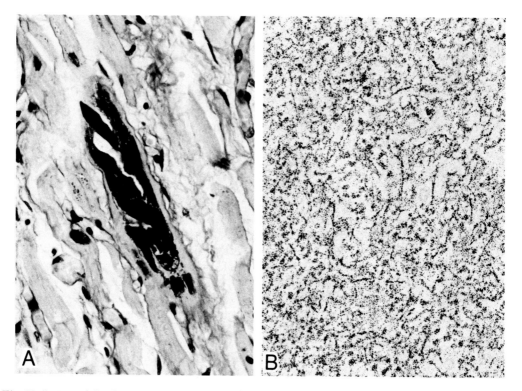

Fig. 29–5. Basophilic degeneration in the heart of a 68-year-old patient with hypertensive heart disease. (**A**) Histologic section showing large mass of darkly stained material in the center of a muscle cell. (PAS, × 600.) (**B**) Electron micrograph of section stained with the periodic acid-thiosemicarbazide-silver proteinate method, showing fibrillar nature of basophilic deposits. (× 90,000.)

poxia.[53] They are located in the outer mitochondrial compartment, that is, the space
between the inner and outer mitochondrial
membranes. They can be composed of β-par-
ticles, of α-particles (rosettes), or of mixtures
of these two constituents and can be removed
by amylase digestion.

Intranuclear Glycogen

Intranuclear glycogen deposits also occur as
nonspecific findings in a small percentage of
cardiac muscle cells in some patients with
myocardial hypertrophy.[135] No relationship to
diabetes mellitus has been found.

Both intramitochondrial and intranuclear
glycogen appear to be synthesized in situ and
probably represent the results of translocation
of enzymes of glycogen synthesis.

Mucopolysaccharidoses

The mucopolysaccharidoses (MPS) are characterized by deficiencies in lysosomal enzymes involved in the degradation of various
acid mucopolysaccharides. The clinical and
pathologic manifestations of these diseases reflect not only the storage of mucopolysaccharides within lysosomes but also complex
abnormalities in the organization of extracellular elements of connective tissue. Normal
formation of these elements involves complex
interactions between acid mucopolysaccharides and connective tissue proteins, especially collagen. Abnormalities in such
interactions probably are the factors responsible for the various anatomic changes that
occur in cardiac valves (and also in skin, cartilage, and bone) in several of these disorders.
Hunter syndrome is transmitted as a sex-
linked recessive disorder; the other mucopolysaccharidoses, as autosomal recessive
disorders. As in the case of the glycogenoses,
the diagnosis should be made on the basis of
clinical and anatomic findings combined with
biochemical demonstration of the enzymatic
defect (in cultured skin fibroblasts) and of abnormal urinary excretion of certain acid mucopolysaccharides.

Mucopolysaccharidosis I

Three clinically distinct subtypes of MPS I (α-
L-iduronidase deficiency) occur: Hurler syn-
drome (MPS I-H), Scheie syndrome (MPS
I-S), and Hurler-Scheie syndrome (MPS I-HS).

Hurler Syndrome

Cardiovascular lesions in Hurler syndrome
involve valves, endocardium, myocardium,
coronary arteries, and large systemic arteries
(Figs. 29–6 and 29–7).[275,356,377] The valves are
considerably thickened, particularly the mitral valve; right-sided cardiac valves are less
severely affected than left-sided valves. The
valvular thickening is most pronounced at the
free margins, which have an irregular, nodular
appearance. Commissures are not fused.
Chordae tendineae of the atrioventricular
valves are moderately shortened and thickened. Calcific deposits occur in the angle just
deep to the basal attachment of the posterior
mitral leaflet (mitral annular calcification), in
the mitral leaflets, and in the aortic aspect of
aortic valve cusps. The endocardium is diffusely thickened, more on the left than on the
right side of the heart. Large extramural coronary arteries are rigid and thickened, and
their lumina are severely narrowed (>75 percent). The aorta and large systemic arteries
have raised intimal plaques. Two patients
have been reported in whom left ventricular
endocardial fibroelastosis was the main manifestation of Hurler syndrome.[441]

The valves, endocardium, myocardium,
and blood vessels contain large, oval, or
rounded connective tissue cells (Hurler cells)
filled with numerous clear vacuoles, which are
the sites of deposition of acid mucopolysaccharide material. It is extremely soluble and
difficult to preserve. In addition, small granular cells that contain membrane-limited electron-dense material associated with fragments
of collagen fibrils are present.[377] The tissue
thickening just cited is due to the presence

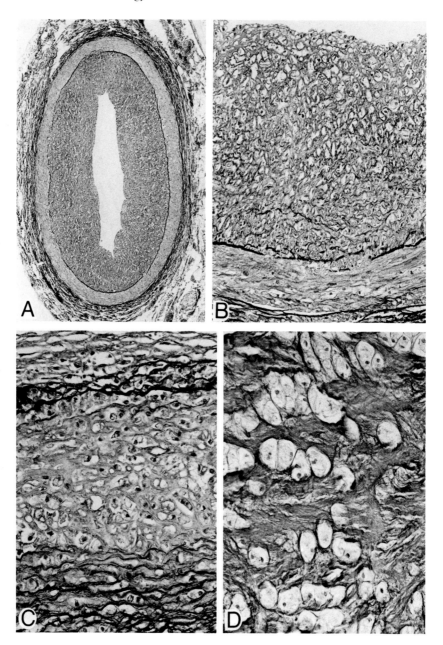

Fig. 29–6. Hurler syndrome (mucopolysaccharidosis I-H). (**A**) Coronary artery showing marked intimal thickening and luminal narrowing. (Movat's pentachrome, × 30.) (**B**) Higher magnification of part of the vessel shown in Fig. A. The intimal thickening is caused by proliferation of vacuolated intimal cells, which on electron microscopic study (Fig. 29–5B) are smooth muscle cells. (Movat's pentachrome, × 160.) (**C**) Section of aorta showing intimal thickening due to proliferation of fibrous connective tissue and vacuolated cells. (Movat's pentachrome, × 250.) (**D**) Section of mitral valve leaflet showing accumulation of large cells with clear cytoplasm. Compare with electron micrograph shown in Fig. 29–5A. (Movat's pentachrome, × 400.)

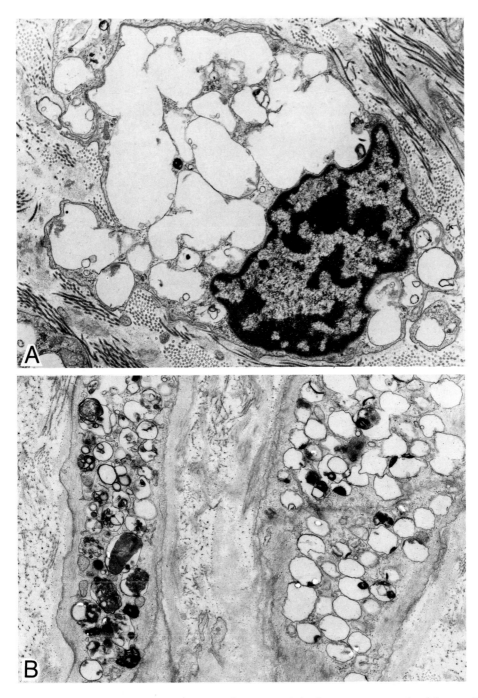

Fig. 29–7. Hurler syndrome (mucopolysaccharidosis I-H). (**A**) Electron micrograph of foam cell in tricuspid valve leaflet. This cell contains large electron-lucent, membrane-limited vacuoles, considered to be altered lysosomes. (Uranyl acetate and lead citrate, × 10,500.) (**B**) Electron micrograph of coronary intima showing two smooth muscle cells that contain electron-lucent vacuoles and vacuoles filled with concentric lamellae. (× 16,000.)

of these cells and an increased amount of fibrous connective tissue. Cardiac muscle cells and both intimal and medial smooth muscle cells of coronary arteries also contain deposits of glycolipid material that appear in the form of concentric or parallel lamellae; such deposits are present in other connective tissues, but only to a very limited extent. In cardiocytes they are located in the perinuclear area and occupy only a small fraction of cell volume. In coronary arterial smooth muscle they are much more extensive. The narrowing of the coronary arteries is produced by marked proliferation of intimal smooth muscle cells and Hurler cells.[356,377] In contrast, lesions in peripheral arteries resemble fibrous atherosclerotic plaques; thus, these lesions do not result from accumulation of masses of clear cells, which are present only in small numbers.[176]

Scheie and Hurler-Scheie Syndromes

Cardiac involvement in the other subtypes has been less well defined, particularly with respect to involvement of the coronary arteries and myocardium. The proper classification of a number of cases of mucopolysaccharidoses reported in the older literature remains uncertain.[321]

In the Scheie syndrome, aortic stenosis and regurgitation have been observed clinically,[276,321] but the only description available of the anatomic lesion reported cardiomegaly, severe right ventricular dilation, thickening and nodularity of all valves, fibrosis and shortening of chordae tendineae, and thickening of coronary arteries, with great reduction in their lumina.[98] Clear cells were present in endocardium, valves, chordae tendineae, and the media and intima of aorta, coronary arteries, and other large arteries.

One patient with Hurler-Scheie syndrome had moderate mitral stenosis, trivial mitral regurgitation, and aortic regurgitation; a similarly affected sister had calcification of mitral and aortic valves.[321] Two other patients showed evidence of mitral stenosis and mitral

annular calcification.[405] Another patient had thickening of the mitral leaflets and shortening and thickening of the chordae tendineae.[501] Vacuolated connective tissue cells were present in the valve, together with increased amounts of collagen and connective tissue ground substance.

Mucopolysaccharidosis II

MPS II (Hunter syndrome) is characterized by a deficiency of iduronate sulfatase. Three patients with MPS II were found to have diminished left ventricular ejection fractions and decreased velocity of circumferential fiber shortening, but no evidence of valvular disease.[405] However, in one necropsy patient, the edges of the mitral and tricuspid valve cusps appeared markedly thickened; the aortic valve was also slightly thickened, but the coronary arteries and aorta were not.[338] The valves contained large clear cells similar to those in patients with Hurler syndrome, as well as small sudanophilic cells (glycolipid deposits?). Clear cells also were present in myocardium and endocardium, but not in coronary arteries. Cardiac muscle cells did not contain abnormal material. Autopsy findings in a 10-year, 8-month-old boy with Hunter syndrome included clear, vacuolated cells in cardiac interstitium and valves, but without involvement of cardiac myocytes.[344] In a 32-year-old man with Hunter syndrome, severe aortic stenosis and mitral regurgitation were present; both valves were thickened and rigid. Histologically, they contained abundant fibrous tissue and clear cells. In addition, there was a left ventricular apical aneurysm, the wall of which contained many clear cells.[348]

Mucopolysaccharidosis III

Two types of MPS III (Sanfilippo syndrome) which differ in enzymatic defect are recognized: deficiency of heparan sulfatase in type A, and of N-acetyl-α-D-glucosaminidase in type B.

Cardiovascular pathologic findings have been described in three patients with type

A.[64,218,503] Two had mitral valvular deformity, which consisted of rigidity and thickening of the leaflets and shortening of the chordae tendineae.[64,218] These changes were attributed to diffuse fibrosis and to intra- and extracellular deposits of acid mucopolysaccharide material. Intracellular deposits were localized in small granular cells; large, clear (Hurler-like) cells were not present. One patient was thought to have narrowing of the mitral orifice.[64] Gross cardiomegaly has not been described. The aorta was normal in one patient[64] and showed minor changes in another.[503] One patient had subendothelial deposits of PAS-positive material in small splenic arteries.[64] The significance of these deposits is unclear.

Necropsy in one patient with biochemically proven Sanfilippo syndrome type B showed slight dilation of both ventricles and numerous tiny nodules on aortic and mitral valves.[422] The nodules were composed of fibrous connective tissue and numerous vacuolated cells. The coronary arteries and aorta were slightly sclerotic. Cardiac muscle cells and medial smooth muscle cells of systemic arteries also were vacuolated. The myocardial interstitium, endocardium, and areas of intimal thickening in large and medium-sized arteries also contained vacuolated cells. Ultrastructural study showed that some vacuoles in the clear cells were electron-lucent, whereas others were filled with laminated osmiophilic material.

Mucopolysaccharidosis IV

MPS IV (Morquio syndrome), due to deficiency of hexosamine-6-sulfatase, is sometimes associated with clinical evidence of aortic regurgitation.

Cardiac anatomic lesions reported in this syndrome include variable degrees of cardiomegaly; calcification of the pulmonary and aortic valve rings; thickening, and nodularity along the free edges, of the mitral, tricuspid, and pulmonary valve leaflets; endocardial thickening; and intimal thickening in the aorta, pulmonary trunk, and coronary arteries.[120,402] The coronary arteries can be significantly narrowed. Ultrastructural study detected clear vacuoles in the cytoplasm of smooth muscle cells in the coronary intima.[120]

One patient with MPS IV who had clinically significant mitral stenosis was found at autopsy to have thickening of the mitral, aortic and tricuspid valves and, to a lesser extent, of the pulmonary valve, in association with deposits of acid mucopolysaccharide material.[238]

Mucopolysaccharidosis VI

MPS VI (Maroteaux-Lamy syndrome), caused by deficiency of aryl sulfatase B, exists in at least three closely related forms. Aortic stenosis and regurgitation are the predominant lesions noted clinically; however, endocardial thickening and mitral valvular calcification have been observed at autopsy in other patients.[172,320,435] One patient with severe aortic valvular disease underwent aortic valvular replacement and was found to have a severely stenosed, calcified valve that contained vacuolated cells.[498]

Two patients with biochemically proven type VI MPS presented with a clinical picture of endocardial fibroelastosis. The diagnosis was confirmed at autopsy in one of them. The myocardium contained fibroblasts in which either parallel electron-dense lamellae or flocculent materials were present.[141]

Mucopolysaccharidosis VII

One patient with MPS VII (β-glucuronidase deficiency) had systemic hypertension, aortic regurgitation, and obstructive lesions in aorta and major blood vessels. His abdominal aorta showed fibromuscular dysplasia associated with vacuolated cells and abundant extracellular deposits of acid mucopolysaccharides.[27]

Mucolipidosis II and III

Mucolipidosis II (I cell disease) is transmitted as an autosomal recessive disorder characterized by a deficiency of multiple lysosomal hydrolases, which are active in the degradation of lipids and mucopolysaccharides, and by an accumulation of large, pleomorphic inclusions in a variety of cell types. Myocardial involvement is clinically prominent. Death frequently results from congestive heart failure.[39,165,168,339,355] Cardiomegaly occurs, sometimes in association with endocardial and pericardial thickening.[114] The mitral, tricuspid, and aortic valves are the sites of fibrous and nodular thickening. Prolapse of mitral, tricuspid, and aortic valve has been described in one patient.[400] Chordae tendineae are shortened and thickened. Lipid plaques are present in the aorta and other major vessels. The coronary arteries are thickened. Clear cells are present in the valves, chordae, and myocardial interstitium and in the intima of the aorta, the coronary, and other systemic arteries. Vacuoles in the clear cells contain flocculent material. Cardiac muscle cells have large, clear central areas; on ultrastructural study they contain pleomorphic inclusions.[339] Concentric lamellae are prominent components of these inclusions.

Patients with mucolipidosis III have been reported to have aortic and mitral murmurs,[262,420] but there are no anatomic descriptions of the cardiovascular lesions in this disorder.

Hyperoxaluria (Oxalosis)

Deposits of oxalate crystals (oxalosis) are found in the myocardium in primary and secondary hyperoxaluria.

Primary Hyperoxaluria

Primary hyperoxaluria is a general term for two rare disorders of glyoxalate metabolism with autosomal recessive transmission.[72] They are clinically indistinguishable from one another and are characterized by nephrocalcinosis and extrarenal deposits of calcium oxalate (oxalosis), which is identified as light yellow-brown, strongly birefringent crystals in routinely prepared sections stained with

H&E. Its insolubility in acetic acid helps differentiate it from other calcium salts.

In type I (glycolic aciduria), the most common form of the disease, deficiency of 2-oxoglutarate:glyoxylate carboligase results in systemic accumulation of glyoxylate and excessive urinary excretion of oxalic, glycolic, and glyoxylic acids. In type II (L-glyceric aciduria), deficiency of D-glyceric dehydrogenase results in accumulation of hydroxypyruvate and in excessive urinary excretion of oxalic and glyceric acids. In both types, the heart is the site of widespread deposits of oxalate crystals (Fig. 29–8), both intra- and extracellularly.[33,82,458,486] This is associated with necrosis, fibrosis, and infiltration with mononuclear and foreign-body-type giant cells. Oxalate deposits also occur in the conduction system, frequently in association with heart block. All arteries are affected to some degree; muscular arteries are more severely affected than elastic ones. Smooth muscle cells of arterial media are the most common site of deposition of oxalate crystals in many organ systems. These deposits are associated with degeneration or necrosis of the smooth muscle cells. Oxalate crystals in arterioles and capillaries often are larger than the vessel wall; they cause part of the wall to protrude into the lumen, which becomes narrowed or occluded. Acrocyanosis or gangrene of the extremities may result.

One patient with primary oxalosis developed massive intracardiac calcification and had an occlusion, presumably caused by emboli of calcific material, of a branch of the right middle cerebral artery.[101]

Secondary Oxalosis

Secondary oxalosis resulting from chronic renal insufficiency causes oxalate deposition in the heart and blood vessels similar to that seen in primary oxalosis.[38,127,198,397] Other causes of secondary oxalosis are

1. Ingestion of oxalic acid, oxalates, or ethylene glycol
2. Intravenous feeding with xylitol or anes-

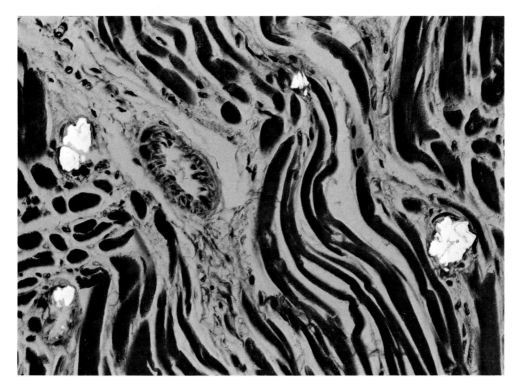

Fig. 29–8. Myocardium of a patient with primary oxalosis. Section viewed with polarized light to demonstrate birefringent crystals of calcium oxalate. (H&E × 400.)

thesia with methoxyflurane (two compounds that are metabolized to oxalate)
3. Enteric hyperoxaluria occurring in patients with extensive disease of the small bowel
4. Pyridoxine deficiency[71]

DISEASES OF AMINO ACID AND PROTEIN METABOLISM

Diseases of Amino Acid Metabolism

Ochronosis

Ochronosis, a manifestation of chronic alkaptonuria, results from the deposition of pigment produced by the oxidation and polymerization of homogentisic acid, an intermediate metabolite of tyrosine and phenylalanine.[156,343] The metabolic defect, a recessive trait, consists of deficient activity of homogentisic acid oxidase. Secondary ochronosis also can result from chronic toxicity of phenol and other compounds.

Ochronotic pigment appears bluish-black on gross examination and brownish in histologic sections. It is deposited in cartilage, intervertebral discs, and, to a lesser extent, in skin and sclera. All heart valves and valvular annuli, especially those of the mitral (Fig. 29–9) and aortic valves, are sites of heavy pigment deposition. Also involved by deposits are the endocardium, particularly at the base and tips of the papillary muscles; areas of endocardial and pericardial thickening; the aorta; the coronary arteries; other elastic and muscular arteries; veins and capillaries; and myocardium, especially in areas of fibrosis[85,156,289,343] and in

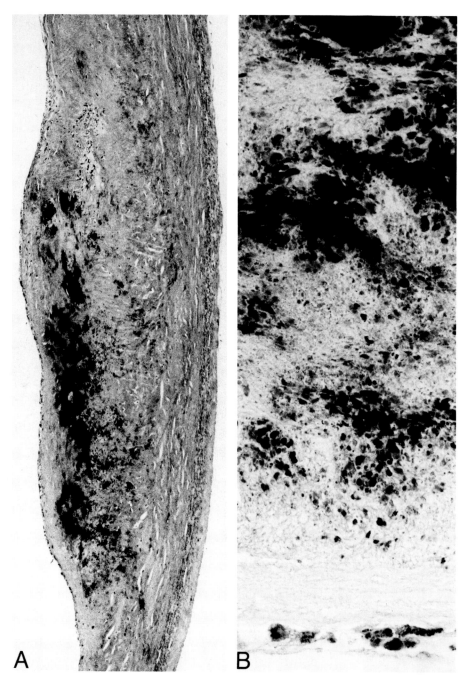

Fig. 29–9. Two views of mitral valve from a patient with ochronosis. (**A**) Low magnification showing distribution of dark deposits of ochronotic pigment. (Movat's pentachrome, × 40.) (**B**) High magnification of ventricular surface of the mitral valve shown in Fig. A. Note the intracellular (bottom) and extracellular (center and top) deposits of ochronotic pigment. (Movat pentachrome stain, × 400.)

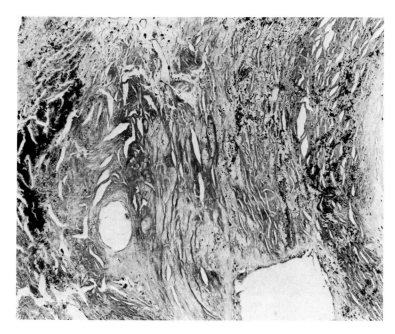

Fig. 29–10. Low magnification of large, extramural coronary artery from patient with ochronosis. The vessel is severely narrowed by plaque, which contains granular deposits of ochronotic pigment. (H&E, × 40.)

scars due to previous myocardial infarcts. Heavy pigmentation in cardiac valves and valvular annuli is frequently associated with calcium deposits.[85,89,290] It has been suggested that the presence of ochronotic pigment predisposes to valvular calcification.[155] Several patients with ochronosis have been reported to have aortic stenosis, with or without fusion of the commissures and with[187,291] or without[154,155] leaflet calcification. Marked pigmentation also has been observed in calcified and noncalcified atheromatous plaques in the aorta and other arteries, including coronary arteries (Fig. 29–10).[85,156,187,291,292]

Ochronotic pigment is deposited both intra- and extracellularly. Intracellular deposits occur in endothelial cells, fibroblasts, smooth muscle cells[154,155] and macrophages. They form small, membrane-bounded inclusions filled with electron-dense particles less than 100 nm in diameter.[354] Extracellular deposits form much larger, homogeneous granules in connective tissue.[18] These deposits, which are thought to resolve from breakdown of pigment-containing cells, affect all three layers of the arterial wall, especially the inner portion of the media. It is difficult to differentiate histochemically between ochronotic pigment and melanin.[343]

Homocystinuria

Homocystinuria, transmitted as an autosomal recessive disorder, is caused by a defect in the activity of cystathionine synthetase, which converts homocysteine to cystathionine. This results in increased plasma levels of homocysteine (which can be reversibly converted to homocystine) and methionine, and in increased urinary excretion of homocystine. A clinically similar syndrome occurs in patients with a defect in the activation of vitamin B12 (which is required to methylate homocysteine). Homocystinuria is manifest by mental retardation, seizures, skeletal deformities and ectopia lentis (similar to those seen in Marfan syndrome), and occlusive vascular disease (the major cause of death).

Lesions related to vascular disease include cerebrovascular accidents, myocardial infarction, peripheral arterial occlusions, venous thromboses, and pulmonary and systemic emboli.[192] Aortic thrombosis and aortic aneurysms also have been reported.[9,67] Veins, including cerebral cortical veins and sinuses, often are the sites of thromboses.[68,164] Histologically, the aorta shows intimal thickening and marked fragmentation of elastic fibers. Muscular arteries, including coronary arteries, demonstrate marked fibromuscular intimal thickening, fragmentation of the internal elastic lamina, and medial fibrosis. These changes lead to severe luminal narrowing. Arterioles show prominent vacuolization of endothelial cells and proliferation of perivascular connective tissue.[229,248,316]

The extraordinary tendency of vessels in patients with homocystinuria to undergo thrombosis seems related to (1) increased platelet consumption, (2) decreased platelet survival time, and (3) pronounced fragility of the endothelium, which tends to desquamate, thus predisposing to platelet thrombus formation on denuded subendothelial connective tissue. The vascular changes in homocystinuria are thought to result from increased plasma levels of homocysteine and can be reproduced in experimental animals by the administration of homocysteine.[199]

Hemoglobinopathies

Cardiovascular pathologic changes in patients with hemoglobinopathies can be classified according to whether they are consequences of anemia or of erythrocyte sickling. Cardiomegaly, hypertrophy, dilation of all cardiac chambers, a flabby consistency of heart muscle, and yellowish patches in the endocardial surfaces (caused by focal fatty degeneration of myocardial cells) are common in all types of severe anemia.[318] Myocardial hemosiderosis may result from multiple blood transfusions.

In addition to the lesions just described, patients with sickle cell disease (SS hemoglobin) often develop pulmonary vascular disease and pulmonary hypertension, related to repeated episodes of sickling and thrombosis in small pulmonary artery branches.[293,393] They also may have cerebrovascular disease, which results from sickling and thrombosis in small cerebral blood vessels and from narrowing and occlusion of large vessels. The latter changes are thought due to organization of thrombi and to fibromuscular proliferation that occurs independently of thrombus formation.[325,442] The types of cerebral/vascular lesions that may occur in sickle cell disease include ischemic and/or hemorrhagic infarction, intracerebral hemorrhage, cortical venous and/or sinus thrombosis, and subarachnoid hemorrhage.[504] Sickling and thrombosis in sickle cell disease also develop in vessels of other organs, including the heart, spleen, kidney, and retina. Conjunctival vessels may show striking tortuosity.[200] Areas of myocardial necrosis and fibrosis have been reported in a few patients with sickle cell disease.[393] Coronary arteries with unusually large diameters have been observed in other patients with the disease.[163] The existence of a type of cardiomyopathy that is specific for sickle cell disease or sickle cell trait continues to be debated.

In comparison with patients with sickle cell disease, those with sickle cell trait (SA hemoglobin) have much milder and infrequent episodes of visceral infarction, and, as a rule, do not show chronic cardiovascular abnormalities.[293] However, sudden cardiac death and myocardial infarction due to coronary thrombosis have been reported in patients with sickle cell trait[46] and in nonanemic patients with sickling associated with less well-defined abnormalities of hemoglobin types.[46,138]

Patients with hemoglobin SC disease are more symptomatic than those with sickle cell trait but have a lower incidence and severity of cardiovascular manifestations than do patients with sickle cell disease.[293] However, they frequently have pulmonary infarction[392] and much more severe retinal vascular occlusive disease than do patients with sickle cell disease.[77]

Amyloidosis

The term amyloidosis describes many disease processes that have as a common feature formation of extracellular deposits of proteins characterized by a β-pleated sheet conformation (amyloid deposits). This conformation is responsible for the distinctive staining characteristics of amyloid.[171] In these disorders are found, in various tissues, deposits of extracellular fibrils that measure 10 nm in diameter, have an affinity for Congo red stain, show a roentgen ray diffraction pattern of a β-pleated sheet, and are derived from soluble circulating proteins that are processed biochemically (involving partial proteolysis and polymerization) to convert them into insoluble deposits: target organs may be remote from the sites of synthesis of these proteins.[169,170] Several major types of amyloidosis, including AA amyloidosis, ASc amyloidosis, and AL amyloidosis, are recognized on the basis of the biochemical nature of the amyloidogenic proteins involved.

AA Amyloidosis

AA (secondary) amyloidosis is most often associated with chronic inflammatory states, including familial Mediterranean fever, rheumatoid arthritis, tuberculosis, and osteomyelitis. In AA amyloidosis, the deposited AA protein is a proteolytic product of serum AA protein, which behaves as an acute-phase reactant.[169,170,185]

ASc Amyloidosis

In the cardiovascular senile form of amyloidosis (isolated cardiac amyloidosis), the involved proteins are known as senile amyloid (ASc) proteins. Two of these proteins, a ventricular and an atrial form, have been iden-tified. The ventricular form has an amino acid sequence similar to that of serum prealbumin.[87,487,488] The pathogenesis of these two forms is unknown.

In other localized types of amyloidosis, the deposited proteins are derived from protein hormone precursors, as in pancreatic islets and in medullary carcinoma of the thyroid.[169,170,184]

AL Amyloidosis

AL amyloidosis, the most common form, occurs in primary amyloidosis and in multiple myeloma.[101] The proliferating plasma cells in both these disorders produce either whole immunoglobulin light chains or fragments thereof; these proteins are found in the plasma or urine or both and are the source of the amyloid deposits. It can be difficult to distinguish between AL amyloidosis related to multiple myeloma and that caused by primary amyloidosis, as bone marrow plasmacytosis occurs in both disorders. In myeloma, many clinical manifestations are related directly to the proliferation of plasma cells, whereas in primary amyloidosis, they are determined mainly by the organ dysfunction caused by the deposits of proteins synthesized by plasma cells.

Morphologic Changes

Cardiac deposits are very frequent in most types of amyloidosis and can be manifested by congestive heart failure, arrhythmias, restrictive cardiomyopathy, or by features mimicking those of ischemic or valvular disease (see Ch. 5).[54,66,432] Several reports have documented clinical features mimicking those of hypertrophic cardiomyopathy,[94,215,244,280,345,417,489] with both the obstructive and nonobstructive forms being reported.

Grossly, the heart in clinically significant cardiac amyloidosis is firm, rubbery, and noncompliant.[54] Amyloid deposits (Fig. 29–11) may occur in myocardial interstitium, con-

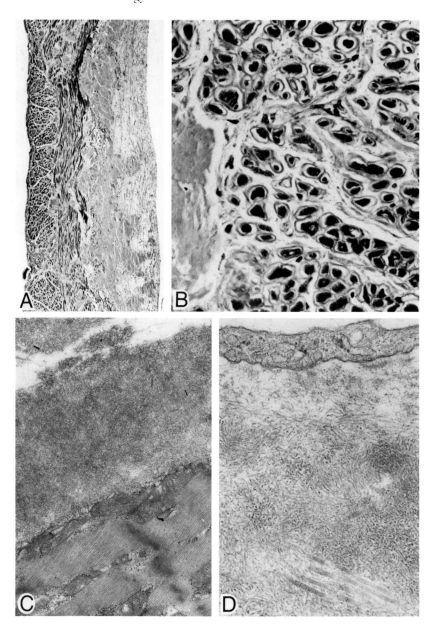

Fig. 29–11. (A, B) Light and **(C, D)** electron micrographs of heart of a patient with amyloidosis. **(A)** Low magnification of right atrial wall showing large deposits between endocardial surface and muscular layer. (H&E, × 40.) **(B)** High magnification of part of area shown in Fig. A. Part of large mass of amyloid is seen at left. Muscle fibers in center and right are surrounded by rings of amyloid material. **(C)** Peripheral region of cardiac muscle cell and surrounding ring composed of amyloid fibrils. (Uranyl acetate and lead citrate, × 16,500.) **(D)** High magnification showing structure of amyloid fibrils surrounding a capillary (endothelial cell is at top). (Uranyl acetate and lead citrate, × 37,500.)

duction tissue, valves, endocardium, pericardium, and in small intramural coronary arteries, veins, and capillaries; epicardial nerves are involved in patients with familial neuropathic syndromes of amyloidosis.[54,248] In the interstitium, amyloid deposits often form rings around cardiac myocytes and capillaries. Valvular deposits are either waxy and glistening or verrucous; only rarely do they significantly impair valvular function. Amyloid deposits localized to the valves have been described.[119] Bioprosthetic heart valves implanted for long periods develop amyloid deposits[175]: their pathogenesis is unknown. Endocardial deposits are tan, waxy-appearing, and can be seen grossly.[54] Deposits in coronary vessels involve all layers and can cause luminal obliteration.[54,432] Amyloid fibrils in myocardial interstitium have been demonstrated by electron microscopic study of necropsy and biopsy material.[54,70,212,234, 413,447] Such fibrils must be distinguished from connective tissue microfibrils, which occur commonly in fibrotic hearts and are larger (13 nm or more in diameter) than amyloid fibrils. The diagnosis of amyloidosis must be confirmed by demonstrating the green (dichroic) birefringence of the deposits, after staining with alkaline Congo red.

In familial neuropathic syndromes, amyloid deposits in blood vessels are prominent in the Portuguese type; myocardial interstitium is involved to a lesser extent. Cardiac interstitial involvement is extremely rare in amyloidosis associated with familial Mediterranean fever, but arterioles throughout the body are sites of amyloid deposition in this disorder.

A distinct syndrome of familial cardiomyopathy with extensive amyloid deposits in all cardiac structures has been reported in Denmark. Two patients had persistent right atrial standstill and familial cardiomyopathy with amyloidosis.[54] A syndrome of cerebral hemorrhage associated with amyloid deposits in cerebral arteries has been described in Iceland.[301]

Light Chain Deposit Disease

Under some circumstances, amyloidogenic proteins (usually immunoglobulin light chains) in the blood of certain patients with amyloidosis-like disorders do not form fibrils but, instead, produce amorphous deposits that do not stain with Congo red or the other usual stains for amyloid. Excessive amounts of either kappa or lambda chains can be synthesized (sometimes together with fragments of heavy chains) in AL amyloidosis; however, kappa light chains are more frequently associated with AL amyloidosis than are lambda light chains.[157,285] Some patients have been described in whom the function of organs, most notably the kidneys and heart, has been compromised by deposits that consists of light chains that do not form amyloid fibrils.[102,157,222,370] These patients are referred to as having "light chain deposit disease." This disorder, which occurs most frequently, but not exclusively, in association with multiple myeloma, is characterized by rapidly progressive renal disease, cardiac involvement manifested by congestive heart failure and restrictive cardiomyopathy, hepatic disease, and polyneuropathy.[157,158,222,285,370]

The mechanism of tissue deposition in most cases of AL amyloidosis is related to postsecretory proteolysis of light chains that are secreted as normal-sized chains but are especially sensitive to proteolysis. Thus, the AL amyloid fibrils contain fragments of light chains that essentially correspond to the "variable" regions of such chains.[157] This mechanism is different from that involved in light chain deposition disease, which involves the synthesis of structurally abnormal immunoglobulin chains. The spectrum of alterations in these chains includes abnormal chain glycosylation, aberrations in chain length, and defects in the "variable" region of the chain, all of which are considered critical for amyloid fibril formation. These biochemical abnormalities favor deposition of amorphous rather

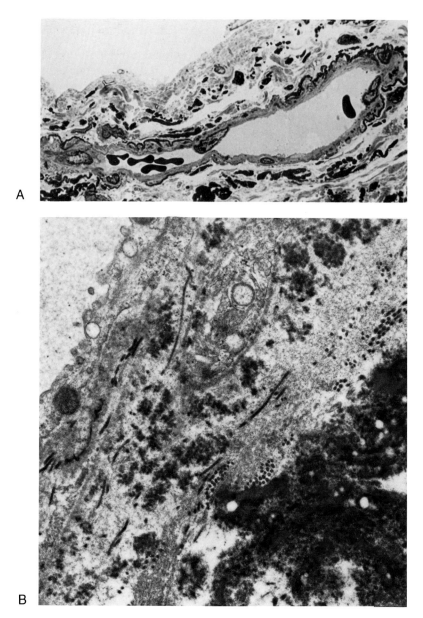

Fig. 29–12. (**A**) Intramyocardial arteriole from patient with light chain deposition disease. Amorphous deposits of light chains are seen in the vascular wall. (1-μm-thick plastic section.) (Alkaline toluidine blue, × 800.) (**B**) Electron microgaph of part of the vessel shown in Fig. A. The light chain deposits are amorphous, electron-dense, and localized in the subendothelial space, around smooth muscle cells, and in the adventitia. (× 20,000.)

than fibrillar material.[157] It has been suggested that deposits in light chain deposition disease contain variously altered "constant" portions of the light chains.[157] An intermediate form, featuring both AL amyloidosis and light chain deposition, has been reported in a patient in whom results of ultrastructural and immunohistochemical studies demonstrated amyloid deposits in the myocardium, tongue, walls of portal vein branches, and synovium from the knee, and light chain deposits in the liver, spleen, and bone marrow.[270] Differences in the therapeutic and prognostic implications of AL amyloidosis and light chain deposition disease remain to be fully assessed.

Light chain deposits occurring in myocardium (Figs. 29–12 and 29–13) as a complication of multiple myeloma were identified ultrastructurally and immunohistochemically in a right ventricular endomyocardial biopsy specimen from a patient who presented with clinical and hemodynamic findings of restrictive cardiomyopathy. These deposits were not evident on routine histopathologic examination; they were Congo red-negative and gave a positive immunoperoxidase reaction for kappa light chains and a negative reaction for lambda chains. They consisted of amorphous, electron-dense granules that formed discontinuous layers adjacent to the plasma membranes of cardiac myocytes, arteriolar endothelial and smooth muscle cells, and neural elements.[313]

Diseases of Protein Metabolism

Included in this section are several genetic disorders related to abnormal synthesis of extracellular connective tissue proteins, particularly those in collagenous and elastic fibers. Synthesis of these components is highly complex and incompletely delineated. Different biochemical defects in these processes lead to various types of structural weaknesses in cardiac valves and blood vessel walls, as well as to diverse extracardiac abnormalities, which often involve the skeletal system. Microscopic findings, which are similar in some of the diseases, must be carefully correlated with gross anatomic findings, which may be more distinctive.

Marfan Syndrome

Marfan syndrome is characterized by musculoskeletal abnormalities, ectopia lentis, and cardiovascular lesions, the most striking of which are dilation of the aortic root and mitral and aortic regurgitation. It is transmitted as an autosomal dominant trait; the biochemical defect is unknown. Expression of the abnormalities varies among different patients. It had been thought unlikely that a single biochemical defect could explain the wide range of phenotypic expression in Marfan syndrome.[193] Recent studies suggest that the basic abnormality may be a defect in the synthesis of microfibrils associated with elastic fibers.[173] Correlation between cardiac and extracardiac lesions is variable. Some patients (said to have a forme fruste of the syndrome) present only part of the spectrum of clinical manifestations.

Roberts[379] identified three patterns of cardiovascular involvement in patients with Marfan syndrome: saccular aneurysms of the ascending aorta, dissection of the entire aorta, and mitral valve prolapse not associated with aortic disease.

Saccular aneurysms involve the sinuses of Valsalva and proximal tubular portion of the ascending aorta. They tend to rupture rather than dissect.[145] Aneurysms in Marfan syndrome also have been reported in the descending thoracic and abdominal aorta,[174,227] pulmonary artery,[319] cerebral vessels,[256] ductus arteriosis,[89] and coronary arteries.[145] The walls of the aneuryms (Fig. 29–14) show severe fragmentation, atrophy and loss of elastic fibers, and an increase in acid mucopolysaccharide material, which forms pools between remaining elastic lamellae.[44,399,449] Increased vascularization of the media also has been described.[145] Ultrastructural studies show that

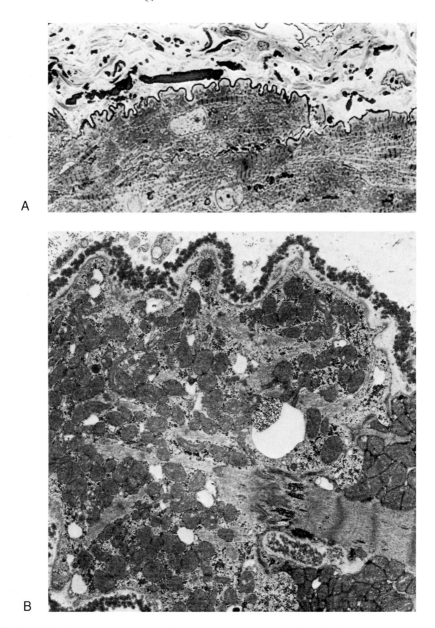

Fig. 29–13. (**A**) Light chain deposition disease. Same tissue as in Fig. 29–12. Semithin section, showing light chain deposits along external surfaces of cardiac myocytes. (Toluidine blue, × 700.) (**B**) Electron micrograph of myocyte shown in Fig. A. Note amorphous deposits of light chains in area of basement membrane. (× 20,000.)

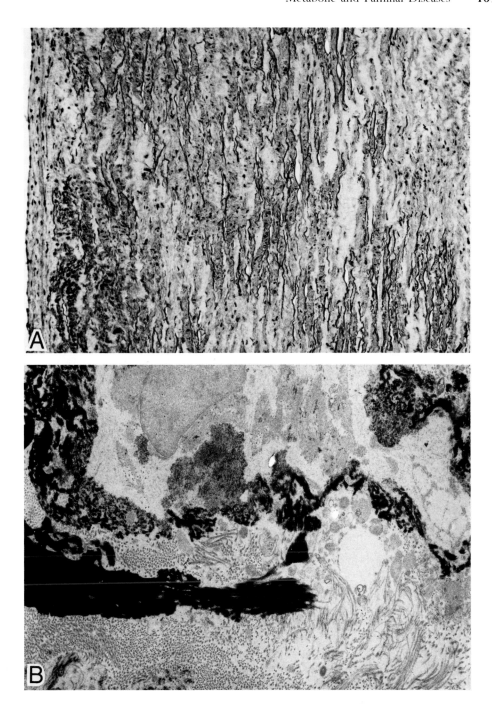

Fig. 29–14. Aorta in Marfan syndrome. (**A**) Histologic section showing loss of elastic fibers and accumulation of pools of acid mucopolysaccharide material in the media. (Movat's pentachrome, × 100.) (**B**) Electron micrograph of media showing one normal elastic fiber (lower left) and two other abnormal, frayed elastic fibers (center and upper right). (Tannic acid-uranyl acetate, × 13,500.)

the accumulations of acid mucopolysaccharide material form a meshwork of fine filaments and star-shaped granules that often are in close relationship to elastic and collagenous fibers.[399,449] Elastic fibers (Fig. 29–9) have a moth-eaten appearance; their amorphous component shows an increase in electron density and appears to degenerate into masses of dark granules. These changes in elastic tissue are nonspecific and have been observed in other conditions, including senile elastoses. To a lesser extent, the changes just described may be found in other arteries, including coronary arteries;[440,449] however, peripheral arterial disease is rarely of clinical significance in Marfan syndrome.[319]

Patients with Marfan syndrome in whom aortic dissection occurs tend to have morphologically normal aortas, which show changes comparable to those in age-matched control patients.[379] Schlatmann and Becker demonstrated that functions of aging in normal aortas include the occurrence of changes of cystic medial necrosis (defined as pooling of acid mucopolysaccharides), elastic tissue fragmentation, fibrosis, and loss of nuclei. Thus, differences with respect to these changes in normal and abnormal aortas are quantitative rather than qualitative.[408,409]

The following factors can contribute to the development of aortic regurgitation in Marfan syndrome: dilation of the sinuses of Valsalva and the aortic annulus (by far the most common causes),[96,338,379] floppiness and myxoid change in aortic valve cusps,[346] aortic dissection displacing a cusp downward,[336] and perforation of a cusp (see also Ch. 27).[379] Aortic lesions in Marfan syndrome are more common in adults; mitral lesions are more common in children.[363,378]

Mitral regurgitation in Marfan syndrome is most commonly due to floppiness of the leaflets and dilation of the mitral annulus;[365] calcification of the annulus[258]; or elongation, contraction, or rupture of chordae tendineae. Papillary muscle dysfunction also can occur (see also Ch. 25).[428] The floppy mitral leaflet and aortic cusps show accumulation of myxoid material, mainly in the spongiosa.[254,346] Severe cardiac hypertrophy can result from the aortic and mitral valvular lesions.

Luminal narrowing due to fibromuscular intimal hyperplasia has been found in small intramural coronary arteries and in arteries supplying the SA and AV nodes.[252] A particularly severe, rapidly progressive form of Marfan syndrome has been reported in small children, in whom aortic dilation and cardiac valvular lesions coexist in association with muscular skeletal deformities and with marked alterations in the aortic structure.[308] The latter shows histologic changes consisting of loss and disruption of elastic fibers and accumulation of acid mucopolysaccharide material. These changes are similar to those observed in adults with Marfan syndrome. A variety of congenital heart malformations have been observed in association with Marfan syndrome; coarctation of the aorta and atrial septal defect are unusually frequent.[116,307,319]

A syndrome of *congenital contractural arachnodactyly* has been reported as being different from Marfan syndrome.[362] It is characterized by arachnodactyly and by contractures of the fingers, elbows, and knees. It was originally thought not to be associated with cardiovascular lesions[209,299]; however, one patient with this syndrome had mitral and tricuspid valvular prolapse and dilation of the aortic and pulmonary root.[194] More recently, several patients with this syndrome were found to have mitral valvular prolapse, thus blurring the distinction between this disorder and Marfan syndrome.[12]

9q34 Duplication Syndrome

Patients with the 9q34 duplication syndrome present with physical findings similar to those observed in Marfan syndrome and in congenital contractile arachnodactyly.[7] However, they have minimal or no cardiovascular complications, and they can be clearly identified on the basis of cytogenetic studies, which show the chromosomal abnormality.

Larsen Syndrome

Larsen syndrome is characterized by skeletal dysplasia with multiple joint dislocation and a characteristic facies. The basis of these abnormalities appears to be a generalized, still unidentified, disorder of connective tissue. More than 80 cases have been reported in the literature with isolated instances of congenital cardiac septal defects and acquired abnormalities of aorta or mitral valve. These abnormalities include dilation of the aorta, aortic insufficiency, mitral valve prolapse, tricuspid valve prolapse, and aortic dissection and aneurysm. One patient had aortic dilation and an aneurysm of the ductus arteriosus.[268] Histologically, the wall at the aneurysm showed myxoid change and disruption of elastic fibers. These changes were thought to resemble those reported in Marfan syndrome.

Fragile X Syndrome (Martin-Bell Syndrome)

A high incidence of mitral valve prolapse and dilation of the aortic root has been found in patients with the fragile X syndrome, a relatively common disorder characterized by mental retardation, a long face, large and prominent ears, macroorchidism, prognathism, and a fragile site on the long arm of the X chromosome. A metabolic defect in connective tissue is suspected but has not been identified. Cardiovascular morphologic findings have been described in only one patient, who showed fragmentation and a decreased number of elastic fibers in the aorta and myxoid change and elastic fiber fragmentation in the mitral valve leaflets.[436]

An 18-year-old mentally retarded male with Martin-Bell syndrome was fragile X positive. He died suddenly with viral pneumonia and myocarditis. At autopsy, generalized tubular hypoplasia of the aorta and a mild coarctation were discovered. The base of the mitral and tricuspid valves showed striking aberrations in elastin distribution and structure by light microscopy. Local collagen alterations were also noted. Comparable changes were seen in skin elastin as well as a severe depletion of acid mucopolysaccharides.[480]

Ehlers-Danlos Syndrome

Ehlers-Danlos syndrome is a heterogeneous group of 12 genetically distinct disorders of connective tissue synthesis, which differ in major clinical features, inheritance patterns, and biochemical defects. The modes of inheritance are autosomal dominant in types I–IV and VIII; X-linked recessive in types V and IX; autosomal recessive in types VI, VII, and X; and undetermined in types XI and XII. Types I, II, and III are due to unknown biochemical defects; type IV, to deficient synthesis of type III collagen (several different defects have been found in different patients); type V, to a lysyl oxidase deficiency; type VI, to lysyl hydroxylase deficiency; type VII, to a procollagen peptidase deficiency; type IX, to defective collagen cross-linking due to decreased lysyl oxidase activity (abnormal cellular handling of copper); type X, to defective fibronectin; and types IX, XI, and XII to unknown defects.[416]

Cardiovascular lesions have been described in most types of Ehlers-Danlos syndrome.[499] Evaluation of cardiovascular findings in many reported patients is complicated because clinical features of approximately half of them are difficult to classify exactly. It has been emphasized that there is poor correlation between the severity of cardiac and extracardiac findings in patients with Ehlers-Danlos syndrome.[423] Dissection of the aorta and tears in peripheral arteries have been reported in type I, the gravis form.[30] One patient with type II, the mitis form, had an atrial septal defect, congenital AV block, and an aneurysm of the ascending aorta.[388] Another patient had aneurysms of the brachial artery and abdominal aorta.[59] Mitral valvular prolapse occurs in type III, the benign hypermobile form.[63] Major vascular complications are most common in patients with type IV, the ecchymotic, arterial, or Sack type.[23,30,412,416,464] These patients are predisposed to sudden death from rupture of the aorta or other major arteries or veins. They frequently have varicose veins, tortuous arteries, arterial aneurysms, and a prominent superficial venous pattern. Affected vessels are easily torn and may appear smaller than normal in size. Histologically, they show thinning of the wall, with a diffuse decrease in elastic tissue in the media, deposition of acid mucopolysaccharide material between medial elastic lamellae, and a decrease in adventitial and medial collagen. They do not show changes of "cystic medial necrosis." Aortic rupture may be mediated by a tear in a previously undamaged but thin and fragile portion of the vessel.

A rare finding associated with Ehlers-Danlos syndrome is the occurrence of multiple congenital aneurysms of elastic and muscular arteries, including coronary arteries. Of four patients reported with these changes (which may represent a variant of type IV Ehlers-Danlos syndrome), three were between the ages of 5 and 8 years, and one was 42-years-old; only two of these patients demonstrated some of the other connective tissue abnormalities associated with Ehlers-Danlos syndrome.[236,424,497] Histologic studies demonstrated a normal internal elastic lamina, distortion and clumping of medial elastic fibers, replacement of the outer third of the media by collagen, and an increased amount of acid mucopolysaccharide material in the media. The media of the aorta and muscular arteries showed a decrease in the total amount of connective tissue, with separation and disruption of collagen fibers. Medial smooth muscle cells in muscular arteries were decreased in number; in the aorta, they varied in size and arrangement. Recent studies indicate that there may be further clinical and biochemical heterogeneity among patients with type IV.[60] A consistent, but not specific, ultrastructural abnormality in this type is the reduction in the diameter of collagen fibrils in the media of muscular arteries.[60]

Cardiovascular lesions reported in other types of Ehlers-Danlos syndromes include mitral valvular prolapse in types V, VI, VIII, X, and XI; aortic rupture in type VI; cor pulmonale in type IX; dilated aortic root in type X; and sinus of Valsalva aneurysms in type XII.[499]

Various congenital heart malformations have been recorded in patients with undetermined types of Ehlers-Danlos syndrome,[13,31,125,481] but it is uncertain whether such abnormalities of cardiac morphogenesis are a consequence of the connective tissue disorder.

Osteogenesis Imperfecta

Osteogenesis imperfecta is the name given to a group of generalized disorders of connective tissue that primarily affects bone, tendons, ligaments, and dentin. It occurs in four forms,[427] which differ in age of onset, associated phenotypic signs, mode of inheritance, severity of bone fragility, and resultant skeletal deformity.[226,366,493,494] Type II is the most devastating form and is lethal in the perinatal period. The presence of broad, as opposed to thin, bones and the fracture pattern of ribs determine the subtype (A, B, or C) of lethal perinatal (type II) osteogenesis imperfecta. Osteogenesis imperfecta results from structural defects in collagen. The defects usually involve the proalpha chains of procollagen I monomers and may result in secondary metabolic derangements such as decreased procollagen secretion.

Aortic valve insufficiency is the most commonly encountered cardiac manifestation of osteogenesis imperfecta type I and is frequently accompanied by dilation of the aortic root. Mitral valve dysfunction has also been reported. Redundant mitral leaflets and dilated valve rings accounted for mitral regurgitation in a few cases. Wood et al.[505] described two patients with ruptured mitral valve chordae tendineae. Myxoid (mucinous) degeneration of the aortic valves and cystic medial necrosis of the aorta have been noted. Criscitiello et al.[88] also described a decrease in the number of elastic lamellae in the aorta and pulmonary artery of a 50-year-old man with osteogenesis imperfecta type I. There seem to be no descriptions of cardiovascular pathology in patients with osteogenesis imperfecta type III or IV.

Overall, the most common valvular problem in osteogenesis imperfecta is aortic regurgitation; less common are mitral regurgitation and combined aortic and mitral regurgitation.[80,92,210,323,364,376,426,439] Aortic regurgitation results from dilation of the aortic root and deformity of the valvular leaflets, which become abnormally translucent, weak, and elongated. Aneurysms of the sinuses of Valsalva also occur. The mitral annulus is dilated; the mitral leaflets are attenuated, redundant, and tend to prolapse, and chordae tendineae may rupture. The coronary arteries usually are normal. The aorta and valves show decreased amounts of fibrous connective tissue and elastic fibers, as well as areas of myxoid change with accumulation of acid mucopolysaccharide material.[88,217,438,484,505]

Cutis Laxa

The term cutis laxa designates a heterogeneous group of disorders that affect elastic fibers and are characterized by loose, redundant, inelastic skin and a high incidence of emphysema, aortic dilation, and multiple hernias. Congenital and acquired types have been described. A deficiency of lysyl oxidase may be involved in the pathogenesis of the congenital type. It can be variously transmitted as an autosomal dominant, autosomal recessive, or sex-linked disorder. The dominant form is not associated with cardiovascular lesions.[32] Emphysema and arterial disease are most prominent in the recessive form, in which the aortic root, the ascending aorta, and major branches of the aortic arch and the vertebral arteries show dilation, elongation, and tortuosity.[32,104,206,478] Dilation of the thoracic aorta also occurs in the acquired type.[201,373] Rupture of the thoracic aorta without aneurysm formation has been described in a patient with the acquired type.[201] Dilation of the pulmonary artery, multiple stenoses in

peripheral pulmonary arterial branches, and tortuosity of pulmonary veins have been reported in the congenital recessive form of cutis laxa.[296,483] Cor pulmonale can result from emphysema or from multiple pulmonary arterial stenoses.[483]

Histologically, affected vessels show a marked decrease in elastic fibers (which often appear fragmented and granular) and an increase in acid mucopolysaccharides.[178,322,401] On ultrastructural study, elastic fibers appear irregular in outline; abundant microfibrils and accumulations of electrodense granular material surround the amorphous (elastin) component. The elastic fibers are not calcified.[178,201,204,401] Both the histologic and ultrastructural changes resemble those found in Marfan syndrome. In one patient with cutis laxa, study of the elastic fibers of the skin revealed normal microfibrils and abnormal, markedly decreased amorphous (elastin) components.[97] Severe coronary arterial narrowing associated with an aortic aneurysm was reported in a small child with the acquired form of cutis laxa (Sweet syndrome).[337] The pathogenesis of this lesion (postinflammatory and elastolysis) remains unknown.

Pseudoxanthoma Elasticum

Pseudoxanthoma elasticum (PXE) is a systemic disorder transmitted as an autosomal recessive trait and manifested by cutaneous lesions, retinal angioid streaks, gastrointestinal hemorrhages, and fragmentation and calcification of elastic fibers. The underlying biochemical defect is unknown.

Cardiovascular manifestations result from enlargement and calcification of elastic fibers in the intima and media of peripheral muscular arteries.[181] These changes may be associated with premature atherosclerosis. The distinctive cardiac lesions (Fig. 29–15A) are yellowish-white endocardial plaques, which are composed of degenerated, calcified elastic fibers located in the deeper areas of the endocardium.[324,402] Endocardium is more frequently affected in the atria than in the

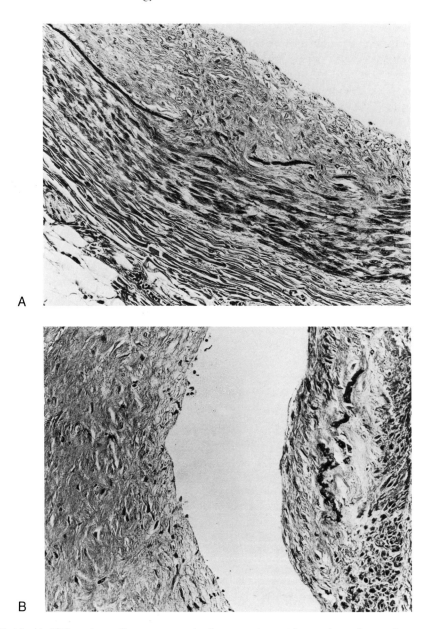

Fig. 29–15. (**A, B**) Two views of coronary arteries from a patient with pseudoxanthoma elasticum, showing areas of calcification and fragmentation of the internal elastic lamina. (H&E, × 160.)

ventricles. Calcification of the posterior leaflet of the tricuspid valve has been described.[324] The femoral, radial, and ulnar arteries are among the most common sites of arterial calcification.[181] Despite its abundant content of elastic fibers, the aorta is infrequently involved; however, almost complete occlusion of the ascending aorta by a calcific mass has been reported.[328] Intimal calcification involves the internal elastic lamina (Fig. 29–

15B) and can progress to irregular, discrete plaques, causing severe luminal narrowing. Atherosclerotic plaques also can contribute to luminal stenosis. Medial calcification is more uniformly distributed, encompasses the entire circumference of the artery, and is not frequently associated with marked luminal narrowing.[181] There is extreme variation in the degree of coronary arterial disease. Sudden death in PXE has been associated with coronary arterial involvement[496] and with encasement of the bundle branches by fibrous tissue.[229] Myocardial infarction is surprisingly infrequent.[90]

On histologic examination, abnormal elastic fibers appear larger than normal, are disorganized and fragmented, and show strong basophilia in preparations stained with hematoxylin and eosin. The basophilia is due to calcific deposits, which involve the amorphous (elastin) component of elastic fibers.[5]

DISEASES OF PURINE AND PYRIMIDINE METABOLISM

Gout

Accelerated atherosclerosis is the most common cardiovascular lesion associated with gout. More direct, but rather uncommon consequences of gout are deposits of urate crystals, sometimes forming large tophi. These are found in the walls of blood vessels (including coronary arteries) and in the myocardial interstitium, pericardium, and conduction system (occasionally causing complete heart block); also, in the mitral annulus and mitral, aortic, and tricuspid valve leaflets.[58,78,216,292,367,459,476] Urate deposits are histochemically identifiable by fixation in absolute ethanol, followed by staining with the de Galantha method. Uric acid crystals must

be differentiated from other types of crystals that can be deposited in myocardial tissues.

Progeria

Patients with progeria (Hutchinson-Gilford syndrome) develop, at a very early age, hypertension, hypercholesterolemia, generalized arteriosclerosis, and ischemic heart disease; death follows cardiac complications during late childhood or adolescence. The heart shows dilation of all chambers. Some patients have multiple, small foci of myocardial necrosis and fibrosis, whereas others have large infarcts. Coronary atherosclerosis is usually severe, and the coronary ostia may be markedly narrowed. Numerous lipofuscin granules may accumulate in cardiac muscle cells. Calcification develops in aortic and mitral valvular leaflets, large extramural coronary arteries, and cerebral arteries. Left ventricular endocardium may be thickened. Atheromatous changes are present in the aorta, pulmonary artery, and large and medium-sized systemic arteries.[16,152,302,303,375,387,450]

The biochemical defect in progeria is unknown, although it has been suggested that defective repair of DNA breaks may be at fault.[118]

DISEASES OF LIPID METABOLISM

Hyperlipoproteinemia

The five types of hyperlipoproteinemia exist both as genetically transmitted disorders (primary hyperlipoproteinemias) and as acquired disorders (secondary hyperlipoproteinemias) related to other systemic diseases. There is evidence indicating that each of the five familial types of hyperlipoproteinemia is biochemically heterogeneous.[148]

Type I Hyperlipoproteinemia

Type I hyperlipoproteinemia is characterized by defective activity of lipoprotein lipase, an enzyme located on the plasma membrane of endothelial cells that hydrolyzes chylomicrons. The defect may involve either the enzyme itself or its activator, apoprotein C-II, and results in greatly delayed clearance of chylomicrons formed from absorption of dietary fat. Because of this, chylomicrons accumulate in large amounts in plasma, from which they are removed by cells of the mononuclear phagocyte system, particularly in bone marrow and spleen.[132,136] These cells become enlarged and filled with chylomicron aggregates and with the products of their degradation (Fig. 29–16). Patients with type I hyperlipoproteinemia have no evidence of accelerated atherosclerosis; the only cardiovascular lesions described in these patients are yellow patches containing foam cells found in the left atrial endocardium.[381]

Type II Hyperlipoproteinemia

Type II hyperlipoproteinemia (familial hypercholesterolemia) is manifested by elevation of plasma low density lipoproteins (LDL) and plasma cholesterol without (type IIa) or with (type IIb) elevation of triglycerides. It is caused by deficiency of LDL receptors. Located on the surfaces of certain cells, these receptors control the intracellular entry of LDL, thus regulating LDL degradation and synthesis of cholesterol.[177]

Type II hyperlipoproteinemia exists in homozygous and heterozygous forms, which differ in the severity and age of onset of clinical symptoms. Symptoms are related to accel-

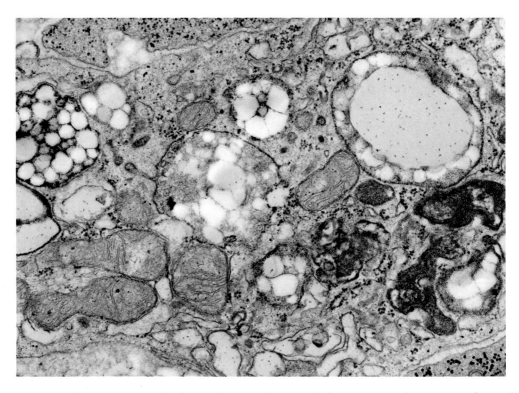

Fig. 29–16. Electron micrograph of part of a macrophage in the bone marrow of a patient with type I hyperlipoproteinemia. The cell contains phagosomes filled with chylomicrons (rounded, electron-lucent particles) embedded in a dense matrix. (Uranyl acetate and lead citrate, × 30,000.)

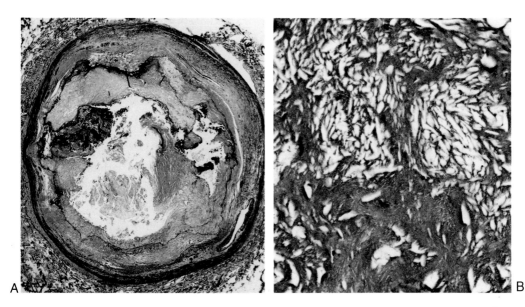

Fig. 29–17. Homozygous type II hyperlipoproteinemia. **(A)** Coronary artery showing severe atheromatosis and calcification. (H&E, × 20.) **(B)** Abundant lipid deposits, seen as "cholesterol clefts" in fibrous connective tissue, are present in endocardium. (Movat's pentachrome, × 250.)

erated atherosclerosis and to deposition of cholesterol in vascular walls, cardiac valves, and xanthomatous lesions (Figs. 29–17 and 29–18). Extremely severe aortic and coronary atherosclerosis (Fig. 29–17) develop in childhood in homozygous patients in association with tuberous and tendinous xanthomas. Aortic valvular disease is frequent. With the exception of the latter, which does not occur in heterozygous patients, these cardiovascular lesions are similar in heterozygous patients but become manifested in adulthood.[378]

The atherosclerotic lesions are more severe in the ascending than in the abdominal aorta (reversal of the usual pattern of distribution of aortic atherosclerotic lesions). The degree of involvement of the ascending aorta in homozygous patients can be so severe as to produce the clinical and angiographic picture of supravalvular aortic stenosis.[383,390,429,437,485] Atherosclerotic plaques can produce severe coronary ostial narrowing and myocardial infarction without significant coronary artery disease.[382] The aortic valve may be markedly stenosed by fibrous tissue, deposits of foam

cells, and cholesterol clefts in the cusps.[24,314] Thickening of the mitral valve (causing both mitral stenosis and mitral regurgitation), pulmonary valve, and endocardium (Fig. 29–12) by foam cells also has been reported.[24,300] The foam cells in xanthomas in type II hyperlipoproteinemia (Fig. 29–18) contain abundant lipid deposits; most are free in the cytoplasm, and only a few are intralysosomal.[56] Similar cells are found in bone marrow.

The coronary arteries show widespread proximal and distal disease, with frequent, clinically significant stenosis in the left main coronary artery.[42] Atherosclerotic plaques also develop in the pulmonary trunk and its branches.[24] The histologic appearance of the atherosclerotic plaques does not differ in patients with type II or type IV hyperlipoproteinemia or than those found in persons with normal lipoprotein patterns.[177,379]

Type III Hyperlipoproteinemia

Type III hyperlipoproteinemia is characterized by increased plasma levels of triglycer-

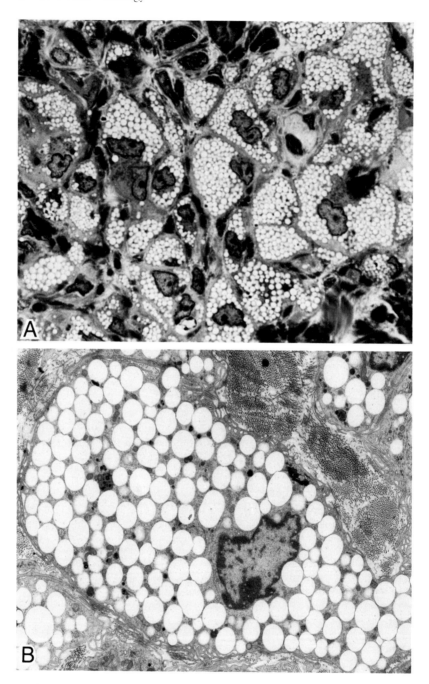

Fig. 29–18. Tuberous xanthoma from the elbow of a patient with homozygous type II hyperlipopro-teinemia. (**A**) Light micrograph showing foam cells with numerous lipid droplets. (1-μm-thick section of plastic-embedded tissue.) (Alkaline toluidine blue, × 1200.) (**B**) Electron micrograph of foam cell in same tissue as in Fig. A, showing irregular, convoluted cell surfaces and lipid deposits composed of spherical droplets. (Uranyl acetate and lead citrate, × 6,300.)

ides and cholesterol; tuberoeruptive xanthomas of the palms, elbows, knees, and buttocks; and premature cardiovascular disease, including coronary artery and peripheral vascular disease.[334] Diseases associated with type III include diabetes mellitus and hypothyroidism. Elevated uric acid values have been reported in 40 percent of patients, although clinical gout is rare.

Three major classes of molecular defects are associated with type III hyperlipoproteinemia: a deficiency in apolipoprotein E, a structural defect in apolipoprotein E, and a functional defect in the liver receptor system. Apolipoprotein E is a major determinant in the hepatic catabolism of intestine-derived chylomicron remnant particles. Most patients with type III have a structural defect in apolipoprotein E, delayed catabolism of chylomicrons remnants, elevated levels of plasma cholesterol and triglycerides, elevated plasma very low-density lipoprotein (VLDL) cholesterol, and reduced plasma LDL cholesterol and high density lipoprotein (HDL) cholesterol.[50,204,207] In type III patients the VLDL and intermediate density lipoproteins are cholesterol-rich and triglyceride-poor compared with VLDL from control subjects.[50]

The first necropsy observations in a patient with type III hyperlipoproteinemia described occlusion of the lumina of major coronary arteries by deposits consisting primarily of foam cells that stained strongly with fat stains.[380,382] However, subsequent reports showed that both coronary arteries (Fig. 29–19) and saphenous vein bypass grafts were occluded by atheromas that were unusual only because they contained a scattering of foam and mononuclear cells.[11,61,188,223,291] Of six patients with type III hyperlipoproteinemia who died from coronary artery disease, all had severe atherosclerosis of the aorta, major coronary arteries, and common iliac arteries; three had severe narrowing (> 75% of the cross-sectional area of the lumen) of the left main coronary artery; and only one had atypical coronary atherosclerotic plaques with increased numbers of foam cells. Immuno-peroxidase staining of coronary plaques from patients with type III showed no difference in the location of apolipoproteins A-I, A-II, B, C-I, and C-III when compared to plaques from patients with type II and IV hyperlipoproteinemia or from those with normal lipoprotein values.[50]

Type IV Hyperlipoproteinemia

Patients with type IV hyperlipoproteinemia have elevated plasma VLDL levels. The condition is associated with a high incidence of coronary artery disease and myocardial infarction. The biochemical defect is unknown. In angiographic studies, Bloch et al.[42] found that patients with type IV hyperlipoproteinemia have less severe coronary artery disease and much less frequent stenosis of the left main coronary artery than patients with type II hyperlipoproteinemia. The atherosclerotic plaques in patients with type IV hyperlipoproteinemia do not differ morphologically from those in patients with type II hyperlipoproteinemia or in patients with normal lipoprotein patterns. As in type III hyperlipoproteinemia, atherosclerosis in type IV hyperlipoproteinemia is more severe in the abdominal than thoracic aorta.

Type V Hyperlipoproteinemia

Primary type V hyperlipoproteinemia is a diverse group of disorders in which exogenous hypertriglyceridemia (chylomicrons are present in the fasting state) is accompanied by endogenous hypertriglyceridemia (increased VLDL levels).[218] The hypertriglyceridemia often is severe (triglyceride levels > 2000 mg/dL) and frequently is accompanied by pancreatitis, abdominal pain, hepatosplenomegaly, eruptive xanthomas, abnormal glucose tolerance, and hyperuricemia.[124,147] The biochemical defect has not been identified.

The rarity of type V hyperlipoproteinemia may account for the paucity of reports of cardiovascular lesions in this disorder and of its association with accelerated atherosclerosis. All major coronary arteries were occluded to

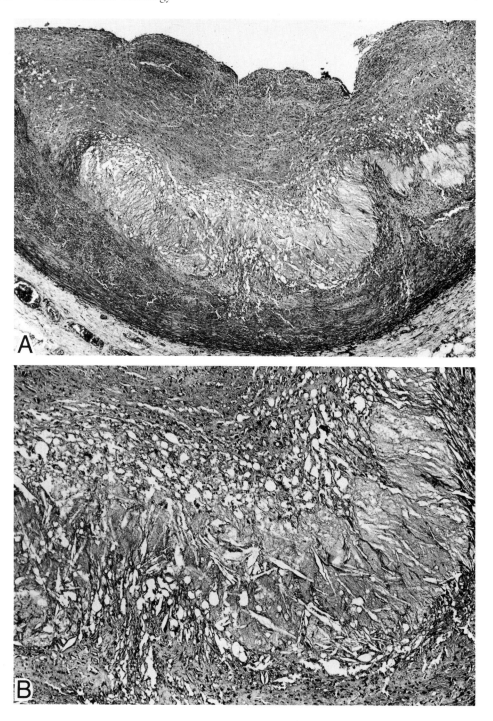

Fig. 29–19. Coronary artery in type III hyperlipoproteinemia. (**A**) Low magnification, showing lipid-rich plaque surrounded by dense fibrous tissue. (H&E, × 40.) (**B**) Higher magnification of plaque in Fig. A, showing foam cells and cholesterol clefts. (H&E, × 100.)

variable degrees in a patient reported with type V hyperlipoproteinemia.[439] Histologically, coronary arteries were thickened by fibrous plaques and frank atheromas, some of which were calcified. Another report described severe coronary atherosclerosis in a 40-year-old man with type V who died of coronary artery disease.[294]

Familial Lipoprotein Deficiency

A significant, independent, inverse relation between HDL cholesterol levels and coronary artery disease has been described in epidemiologic studies of a general population.[69,183] Several reports have characterized a group of inherited dyslipoproteinemias in which low levels of HDL cholesterol are associated with accelerated atherosclerosis.[133,196,221,280] These disorders are familial apo A-I and apo C-III deficiency, Tangier disease, HDL deficiency with planar xanthomas, apo A-I Milano, fish-eye disease, and familial hypoalphalipoproteinemia.[403]

The mechanisms of accelerated atherosclerosis in these disorders are not clear. It has been speculated that low HDL cholesterol levels predispose to endothelial injury, which may be followed by localized thrombosis and initiation of atherosclerosis. Cholesterol may accumulate in arterial smooth muscle cells because of faulty transport to the liver.[280]

Coronary artery disease before 60 years of age has been observed in most HDL-deficient kindreds, but not in patients with apo A-I Milano or fish-eye disease. In the last-named condition, coronary artery disease has been observed in persons over 60 years of age. In the proband for familial apolipoprotein A-I and C-II deficiency, necropsy examination of the coronary arteries revealed typical atherosclerosis. No premature coronary artery disease or cerebrovascular disease has been noted in Tangier heterozygotes or homozygotes before age 40.

Tangier Disease

Tangier disease is characterized clinically by enlarged, yellow-orange tonsils, corneal opacities, relapsing peripheral neuropathy, low levels of plasma cholesterol, and storage of cholesteryl esters in various tissues.[133] The only cardiac abnormalities thus far described in this rare disorder are

1. Congenital pulmonary stenosis, which occurred in one patient[479] and probably represented a coincidental finding. (Study of operatively obtained biopsies revealed a few small deposits of lipid in the wall of the pulmonary artery but not in right atrial myocardium.)
2. Yellow patches containing foam cells on the endocardial surfaces of the mitral and tricuspid valves in one patient.[22]
3. Of eight Tangier homozygotes older than 40 years, five had evidence of coronary artery or cerebrovascular disease.[272] Seven of 14 Tangier heterozygotes over age 40 had premature coronary artery disease. Premature atherosclerosis also has been reported in the probands for HDL deficiency with planar xanthomas and for familial hypoalphalipoproteinemia. The latter also has been associated with strokes in children.[403]

Familial Disorders Associated with Low Levels of Low-Density Lipoproteins

Very low levels of LDL cholesterol have been found in patients with hypobetalipoproteinemia and abetalipoproteinemia (Bassen-Kornzweig syndrome).

Hypobetalipoproteinemia

Hypobetalipoproteinemia is rarely accompanied by clinical symptoms and has received attention because of its association with increased longevity and decreased coronary artery disease.[280] Myocardial infarction was reported in a 45-year-old woman with familial hyperalpha- and hypobetalipoproteinemia; however, the coronary arteries appeared angiographically normal, suggesting that this myocardial infarct was due to factors other than atherosclerosis.[369]

Bassen-Kornzweig Syndrome

Bassen-Kornzweig syndrome (abetalipoproteinemia) is characterized by acanthocytosis; absence of chylomicrons; very low density lipoproteins and high density lipoproteins; malabsorption of fat; retinitis pigmentosa, external opthalmoplegia, and oropharyngeal weakness; and degenerative central nervous system disease that involves the cerebellum, long tracts, and peripheral nerves and that clinically resembles that seen in Friedreich's ataxia. Cardiac autopsy observations have been reported on only two patients with Bassen-Kornzweig syndrome. One had ventricular dilation and an organized mural thrombus.[434] The other had considerable cardiomegaly, severe fibrosis of the myocardium, endocardium and trabeculae carneae, and increased amounts of lipofuscin in cardiac muscle cells. The coronary arteries showed fragmentation of the internal elastic lamina and marked intimal fibrous thickening, but without luminal occlusion.[105] Cardiomyopathy also has been reported in a patient with acanthocytosis and amyotrophic chorea.[122]

Diseases Involving Storage of Cholesterol, Other Sterols, and Phytanic Acid

Acid Cholesteryl Ester Hydrolase Deficiency

Wolman's disease and cholesteryl ester storage disease are two diseases in which cholesteryl ester and triglycerides accumulate in lysosomes in a variety of tissues. These two disorders are allelic, involving mutations at loci controlling the activity of acid cholesteryl ester hydrolase, a lysosomal esterase.[148]

Wolman's Disease

Wolman's disease is the more severe form of acid cholesteryl ester hydrolase deficiency. It is associated with hypersplenism and calcification of the adrenals; death occurs in infancy in Wolman's disease, the heart appears grossly normal, but lipid droplets may be seen in muscle cells and vascular endothelium.[91,195] Lipid deposition may be extensive in the aorta,[298] but atherosclerotic changes have not been described.

Cholesteryl Ester Storage Disease

Unlike Wolman's disease, cholesteryl ester storage disease is more benign and is compatible with adult life. Patients known to have cholesteryl ester storage disease, including two in their fourth decade of life, have had clinical evidence of atherosclerosis. Nevertheless, at autopsy, two patients had anatomic evidence of accelerated atherosclerosis. One, who died at age 21, had aortic valvular stenosis as well as severe coronary arterial luminal narrowing and less severe lesions in the circle of Willis, abdominal aorta, and common iliac arteries[148]; the other patient, who died at age 9, had a few elevated plaques in the ascending aorta.[28] Patients with cholesteryl ester storage disease often have hypercholesterolemia and hyperbetalipoproteinemia, but they do not develop xanthomas of the type seen in familial hypercholesterolemia.

Familial Lecithin-Cholesterol Acyltransferase Deficiency

The clinical features of familial deficiency of lecithin-cholesterol acyltransferase (the enzyme that controls formation of cholesteryl esters in plasma) are corneal opacity with arcus formation, anemia with target cells, proteinuria and progressive renal disease, and lipid deposits in bone marrow, renal glomeruli, and other organs. The chemical composition of atheromatous lesions was found to be unusual in one patient with familial lecithin-cholesterol acyltransferase deficiency; the percentage of free cholesterol was high, while the percentage of esterified cholesterol was low, and the percentage composition of fatty acids esterified to cholesterol reflected the abnormal pattern found in plasma.[443]

Deposition of lipid occurs in larger muscular arteries in association with hyalinization of the vessel wall and proliferation of intimal muscle cells. Lipid deposits form in layers, but especially in the subendothelial space, and consist of lucent lipid droplets and irregularly shaped groups of electron-dense lamellae; these deposits contain free cholesterol and phospholipids.[228]

Cerebrotendinous Xanthomatosis

Cerebrotendinous xanthomatosis, transmitted as an autosomal recessive disorder, is characterized by xanthomas in tendons, lungs, and brain; cataracts; subnormal intelligence; progressive cerebellar ataxia, dementia, and spinal cord paresis; and normal or low-plasma cholesterol levels. Large amounts of cholestanol accumulate in various tissues. Premature atherosclerosis, including coronary artery disease, has been found in a few patients with cerebrotendinous xanthomatosis; however, no detailed descriptions of the lesions have been reported.[396,407]

Refsum's Disease

Refsum's disease (phytanic acid storage disease) is transmitted as an autosomal recessive trait. It is characterized by the absence of phytanic acid α-hydroxylase, which converts phytanic acid to α-hydroxyphytanic acid[6] and manifest by peripheral neuropathy external ophthalmoplegia, ataxia, retinitis pigmentosa, and changes in skin and bones. Arrhythmias and sudden cardiac death are common, but the disease is not associated with premature atherosclerosis.[257,374] Cardiac pathologic changes consist of moderate cardiac enlargement, widespread myocardial fibrosis, variation in size of myocardial fibers and nuclei, and deposition of fine fat droplets around nuclei of muscle cells. High levels of phytanic acid have been found in heart muscle.[66,182] Aortic cystic medial necrosis was reported in two patients.[8]

The Sphingolipidoses

Fabry's Disease

Fabry's disease (angiokeratoma corporis diffusum universale) is caused by deficiency of a lysosomal galactosidase A (ceramide trihexosidase) and has an X-linked recessive mode of inheritance. Recent studies have shown the complexity and heterogenicity of the genetic defect in Fabry's disease.[36,273,284] Among diseases caused by deficiencies of lysosomal hydrolases active in lipid metabolism, Fabry's disease is the one in which cardiovascular involvement is most important both clinically and pathologically.

Fabry's disease is manifested by skin lesions (angiokeratomas), pain and paresthesias in the extremities, and progressive renal and cardiovascular disease. The last-named causes cardiac hypertrophy and dilation, congestive heart failure, anginal pain, and hypertension, all of which are related to the presence of deposits of ceramide trihexoside in lysosomes in endothelial, smooth muscle, and perithelial cells throughout the vascular system, especially in the coronary arteries, as well as in renal glomeruli and tubules, cardiac muscle cells, specialized tissues of the atrioventricular conduction system, and valvular fibroblasts. Myocardial infarction at an early age has been reported in several patients with Fabry's disease.[123,354,502] Hypertrophic cardiomyopathy with or without obstruction to left ventricular outflow has been documented by hemodynamic echocardiographic and autopsy studies in some patients with Fabry's disease.[83,115,150,451] In addition to the vascular lesions already mentioned, areas of ectasia develop in small blood vessels in the skin and other organs, and microaneurysms are prominent in ocular vessels.[286] The aorta in one patient showed changes suggestive of cystic medial necrosis.[29] Cardiac valvular lesions have been described in some patients with Fabry's disease and include mitral stenosis,[287] aortic regurgitation,[107] and pulmonary regurgitation[310] (no anatomic studies were made of these valves); aortic stenosis associated with calcification of the cusps[100]; and mitral regurgitation.[100,134] The last-named lesions were thought to be due to cardiac dilation in one patient,[134] to thickening of the leaflets and papillary muscles and interchordal hooding in two (the chordae tendineae were normal in both these patients[100]) and to attenuation of the chordae and thickening, ballooning, and overshooting of the leaflets in another patient.[29]

In ordinary histologic sections, deposits of ceramide trihexoside appear as vacuoles; in frozen sections, they are sudanophilic, PAS-positive, and strongly birefringent. In cardiac muscle cells these deposits occupy the central, perinuclear areas, displacing the contractile elements toward the periphery.[29,100,108,134] This results in a histologic appearance (lacework) similar to that in type II glycogenosis (Fig. 29–20). Ultrastructural study reveals that the ceramide trihexoside deposits form intralysosomal aggregates of concentric or parallel lamellae spaced 4 to 5.5 nm apart.[29,108,134,310,389] These lamellae show a positive reaction with the periodate-thiosemicarbazide-silver proteinate[129] and periodate-thiosemicarbazideosmium tetroxide[471] methods of demonstrating carbohydrate materials ultrastructurally. The lamellar structure of the deposits is also demonstrable on free-fractured preparations.[389] Their birefringence in frozen sections and highly organized substructure differentiate the lamellar deposits in Fabry's disease from the irregular arrays of concentric lamellae that often are encountered as nonspecific findings in degenerated cardiac muscle cells.

Gaucher's Disease

Several patients with the adult form of Gaucher's disease (glucosyl ceramide lipidosis, caused by deficiency of a lysosomal glucocerebrosidase) have developed pulmonary hypertension and cor pulmonale as a consequence of occlusion of alveolar capillaries by Gaucher cells derived from the bone marrow.[381] In a few other patients, constrictive calcific pericarditis resulted from intrapericardial hemorrhage related to the bleeding diathesis that is frequent in Gaucher's disease.[34,203] Marked infiltration of the myocardial interstitium (but not of the conduction system) by typical Gaucher cells, causing decreased left ventricular compliance and decreased cardiac output, has been reported in one adult patient.[433] This constitutes a clear exception to the usual lack of significant involvement of the heart muscle in any of the types (infantile, juvenile, or adult) of Gaucher's disease.

Niemann-Pick Disease

The metabolic defect in types A, B, and C of Niemann-Pick disease involves the lysosomal enzyme sphingomyelinase; the activity of this enzyme is normal in types D and E. As a rule, the heart and blood vessels show no significant involvement in any type of Niemann-Pick disease, although occasional foam cells can be found in the myocardial interstitium. Two reports have described cardiac lesions in patients considered to have Niemann-Pick disease on the basis of morphologic studies and measurements of sphingomyelin levels in tissues (enzymatic deficiency was not demonstrated biochemically). One patient, an infant, had cardiomegaly and left ventricular endocardial fibroelastosis; however, no foam cells were observed in endocardium.[490] The other patient, a 54-year-old woman, had pericardial nodules composed of aggregates of foam cells.[71]

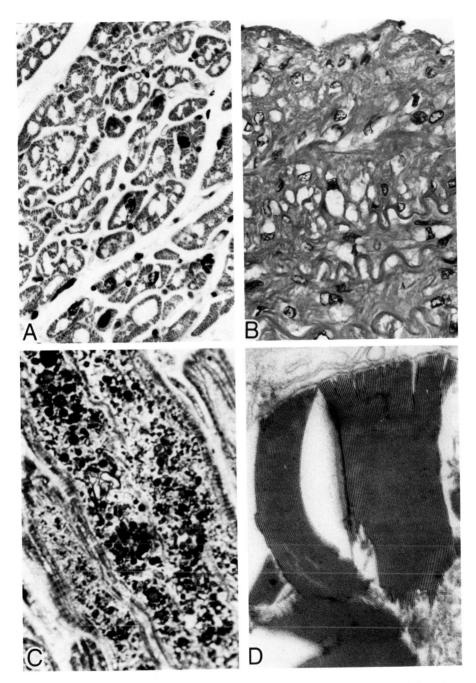

Fig. 29–20. Fabry's disease. Histologic sections showing marked vacuolization of (**A**) cardiac muscle cells and (**B**) smooth muscle cells in the wall of an artery. (H&E, each × 250.) (**C**) Darkly stained lamellae composed of glycolipid material fill the cytoplasm of the cardiac muscle cells. (1 μm-thick section of plastic-embedded tissue.) (Alkaline toluidine blue, × 1000.) (**D**) Electron micrograph showing membrane-limited group of lamellae composed of alternating dense and light bands. (Uranyl acetate and lead citrate, × 92,000.)

Farber's Disease

Farber's disease (lipogranulomatosis) is transmitted as an autosomal recessive disorder that exists in two forms, clinically severe and clinically mild, which differ in the severity and age of onset of symptoms. In the severe form, the defect involves the activity of ceramidase, a lysosomal enzyme that hydrolyzes ceramide to sphingosine and a free fatty acid. Biochemical data on the mild form are lacking. Both forms of the disease are manifested by accumulation of ceramide and acid mucopolysaccharides in a variety of cell types and by the formation of granulomas with lipid-filled histiocytes. These granulomas give rise to clinical symptoms of hoarseness, swollen joints, periarticular subcutaneous nodules, and pulmonary infiltrates. Clinical cardiac manifestations are prominent in some patients and are related to the presence of yellow plaques on the pericardium, on the aortic, mitral, and tricuspid valves, on chordae tendineae, and in coronary arteries, the aorta, and pulmonary artery.[2,26,126,331] These plaques are the sites of formation of granulomas similar to those in other tissues. Ultrastructural studies of the granulomas have described pleomorphic inclusions containing either parallel lamellae or curvilinear tubules in a matrix.[109] These tubules resemble those seen in Batten's disease.[93]

The Gangliosidoses

GM1 Gangliosidosis

Generalized GM1 gangliosidosis (β-galactosidase deficiency) exists in two clinically distinct forms: infantile (type I) and juvenile (type II). Both forms are associated with the accumulation of GM1 ganglioside and its asialo derivative in the central nervous system and the accumulation of a keratin sulfate-like proteoglycan in visceral organs.

Infantile Form

Type I generalized GM1 gangliosidosis is characterized by coarse facial features, hepatosplenomegaly, dysostosis multiplex, and progressive mental and motor retardation. Death is usual, during the first two years of life. Cardiovascular lesions include cardiomegaly and diffuse, nodular thickening of the mitral and tricuspid valves, especially their free margins, by swollen histiocytes containing PAS-positive cytoplasmic granules; similar cells have been found in the aortic valve, which is only slightly thickened.[179,197] Two patients were reported to have foam cells in the myocardial interstitium.[281]

Juvenile Form

In type II generalized GM1 gangliosidosis, visceromegaly is much less pronounced than in type I, and survival may extend for up to 10 years. Cardiovascular lesions include cardiomegaly and aortic and mitral regurgitation. The valvular leaflets are opaque, nodular, markedly thickened, deformed, and contain numerous vacuolated cells with the PAS, oil red O, and Alcian blue methods, thus indicating the presence of lipids and acidic carbohydrates.[166] On ultrastructural study, these cells appear filled with two types of deposits: concentric, electron-dense lamellae and membrane-bound vacuoles containing reticulogranular material.[166] Such deposits have been described in cardiac muscle cells in patients with proven type II GM1 gangliosidosis.

In patients with generalized GM1 gangliosidosis of *undetermined type*, cardiac muscle cells contain membrane-limited vacuoles filled with granular or flocculent substances. The endothelial cells, interstitial cells, and unmyelinated nerves contain membrane-bound vacuoles filled with electron-dense material without discernible substructure; nonmyelinated nerve fibers also contain inclusions composed of parallel or concentric lamellae.[20]

GM2 Gangliosidosis

The two types of generalized GM2 gangliosidosis, Tay-Sachs disease and Sandhoff's disease, are clinically very similar; however, in Sandhoff's disease there is reduction in the activity of both the A and B forms of β-N-acetyl hexosaminidase, whereas in Tay-Sachs disease only the A form is affected.

Tay-Sachs Disease

Patients with Tay-Sachs disease have no clinical manifestations of cardiovascular disease but show nonspecific electrocardiographic changes and accumulations in heart tissue of a GM2 ganglioside similar to that found in excessive amounts in the brain.[378] Their hearts are normal grossly and histologically, but have not been examined by electron microscopy. Thus, the question of the localization of ganglioside storage in lysosomes in the heart remains to be clarified.

Sandhoff's Disease

Cardiomegaly and mitral regurgitation are clinically prominent in some patients with Sandhoff's disease. Anatomic studies of the heart in this disease have shown (1) left atrial and ventricular enlargement associated with endocardial fibroelastosis, and (2) thickening of the mitral and tricuspid valve leaflets, with thickening and fusion of chordae tendineae and thickening of the aortic and pulmonary valves.[41,106,274] The coronary arteries are smaller than usual and have focal areas of luminal narrowing caused by fibromuscular intimal proliferation; the media shows focal degenerative changes consisting of extracellular accumulations of basophilic material. Histologic and ultrastructural studies have disclosed lipid deposits, composed of membrane-bound, electron-dense lamellae, arranged either concentrically or parallel, in endocardial fibroblasts; connective tissue cells in all heart valves; endothelial cells; vascular smooth muscle cells; cardiac muscle cells; neural elements in epicardium; and foam cells in small cardiac nerve trunks.[41,106,274]

Carnitine Deficiency

Carnitine deficiency is thought to result in at least two syndromes of skeletal muscle myopathy associated with lipid storage phenomena and with cardiomyopathy. In the first, the deficiency of carnitine is generalized, due to defective hepatic biosynthesis, and carnitine levels are decreased in plasma and muscle.[48,116,333] In the second syndrome, carnitine levels are normal in plasma but decreased in muscle, and the mechanism of active transport of carnitine into skeletal and cardiac muscle is believed to be defective.[48,116,333] Carnitine is necessary for the transport of long-chain fatty acids into the inner mitochondrial compartment, where they undergo β-oxidation and become a major source of energy.

The *generalized form* of carnitine deficiency is characterized clinically by a premyopathic phase in which the patients have recurrent, spontaneous episodes of nausea, vomiting, adynamia, acidosis, and stupor. This is followed by a later phase of muscular weakness, atrophy, and hepatic insufficiency. The *muscular form* is manifested mainly by muscular weakness and atrophy.[86,202]

The histologic and ultrastructural appearance of skeletal muscle is similar in both forms, with lipid storage (in the form of numerous droplets free in the sarcoplasm) in type I fibers and atrophy in type II fibers. Lipid deposits also have been found in the cytoplasm of pericytes, fibroblasts, and endothelial cells in capillaries and venules.[116] Crystalline inclusions and other nonspecific abnormalities have been observed in skeletal muscle mitochondria.[48] Lipid deposits also occur in kidney and liver in the generalized form.[48,86] The lipid deposits in skeletal muscle consist mainly of triglycerides and smaller amounts of diglycerides and free fatty acids.[86]

Clinical evidence of cardiac involvement has been found in some patients with either form of carnitine deficiency.[333] At least two patients had extensive deposits of lipid in cardiac muscle cells[48,86]; in another patient, the cardiac muscle cells were vacuolated and the myofibrils widely separated by aggregates of mitochondria (a nonspecific finding), but lipid deposits were not found.[202] More recently, some patients have been found to have endocardial fibroelastosis associated with carnitine deficiency.[460] Furthermore, some had a favorable clinical response to treatment with carnitine.[460]

DISEASES OF IRON, COPPER, AND CALCIUM METABOLISM

Hemochromatosis and Hemosiderosis

Cardiac iron deposits occur in idiopathic (familial) hemochromatosis as well as in hemosiderosis secondary to iron overloading (due to multiple transfusions or excessive dietary intake). Cardiac iron deposits in these disorders are morphologically similar and have the same distribution; they are always accompanied by deposits in other organs.[55] Iron deposits (Fig. 29–21) are more extensive in the ventricles than in the atria, and least extensive in the conduction system (especially in the sinoatrial node).[55] The amount of iron in the ventricles is greatest in the epicardial third, intermediate in the subendocardial third, and least in the middle third.[55,247] The amount of iron in the heart correlates with the presence and severity of congestive heart failure, which has been reported to occur in 31 percent of patients with hemochromatosis.[137] The presence of supraventricular arrhythmias correlates with the extent of iron deposition in the atrial myocardium.[55] The heart is brownish and may show hypertrophy and dilation. The coronary arteries and valves are not involved.[287,446,461] There is no correlation between the amount of iron and the degree of myocardial fibrosis. In milder degrees of severity, deposits are located mostly in the perinuclear areas of the muscle and occupy a small portion of the cell volume. In cases of more severe deposition, a greater number of myocytes contain iron; the deposits occupy a larger portion of the cytoplasmic volume and extend toward the periphery of the cell.[55] Iron is always present in both myocardial connective tissue cells and myocytes. Cardiac muscle has a greater affinity for iron than does skeletal or smooth muscle. The iron deposits are localized, mostly in membrane-bound "siderin" granules, which are thought to be altered lysosomes and contain electron-dense particles, 6 nm in diameter, embedded in an electron-lucent matrix. These particles also may be found free in the sarcoplasm.[55] Iron deposits are readily identified by histochemical staining and by energy dispersive radiographic microanalysis.

Diseases of Copper Metabolism

Wilson's Disease

Wilson's disease (hepatolenticular degeneration) is transmitted as an autosomal recessive trait and is characterized by cirrhosis of the liver; degenerative changes in the brain, especially in the basal ganglia; and Keyser-Fleischer corneal rings. Low serum copper concentrations, decreased serum ceruloplasmin levels, and increased urinary copper excretion are observed, together with increased copper deposition in various tissues. Two boys with Wilson's disease were shown (one by autopsy study,[47] the other by myocardial biopsy[19]) to have cardiac hypertrophy and increased copper concentrations in the heart. The latter finding was also demonstrated in one of the patients by the rubeanic acid stain, used to detect copper in tissue sections.[19] Of

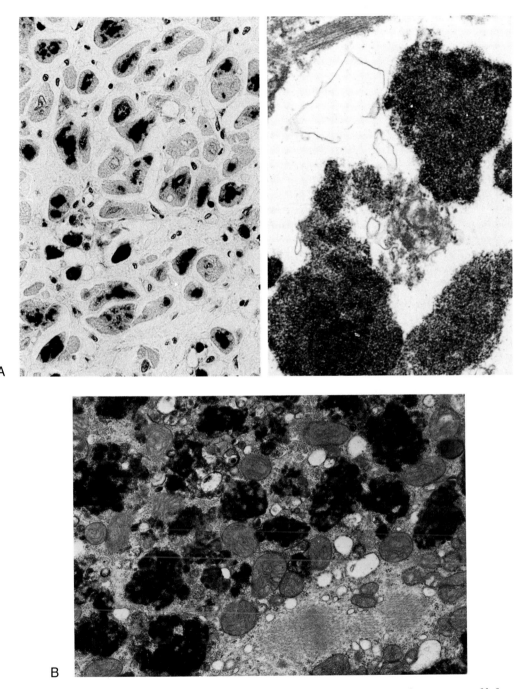

Fig. 29–21. (**A**) Cardiac hemosiderosis after multiple blood transfusions. Histologic section of left ventricle, showing prominent, darkly stained iron deposits. (Perls' reaction, × 400.) (**B**) Intralysosomal iron particles are present in a cardiac myocyte in a myocardial biopsy from a patient with idiopathic hemochromatosis. (× 40,000.)

nine patients with Wilson's disease studied at necropsy by Factor et al.[122] all had evidence of interstitial and replacement fibrosis, intramyocardial small vessel sclerosis, and focal inflammatory cell inflammation to a variable degree. One patient had AV nodal degeneration, and a 15-year-old boy had severe atherosclerosis of the left main coronary artery. Two patients died suddenly, presumably secondary to an arrhythmia; one of these patients had the most marked myocardial alterations. These changes could not be correlated, specifically, with tissue levels of copper, treatment with D-penicillamine, or the presence of cirrhosis. Kuan[277] observed a number of clinical and ECG abnormalities in 34 percent of 53 patients with Wilson's disease. Two of these patients died, and at autopsy one had increased levels of copper in the myocardium and bundle His; the other patient had changes of dilated cardiomyopathy.

Menkes Syndrome

Menkes kinky hair syndrome is a sex-linked, recessively transmitted copper deficiency state related to impaired absorption of copper from the gastrointestinal tract. Cardiovascular lesions in this syndrome are characterized by widespread but patchy, degenerative changes in the arterial walls.[95,332,347,466] Copper is a cofactor required for lysyl oxidase, the enzyme responsible for forming crosslinks between lysine residues in elastin and collagen.

Grossly, the heart in Menkes syndrome is normal, but superficial vessels often appear tortuous or dilated; aneurysm formation often involves major arteries and veins. Arterial wall changes consist of fragmentation, splitting, and reduplication of the internal elastic lamina, an abnormal increase in the amount of collagen throughout the vessel wall, and a marked reduction in the number of smooth muscle cells. Involvement of coronary arteries is variable. The vascular lumina often are compromised and occasionally are obliter-

ated.[305,492] The resultant vascular insufficiency is regarded as a principal factor in the changes seen in the central nervous system in Menkes syndrome. Aneurysm formation is associated with subintimal edema, marked collagenous thickening of the media, and extensive loss of elastin and smooth muscle cells.

Ultrastructural study of the aorta in a patient with Menkes syndrome showed that the elastic lamellae were poorly formed and were composed of clumps of elastin surrounded by large numbers of connective tissue microfibrils. Aortic smooth muscle cells contained large aggregates of loosely arranged, flocculent material that showed marked metachromasia. The composition of this material is unknown.[342]

Idiopathic Infantile Hypercalcemia

The syndrome of idiopathic infantile hypercalcemia, manifested by mental and physical retardation, a typical facies, and dental malformations, is now known to be associated with a number of cardiovascular anomalies. The most common is supravalvular aortic stenosis.[140,159,235] Other anomalies observed are aortic regurgitation,[14,160] pulmonary valvular stenosis,[14,160,254] peripheral stenoses of the pulmonary arteries,[11,352] atrial septal defect,[254] ventricular septal defect,[214,254] mitral regurgitation,[140,235] calcification of the mitral annulus,[352] bicuspid aortic valve,[14] hypoplasia of the aorta,[14] aortic coarctation,[279] coarctation of systemic arteries other than the aorta,[279,351] dilated and tortuous coronary arteries,[14,160] and disarray of elastic lamellae and smooth muscle cells of the aortic media.[235] The total length of the ascending aorta is reduced, and the extent of this reduction is not related to the severity of supravalvular aortic stenosis.[140] The pathogenesis of this syndrome is unclear (see also Chs. 10 and 21).

NUTRITIONAL HEART DISEASE

The study of cardiovascular anatomic changes produced by nutritional deficiencies presents considerable difficulties. Isolated deficiency of a single nutrient seldom occurs in humans without the complicating factors of other forms of dietary deficiencies; proper biochemical documentation of the deficiency state is seldom obtained; relatively few morphologic studies have been made of the hearts of patients with carefully investigated biochemical lesions; and the findings in most studies have been nonspecific. Thus, the morphologic diagnosis of cardiac lesions related to nutritional deficiencies must be verified by clinical and biochemical evidence.

Deficiencies

No cardiovascular anatomic lesions have been shown to develop in humans as the result of deficiencies of vitamin A, vitamin D, niacin, pyridoxine, biotin, pantothenic acid, cyanocobalamin, riboflavin, vitamin E, or folic acid, even though deficiency of these compounds is known to cause a variety of cardiac lesions either in experimental animals or their offspring.[142,482,465]

Thiamine Deficiency (Beriberi Heart Disease) (See also Ch. 33)

Thiamine pyrophosphate (cocarboxylase) constitutes a cofactor for two separate decarboxylases, which act on pyruvic acid and α-ketoglutaric acid; it is also a cofactor for transketolase, an enzyme that carries out several oxidative decarboxylation steps in the pentose shunt. Thus, the reduction in cocarboxylase impairs energy production; however, the high cardiac output state in some patients with thiamine deficiency is thought to be due to high levels of circulating catecholamines and to decreased peripheral vascular resistance. Thiamine deficiency can be manifested as *dry* beriberi, in which cardiac manifestations are minimal and the clinical picture is dominated by neurologic manifestations; *wet* beriberi, in which cardiac involvement is prominent; and *Shoshin* beriberi, which is a very acute form associated with fulminating cardiac failure, metabolic acidosis, peripheral cyanosis, and vascular collapse.[4,17,40,477]

Cardiac gross anatomic findings in beriberi consist of hypertrophy and dilation, both of which involve the right side of the heart to a greater degree than the left. Petechiae have been described in the epicardium; the endocardial surfaces are normal. Microscopic changes are interstitial and intracellular edema, fatty infiltration, and other degenerative changes in the muscle cells. Fatty infiltration is most pronounced in the left ventricular subendocardium.[40,237,474] These microscopic changes are nonspecific and resemble those in patients with alcoholic cardiomyopathy.[131]

A long-standing controversy persists about the reversibility of chronic cardiomyopathy due to thiamine deficiency in humans, although a dramatic clinical improvement with thiamine treatment has been observed in the Shoshin form. Thiamine deficiency in the Western world is seen most frequently in patients who also have chronic alcoholism.[17] However, the cardiac disease in the majority of such patients does not respond to therapy with thiamine, although in some patients the administration of thiamine has caused cardiac manifestations to change from those of the high-output state of thiamine deficiency to those of the low-output state of congestive cardiomyopathy associated with alcoholism.[4,477] Ultrastructural study of thiamine deficiency induced experimentally in rats has demonstrated a marked increase in the size and volume fraction of mitochondria in cardiac muscle cells.[49] These changes, which are reversible on replacement therapy with thiamine, have not been demonstrated in the human disease.

Vitamin C Deficiency (Scurvy)

Ascorbic acid has many antioxidant functions and also plays a role in proline hydroxylation, an important step in collagen synthesis. Cardiovascular lesions reported in ascorbic acid deficiency consist of hemorrhagic phenomena—which have been shown in animals to result from disruption of capillary basal laminae, depletion of pericapillary collagen, and separation of endothelial cell junctions[184] and right ventricular hypertrophy, which has been observed in several necropsy studies of children with scurvy.[141] The mechanism by which this hypertrophy develops is unknown.

Deficiency of Minerals and Trace Elements

Numerous minerals and trace elements have been shown to be of importance in various aspects of cardiovascular diseases; however, morphologically distinct cardiovascular lesions related to deficiency states involving these elements have not been unequivocally documented in humans, except in the case of selenium.[142] Selenium deficiency (Keshan disease), with or without associated deficiency of vitamin E, causes cardiomyopathy, vascular lesions, and myocardial hemorrhages in various animals and cardiomyopathy in humans.[472,473]

Keshan Disease

Keshan disease is a type of ventricular-dilated cardiomyopathy that occurs in China, in a zone that extends from the northeast to the southwest that has a very low selenium content in the soil.[264,418] The disease is manifested by the insidious onset of congestive heart failure or, less frequently, by sudden death or by embolic strokes related to cardiac mural thrombi.

The heart has a globular shape and shows biventricular dilation. Microscopically, edema, nonspecific degenerative changes, mitochondrial swelling, hypercontraction bands, and widespread foci of myocytolysis are prominent in myocardium (Fig. 29–22). Inflammatory reaction is largely absent. The fibrosis is variable but can be extensive.[76,162,507]

The concept that Keshan disease is related to selenium deficiency is based on three observations: (1) the geographic distribution of Keshan disease in northern China is similar to that of "white muscle disease"[264,418]; (2) the content of selenium in hair of patients with Keshan disease is very low[263]; and (3) children treated prophylactically with sodium selenite had a much lower incidence of Keshan disease than did children treated with placebos.[265] In Western countries, selenium deficiency has been reported to cause fatal cardiomyopathy in patients maintained for prolonged periods on parenteral alimentation.[21,81,139,253,269]

Deficiencies of Other Minerals

Magnesium deficiency causes myocardial fiber calcification in rats.[213,214] Copper deficiency (Fig. 29–23) and iron deficiency cause myocardial hypertrophy in rats.[180] In experimental animals, copper deficiency, because of its need for the function of lysyl oxidase, also causes lesions characterized by disruption of elastic tissue; they lead to rupture of the aorta and other major vessels.[422] These lesions resemble those in Menkes syndrome in humans.[95,342] The role of dietary deficiency of iron in producing heart disease is discussed in Chapter 33.

Focal areas of myocardial necrosis and fibrosis have been observed in patients with hypokalemia associated with other (usually gastrointestinal) disorders.[266,313,357] Such necroses resemble lesions induced by experimental potassium deficiency in rats.[312]

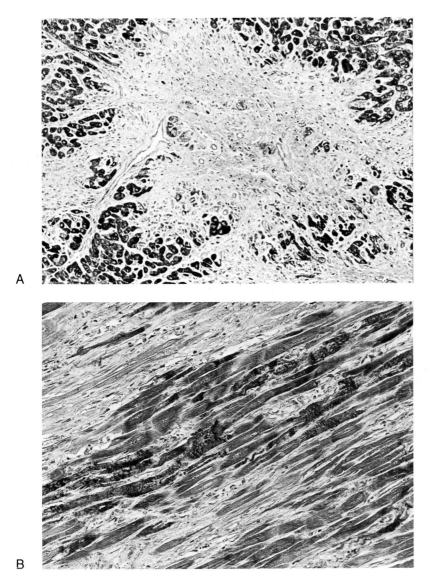

A

B

Fig. 29–22. (**A**) Section of left ventricular wall from a patient with the acute, initial stage of Keshan disease, showing myocytolysis and acute necrosis of the contraction band type. (× 200.) (**B**) Appearance of left ventricle in a more chronic case of Keshan disease, showing extensive fibrosis. (× 100.)

Protein Malnutrition

The clinical spectrum of protein-caloric malnutrition includes marasmus and kwashiorkor in children, starvation with greatly subnormal body weight, and liquid protein diet syndrome in obese adults undergoing weight reduction.

Marasmus is a state of emaciation in young children, usually under one year of age, who have been fed diets extremely low in calories, protein, and other nutrients. Severe skeletal muscle wasting, loss of subcutaneous fat, and

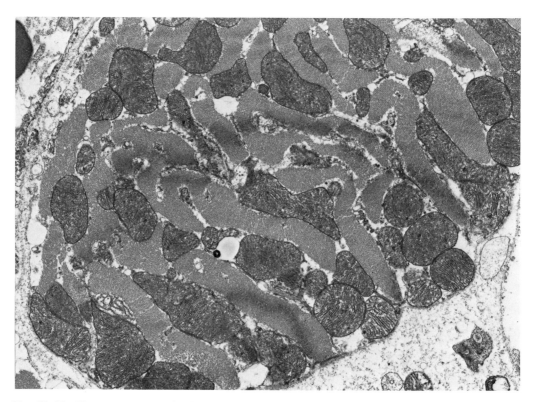

Fig. 29–23. Electron micrograph of myocardium of a rat with cardiac hypertrophy due to copper deficiency. Marked enlargement of mitochondria is evident. (× 10,000.)

atrophy of most organs, including the heart, usually occur. Kwashiorkor occurs in children older than one year of age fed diets that may be adequate in calories but deficient in protein (see also Ch. 33). Muscle atrophy occurs but may be masked by generalized edema, which usually is marked; hepatic enlargement and fatty infiltration also are prominent.[189,495] In both syndromes, clinical deterioration often follows episodes of diarrhea or infection.

In kwashiorkor the heart is pale and flabby. In some patients it is dilated, whereas in others it has a normal size.[318,365,491] The relationship between heart weight and body weight is variable. Epicardial fat is absent, and the endocardium may be focally thickened. Microscopic changes include patchy myocardial necrosis and fibrosis; inflammatory cell infiltrates; deposition of lipid in the cytoplasm of cardiac and muscle cells; cellular atrophy, vacuolization, and loss of

striations; and interstitial and intracellular edema.[318,365,491] Electron microscopic studies have shown disorganization of myofibrils and Z bands, loss of myofibrils, and prominent intracellular edema.[365] Atrophy and myocytolysis have been observed in the cardiac conduction tissue.[429] Changes of myocardial atrophy and extracellular edema have been reproduced in animal models of protein-calorie malnutrition.[1,75]

In severe starvation, with massive loss of body weight, such as is seen in prisoners in concentration camps, reduction in the heart size is proportional to the loss of total body weight. Reduction in epicardial fat is more striking; however, uniform atrophy of cardiac muscle cells in all four chambers is responsible for most of the loss of cardiac weight. In addition to a reduction in the size of muscle fibers, microscopic changes (Fig. 29–24) include increased pigmentation, vacuolization,

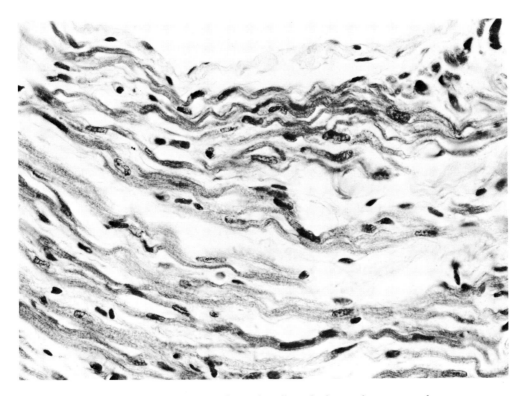

Fig. 29–24. Thin, atrophic, widely separated muscle cells in the heart of a patient with severe starvation (H&E, × 400.)

cloudy swelling, loss of striations, and brown atrophy.[267,294]

Therapeutic starvation to treat severe obesity has been associated with sudden cardiac death (see also Ch. 21) and with myofibrillar changes of uncertain significance.[161,242,326] Sudden death caused by well-documented ventricular arrhythmias related to prolongation of the QT interval has occurred in patients who were receiving liquid protein diets (containing mostly a hydrolysate of collagenous proteins) as part of their weight-reduction regimen.[242] Right ventricular endomyocardial biopsy in one of these patients disclosed fibrosis, mononuclear cell infiltrates, focal necrosis, and degeneration.[385] However, histologic study of left ventricular myocardium obtained at necropsy in 16 other patients disclosed attenuated myocardial fibers in 12, increased lipofuscin pigment in 11, and mononuclear cell myocarditis in 1. Similar histologic findings were observed in 16 cachectic control subjects studied in similar fashion. ECGs in the control patients did not show prolongation of the QT interval or episodes of ventricular tachycardia. Thus, the morphologic findings in the patients dying suddenly while on the liquid protein diet probably were related to the extent of the weight loss rather than to the use of a particular liquid protein product.[242]

Some investigators consider protein malnutrition a contributory factor in the pathogenesis of idiopathic congestive cardiomyopathy, alcoholic cardiomyopathy, cobalt-beer cardiomyopathy, endomyocardial fibrosis, and the cardiomyopathy that occurs in association with hepatic iron overloading among the Bantu. (These disorders are discussed in Ch. 20.)

A low-protein, high-carbohydrate diet based on cassava starch induces a mucoid vasculopathy when in bonnet monkeys. It resembles a similar vasculopathy seen in humans in southern India. (See the addendum to Ch. 10.)

Heart Disease Related to Obesity

In a study of the cardiac pathology of chronic exogenous obesity, Amad et al.[10] found that the heart weight in each of 12 subjects was considerably increased over the value predicted for ideal body weight. Of the 12 subjects, nine were found to have an increased ventricular wall thickness, and two were found to have an increased right ventricular wall thickness. The increases in heart weight and ventricular wall thickness were due to muscle hypertrophy involving the left ventricle or both left and right ventricles. Neither isolated nor predominant right ventricular hypertrophy was observed. These authors concluded that myocardial hypertrophy is a more specific and significant anatomic alteration in the hearts of very obese subjects than are the previously reported findings of excess epicardial fat and fatty infiltration of the myocardium. In one patient with marked obesity and the Pickwickian syndrome, atrial fibrillation, and right bundle branch block, James et al.[251] found extensive fatty replacement of the sinoatrial node, lesser but still significant fatty replacement and fibrosis in the atrioventricular node and His bundle, and extensive destruction of the right bundle branch.

NEUROMUSCULAR DISEASES

Heredofamilial neuromuscular diseases showing cardiac involvement will be considered according to the following categories: (1) myotonic dystrophy, (2) nonmyotonic muscular dystrophies, (3) myopathies, including mitochondrial myopathies and the syndrome of ophthalmoplegia plus, and (4) other conditions, including tuberous sclerosis (Bourneville's disease), neurofibromatosis (von Recklinghausen's disease), and Kugelberg-Welander syndrome. Many other neuromuscular disorders are associated with clinical or laboratory evidence of cardiovascular disease, but cardiac anatomic observations in such disorders are lacking.

Myotonic Dystrophy

Myotonic dystrophy (Steinert's disease) is transmitted as an autosomal dominant disorder, the cardiac clinical manifestations of which include a high frequency of ECG abnormalities (prolongation of PR interval, widening of QRS complex, left bundle branch block sinus bradycardia, atrial flutter, and atrial fibrillation) but only a low frequency of overt heart failure.[358] Cor pulmonale may occur as a consequence of alveolar hypoventilation. Cardiac manifestations may be recognized clinically before neurologic changes become evident. The myotonic phenomenon appears not to be directly related to cardiac changes, as patients with myotonia congenita show no cardiac involvement.[330]

On gross examination, some hearts appear normal, whereas others show cardiomegaly and focal fibrosis. Coronary arteries are not affected by the disease. Mitral valve prolapse has been described in myotonic dystrophy, in association with the usual myxoid changes in valve tissue.[84] Histologic abnormalities in the heart differ from those in skeletal muscle. The "ring-binden," which are prominent in skeletal muscle, have not been described in cardiac muscle. Changes in the latter consist of patchy interstitial fibrosis, often accompanied by focal fatty infiltration and evidence of hypertrophy.[454,463] Similar fibrofatty changes affect the SA and AV nodes and the bundle of His and its proximal branches.[263] Focal disarray of right and left ventricular muscle fibers has been observed.[146] Electron microscopy has revealed nonspecific changes such as rupture and distortion of the Z bands, focal loss of myofilaments with replacement by mitochondria, an increase in interstitial collagen, vacuolization of the sarcoplasmic reticulum, and degeneration of mitochondria with disorganization of their internal structure.[57,298]

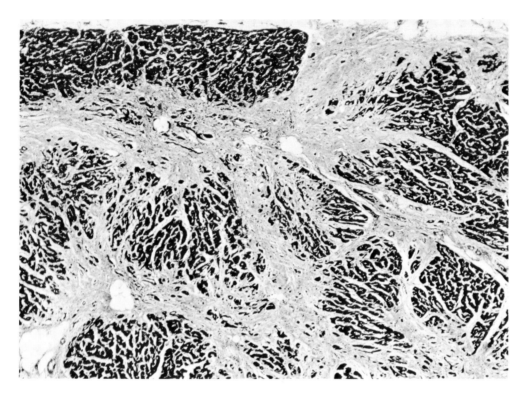

Fig. 29–25. Severe subepicardial fibrosis in the left ventricle of a patient with progressive muscular dystrophy of Duchenne type. (Masson's trichrome, × 40.)

Duchenne-type Muscular Dystrophy

Progressive muscular dystrophy of the Duchenne type[151] can be classified into two types: (1) a rapidly progressive form (the classic form) transmitted as a sex-linked recessive trait, and (2) a slowly progressive form, which can be either of early onset and transmitted as an autosomal recessive trait or later onset and transmitted as a sex-linked recessive trait.

Rapidly Progressive Form

In the rapidly progressive form of Duchenne type muscular dystrophy (Fig. 29–25), cardiomegaly is usually present, with dilation and hypertrophy, fibrosis, and degenerative changes in both ventricles.[145,310,394] These changes are more severe in the left ventricle, especially in the posterobasal region of the free wall.[360] It has been suggested that this selective distribution accounts for the ECG changes characteristic in muscular dystrophy of Duchenne type; however, this is uncertain.[262] Similar ECG changes occur in a small percentage of female carriers.[298] The fibrosis usually involves the subepicardial areas, in contrast to the fibrosis that occurs in most other types of cardiac disease; however, foci of subendocardial fibrosis also are present. The areas of myocardial fibrosis show no inflammatory changes. Endocardial fibrous thickening also has been reported.[444] One patient was found to have asymmetric septal hypertrophy, thought to be due to a combination of septal hypertrophy and thinning of the posterobasal free wall of the left ventricle.[394] Large extramural coronary arteries are normal, although small intramural coronary arteries show luminal narrowing due to fibromuscular intimal proliferation; these changes may be pronounced in arteries to the sinoatrial atrioventricular nodes.[246,360] Ultrastructural study of myocardium showed myofibrillar lysis, with loss of actin and myosin filaments, disorganization of Z-band material, and preservation of the structure of the transverse tubular system.[398]

Ultrastructural studies using freeze-fracture techniques have disclosed abnormalities in the plasma membranes of skeletal muscle and other cell types in patients with Duchenne-type muscular dystrophy, suggesting that this should be considered a systemic disease of cell membranes.[151] It has not been determined whether such abnormalities occur in the myocardium of these patients.

Slowly Progressive Form

Cardiac morphologic changes have been reported in detail in only one patient with the slowly progressive form of Duchenne-type progressive muscular dystrophy. This patient, who had complete heart block, had at necropsy, widespread fibrosis in both ventricles, extensive hyalinization of the bundle of His, prominent fatty replacement of myocardium in the right ventricle, and moderate medial fibrosis causing thickening of some small intramural coronary arteries.[359]

Cardiac involvement is rare and clinically unimportant in *facioscapulohumeral dystrophy of Landouzy-Dejerine*, and conduction disturbances occur in the *Erb type of limb-girdle dystrophy*. However, pathologic studies of the heart in these two diseases have not been reported in detail.[360]

Congenital Myopathies

Congenital myopathies are present at birth and are either nonprogressive or slowly progressive. In severe cases of congenital myopathies there is significant weakness at birth

leading to death in infancy, childhood, or adolescence. However, most patients with mild forms of these diseases remain almost asymptomatic in early childhood.[316] These myopathies seem to affect specific muscular structures, without the destructive changes of other myopathies. They derive their names from some of their pathologic changes. Included among these disorders are nemaline myopathy, centronuclear myopathy, Leigh's disease and other mitochondrial myopathies, and a group of syndromes of external ophthalmoplegia plus (Kearns-Sayre syndrome, Refsum's syndrome, progressive external ophthalmoplegia, abetalipoproteinemia).

Nemaline Myopathy

Bicuspid aortic valve regurgitation, left ventricular hypertrophy, dilated cardiomyopathy, and biventricular failure have been reported in nemaline myopathy.[316,386] In a patient with nemaline myopathy and left ventricular hypertrophy who died of congestive heart failure, autopsy revealed a patent ductus arteriosus, mild infundibular pulmonic stenosis, anomalous papillary muscles, and myocardial scarring.[316] There are few reports of adult-onset nemaline myopathy presenting with diaphragmatic paralysis. Nemaline myopathy is characterized morphologically by the presence of nemaline rods in cardiac myocytes. These rods represent accumulation of Z-band material with a periodic substructure and a transverse periodicity of about 20 nm. Nemaline rods need to be distinguished from focal accumulations of Z-band material that are often seen in the myocardium as a nonspecific finding, especially in dilated atria.

Centronuclear Myopathy

Centronuclear (myotubular) myopathy may either be sporadic or have a sex-linked autosomal recessive or autosomal dominant mode of inheritance.[211] Central nuclei are present in fetal muscle through the first 15 weeks of gestation, suggesting that centronuclear myopathy may represent an arrest of muscle development.[186] Although most patients do not have an associated cardiomyopathy, cardiac fibrosis with dilation and focal hypertrophy does occur.[186,475]

Leigh's Disease

A number of patients with symptoms of skeletal muscle myopathy and cardiomyopathy have been described as having abnormalities of mitochondrial structure and function in both types of muscle, sometimes in association with encephalopathy.[329] Prominent among these disorders is Leigh's disease (progressive subacute necrotizing encephalomyelopathy), an autosomal recessive condition with clinical manifestations that appear in infancy and are mainly neurologic; cardiac manifestations are those of hypertrophic cardiomyopathy.[271,283,395,475] The biochemical defect is thought to be heterogeneous, with low levels of pyruvate decarboxylase in the central nervous system, liver, skeletal muscle and heart; in some cases there is also deficiency of cytochrome oxidase. The disease is usually fatal in infancy; however, some patients have survived to adolescence or adulthood.

The heart in Leigh's disease shows massive hypertrophy, with an increase in weight of up to twice that expected for the patient's age. Grossly, the hypertrophy may resemble that seen in the usual form of hypertrophic cardiomyopathy. Asymmetric septal thickening and myocardial fiber disarray have been observed. Ultrastructurally, there is a paucity of myofibrils and a marked increase in the numbers of mitochondria, which may be abnormally shaped and have tubular cristae. This disease has been thought to represent a "mitochondrial cardiomyopathy." However, quantitative parameters for establishing this diagnosis have not been determined. It is of interest that one patient with aniridia and catalase deficiency was found to have a very severe degree of hypertrophic cardiomyopathy.[167] Also associated with hypertrophic cardiomyopathy is a syndrome of congenital cataracts, mitochondrial myopathy affecting skeletal and cardiac muscle, and exercise-induced lactic acidosis. Some patients with this syndrome have asymmetric ventricular septal thickening and a marked degree of myocardial fiber disarray.[92,419,470] Nevertheless, mitochondrial cardiomyopathies are not always associated with the gross anatomic features of hypertrophic cardiomyopathy; other disorders of unknown etiology, including some rare cases of dilated cardiomyopathy, have been reported to occur in association with marked increases in the number of mitochondria in cardiac myocytes.[191,231,415]

Ophthalmoplegia Plus Syndrome

Ophthalmoplegia combined with cardiac disease is an important feature of several disease states, including Kearns-Sayre syndrome, progressive ophthalmoplegia, Refsum's disease, and abetalipoproteinemia (Bassen-Kornzweig syndrome). The last-named two disorders have been discussed in the section on lipid metabolism.

Kearns-Sayre Syndrome

Kearns-Sayre syndrome features external ophthalmoplegia, retinitis pigmentosa, and varying degrees of atrioventricular block (see also Ch. 37).[340] Additional clinical abnormalities include subnormal mentation, hearing loss, impaired growth, proximal weakness of the extremities, cerebellar abnormalities, and increased protein in the cerebrospinal fluid. Biopsy specimens of skeletal muscle show ultrastructural mitochondrial abnormalities.[349] "Ragged-red fibers" are recognized with modified Gomori trichrome stain. Some patients with Kearns-Sayre syndrome also have hypertrophic cardiomyopathy. Evidence is accumulating that Kearns-Sayre syndrome is a metabolic disease caused by defective mitochondrial function (see later discussion also).[415]

Progressive External Ophthalmoplegia

Progressive external ophthalmoplegia is manifested by progressive weakness of the external ocular muscles and ptosis. When the pharyngeal muscles are also involved, the syndrome is called oculopharyngeal dystrophy. The most common ECG abnormalities are atrioventricular conduction defects. Cardiovascular morphologic abnormalities have not been defined.

Other Neurologic Disorders

Friedreich's Ataxia

Most commonly transmitted as an autosomal recessive and rarely as a sex-linked abnormality, Friedreich's ataxia chiefly involves the spinocerebellar and pyramidal tracts and dorsal columns. It is manifested by skeletal deformities, ataxia, speech disturbances, and cardiovascular disease. One-third of patients have physical signs and symptoms of heart disease (progressive heart failure and precordial pain); 90 percent eventually develop ECG abnormalities, and 100 percent show cardiac involvement at autopsy.[358]

The severity of the CNS disease does not parallel that of cardiac involvement.[456] Left ventricular hypertrophy is more common in slightly to moderately disabled patients, while right ventricular hypertrophy is more common in severely affected patients.[457] Gross anatomic changes in the heart include cardiomegaly, with or without dilation; patchy or diffuse interstitial fibrosis; and, less frequently, endocardial thickening with mural thrombosis.[220,243,406] A high incidence of hypertrophic cardiomyopathy with asymmetric hypertrophy of the ventricular septum has been shown by echocardiographic and hemodynamic studies, to occur in Friedreich's ataxia.[25,153,361,436] Both obstructive and nonobstructive forms of hypertrophic cardiomyopathy have been described.[25,153,361,430] Fibrous replacement of myocardium is widespread, especially in subendocardial and subepicardial areas. Fatty infiltration may be prominent. The cardiac muscle cells show hypertrophy; disarray of septal muscle has not been described. The valves and conduction system usually are normal. The large extramural coronary arteries usually are not affected, but may be involved in all stages of intimal proliferation. Small intramural coronary arteries are frequently the site of marked intimal thickening, which may be occlusive.[250]

Peroneal Muscular Atrophy

Peroneal muscular atrophy is a slowly progressive neurogenic atrophy affecting mainly the distal muscles of the legs and sometimes the intrinsic muscles of the hands. It is related to Friedreich's ataxia. Isolated cases of Friedreich's ataxia occur in families with peroneal muscular atrophy, and the two diseases have been described in the same person.

Cardiomyopathy is not characteristically associated with peroneal muscular atrophy.[110] But there are a few reports associating peroneal muscular atrophy with heart disease.[241,259,295] A myocardial biopsy specimen from a 42-year-old man with familial heart block and peroneal muscular atrophy revealed ultrastructural changes similar to those described in simple myocardial hypertrophy and hypertrophic obstructive cardiomyopathy.[259] Littler[296] described the coexistence of cardiac conduction defect and peroneal muscular atrophy in a family in which 10 members of three generations were affected (three manifested both conditions, six had the cardiac defect alone, and one had only the neurologic disorder). Thus, it seems likely that some cases of peroneal muscular atrophy have conductive cardiac defects and cardiomyopathy.

Tuberous Sclerosis

The inheritance of this disease fits an autosomal dominant pattern. A commonly encountered triad of adenoma sebaceum, seizures, and mental retardation are the clinical characteristics of this disease, but visceral anomalies are not uncommon. In this regard tuberous sclerosis is associated with cardiac rhabdomyoma in about 37 to 50 percent of cases. The tumor can be single or multiple and intracavitary or intramural.

Neurofibromatosis

The incidence of pheochromocytoma in patients with neurofibromatosis is greater than that in the general population. It is possible that patients with both conditions can develop cardiac ailments due to systemic arterial hypertension. Myocardial rhabdomyosarcomas producing systemic and cerebral emboli also have been reported in patients with neurofibromatosis (see also Ch. 10).[307]

Kugelberg-Welander Syndrome

The Kugelberg-Welander syndrome, also known as the juvenile form of progressive spinal muscular atrophy, is associated with atrial arrhythmias, atrioventricular conduction disturbances, and congestive heart failure; cardiomegaly is usually present. No autopsy data have been reported in patients with this syndrome. Endomyocardial biopsy in three patients has shown right atrial[445] and right ventricular[452,453] fibrosis as well as degenerative changes in right ventricular muscle cells.[452] Some of the latter changes (preferential loss of myosin filaments and mitochondrial and Z-band alterations) were of a nonspecific nature. The significance of the leptofibrils found in a patient[452] is unknown.

Kearns-Sayre Syndrome

The Kearns-Sayre syndrome typically manifests before the twentieth year of life, involves both sexes equally, and is characterized by external ophthalmoplegia, retinitis pigmentosa, and heart block.[378] Cardiac conduction abnormalities, most frequently right bundle branch block with left axis deviation, are present in most patients. These abnormalities most frequently develop after the ocular manifestations and may progress to complete heart block with Adams-Stokes attacks and sudden death.[35,260,267,378,467]

In one patient, detailed postmortem examination of the conduction system revealed infiltration of the distal portion of the bundle of His and its two branches by fibrous and adipose tissue[79]; however, less detailed necropsy studies in other patients have failed to show abnormalities of the conduction system.[260,382] Direct myocardial involvement has not been reported, although left ventricular hypertrophy was noted at autopsy in a patient with complete heart block (see also Ch. 37).[261]

GENETIC DISEASES ASSOCIATED WITH CONGENITAL CARDIOVASCULAR MALFORMATIONS

There is a rapidly increasing number of syndromes of genetic disorders in which various congenital cardiac malformations are associated with chromosomal aberrations and/or with extracardiac anomalies.[73,341,391,455] Information concerning these disorders and their associated lesions is presented in Tables 29-1 (chromosomal aberrations), 29-2 (skeletal anomalies), 29-3 (deafness), 29-4 (cutaneous anomalies), and 29-5 (other extracardiac anomalies).

Table 29-1.   Syndromes of Congenital Heart Disease Associated with Chromosomal Aberrations

Syndrome	Usual Cardiovascular Anomalies	Extracardiac Anomalies
Trisomy 21 (Down syndrome)	Atrioventricularis communis, ventricular septal defect, atrial septal defect, tetralogy of Fallot, patent ductus arteriosus	Mental retardation, mongoloid facies
Trisomy D (Patau syndrome or trisomy 13–15)	Complex ventricular septal defect, patent ductus arteriosus, atrial septal defect, dextrocardia, transposition of great vessels	Microphthalmos, cataracts, low-set ears, cleft lip, polydactyly
Trisomy E (Edward syndrome or trisomy 18)	Ventricular septal defect, patent ductus arteriosus, aortic and pulmonic stenosis (variable)	Low-set ears, syndactyly, rocker-bottom feet, flexion of fingers, horseshoe kidney
Trisomy 22	Atrial septal defect, ventricular septal defect, patent ductus arteriosus	Mental and growth retardation, micrognathia, microcephaly, deformed lower extremities
Cat eye syndrome	Total anomalous pulmonary venous return, tetralogy of Fallot, tricuspid atresia, atrial septal defect, ventricular septal defect	Anal atresia, choroidal and iridal colobomata
4p- (Wolf syndrome)	Atrial septal defect, ventricular septal defect	Psychomotor retardation, seizures, cleft palate, hypospadias, midline scalp defect
5p- (Cri-du-chat syndrome)	Patent ductus arteriosus, aortic stenosis, ventricular septal defect (variable)	Cat-like cry, mental retardation, hypertelorism, low-set ears, epicanthus, visceral anomalies
13q-	Tetralogy of Fallot, ventricular septal defect	Mental retardation, microcephaly, hypertelorism, microphthalmia, hip dysplasia, hypoplastic or absent thumbs
18q- (Carp mouth syndrome)	Variable	Psychomotor retardation, microcephaly, hypoplastic ear canals, ocular anomalies, fusiform fingers
XXY (Klinefelter syndrome)	Ebstein's malformation, tetralogy of Fallot	Small testes, gynecomastia
XO (Turner syndrome)	Coarctation, aortic stenosis, ventricular septal defect	Short stature, absent sexual maturation, web neck, skeletal changes

Table 29-2.   Syndromes of Congenital Heart Disease Associated with Skeletal Anomalies

Syndrome	Usual Cardiovascular Anomalies	Extracardiac Anomalies
Ellis-van Creveld syndrome	Single atrium, ventricular septal defect, atrial septal defect	Dwarfism, chondroectodermal dysplasia, polydactyly
Fanconi syndrome	Patent ductus arteriosus, ventricular septal defect	Hypoplastic thumb or radius, hyperpigmentation pancytopenia
Thrombocytopenia—absent radius syndrome	Atrial septal defect, tetralogy of Fallot, dextrocardia	Radial aplasia, thrombocytopenia with megakaryocytopenia
Rubinstein-Taybi syndrome	Patent ductus arteriosus	Broad thumbs and toes, maxillary hypoplasia, slanting palpebral fissures
Holt-Oram syndrome	Atrial septal defect, ventricular septal defect	Absent or triphalangeal thumb, variable upper limb anomalies
de Lange syndrome	Variable; ventricular septal defect most common	Mental retardation, synophrys, malformed limbs
Klippel-Feil syndrome	Ventricular septal defect	Cervical synostosis, short neck
Lawrence-Moon-Biedl syndrome	Tetralogy of Fallot, ventricular septal defect	Retinitis pigmentosa, mental retardation, hypogonadism, polydactyly
Carpenter syndrome	Patent ductus arteriosus, ventricular septal defect	Craniostenosis
Apert syndrome	Ventricular septal defect, tetralogy of Fallot	Craniosynostosis with midface hypoplasia, syndactyly
Marchesani syndrome	Patent ductus arteriosus, pulmonary valve stenosis (variable)	Brachymorphia, spherophakia, subluxation of lens

Table 29-3.   Syndromes of Congenital Heart Disease Associated with Deafness

Syndrome	Usual Cardiovascular Anomalies	Extracardiac Anomalies
Cardioauditory syndrome	Left ventricular hypertrophy	Deafness, increased digital whorls
Familial pulmonic stenosis and deaf-mutism	Pulmonic stenosis	Deafness
Forney syndrome	Mitral insufficiency	Deafness, freckles, growth retardation, cervical fusion
LEOPARD syndrome	Pulmonic stenosis, heart block	Deafness, lentigines, ocular hypertelorism, growth retardation
Rubella syndrome	Patent ductus arteriosus, peripheral pulmonic stenoses	Deafness, cataracts, microcephaly, microphthalmos

Table 29-4.   Syndromes of Congenital Heart Disease Associated with Cutaneous Manifestations

Syndrome	Usual Cardiovascular Anomalies	Extracardiac Anomalies
Block-Sulzberger incontinentia pigmenti	Patent ductus arteriosus	Irregular skin pigmentation, variable dental, ocular, and skeletal anomalies
Neurofibromatosis	Pulmonic stenosis, renal artery stenosis, coarctation of the aorta	Hamartoma
Osler-Rendu-Weber syndrome	Pulmonary arteriovenous fistulas	Telangiectasia
Sturge-Weber syndrome	Coarctation of the aorta	Trigeminal distribution of facial hemangioma with seizures
Tuberous sclerosis	Rhabdomyoma, cardiac arrhythmias, pulmonary hypertension	Adenoma sebaceum, epilepsy, mental retardation
Watson syndrome	Pulmonic stenosis	Mental retardation, café-au-lait spots

Table 29-5.   Syndromes of Congenital Heart Disease Associated with Other Extracardiac Anomalies

Syndrome	Usual Cardiovascular Anomalies	Extracardiac Anomalies
Absent spleen	Complex intracardiac lesions	Absent spleen, organ symmetry and multiple defects, changes in red blood cell structure
Cardial-facial syndrome	Ventricular septal defect	Lower facial paralysis
DiGeorge syndrome	Truncus arteriosus, tetralogy of Fallot, right aortic arch	Thymic aplasia
Facial dysmorphism	Right aortic arch, patent ductus arteriosus	Mental retardation
Kartagener syndrome	Dextrocardia	Situs inversus, bronchiectasis
Noonan syndrome	Pulmonic stenosis (dysplastic pulmonic valve), atrial septal defect	Hypertelorism, proximal pectus carinatum, low-set ears, webbing of neck
Pierre Robin syndrome	Ventricular septal defect	Hypoplasia of mandible and glossoptosis
Smith-Lemli-Opitz syndrome	Ventricular septal defect, patent ductus arteriosus	Mental retardation, microcephaly, disorders of neuromuscular system, micrognathia

REFERENCES

1. Abel RM, Grimes JB, Alonso D, et al: Adverse hemodynamic and ultrastructural changes in dog hearts subjected to protein-calorie malnutrition. Am Heart J 97:733, 1979

2. Abul-Haj SK, Martz DG, Douglas WF, Geppert LJ: Farber's disease. Report of a case with observations on its histogenesis and notes on the nature of the stored material. J Pediatr 61:221, 1962

3. Akamatsu A, Nomoto R, Nagao H, et al: Adult form acid maltase deficiency. A case report. Jpn J Med 21:203, 1982

4. Akbarian M, Yankopoulos NA, Abelmann WH: Hemodynamic studies in beriberi heart disease. Am Heart J 41:197, 1966

5. Akhtar M, Brody H: Elastic tissue in pseudoxanthoma elasticum. Ultrastructural study of endocardial lesions. Arch Pathol 99:667, 1975

6. Alexander WS: Phytanic acid in Refsum's syndrome. J Neurol Neurosurg Psychiatry 29:412, 1966

7. Allderdice PW, Eales B, Onyett H, et al: Duplication 9q34 syndrome. Am J Hum Genet 35:1005, 1983

8. Allen IV, Swallow M, Nevin NC, McCormick D: Clinicopathological study of Refsum's disease with particular reference to fatal complications. J Neurol Neurosurg Psychiatry 41:323, 1978

9. Almgren B, Eriksson I, Hemmingsson A, et al: Abdominal aortic aneurysm in homocystinuria. Acta Chir Scand 114:545, 1978

10. Amad KH, Brennan JC, Alexander JK: The cardiac pathology of chronic exogenous obesity. Circulation 32:740, 1965

11. Amatruda JM, Margolis S, Hutchins GM: Type III hyperlipoproteinemia, with mesangial foam cells in renal glomeruli. Arch Pathol 98:51, 1974

12. Anderson RA, Koch S, Camerini-Otero RD: Cardiovascular findings in congenital contractural arachnodactyly: Report of an affected kindred. Am J Med Genet 18:265, 1984

13. Antani J, Srinivas HV: Ehlers-Danlos syndrome and cardiovascular abnormalities. Chest 63:214, 1973

14. Antia AU, Wiltse HE, Rowe RD, et al: Pathogenesis of the supravalvular aortic stenosis syndrome. J Pediatr 71:431, 1967

15. Antopol W, Boas EP, Levison W, Tuchman LR: Cardiac hypertrophy caused by glycogen storage in a fifteen-year-old boy. Am Heart J 20:546, 1940

16. Atkins L: Progeria. Report of a case with postmortem findings. N Engl J Med 250:1065, 1954

17. Attas M, Hanley HG, Stultz D, et al: Fulminant beriberi heart disease with lactic acidosis: Presentation of a case with evaluation of left ventricular function and review of pathophysiologic mechanisms. Circulation 58:566, 1978

18. Attwood HD, Clifton S, Mitchell RE: A histological histochemical and ultrastructural study of dermal ochronosis. Pathology 3:115, 1971

19. Azevedo EM, Scaff M, Barbosa ER, et al: Heart involvement in hepatolenticular degeneration. Acta Neurol Scand 58:296, 1978

20. Backwinkel KP, von Bassewitz DB, Diekmann L, Themann H: Ultrastructure of heart muscle in generalized gangliosidosis GMI. Z Kinderheilk 110:104, 1971

21. Baker SS, Lerman RH, Krey SH, et al: Selenium deficiency with total parenteral nutrition: Reversal of biochemical and functional abnormalities by selenium supplementation: A case report. Am J Clin Nutr 37:319, 1983

22. Bale PM, Clifton-Bligh P, Benjamin BNP, Whyte HM: Pathology of Tangier disease. J Clin Pathol 24:609, 1971

23. Barabas AP: Vascular complications in the Ehlers-Danlos syndrome. With special reference to the "arterial type" or Sack's syndrome. J Cardiovasc Surg (Torino) 13:160, 1972

24. Barr DP, Rothbard S, Eder HA: Atherosclerosis and aortic stenosis in hypercholesteremic xanthomatosis. JAMA 156:943, 1954

25. Barrillon A, Bensaid J, Coirault R, et al: Myocardiopathie obstructive et maladie de Friedreich. Arch Mal Coeur 66:1525, 1973

26. Battin J, Vital C, Azanza X: Une neuro-lipidose rare avec lesions nodulaires sous-cutanees et articularies: La lipogranulomatose disseminee de Farber. Ann Dermatol Venerol 97:241, 1970

27. Beaudet AL, Diferrante NM, Ferry GD, et al: Variation in the phenotypic expression of β-glucuronidase deficiency. J Pediatr 86:388, 1975

28. Beaudet AL, Ferry GD, Nichols BL, Rosenberg HS: Cholesterol ester storage disease: Clinical, biochemical, and pathological studies. J Pediatr 90:910, 1979

29. Becker AE, Schoorl R, Balk AG, van der Heide RM: Cardiac manifestations of Fabry's disease. Report of a case with mitral insufficiency and electrocardiographic evidence of myocardial infarction. Am J Cardiol 36:829, 1975

30. Beighton P: Lethal complications of the Ehlers-Danlos syndrome. Br Med J 3:656, 1968

31. Beighton P: Cardiac abnormalities in the Ehlers-Danlos syndrome. Br Heart J 31:227, 1969

32. Beighton P: The dominant and recessive forms of cutis laxa. J Med Genet 9:216, 1972

33. Beil E, Seibel K, Riecker G: Herzerkrankung bei primarer Oxalose. Klin Wochenschr 47:513, 1969

34. Benbassat J, Bassan H, Milwidsky H, et al: Constrictive pericarditis in Gaucher's disease. Am J Med 44:647, 1968

35. Berenberg RA, Pellock JM, DiMauro S, et al: Lumping or splitting? "ophthalmoplegia-plus" or Kearns-Sayre syndrome? Ann Neurol 1:37, 1977

36. Bernstein HS, Bishop DF, Astrin KH, et al: Fabry disease: Six gene rearrangements and an exonic point mutation in the α-galactosidase gene. J Clin Invest 83:1390, 1989

37. Bharati S, Serratto M, DuBrow I, et al: The conduction system in Pompe's disease. Pediatr Cardiol 2:25, 1982

38. Blackburn WE, McRoberts JW, Bhathena D, et al: Severe vascular complications in oxalosis after bilateral nephrectomy. Ann Intern Med 82:44, 1975

39. Blank E, Linder D: I-cell disease (mucolipidosis II): A lysosomopathy. Pediatrics 54:797, 1974

40. Blankenhorn MA, Vilter CF, Scheinker IM, Austin RS: Occidental beriberi heart disease. JAMA 131:717, 1946

41. Blieden LC, Desnick RJ, Carter JB, et al: Cardiac involvement in Sandhoff's disease. Inborn error of glycosphingolipid metabolism. Am J Cardiol 34:83, 1974

42. Bloch A, Dinsmore RE, Lees RS: Coronary arteriographic findings in type II and type IV hyperlipoproteinaemia. Lancet 1:928, 1976

43. Bloom KR, Hug G, Schubert WK, Kaplan S: Pompe's disease and the heart. Circulation, 49, 50 (suppl. 3): 56, 1974

44. Bolande RP: The nature of the connective tissue abiotrophy in the Marfan syndrome. Lab Invest 12:1087, 1963

45. Bordiuk JM, Legato MJ, Lovelace RE, Blumenthal S: Pompe's disease. Electromyographic, electron microscopic, and cardiovascular aspects. Arch Neurol 23:113, 1970

46. Botreau-Roussel P, Drobinski G, Levy, et al: Infarctus du myocarde et drepanocytose heterozygote. A propos de 2 cas. Arch Mal Coeur 70:141, 1977

47. Bottiger LE, Mollerberg H: Increased copper content of hypertrophic myocardium. Acta Med Scand 165:413, 1959

48. Bouding G, Mikol J, Guillard A, Engel AG: Fatal systemic carnitine deficiency with lipid storage in skeletal muscle, heart, liver and kidney. J Neurol Sci 30:313, 1976

49. Bozner A, Knieriem HJ, Meesen H, Reinauer H: Die Ultrastruktur und Biochemie des Herzmuskels der Ratte im Thiaminmangel und nach einer Gabe von Thiamin. Virchows Arch Zellpath 2:125, 1969

50. Brewer HB, Jr, Zech LA, Gregg RE, et al: Type III hyperlipoproteinemia: Diagnosis, molecular defects, pathology, and treatment. Ann Intern Med 98:623, 1983

51. Brown BI, Brown DH: Glycogen storage diseases: Types I, III, IV, V, VII and unclassified glycogenoses. p. 123. In Dickens F, Randle PJ, Whelan WJ: Carbohydrate Metabolism and Its Disorders. Vol. 2. Academic Press, London, 1968

52. Bruni CB, Paluello FM: A biochemical and ultrastructural study of liver, muscle, heart and kidney in type II glycogenosis. Virchows Archiv (Cell Pathol) 4:196, 1970

53. Buja LM, Ferrans VJ, Levitsky S: Occurrence of intramitochondrial glycogen in anine myocardium after prolonged anoxic cardiac arrest. J Mol Cell Cardiol 4:237, 1972

54. Buja LM, Khoi NB, Roberts WC: Clinically significant cardiac amyloidosis. Clinicopathologic findings in 15 patients. Am J Cardiol 26:394, 1970

55. Buja LM, Roberts WC: Iron in the heart. Etiology and clinical significance. Am J Med 51:209, 1971

56. Bulkley BH, Buja LM, Ferrans VJ, et al: Tuberous xanthoma in homozygous type II hyperlipoproteinemia. A histologic, histochemical and electron microscopic study. Arch Pathol 99:293, 1975

57. Bulloch RT, Davis JL, Hara M: Dystrophia myotonica with heart block. A light and electron microscopic study. Arch Pathol 84:130, 1967

58. Bunim JJ, McEwen C: Tophus of the mitral valve in gout. Arch Pathol 29:700, 1940

59. Burnett HF, Bledsoe JH, Char F, Williams GD: Abdominal aortic aneurysmectomy in a 17-year-old patient with Ehlers-Danlos syndrome: Case report and review of the literature. Surgery 74:617, 1973

60. Byers PH, Holbrook KA, McGillivray B, et al: Clinical and ultrastructural heterogeneity of type IV Ehlers-Danlos syndrome. Hum Genet 47:141, 1979

61. Cabin HS, Schwartz DE, Virmani R, et al: Type III hyperlipoproteinemia. Quantification, distribution, and nature of atherosclerotic coronary arterial narrowing in five necropsy patients. Am Heart J 102:830, 1981

62. Caddell JL, Whittemore R: Observations on generalized glycogenosis with emphasis on electrocardiographic changes. Pediatrics 29:743, 1962

63. Caheen WR, Jr, Reza MJ, Kovick RB, Stern MS: Mitral valve prolapse and conduction defects in Ehlers-Danlos syndrome. Arch Intern Med 137:1227, 1977

64. Cain H, Egner E, Kresse H: Mucopolysaccharidosis III A (Sanfilippo disease type A). Histochemical, electron microscopical and biochemical findings. Beitr Pathol 160:58, 1977

65. Caplan H: A case of endocardial fibro-elastosis with features of glycogen-storage disease. J Pathol 76:77, 1958

66. Capone R, Amsterdam EA, Mason DT, Zelis R: Systemic amyloidosis, functional coronary insufficiency, and autonomic impairment. Ann Intern Med 76:599, 1972

67. Carey MC, Donovan DE, Fitzgerald O, McAuley FD: Homocystinuria. I. A clinical and pathological study of nine subjects in six families. Am J Med 45:7, 1968

68. Carson NAJ, Dent CE, Field CMB, Gaull GE: Homocystinuria. Clinical and pathological review of ten cases. J Pediatr 66:565, 1965

69. Castelli WP, Doyle JT, Gordon T, et al: HDL cholesterol levels (HDL-C) in coronary heart disease (CHD)—A cooperative lipoprotein phenotyping study. Circulation 55:767, 1977

70. Chan W, Ikram H: Primary amyloidosis with cardiac involvement diagnosed by left ventricular endomyocardial biopsy. Aust NZ J Med 7:427, 1977

71. Chan WC, Lai KS, Todd D: Adult Niemann-Pick disease—a case report. J Pathol 121:177, 1977

72. Chaplin AJ: Histopathological occurrence and characterisation of calcium oxalate: A review. J Clin Pathol 30:800, 1977

73. Char F: Tables of heritable cardiovascular conditions and associated syndromes. Birth Defects 8:313, 1972

74. Charrow J, Hvizd MG: Cardiomyopathy and skeletal myopathy in an unusual variant of G_{M1} gangliosidosis. J Pediatr 108:729, 1986

75. Chauhan S, Nayak NC, Ramalingaswami V: The heart and skeletal muscle in experimental protein malnutrition in rhesus monkeys. J Pathol Bact 90:301, 1965

76. Chen X, Yang G, Chen J, et al: Studies on the relations of selenium and Keshan disease. Biol Trace Element Res 2:91, 1980

77. Chopdar A: Multiple major retinal vascular occlusions in sickle cell haemoglobin C disease. Br J Ophthalmol 59:493, 1975

78. Chung EB: Histologic changes in gout. Georgetown Med Bull 5:269, 1962

79. Clark DS, Myerburg RJ, Morales RR, et al: Heart block in Kearns-Sayre syndrome, electrophysiologic pathologic correlation. Chest 68:727, 1975

80. Cohen IM, Vieweg WVR, Alpert JS, et al: Osteogenesis imperfecta tarda. Cardiovascular pathology. West J Med 126:228, 1977

81. Collip PJ, Chen SY: Cardiomyopathy and selenium deficiency in a two-year old girl. N Engl J Med 304:1304, 1983

82. Coltart DJ, Hudson REB: Primary oxalosis of the heart: A cause of heart block. Br Heart J 33:315, 1971

83. Colucci WS, Lorell BH, Schoen FJ, et al: Hypertrophic obstructive cardiomyopathy due to Fabry's disease. N Engl J Med 307:926, 1982

84. Cook AW, Bid TD, Spence AM, et al: Myotonic dystrophy, mitral-valve prolapse, and stroke. Lancet 1:335, 1978

85. Cooper JA, Moran TJ: Studies on ochronosis. I. Report of case with death from ochronotic nephrosis. Arch Pathol 64:46, 1957

86. Cornelio F, Di Donato S, Peluchetti D, et al: Fatal cases of lipid storage myopathy with carnitine deficiency. J Neurol Neurosurg Psychiatry 40:170, 1977

87. Cornwell GG, III, Natvig JB, Westermark P: Senile cardiac amyloid: Demonstration of a unique fibril protein in tissue sections. J Immunol 120:1385, 1978

88. Criscitiello MG, Ronan JA, Jr, Besterman EMM, Schoenwetter W: Cardiovascular abnormalities in osteogenesis imperfecta. Circulation 31:255, 1965

89. Crisfield RJ: Spontaneous aneurysm of the ductus arteriosus in a patient with Marfan's syndrome. J Thorac Cardiovasc Surg 62:243, 1971

90. Cristol R, Debray J, Aron M: Les manifestations cardiovasculaires du pseudo-xanthome elastique à propos d'un cas typique avec infarctus myocardique. Ann Med Interne (Paris) 123:771, 1972

91. Crocker AC, Vawter GF, Neuhauser EB, Rosowsky A: Wolman's disease: Three new patients with a recently described lipidosis. Pediatrics 35:627, 1965

92. Cruysberg JRM, Sengers RCA, Pinckers A, et al: Features of a syndrome with congenital cataract and hypertrophic cardiomyopathy. Am J Ophthalmol 102:740, 1986

93. Dal Canto MC, Rapin I, Suzuki K: Neuronal storage disorder with chorea and curvilinear bodies. Neurology (Minneap) 24:1026, 1974

94. Daniels RA, Weinberg R, Rangwala AF, Mintz G: Cardiac amyloidosis and idiopathic hypertrophic subaortic stenosis. J Med Soc N J 81:481, 1984

95. Danks DM, Campbell PE, Stevens BJ, et al: Menkes's kinky hair syndrome. An inherited defect in copper absorption with widespread effects. Pediatrics 50:188, 1972

96. Davis Z, Pluth JR, Giuliani ER: The Marfan syndrome and cardiac surgery. J Thorac Cardiovasc Surg 75:505, 1978

97. De Anda G, Vignale RA: Cutis laxa connatal. Med Cutan Iber Lat Am 12:1, 1984

98. Dekaban AS, Constantopoulos G, Herman MM: Mucopolysaccharidosis type V (Scheie syndrome). A postmortem study by multidisciplinary techniques with emphasis on the brain. Arch Pathol Lab Med 100:237, 1976

99. De los Arcos E, Urquia M, Torrano E, et al: Osteogenesis imperfecta e insuficiencia aortica. Rev Clin Esp 133:531, 1974

100. Desnick RJ, Blieden LC, Sharp HL, et al: Cardiac valvular anomalies in Fabry disease. Clinical, morphologic, and biochemical studies. Circulation 54:818, 1976

101. Di Pasquale G, Ribani M, Andreoli A, et al: Cardioembolic stroke in primary oxalosis with cardiac involvement. Stroke 20:1403, 1989

102. Diebold J: Letters to the case. Pathol Res Pract 180:200, 1985

103. Dincsoy MY, Dincsoy HP, Kessler AD, et al: Generalized glycogenosis and associated endocardial fibroelastosis. Report of 3 cases with biochemical studies. J Pediatr 67:728, 1965

104. Dingman RO, Grabb WC, O'Neal RM: Cutis laxa congenita. Generalized elastosis. Plast Reconstr Surg 44:431, 1969

105. Dische MR, Porro RS: The cardiac lesions in Bassen-Kornzweig syndrome. Report of a case, with autopsy findings. Am J Med 49:568, 1970

106. Dolman CL, Chang E, Duke RJ: Pathologic findings in Sandhoff disease. Arch Pathol 96:272, 1973

107. Dubach UC, Gloor F: Fabry-Krankheit (Angiokeratoma corporis diffusum universale). Phosphatidspeicherkrankheit bei zwei Familien. Duetsche Med Wehnschr 91:241, 1966

108. Duncan C, McLeod GM: Angiokeratoma corporis diffusum universale (Fabry's disease): A case with gross myocardial involvement. Aust NZ J Med 1:58, 1970

109. Dustin P, Tondeur M, Jonniaux G, et al: La maladie de Farber. Etude anatomo-clinique et ultrastructurale. Bull Mem Acad R Med Belg 128:733, 1973

110. Dyck PJ, Swanson CJ, Nishimura RA, et al: Cardiomyopathy in patients with hereditary motor and sensory neuropathy. Mayo Clin Proc 62:672, 1987

111. Ehlers KH, Engle MA: Glycogen storage disease of myocardium. Am Heart J 65:145, 1963

112. Ehlers KH, Hagstrom JWC, Lukas DS, et al: Glycogen-storage disease of the myocardium with obstruction to left ventricular outflow. Circulation 25:96, 1962

113. Eishi Y, Takemura T, Sone R, et al: Glycogen storage disease confined to the heart with deficient activity of cardiac phosphorylase kinase: A new type of glycogen storage disease. Hum Pathol 16:193, 1985

114. Eldridge R: Coarctation in the Marfan syndrome. Arch Intern Med 113:342, 1964

115. Elleder M, Dorazilovaa V, Bradova V, et al: Fabry's disease with isolated disease of the cardiac muscle, manifesting as hypertrophic cardiomyopathy. Cas Lek Cesk 129:369, 1990

116. Engel AG, Banker BQ, Eiben RM: Carnitine deficiency: Clinical, morphological and biochemical observations in a fatal case. J Neurol Neurosurg Psychiatry 40:313, 1977

117. Engel AG, Gomez MR, Seybold ME, Lambert EH: The spectrum and diagnosis of acid maltase deficiency. Neurology (Minneap) 23:95, 1973

118. Epstein J, William JR, Little JB: Deficient DNA repair in human progeroid cells. Proc Natl Acad Sci USA 70:977, 1973

119. Eriksson A, Olofsson BO, Eriksson P: Heart valve involvement in familial amyloidosis with polyneuropathy. Pathol Res Pract 181:563, 1986

120. Factor SM, Biempica L, Goldfischer S: Coronary intimal sclerosis in Morquio's syndrome. Virchows Arch (Pathol Anat) 379:1, 1978

121. Factor SM, Cho S, Sternlieb I, et al: The cardiomyopathy of Wilson's disease. Myocardial alterations in nine cases. Virchows Arch 397:301, 1982

122. Faillace RT, Kingston WJ, Nanda NC, Griggs RC: Cardiomyopathy associated with the syndrome of amyotrophic chorea and acanthocytosis. Ann Intern Med 96:616, 1982

123. Falck I: Angiokeratoma corporis diffusum Fabry mit vasorenalem Symptomenkomplex. Samml Selt Klin Falle 9:20, 1955

124. Fallat RW, Glueck CJ: Familial and acquired type V hyperlipoproteinemia. Atherosclerosis 23:41, 1976

125. Fantl P, Morris KN, Sawyers RJ: Repair of cardiac defect in patient with Ehlers-Danlos syndrome and deficiency of Hageman factor. Br Med J 1:1202, 1961

126. Farber S, Cohen J, Uzman LL: Lipogranulomatosis. A new lipoglyco-protein "storage" disease. Mt Sinai J Med NY 24:816, 1957

127. Fayemi AO, Ali M, Braun EV: Oxalosis in hemodialysis patients. A pathologic study of 80 cases. Arch Pathol Lab Med 103:58, 1979

128. Ferrans VJ, Boyce SW: Metabolic and familial diseases, p. 945. In Silver MD (ed): Cardiovascular Pathology. Churchill Livingstone, New York, 1983

129. Ferrans VJ, Buja LM: Application of periodate-thiocarbohydrazide-silver proteinate method for the ultrastructural cystochemistry of stored materials in diseases of carbohydrate and glycolipid metabolism. p. 231. In Takeuchi T, Ogawa K, Fujita S (eds): Histochemistry and Cytochemistry. Proceedings of the 4th International Congress of Histochemistry and Cytochemistry. Nakanishi Printing Co, Kyoto, Japan, 1972

130. Ferrans VJ, Buja LM, Jones M: Ultrastructure and cytochemistry of glycogen in cardiac diseases. p. 97. In Dhalla NS (ed): Recent Advances in Studies on Cardiac Structure and Metabolism. Myocardial Metabolism. Vol. 3. University Park Press, Baltimore, 1973

131. Ferrans VJ, Buja LM, Roberts WC: Cardiac morphologic changes produced by ethanol. p. 139. In Rothschild MA, Oratz M, Schreiber S (eds): Alcohol and Abnormal Protein Biosynthesis. Pergamon Press, New York, 1974

132. Ferrans VJ, Buja LM, Roberts WC, Fredrickson DS: The spleen in type I hyperlipoproteinemia. Histochemical, biochemical, microfluorimetric and electron microscopic observations. Am J Pathol 64:67, 1971

133. Ferrans VJ, Fredrickson DS: The pathology of Tangier disease. A light and electron microscopic study. Am J Pathol 78:101, 1975

134. Ferrans VJ, Hibbs RG, Burda CD: The heart in Fabry's disease. A histochemical and electron microscopic study. Am J Cardiol 24:95, 1969

135. Ferrans VJ, Maron BJ, Buja LM, et al: Intranuclear glycogen deposits in human cardiac muscle cells: Ultrastructure and cytochemistry. J Mol Cell Cardiol 7:373, 1975

136. Ferrans VJ, Roberts WC, Levy RI, Fredrickson DS: Chylomicrons and the formation of foam cells in type I hyperlipoproteinemia. A morphologic study. Am J Pathol 70:253, 1973

137. Finch SC, Finch CA: Idiopathic hemochromatosis, an iron storage disease. Medicine (Baltimore) 34:381, 1955

138. Fleischer RA, Rubler S: Primary cardio-

myopathy in nonanemic patients. Association with sickle cell trait. Am J Cardiol 22:532, 1968

139. Flemming CR, Lie JT, McCall JT, et al: Selenium deficiency and fatal cardiomyopathy in a patient on home parenteral nutrition. Gastroenterology 83:683, 1982

140. Folger GM, Jr: Further observations on the syndrome of idiopathic infantile hypercalcemia associated with supravalvular aortic stenosis. Am Heart J 93:455, 1977

141. Follis RH, Jr: Sudden death in infants with scurvy. J Pediatr 20:347, 1942

142. Follis RH, Jr: The effects of nutritional deficiency on the heart: A review. Am J Clin Nutr 4:107, 1956

143. Fong LV, Menahem S, Wraith JE, Chow CW: Endocardial fibroelastosis in mucopolysaccharidosis type VI. Clin Cardiol 10:362, 1987

144. Fournier C: Les lesions cardio-vasculaires du syndrome de Marfan. Coeur Med Interne 16:331, 1977

145. Frankel KA, Rosser RJ: The pathology of the heart in progressive muscular dystrophy: Epimyocardial fibrosis. Hum Pathol 7:375, 1976

146. Franks AJ: Cardiac pathology in chronic myopathy, with particular reference to dystrophia myotonia. Pathology 125:213, 1978

147. Fredrickson DS, Ferrans VJ: Acid cholesteryl ester hydrolase deficiency. (Wolman's disease and cholesteryl ester storage disease). p. 670. In Stanbury JB, Wyngaarden JB, Fredrickson DS (eds): The Metabolic Basis of Inherited Disease, 4th Ed. McGraw-Hill, New York, 1978

148. Fredrickson DS, Goldstein JL, Brown MS: The familial hyperlipoproteinemias. p. 604. In Stanbury JB, Wyngaarden JB, Fredrickson DS (eds): The Metabolic Basis of Inherited Disease, 4th ed. McGraw-Hill, New York, 1978

149. Friedman WF: Vitamin D and the supravalvular aortic stenosis syndrome. Adv Teratol 3:85, 1968

150. Fritz P, Schneider H, Heimburg P, Wegner G: Sekundare hypertrophe obstruktive Kardiomyopathie bei Morbus Fabry Med Welt 29:1851, 1978

151. Furukawa T, Peter JB: The muscular dystrophies and related disorders. I. The muscular dystrophies. JAMA 239:1537, 1978

152. Gabr M, Hashem N, Hashem M, et al: Progeria, a pathologic study. J Pediatr 57:70, 1960

153. Gach JV, Andriagne M, Franck G: Hypertrophic obstructive cardiomyopathy and Friedreich's ataxia. Report of a case and review of literature. Am J Cardiol 27:436, 1971

154. Gaines JJ, Jr: The pathology of alkaptonuric ochronosis. Hum Pathol 20:40, 1989

155. Gaines JJ, Jr, Pai GM: Cardiovascular ochronosis. Arch Pathol Lab Med 111:991, 1987

156. Galdston M, Steele JM, Dobriner K: Alcaptonuria and ochronosis. With a report of three patients and metabolic studies in two. Am J Med 13:432, 1952

157. Ganeval D, Mignon FY, Preud'homme JL: Depots de chaines légères et d'Immunonoglubulines monoclonales: Aspects nephrologiques et hypotheses physiopathologiques. Actualites Nephrologiques de l'Hôpital Necker. Flammarion Medecine-Sciences, Paris, p. 179, 1981

158. Ganeval D, Noel LH, Homme JLP: Lightchain deposition disease: Its relation with AL-type amyloidosis. Kidney Int 26:1, 1984

159. Garancis JC: Type II glycogenosis. Biochemical and electron microscopic study. Am J Med 44:289, 1968

160. Garcia RE, Friedman WF, Kaback MM, Rowe RD: Idiopathic hypercalcemia and supravalvular aortic stenosis. Documentation of a new syndrome. N Engl J Med 271:117, 1964

161. Garnett ES, Barnard DL, Ford J, et al: Gross fragmentation of cardiac myofibrils after therapeutic starvation for obesity. Lancet 1:914, 1969

162. Ge K, Xue A, Bai J, Wang S: Keshan disease—an endemic cardiomyopathy in China. Virchows Arch Pathol Anat 401:1, 1983

163. Gerry JL, Jr, Bulkley BH, Hutchins GM: Clinicopathologic analysis of cardiac dysfunction in 52 patients with sickle cell anemia. Am J Cardiol 42:211, 1978

164. Gibson JB, Carson NAJ, Neill DW: Pathological findings in homocystinuria. J Clin Pathol 17:427, 1964

165. Gilbert EF, Dawson G, Zu Rhein GM, et al: I-cell disease, mucolipidosis II. Pathological, histochemical, ultrastructural and biochemical observations in four cases. Z Kinderheilk 114:259, 1973

166. Gilbert EF, Varakis J, Opitz JM, et al: Gen-

eralized gangliosidosis type II (juvenile GM1 gangliosidosis). A pathological, histochemical and ultrastructural study. Z Kinderheilk 120:151, 1975

167. Gilgenkrantz S, Vigneron C, Gergoire MJ, et al: Association of del (11) (p 15.1, p12), aniridia, catalase deficiency, and Ca. Am J Med Genetics 13:39, 1982

168. Glaser JH, McAlister WH, Sly WS: Genetic heterogeneity in multiple lysosomal hydrolase deficiency. J Pediatr 85:192, 1974

169. Glenner GG: Amyloid deposits and amyloidosis: I. The fibrilloses. N Engl J Med 302:1283, 1980

170. Glenner GG: Amyloid deposits and amyloidosis: II. The fibrilloses. N Engl J Med 302:1333, 1980

171. Glenner GG, Ignaczak TF, Page DL: The inherited systemic amyloidoses and localized amyloid deposits. p. 1308. In Stanbury JB, Wyngaarden JB, Fredrickson DS (eds): The Metabolic Basis of Inherited Disease. 4th Ed. McGraw-Hill, New York, 1978

172. Glober GA, Tanaka KR, Turner JA, Liu CK: Mucopolysaccharidosis, an unusual cause of cardiac valvular disease. Am J Cardiol 22:133, 1968

173. Godfrey M, Menashe V, Weleber RG, et al: Cosegregation of elastin-associated microfibrillar abnormalities with the Marfan phenotype in families. Am J Hum Genet 46:652, 1990

174. Goertz K, Diehl AM, Vaseenon T, Mattioli L: A catastrophic complication. Acute dissection of an aortic aneurysm in a child with Marfan's syndrome. J Kans Med Soc 79:115, 1978

175. Goffin YA, Gruys E, Sorenson GD, Wellens F: Amyloid deposits in bioprosthetic cardiac valves after long-term implantation in man. A new localization of amyloidosis. Am J Pathol 114:431, 1984

176. Goldfischer S, Coltoff-Schiller B, Biempica L, Wolinsky H: Lysosomes and the sclerotic arterial lesion in Hurler's disease. Hum Pathol 6:633, 1975

177. Goldstein JL, Brown MS: Familial hypercholesterolemia: Pathogenesis of a receptor disease. Johns Hopkins Med J 143:8, 1978

178. Goltz RW, Hult AM, Goldfarb M, Gorlin RJ: Cutis laxa. A manifestation of generalized elastolysis. Arch Dermatol 92:373, 1965

179. Gonatas NK, Gonatas J: Ultrastructural and biochemical observations on a case of systemic late infantile lipidosis and its relationship to Tay-Sachs disease and gargoylism. J Neuropathol Exp Neurol 24:318, 1965

180. Goodman JR, Warshaw JB, Dallman PR: Cardiac hypertrophy in rats with iron and copper deficiency: Quantitative contribution of mitochondrial enlargement. Pediatr Res 4:244, 1970

181. Goodman RM, Smith EW, Paton D, et al: Pseudoxanthoma elasticum: A clinical and histopathological study. Medicine 42:297, 1963

182. Gordon N, Hudson REB: Refsum's syndrome. Heredopathia atactica polyneuritiformis. A report of three cases, including a study of the cardiac pathology. Brain 82:41, 1959

183. Gordon T, Castelli WP, Hjortland MD, et al: High density lipoprotein as a protective factor against coronary heart disease. Am J Med 62:707, 1977

184. Gore I, Wada M, Goodman ML: Capillary hemorrhage in ascorbic-acid-deficient guinea pigs. Ultrastructural basis. Arch Pathol Lab Med 85:493, 1968

185. Gorevic PD, Franklin EC: Amyloidosis. Annu Rev Med 32:261, 1981

186. Gospe SM, Armstrong DL, Gresik MV, Hawkins HK: Life-threatening congestive heart failure as the presentation of centronuclear myopathy. Pediatr Neurol 3:117, 1987

187. Gould L, Reddy CVR, DePalma D, et al: Cardiac manifestations of ochronosis. J Thorac Cardiovasc Surg 72:788, 1976

188. Gown AM, Hazzard WR, Benditt EP: Type III hyperlipoproteinemia and atherosclerosis. A case report and reevaluation. Human Pathol 13:506, 1982

189. Graham GG: Deficiencies of calories and protein. p. 211. In Rudolph AM, Barnett HL, Einhorn AH (eds): Pediatrics, 16th Ed. Appleton-Century-Crofts, East Norwalk, CT, 1977

190. Grantzow R, Hubner G: Mitochondrial cardiomyopathy with a high degree of heart muscle hypertrophy. Monatsschr Kinderheilkd 130:909, 1982

191. Greene GM, Weldon DC, Ferrans VJ, et al: Juvenile polysaccharidosis with cardioskeletal myopathy. Arch Pathol Lab Med 111:977, 1987

192. Grieco AJ: Homocystinuria: Pathogenetic mechanisms. Am J Med Sci 273:120, 1977

193. Gross DM, Robinson LK, Smith LT, et al: Severe perinatal Marfan syndrome. Pediatrics 84:83, 1989

194. Gruber MA, Graham TP, Jr, Engel E, Smith C: Marfan syndrome with contractural arachnodactyly and severe mitral regurgitation in a premature infant. J Pediatr 93:80, 1978

195. Guazzi GC, Martin JJ, Philippart M, et al: Wolman's disease. Eur Neurol 1:334, 1968

196. Haas LF, Bergin JD: Alpha lipoprotein deficiency with neurological features. Aust Ann Med 19:76, 1970

197. Hadley RN, Hagstrom JWC: Cardiac lesions in a patient with familial neurovisceral lipidosis (generalized gangliosidosis). Am J Clin Pathol 55:237, 1971

198. Hahlweg G, Orf G: Sog. fibroplastische Myocarditis bei Oxalose. Pathol Microbiol (Basel) 29:1, 1966

199. Harker LA, Slichter SJ, Scott CR, Ross R: Homocystinemia. Vascular injury and arterial thrombosis. N Engl J Med 291:537, 1974

200. Harley RD: Pediatric Ophthalmology. WB Saunders, Philadelphia, 1975, p 593

201. Harris RB, Heaphy MR, Perry HO: Generalized elastolysis (cutis laxa). Am J Med 65:815, 1978

202. Hart ZH, Change C, Di Mauro S, et al: Muscle carnitine deficiency and fatal cardiomyopathy. Neurology 28:147, 1978

203. Harvey PKP, Jones MC, Anderson EG: Pericardial abnormalities in Gaucher's disease. Br Heart J 31:603, 1969

204. Hashimoto K, Kanzaki T: Cutis laxa: Ultrastructural and biochemical studies. Arch Dermatol 111:861, 1975

205. Havel RJ, Kottle L, Vigne JL, et al: Radioimmunoassay of human arginine-rich apolipoprotein E: Concentration in blood plasma and lipoproteins as affected by apoprotein E-3 deficiency. J Clin Invest 66:1351, 1980

206. Hayden JG, Talner NS, Klaus SN: Cutis laxa associated with pulmonary artery stenosis. J Pediatr 72:506, 1968

207. Hays AP, Hallett M, Delfs J: Muscle phosphofructokinase deficiency: Abnormal polysaccharide in a case of late-onset myopathy. Neurology 31:1077, 1981

208. Hazzard WR: Type III hyperlipoproteinemia. p. 137. In Rifkind BM, Levy RI (eds): Hyperlipidemia: Diagnosis and Therapy. Grune & Stratton, Orlando, FL, 1977

209. Hecht F, Beals RK: "New" syndrome of congenital contractural arachnodactyly originally described by Marfan in 1896. Pediatrics 49:574, 1972

210. Heckman BA, Steinberg I: Congenital heart disease (mitral regurgitation) in osteogenesis imperfecta. AJR 103:601, 1968

211. Heckmatt JZ, Sewry CA, Hodes D, Dubowitz V: Congenital centronuclear (myotubular) myopathy. A clinical, pathological, and genetic study in eight children. Brain 108:941, 1985

212. Hedner P, Rausing A, Steen K, Torp A: Diagnosis of cardiac amyloidosis by myocardial biopsy. Acta Med Scand 198:525, 1975

213. Heggtveit HA, Herman L, Mishra RK: Cardiac necrosis and calcification in experimental magnesium deficiency. A light and electron microscopic study. Am J Pathol 45:757, 1964

214. Heggtveit HA, Nadkarni BB: Ultrastructural pathology of the myocardium. Methods Achiev Exp Pathol 5:474, 1971

215. Hemmingson LO, Eriksson P: Cardiac amyloidosis mimicking hypertrophic cardiomyopathy. Acta Med Scand 219:421, 1986

216. Hench PS, Darnall CM: A clinic on acute, old-fashioned gout; with special reference to its inciting factors. Med Clin North Am 16:1371, 1933

217. Heppner RL, Babitt HI, Bianchine JW, Warbasse JR: Aortic regurgitation and aneurysm of sinus of valsalva associated with osteogenesis imperfecta. Am J Cardiol 31:654, 1973

218. Herd JK, Subramanian S, Robinson H: Type III mucopolysaccharidosis: Report of a case with severe mitral valve involvement. J Pediatr 82:101, 1973

219. Hers HG, de Barsy T: Type II glycogenosis (acid maltase deficiency). p. 197. In Hers HG, Van Hoof F (eds): Lysosomes and Storage Disorders. Academic Press, San Diego, 1973

220. Hewer RL: The heart in Friedreich's ataxia. Br Heart J 31:5, 1969

221. Hoffman HN, Fredrickson DS: Tangier disease (familial DHL deficiency): Clinical and genetic features in two adults. Am J Med 39:582, 1965

222. Hoffman-Guilaine C, Nochy D, Tricottet V: La maladie des dépôts de chaines léagères:

Une entite anatomopathologique. Ann Pathol 4:105, 1984

223. Hohn AR, Lowe CU, Sokal JE, Lambert EC: Cardiac problems in the glycogenoses with specific reference to Pompe's disease. Pediatrics 35:313, 1965

224. Holimon JL, Wasserman AJ: Autopsy findings in type 3 hyperlipoproteinemia. Arch Pathol 92:415, 1971

225. Holmes JM, Houghton CR, Woolf AL: A myopathy presenting in adult life with features suggestive of glycogen storage disease. J Neurol Neurosurg Psychiatry 23:302, 1960

226. Hortop J, Tsipouras P, Hanley JA, et al: Cardiovascular involvement in osteogenesis imperfecta. Circulation 73:54, 1986

227. Houston HE: Abdominal aortic aneurysm in Marfan's syndrome. J Ky. Med Assoc 76:492, 1978

228. Hovig T, Gjone E: Familial lecithin: Cholesterol acyltransferase deficiency. Ultrastructural studies on lipid deposition and tissue reactions. Scand J Clin Lab Invest 33:135, 1974

229. Huang S, Kumar G, Steele HD, Parker JO: Cardiac involvement in pseudoxanthoma elasticum. Report of a case. Am Heart J 74:680, 1967

230. Hubert JP, Retif J, Brihaye J, Flament-Durand J: Étude anatomopathologique d'un cas d'homocystinurie. Pathol Eur 8:113, 1973

231. Hubner G, Grantzow R: Mitochondrial cardiomyopathy with involvement of skeletal muscles. Virchows Arch 399:115, 1973

232. Hudgson P, Gardner-Medwin D, Worsfold M, et al: Adult myopathy from glycogen storage disease due to acid maltase deficiency. Brain 91:435, 1968

233. Hug G, Schubert WK: Glycogenosis type II. Glycogen distribution in tissues. Arch Pathol 84:141, 1967

234. Husband EM, Lannigan R: Electron microscopy of the heart in a case of primary cardiac amyloidosis. Br Heart J 30:265, 1968

235. Hutchins GM, Mirvis SE, Mendelsohn G, Bulkley BH: Supravalvular aortic stenosis with parafollicular cell (C-cell) hyperplasia. Am J Med 64:967, 1978

236. Imahori S, Bannerman RM, Graf CJ, Brennan JC: Ehlers-Danlos syndrome with multiple arterial lesions. Am J Med 47:967, 1969

237. Inouye K, Katsura E: Etiology and pathology of beriberi. p. 1. In Shimazono N, Katsura E (eds): Review of Japanese Literature on Beriberi and Thiamine. Igaku Shoin, Tokyo, 1965

238. Ireland MA, Rowlands DB: Mucopolysaccharidosis type IV as a cause of mitral stenosis in an adult. Br Heart J 46:113, 1981

239. Ishihara T, Uchino F, Adachi H, et al: Type IV glycogenosis. A study of two cases. Acta Pathol Jpn 25:613, 1975

240. Ishihara T, Yokota T, Yamashita Y, et al: Comparative study of the intracytoplasmic inclusions in Lafora disease and type IV glycogenosis by electron microscopy. Acta Pathol Jpn 37:1591, 1987

241. Isner JM, Hawley RJ, Weintraub AM, Engel K: Cardiac findings in Charcot-Marie-Tooth disease: A prospective study of 68 patients. Arch Intern Med 139:1161, 1979

242. Isner JM, Sours HE, Paris AL, et al: Sudden unexpected death in avid dieters using the liquid-protein-modified-fast diet: Observations in 17 patients and the role of the prolonged Q-T interval. Circulation 60:1401, 1979

243. Ivemark B, Thoren C: The pathology of the heart in Friedreich's ataxia. Changes in coronary arteries and myocardium. Acta Med Scand 175:227, 1964

244. Iwata T, Nakamura H, Nagasawa T, et al: Amyloid deposits in heart valves. Acta Pathol Jpn 32:23, 1982

245. Jadro-Santel D: Zahacenost vaskularnih, mezenhimalnih struktura u misicu bolesnika od Pompeove bolesti (glikogenoze tip II). (Elektronsko-mikroskopska studija). Acta Med Yugosl 30:203, 1976

246. James TN: Observations on the cardiovascular involvement, including the cardiac conduction system, in progressive muscular dystrophy. Am Heart J 63:48, 1962

247. James TN: Pathology of the cardiac conduction system in hemochromatosis. N Engl J Med 271:92, 1964

248. James TN: Pathology of the cardiac conduction system in amyloidosis. Ann Intern Med 65:28, 1966

249. James TN, Carson NAJ, Froggatt P: De subitaneis mortibus. IV. Coronary vessels and conduction system in homocystinuria. Circulation 49:367, 1974

250. James TN, Fisch C: Observations on the car-

diovascular involvement in Friedreich's ataxia. Am Heart J 66:164, 1963

251. James TN, Frame B, Coates EO: De subitaneis mortibus. III. Pickwickian syndrome. Circulation 48:1311, 1973

252. James TN, Frame B, Schatz IJ: Pathology of cardiac conduction system in Marfan's syndrome. Arch Intern Med 114:339, 1964

253. Johnson RA, Baker SS, Fallon JT, et al: An occidental case of cardiomyopathy and selenium deficiency. N Engl J Med 304:1210, 1981

254. Jones KL, Smith DW: The Williams elfin facies syndrome. A new perspective. J Pediatr 86:718, 1975

255. Jortner R, Shahin W, Eshkol D, et al: Cardiovascular manifestations and surgery for Marfan's syndrome. Chest 56:24, 1969

256. Julien J, de Boucaud D: Aneurysme dans le systeme de la veine de Galien et syndrome de Marfan. Bordeaux Med 11:3245, 1971

257. Kahlke W: Heredopathia atactica polyneuritiformis (Refsum's disease). p. 352. In Schettler G (ed): Lipids and Lipidoses. Springer-Verlag, New York, 1967

258. Kasper W, Limbourg P, Just H: Verkalkung des Mitralklappenringes als kardiale Manifestation des Marfan-Syndroms. Z Kardiol 66:116, 1977

259. Kay JM, Littler WA, Meade JB: Ultrastructure of myocardium in familial heart block and peroneal muscular atrophy. Br Heart J 34:1081, 1972

260. Kearns TP: External ophthalmoplegia, pigmentary degeneration of the retina and cardiomyopathy. A newly recognized syndrome. Trans Am Ophthalmol Soc 63:559, 1965

261. Kearns TP, Sayre GP: Retinitis pigmentosa, external ophthalmoplegia and complete heart block. Arch Ophthalmol 60:280, 1958

262. Kelly TE, Thomas GH, Taylor HA, et al: Mucolipidosis III (pseudo-Hurler polydystrophy): Clinical and laboratory studies in a series of patients. Johns Hopkins Med J 137:156, 1975

263. Kennel AJ, Titus JL, Merideth J: Pathologic findings in the atrioventricular conduction system in myotonic dystrophy. Mayo Clin Proc 49:838, 1974

264. Keshan Disease Research Group of the Chinese Academy of Medical Sciences, Beijing: Epidemiologic studies on the etiologic rela-

tionship of selenium and Keshan disease. Chin Med J 92, 477, 1979

265. Keshan Disease Research Group of Chinese Academy of Medical Sciences, Beijing; Antiepidemic Station of Sichuan Province, Chengdu; Antiepidemic Station of Xichang District, Sichuan; Antiepidemic Station of Mianning County, Sichuan: Observations on effect of sodium selenite in prevention of Keshan disease. Chin Med J 92:471, 1979

266. Keye JD Jr: Death in potassium deficiency. Report of a case including morphologic findings. Circulation 5:766, 1952

267. Keys A: Cardiovascular effects of undernutrition and starvation. Mod Concepts Cardiovasc Dis 17:21, 1948

268. Kiel EA, Frias JL, Victorica BE: Cardiovascular manifestations in the Larsen syndrome. Pediatrics 71:942, 1983

269. Kien CL, Ganther HE: Manifestations of chronic selenium deficiency in a child receiving total parenteral nutrition. Am J Clin Nutr 37:319, 1983

270. Kirkpatrick CJ, Curry A, Galle J: Systemic kappa light chain deposition and amyloidosis in multiple myeloma: Novel morphological observations. Histopathology 10:1065, 1986

271. Kluitmann G, Braumann HG, Kratz HW, et al: Akuter Verlauf des Leigh-Syndroms mit hypertropher Kardiomyopathie bei einem weiblichen Saugling. Monatsschr Kinderheilkd 133:688, 1985

272. Kocen RS, King RHM, Thomas PK, Haas LF: Nerve biopsy findings in two cases of Tangier disease. Acta Neuropathol 26:317, 1973

273. Kornreich R, Bishop, Desnick RJ: α-Galactosidase A gene rearrangements causing Fabry disease. J Biol Chem 265:9319, 1990

274. Krivit W, Desnick RJ, Lee J, et al: Generalized accumulation of neutral glycospingolipids with GM2 ganglioside accumulation in the brain. Sandhoff's disease (variant of Tay-Sachs disease). Am J Med 52:763, 1972

275. Krovetz LJ, Lorincz AE, Schiebler GL: Cardiovascular manifestations of the Hurler syndrome. Hemodynamic and angiocardiographic observations in 15 patients. Circulation 31:132, 1965

276. Krovetz LJ, Schiebler GL: Cardiovascular manifestations of the genetic mucopolysaccharidoses. Birth Defects 8:192, 1972

277. Kuan P: Cardiac Wilson's disease. Chest 91:579, 1987

278. Kuhn H, Kohler E, Hort W, Frenzel H: Concealed myocardial storage disease (Fabry's disease): Pitfalls in the diagnosis of hypertrophic nonobstructive cardiomyopathy. Circulation 66:II–117, 1982

279. Kurlander GJ, Petry EL, Taybi H, et al: Supravalvar aortic stenosis. Roentgen analysis of twenty-seven cases. AJR 98:782, 1966

280. Kwiterovich PO Jr, Sniderman AD: Atherosclerosis and apoproteins B and A-I. Prev Med 12:815, 1983

281. Ladefoged C, Rohr N: Amyloid deposits in aortic and mitral valves. A clinicopathological investigation of material from 100 consecutive heart valve operations. Virchows Arch 404:301, 1984

282. Landing BH, Silverman FN, Craig JM, et al: Familial neurovisceral lipidosis. Am J Dis Child 108:503, 1964

283. Langes K, Frenzel H, Seitz RJ, Kluitmann G: Cardiomyopathy associated with Leigh's disease. Virchows Arch Pathol Anat 407:97, 1985

284. Laszlo A, Torok L, Hauess Z, Bartos Z: Manifestation of angiokeratoma diffusum in a girl patient with heterozygous genotype for Fabry's disease. Acta Peadiatr (Hung) 24:331, 1988–1989

285. Laurent M, Toulet R, Ramee MP: Maladie des chaines légères avec myocardiopathie terminale. Arch Mal Coeur 78:943, 1984

286. Le Bodic MF, Le Bodic L, Buzelin F, et al: Les lesions vasculaires de la maladie de Fabry. Études optique, histo-chimique et ultrastructurale. Ann Anat Pathol (Paris) 23:23, 1978

287. Leder AA, Bosworth WC: Angiokeratoma corporis diffusum universale (Fabry's disease) with mitral stenosis. Am J Med 38:814, 1965

288. Lewis HP: Cardiac involvement in hemochromatosis. Am J Med Sci 227:544, 1954

289. Levin S, Moses SW, Chayoth R, et al: Glycogen storage disease in Israel. A clinical, biochemical and genetic study. Isr J Med Sci 3:397, 1967

290. Levine HD, Parisi AF, Holdsworth DE, Cohn LH: Aortic valve replacement for ochronosis of the aortic valve. Chest 74:466, 1978

291. Lichtenstein L, Kaplan L: Hereditary ochronosis. Pathologic changes observed in two necropsied cases. Am J Pathol 30:99, 1954

292. Lichtenstein L, Scott HW, Levin MH: Pathologic changes in gout. Survey of eleven necropsied cases. Am J Pathol 32:871, 1956

293. Lindsay J, Jr, Meshel JC, Patterson RH: The cardiovascular manifestations of sickle cell disease. Arch Intern Med 133:643, 1974

294. Linzbach AJ: Mikrometrische und histologische Analyse menschlicher Hungerherzen. Virchows Arch (Pathol Anat) 314:600, 1947

295. Lithell H, Vessby B, Walldius G, Carlson LA: Hypertriglyceridemia-acute pancreatitis-ischemic heart disease. A case study in a pair of monozygotic twins. Acta Med Scand 221:311, 1987

296. Littler WA: Heart block and peroneal muscular atrophy: A family study. Q J Med 39:431, 1970

297. Lowden JA, Barson AJ, Wentworth P: Wolman's disease: A microscopic and biochemical study showing accumulation of ceroid and esterified cholesterol. Can Med Assoc J 102:402, 1970

298. Ludatscher RM, Kerner H, Amikam S, Gellei B: Myotonia dystrophica with heart involvement: An electron microscopic study of skeletal, cardiac, smooth muscle. J Clin Pathol 31:1057, 1978

299. Lukasik E: Electrocardiographic studies in female carriers of Duchenne muscular dystrophy. J Neurol 209:279, 1975

300. MacLeod PM, Fraser FC: Congenital contractural arachnodactyly. A heritable disorder of connective tissue distinct from Marfan's syndrome. Am J Dis Child 126:810, 1973

301. Maher JA, Epstein FH, Hand EA: Xanthomatosis and coronary heart disease. Necropsy studies of two affected siblings. Arch Intern Med 102:437, 1958

302. Mahloudji M, Teasdall RD, Adamkiewicz JJ, et al: The genetic amyloidoses. With particular reference to hereditary neuropathic amyloidosis, Type II (Indiana or Rukavina type). Medicine 48:1, 1969

303. Makous N, Friedman S, Yakovac W, Maris EP: Cardiovascular manifestations in progeria. Report of clinical and pathologic findings in a patient with severe arteriosclerotic heart disease and aortic stenosis. Am Heart J 64:334, 1962

304. Manschot WA: A case of progeronanism (pro-

geria of Gilford). Acta Pediatr Scand 39:158, in press

305. Maron BJ, Ferrans VJ: Intramitochondrial glycogen deposits in hypertrophied human myocardium. J Mol Cell Cardiol 7:697, 1975

306. Martin JJ, Flament-Durand J, Farriaux JP, et al: Menkes kinky-hair disease. A report on its pathology. Acta Neuropathol (Berl) 42:25, 1978

307. Marvel RJ, Genovese PD: Cardiovascular disease in Marfan's syndrome. Am Heart J 42:814, 1951

308. Mata M, Wharton M, Geisinger K, Pugh JE: Myocardial rhabdomyosarcoma in multiple neurofibromatosis. Neurology 31:1549, 1981

309. Mathieu M, Labeille B, Sevestre H, et al: Marfan disease presenting in neonates with rapid cardiovascular failure. Apropos of 2 cases. Ann Pediatr (Paris) 36:469, 1989

310. Matsuda M, Akatsuka N, Yamaguchi T, et al: Systolic time intervals in patients with progressive muscular dystrophy of the Duchenne type. Jpn Heart J 18:638, 1977

311. Matsui S, Murakami E, Takekoshi N, et al: Cardiac manifestations of Fabry's disease. Report of a case with pulmonary regurgitation diagnosed on the basis of endomyocardial biopsy findings. Jpn Circ J 41:1023, 1977

312. Maurat JP, Mercier NN, Ledoux C, Hatt PY: Le myocarde dans les depletions experimentales en potassium chez le rat. Étude au microscope electronique. Arch Mal Coeur 58:1004, 1965

313. McAllen PM: Myocardial changes occurring in potassium deficiency. Br Heart J 17:5, 1955

314. McAllister HA, Jr, Seger J, Bossart M, Ferrans VJ: Restrictive cardiomyopathy with kappa light chain deposits in myocardium as a complication of multiple myeloma. Arch Pathol Lab 112:1151, 1988

315. McCleary JE, Brunsting LA, Kennedy RLJ: Primary xanthoma tuberosum in children. With classification of xanthomas. Pediatrics 23:67, 1959

316. McComb RD, Markesbery WR, O'Connor WN: Fatal neonatal nemaline myopathy with multiple congenital abnormalities. J Pediatr 94:47, 1979

317. McCully KS: Vascular pathology of homocysteinemia. Implications for the pathogenesis of arteriosclerosis. Am J Pathol 56:111, 1969

318. McKinney B: Pathology of the Cardiomyopathies. Butterworths (Publishers), London, 1974

319. McKusick VA: The cardiovascular aspects of Marfan's syndrome: A heritable disorder of connective tissue. Circulation 11:321, 1955

320. McKusick VA: Heritable Disorders of Connective Tissue. 4th Ed. CV Mosby, St. Louis, 1972

321. McKusick VA, Neufeld EF, Kelley TE: The mucopolysaccharide storage diseases. p. 1282. In Stanbury JB, Wyngaarden JB, Fredrickson DS (eds): The Metabolic Basis of Inherited Disease. 4th Ed. McGraw-Hill, New York, 1978

322. Mehregan AH, Lee SC, Nabai H: Cutis laxa (generalized elastolysis). A report of four cases with autopsy findings. J Cutan Pathol 5:116, 1978

323. Melamed R, Aygen MM, Lowenstein A: Osteogenesis imperfecta with mitral insufficiency due to ballooning of the mitral valve. A case report. Isr J Med Sci 12:1325, 1976

324. Mendelsohn G, Bulkley BH, Hutchins GM: Cardiovascular manifestations of pseudoxanthoma elasticum. Arch Pathol Lab Med 102:298, 1978

325. Merkel KHH, Ginberg PL, Parker JC Jr, Post MJD: Cerebrovascular disease in sickle cell anemia: A clinical, pathological and radiological correlation. Stroke 9:45, 1978

326. Michiel RR, Sneider JS, Dickstein RA, et al: Sudden death in a patient on a liquid protein diet. N Engl J Med 298:1005, 1978

327. Miller CG, Alleyne GA, Brooks SEH: Gross cardiac involvement in glycogen storage disease type III. Br Heart J 34:862, 1972

328. Milstoc M: An unusual anatomopathologic aspect of a case with pseudoxanthoma elasticum. Dis Chest 55:431, 1969

329. Miyabayashi S, Ito T, Narisawa K, et al: Biochemical study in 28 children with lactic acidosis, in relation to Leigh's encephalomyelopathy. Eur J Pediatr 143:278, 1985

330. Miyamoto Y, Etoh Y, Joh R, et al: Adult-onset acid maltase deficiency in siblings. Acta Pathol Jpn 35:1533, 1985

331. Molz G: Farbersche Krankheit. Pathologisch-anatomische Befunde. Virchows Arch (Pathol Anat) 344:86, 1968

332. Moon HR, Chi JG, Yeon KM, et al: Menkes disease—an autopsy case with metal analysis of hair. J Korean Med Sci 2:75, 1987

333. Morand P, Despert F, Carrier HN, et al: Myopathie lipidique avec cardiomyopathie sévère par deficit generalise en carnitine. Arch Mal Coeur 72:536, 1979

334. Morganroth J, Levy RI, Fredrickson DS: The biochemical, clinical, and genetic features of type III hyperlipoproteinemia. Ann Intern Med 82:158, 1975

335. Moses SW, Gadoth N, Bashan N, et al: Neuromuscular involvement in glycogen storage disease type III. Acta Paediatr Scand 75:289, 1986

336. Murdoch JL, Walker BA, Halpern BL, et al: Life expectancy and causes of death in the Marfan syndrome. N Engl J Med 286:804, 1972

337. Muster AJ, Bharati S, Herman JJ, et al: Fatal cardiovascular disease and cutis laxa following acute febrile neutrophilic dermatosis. J Pediatr 102:243, 1983

338. Nagashima K, Endo H, Sakakibara K, et al: Morphological and biochemical studies of a case of mucopolysaccharidosis II (Hunter's syndrome). Acta Pathol Jpn 26:115, 1976

339. Nagashima K, Sakakibara K, Endo H, et al: I-cell disease (mucolipidosis II). Pathological and biochemical studies of an autopsy case. Acta Pathol Jpn 27:251, 1977

340. Nigel KR, Perloff JK, Kark AP: Cardiac conduction in Kearns-Sayre syndrome. Am J Cardiol 44:1396, 1979

341. Noonan JA: Association of congenital heart disease with syndromes or other defects. Pediatr Clin North Am 25:797, 1978

342. Oakes BW, Banks DM, Campbell PE: Human copper deficiency: Ultrastructural studies of the aorta and skin in a child with Menkes' syndrome. Exp Mol Pathol 25:82, 1976

343. O'Brien WM, La Du BN, Bunim JJ: Biochemical, pathologic and clinical aspects of alcaptonuria, ochronosis and ochronotic arthropathy. Am J Med 34:813, 1963

344. Oda H, Sasaki Y, Nakatani Y, et al: Hunter's syndrome: An ultrastructural study of an autopsy case. Acta Pathol Jpn 38:1175, 1988

345. Oh JK, Tajik AJ, Edwards WD, et al: Dynamic left ventricular outflow tract obstruction in cardiac amyloidosis detected by continuous-wave Doppler echocardiography. Am J Cardiol 59:1008, 1987

346. Olinger GN, Korns ME, Bonchek LI: Acute aortic valvular insufficiency due to isolated myxomatous degeneration. Ann Intern Med 88:807, 1978

347. Olivares L, Opez JL, Tosao S, et al: Menkes syndrome: Study of 2 new cases. Ann Esp. Pediatr 31:380, 1989

348. Oliver J, Fernandez FG, Cerdan SA, et al: Insuficiencia mitral y estenosis aortica severa en un paciente con sindrome de Hunter. Rev Esp Cardiol 35:465, 1982

349. Olson W, Engel WC, Walsh GO, et al: Oculocraniosomatic neuromuscular disease with "ragged-red" fibers. Arch Neurol 26:193, 1972

350. Orndahl G, Thulesius O, Enestrom S, Dehlin O: The heart in myotonic disease. Acta Med Scand 176:479, 1964

351. Ottesen OE, Antia AU, Rowe RD: Peripheral vascular anomalies associated with the supravalvular aortic stenosis syndrome. Radiology 86:430, 1966

352. Page HL Jr, Vogel JHK, Pryor R, Blount SG, Jr: Supravalvular aortic stenosis. Unusual observations in three patients. Am J Cardiol 23:270, 1969

353. Pages A, Baldet P: Ochronose: Aspects anatomo-cliniques et ultrastructuraux. Ann Anat Pathol (Paris), 16:27, 1971

354. Parkinson JE, Sunshine A: Angiokeratoma corporis diffusum universale (Fabry) presenting as suspected myocardial infarction and pulmonary infarcts. Am J Med 31:951, 1961

355. Patriquin HB, Kaplan P, Kind HP, Giedion A: Neonatal mucolipidosis II (I-cell disease): Clinical and radiologic features in three cases. AJR 129:37, 1977

356. Perkins DG, Haust MD: Ultrastructure of myocardium in the Hurler syndrome: Possible relation to cardiac function. Virchows Arch Pathol Anat 394:195, 1982

357. Perkins JG, Petersen AB, Riley JA: Renal and cardiac lesions in potassium deficiency due to chronic diarrhea. Am J Med 8:115, 1950

358. Perloff JK: The myocardial disease of heredofamilial neuromyopathies. p. 319. In Fowler NO (ed): Myocardial Diseases. Grune & Stratton, Orlando, FL, 1973

359. Perloff JK, DeLeon AC, Jr, O'Doherty D:

The cardiomyopathy of progressive muscular dystrophy. Circulation 33:625, 1966

360. Perloff JK, Roberts WC, DeLeon AC, Jr, O'Doherty D: The distinctive electrocardiogram of Duchenne's progressive muscular dystrophy. Am J Med 42:179, 1967

361. Pernot C: La myocardiopathie de la maladie de Friedreich. À propos d'une serie de 17 observations. Arch Fr Pediatr 36:11, 1979

362. Philip N, Garcia-Meric P, Wernert F: Syndrome de Beals-Hecht (Congenital contractural arachnodactyly) a revelation noenatale. Pediatrie 43:609, 1988

363. Phornphutkul C, Rosenthal A, Nadas AS: Cardiac manifestations of Marfan syndrome in infancy and childhood. Circulation 57:587, 1973

364. Pijoan de Beristain C: Asociacion de insuficiencia aortica con osteogenesis imperfecta, en dos sujetos de la misma familia. Rev Esp Cardiol 26:405, 1973

365. Piza J, Troper L, Cespedes R, et al: Myocardial lesions and heart failure in infantile malnutrition. Am J Trop Med Hyg 20:343, 1971

366. Pope FM, Daw CM, Narcisi P, Richarda AR: Prenatal diagnosis and prevention of inherited abnormalities of collagen. J Inher Metab Dis 12:135, 1989

367. Pund EE Jr, Hawley RL, McGee HJ, Blount SG Jr: Gouty heart. N Engl J Med 263:835, 1960

368. Pyeritz RE, McKusick VA: The Marfan syndrome: Diagnosis and management. N Engl J Med 300:772, 1979

369. Rabkin SA, Ledwich R, Mymin D: Myocardial infarction in familial hyperalpha and hypo-beta-lipoproteinemia. Postgrad Med J 57:385, 1981

370. Randall RE, Williamson WC, Mullinas F: Manifestations of systemic light chain deposition. Am J Med 60:293, 1976

371. Reed GB Jr, Dixon JFP, Neustein HB, et al: Type IV glycogenosis. Patient with absence of a branching enzyme α-1,4-glucan: α-1,4-glucan 6-glycosyl transferase. Lab Invest 19:546, 1968

372. Reed WB, Horowitz RE, Beighton P: Acquired cutis laxa. Primary generalized elastolysis. Arch Dermatol 103:661, 1971

373. Rees A, Elbl F, Minhas K, Solinger R: Echocardiographic evidence of outflow tract obstruction in Pompe's disease (glycogen storage disease of the heart). Am J Cardiol 37:1103, 1976

374. Refsum S: Heredopathia atactica polyneuritiformis. Phytanic acid storage disease (Refsum's disease). p. 181. In Vinken PJ, Bruyn GW (eds): Handbook of Clinical Neurology. Vol. 21. System Disorders and Atrophies. Part 1. Elsevier Science Publishing, New York, 1975

375. Reichel W, Garcia-Bunuel R: Pathologic findings in progeria: Myocardial fibrosis and lipofuscin pigment. Am J Clin Pathol 53:243, 1970

376. Remigio PA, Grinvalsky HT: Osteogenesis imperfecta congenita. Association with conspicuous extraskeletal connective tissue dysplasia. Am J Dis Child 119:524, 1970

377. Renteria VG, Ferrans VJ, Roberts WC: The heart in the Hurler syndrome. Gross, histologic and ultrastructural observations in five necropsy cases. Am J Cardiol 38:487, 1976

378. Roberts NK, Perloff JK, Kark RAP: Cardiac conduction in the Kearns-Sayre syndrome (a neuromuscular disorder associated with progressive external ophthalmoplegia and pigmentary retinopathy). Am J Cardiol 44:1396, 1979

379. Roberts WC: Congenital cardiovascular abnormalities usually "silent" until adulthood: Morphologic features of the floppy mitral valve, valvular aortic stenosis, discrete subvalvular aortic stenosis, hypertrophic cardiomyopathy, sinus of Valsalva aneurysm, and the Marfan syndrome. p. 407. In Roberts WC (ed): Congenital Heart Disease in Adults. FA Davis, Philadelphia, 1979

380. Roberts WC, Ferrans VJ, Levy RI, Fredrickson DS: Cardiovascular pathology in hyperlipoproteinemia. Anatomic observations in 42 necropsy patients with normal or abnormal serum lipoprotein patterns. Am J Cardiol 31:557, 1973

381. Roberts WC, Fredrickson DS: Gaucher's disease of the lung causing severe pulmonary hypertension with associated acute recurrent pericarditis. Circulation 35:783, 1967

382. Roberts WC, Levy RI, Fredrickson DS: Hyperlipoproteinemia. A review of the five types with first report of necropsy findings in type 3. Arch Pathol 90:46, 1970

383. Rodriguez-Torres R, Schneck L, Kleinberg

W: Electrocardiographic and biochemical abnormalities in Tay-Sachs disease. Bull NY Acad Med 47:717, 1971

384. Rosai J, Lascano EF: Basophilic (mucoid) degeneration of myocardium. A disorder of glycogen metabolism. Am J Pathol 61:99, 1970

385. Rose M, Greene RM: Cardiovascular complications during prolonged starvation. West J Med 130:170, 1979

386. Rosenson RS, Mudge GH, Jr, Sutton MG: Nemaline cardiomyopathy. Am J Cardiol 58:175, 1986

387. Rosenthal IM, Bronstein IP, Dallenbach FD, et al: Progeria. Report of a case with cephalometric roentgenograms and abnormally high concentrations of lipoproteins in the serum. Pediatrics 18:565, 1956

388. Rotberg T, Sanagustin MT, Salinas L, Macias R: Sindrome de Ehlers-Danlos asociado a comunicacion interauricular, bloqueo A-V completo, aneurisma de aorta y crecimiento del ventriculo izquierdo (miocardiopatia). Arch Inst Cardiol Mex 47:562, 1977

389. Roth J, Roth H: Elektronenmikroskopische Befunde an inneren Organen bei Morbus Fabry. Virchows Arch (Pathol Anat) 378:75, 1978

390. Rothbard S, Hagstrom JWC, Smith JP: Aortic stenosis and myocardial infarction in hypercholesterolemic xanthomatosis. Am Heart J 73:687, 1967

391. Rowe RD, Uchida IA, Char F: Heart disease associated with chromosomal abnormalities. p. 897. In Keith JD, Rowe RD, Vlad P (eds): Heart Disease in Infancy and Childhood. 3rd Ed. Macmillan, New York, 1978

392. Rowley PT, Enlander D: Hemoglobin S-C disease presenting as acute cor pulmonale. Am Rev Respir Dis 98:494, 1968

393. Rubler S, Fleischer RA: Sickle cell states and cardiomyopathy. Sudden death due to pulmonary thrombosis and infarction. Am J Cardiol 19:867, 1967

394. Rubler S, Perloff JK, Roberts WC: Duchenne's muscular dystrophy. Am Heart J 94:776, 1977

395. Rutledge JC, Haas JE, Monnat R, Milstein JM: Hypertrophic cardiomyopathy as a component of subacute necrotizing encephalomyelopathy. J Pediatr 101:706, 1982

396. Salen G: Cholestanol deposition in cerebrotendinous xanthomatosis. A possible mechanism. Ann Intern Med 75:843, 1971

397. Salyer WR, Hutchins GM: Cardiac lesions in secondary oxalosis. Arch Intern Med 134:250, 1974

398. Sanyal SK, Johnson WW, Thapar MK, Pitner SE: An ultrastructural basis for electrocardiographic alterations associated with Duchenne's progressive muscular dystrophy. Circulation 57:1122, 1978

399. Saruk M, Eisenstein R: Aortic lesions in Marfan syndrome. The ultrastructure of cystic medial degeneration. Arch Pathol Lab Med 101:74, 1977

400. Satoh Y, Sakamoto K, Fujibayashi Y, et al: Cardiac involvement in mucolipidosis importance of noninvasive studies for detection of cardiac abnormalities. Jpn Heart J 24:149, 1983

401. Sayers CP, Goltz RW, Mottaz J: Pulmonary elastic tissue in generalized elastolysis (cutis laxa) and Marfan's syndrome. A light and electron microscopic study. J Invest Dermatol 65:451, 1975

402. Schachner L, Young D: Pseudoxanthoma elasticum with severe cardiovascular disease in a child. A J Dis Child 127:571, 1974

403. Schaefer EJ: Clinical, biochemical and genetic features in familial disorders of high density lipoprotein deficiency. Arteriosclerosis 4:303, 1984

404. Schenk EA, Haggerty J: Morquio's disease. A radiologic and morphologic study. Pediatrics 34:839, 1964

405. Schieken RM, Kerber RE, Ionasescu VV, Zellweger H: Cardiac manifestations of the mucopolysaccharidoses. Circulation 52:700, 1975

406. Schilero AJ, Antzis E, Dunn J: Friedreich's ataxia and its cardiac manifestations. Am Heart J 44:805, 1952

407. Schimschock JR, Alvord EC, Jr, Swanson PD: Cerebrotendinous xanthomatosis. Clinical and pathological studies. Arch Neurol 18:688, 1968

408. Schlatmann TJM, Becker AE: Histologic changes in the normal aging aorta: Implications for dissecting aortic aneurysm. Am J Cardiol 39:13, 1977

409. Schlatmann TJM, Becker AE: Pathogenesis of dissecting aneurysm of aorta. Comparative histopathologic study of significance of medial changes. Am J Cardiol 39:21, 1977

410. Schlenska GK, Heene R, Spalke G, Seiler D:

The symptomatology, morphology and biochemistry of glycogenosis type II (Pompe) in the adult. J Neurol 212:237, 1976

411. Schochet SS, Jr, McCormick WF, Zellweger H: Type IV glycogenosis (amylopectinosis). Light and electron microscopic observations. Arch Pathol 90:354, 1970

412. Schoolman A, Kepes JJ: Bilateral spontaneous carotid-cavernous fistulae in Ehlers-Danlos syndrome. Case report. J Neurosurg. 26:82, 1967

413. Schroeder JS, Billingham ME, Rider AK: Cardiac amyloidosis. Diagnosis by transvenous endomyocardial biopsy. Am J Med 59:269, 1975

414. Schulz R, Vogt J, Voss W, Hanefeld F: Mucolipidose Type II (I-cell disease) mit ungewohnlich ausgepragter Herzbeteiligung. Moratsschr Kinderheilkd 135:708, 1987

415. Schwartzkopff B, Frenzel H, Losse B, et al: Heart involvement in progressive external ophthalmoplegia (Kearns-Sayre syndrome): Electrophysiologic, hemodynamic and morphologic findings. Z Kardiol 75:161, 1986

416. Scully RE, Galdabini JJ, McNeely BU: Case 3–1979, presentation of case. (Case Records of the Massachusetts General Hospital). N Engl J Med 300:129, 1979

417. Sedlis SP, Saffitz JE, Schwob VS, Jaffe AS: Cardiac amyloidosis simulating hypertrophic cardiomyopathy. Am J Cardiol 53:969, 1984

418. Selenium in the heart of China (unsigned editorial). Lancet 27:889, 1979

419. Sengers RCA, Stadhouders AM, van Lakwijk-Vondrovicova E, et al: Hypertrophic cardiomyopathy associated with a mitochondrial myopathy of voluntary muscles and congenital cataract. Br Heart J 54:543, 1985

420. Sensenbrenner JA: Pseudo-Hurler polydystrophy (mucolipidosis III) with aortic regurgitation. Birth Defects 8:295, 1972

421. Shapir Y, Roguin N: Echocardiographic findings in Pompe's disease with left ventricular obstruction. Clin Cardiol 8:181, 1985

422. Shimamura K, Hakozaki H, Takahashi K, et al: Sanfilippo B syndrome. A case report. Acta Pathol Jpn 26:739, 1976

423. Shohet I, Rosenbaum I, Frand M, et al: Cardiovascular complications in the Ehlers-Danlos syndrome with minimal external findings. Clin Genet 31:148, 1987

424. Short DW: Multiple congenital aneurysms in childhood: Report of a case. Br J Surg 65:509, 1978

425. Sidbury JB Jr, Mason J, Burns WB Jr, Ruebner BH: Type IV glycogenosis. Report of case proven by characterization of glycogen and studied at necropsy. Johns Hopkins Med J 111:157, 1962

426. Siggers DC: Osteogenesis imperfecta with aortic valve replacement. Birth Defects 10:495, 1974

427. Sillence D: Osteogenesis imperfecta: An expanding panorama of variants. Clin Orthop 159:11, 1981

428. Simpson JW, Nord JJ, McNamara DG: Marfan's syndrome and mitral valve disease: Acute surgical emergencies. Am Heart J 77:96, 1969

429. Sims BA: Conducting tissue of the heart in kwashiorkor. Br Heart J 34:828, 1972

430. Smith ER, Sangalang VE, Hoffernan LP, et al: Hypertrophic cardiomyopathy: The heart disease of Friedreich's ataxia. Am Heart J 94:428, 1977

431. Smith HL, Amick LD, Sidbury JB: Type II glycogenosis: Report of a case with 4 year survival and absence of acid maltase associated with an abnormal glycogen. Am J Dis Child 111:475, 1966

432. Smith RRL, Hutchins GM: Ischemic heart disease secondary to amyloidosis of intramyocardial arteries. Am J Cardiol 44:413, 1979

433. Smith RRL, Hutchins GM, Sack GH Jr, Ridolfi RL: Unusual cardiac, renal and pulmonary involvement in Gaucher's disease. Interstitial glucocerebroside accumulation, pulmonary hypertension and fatal bone marrow embolization. Am J Med 65:352, 1978

434. Sobrevilla LA, Goodman ML, Kane CA: Demyelinating central nervous system disease, macular atrophy and acanthocytosis (Bassen-Kornzweig syndrome). Am J Med 37:821, 1964

435. Spranger JW, Koch F, McKusick VA, et al: Mucopolysaccharidosis VI (Maroteaux-Lamy's disease). Helv Paediatr Acta 25:337, 1970

436. Sreeram N, Wren C, Bhate M, et al: Cardiac abnormalities in the fragile X syndrome. Br Heart J 61:289, 1989

437. Stanley P, Chartrand C, Davignon A: Acquired aortic stenosis in a twelve-year-old girl

with xanthomatosis. N Engl J Med 273:1378, 1965

438. Stein D, Kloster FE: Valvular heart disease in osteogenesis imperfecta. Am Heart J 94:637, 1977

439. Steiner G, Adelman AG, Silver MD: Early coronary atherosclerosis in primary type V hyperproteinemia. Can Med Assoc J 105:1172, 1971

440. Stelzig HH, Kossling FK: Zur Pathologie der Aorta und der grossen Arterien beim Marfansyndrome. Frankfurter Z Pathol 76:201, 1967

441. Stephan MJ, Stevens EL, Jr, Wenstrup RJ, et al: Mucopolysaccharidosis I presenting with endocardial fibroelastosis of infancy. Am J Dis Child 143:782, 1989

442. Stockman JA, Nigro MA, Mishkin MM, Oski FA: Occlusion of large cerebral vessels in sickle-cell anemia. N Engl J Med 287:846, 1972

443. Stokke KT, Bjerve KS, Blomhoff JP, et al: Familial lecithin: Cholesterol acyltransferase deficiency. Studies on lipid composition and morphology of tissues. Scand J Clin Lab Invest 33:93, 1974

444. Storstein O: The heart in progressive muscular dystrophy. Exp Med Surg 22:13, 1964

445. Sugimura F, Iijima M, Ozawa Y, et al: Two cases of Kugelberg-Welander's disease with cardiopathy. Clin Neurol 13:79, 1973

446. Swan WGA, Dewar HA: The heart in haemochromatosis. Br Heart J 14:117, 1952

447. Swanton RH, Brooksby IAB, Davies MJ, et al: Systolic and diastolic ventricular function in cardiac amyloidosis. Studies in six cases diagnosed with endomyocardial biopsy. Am J Cardiol 39:658, 1977

448. Tachi N, Tachi M, Sasaki K, et al: Glycogen storage disease with normal acid maltase: Skeletal and cardiac muscles. Pediatr Neurol 5:60, 1989

449. Takebayashi S, Kubota I, Takagi T: Ultrastructural and histochemical studies of vascular lesions in Marfan's syndrome, with report of 4 autopsy cases. Acta Pathol Jpn 23:847, 1973

450. Talbot NB, Butler AM, Pratt EL, et al: Progeria. Clinical, metabolic and pathologic studies on a patient. Am J Dis Child 69:267, 1945

451. Tanaka H, Adachi K, Yamashita Y, et al: Four cases of Fabry's disease mimicking hypertrophic cardiomyopathy. J Cardiol 18:705, 1988

452. Tanaka H, Nishi S, Nuruki K, Tanaka N: Myocardial ultrastructural changes in Kugelberg-Welander syndrome. Br Heart J 39:1390, 1977

453. Tanaka H, Uemura N, Toyama Y, et al: Cardiac involvement in the Kugelberg-Welander syndrome. Am J Cardiol 38:528, 1976

454. Tanaka N, Tanaka H, Takeda M, et al: Cardiomyopathy in myotonic dystrophy. A light and electron microscopic study of the myocardium. Jpn Heart J 14:202, 1973

455. Taylor WJ: Genetics and the cardiovascular system. p. 753. In Hurst JW (ed): The Heart. 4th Ed. McGraw-Hill, New York, 1978

456. Thilenius OG, Gross BJ: Friedreich's ataxia with heart disease in children. Pediatrics 27:246, 1961

457. Thoren C: Cardiomyopathy in Friedreich's ataxia. Acta Paediatr, suppl. 153:1, 1964

458. Tonkin AM, Mond HG, Mathew TH, Solman JG: Primary oxalosis with myocardial involvement and heart block. Med J Aust 1:873, 1976

459. Traut EF, Knight AA, Szanto PB, Passerelli EW: Specific vascular changes in gout. JAMA 156:591, 1954

460. Tripp ME, Katcher ML, Peters HA, et al: Systemic carnitine deficiency presenting as familial endocardial fibroelastosis. A treatable cardiomyopathy. N Engl J Med 305:385, 1981

461. Tucker HS, Jr, Moss LF, Williams JP: Hemochromatosis with death from heart failure. Am Heart J 35:993, 1948

462. Tunon T, Bengoechea O, Narbona J: Glycogenosis with amylopectinoid deposits in a 13-year-old girl. Clin Neuropathol 7:100, 1988

463. Uemura N, Tanaka H, Niimura T, et al: Electrophysiological and histological abnormalities of the heart in myotonic dystrophy. Am Heart J 86:616, 1973

464. Umlas J: Spontaneous rupture of the subclavian artery in the Ehlers-Danlos syndrome. Hum Pathol 3:121, 1972

465. Underwood EJ: Trace Elements in Human and Animal Nutrition. Academic Press, San Diego, 1971

466. Uno H, Arya S, Laxova R, Gilbert EF: Menkes syndrome with vascular and adrenergic nerve abnormalities. Arch Pathol Lab Med 107:286, 1983

467. Uppal SC: Kearns' syndrome, a new form of cardiomyopathy. Br Heart J 35:766, 1973

468. Van Creveld S, Huijing F: Glycogen storage disease. Biochemical and clinical data in sixteen cases. Am J Med 38:554, 1968

469. Van der Walt JD, Swash M, Leake J, Cox EL: The pattern of involvement of adult-onset acid maltase deficiency at autopsy. Muscle Nerve 10:272, 1987

470. Van Ekeren GJ, Stadhouders AM, Egberink GJM, et al: Hereditary mitochondrial hypertrophic cardiomyopathy with mitochondrial myopathy of skeletal muscle, congenital cataract and lactic acidosis. Virchows Arch 412:47, 1987

471. Van Mullen PJ, Ruiter M: Histochemische Untersuchungen anlasslich der Lipoidspeicherung bei der sogenannten Fabryschen Krankheit (Angiokeratoma corporis diffusum). Arch Klin Exp Dermatol 232:148, 1968

472. Van Vleet JF, Ferrans VJ, Ruth GR: Ultrastructural alterations in nutritional cardiomyopathy of selenium-vitamin E deficient swine. I. Fiber lesions. Lab Invest 37:188, 1977

473. Van Vleet JF, Ferrans VJ, Ruth GR: Ultrastructural alterations in nutritional cardiomyopathy of selenium-vitamin E deficient swine. II. Vascular lesions. Lab Invest 37:301, 1977

474. Vedder EYB: The pathology of beriberi. JAMA 110:893, 1978

475. Verhiest W, Brucher JM, Goddeeris P, et al: Familial centronuclear myopathy associated with "cardiomyopathy." Br Heart J 38:504, 1976

476. Virtanen KSI, Halonen PI: Total heart block as a complication of gout. Cardiologia 54:359, 1969

477. Wagner PI: Beriberi heart disease. Physiologic data and difficulties in diagnosis. Am Heart J 69:200, 1965

478. Wagstaff LA, Firth JC, Levin SE: Vascular abnormalities in congenital generalized elastolysis (cutis laxa). Report of a case. S Afr Med J 44:1125, 1970

479. Waldorf DS, Levy RI, Fredrickson DS: Cutaneous cholesterol ester deposition in Tangier disease. Arch Dermatol 95:161, 1967

480. Waldstein G, Hagerman R: Aortic hypoplasia and cardiac valvular abnormalities in a boy with fragile X syndrome. Am J Med Genet 30:83, 1988

481. Wallach EA, Burkhart EF: Ehlers-Danlos syndrome associated with the tetralogy of Fallot. Arch Dermatol Syphil 61:750, 1950

482. Walsh JJ, Burch GE: Nutritional heart disease. Bull Tulane Univ Med Fac 20:121, 1961

483. Weir EK, Joffe HS, Blaufuss AH, Beighton P: Cardiovascular abnormalities in cutis laxa. Eur J Cardiol 5:255, 1977

484. Weisinger B, Glassman E, Spencer FF, Berger A: Successful aortic valve replacement for aortic regurgitation associated with osteogenesis imperfecta. Br Heart J 37:475, 1975

485. Wennevold A, Jacobsen JG: Acquired supravalvular aortic stenosis in familial hypercholesterolemia. A hemodynamic and angiographic study. Am J Med 50:823, 1971

486. West RR, Salyer WR, Hutchins GM: Adult-onset primary oxalosis with complete heart block. Johns Hopkins Med J 133:195, 1973

487. Westermark P, Cornwell GG, III, Johansson B: Senile cardiac amyloidosis. p. 217. In Glenner GG (ed): Symposium on Amyloidosis. Excerpta Medica, Princeton, NJ, 1980

488. Westermark P, Natvig JB, Johansson B: Characterization of an amyloid fibril protein from senile cardiac amyloid. J Exp Med 146:631, 1977

489. Weston LT, Raybuck BD, Robinowitz M, et al: Primary amyloid heart disease presenting as hypertrophic obstructive cardiomyopathy. Cathet Cardiovasc Diagn 12:176, 1986

490. Westwood M: Endocardial fibroelastosis and Niemann-Pick disease. Br Heart J 39:1394, 1977

491. Wharton BA, Balmer SE, Somers K, Templeton AC: The myocardium in kwashiorkor. Q J Med 38:107, 1969

492. Wheeler EM, Roberts PF: Menkes's steely hair syndrome. Arch Dis Child 51:269, 1976

493. Wheeler VR, Cooley NR, Blackburn WR: Cardiovascular pathology in osteogenesis imperfecta type IIA with a review of the literature. Pediatric Pathol 8:55, 1988

494. White NJ, Winearls CG, Smith R: Cardiovascular abnormalities in osteogenesis imperfecta. Am Heart J 106:1416, 1983

495. Whittemore R, Caddell JL: Metabolic and

nutritional diseases. p. 579. In Moss AJ, Adams FH, Emmanouilides GC (eds): Heart Disease in Infants, Children and Adolescents. 2nd Ed. Williams & Wilkins, Baltimore, 1977

496. Wilhelm K, Paver K: Sudden death in pseudoxanthoma elasticum. Med J Aust 2:1363, 1972

497. Williams JL: Multiple aneurysms in a child. Proc R Soc Med 68:523, 1975

498. Wilson CS, Mankin HT, Pluth JR: Aortic stenosis and mucopolysaccharidosis. Ann Intern Med 92:496, 1980

499. Wilson JH, Moodie DS: Cardiac amyloidosis in a patient with Ehlers-Danlos syndrome type IV[1]. Cleve Clin Q 53:205, 1986

500. Wilson RA, Clark N: Endocardial fibroelastosis associated with generalized glycogenosis. Occurrence in siblings. Pediatrics 26:86, 1960

501. Winters PR, Harrod MJ, Molenich-Heetred SA, et al: α-L-iduronidase deficiency and possible Hurler-Scheie genetic compound. Clinical, pathologic, and biochemical findings. Neurology 26:1003, 1976

502. Wise D, Wallace HJ, Jellinek EH: Angiokeratoma corporis diffusum. A clinical study of eight affected families. Q J Med 31:177, 1962

503. Witting C, Muller KM, Kresse H, et al: Morphological and biochemical findings in a case of mucopolysaccharidosis type III A (Sanfilippo's disease type A). Beitr Pathol 154:324, 1975

504. Wood DH: Cerebrovascular complications of sickle cell anemia. Stroke 9:73, 1978

505. Wood SJ, Thomas J, Braimbridge MV: Mitral valve disease and open heart surgery in osteogenesis imperfecta tarda. Br Heart J 35:103, 1973

506. Yokota T, Ishihara T, Kawano H, et al: Immunological homogeneity of Lafora body, corpora amylacea, basophilic degeneration in heart, and intracytoplasmic inclusions of liver and heart in type IV glycogenosis. Acta Pathol Jpn 37:941, 1987

507. Yu WH: A study of nutritional and bio-geochemical factors in the occurrence and development of Keshan disease. The 6th conference on prevention for rheumatic fever and rheumatic heart disease. Jpn Circ J 46:1201, 1982

30

Collagen Vascular Diseases and the Cardiovascular System

Hugh A. McAllister, Jr.

MECHANISMS AND MANIFESTATIONS OF THE IMMUNE RESPONSE IN THE COLLAGEN VASCULAR DISEASES

Several disorders are grouped as collagen vascular diseases because they have in common morphologically similar lesions of connective tissue.[61] These lesions are characterized by alterations of collagen or ground substance, usually with the finding of fibrinoid material at some stage of the disease. In the typical lesion of fibrinoid necrosis, an increase in ground substance with swollen, fragmented collagen fibers and necrosis produces a structureless eosinophilic area histochemically resembling fibrin.[90] The collagen vascular diseases include rheumatic fever (see Ch. 24), rheumatoid arthritis, systemic lupus erythematosus (SLE), progressive systemic sclerosis (scleroderma), dermatomyositis (polymyositis), panarteritis nodosa, and thrombotic thrombocytopenic purpura.[112] Although not classically included in the list of collagen vascular diseases, the lesions of Wegener's granulomatosis, ankylosing spondylitis, Reiter syndrome, psoriatic arthritis, and relapsing polychondritis are most likely immunologically mediated as well.[8]

There is no unequivocal evidence that allergic reactions cause collagen vascular diseases but most of the lesions observed may be explained by immune complex-mediated mechanisms.[8] Toxic complexes are almost certainly responsible for most of the lesions of panarteritis nodosa, rheumatoid arthritis, and SLE.[118] The toxic complexes causing the last two diseases are formed by autoantibodies to the patient's own tissues.[118]

Collagen vascular diseases vary markedly in their clinical features, time course, location of lesions, pathologic picture, and immune findings, but there is considerable overlap of pathologic features within the disease group. Many individuals with a collagen vascular disease have associated angiitis or glomerulonephritis, immunoglobulin abnormalities, and autoantibodies with varied specificity of reactivity. Autoimmunity may be considered a tertiary manifestation of the immune response directed at antigen whose inappropriate processing leads to destruction of host tissues.[8]

Three hypotheses are proposed to explain

the mechanism and manifestations of autoimmune disease: the first, the *forbidden clone theory*, postulates a clone of mutant lymphocytes arising through somatic mutation.[8] Normally, mutant cells that carry a surface antigen recognized as foreign would be destroyed; however, according to this theory, mutant cells that lack surface antigen would not be destroyed. With a proliferation of antigen-deficient mutants (forbidden clones), these cells would be capable of reacting with target tissues because of genetic dissimilarity.

The second hypothesis, the *sequestered antigen theory*, is based on the phenomenon of tolerance induction in the fetus. This theory proposes that during embryonic development, tissues exposed to the lymphoreticular system are recognized as "self."[8] Those that are anatomically separated or sequestered from the lymphoreticular system are not identified as "self." In later life, exposure, through trauma or infection, of the sequestered antigens to the lymphoreticular system results in autoimmune disease. Both concepts are based on the premise of hyperactivity of the immune response which, through autoantibody formation, or sensitized lymphocytes (delayed hypersensitivity), leads to the production of an autoimmune disease.[8,118]

The third hypothesis, the *immunologic deficiency theory*, is based on a hypoactive or deficient immunologic system.[8] It derives support from the clinically observed relationship between immunologic deficiency syndromes and an increased incidence of autoimmune abnormalities. Tissue injury would occur through the emergent mutant lymphocytes or as a consequence of persistent microbial antigen. From these observations, it has been postulated that otherwise normal persons in whom autoimmune disease develops may, in fact, have a more subtle form of underlying immune deficiency, predisposing them to autoimmune states.[8,118]

Any concept formed to explain the development of the autoimmune state must take into account genetic control of the immune system.[100] Familial patterns and sex distribution characterize most autoimmune disorders.[8] The discovery of the association of certain histocompatibility antigens with a variety of diseases suggest that the autoimmune response (Ir) gene in humans may be closely linked to the HLA loci on the sixth chromosome.[8,9,13] The most notable association is the relatively high risk of developing ankylosing spondylitis or Reiter syndrome in HLA-B27-positive persons who have inherited a susceptibility for the development of these conditions from a variety of antigen stimuli.[13,18,60] Psoriatic arthritis with or without aortitis occurs most commonly in HLA-B13- or B27-positive persons, whereas rheumatoid disease most frequently occurs in those with DRW4 antigen.[8,91]

Rheumatoid Arthritis

Although several etiologies have been postulated, including metabolic derangements and infectious agents (viruses, bacteria, and mycoplasma), the etiology of rheumatoid arthritis remains unknown.[8,112] Families of probans affected with rheumatoid arthritis show an increased incidence of connective tissue disorders.[112] Paradoxically, children with immune deficiency (hypogammaglobulinemia) have an increased incidence of connective tissue diseases, including rheumatoid arthritis.[6,8] Therefore, underlying genetic factors may exist that determine the susceptibility of individual patients to rheumatoid arthritis, but they are complex and ill understood.

Rheumatoid factor (RF) is an IgM globulin that has the capacity to react with IgG globulins in vitro.[7,125] The stimulus for its production is not known. This factor is found in the sera and synovial fluid of adult patients with established rheumatoid arthritis but is seldom present in patients with juvenile rheumatoid arthritis.[112] Children with rheumatoid arthritis, unlike adults, are more likely to have IgG (than IgM RF), which is not detectable by the usual agglutination tests, such as latex fixation.[8] Although RF is diagnostically useful, it is not specific for the disease and is found in a variety of other diseases, including connective tissue disorders.[112] Because the rheumatoid factor-gammaglobulin-complement complex has been found in synovial fluids, RF has been implicated as a causative factor of the chronic inflammatory joint disease of rheumatoid arthritis.[115,121] Unlike SLE, a lowered serum complement level is rarely present in the sera of patients with rheumatoid arthritis unless the patient is in a phase of necrotizing arthritis accompanied by rheumatic vasculitis.[38,112] These patients with rheumatoid vasculitis and extraarticular disease are also distinguished by having large amounts of low-molecular-weight (7S) IgM in their serum.[112] The demonstration of IgG, IgM, and complement components in the walls of affected blood vessels supports the view that vascular disease is related to the deposition of soluble immune complexes.[112]

Ankylosing Spondylitis

Ankylosing spondylitis is a chronic, progressive form of arthritis distinguished by involvement of the sacroiliac joints, the spinal apophyseal joints, and the paravertebral soft tissues. Onset is usually in the second or third decade of life and the disease is relatively uncommon after 30 years of age. Approximately 90 percent of patients are males.[112]

Although the precise etiology of ankylosing spondylitis is uncertain, the finding of an unusually high frequency of the inherited antigen HLA-B27 in up to 95 percent of patients and in 50 percent of first-degree relatives provides overwhelming evidence of a genetic linkage in this disorder.[13,18] The frequent associations between ankylosing spondylitis and such seemingly unrelated disorders as ulcerative colitis, regional enteritis, Reiter syndrome, and psoriasis have, until recently, been unexplained. It now appears that among these underlying disorders, patients with the B27 antigen are those who are primarily destined to develop ankylosing spondylitis.[8,82] Precisely how this genetic relationship links the susceptible individual to the eventual development of ankylosing spondylitis is un-

known. Variable inciting factors such as ulcerative colitis might precipitate the evolution of spondylitis in a genetically predisposed individual having the B27 marker. The disease may then be perpetuated by a self-destructive attack of the immune response against "altered self." In addition, there is evidence of antibody formation and immune complex deposition in ankylosing spondylitis.[8] Relapsing polychondritis is also thought to have an immunologic basis, and immunofluorescence studies have suggested that antibodies to cartilage are present in the lesions.[32]

Systemic Lupus Erythematosus

Systemic lupus erythematosus is a complex syndrome caused by autoantibodies produced to a wide variety of a patient's own cellular antigens, particularly nuclear antigens. This disease appears most frequently in women of child-bearing age and characteristically involves many different tissues.[112] The extensive antibody formation is reflected by a hypergammaglobulinemia characteristic of many of the autoimmune diseases. Except for damaging blood cells, the autoantibody alone does not seem to initiate tissue injury directly. Rather, tissue damage is thought to occur primarily through the deposition of antigen-antibody complexes with components of complement.[8] As in many immune complex-induced vascular disorders, certain tissues are more vulnerable to injury than others. These include small blood vessels, glomeruli, joints, spleen, heart valves, and the pericardium.

A genetic predisposition termed *lupus diathesis* has been implicated, on the basis of an increased incidence in twins and the existence of autoimmune disease in families of patients with SLE.[8,31,65] A relationship of maternal anti-Ro (SS-A) to neonatal SLE has been established.[106] In the genetically susceptible individual, certain exogenous factors such as ultraviolet light, some drugs, and a variety of infectious agents may serve as antigens or produce antigens that trigger self-destructive immunologic responses. Evidence obtained from experimental animals also suggests a genetic etiology. In inbred New Zealand black (NZB) strains of mice a lupuslike syndrome occurs, consisting of lupus erythematosus (LE) cells and glomerular lesions.[63,126] In addition to a genetic predisposition, the finding of viruslike particles in these mice raises the possibility of an infectious etiology leading to the autoimmune state.[84] There is also evidence that suppressor T cells or a soluble immune response suppressor substance may be deficient in NZB mice.[118] Although the precise function of suppressor T cells in the human is unknown, they play an important role in immunologic regulation and in the prevention of autoantibody production. A deficiency of suppressor cell function might allow B cells to escape from this normal regulatory mechanism and proceed to produce autoantibodies.[8] Although descriptions of myxovirus-like subparticles in renal biopsy material from human cases of SLE have been made, the significance of these findings is, as yet, unknown.[48,101,128] These tubuloreticular inclusions (TRI), although found in many tissues and disorders, are strongly associated with SLE and with viral infections.[45,47]

Tubuloreticular inclusions are intracytoplasmic membranous tubules approximately 25 nm in diameter, usually present within the cisternae of rough endoplasmic reticulum. They are closely linked to α-interferons and are commonly found in patients with acquired immune deficiency syndrome (AIDS) and SLE, both of which are associated with an acid-labile form of α-interferon.[103,107]

A principal diagnostic finding is the presence of the LE cell, a polymorphonuclear neutrophil that has phagocytized nuclear material. Its formation depends on the presence of an antibody capable of reacting with DNA. A variety of antinuclear antibodies have been identified in the sera of patients with SLE, and their identification has largely replaced the LE cell test in the clinical laboratory.

These include anti-DNA, antinucleoprotein, antihistones, antiacidic nuclear proteins, antinucleolar RNA, and antibodies to fibrous or particulate nucleoprotein.[118] Anti-DNA antibody and DNA-binding are newer tests that have a high specificity for SLE. They are used serially to assess disease activity. These tests are usually negative in drug-induced and discoid lupus.[8]

Scleroderma

Scleroderma (progressive systemic sclerosis) is a generalized disorder of connective tissue characterized by inflammatory, fibrotic, and degenerative changes accompanied by vascular lesions in the skin, synovium, and certain internal organs, notably the esophagus, intestinal tract, heart, lung, and kidney. Females are affected approximately two to three times as frequently as males.[112] Although the etiology of scleroderma remains obscure, the demonstration of serologic abnormalities in a high proportion of cases, together with certain morphologic and other findings, has engendered suspicion that aberrant immunity has a role in its pathogenesis.[8] Hypergammaglobulinemia (IgG) of a mild degree is a frequent finding, and one-quarter to one-third of patients have positive tests for rheumatoid factor.[113] Occasionally, there are false-positive tests for syphilis and positive LE cell reactions. Antinuclear antibodies are found in at least three-quarters of patients with scleroderma.[113] In most cases, the titers are relatively low compared with those present in SLE. Nucleolar immunofluorescence has been observed in 10 to 54 percent of patients and is seen more often in scleroderma than in any other connective tissue disease.[110] The pattern of nuclear immunofluorescence is commonly that of fine or large speckles.[112] In vitro examination of skin fibroblasts from patients with scleroderma demonstrates an increase in collagen synthesis, suggesting that the basic defect in scleroderma is one of disordered regulation or activation of the fibroblasts.[66]

Dermatomyositis (Polymyositis)

Polymyositis is a systemic autoimmune disorder characterized pathologically by degeneration and inflammation of skeletal muscle. Dermatomyositis is a form of polymyositis in which there is also involvement of the skin. The incidence of these disorders is increased in association with malignant tumors, lymphoproliferative syndromes, and certain autoallergic diseases. Females are affected twice as commonly as males.[112] The etiology of these conditions is obscure, although evidence for a cell-mediated mode of immune injury of muscle continues to mount.[136] Search for a circulating antibody directed against muscle tissue has been unrewarding.[21] However, deposits of IgG, IgM, and C3 alone or in combination have been demonstrated in the blood vessel walls of skeletal muscle in 17 of 39 patients with polymyositis.[138] These deposits were particularly common in children with dermatositis (9 of 11). Other studies suggest that certain types of polymyositis may be due to cell-mediated immune reactions.[30,57] Activated lymphocytes from patients with polymyositis are cytotoxic to fetal muscle cells in culture.[57] This has been traced to the production of a lymphotoxin, the action of which is inhibited by the addition of prednisolone. Picornavirus-like structures have been observed in muscle cells of a few patients with polymyositis[24]; in many more, tubuloreticular inclusions resembling nucleocapsid of paramyxovirus have been found in myocytes and in endothelial cells of blood vessels in skin and muscle[94] (see the section on systemic lupus erythematosus). Experimental allergic myositis may be produced in animals by immunization with xenogeneic muscle tissue in complete Freund's adjuvant; the inflammatory lesions in the muscles of patients with myositis are also consistent with a delayed hypersensitivity reaction.[118]

Panarteritis Nodosa

Panarteritis nodosa is a form of necrotizing arteritis that chiefly affects medium-sized muscular arteries. It affects males most often. Gammaglobulin may be identified in the areas of fibrinoid necrosis.[118] Many patients with panarteritis nodosa also have hepatitis B antigenemia, suggesting that panarteritis occurring naturally may be caused by an immune response to viral hepatitis infection with HB antigen release.[119] The presence of immune complexes of the hepatitis B surface antigen in affected tissues has been demonstrated in 30 to 40 percent of patients with panarteritis nodosa.[5] Otherwise, the etiology of this condition remains unknown. The immunopathologic hallmark, however, is an arteritis similar to an immune complex-type injury.

Wegener's Granulomatosis

Wegener's granulomatosis is a disease that has a distinctive clinicopathologic complex of necrotizing granulomatous vasculitis of the upper and lower respiratory tracts, glomerulonephritis, and variable degrees of disseminated small vessel vasculitis. The etiology is unclear, although a hypersensitivity reaction to an as yet unidentified antigen is highly suspect.[139] Circulating immune complexes have been described in patients with active disease; immune reactants and complexlike deposits were present in some but not all renal biopsies from a group of patients with Wegener's granulomatosis.[55] The precise role of immune complexes in the pathogenesis of the disease is not clear; it is uncertain whether they have a primary role in tissue damage or are only associated or secondarily involved. It is possible that the type or properties of immune complexes in Wegener's granulomatosis are partly responsible for triggering the granulomatous reactivity seen in this disease.[35] By contrast, a delayed hypersensitivity-like response to the hypothetical antigen itself may elicit the granulomatous responses, with immune complex formation being a secondary phenomenon that may or may not contribute to the pathogenesis of the disease.[35]

Thrombotic Thrombocytopenic Purpura

Thrombotic thrombocytopenic purpura is a multisystem disease that usually occurs in young women. It is ordinarily fulminant and fatal but may remit completely. This rare disorder has been linked to the collagen diseases because of certain clinical similarities to SLE.[112] The acute onset and other features have raised the question of a hypersensitivity reaction, although only a few patients have histories of prior immunization or drug ingestation.[112] The disease has also been associated with infection, rheumatoid arthritis, carcinoma, and pregnancy.[112] Histochemical and immunopathologic studies have failed to demonstrate either immunoglobulin or complement in lesions, as would be expected if they were induced by immune complex deposition. Instead, the bland hyaline deposits consist almost entirely of fibrinogen or fibrin.[36] Coagulation studies reveal platelet consumption greatly in excess of fibrinogen utilization, a pattern compatible with some form of vascular damage, rather than with intravascular coagulation in which the reverse is observed.[51] The pathogenesis of this disorder is unknown.

Mixed Connective Tissue Disease

The designation *mixed connective tissue disease* is reserved for patients with combined clinical features of rheumatoid arthritis, SLE, scleroderma, and polymyositis.[120] These patients exhibit polyarthritis, diffusely swollen hands, Reynaud's phenomenon, disturbed esophageal motility, myositis, lymphadenopathy, and hypergammaglobulinemia in varying combinations and in varying degrees of severity. Typically, patients have positive ANA of the speckled pattern.[8] Diagnosis is confirmed by the demonstration of high titers of antibody to extractable nuclear antigen (ENA).[120] Mixed connective disease serum antibody does not react with the antigen when treated with ribonuclease, unlike the situation in SLE.[8] Long-term follow-up of these patients to determine the incidence and types of cardiovascular involvement has not yet been possible.

MORPHOLOGY OF COLLAGEN VASCULAR DISEASES

Rheumatoid Arthritis

Approximately 50 percent of patients dying with rheumatoid arthritis will have morphologic evidence of heart disease at autopsy.[22,64,123,124] There is a marked disparity between clinical and pathologic evidence in that only 10 to 20 percent of these patients develop clinical signs or symptoms.[64] Approximately 30 percent of those with rheumatoid arthritis have fibrous obliterative pericarditis at autopsy.[71] Less often, an acute fibrinous exudate is present; rarely is there calcific or cholesterol pericardial disease. Usually, no functional consequences result from the obliterative pericarditis; however, a small number of patients develop a constrictive pericarditis. The fibrous pericarditis is usually nonspecific, but in approximately 20 percent, diagnostic rheumatoid granulomas are present[71] (Fig. 30–1).

A myocarditis, which may be either nonspecific or granulomatous, may also be found

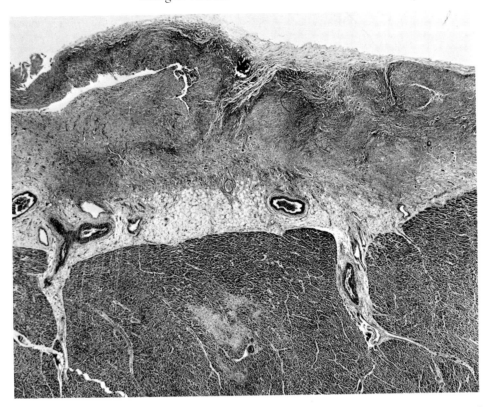

Fig. 30–1. Fibrous pericarditis in a patient who died with rheumatoid arthritis after many years. There is a rheumatoid granuloma in the pericardium adjacent to the epicardial fat. (H&E, × 40.)

in the hearts of patients dying with rheumatoid arthritis. The nonspecific form, reported in 4 to 30 percent of autopsy cases, usually consists of focal, interstitial aggregates of lymphocytes, histiocytes, and plasma cells.[22,64,124] It is rarely of clinical significance; however, severe, diffuse myocarditis with myocardial degeneration has also been reported.[22,64,124] It is not clear whether these nonspecific forms of myocarditis are actually a manifestation of rheumatoid disease or the result of a patient's increased susceptibility to infection. The specific lesions are granulomas identical in appearance to the subcutaneous nodules of rheumatoid arthritis (Fig. 30–2). They have been described in 5 to 32 percent of patients and are most frequently located in the left ventricular myocardium.[64,71,123,124] When they involve the conduction system,

varying degrees of heart block may be encountered clinically.[64,109] Rheumatoid granulomas in the myocardium may be macroscopic or microscopic. Macroscopically, they appear as foci of yellow or gray necrosis, which may be extensive[75,109] (Fig. 30–3). Perforation resulting in an aortic–right atrial fistula has been described.[54] Microscopically, the granulomas consist of a central zone of fibrinoid necrosis in which gammaglobulin has been identified.[131] The fibrinoid necrosis is surrounded by palisaded histiocytes and fibroblasts, occasionally with multinucleated giant cells and an outer zone of fibrosis containing chronic inflammatory cells.

Rheumatoid granulomas may occur in any of the cardiac valves (approximately 10 percent of autopsied patients) but are most common in the mitral and aortic valves[20,37,75,76,109]

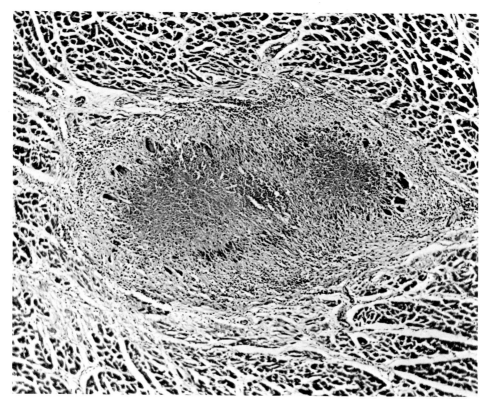

Fig. 30–2. Section of myocardium containing a rheumatoid granuloma with a central zone of fibrinoid necrosis surrounded by palisaded histiocytes and fibroblasts, occasionally with multinucleated giant cells, and an outer zone of fibrosis containing chronic inflammatory cells. (H&E, × 35.)

(Fig. 30–4). Involvement may be focal or diffuse and is usually most prominent in the midportion or base of the valve. Diffuse involvement may result in valvular incompetence or stenosis. The chordae tendineae are usually uninvolved, but occasionally they may be fibrotic and shortened. Commissural fusion is rare. Rheumatoid nodules are most commonly located within the valve leaflets and are enclosed by fibrous tissue; rarely, a rheumatoid nodule erodes the surface of the valve so that the necrotic center of the nodule communicates with a cardiac cavity. In these unusual occurrences, there may be superimposed thrombus or infective endocarditis.[71] Verrucae of fibrinoid necrosis common in rheumatic valvulitis and SLE are not a feature of pure rheumatoid valvulitis. Typical rheumatic-type valve disease undoubtedly occurs in patients with rheumatoid disease but is no more frequent than in controls.[10,102] Indeed, there is no evidence of an increased susceptibility to rheumatic carditis in patients with rheumatoid arthritis.

Several types of vascular lesions occur in rheumatoid arthritis and are recognized as a cardinal feature of the disease (see Ch. 11). These have been classified into three main groups according to pathologic findings, which probably represent a spectrum of changes evolving over the course of time.[112,116]

1. Bland, obliterative intimal proliferation of the digital arteries, sometimes accompanied by similar involvement of mesenteric, coronary, and other arteries
2. Subacute lesions in the small vessels of the

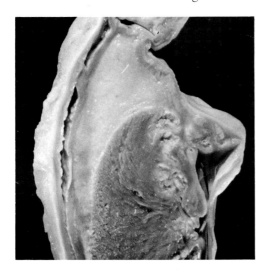

Fig. 30–3. Two macroscopic rheumatoid granulomas are evident in this section—one in the basal portion and annulus of the mitral valve and one serpinginous granuloma in the adjacent myocardium. They appear as foci of yellow or gray necrosis and may be extensive.

muscles, heart, nerves, and other tissues
3. Fulminant, widespread necrotizing arteritis affecting medium-sized and large vessels, occasionally indistinguishable from panarteritis nodosa

Vasculitis associated with rheumatoid arthritis most commonly appears as a typical leukoclastic vasculitis of small venules, predominantly involving the skin, as is characteristic of classic hypersensitivity vasculitidies.[35] Less often, patients with rheumatoid arthritis (usually those with severe erosive and nodular disease and seropositivity for rheumatoid factor) develop a fulminant disseminated vasculitis involving arterioles, medium-sized muscular arteries, and large veins.[88] It was previously believed that administration of corticosteroids either precipitated the development of rheumatoid arthritis or worsened the systemic vasculitis associated with it; it is now generally believed that this is not the case, and that systemic vasculitis merely reflects markedly severe rheumatoid arthritis, a condition that probably would evoke corticosteroid therapy.[80] The mechanism of vasculitis is probably immune complex deposition, as circulating immune complexes have been clearly shown in the serum of patients and immune deposits have been demonstrated in the walls of involved vessels.[35]

Approximately 10 percent of patients have rheumatoid granulomas in epicardial coronary arteries, and in 10 percent the aorta will be involved as well[27,71,132,135] (Fig. 30–5). Coronary artery involvement may lead to myocardial infarction in the absence of atherosclerosis.[23,59] When the aorta contains rheumatoid nodules, they are most common in the proximal 3 cm of the ascending portion. Occasionally, the entire length of the aorta is involved, either continuously or with clearly demarcated skip areas.[27,78]

Systemic amyloidosis, which may affect the heart, has been reported in 14 to 26 percent of autopsied patients with rheumatoid arthritis.[19,86] Indeed, rheumatoid arthritis is probably the most frequent predisposing disease for amyloidosis.[56] Amyloidosis is also an important cause of morbidity and mortality in juvenile rheumatoid arthritis, occuring in approximately 4 percent of patients.[122] The onset of systemic amyloidosis occurs at a mean of 8.2 years after the diagnosis of juvenile arthritis.[122] Amyloidosis has also been reported in ankylosing spondylitis, Reiter syndrome, psoriatic arthritis, chronic rheumatic heart disease, dermatomyositis, scleroderma, Behçet syndrome and, rarely, SLE.[41]

Ankylosing Spondylitis

The main cardiovascular dysfunction encountered in patients with ankylosing spondylitis is aortic insufficiency secondary to aortic dilation (see Ch. 27). The aortic valve cusps are shortened and thickened at their basal attachments and distal margins. Focal calcific deposits may be present along the bases of the cusps and occasionally extend to the anterior mitral leaflet and membranous septum. Thickening of the aortic wall is usually limited to the proximal 3 cm of the ascending aorta,

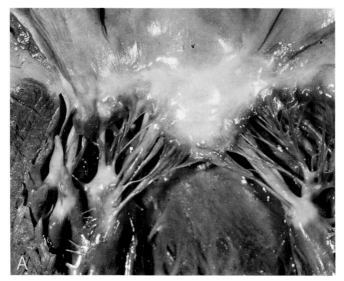

Fig. 30–4. (A) Diffuse fibrous thickening of the mitral valve of a 54-year-old man with a long history of rheumatoid arthritis. Rheumatoid granulomas may occur in any of the cardiac valves, usually in mid-portion or base. Note the relative sparing of the chordae tendineae and absence of commissural fusion. (B) Section of myocardium, aorta, and aortic valve from the heart of the same patient illustrated in Fig. A. The aortic valve and ascending aorta exhibit diffuse fibrous thickening. The myocardium contains numerous rheumatoid granulomas. (H&E, × 4.)

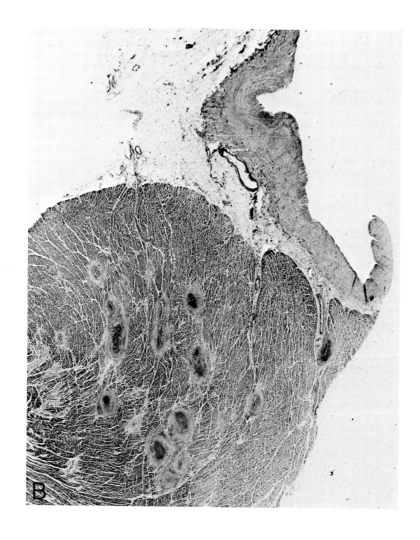

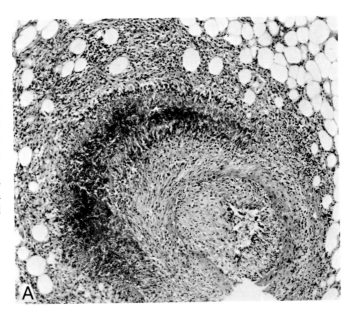

Fig. 30–5. (A) Section of left anterior descending coronary artery illustrating marked intimal thickening with fibrous tissue and chronic inflammatory cells. A classic rheumatoid granuloma involves the media and adventitia. (H&E, × 70.) (B) Rheumatoid granuloma in the media of the ascending aorta in a patient dying with advanced rheumatoid arthritis. (H&E, × 80.)

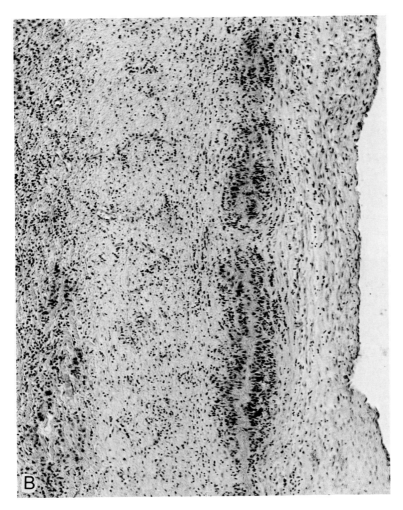

including the portion within the sinuses of Valsalva[3,29,44] (see Ch. 9). This thickening arises from dense connective tissue in the adventitia of the aorta, which is frequently contiguous with dense fibrous scarring in the groove between the anterior mitral leaflet and the aortic valve cusps, producing a fibrous ridge between the base of the aortic valve cusps and the anterior mitral leaflet.[16] The media of the involved segment of aorta is markedly degenerated with loss of elastic fibers and smooth muscle and with fibrous tissue replacement. The overlying intima is thickened by proliferated fibrous tissue (Fig. 30–6). There is extensive intimal proliferation and medial hypertrophy of the vasa vasorum; scattered mononuclear cells may be present in the adventitia adjacent to them.[102,134] The coronary ostia may be narrowed by this fibrotic process.[102] No granulomatous lesions, as are seen in rheumatoid disease, have been

described in the aortic lesions of ankylosing spondylitis. Extension of the aortic adventitial fibrosis beyond the aortic valve occasionally causes conduction disturbances because of the close proximity of the atrioventricular node to the membranous ventricular septum.[12,58,69,137] Mitral regurgitation may also develop, because of involvement of the anterior mitral leaflet.[15] The reported incidence of aortic involvement in ankylosing spondylitis has varied from 1 to 10 percent. It appears to be related to the duration and severity of the spondylitis.[44]

Aortic lesions identical to those of ankylosing spondylitis have been reported in patients with psoriatic arthritis associated with spondylitis.[25,91,105] and in patients with Reiter syndrome.[42,98,111] Some patients with Reiter syndrome will develop pericardial friction rub, heart block and various cardiac abnormalities that have been attributed to pericarditis and

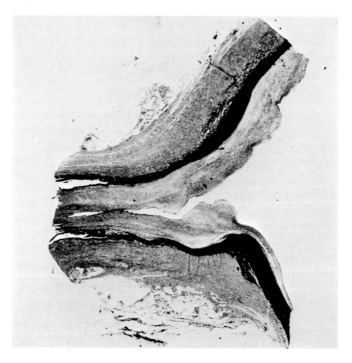

Fig. 30–6. The histologic changes in the aorta in ankylosing spondylitis are nonspecific in that they are identical to other forms of granulomatous-sclerosing aortitis. There is intimal and adventitial fibrosis with fibrous replacement of the central portion of the media. In this case, the proximal portion of the left main coronary artery was also involved. (Movat's pentachrome, × 10.)

myocarditis.[26,28,111,112] The incidence of complete heart block in patients with Reiter syndrome may be unusually high.[12,93]

Aortic insufficiency in patients with relapsing polychondritis is not uncommon.[50,97] The aortic lesions have varied, microscopically, from those identical to ankylosing spondylitis[99] to cystic medial degeneration with or without aortic dissection.[50,117] Mitral and aortic insufficiency with myxomatous degeneration of valve leaflets has also been described in this condition.[2]

Systemic Lupus Erythematosus

Some type of cardiac abnormality is observed in more than 50 percent of patients with clinical SLE and in at least that percentage of autopsy cases of SLE.[4] On the basis of combined clinical and autopsy observations, pericarditis is the most frequent lesion associated with SLE.

Approximately 50 percent of patients with SLE will have some form of pericarditis at autopsy.[17] The most common form is fibrous pericarditis; however, either fibrinous pericarditis, with or without adhesions, or purulent pericarditis may occasionally be encountered. Fibrinous pericarditis is especially common in those with lupus nephritis and uremia.[71] Lupus pericarditis may or may not be asymptomatic; however, progression to constrictive pericarditis is rare.[130] Histologically, fibrinoid necrosis with a mixed inflammatory cell infiltrate and granulation tissue with occasional hematoxylin bodies are present in varying combinations. There is a high correlation between the presence of lupus pericarditis and atypical verrucous endocarditis of Libman and Sacks[17] (see Ch. 18).

Pericarditis, with or without effusion, has been reported in patients with drug-induced SLE. It is rare, however, for patients with drug-induced SLE to present with pericarditis as the major initial manifestation, and cardiac tamponade is exceptional.[39,71] When the offending drug is discontinued, signs and symptoms of pericarditis disappear, but they may recur promptly on readministration. There has been a steady accumulation of reports describing the induction of lupus-like syndromes by various drugs.[112] In many the evidence linking drugs to disease is often highly circumstantial and, in some cases, symptoms suggestive of SLE have antedated use of the drug in question. The syndromes that have been most extensively investigated and that are most firmly established have been those that followed use of hydralazine and procainamide. Lupus-like syndromes with pericarditis usually occur only after prolonged treatment with large doses and only affect a small group of the patients exposed to the drug. As in spontaneously occurring SLE, women are affected more commonly than men.[112]

Some patients with active drug-induced SLE secondary to hydralazine possess circulating antibodies to the drug and show evidence of delayed hypersensitivity (lymphocyte transformation upon exposure to hydralazine), as well as antibodies to native human DNA.[49] In patients receiving procainamide for an appreciable length of time, antinuclear antibodies develop in 75 percent.[87] Only a small percentage of these patients, however, develop a lupus-like reaction. Nevertheless, procainamide is currently the most commonly recognized offender in drug-induced SLE.

Nonspecific interstitial myocarditis has been observed in SLE.[14,52,62,72,127] The lesions are focal collections of inflammatory cells, including polymorphonuclear leukocytes, lymphocytes, plasma cells, and macrophages with interstitial edema. Often, adjacent myofibers are damaged. Occasionally fibrinoid necrosis is found in interstitial locations, especially adjacent to small blood vessels; it is usually associated with an exudative reaction (Fig. 30–7). Vascular lesions in the myocardium are frequent with small arteries, arterioles, and venules being principally affected.[14,62] These vascular lesions consist of fibrinoid changes in

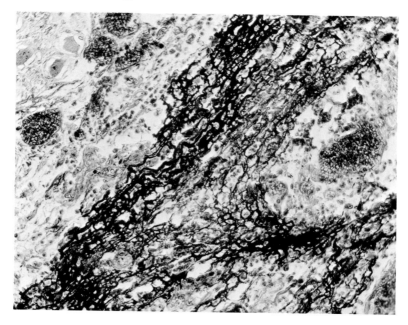

Fig. 30–7. Fibrinoid necrosis in the myocardial interstitium in a patient dying of systemic lupus erythematosus and nonspecific interstitial myocarditis. (Movat's pentachrome, × 160.)

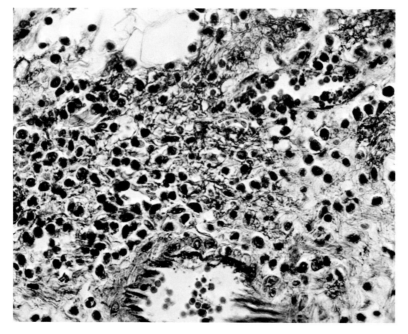

Fig. 30–8. In patients dying of SLE myocarditis, interstitial fibrinoid necrosis often is most prominent adjacent to small blood vessels and is usually associated with an exudative reaction consisting mainly of mononuclear cells. Occasionally, small arteries, arterioles, and venules may also be affected. (H&E, × 300.)

the vessel wall, varying amounts of inflammatory exudate, and granular or hyaline thrombi in the lumen (Fig. 30–8). Clinically, heart failure has been ascribed to the myocardial lesions.[52,112] Endomyocardial biopsy has proved helpful in diagnosing lymphocytic myocarditis in these patients and in the identification of toxic damage to myocytes by drugs used to treat this disorder.[77,104]

Less well recognized is the occasional report of myocardial infarction in young patients with SLE and coronary arteritis.[11,23] In addition to myocardial infarction secondary to arteritis of the extramural coronary arteries, premature severe atherosclerosis resulting in myocardial infarction has been reported in some young women, raising the question whether SLE predisposes a patient to early atherosclerosis, possibly as a complication of the arteritis.[129] Another potential factor for accelerated atherosclerosis in these patients is prolonged corticosteroid therapy with its associated alterations in carbohydrate metabolism.[80]

Atypical verrucous endocarditis of Libman and Sacks is recognized as a specific valvular abnormality occurring in SLE. It is encountered in 25 to 60 percent of autopsied patients[62,68] (Fig. 30–9). The lesions are small, usually ranging from 1 to 4 mm in diameter but rarely achieve a size of 8 to 10 mm.[4] They are sterile, dry, granular pink vegetations that may be single or multiple and conglomerate. They have no special tendency to occur along the lines of closure of valves and may be scattered on the valvular endocardium, on the chordae tendineae and on the mural endocardium of the atria or ventricles. Most frequently, the lesions are located on the undersurface of the atrioventricular valves. Any valve may be involved, but the mitral and tricuspid valves are most often affected.[4,46,68] Clinical manifestations of atypical verrucous endocarditis are considerably less frequent than the morphologic lesions observed at autopsy and have been described in 6 to 20 percent of patients with SLE.[4,14] This discrepancy between the clinical and autopsy

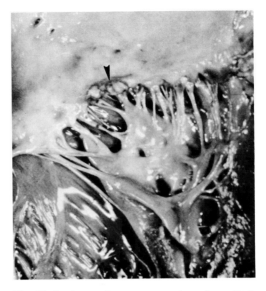

Fig. 30–9. Atypical verrucous endocarditis of Libman and Sacks usually consists of small vegetations ranging from 1 to 4 mm in diameter (arrowhead). They have no special tendency to occur along the lines of closure of the valves and may even involve the mural endocardium.

incidence of this lesion supports the view that atypical verrucous endocarditis rarely causes significant valvular dysfunction.[14] Histologically, the verrucae consist of a finely granular eosinophilic material which is fibrinous and may contain hematoxylin bodies.[4,46] In a general sense, such hematoxylin bodies are the tissue equivalent of the LE cell of the blood and bone marrow. The verrucous endocardial lesions result from degenerative and inflammatory processes of the endocardium and deeper layers of the valves. An intense valvulitis is present, characterized by fibrinoid necrosis of the valve substance that is often contiguous with the vegetation (Fig. 30–10). The fibrinoid necrosis may erode the endothelium and extrude into a cardiac cavity, forming a nidus for superimposed fibrin and platelet thrombi. Exudative and proliferative cellular reactions, which may be extensive, are present in the deeper layers of the valve.[14,46] Healing may produce foci of granulation tissue which develop into focal fibrous

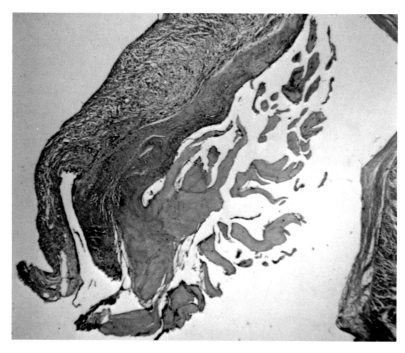

Fig. 30–10. This Libman-Sacks vegetation involves the ventricular surface of the mitral valve in a young woman with SLE. An intense valvulitis is present. It is characterized by fibrinoid necrosis of valve substance. The fibrinoid necrosis has eroded the endothelium and extrudes into the ventricular cavity. (H&E, × 200.)

thickenings in the valves or the mural endocardium. Also, with healing, the posterior mitral leaflet may become adherent to the posterior ventricular wall, causing valvular incompetence (see Ch. 25). Rarely, bacterial endocarditis has been superimposed on the Libman-Sacks lesion.[14,52,62]

In as many as 20 percent of patients with SLE dermal vasculitis develops during the course of their disease.[33] This is predominantly a small vessel vasculitis; however, diffuse central nervous system (CNS) vasculitis and systemic vasculitis involving medium-sized muscular arteries in a manner similar to panarteritis nodosa may also occur.[33,85] There is ample evidence of immune complex-mediated tissue injury in lupus vasculitis.[35,40]

Scleroderma

In scleroderma (progressive systemic sclerosis), myocardial scarring that cannot be attributed to any other cause is the most fre-

quent finding correlated with cardiac dysfunction.[4,15,96,114] Although the incidence of myocardial fibrosis in patients with scleroderma has varied in different studies, the results of two large autopsy series indicate an incidence of approximately 50 percent.[15,96] Unlike myocardial scarring associated with atherosclerotic coronary artery disease, that in scleroderma is usually as severe in the right ventricle as in the left. This scarring has no particular relationship to blood vessels and cannot be correlated with the presence of intramyocardial coronary artery intimal lesions, which exist in the form of mucoid degeneration or fibrinoid or both, and which are even less common in the heart than fibrosis.[15,96] In contrast to the myocardial lesions of dermatomyositis, there is only a minimal infiltrate of lymphocytes and plasma cells (Fig. 30–11). Areas of morphologically normal myocardium are interspersed among the foci of fibrosis. In other areas, contraction band necrosis may be prominent.[15] Whether the myocardial fibrosis

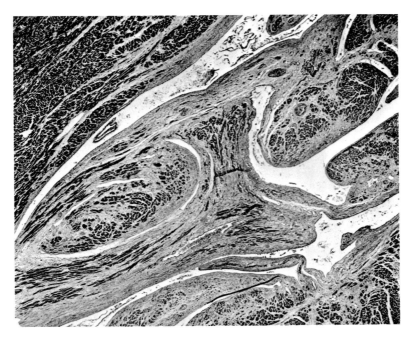

Fig. 30–11. In scleroderma, myocardial scarring that cannot be attributed to any other cause is frequently present. Scarring in the myocardium of the right ventricle is usually as severe as that in the left ventricle. In contrast to the myocardial lesions of dermatomyositis there is only a minimal infiltrate of lymphocytes and plasma cells. (H&E, × 150.)

is primary or secondary to degeneration of myofibers has not been established. Although congestive heart failure may result from myocardial lesions, it is more frequently associated with cor pulmonale secondary to scleroderma pulmonary disease, or to systemic hypertension secondary to scleroderma renal disease.[96] Fibrous replacement of the conducting tissue may also occur, resulting in varying degrees of heart block, including complete heart block.[67]

Although uncommon clinically, pericardial heart disease is found commonly at autopsy in patients with scleroderma.[96] Fibrous obliterative pericarditis is the most frequent. Fibrinous pericarditis is less common and may result from associated renal failure with uremia as well as primary scleroderma involvement of the pericardium.[83,92]

Valvular lesions in scleroderma are distinctly rare, but when present the most common is nonbacterial thrombotic endocarditis. Mitral and aortic valves are most commonly involved.[71]

Dermatomyositis (Polymyositis)

Cardiac involvement is unusual in patients with dermatomyositis; however, some develop pericarditis and various nonspecific electrocardiographic (ECG) changes.[43,53,70] At autopsy, this pericarditis may be either fibrinous or fibrous. Less frequently, the myocardium may be involved with a myocarditis resembling the degenerative and inflammatory changes present in skeletal muscle.[53] These myocardial lesions include focal or extensive primary degeneration of muscle fibers; necrosis of parts of or entire muscle fibers; focal or diffuse infiltrates of chronic inflammatory cells that are mainly small lymphocytes with lesser numbers of plasma cells; interstitial fibrosis which varies in severity, especially with the duration of the disease; and a variation in cross-sectional diameter of myocardial fibers, especially in disease of a relatively long duration (Fig. 30–12). Primary valvulitis is not a feature of dermatomyositis,

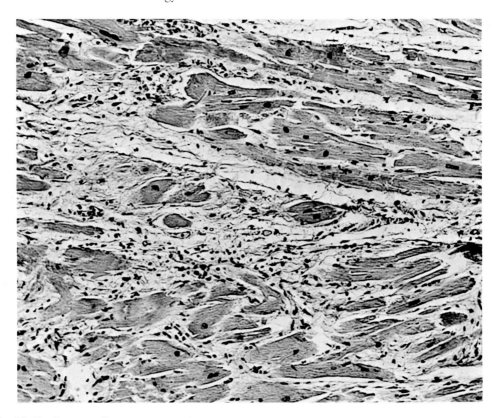

Fig. 30–12. Occasionally in patients with dermatomyositis the myocarditis resembles the degenerative and inflammatory changes present in skeletal muscle. There is focal or extensive degeneration of myofibers with an infiltrate of chronic inflammatory cells, consisting mainly of small lymphocytes with lesser numbers of plasma cells. (H&E, × 200.)

although nonbacterial thrombotic endocarditis may occur, especially in those patients with an associated mucinous adenocarcinoma.[112]

Panarteritis Nodosa

Panarteritis nodosa is a form of necrotizing arteritis that chiefly affects medium-sized muscular arteries, the coronary arteries being no exception[1,89,140] (Fig. 30–13). The active lesion of panarteritis nodosa consists of segmental necrosis and inflammation of all layers of the arterial wall. The inflammatory cell population is mixed, but in the active lesion polymorphonuclear leukocytes are the most common. Fibrinoid necrosis is usually present in the intima and inner one-third of the media, and a superimposed thrombus is frequently encountered (Fig. 30–14).[1,73] These lesions are usually present in varying stages of evolution and devolution and the arterial lumen may be occluded by fresh thrombus or by formation of granulation tissue with fibrosis and recanalization in varying combinations. The myocardial lesions in panarteritis nodosa are usually secondary to involvement of the epicardial coronary arteries, resulting in myocardial infarction. Occasionally, however, there is a nonspecific myocarditis consisting mainly of polymorphonuclear leukocytes with focal myofiber necrosis.[89] Because of the variety of lesions in the epicardial arteries, the

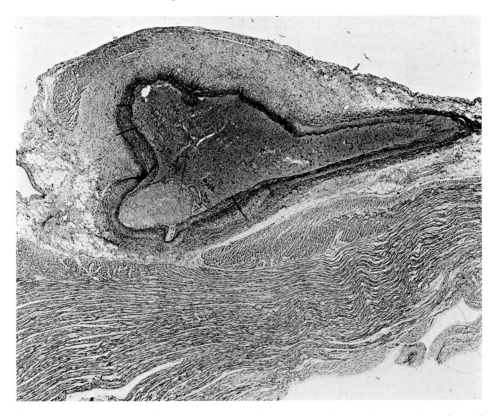

Fig. 30–13. Left anterior descending coronary artery from a patient dying of panarteritis nodosa. There is segmental necrosis of the arterial wall with aneurysm formation (top). A thrombus completely occludes the artery. (H&E, × 16.)

myocardial infarcts will also be of various sizes and in different stages of evolution, ranging from healed infarcts with fibrous scarring to acute myocardial infarction.[69,71] Other morphologic findings include cardiac hypertrophy and fibrinous pericarditis. In most instances, cardiac hypertrophy is related to hypertension,[4] whereas pericarditis may be related to uremia and not to primary cardiac disease.[69,71] Clinically, congestive heart failure is the most frequent manifestation of cardiac involvement in panarteritis nodosa[4] (see also Ch. 11).

Wegener's Granulomatosis

Wegener's granulomatosis often is confused with panarteritis nodosa, since both diseases are characterized by disseminated vasculitis and both renal and cardiac disease. As previously discussed, classic panarteritis nodosa involves medium-sized muscular arteries; by contrast, Wegener's granulomatosis involves predominantly small arteries, arterioles, and venules. In addition, pulmonary arteries are not usually involved in classic panarteritis nodosa, whereas pulmonary disease is common in Wegener's granulomatosis.[34] Necrotizing granulomata and upper airway disease so characteristic of Wegener's granulomatosis are not features of panarteritis nodosa.[34] These necrotizing granulomata consist of foci of necrosis surrounded by a zone of fibroblastic proliferation, with giant cells of the Langhans or foreign body type and a mixed inflammatory cell infiltrate (Fig. 30–15). Often the acute necrosis produces a total granular disintegration of the background tissue. The lesions un-

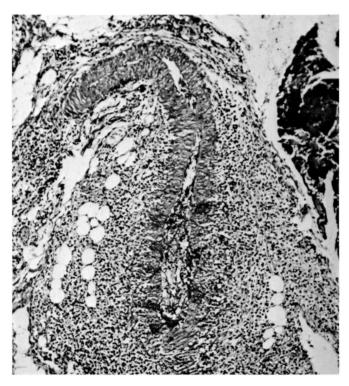

Fig. 30–14. The active lesion of panarteritis nodosa consists of segmental necrosis and inflammation of all layers of the arterial wall. The inflammatory cell infiltrate is mixed, but in the active lesion polymorphonuclear leukocytes are most common. Fibrinoid necrosis is usually present in the intima and inner one-third of the media. (H&E, × 80.)

dergo progressive fibrosis and organization. Myocardial destruction may be extensive. At autopsy, cardiac pathology is present in approximately 30 percent of patients with Wegener's granulomatosis.[34] The disease can affect the heart in any number of forms, including pericarditis, which is usually fibrinous, pancarditis, or coronary arteritis with acute myocardial infarction.[23] Although fibrinous pericarditis is the most common lesion encountered, myocarditis and coronary arteritis are the most devastating. Valvulitis is most unusual in Wegener's granulomatosis; the mitral valve is most commonly involved by the inflammatory process, which may result in subsequent fibrosis with commissural fusion resembling rheumatic mitral stenosis.[81] The clinical manifestations of cardiac involvement include chest pain, intractable arrhythmias, and congestive heart failure[34] (see also Ch. 11).

Thrombotic Thrombocytopenic Purpura

Thrombotic thrombocytopenic purpura is regarded by many as a collagen vascular disease.[112] This condition is characterized by endothelial damage to arterioles, and formation of hyaline deposits that may obstruct the vessels.[36] Endomyocardial biopsy may be helpful in identifying these vascular lesions as an indication for therapeutic plasmaphoresis. The lesions are usually widespread. Cardiac involvement is secondary to vascular lesions of the coronary arterioles, the obstruction of which may lead to focal areas of myocardial

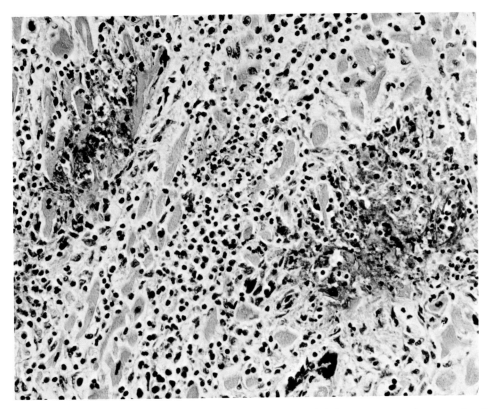

Fig. 30–15. In patients with Wegener's granulomatosis, myocardial destruction may be extensive. The affected myocardium contains necrotizing granulomata consisting of foci of necrosis surrounded by a zone of fibroblastic proliferation with Langhans, myogenic, or foreign body giant cells and a mixed inflammatory cell infiltrate. Often the acute necrosis produces granular disintegration of the background tissues. (H&E, × 115.)

necrosis (Fig. 30–16).[4] Although the most common cardiac involvement in thrombotic thrombocytopenic purpura is focal myocardial necrosis, nonbacterial thrombotic endocarditis is not uncommon. The valves most frequently involved are the mitral and aortic, although any valve may be affected. Embolization from these lesions is extremely common.

Diseases Simulating Collagen Vascular Diseases

Although not classically considered as collagen vascular diseases, three entities that may result in pancarditis, including fibrous thick-

ening of the cardiac valves and thickening and fusion of chordae tendineae, are Whipple's disease, endomyocardial fibrosis with eosinophilia and radiation.

Whipple's Disease

In an autopsy study of 19 patients dying with Whipple's disease (intestinal lipodystrophy), 58 percent had clinical cardiac findings and 79 percent had gross cardiac lesions at autopsy.[74] Histologically, there were PAS-positive macrophages in the pericardium, myocardium, and valves of each patient. These collections of macrophages were associated with chronic inflammatory cells and foci of fibrosis with resultant fibrous adhesive peri-

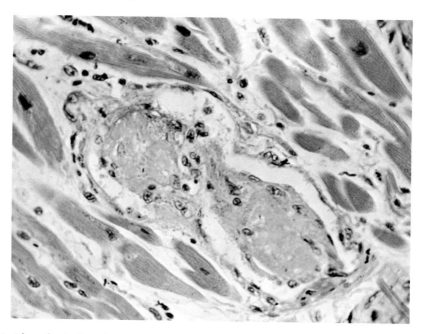

Fig. 30–16. Thrombotic thrombocytopenic purpura is characterized by endothelial damage to arterioles and formation of hyaline deposits which may obstruct these vessels. Obstruction of coronary arterioles, as illustrated here, may lead to focal necrosis of myocardial fibers. (H&E, × 300.)

carditis, focal myocardial fibrosis similar to the fibrosis of idiopathic cardiomyopathy, and valvular fibrosis with deformity grossly resembling the valvular lesions of chronic rheumatic heart disease. Four of the patients with mitral valvular deformity had cardiac murmurs, and ECG changes were noted in six patients with extensive focal myocardial fibrosis. In addition, pericardial friction rubs were heard in two patients. Diagnostic PAS-positive macrophages in areas of fibrosis were present in the pericardium in all 19 patients, and microscopic foci of fibrosis were noted throughout the myocardium in 89 percent of these patients.[74] Areas of fibrosis within the myocardium are primarily stellate or intermysial and are associated with focal myofiber loss and collections of PAS-positive macrophages, lymphocytes, and Anitschkow cells (Fig. 30–17). Occasionally the areas of fibrosis and myocarditis are perivascular; however, no Aschoff nodules or foci of lamellar fibrosis suggestive of healed Aschoff nodules are present.

The valve most commonly involved in Whipple's disease is the mitral, followed by the tricuspid and aortic.[76] The gross deformity closely resembles that seen in chronic rheumatic heart disease with diffuse thickening and fibrosis of valve leaflets and chordae tendineae and rolling of the free edges of the leaflets (Fig. 30–18). Microscopically, large macrophages filled with PAS-positive granules identical to those found in the small intestine of patients with Whipple's disease are present in the valve substance. Proliferating fibrous tissue and chronic inflammatory cells are commonly associated with the PAS-positive macrophages. Scattered rod-shaped bodies 1.5 to 2.0 μm long and 0.2 to 0.4 μm in diameter are present intracellularly and extracellularly in the affected valve, myocardium, and pericardium. These bodies, as well as membrane-bound masses of fibrillar material within the macrophages, are identical to those described in jejunal biopsies of those with Whipple's disease.[74]

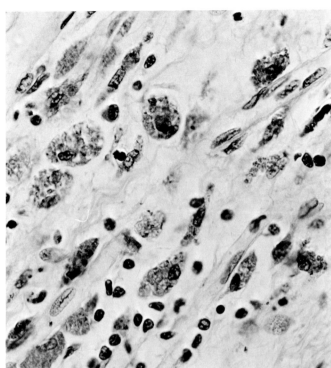

Fig. 30–17. In patients dying of untreated Whipple's disease (intestinal lipodystrophy) there are macrophages containing PAS-positive granules in the pericardium, myocardium, and cardiac valves. These collections of macrophages are associated with chronic inflammatory cells and fibrosis with resultant fibrous adhesive pericarditis, focal myocardial fibrosis, and valvular fibrosis. This section, illustrating PAS-positive macrophages and chronic inflammatory cells, is from the left ventricular myocardium. (PAS, × 300.)

Endomyocardial Fibrosis with Eosinophilia

In endomyocardial fibrosis with eosinophilia (Löffler's fibroplastic parietal endocarditis with blood eosinophilia, disseminated eosinophilic collagen vascular disease) there is endocardial fibrosis of one or both ventricles, an increased number of eosinophils in the peripheral blood and usually mitral regurgitation.[95] Rarely, constrictive pericarditis may also be present.[133] Death characteristically results from congestive heart failure. The endocardial thickening is located primarily in the inflow tracts of the ventricles and commonly extends into the adjacent myocardium. It usually begins in the apices and progresses to involve the endocardium deep to the posterior mitral leaflet and/or the endocardium deep to the posterior or septal tricuspid valve leaflets.[95] Fibrin thrombus is frequently superimposed on the fibrotic mural endocardium. This endomyocardial fibrosis frequently re-

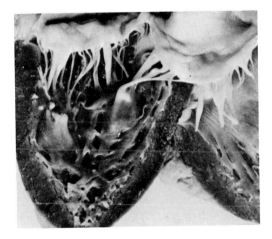

Fig. 30–18. Heart from a 52-year-old man who developed diarrhea and symptoms of malabsorption 3 years before death. A diagnosis of Whipple's disease was established postmortem. The mitral valve is diffusely thickened, with rolling of the free margin; the chordae tendineae are fused and shortened. The resultant valvular deformity resembles that seen in chronic rheumatic heart disease.

sults in decreased diastolic compliance of the ventricles; also, the volume of the ventricular cavities may be considerably decreased by thrombus.[108] The cardiac valves most commonly involved are the mitral and tricuspid, with a less frequent involvement of the aortic valve.[95,108] The posterior mitral leaflet or the posterior or septal tricuspid leaflets may become adherent to the underlying mural endocardium, with resulting regurgitation (Fig. 30–19) (see Ch. 25). The aortic valve cusps are occasionally thickened by vascularized fibrous tissue with superimposed fibrin thrombus.[108] Eosinophilic leukocytes in varying numbers are usually present at the periphery of the fibrous lesions.

Irradiation

Irradiation may produce several morphologic changes in the heart; the most frequent is thickening of the parietal and visceral peri-

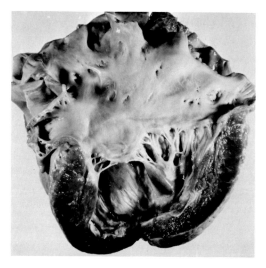

Fig. 30–19. In endomyocardial fibrosis with eosinophilia (Löffler's fibroblastic parietal endocarditis) there is endocardial fibrosis, an increased number of eosinophils in the peripheral blood and usually mitral regurgitation, as in this patient. The posterior mitral leaflet adheres to the underlying mural endocardium, as a result of progressive fibrosis with superimposed organizing thrombus, resulting in an incompetent valve.

cardia, with or without associated pericardial effusion or tamponade.[108] The second most frequent change is interstitial and perivascular myocardial fibrosis of varying degrees.[108] Focal endocardial fibrosis may also occur. Rarely, in patients receiving mediastinal irradiation, lesions of the cardiac valves may develop. Those most commonly involved are the tricuspid and mitral, followed by the aortic and pulmonic.[108] The fibrous valvular thickenings are focal, and the anterior tricuspid leaflet and anterior mitral leaflet are usually more markedly involved than the posterior leaflets.[79] The chordae tendineae also may be focally thickened with fibrous tissue.[108] Prematurely developed coronary atherosclerosis and its sequelae are also complications.

REFERENCES

1. Alarcon-Segovia D, Brown AL Jr: Classification and etiologic aspects of necrotizing angiitides: An analytical approach to a confused subject, with a critical review of the evidence for hypersensitivity in polyarteritis nodosa. Proc Staff Meet Mayo Clin 39:205, 1964
2. Alexander CS, Derr RF, Sako Y: Abnormal amino acid and lipid composition of aortic valve in relapsing polychondritis. Am J Cardiol 28:337, 1971
3. Ansell BM, Bywaters EGL, Doniach I: The aortic lesion of ankylosing spondylitis. Br Heart J 20:507, 1958
4. Baggenstoss AH, Titus JL: Rheumatic and collagen disorders of the heart. p. 701. In Gould SE (ed): Pathology of the Heart and Blood Vessels. 3rd Ed. Charles C Thomas, Springfield, 1968
5. Baker AL, Marshall MK, Wendy CB, et al: Polyarteritis associated with Australia antigen-positive hepatitis. Gastroenterology 62:105, 1972
6. Barnett EV, Winkelstein A, Weinberger AJ: Agammaglobulinemia with polyarthritis and subcutaneous nodules. Am J Med 48:40, 1970
7. Bartfeld H, Epstein WV (eds): Rheumatoid factors and their biological significance. Ann NY Acad Sci 168:1, 1969

8. Bellanti JA, Calabro JJ, Gelfand MC: Immunologically mediated disease involving autologous antigens. p. 565. In Bellanti JA (ed): Immunology. Vol. II. WB Saunders, Philadelphia, 1978

9. Benacerraf B, McDevitt HO: Histocompatibility-linked immune response genes. Science 175:273, 1972

10. Bonfiglio T, Atwater EC: Heart disease in patients with seropositive rheumatoid arthritis. Arch Intern Med 124:714, 1969

11. Bonfiglio TA, Botti RE, Hagstrom JWC: Coronary arteritis, occlusion, and myocardial infarction due to lupus erythematosus. Am Heart J 83:153, 1972

12. Böttiger LE, Edhag O: Heart block in ankylosing spondylitis and uropolyarthritis. Br Heart J 34:487, 1972

13. Brewerton DA, James DC: The histocompatibility antigen (HL-A27) and disease. Semin Arthritis Rheum 4:191, 1975

14. Brigden W, Bywaters EGL, Lessof MH, Ross JP: The heart in systemic lupus erythematosus. Br Heart J 22:1, 1960

15. Bulkley BH, Ridolfi RL, Salyer WR, et al: Myocardial lesions of progressive systemic sclerosis. A cause of cardiac dysfunction. Circulation 53:483, 1976

16. Bulkley BH, Roberts WC: Ankylosing spondylitis and aortic regurgitation. Circulation 48:1014, 1973

17. Bulkley BH, Roberts WC: The heart in systemic lupus erythematosus and the changes induced in it by corticosteroid therapy. A study of 36 necropsy patients. Am J Med 58:253, 1975

18. Calin A, Fries JF: Striking prevalence of ankylosing spondylitis in "healthy" W27-positive males and females. N Engl J Med 293:835, 1975

19. Calkins E, Cohen AS: Diagnosis of amyloidosis. Bull Rheum Dis 10:215, 1960

20. Carpenter DF, Golden A, Roberts WC: Quadrivalvular rheumatoid heart disease associated with left bundle branch block. Am J Med 43:922, 1967

21. Caspary EA, Gubbary SS, Stern GM: Circulating antibodies in polymyositis and other muscle-wasting disorders. Lancet 2:941, 1964

22. Cathcart ES, Spodick DH: Rheumatoid heart disease: A study of the incidence and nature of cardiac lesions in rheumatoid arthritis. N Engl J Med 266:959, 1962

23. Cheitlin MD, McAllister HA, De Castro C: Myocardial infarction without atherosclerosis. JAMA 231:951, 1975

24. Chou SM, Gutman L: Picornavirus-like crystals in subacute polymyositis. Neurology (NY) 20:205, 1970

25. Clark WS, Kulka JP, Bauer W: Rheumatoid aortitis with aortic regurgitation. An unusual manifestation of rheumatoid arthritis (including spondylitis). Am J Med 22:580, 1957

26. Cliff JM: Spinal bony bridging and carditis in Reiter's disease. Ann Rheum Dis 30:171, 1971

27. Cruickshank B: Heart lesions in rheumatoid disease. J Pathol 76:223, 1958

28. Csonka GW, Litchfield JW, Oates JW, Cillcox RR: Cardiac lesions in Reiter's disease. Br Med J 1:243, 1961

29. Davidson P, Baggenstoss AH, Slocomb CH, Daugherty GH: Cardiac and aortic lesions in rheumatoid spondylitis. Proc Staff Meet Mayo Clin 38:427, 1963

30. Dawkins RL, Mastaglia FL: Cell-mediated cytotoxicity to muscle in polymyositis. N Engl J Med 288:434, 1973

31. DeHoratius R, Pillarisetty RJ, Messner RP, et al: Antinucleic acid antibodies in systemic lupus erythematosus patients and their families—incidence and correlation with lymphocytotoxic antibodies. J Clin Invest 56:1149, 1975

32. Dolan DL, Lemmon GB, Teitelbaum SL: Relapsing polychondritis. Analytical literature review and studies on pathogenesis. Am J Med 41:285, 1966

33. Estes D, Christian CL: The natural history of systemic lupus erythematosus by prospective analysis. Medicine (Baltimore) 50:85, 1971

34. Fauci AS, Wolff SM: Wegener's granulomatosis and related diseases. DM 23(7):1, 1977

35. Fauci AS, Haynes BF, Katz P: The spectrum of vasculitis-clinical, pathologic, immunologic, and therapeutic considerations. Ann Intern Med 89(part 1):660, 1978

36. Feldman JD, Mardinay MR, Unanne ER, Cutting H: The vascular pathology of thrombotic thrombocytopenic purpura: Immunohistochemical and ultrastructural study. Lab Invest 15:927, 1966

37. Ferrans VJ, Rodriguez ER, McAllister HA Jr: Grannulomatous inflammation of the heart. Heart Vessels 1:262, 1985

38. Franco AE, Schur PH: Hypocomplementemia in rheumatoid arthritis. Arthritis Rheum 14:231, 1971

39. Ghose MJ: Pericardial tamponade. A presenting manifestation of procainamide-induced lupus erythematosus. Am J Med 58:581, 1975

40. Gilliam JN, Smiley JD: Cutaneous necrotizing vasculitis and related disorders. Ann Allergy 37:328, 1976

41. Glenner GG: Amyloid deposits and amyloidosis, the B-fibrilloses. N Engl J Med 302:1333, 1980

42. Good AE: Reiter's disease: A review with special attention to cardiovascular and neurologic sequelae. Semin Arthritis Rheum 3:253, 1974

43. Gottdiener JS, Sherber HS, Hawley RJ, Engel WK: Cardiac manifestations in polymyositis. Am J Cardiol 41:1141, 1978

44. Graham DC, Smythe HA: The carditis and aortitis of ankylosing spondylitis. Bull Rheum Dis 9:171, 1958

45. Grimley PM, Schaff Z: Significance of tubuloreticular inclusions in the pathobiology of human diseases. Pathobiol Annu 6:221, 1976

46. Gross L: Cardiac lesions in Libman-Sacks disease, with consideration of its relationship to acute diffuse lupus erythematosus. Am J Pathol 16:375, 1940

47. Gyorkey F, Sinkovics JG, Min KW, Gyorkey P: A morphologic study on the occurrence and distribution of structures resembling viral nucleocapsids in collagen diseases. Am J Med 53:148, 1972

48. Haas JE, Yunis EJ: Tubular inclusions of systemic lupus erythematosus: Ultrastructural observations regarding their possible viral nature. Exp Mol Pathol 12:257, 1970

49. Hahn BH, Shapp GC, Irvin WS, et al: Immune responses to hydralazine and nuclear antigens in hydralazine-induced lupus erythematosus. Ann Intern Med 76:365, 1972

50. Hainer JW, Hamilton GW: Aortic abnormalities in relapsing polychondritis: Report of a case with dissecting aortic aneurysm. N Engl J Med 280:116, 1969

51. Harker L: Studies of platelet and fibrinogen consumption. J Clin Invest 49:392, 1970

52. Hejmancik MR, Wright JC, Quint R, Jennings FL: The cardiovascular manifestations of systemic lupus erythematosus. Am Heart J 68:119, 1964

53. Hill DL, Barrows HS: Identical skeletal and cardiac muscle involvement in a case of fatal polymyositis. Arch Neurol 19:545, 1968

54. Howell A, Say J, Hedworth-Whitty R: Rupture of the sinus of Valsalva due to severe rheumatoid heart disease. Br Heart J 34:537, 1972

55. Howell SB, Epstein WV: Circulating immunoglobulin complexes in Wegener's granulomatosis. Am J Med 60:259, 1976

56. Husby G: Amyloidosis in rheumatoid arthritis. Ann Clin Res 7:154, 1975

57. Johnson RL, Fink CW, Ziff M: Lymphotoxin formation by lymphocytes and muscle in polymyositis. J Clin Invest 51:2435, 1972

58. Julkunen H: Atrioventricular conduction defect in ankylosing spondylitis. Geriatrics 21:129, 1966

59. Karten I: Arteritis, myocardial infarction and rheumatoid arthritis. JAMA 210:1717, 1969

60. Kemple K, Bluestone R: The histocompatibility complex and rheumatic diseases. Med Clin North Am 61:331, 1977

61. Klemperer P: The concept of collagen disease. Am J Pathol 26:505, 1950

62. Klemperer P, Pollack AD, Baehr GG: Pathology of disseminated lupus erythematosus. Arch Pathol 32:569, 1941

63. Lambert PH, Dixon FJ: Pathogenesis of glomerulonephritis of NZB/W mice. J Exp Med 127:507, 1968

64. Lebowitz WB: The heart in rheumatoid arthritis (rheumatoid disease): A clinical and pathological study of sixty-two cases. Ann Intern Med 58;102, 1963

65. Leonhardt T: Family studies in systemic lupus erythematosus. Acta Med Scand 416(suppl):1, 1964

66. LeRoy EC: Increased collagen synthesis by scleroderma skin fibroblasts in vitro. A possible defect in the regulation or activation of the scleroderma fibroblast. J Clin Invest 54:880, 1974

67. Lev M, Landowne M, Matchar JC, Wagner JA: Systemic scleroderma with complete heart block. Report of a case with comprehensive study of the conduction system. Am Heart J 72:13, 1966

68. Libman E, Sacks B: A hitherto undescribed

form of valvular and mural endocarditis. Arch Intern Med 33:701, 1924

69. Liu SM, Alexander CS: Complete heart block and aortic insufficiency in rheumatoid spondylitis. Am J Cardiol 23:888, 1969

70. Lynch PG: Cardiac involvement in chronic polymyositis. Br Heart J 33:416, 1971

71. McAllister HA Jr: Pathology of the cardiovascular system in chronic renal failure. p. 1. In Lowenthal DT, Pennock RL (eds): Management of Cardiovascular Disease in Renal Failure. FA Davis, Philadelphia, 1981

72. McAllister HA Jr: Myocarditis: Some current perspectives and future directions. Texas Heart Inst J 14:331, 1987

73. McAllister HA Jr: An overview of human arterial pathology. Toxicol Pathol 17:219, 1989

74. McAllister HA Jr, Fenoglio JJ Jr: Cardiac involvement in Whipple's disease. Circulation 52:152, 1975

75. McAllister HA Jr, Ferrans VJ: Granulomas of the heart and major blood vessels. p. 75. In Ioachim HL (ed): Differential Diagnosis of Granulomas. Raven Press, New York, 1982

76. McAllister HA Jr, Ferrans VJ: Eosinophilic and granulomatous inflammation of the heart. p. 246. In Kapour AS (ed): Cancer and the Heart—A Textbook of Cardiac Oncology. Springer-Verlag, New York, 1986

77. McAllister HA Jr, Ferrans VJ, Bossart M, Hall RJ: Chloroquine cardiomyopathy. Arch Pathol Lab Med 10:953, 1987

78. McAllister HA Jr, Ferrans VJ: The cardiovascular system. p. 787. In Silverberg SG (ed): Principles and Practice of Surgical Pathology. 2nd Ed. Churchill Livingstone, New York, 1990

79. McAllister HA Jr, Hall RJ: Iatrogenic heart disease. p. 871. In Cheng TS (ed): The International Textbook of Cardiology. Pergamon Press, New York, 1986

80. McAllister HA Jr, Mullick FG: The cardiovascular system. p. 201. In Riddell R (ed): Pathology of Drug-Induced and Toxic Diseases. Churchill Livingstone, New York, 1982

81. McCrea PC, Childers RW: Two unusual cases of giant cell myocarditis associated with mitral stenosis and with Wegener's syndrome. Br Heart J 26:490, 1964

82. McEwen C, Di Tata D, Lingg C, et al: Ankylosing spondylitis and spondylitis accompanying ulcerative colitis, regional enteritis, psoriasis and Reiter's disease. A comparative study. Arthritis Rheum 14:291, 1971

83. McWhorter JE, LeRoy EC: Pericardial disease in scleroderma (systemic sclerosis). Am J Med 57:566, 1974

84. Mellors RC, Huang CY: Immunopathology of NZB/BL mice. V. Virus-like (filterable) agent separable from lymphoma cells and identifiable by electron microscope. J Exp Med 124:1031, 1966

85. Mintz G, Fraga A: Arteritis in systemic lupus erythematosus. Arch Intern Med 116:55, 1965

86. Missen GAK, Taylor JD: Amyloidosis in rheumatoid arthritis. J Pathol 71:179, 1956

87. Molina J, Dubois E, Bilitch M, et al: Procainamide-induced serologic changes in asymptomatic patients. Arthritis Rheum 12:608, 1969

88. Mongan ES, Cass RM, Jacox RF, Vaughan JH: A study of the relation to seronegative and seropositive rheumatoid arthritis to each other and to necrotizing vasculitis. Am J Med 47:23, 1969

89. Moskowitz RW, Baggenstoss AH, Slocumb CH: Histopathologic classification of periarteritis nodosa: A study of 56 cases confirmed at necropsy. Mayo Clin Proc 38:345, 1963

90. Movat HZ: The concept of fibrinoid. Am J Med Sci 236:373, 1958

91. Muna WF, Roller DH, Craft J, et al: Psoriatic arthritis and aortic regurgitation. JAMA 244:363, 1980

92. Nasser WK, Mishkin MD, Rosenbaum D, Genovese P: Pericardial and myocardial disease in progressive systemic sclerosis. Am J Cardiol 22:538, 1968

93. Neu LT, Reider RA, Mack RE: Cardiac involvement in Reiter's disease: Report of case with review of literature. Ann Intern Med 53:215, 1960

94. Norton WL, Velayos E, Robisan L: Endothelial inclusions in dermatomyositis. Ann Rheum Dis 29:67, 1970

95. Olsen EGJ, Spry CJF: The pathogenesis of Löffler's endomyocardial disease, and its relationship to endomyocardial fibrosis. Progress in Cardiology 8:281, 1979

96. Oram S, Stokes W: The heart in scleroderma. Br Heart J 23:243, 1961

97. Owen DS, Irby R, Toone E: Relapsing polychondritis with aortic involvement. Arthritis Rheum 13:877, 1970

98. Paulus HE, Pearson CM, Pitts W: Aortic insufficiency in five patients with Reiter's syndrome. A detailed clinical and pathological study. Am J Med 53:464, 1972

99. Pearson CM, Kroening R, Verity MA, Getzen JH: Aortic insufficiency and aortic aneurysm in relapsing polychondritis. Trans Assoc Am Physicians 80:71, 1967

100. Peterson RD, Good RA: Interrelationships of the mesenchymal diseases with consideration of possible genetic mechanisms. Annu Rev Med 14;1, 1963

101. Phillips PE: The role of viruses in systemic lupus erythematosus. Clin Rheum Dis 1:505, 1975

102. Pomerance A: Cardiac involvement in rheumatic and "collagen" diseases. p. 279. In Pomerance A, Davies MJ (eds): The Pathology of the Heart. Blackwell Scientific Publications, Oxford, 1975

103. Preble OT, Black RJ, Friedman RM, et al: Systemic lupus erythematosus: Presence in human serum of an unusual acid-labile leukocyte interferon. Science 216:429, 1982

104. Ratliff NB, Estes ML, Myles JL, et al: The diagnosis of chloroquine cardiomyopathy by endomyocardial biopsy. N Engl J Med 316:191, 1987

105. Reed WB: Psoriatic arthritis: A complete clinical study of 86 patients. Acta Dermatovener (Stockh) 41:396, 1961

106. Reichlin M, Wasicek CA: Clinical and biologic significance of antibodies to Ro/SSA. Hum Pathol 14:401, 1983

107. Rich SA: Human lupus inclusions and interferon. Science 213:772, 1981

108. Roberts WC, Dangel JC, Bulkley BH: Nonrheumatic valvular cardiac disease: A clinicopathologic survey of 27 different conditions causing valvular dysfunction. Cardiovasc Clin 5:333, 1973

109. Robinowitz M, Virmani R, McAllister HA Jr: Rheumatoid heart disease: A clinical and morphologic analysis of 34 autopsy patients. J Lab Invest 42:49, 1980

110. Rodnan GP: Progressive systemic sclerosis (scleroderma). p. 962. In Hollander JL, McCarty DJ Jr (eds): Arthritis and Allied Conditions, 8th Ed. Lea & Febiger, Philadelphia, 1972

111. Rodnan GP, Benedek TG, Shaver JA, Fennell RH: Reiter's syndrome and aortic insufficiency. JAMA 189:889, 1964

112. Rodnan GP, McEwen C, Wallace SL: Primer on the rheumatic diseases. JAMA 224(suppl):662, 1973

113. Rothfield NF, Rodnan GP: Serum antinuclear antibodies in progressive systemic sclerosis (scleroderma). Arthritis Rheum 11:607, 1968

114. Rottenberg EN, Slocumb CH, Edwards JE: Cardiac and renal manifestations in progressive systemic scleroderma. Proc Staff Meet Mayo Clin 34:77, 1959

115. Ruddy S, Austen JK: The complement system in rheumatoid synovitis. I. an analysis of complement component activities in rheumatoid synovial fluids. Arthritis Rheum 13:713, 1970

116. Scott JT, Hourihame DO, Doyle FH, et al: Digital arteritis in rheumatoid disease. Ann Rheum Dis 20:224, 1961

117. Self J, Hammersten JF, Lyne B, Peterson DA: Relapsing polychondritis. Arch Intern Med 120:109, 1967

118. Sell S: Immunopathology. Am J Pathol 90:215, 1978

119. Sergent JS, Lockshin MD, Christian CL, et al: Vasculitis with hepatitis B antigenemia: long-term observations in nine patients. Medicine (Baltimore) 55:1, 1976

120. Sharp GC: Mixed connective tissue disease—Overlap syndromes. Clin Rheum Dis 1:561, 1975

121. Smiley JD, Sachs C, Ziff M: In vitro synthesis of immunoglobulin by rheumatoid synovial membrane. J Clin Invest 47:624, 1968

122. Smith ME, Ansell BM, Bywaters EGL: Mortality and prognosis related to the amyloidosis of Still's disease. Ann Rheum Dis 27:137, 1968

123. Sokoloff L: The heart in rheumatoid arthritis. Am Heart J 45:635, 1953

124. Sokoloff L: Cardiac involvement in rheumatoid arthritis and allied disorders: Current concepts. Mod Concepts Cardiovasc Dis 33:847, 1964

125. Stage DE, Mannik M: Rheumatoid factors in rheumatoid arthritis. Bull Rheum Dis 23:720, 1973

126. Talal N: Autoimmunity and lymphoid malignancy in New Zealand black mice. Prog Clin Immunol 2:101, 1974

127. Taylor RT: Systemic lupus erythematosus. Br J Med 4:653, 1970

128. Tisher CC, Kelso HB, Robinson RR: Intraendothelial inclusions in kidneys of patients with systemic lupus erythematosus. Ann Intern Med 75:537, 1971

129. Tsakraklides VG, Bliden LC, Edwards JE: Coronary atherosclerosis and myocardial infarction associated with lupus erythematosus. Am Heart J 87:637, 1974

130. Urchak PM, Levine SA, Gorlin R: Constrictive pericarditis complicating disseminated lupus erythematosus. Circulation 31:113, 1965

131. Vazquez JJ, Dixon FJ: Immunohistochemical study of lesions in rheumatic fever, systemic lupus erythematosus, and rheumatoid arthritis. Lab Invest 6:205, 1957

132. Virmani R, McAllister HA Jr: The pathology of aorta and major arteries. p. 7. In Lande A, Berkmen Y, McAllister HA Jr (eds): Aortitis: Clinical, Pathologic, and Radiographic Aspects. Raven Press, New York, 1986

133. Virmani R, Chun PKC, McAllister HA Jr, et al: Eosinophilic constrictive pericarditis: Report of 3 patients and a review of the spectrum of hypereosinophilic damage. Am Heart J 107:803, 1984

134. Virmani R, Lande A, McAllister HA Jr: Pathologic aspects of Takayasu's arteritis. p. 55. In Lande A, Berkmen Y, McAllister HA Jr (eds): Aortitis: Clinical, Pathologic, and Radiographic Aspects. Raven Press, New York, 1986

135. Virmani R, Robinowitz M, McAllister HA Jr: Aortitis: A clinical and pathologic study of 77 patients. Am J Clin Pathol 77:240, 1982

136. Walton JN: Polymyositis: New light on pathogenesis and treatment. Proc Aust Assoc Neurol 9:1, 1973

137. Weed CL, Kulander B, Mazzarella JA, Decker JL: Heart block in ankylosing spondylitis. Arch Intern Med 117:800, 1966

138. Whitaker JN, Engel WK: Vascular deposits of immunoglobulin and complement in inflammatory myopathy. N Engl J Med 286:333, 1972

139. Wolff SM, Fauci AS, Horn RG, et al: Wegener's granulomatosis. Ann Intern Med 81:513, 1974

140. Zeek PM: Medical progress. Periarteritis nodosa and other forms of necrotizing angiitis. N Engl J Med 248:764, 1953

31

Endocrine Diseases and the Cardiovascular System

Hugh A. McAllister, Jr.

ACROMEGALY

Acromegaly is almost invariably the result of a growth hormone-producing eosinophilic or chromophobe pituitary adenoma; however, it may occur as a component of multiple endocrine syndromes, with or without concomitant cardiac myxoma.[24,119] The disease is usually slowly progressive, with signs and symptoms often predating diagnosis by more than a decade.[157] The physical features of the acromegalic patient are the result of growth hormone effects on bone, muscle, and connective tissue, resulting in broadening of the hands and feet, and organomegaly. Disproportionate cardiomegaly, compared with other types of organomegaly, occurs in approximately 75 percent of affected patients.[5,35,45,57,78] Although the enlarged heart seldom exceeds twice the expected weight, hearts weighing more than 1,000 g have been reported.[37,59,61,95] Cardiomegaly appears to be related to the duration of acromegaly and is present in both hypertensive and nonhypertensive patients.[78]

Although the cardiomegaly may be related to the generalized effect of growth hormone (somatotropin) on protein synthesis, some data suggest that other etiologic factors may be active, especially in light of evidence that there is no direct relationship between the degree of cardiomegaly and the level of circulating growth hormone.[91] The frequency of other cardiovascular disorders, including hypertension, congestive heart failure, cardiac arrhythmias (including premature ventricular contractions and atrioventricular conduction defects), and perhaps accelerated atherosclerosis, is increased in acromegaly. In addition, 15 to 20 percent of patients with acromegaly develop diabetes mellitus.[28] Because of the frequent occurrence of congestive heart failure and cardiac arrhythmias in patients who otherwise have no predisposing factors such as hypertension or atherosclerosis, it has been suggested that a specific acromegalic cardiomyopathy exists.[3,19,30,63,104] Although many acromegalics also have atherosclerosis, it is usually not severe and its incidence does not seem inordinately high; moreover, myocardial ischemia from coronary insufficiency does not adequately explain the cardiomyopathy.[3,157] Another possible explanation for acromegalic cardiomyopathy is that pituitary products other than growth hormone may be responsible. In a preliminary survey of 35 hyperprolactinemic patients, five were identified with elevated blood pressure and four, two of whom were normotensive, had cardiomegaly on chest radiographs.[34]

Since prolactin exerts a metabolic growth hormone-like effect in animals and man, the possibility that prolactin hypersecretion might induce or maintain cardiomegaly in patients with pituitary tumors has been conjectured.[34]

In acromegalic heart disease, all chambers are hypertrophied and dilated, and the myocardium of both ventricles is greatly thickened. Although these hearts are usually enlarged to an extent out of proportion to the general visceral enlargement, their configuration is usually normal (Fig. 31–1). Echocardiographic evidence of asymmetric septal hypertrophy has been reported as a frequent finding in these patients; however, morphologic studies have not confirmed this observation.[78,136] Indeed, the most common morphologic type of left ventricular hypertrophy is concentric. Microscopically the most striking feature is a moderate to marked increase in interstitial fibrous tissue (Fig. 31–2). It has been demonstrated that acromegalic myocar-

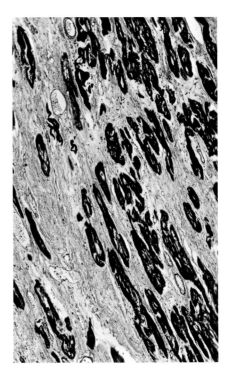

Fig. 31–2. Microscopically, the most striking feature in the myocardium in acromegalic heart disease is a moderate to marked increase in interstitial fibrous tissue. In addition, there is hypertrophy of individual cardiac muscle cells, as well as focal myofibrillar degeneration. (Masson's trichrome, × 200.)

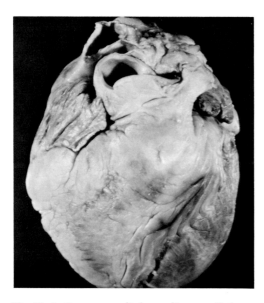

Fig. 31–1. In acromegalic heart disease, all chambers are hypertrophied and dilated. Although these hearts are usually somewhat disproportionately enlarged in relationship to the general visceral enlargement, their configuration is usually normal.

dial muscle contains 10 percent more collagen per gram than does myocardial muscle from normal hearts.[3,118] In addition, there is hypertrophy of the individual cardiac muscle cells, as well as focal myofibrillar degeneration similar to that observed in patients dying with pheochromocytoma.[78]

Occasionally there may be intimal and medial fibromuscular hyperplasia involving intramural coronary arterioles.[78] (Fig. 31–3). Sudden death has been associated with inflammatory and degenerative changes in the sinoatrial perinodal nerve plexes and with degeneration of the atrioventricular node.[118]

The diagnosis of acromegaly is established by documenting the nonsuppressibility of serum growth hormone levels following glucose

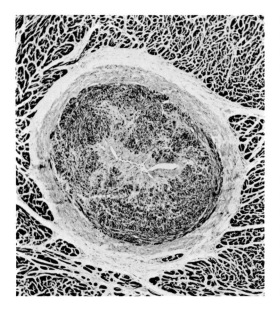

Fig. 31–3. Occasionally, the acromegalic heart contains intramural coronary arterioles with extensive intimal and medial fibromuscular hyperplasia. (Masson's trichrome, × 120.)

loading. The functional status of other pituitary products should also be established.[157]

HYPOPITUITARISM

Hypopituitarism is not a distinct pathophysiologic entity, since the disorder is attributable to diverse causes and may vary from a unihormonal deficiency to panhypopituitarism.[129] The effects on the cardiovascular system depend on the degree of individual hormone deficit and on hormonal interaction. Growth hormone is most commonly decreased in hypopituitarism.[3] The clinical course of these patients is usually not marked by cardiac disorders. Radiographically, however, the heart is usually small and vertical, similar to that seen in patients with Addison's disease.[129] Cardiac muscle fibers appear thin and atrophic on histologic examination. In occasional patients with secondary myxedema, cholesterol pericarditis and congestive heart failure may develop.[27,142] Patients with Werner syndrome (progeria of the adult) will not uncommonly have hypopituitarism contributing to this complex condition.[43]

HYPERTHYROIDISM

Hyperthyroidism is the clinical condition that results from increased production of thyroxine, triiodothyronine, or both, usually as a consequence of a diffuse toxic goiter.[157] The second most common cause of hyperthyroidism is nodular toxic goiter. Rarely, hyperthyroidism may occur as a result of thyroid carcinoma or the production of thyroid hormone from ectopic thyroid tissue.[157]

Cardiovascular signs and symptoms are important clinical features of hyperthyroidism and include palpitations, dyspnea, tachycardia, and systolic hypertension. Diastolic hypertension occurs in approximately 30 percent of these patients.[157] Although many of the changes in cardiac function are secondary to increased metabolic demands of peripheral tissues, there is evidence that thyroid hormone exerts a direct stimulant action on the heart, independent of its effect on general tissue metabolism.[21,23,84,96,99,122] Available data suggest that the direct effect of thyroid hormone on the heart is mediated via a change in protein synthesis.[10,33,105,149,159] Although the development of clinical manifestations of congestive heart failure or myocardial ischemia in patients with hyperthyroidism usually signifies the presence of underlying cardiac or coronary artery disease, there is evidence that severe thyrotoxicosis can overtax even the normal heart. Congestive heart failure has been produced in experimental animals by administration of thyroxine.[157] Also, it has been documented that in infants with neonatal thyrotoxicosis but without underlying cardiac disease, congestive heart failure may develop.[128]

Myocardial hypertrophy, especially concentric left ventricular hypertrophy, is present in many patients dying with prolonged thyroxoticosis but no characteristic lesion is produced in the human heart by hyperthyroidism.[60,154,155] In a few instances, myofiber necrosis, increased amounts of fat in cardiac muscle cells, and interstitial myocarditis have been reported but have not been established as being secondary to thyroid hormone.[60,154] Although an association of hyperthyroidism with mitral valve prolapse has been suggested, the simultaneous occurrence of these disorders appears to be coincidental.[82,161]

The diagnosis of hyperthyroidism is made by identifying elevated levels of thyroid hormone in the blood. Because only serum triidothyronine is elevated in some individuals, it is important to obtain serum levels of both triiodothyronine and thyroxine as well as an index of the thyroid-binding capacity of the patient's serum.[157]

HYPOTHYROIDISM

Hypothyroidism is the clinical condition that results from reduced secretion of thyroxine and triiodothyronine, usually as a consequence of destruction of the thyroid gland by an inflammatory process.[157] In some cases it is secondary to decreased secretion of thyrotropin secondary to either pituitary or hypothalamic disease. In secondary hypothyroidism, the signs and symptoms associated with deficiency of other pituitary hormones are also usually present.[157] The incidence of hypothyroidism peaks between the ages of 30 and 60 years and is twice as common in women as in men.[157] Infants with congenital hypothyroidism may have a cardiac murmur, pallor, hepatomegaly, and edema appearing before the signs of congenital hypothyroidism, which may not be apparent until 1 to 3 months of age.[156]

With the development of methods that accurately measure circulating levels of thyroid hormones, the diagnosis of hypothyroidism is being made with increasing frequency and at an earlier stage of the disease. Treatment is therefore initiated earlier, resulting in a reduction of the incidence of cardiovascular signs and symptoms, including the classic findings of cardiac enlargement, cardiac dilation, bradycardia, weak arterial pulses, hypotension, distant heart sounds, low cardiographic voltage, and nonpitting facial and peripheral edema. Sufficient data on the pathologic changes in mild hypothyroidism or in hypothyroidism that has been recognized and treated early are not available, since few such patients with an established diagnosis come to autopsy.[157]

In severe myxedema, the heart is usually markedly enlarged and all chambers are dilated. The myocardium appears pale and flabby; however, unless the patient has coexisting hypertension, the ventricular walls exhibit little if any hypertrophy.[56] Hypertension correctable by thyroid hormone replacement occurs in a significant fraction of hypothyroid patients.[92]

Although microscopic changes similar to those occurring in the subcutaneous tissue or skeletal muscle may be present in the myocardium, specific myocardial changes warranting a diagnosis of either "myocarditis" or "myxedema heart" are lacking. The histologic changes most frequently encountered are swelling of myocardial cells, some of which are pale while others are deeply stained and contain small pyknotic nuclei; vacuolization; degeneration of myofibers with a relative loss of cross-striations; and, occasionally, fatty infiltration and interstitial edema.[135] The interstitium may contain accumulations of mucoprotein that is weakly acidic and is periodic acid-Schiff (PAS)-positive. In addition, the myocardial fibers contain an increased amount of basophilic mucoid degeneration over agematched controls.[83] Basophilic mucoid degeneration consists of accumulations of finely granular material in the cytoplasm of isolated individual myofibers and is most commonly present in the myocardium of the left ventricle and ventricular septum[83] (Fig. 31–4). The material stains blue-gray with hematoxylin and

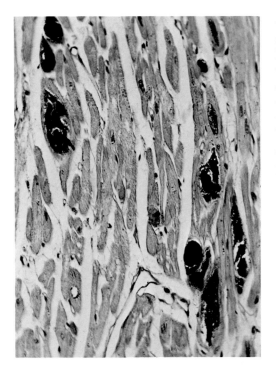

Fig. 31–4. In hypothyroidism, the myocardial fibers contain an increased amount of basophilic mucoid degeneration compared with age-matched controls. Basophilic mucoid degeneration consists of accumulations of finely granular material in the cytoplasm of isolated myofibers. The material stains blue-gray with H&E and is PAS positive. (PAS, × 300.)

eosin (H&E) and is PAS-positive. Ultrastructurally, it consists of fibrils similar to those of glycogen in type IV glycogen storage disease and can be digested, although slowly, by amylase[40,117] (see Ch. 5). The biochemical disorders responsible for these lesions have not been identified. Thickening of the basement membranes of myocardial capillaries with PAS-positive staining has been reported in myxedematous as well as diabetic patients.[130]

Myxedema is associated with increased capillary permeability and subsequent leakage of protein into the interstitial space. This results in pericardial effusion, a common clinical finding in overt myxedema. It occurs in approximately one-third of all patients.[67] In addition

to having a high protein content, the pericardial effusion in myxedema is rich in cholesterol that may occasionally be so concentrated as to give the effusion the appearance of "gold paint."[36] There may be large quantities of fluid (sometimes in excess of 1 L) in the pericardial sac of patients with myxedema, but tamponade is rare, presumably because of a slow rate of accumulation.[4,36,137] In most patients with hypothyroidism and pericardial effusion, sections of the pericardium are histologically normal. However, in patients with large effusions with high levels of cholesterol, "cholesterol pericarditis" may occur as a secondary phenomenon. In cholesterol pericarditis, the parietal and visceral pericardium may become markedly thickened. Histologically, there are giant cells containing cholesterol clefts, mononuclear cells (including foam cells), and fibrous tissue (Fig. 31–5). The pericarditis in hypothyroid patients appear to be a secondary phenomenon, whereas cholesterol pericarditis in euthyroid patients must be associated with an actual pericardial inflammation for cholesterol to accumulate.[114] The cholesterol crystals incite a vigorous cellular reaction enhancing fluid production and pericardial thickening.[114] Chronic exudation and diminished reabsorption of cholesterol might increase its concentration and allow crystalization. The total lipid content of the pericardial fluid, however, is approximately the same as that of the serum.[20] (See Ch. 19, also.)

The sluggish cardiac action in myxedematous patients with feeble pulsations and muffled or distant heart sounds is related to decreased contractile force as well as pericardial effusion. There is little evidence, however, from either experimental or clinical studies, that congestive heart failure is common in myxedema or that it occurs in the absence of other cardiac disease.[1] Presumably the depressed myocardial contractility is sufficient to sustain the reduced workload placed on the heart in hypothyroidism.[157]

Hypertension is one of the more mysterious features of hypothyroidism in that it would

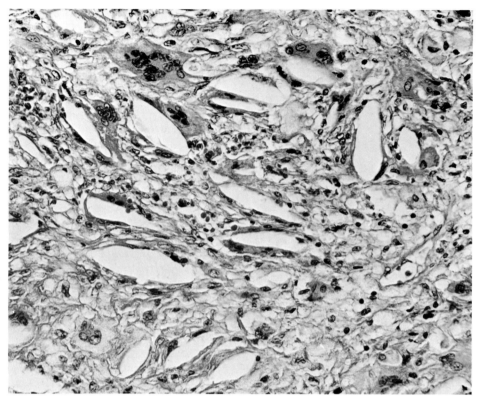

Fig. 31–5. Occasionally, hypothyroid patients with large pericardial effusions and high levels of cholesterol develop cholesterol pericarditis. Multinucleated giant cells, chronic inflammatory cells, and large cholesterol clefts are present in the pericardium of this patient with longstanding untreated myxedema and pericardial effusion containing cholesterol crystals ("gold paint" effusion). (H&E, × 160.)

appear paradoxical that a condition characterized by decreased cardiac output should also produce hypertension. Hyperthyroidism produces systolic hypertension and a widened pulse pressure, whereas the hypertension occasionally seen in hypothyroid patients is both systolic and diastolic and reverts to normal following thyroid hormone replacement.[143] The mechanism for hypertension in these patients is speculative but is believed to be related to changes in arteriolar wall composition.[143]

The view that hypothyroidism accelerates atherogenesis has been disputed by those who maintain that the association is coincidental because the patients are usually in the age group in which significant atherosclerosis is expected.[79,141,143,152] However, hypercholesterolemia, hypertriglyceridemia, and impairment of free fatty acid mobilization, all of which are associated with the development of premature coronary artery disease, are present in patients with hypothyroidism.[157] In those with myxedema, coronary atherosclerosis occurs with twice the frequency of age- and sex-matched controls.[150] Development of atherosclerosis in cholesterol-fed animals is enhanced by hypothyroidism and reduced when thyroid hormone is administered.[97] Hypertension in the presence of lipid abnormalities associated with hypothyroidism may play an important role in accelerating atherosclerosis. Despite the evidence suggesting accelerated atherosclerosis, myocardial infarction and angina are relatively uncommon in patients with hypothyroidism.[66,79,97] It has been suggested that the low frequency of cardiac complications from atherosclerosis is simply a reflection of decreased metabolic demands on the myocardium in hypothyroidism.[157] Indeed, angina pectoris may be precipitated by the institution of thyroid therapy given too rapidly or in excessive dosage.[157]

HYPERPARATHYROIDISM

Hyperparathyroidism, an excess production of parathyroid hormone, is usually secondary to a parathyroid adenoma. Occasionally, generalized parathyroid hyperplasia exists, and infrequently, carcinoma of the parathyroid gland is present. The signs and symptoms of hyperparathyroidism are related to its direct effects on kidney or bone or to those associated with hypercalcemia. Nearly one-half the patients have signs or symptoms of renal dysfunction and, in severe cases, nephrocalcinosis and uremia may occur.[157] Renal failure and uremia from other causes may result in secondary hyperparathyroidism.

The electrocardiographic (ECG) abnormalities, including varying degrees of atrioventricular block, are usually ascribed to hypercalcemia.[81,151] However, several features of hyperparathyroidism other than hypercalcemia per se could possibly cause atrioventricular conduction disturbance. Among them are scattered subendocardial petechiae,[140] focal myocardial necrosis,[62] and focal or diffuse myocardial calcification.[87,148] Hypercalcemia is probably instrumental in the development of these lesions; indeed, an increased incidence of calcification of cardiac valves and the ventricular septum sometimes accompanied by complete heart block has been demonstrated in other disorders resulting in hypercalcemia, such as generalized Paget's disease of bone.[53,69]

Although hypertension is not a frequent presenting sign of primary hyperparathyroidism, it is present in some patients, especially when there is significant renal impairment.[29,81] Hypertension is more frequent when primary renal disease results in secondary hyperparathyroidism.[81] Calcification of the myocardium and blood vessels occurs more frequently and to a greater extent with secondary hyperparathyroidism due to renal disease than with primary hyperparathyroidism.[81,87]

Metastatic calcification involving the coronary arteries has been well documented in hyperparathyroidism and may lead to myocardial fibrosis with congestive heart failure[87] (Fig. 31–6). In addition to calcification of cor-

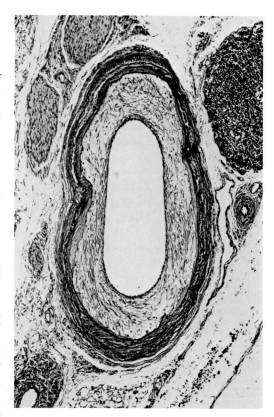

Fig. 31–6. The arterial calcification of hyperparathyroidism characteristically involves the internal elastic membrane and adjacent media. Although the large elastic arteries are commonly affected by metastatic calcification, medium-sized muscular arteries, as well as arterioles, capillaries, and venules may be involved. Metastatic calcification of coronary arteries is a common finding. The associated intimal proliferation may be sufficient to cause ischemic myocardial damage. (Movat's pentachrome, × 40.)

onary arteries, there may be myocardial calcification, which is particularly ominous when it involves the conduction system (Fig. 31–7). Calcified nodules situated high in the bundle of His may cause complete heart block. In uremic patients, calcification and fibrosis of the sinoatrial and atrioventricular nodes are not uncommon.[87] In the myocardium, metastatic calcification first appears as a fine basophilic granulation in small groups of otherwise normal myofibers. Later, myofiber degeneration becomes apparent, and eventually confluent areas of calcification completely replace large areas of myocardium and are commonly surrounded by dense fibrous tissue.[87]

Uremia may influence the development of multiple, minute foci of myocardial necrosis that subsequently calcify. The laws of mass action and of ionic equilibrium of saturated solutions of poorly soluble salts explain, in the case of tricalcium phosphate, the ease with which precipitation may be induced by increases of calcium or phosphate.[12] Massive calcification of the myocardium may be revealed in radiographs during a patient's life.[12]

The arterial calcification of hyperparathyroidism characteristically involves the internal elastic membrane and adjacent media. Although the large elastic arteries (the aorta and pulmonary artery) are commonly affected in metastatic calcification, medium-sized muscular arteries, as well as arterioles, capillaries, and venules, may also be involved.[87] Metastatic calcification of coronary arteries and arterioles with luminal narrowing is a common finding; the intimal proliferation associated with this calcification may occasionally be sufficient to cause ischemic myocardial damage.[26] The myocardial and vascular pathology of advanced secondary hyperparathyroidism clearly plays a prominent role in the increased death rate in patients with chronic renal failure.[55,87]

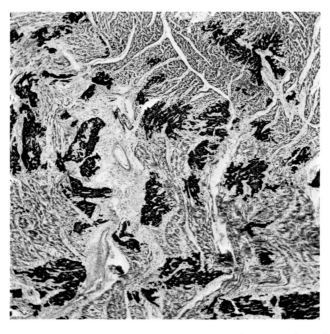

Fig. 31–7. In addition to calcification of the coronary arteries in hyperparathyroidism, there may be myocardial calcification. Such metastatic calcification appears first as a fine basophilic granulation in small groups of otherwise normal myofibers. Later, myofiber degeneration becomes apparent; eventually confluent areas of calcification completely replace large areas of myocardium. (H&E, × 80.)

In addition to myocardial and vascular metastatic calcification, there is evidence that hyperparathyroidism may contribute to risk factors associated with accelerated atherosclerosis. Hyperparathyroidism seems to have a minor role in abnormal carbohydrate metabolism and a minimal effect on hyperlipidemia.[55,72]

In addition to myocardial and arterial lesions, patients with hyperparathyroidism often have endocardial calcification, especially in the presence of uremia. Valvular calcification due to hyperparathyroidism may follow or accentuate pre-existing valvular disease. When valvular calcification occurs in the uremic patient with secondary hyperparathyroidism, the aortic valve is most commonly involved.[87] Mitral annular calcification is more common in patients with chronic renal failure and secondary hyperparathyroidism than in other patients of similar age.[42]

Hypoparathyroidism causes no specific cardiac disease other than ECG abnormalities secondary to hypocalcemia and impaired cardiac contractility, resulting in a potentially reversible dilated cardiomyopathy.[42,44,76,81,110]

CUSHING SYNDROME, ALDOSTERONISM, AND ADDISON'S DISEASE

Cushing Syndrome

Cushing syndrome is characterized by truncal obesity, hypertension, fatigue, weakness, amenorrhea, hirsutism, purple abdominal striae, glucosuria, edema, and osteoporosis. Hypertension is present in 80 to 90 percent of these patients, and diabetes mellitus in approximately 20 percent.[77,158] There is both clinical and laboratory evidence of excess production of glucocorticoids and androgens in most cases.[157]

Cushing syndrome has several causative mechanisms. The most common is an excess production of glucocorticoids and androgens

from bilateral adrenal hyperplasia.[77] Other causes are secondary to adenocorticotrophic hormone (ACTH)-producing tumors, either nonendocrine carcinomas (ectopic ACTH syndrome), or by a pituitary tumor. Occasional cases may be caused by a primary adrenal adenoma or carcinoma. Cushing syndrome may also occur as a component of multiple endocrine syndromes, with or without concomitant cardiac myxoma.[24]

The most common cardiac structural alterations in Cushing syndrome are secondary to the effects of hypertension and accelerated atherosclerosis. The pathogenesis of hypertension in Cushing syndrome is most likely multifactorial, including volume expansion, glucocorticoid potentiation of vascular smooth muscle response to vasoconstrictive agents, and ACTH- or cortisol-induced increases in renin substrate.[157] The mineralocorticoid activity of cortisol, in addition to the excess production of mineralocorticoid from the adrenal cortex, probably plays a dominant role in producing sodium retention, hypertension, and hypokalemic alkalosis.[15] Although hypertension probably has a major role in the development of accelerated atherosclerosis in these patients, other factors known to stimulate atherogenesis are also present. Chronic excess production of cortisol leads to hyperlipidemia, hypercholesterolemia, and an increased distribution of adipose tissues. Hypercholesterolemia is common,[138] and advanced atherosclerosis has been described in children with this syndrome.[121]

The mineralocorticoid excess present in patients with Cushing syndrome may also contribute to the cardiac pathology by enhancing the effects of catecholamines on the myocardium, resulting in the production of focal myocardial lesions consisting of myofibrillar degeneration, identical to those present in the myocardium of patients dying with pheochromocytoma.[126] The focal vacuolization and hyalinization of cardiac muscle cells in some patients dying with Cushing syndrome may be secondary to chronic hypokalemia (Fig. 31–8).

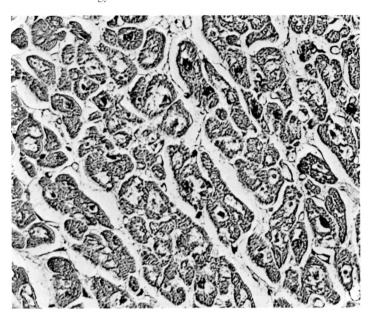

Fig. 31–8. Focal vacuolization of cardiac muscle cells may be found in patients dying of Cushing syndrome. The vacuolization is nonspecific and is similar to that occasionally seen in patients receiving glucocorticoid therapy or in those with chronic hypokalemia. (H&E, × 300.)

The diagnosis of Cushing syndrome requires laboratory confirmation of both high cortisol production and disturbed physiologic control mechanisms. The diagnosis is established by the lack of appropriate suppression of cortisol secretion by dexamethasone.[157]

Aldosteronism

Aldosteronism is the syndrome associated with increased secretion of aldosterone. When the stimulus for the excess production originates within the adrenal, the syndrome is termed *primary* aldosteronism. When the stimulus is of extra-adrenal origin, the term *secondary* aldosteronism applies. Both conditions result in excess mineralocorticoid secretion with retention of sodium and loss of potassium.[157] The most common cardiac structural alterations in aldosteronism are secondary to the effects of hypertension and hypokalemic alkalosis, described previously under Cushing syndrome.

The diagnosis of primary aldosteronism is established by diastolic hypertension without edema, hypersecretion of aldosterone that fails to suppress appropriately during volume expansion, hyposecretion of renin, and hypokalemia with inappropriate urinary potassium loss during salt loading.[157] Secondary aldosteronism may be distinguished from primary aldosteronism by the plasma renin activity that is elevated in the former and reduced in the latter.[157]

Addison's Disease

Addison's disease (primary adrenal insufficiency) may result from idiopathic atrophy, destruction of the adrenals by granulomatous processes (such as tuberculosis or histoplasmosis), replacement of the adrenal gland by amyloid or neoplastic tumors, and acute hemorrhagic necrosis due to infection or during anticoagulant therapy.[15] Other causes include selective hypoaldosteronism, enzyme deficiency (congenital adrenal hyperplasia) and secondary adrenal insufficiency due to a lack of ACTH.[157] The metabolic abnormalities in Addison's disease are secondary to deficiencies in both cortisol and aldosterone production, resulting in hemoconcentration, hypoglycemia, azotemia, hyperkalemia, hyponatremia, mild acidosis, and occasionally hypercalcemia.[15]

The most common cardiovascular finding in adrenal insufficiency is arterial hypotension with a decrease in peripheral pulses and heart size. The heart in Addison's disease is characteristically small and hypodynamic. The small size is due to the combined influence of relative disuse atrophy and hypovolemia, as well as deprivation of the direct effects of adrenal steroids.[15] In patients dying with adrenal insufficiency over a prolonged time, there is an actual decrease in heart mass, and the cardiac muscle fibers appear thin and atrophic histologically.[11,120]

PHEOCHROMOCYTOMA

Pheochromocytomas are catecholamine-producing tumors derived from chromaffin cells. When they arise from extra-adrenal chromaffin cells, they are termed nonadrenal pheochromocytomas, or paragangliomas. Although most of these tumors occur sporadically, approximately 5 percent are inherited as an autosomal trait and may be part of a pluriglandular neoplastic syndrome, which may include medullary carcinoma of the thyroid, hyperparathyroidism, and retinal or cerebellar hemangioblastomas.[157] Rarely, a multiendocrine syndrome may be associated with cardiac myxoma.[24] Pheochromocytomas are usually solitary adrenal tumors; however, approximately 10 percent are bilateral and 10 percent are nonadrenal. In the familial form of pheochromocytoma, approximately half the patients have bilateral adrenal tumors.[157] Tumors secreting increased quantities of norepinephrine only and various mixtures of nor-

epinephrine and epinephrine are well known. Rarely, pure elevations of epinephrine and its primary metabolite, metanephrine, have been documented.[54]

Hypertension is the major cardiovascular manifestation of pheochromocytoma. Although paroxysmal attacks of hypertension are a hallmark of pheochromocytoma, more than half of the patients have fixed hypertension and nearly 10 percent are normotensive.[157] Many of the clinical features are similar to those of hyperthyroidism; therefore, only a clinical awareness of the entity and specific laboratory testing permit proper diagnosis.

In addition to the structural alterations induced by hypertension, at least 50 percent of patients dying with pheochromocytoma will have foci of myocardial necrosis with contraction bands (myofibrillar degeneration)[133] (see Ch. 16). Early lesions consist of myocardial hemorrhages, most conspicuous on the endocardial surfaces, with minimal to no involvement of the heart valves.[70] These subendocardial hemorrhages are chiefly found in the left ventricle, characteristically along the papillary muscles.[109] Microscopically, there is loss of definition of the linear arrangement of myofibrils with cross-striations and the appearance of areas of dense eosinophilic transverse banding, alternating with lighter-staining granular zones within the cytoplasm[108] (Fig. 31–9). This characteristic becomes less prominent with the passage of time, as macrophages infiltrate and phagocytose necrotic cell debris. In some instances areas of cytoplasmic bands are occasionally seen immediately adjacent to intercalated discs, and there is retention of cross-striation in the remainder of the cell cytoplasm. More frequently, there is no special intracellular localization and several separate bands can be seen within a single myofiber.[41] A basophilic, finely granular material is often present between the eosinophilic bands and represents translocated mitochondria initially containing amorphous calcium phosphate and later calcium hydroxiapatite. These calcific deposits are regarded as evidence of irreversible mi-

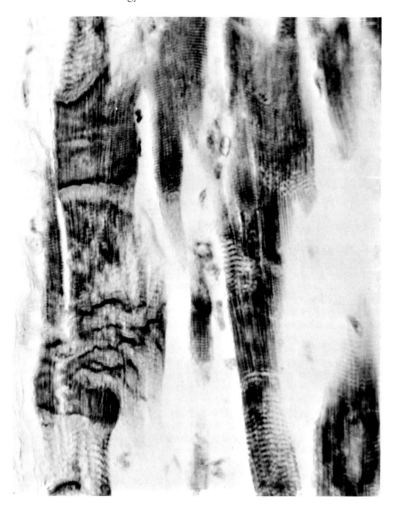

Fig. 31–9. Myocardial necrosis with contraction bands is usually present in the myocardium of patients dying with pheochromocytoma. There is loss of definition of the linear arrangement of myofibrils with cross-striations and appearance of areas of dense eosinophilic transverse banding, alternating with lighter-staining granular zones within the cytoplasm. (H&E, × 400.)

tochondrial damage.[22] Progression of necrosis with contraction bands to a stage of myocytolysis is mediated through lysis of the myofilaments, a change that results in an empty appearance of the cells[125] (Fig. 31–10). In later stages, stromal condensation of fibrosis may become evident, resulting in focal myocardial fibrosis[109] (Fig. 31–11). Polymorphonuclear leukocytes surrounding the injured myocardial cells are scarce or absent and never be-

come prominent among the cells reacting in this type of injury (in contrast to the cellular reaction that occurs in a myocardial infarction). This type of myocardial damage is not specific for pheochromocytoma. Indeed, it can be found regularly in patients dying after cardiovascular surgery,[98,108,146] subarachnoid hemorrhage,[48] or hypovolemic shock,[85] and at the periphery of areas of typical ischemic coagulation necrosis in patients dying of

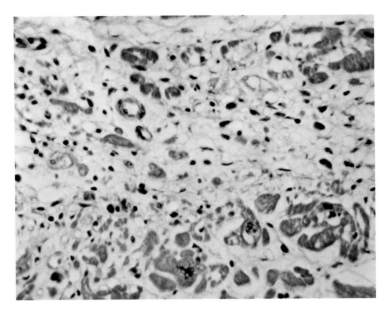

Fig. 31–10. Progression of necrosis with contraction bands to a stage of myocytolysis is mediated through lysis of the myofilaments, a change that results in an empty appearance of the cells. (Movat's pentachrome, × 300.)

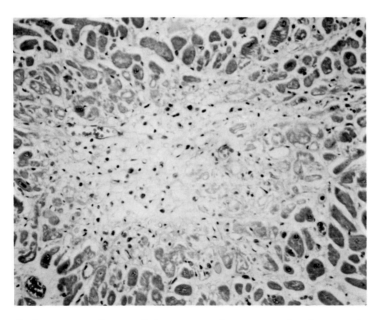

Fig. 31–11. In the later stages of myocardial necrosis with contraction bands, stromal condensation and fibrosis may become evident, resulting in focal myocardial fibrosis. Usually early, intermediate, and late stages of this lesion are evident microscopically in the myocardium of patients with longstanding pheochromocytoma. (Movat's pentachrome, × 195.)

myocardial infarction.[108] The lesion can also be produced in experimental animals by many different means.[109]

The diagnosis of pheochromocytoma is established by documenting increased urinary levels of catecholamines or catecholamine metabolites, such as vanillyl mandelic acid (VMA) or metanephrine. In screening for pheochromocytoma, it is prudent to measure both the catecholamine level and one of the two metabolites, preferably metanephrine.[157]

Paragangliomas (intrapericardial pheochromocytomas) may involve the base of the heart, especially the posterior wall of the left atrium. They are usually invasive and are extremely vascular, making surgical resection difficult. In one reported case, a paraganglioma was resected during a procedure that involved removal and reimplantation of the entire heart.[58]

DIABETES MELLITUS

Diabetes mellitus is a metabolic disorder characterized by an absolute or relative lack of insulin, which results in impaired utilization of carbohydrates and altered lipid and protein metabolism. Most cases of adult-onset diabetes mellitus are probably the result of genetic predisposition; however, many cases of the juvenile form may be infectious in origin.[31,111] Other forms of nonhereditary diabetes mellitus include destruction of a significant portion of the pancreas and its islets (either surgically or by disease) and other endocrinopathies, including hyperadrenalism, acromegaly, and pheochromocytoma. While these endocrinopathies affect carbohydrate metabolism and induce hyperglycemia and diabetes, control of the basic endocrine dysfunction corrects the metabolic derangement. The impaired carbohydrate, fat, and protein metabolism of the diabetic patient eventually involves all the endocrine glands, but primarily the anterior pituitary and the adrenal glands.[112] Growth hormone is necessary for

the mobilization of triglycerides; however, the liberated fatty acids act as insulin inhibitors. Adrenal steroids are involved in the process of gluconeogenesis. Therefore, diabetes mellitus is a complex metabolic pluriglandular systemic disorder manifested primarily by glycosuria, hypercholesterolemia, and frequently ketoacidosis.[112]

Although metabolic derangements are significant to the survival of the diabetic, they usually can be controlled medically by proper diet or by the use of insulin or oral hypoglycemia agents, as indicated. A greater threat to health is the increased susceptibility to generalized vascular disease, mainly atherosclerosis and small vessel disease (microangiopathy) (see Chs. 11, 12, and 13). Atherosclerosis usually appears in diabetic patients at an earlier age than in nondiabetics and is often more severe, progresses more rapidly, and produces greater disability.[7] Accelerated atherosclerosis accounts for the increased frequency of myocardial infarction, cerebral vascular disease, and peripheral vascular disease. The incidence of coronary heart disease, the leading cause of death among adult diabetics, appears to correlate more closely with the duration of diabetes than with the severity.[157] However, it is suggested that patients with juvenile diabetes have less clinical evidence of vascular disease when episodes of ketoacidosis are absent.[103,115,116] In addition, the presence of diabetes mellitus beginning early in life does not always indicate the presence of coronary heart disease, either clinically or at autopsy, 20 or more years later.[32] There is evidence that the role of diabetes mellitus as a cardiovascular risk factor does not derive from an altered ability to contend with other known risk factors.[64]

Diabetic patients have an increased risk of cerebrovascular disease, with a greater incidence of cerebral infarction but not cerebral hemorrhage.[2] Accelerated atherosclerosis in the peripheral blood vessels may result in renal failure, mesenteric artery occlusion with intestinal infarction, and gangrene of the lower extremities. The smaller arteries below the knee are more likely to be involved in patients with diabetes, in contrast to iliac or femoral artery disease in nondiabetic patients[144] (see Ch. 10). The vascular changes affecting the kidney, often in combination with parenchymal damage secondary to pyelonephritis, result in a variety of renal disorders including hypertension and uremia, both of which also accelerate atherosclerosis.[87,157]

Pathologically, diabetic microangiopathy manifests itself by thickening of the basement membrane of precapillaries, capillaries, and venules in many parts of the body[13,14,131,139,153] (see also Ch. 12). The lesion is largely the consequence of uneven thickening and splitting of the basement membrane of the small vessels accompanied by the deposition of a PAS-positive material rich in mucopolysaccharide. In addition, immunoglobulins and complement have been identified in some thickened capillaries.[16] Microangiopathy is responsible for the clinical manifestations of diabetic retinopathy and diabetic glomerulosclerosis. Other manifestations of microangiopathy are controversial. The basement membranes of myocardial capillaries have been reported thicker in diabetic than in control patients.[17,50,52,73–75,123,130,160] In addition to PAS-positive staining of the basement membrane, subintimal deposits of PAS-positive material may be present.[49,106] Some of the affected vessels may exhibit an increase in periarterial collagen, which occasionally extends between the cardiac muscle cells.[106,107] Although microaneurysms have been demonstrated in the hearts of diabetics by postmortem injection studies, histologic verification of their presence is lacking, and their significance is unclear.[38]

Proliferation of intimal and endothelial cells of small arterioles leading to luminal compromise has been described with greater frequency in diabetics than in nondiabetics, and is considered by some a manifestation of small vessel disease.[16,17] Such blood vessel changes are similar to those found in various "immune" disorders and have been

postulated to result from an autoimmune process initiated by insulin.[16] However, others interpret these changes as merely reflecting increased permeability of damaged vessels.[71]

The risk of diabetic patients developing congestive heart failure is increased substantially over the nondiabetic population.[65] This increased risk persists after taking into account age, blood pressure, weight, cholesterol values, and coronary heart disease. One suggested possibility for this increased incidence of congestive heart failure is a diabetes-induced cardiomyopathy[52,106,107,127] (see Ch. 21). Although congestive cardiomyopathy has been reported in association with diabetes mellitus, the morphologic findings have been variable and nonspecific; they include PAS-positive staining material in the interstitium, increased perivascular and interstitial collagen, and increased amounts of triglyceride and cholesterol in cardiac muscle cells, in addition to intramyocardial microangiopathy. No lesion specific for diabetic cardiomyopathy has been identified.[145]

THE CARCINOID SYNDROME

Carcinoid tumors arise from enterochromaffin cells (Kultchitsky cells), which are found throughout the gastrointestinal tract. These cells, which contain granules that often stain with silver either directly (argentaffin cells) or upon addition of a reducing agent (argyrophilic cells), are also found normally in the bronchi, bile duct, and pancreatic ducts.[80] Primary functioning carcinoid tumors arising in the pancreatic ducts have been described. Carcinoid tumors in ovarian or testicular teratomas have also been reported.[9,124] Most commonly, primary carcinoid tumors arise in the small intestine (chiefly in the terminal ileum) or in the appendix. Usually, appendiceal carcinoids are localized and seldom metastasize to produce the carcinoid syndrome.[68]

The functional carcinoid syndrome most frequently occurs with carcinoid tumors of the small intestine after metastases to regional lymph nodes and liver have occurred. Carcinoid tumors of the stomach and bronchi produce syndromes that may differ from the classic syndrome associated with ileal carcinoids.[93,100,132] The tumor produces several biologically active substances, including serotonin (5-hydroxytryptamine), histamine, and kinin peptides (bradykinin). Dermal flushing and diarrhea occur in almost all patients with the syndrome; wheezing occurs in approximately one-third, and thickening of valvular and mural endocardium of the heart is present in more than one-half of affected patients.[39,46] Telangiectasia may develop in the skin over the nasal bridge, malar area, and upper chest. Rarely, a permanent cyanotic hue may result in the flush area.[80]

In carcinoid heart disease, there is either focal or diffuse plaquelike thickening of valvular and mural endocardium, and occasionally of the intima of the great veins, coronary sinus, pulmonary trunk, and main pulmonary arteries.[39,51] These plaques usually appear only in patients with hepatic metastases or when the venous blood from the tumor bypasses the liver, as with bronchial or ovarian carcinoids. The fibrous tissue is atypical and is limited in most instances to the right side of the heart.[39] When the pulmonary valve is involved, deposition is almost exclusively on the arterial aspect of the valve cusps (Fig. 31–12). The fibrous tissue is located predominantly on the ventricular aspect of the posterior and septal leaflets of the tricuspid valve, and about equally on the ventricular and atrial aspect of the anterior leaflet when the latter is affected.[39,80,88] Involvement of the tricuspid valve often causes the leaflets to adhere to the adjacent ventricular wall, producing regurgitation as the principal functional defect. The pulmonic valve becomes predominantly stenotic, although some regurgitation may occur.[25] These carcinoid fibrous plaques are also deposited on the endocardial surface of the right atrium, especially on the atrial septum

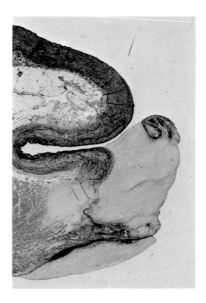

Fig. 31–12. In carcinoid heart disease, there is either focal or diffuse plaquelike thickening of valvular and mural endocardium. When the pulmonary valve is involved, as was the case in this patient, deposition of fibrous tissue is almost exclusively on the arterial aspect of valve cusps. (Movat's pentachrome, × 10.)

immediately proximal to the junction of the septal and anterior tricuspid leaflets (Fig. 31–13). When there is diffuse deposition of fibrous tissue on the endocardium of the right atrium, its walls become relatively noncompliant.[88] Fibrous plaques are less extensive in the right ventricle than in the atrium, and usually consist of capping of the papillary muscles, most commonly resulting in no functional significance.[80]

Similar lesions may be observed in the mitral and aortic valves in patients with predominantly right-sided carcinoid heart disease and a patent foramen ovale, or in those with a functioning bronchial carcinoid tumor, or with pulmonary metastases.[6,94,113] In some patients with predominant right-sided carcinoid heart disease, the mitral and aortic valves also may be involved to a lesser degree.[88] Involvement of the left side of the heart appears to be a late development of the disease, except

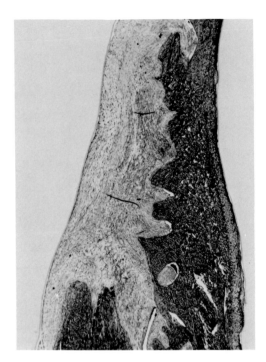

Fig. 31–13. Carcinoid fibrous plaques are also deposited on the endocardial surface of the right atrium, especially on the atrial septum. Microscopically, the lesions contain fibroblasts, myofibroblasts, and smooth muscle cells embedded in a distinctive stroma rich in collagen and proteoglycans but lacking elastic fibers. The mural endocardium and valve cusps, per se, are morphologically normal and clearly separated from the atypical fibrous tissue by intact elastic lamellae. (Movat's pentachrome, × 13.)

in the presence of a right-to-left shunt or a bronchial carcinoid.[80] When the mitral valve is extensively involved, the posterior mitral leaflet may adhere to the underlying mural endocardium, resulting in mitral regurgitation. When the aortic valve is extensively involved, the fibrous plaquing is usually on the arterial surface within the sinuses of Valsalva, predisposing the valve to stenosis or insufficiency.[39]

Microscopically, these lesions contain fibroblasts, myofibroblasts, and smooth muscle cells embedded in a distinctive stroma rich in collagen and proteoglycans but lacking in elas-

tic fibers.[39] The cellular elements are narrow, elongated, arranged parallel to the surface of the plaque, and stain intensely with phosphotungstic acid hematoxylin. The valvular cusps and the mural endocardium, per se, are morphologically normal and clearly separated from the atypical fibrous tissue by intact elastic lamellae.[39] Blood vessels, often thick-walled, may be immediately adjacent to the valve leaflets. Lymphocytes, plasma cells, and occasionally mast cells are frequently located adjacent to these blood vessels.[88]

The pathogenesis of the carcinoid plaque is uncertain. It has not been possible to produce the valvular and endocardial lesions in animals by giving serotonin, and urinary levels of the breakdown product of serotonin, 5-hydroxyindoleacetic acid (5-HIAA), and blood serotonin levels have been similar in patients with the carcinoid syndrome with and without cardiac involvement.[134,147] However, serotonin does stimulate fibroblast growth in tissue culture.[18] Initially serotonin was also believed to be responsible for the dermal flush in this syndrome, but this hypothesis has been challenged.[101,102] A kinin peptide such as bradykinin appears the more likely cause of the flush and may also participate in the development of the carcinoid endocardial lesions, although this has not been demonstrated.[101,102]

Although the valvular and endocardial lesions were once believed pathognomonic of this condition, identical lesions lacking in elastic fibers have been described in patients being treated with methysergide and, less commonly, with ergotamine tartrate.[8,47,86,89,90] The similarity of the chemical structure of methysergide to that of serotonin to which it is an antagonist is striking.[47] The major difference between the cardiac lesions in carcinoid syndrome and those associated with methysergide is the predominant right-sided cardiac involvement in the carcinoid syndrome, compared with the preponderance of left-sided disease associated with methysergide.[90] When the atrioventricular valves are involved with methysergide-associated fibrosis, the fibrous thickening not uncommonly involves the chordae tendineae and the tips of the papillary muscles. The chordae tendineae may be thickened and fused.[86] The endocardium may contain similar lesions with or without contiguity with the valvular lesions. Occasionally, extensive endocardial fibrosis is associated with adjacent intramyocardial fibrosis.[86]

Even though neither serotonin nor its byproduct (5-HIAA) has been unequivocally implicated in the pathogenesis of the valvular and endocardial lesions in carcinoid heart disease, the excessive production of serotonin resulting in increased levels of 5-HIAA excreted in the urine has offered a useful noninvasive diagnostic test. Increased urinary levels of 5-HIAA occur only in those patients with hepatic metastases or if the venous blood from the neoplasm bypasses the liver. Urinary 5-HIAA levels may also be elevated by eating serotonin-containing foods, such as bananas or pineapples. Drugs such as phenothiazines, glyceryl guaiacolate, and methocarbamol compounds may also interfere with the nitrosonaphthol method for 5-HIAA determination.

REFERENCES

1. Aber CP, Thompson GS: The heart in hypothyroidism. Am Heart J 68:429, 1964
2. Alex M, Baron EK, Goldenberg S, Blumenthal HT: An autopsy study of cerebrovascular accident in diabetes mellitus. Circulation 25:663, 1962
3. Aloia JF, Field RA: The heart and the endocrine system. p. 1252. In Conn HL Jr, Horwitz O (eds): Cardiac and Vascular Disease. Vol. II. Lea & Febiger, Philadelphia, 1971
4. Alsever RN, Stjernholm MR: Cardiac tamponade in myxedema. Am J Med Sci 269:117, 1975
5. Atkinson FRB: Acromegaly. John Bale Sons and Danielsson, London, 1932
6. Azzopardi JG, Bellau AR: Carcinoid syndrome and oat-cell carcinoma of the bronchus. Thorax 20:393, 1965
7. Balodimos MC, Cahill GF Jr: Diabetes and vascular disease. Part IV. p. 1284. In Conn HL Jr, Horwitz O (eds): Cardiac and Vascular Disease. Vol. II. Lea & Febiger, Philadelphia, 1971
8. Bana DS, McNeal PS, LeCompte PM, et al: Cardiac murmurs and endocardial fibrosis associated with methysergide therapy. Am Heart J 88:640, 1975
9. Bancroft JHJ, O'Brien DJ, Tickner A: Carcinoid syndrome due to carcinoid tumour of the ovary. Br Med J 2:1440, 1964
10. Banerjee SK, Flink IL, Morkin E: Enzymatic properties of native and N-ethylmaleimide-modified cardiac myosin from normal and thyrotoxic rabbits. Circ Res 39:319, 1976
11. Barker NW: The pathological anatomy in 28 cases of Addison's disease. Arch Pathol 8:432, 1929
12. Batsakis JG: Degenerative lesions of the heart. p. 483. In Gould SE (ed): Pathology of the Heart and Blood Vessels. 3rd Ed. Charles C Thomas, Springfield, IL, 1968
13. Beisswenger PJ, Spiro RG: Human glomerular basement membrane: Chemical alteration in diabetes mellitus. Science 168:596, 1970
14. Berkman J, Rifkin H: Newer aspects of diabetic microangiopathy. Annu Rev Med 17:83, 1966
15. Bledsoe T: Cardiovascular abnormalities in disorders of the adrneal cortex. Part V. p. 1295. In Conn HL Jr, Horwitz O (eds): Cardiac and Vascular Diseases, Vol. II. Lea & Febiger, Philadelphia, 1971
16. Blumenthal HT: The relation of microangiopathies to arteriosclerosis, with special reference to diabetes. Ann NY Acad Sci 149:834, 1968
17. Blumenthal HT, Alex M, Goldenberg S: A study of lesions of the intramural coronary artery branches in diabetes mellitus. Arch Pathol 70:27, 1960
18. Bowcek RJ, Alvarez TR: 5-hydroxytryptamine: A cytospecific growth stimulator of cultured fibroblasts. Science 167:898, 1970
19. Brigden W: Uncommon myocardial diseases: The noncoronary cardiomyopathies. Lancet 2:7007, 1957
20. Brown AK: Chronic idiopathic pericardial effusion. Br Heart J 28:609, 1966
21. Buccino RA, Spann JF, Pool PE, Braunwald

E: Influence of the thyroid state on the intrinsic contractile properties and the energy stores of the myocardium. J Clin Invest 46:1669, 1967

22. Buja LM, Dees JH, Harling DF, Willerson JT: Analytical electron microscopic study of mitochondrial inclusions in canine myocardial infarcts. J Histochem Cytochem 24:508, 1976

23. Cairoli VJ, Crout JR: Role of the autonomic nervous system in the resting tachycardia of experimental hyperthyroidism. J Pharmacol Exp Ther 158:55, 1967

24. Carney JA, Gordon H, Carpenter PC, et al: The complex of myxomas, spotty pigmentation, and endocrine overactivity. Medicine (Baltimore) 64:270, 1985

25. Carpena C, Kay JH, Mendez AM, et al: Carcinoid heart disease. Surgery for tricuspid and pulmonary valve lesions. Am J Cardiol 32:229, 1973

26. Cheitlin MD, McAllister HA Jr, de Castro CM: Myocardial infarction without atherosclerosis. JAMA 231:951, 1975

27. Cluxoon HE Jr, Bennett WA, Kepler EJ: Anterior pituitary insufficiency (panhypopituitarism-Simmond's disease), pituitary myxedema, and congestive heart failure (myxedema heart). Report of a case and findings at necropsy. Ann Intern Med 29:732, 1948

28. Coggeshall C, Root HF: Acromegaly and diabetes mellitus. Endocrinology 26:1, 1940

29. Cope O: The story of hyperparathyroidism at the Massachusetts General Hospital. N Engl J Med 274:1174, 1966

30. Courville C, Mason VR: The heart in acromegaly. Arch Intern Med 61:704, 1938

31. Craighead JE: Viral diabetes mellitus in man and experimental animals. Am J Med 70:127, 1981

32. Crall FV Jr, Roberts WC: The extramural and intramural coronary arteries in juvenile diabetes mellitus. Analysis of nine necropsy patients aged 19 to 38 years with onset of diabetes before age 15 years. Am J Med 64:221, 1978

33. Curfman GD, Crowley TJ, Smith TW: Thyroid-induced alterations in myocardial sodium- and potassium-activated adenosine triphosphatase, monovalent cation active transport and cardiac glycoside binding. J Clin Invest 59:586, 1977

34. Curtarelli G, Ferri C: Cardiomegaly and heart failure in a patient with prolactin secreting pituitary tumor. Thorax 34:328, 1979

35. Cushing H, Davidoff LM: The pathologic findings in four autopsied cases of acromegaly with a discussion of their significance. Monograph 22. The Rockefeller Institute for Medical Research, New York, 1927, p. 1

36. David PJ, Jacobson S: Myxedema with cardiac tamponade and pericardial effusion of "gold paint" appearance. Arch Intern Med 120:615, 1967

37. Epstein CC: Extreme cardiac enlargement. Ann Intern Med 48:1387, 1958

38. Factor SM, Okin EM, Minase T: Capillary microaneurysms in the human diabetic heart. N Engl J Med 14:384, 1980

39. Ferrans VJ, Roberts WC: The carcinoid endocardial plaque. An ultrastructural study. Hum Pathol 7:387, 1976

40. Ferrans VJ, Buja LM, Jones M: Ultrastructure and cytochemistry of glycogen in cardiac diseases. p. 97. In Dhalla NS (ed): Recent Advances in Studies on Cardiac Structure and Metabolism. Myocardial Metabolism. Vol. 3. University Park Press, Baltimore, 1973

41. Ferrans VJ, Hibbs RG, Black WC, Weilbaecher DG: Isoproterenol-induced myocardial necrosis. A histochemical and electron microscopic study. Am Heart J 68:71, 1964

42. Forman MB, Virmani R, Robertson RM, Stone WJ: Mitral annular calcification in chronic renal failure. Chest 85:367, 1984

43. Gibbs DD: Werner's syndrome ("Progeria of the Adult"). Proc R Soc Med 60:135, 1967

44. Giles TD, Iteld BJ, Rives HL: The cardiomyopathy of hypoparathyroidism: Another reversible form of heart muscle disease. Chest 79:225, 1981

45. Gordon DA, Hill FM, Ezrin C: Acromegaly: A review of 100 cases. Can Med Assoc J 87:1106, 1962

46. Grahame-Smith DG: The carcinoid syndrome. p. 1703. In Bondy PK, Rosenberg LE (eds): Metabolic Control and Disease. 9th Ed. WB Saunders, Philadelphia, 1980

47. Grahan JR: Cardiac and pulmonary fibrosis during methysergide therapy for headache. Am J Med Sci 254:1, 1967

48. Greenhoot JH, Reichenbach DD: Cardiac injury and subarachnoid hemorrhage. A clinical, pathological, and physiological correlation. J Neurosurg 30:521, 1969

49. Haerem JW: Cushion-like intimal lesions in intramyocardial arteries of man: Their relation to age, sex, coronary atherosclerosis, and certain diseases. Acta Pathol Microbiol Scand 77:598, 1969

50. Halkin H, Ravid M: Involvement of the intramural coronary circulation in diabetic angiopathy. Isr J Med Sci 8:733, 1972

51. Hall RJ, McAllister HA Jr, Cooley DA, Frazier OH: Neoplastic heart disease. p. 1382. In Hurst JW (ed): The Heart. 7th Ed. McGraw-Hill, New York, 1990

52. Hamby RI, Zoneraich S, Sherman L: Diabetes cardiomyopathy. JAMA 229:1749, 1974

53. Harrison CV, Lennox B: Heart block in osteitis deformans. Br Med J 10:167, 1948

54. Harrison TS, Bartlett JD Jr, Seaton JF: Current evaluation and management of pheochromocytoma. Ann Surg 168:701, 1968

55. Herrmann G, Hehrmann R, Scholz HC, et al: Parathyroid hormone in coronary artery disease—Results of a prospective study. J Endocrinol Invest 9:265, 1986

56. Higgins WH: The heart in myxedema. Am J Med Sci 191:80, 1936

57. Hinsdale G: Acromegaly (reprinted). William M Warren, Detroit, 1898

58. Hui G, McAllister HA Jr, Angelini P: Left atrial paraganglioma: Report of a case and review of the literature. Am Heart J 113:1230, 1987

59. Humphry L, Dixon WE: A case of acromegaly with hypertrophied heart: Pressor substances in the urine. Br Med J 2:1047, 1910

60. Hurxthal LM: Heart failure and hyperthyroidism, with special reference to etiology. Am Heart J 4:103, 1928

61. Hurxthal LM, Dee JF: Acromegaly. Lahey Clin Bull 3:196, 1944

62. James PR, Richards PG: Parathyroid crisis. Arch Surg 72:553, 1956

63. Jonas EA, Aloia JR, Lane FJ: Evidence of subclinical heart muscle dysfunction in acromegaly. Chest 67:190, 1975

64. Kannel WB, McGee DL: Diabetes and cardiovascular risk factors: The Framingham study. Circulation 59:8, 1979

65. Kannel WB, Hjortland M, Castelli WP: The role of diabetes in congestive heart failure: The Framingham study. Am J Cardiol 34:29, 1974

66. Keating FR, Parkin TW, Selby JB, Dickson LS: Treatment of heart disease associated with myxedema. Prog Cardiovasc Dis 3:364, 1960

67. Kerber RE, Sherman B: Echocardiographic evaluation of pericardial effusion in myxedema. Incidence and biochemical and clinical correlations. Circulation 52:823, 1975

68. Kieraldo J, Eversole S, Allen R: Carcinoid tumor of vermiform appendix with distant metastasis: Review of the literature and report of two cases, one in a 14-year-old girl. Calif Med 99:161, 1963

69. King M, Huang J, Glassman E: Paget's disease with cardiac calcification and complete heart block. Am J Med 46:302, 1969

70. Kline IK: Myocardial alterations associated with pheochromocytoma. Am J Pathol 38:539, 1961

71. Larsson O: studies of small vessels in patients with diabetes. Acta Med Scand 480 (suppl):5, 1967

72. Lazarus JM, Lowrie EG, Hampers CL, Merrill JP: Cardiovascular Disease in Uremic Patients on Hemodialysis. Kidney Int (suppl)2: S167, 1975

73. Ledet T: Histological and histochemical changes in the coronary arteries of old diabetic patients. Diabetologia 4:268, 1968

74. Ledet T: Diabetic cardiopathy. Quantitative histological studies of the heart from young juvenile diabetics. Acta Pathol Microbiol Scand [A] 84:421, 1976

75. Ledet T, Neubauer B, Christensen NJ, Lundbaek K: Diabetic cardiopathy. Diabetologia 16:207, 1979

76. Levine SN, Rheams CN: Hypocalcemic heart failure. Am J Med 78:1033, 1985

77. Liddle GW: Pathogenesis of glucocorticoid disorders. Am J Med 53:638, 1972

78. Lie JT, Grossman SJ: Pathology of the heart in acromegaly: Anatomic findings in 27 autopsied patients. Am Heart J 100:41, 1980

79. Littman DS, Jeffers WA, Rose E: The infrequency of myocardial infarction in patients with thyrotoxicosis. Am J Med Sci 233:10, 1957

80. Ludwig GD: Carcinoid heart disease. Part 4. p. 1309. In Conn HL Jr, Horwitz O (eds): Cardiac and Vascular Diseases. Vol. II. Lea & Febiger, Philadelphia, 1971

81. Ludwig GD, Cushard WG Jr: Parathyroid disease and the heart. Part II. p. 1267. In

Conn HL Jr, Horwitz O (eds): Cardiac and Vascular Diseases. Vol. II. Lea & Febiger, Philadelphia, 1971

82. Malcolm AD: Mitral valve prolapse associated with other disorders. Casual coincidence, common link, or fundamental genetic disturbance? Br Heart J 53:353, 1985

83. Manion WC: Basophilic mucoid degeneration of the heart. Med Ann DC 34:60, 1965

84. Markowitz C, Yater WM: Response of explanted cardiac muscle to thyroxine. Am J Physiol 100:162, 1932

85. Martin AM Jr, Hackel DB: The myocardium of the dog in hemorrhagic shock. Lab Invest 12:77, 1963

86. Mason JW, Billingham ME, Friedman JP: Methysergide-induced heart disease. A case of multivalvular and myocardial fibrosis. Circulation 56:889, 1977

87. McAllister HA Jr: Pathology of the cardiovascular system in chronic renal failure. In Lowenthal DT, Pennock RL, Likoff W, Onesti G (eds): Management of Cardiovascular Disease in Renal Failure. FA Davis, Philadelphia, 1981

88. McAllister HA Jr, Ferrans VJ: The Cardiovascular System. p. 787. In Silverberg SG (ed): Principles and Practice of Surgical Pathology. 2nd Ed. Churchill Livingstone, New York, 1990

89. McAllister HA Jr, Hall RJ: Iatrogenic heart disease. p. 871. In Cheng TO (ed): The International Textbook of Cardiology. Pergamon Press, New York, 1986

90. McAllister HA Jr, Mullick FG: Pathology of drug-induced and toxic diseases in the cardiovascular system. In Riddell R (ed): Pathology of Drug-Induced and Toxic Diseases. Churchill Livingstone, New York, 1982

91. McGuffin WL, Sherman BM, Roth J, et al: Acromegaly and cardiovascular disorders. Ann Intern Med 81:11, 1974

92. Means JH, DeGrott LJ, Stanbury JB: The Thyroid and Its Diseases. McGraw-Hill, New York, 1963

93. Melmon KL, Sjoerdsma A, Mason DT: Distinctive clinical therapeutic aspects of the syndrome associated with bronchial carcinoid tumors. Am J Med 39:568, 1965

94. Mengel CE: Carcinoid and the heart. Mod Concepts Cardiovasc Dis 35:75, 1966

95. Mihailescu V, Vereanu I, Alinescu R: Insuficienta cardiaca la acromegali. Med Interne 13:929, 1961

96. Murayama M, Goodkind MJ: Effect of thyroid hormone on the frequency-force relationship of atrial myocardium from the guinea pig. Circ Res 23:743, 1968

97. Myasnikov AL, Zaitsev VF: The influence of thyroid hormones on cholesterol metabolism in experimental atherosclerosis in rabbits. J Atheroscler Res 3:295, 1963

98. Najafi H, Heson D, Dye WS, et al: Left ventricular hemorrhagic necrosis. Ann Thorac Surg 7:550, 1969

99. Nishizawa Y, Hamada N, Fujii S, et al: Serum dopamine-beta-hydroxylase activity in thyroid disorders. J Clin Endocrinol Metab 39:599, 1974

100. Oates JA, Sjoerdsma A: A unique syndrome associated with secretion of 5-hydroxytryptophan by metastatic gastric carcinoids. Am J Med 32:333, 1962

101. Oates JA, Melmon K, Sjoerdsma A, et al: Release of a kinin peptide in the carcinoid syndrome. Lancet 1:514, 1964

102. Oates JA, Pettinger WA, Doctor RR: Evidence for the release of bradykinin in carcinoid syndrome. J Clin Invest 45:173, 1966

103. Paz-Guevara AT, Tah-Hsiung H, White P: Juvenile diabetes mellitus after 40 years. Diabetes 24:559, 1975

104. Pepine CJ, Alcia J: Heart muscle disease in acromegaly. Am J Med 48:530, 1970

105. Philipson KD, Edelman IS: Thyroid hormone control of Na^+-K^+-ATPase and K^+-dependent phosphatase in rat heart. Am J Physiol 232:C196, 1977

106. Regan TJ, Ahmed SS, Levinson GE, et al: Cardiomyopathy and regional scar in diabetes mellitus. Trans Assoc Am Physicians 88:217, 1975

107. Regan TJ, Lyons MM, Ahmed SS, et al: Evidence for cardiomyopathy in familial diabetes mellitus. J Clin Invest 60:885, 1977

108. Reichenbach DD, Benditt EP: Myofibrillar degeneration, a response of myocardial cell to injury. Arch Pathol 85:189, 1968

109. Reichenbach DD, Benditt EP: Catecholamines and cardiomyopathy: The pathogenesis and potential importance of myofibrillar degeneration. Hum Pathol 1:25, 1970

110. Rimailho A, Burchard P, Schaison G, et al:

Improvement of hypocalcemic cardiomyopathy by correction of serum calcium level. Am Heart J 109:611, 1985

111. Rimoin DL: Inheritance in diabetes mellitus. Med Clin North Am 55:807, 1971

112. Robbins SL: Systemic diseases. p. 259. In Robbins SL (ed): Pathologic Basis of Disease. WB Saunders, Philadelphia, 1974

113. Roberts WC, Sjoerdsma A: The cardiac disease associated with the carcinoid syndrome (carcinoid heart disease). Am J Med 36:5, 1969

114. Roberts WC, Spray TL: Pericardial heart disease. In Harvey WP (ed): Current Problems in Cardiology. Vol. II. No. 3. Year Book Medical Publishers, Chicago, 1977

115. Root HF: Diabetes and arteriosclerosis in youth. Am Heart J 35:860, 1948

116. Root HF, Barclay P: Diabetes of 35 years duration. JAMA 161:801, 1956

117. Rosai J, Lascano EF: Basophilic (mucoid) degeneration of myocardium. A disorder of glycogen metabolism. Am J Pathol 61:99, 1970

118. Rossi L, Thiene G, Caregaro L, et al: Dysrhythmias and sudden death in acromegalic heart disease. A clinicopathologic study. Chest 72:495, 1977

119. Roth KA, Wilson DM, Eberwine J, et al: Acromegaly and pheochromocytoma: A multiple endocrine syndrome caused by a plurihormonal adrenal medullary tumor. J Clin Endocrinol Metab 63:1421, 1986

120. Roundtree LG, Snell AM: A Clinical Study of Addison's Disease. Mayo Clinic Monographs. WB Saunders, Philadelphia, 1931

121. Ruggieri A: Die bedeutung der hypophyse fur die pathologie der blutgefaze. Ergeb Inn Med Kinderheilkd 49:262, 1935

122. Rutherford JP, Vatern SF, Braunwald E: Adrenergic control of the myocardial contractility in conscious hypertrophied dogs. Am J Physiol 237:590, 1980

123. Saphir O, Ohringer L, Wong R: Changes in the intramural coronary branches in coronary arteriosclerosis. Arch Pathol 62:159, 1956

124. Sauer WG, Dearing WH, Flock EV, et al: Functioning carcinoid tumors. Gastroenterology 34:216, 1958

125. Schlesinger MJ, Reiner L: Focal myocytolysis of the heart. Am J Pathol 31:443, 1955

126. Selye H, Bajusz E: Conditioning by corticoids for the production of cardiac lesions with noradrenaline. Acta Endocrinol (Copenh) 30:183, 1959

127. Seneviratne BIB: Diabetic cardiomyopathy: The preclinical phase. Br Med J 1:1444, 1977

128. Shapiro S, Steier M, Dimich I: Congestive heart failure in neonatal thyrotoxicosis. A curable cause of heart failure in the newborn. Clin Pediatr 14:1155, 1975

129. Sheehan HL, Summers VK: The syndrome of hypopituitarism. Q J Med 18:319, 1949

130. Silver MD, Huckell VF, Lorber M: Basement membranes of small cardiac vessels in patients with diabetes and myxedema: Preliminary observations. Pathology 7:213, 1977

131. Siperstein MD, Unger RH, Madison LL: Studies of muscle capillary basement membranes in normal subjects, diabetic and prediabetic patients. J Clin Invest 47:1973, 1968

132. Sjoerdsma A, Melmon K: The carcinoid spectrum. Gastroenterology 47:104, 1964

133. Sjoerdsma A, Engelman K, Waldmann TA: Pheochromocytoma: Current concepts of diagnosis and treatment. Ann Intern Med 65:1302, 1966

134. Sjoerdsma A, Weissbach H, Terry LL, Undenfriend S: Further observations on patients with malignant carcinoid. Am J Med 23:5, 1957

135. Skelton CL, Sonnenblick EH: Cardiovascular system in hypothyroidism. p. 873. In Werner SC, Ingbar SH (eds): The Thyroid. 2nd Ed. Harper & Row, New York, 1962

136. Smallridge RC, Rajfer S, Davia J, Schaaf M: Acromegaly and the heart: An echocardiographic study. Am J Med 66:22, 1979

137. Smolar EN, Rubin JE, Avramides A, Carter AC: Cardiac tamponade in primary myxedema and review of the literature. Am J Med Sci 272:345, 1976

138. Soffer LJ, Iannaecone A, Gabrilove JL: Cushing's syndrome (Study of 50 patients). Am J Med 45:116, 1968

139. Stary HC: Disease of small blood vessels in diabetes mellitus. Am J Med Sci 252:357, 1966

140. Staub W, Grayzel DM, Rosenblatt P: Mediastinal parathyroid adenoma. Arch Intern Med 85:765, 1950

141. Steinberg AD: Myxedema and coronary artery disease—A comparative autopsy study. Ann Intern Med 68:338, 1968

142. Stephan E, Laham E, Panier M, Saleh J:

Coeur et hypopituitarisme. 1. Anomalies electrocardiographies constantes. 2. Une complication rare: l'épanchement pericardique (À propos de 10 cas). Arch Mal Coeur 58:1493, 1965

143. Sterling FH: The heart in hypothyroidism. Part III. p. 1275. In Conn HL Jr, Horwitz O (eds): Cardiac and Vascular Diseases. Vol. II. Lea & Febiger, Philadelphia, 1971

144. Strandness DE Jr, Priest RE, Gibbons EG: Combined clinical and pathologic study of diabetic and nondiabetic peripheral arterial disease. Diabetes 13:366, 1964

145. Sunni S, Bishop SP, Kent SP, Geer JC: Diabetic cardiomyopathy. A morphological study of intramyocardial arteries. Arch Pathol Lab Med 110:375, 1986

146. Taber RE, Morales AR, Fine G: Myocardial necrosis and the postoperative low cardiac output syndrome. Ann Thorac Surg 4:12, 1967

147. Tammes AR: Exogenous serotonin administered to rats with liver damage. Arch Pathol 79:626, 1965

148. Thomas WC: Hypercalcemia crisis due to hyperparathyroidism. Am J Med 24:229, 1958

149. Thyrum PT, Kritcher EM, Luchi RJ: Effect of l-thyroxine on the primary structure of cardiac myosin. Biochim Biophys Acta 197:335, 1970

150. Vanhaelst L, Neve P, Chailly P, Bastenie PA: Coronary-artery disease in hypothyroidism. Lancet 2:800, 1967

151. Voss DM, Drake EH: Cardiac manifestations of hyperparathyroidism with presentation of previously unreported arrhythmia. Am Heart J 73:235, 1967

152. Walter KW: The significance of alterations in serum lipids in thyroid dysfunction. II. Alterations in the metabolism and turnover of I^{131} low-density lipoproteins in hypothyroidism and thyrotoxicosis. Clin Sci 29:217, 1965

153. Warren S, LeCompte PM, Legg MA: The Pathology of Diabetes Mellitus. 4th Ed. Lea & Febiger, Philadelphia, 1966

154. Weller CV, Wanstrom RC, Gordon H, Bugher JC: Cardiac histopathology in thyroid disease. Am Heart J 8:8, 1932

155. White PD: Heart Disease, 4th Ed. MacMillan, New York, 1951

156. Whittemore R, Caddell JL: Metabolic and nutritional diseases. p. 887. In Moss A, Adams FH, Emmanouilides GC (eds): Heart Disease in Infants, Children and Adolescents. Williams & Wilkins, Baltimore, 1977

157. Williams GH, Braunwald E: Endocrine and nutritional disorders and heart disease. p. 1825. In Braunwald E (ed): Heart Disease. A Textbook of Cardiovascular Medicine. Vol. 2. WB Saunders, Philadelphia, 1980

158. Williams GH, Dluhy RG, Thorn GW: Diseases of the adrenal cortex. p. 520. In Thorn GW, Adams RD, Braunwald E, et al (eds): Harrison's Principles of Internal Medicine. 8th Ed. McGraw-Hill, New York, 1977

159. Yazaki Y, Raben MS: Effect of thyroid state on the enzymatic characteristics of cardiac myosin. Circ Res 36:208, 1975

160. Zoneraich S, Silverman G, Zoneraich O: Small stiff heart in diabetes mellitus. Am J Cardiol 41:426, 1978

161. Zullo MA, Devereux RB, Kramer-Fox R, et al: Mitral valve prolapse and hyperthyroidism: Effect of patient selection. Am Heart J 110:977, 1985

32

Effects of Drugs on the Cardiovascular System

John J. Fenoglio, Jr.[*]
Malcolm D. Silver

Adverse reactions to drugs are an increasingly important medical problem. Although their exact incidence is not known, it has been estimated that as many as 5 percent of medical hospital admissions are due to drug reactions and that 15 to 40 percent of patients in hospitals experience at least one adverse drug reaction.[48] Drug reactions may be secondary to (1) allergy, (2) pharmacologic idiosyncrasy, (3) direct toxicity, (4) overdosage, or (5) side effects or interactions between drugs.[103] Disease induced as a result of such reactions may mimic systemic diseases or present with organ-specific signs and symptoms. Currently, knowledge of drug reactions is mainly derived from analysis of clinical signs and symptoms. However, attention has focused on the structural basis of adverse drug reactions.

That drugs cause cardiovascular disease by altering cardiac structure has been known since 1905, when Lewitzky found that large doses of digitalis extract produced myocardial necrosis in experimental animals.[90] Subsequently, other drugs were shown to induce cardiovascular disease in experimental animals, although there was no evidence that they (epinephrine,[68] digitalis extract,[41] and thyroid extract[36]) produced morphologic changes in therapeutic dosages. Isolated examples of drug-induced cardiovascular disease in humans were reported in the 1920s and 1930s, but documentation of morphologic changes was inconclusive. In that era drug-induced diseases were considered secondary to alterations in function rather than in structure. In 1942, French and Weller[44] documented the relationship between sulfonamide administration and the occurrence of myocarditis in a large retrospective autopsy study. This and a subsequent report linking vasculitis and sulfonamide therapy[43] clearly demonstrated that drugs could produce cardiovascular disease by causing structural changes in the heart and/or blood vessels.

However, the recognition of structural changes caused by drug-induced diseases is hampered by difficulty in differentiating drug-induced from naturally occurring cardiovascular disease. Our knowledge of both morphologic changes induced by drugs and the magnitude of these structurally based adverse drug reactions is primarily derived from case reports. Morphologic changes are fre-

[*]Deceased.

quently assumed, on the basis of previous reports, but are less frequently documented. Use of the endomyocardial biopsy is changing that situation and will continue to do so.

Another problem of recognizing drug-induced disease relates to the identification of the drug responsible. To correlate a drug and morphologic changes, a link must be established between the two. This requires that the drug be eligible temporally. The linkage may be established by one of several methods: exclusion, dechallenge, rechallenge, singularity of the drug, pattern, and quantitative determination of the drug. The methodology has been well defined by Irey,[61] although it is frequently not rigorously applied, especially in case reports. In many suspected drug-induced diseases, a relationship to a drug is not documented or the morphologic changes are not clearly defined. A clear, causative relationship between a drug and an adverse tissue reaction is established either by reproducing the reaction in an experimental animal model or by rechallenging the patient. Although rechallenge may be used to document adverse reactions, its applicability is not only limited but often contraindicated medically. The relationship of a drug to an adverse tissue reaction is usually based on presumptive evidence. Proof of the relationship rests on the weight of accumulated evidence that a specific morphologic change is associated with a specific drug.

This subject has been reviewed previously.[11,12,22,100,133] We believe that adverse tissue reactions in the cardiovascular system are best grouped on the basis of morphologic changes, rather than by diseases associated with specific drugs. Morphologic changes in the heart include hypersensitivity (allergic) myocarditis, toxic myocarditis, cardiomyopathy, and endocardial fibrosis. Vascular changes include drug-related (hypersensitivity) vasculitis, necrotizing vasculitis, fibromuscular hyperplasia, and thromboembolism.

HYPERSENSITIVITY MYOCARDITIS

Myocarditis associated with drug therapy was first recognized by French and Weller,[44] who reported it associated with sulfonamide administration (see also Ch. 19).

Pathology

The myocarditis is characterized by all of the lesions having a similar morphology,[37] suggesting a comparable age. Histologically, there are prominent numbers of eosinophils admixed with mononuclear cells, mainly lymphocytes and plasma cells (Fig. 32–1). The cellular infiltrate may be focal or diffuse and is most prominent interstitially. Focal myocytolysis is always present (Fig. 32–2), although such foci are frequently sparse and obscured by the interstitial infiltrate. Foci of cellular necrosis are rarely seen. Evidence of interstial or replacement fibrosis is uniformly absent. True granulomatous lesions are not a feature of hypersensitivity myocarditis, although isolated giant cells, presumably of myocardial origin, are occasionally seen. Vascular involvement is frequent in areas of extensive interstitial infiltrates and is identical to that seen in drug-related vasculitis. It is characterized by a bland-appearing vasculitis involving small arteries, arterioles, and venules. Necrotizing vascular lesions are not associated with hypersensitivity myocarditis.

Drug-related hypersensitivity myocarditis is distinguished from other forms of myocarditis in which eosinophils are prominent by the absence of extensive myocardial necrosis and of replacement fibrosis. The lack of extensive necrosis or interstitial fibrosis suggests that the drug-induced disease is self-limiting. Once the offending agent is withdrawn, the myocarditis presumably resolves

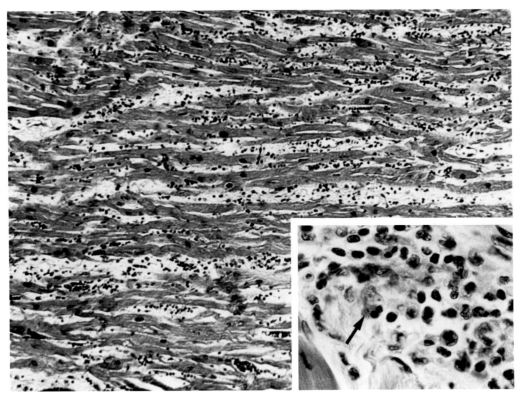

Fig. 32–1. Hypersensitivity myocarditis associated with penicillin. Hypersensitivity myocarditis is characterized by a diffuse interstitial inflammatory infiltrate and separation of myocardial cells by edema. Foci of acute cell death are not usually present. The inflammatory infiltrate (insert) is composed of lymphocytes, plasma cells, and prominent eosinophils (arrow). (H&E, × 140; insert × 575.)

without residual cardiac damage. There are no reports of cardiac fibrosis or of a cardiomyopathy following drug-induced hypersensitivity myocarditis.

Incidence

The exact incidence of hypersensitivity myocarditis is unknown, although it probably represents the most prevalent form of drug-induced heart disease. Our knowledge of this entity is based primarily on isolated case reports and clinical reviews. Clinically, criteria for diagnosing drug hypersensitivity reactions are well established.[91] They are

1. Previous use of the drug without incident.
2. The hypersensitivity reaction bears no relationship to drug dosage.
3. The reaction is neither the pharmacologic nor the toxic effect of the drug.
4. The reaction is characterized by classic allergic symptoms, symptoms of serum sickness, or syndromes suggesting infectious disease.
5. Immunologic confirmation.
6. Persistence of symptoms until the drug is discontinued.

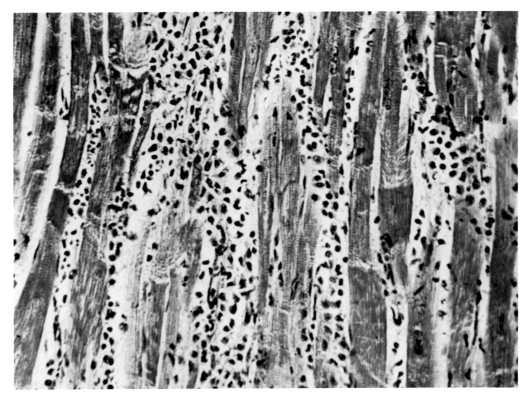

Fig. 32–2. Hypersensitivity myocarditis associated with methyldopa. Myocytolysis is always present in hypersensitivity myocarditis although extensive cellular necrosis is distinctly unusual. Foci of myocytolysis are usually most prominent in areas of extensive interstitial infiltrate. (H&E, × 560.)

Clinical Features

The clinical diagnosis of drug-induced hypersensitivity myocarditis is made on the basis of these criteria, plus signs and symptoms of cardiac disease that abate when the drug is withdrawn. It is presumed that the symptoms are secondary to drug-induced myocarditis. Clinical impression may be confirmed by endomyocardial biopsy (see Ch. 39).

Etiology

Many drugs have been implicated to cause hypersensitivity myocarditis.[125,134] Some that do so regularly are listed in Table 32–1. A similar, presumably hypersensitivity myocarditis, can also occur following injection of

horse serum,[27] tetanus toxoid,[30] and smallpox vaccination.[31,40] The exact pathogenesis of these myocardial lesions is elusive. There is evidence that allergic reactions to penicillin are immunologically mediated,[103] and that a myocarditis, identical to that associated with drugs, can be produced in the rabbit by the injection of rat antiheart antisera.[69] This fa-

Table 32–1. Drugs Associated with Hypersensitivity Myocarditis

Methyldopa[99]
Penicillin[6,55,106,131]
Phenindione[76]
Phenylbutazone[56]
Streptomycin[25]
Sulfonamides[44]
Sulfonylureas[39,78]
Tetracyclines[78,83]

vours the viewpoint that the myocarditis associated with drug therapy is a delayed hypersensitivity phenomenon.

Pathogenic Mechanisms

Hypersensitivity drug reactions are *not mediated through the drug itself, directly, but through chemically reactive metabolites.*[103] The metabolites, now acting as haptens, combine with endogeneous macromolecules, especially proteins; it is the combination of the two molecules that is antigenic. The protein carrier is able to interact with T lymphocytes, initiating the immune response. Once T cells are activated, hapten-specific activation is produced in B lymphocytes and antihapten antibodies are formed. The antigen must have multiple combining sites, permitting it to form a bridge between antibody molecules to elicit symptoms of hypersensitivity. This permits soluble antibody molecules to react with complement and release cytoactive peptides. Bridging between cell-bound antibody molecules or antigen receptors on lymphocytes produces the change in cell membrane conformation required for mediator release or lymphocyte transformation. The requirement of multivalent haptens to initiate antihapten antibodies is one explanation for the relative infrequency of allergic drug reactions. Most drugs and drug metabolites are univalent haptens that compete with multivalent antigens for antibody and thus inhibit the response. The organ-specific allergic reactions can also be explained by this theory. Conjugation of hapten with an organ-specific protein could produce an immunologic response with specificity for the protein as well as the haptenic group.

CARDIOTOXICITY

In addition to eliciting an allergic response, drugs can cause myocardial damage by *direct* toxic effects on myocardial cells. This results in cell death, expressed clinically as an acute myocarditis or as a cardiomyopathy. The clinical expression depends on the extent of cell death and the speed with which it occurs. In acute myocarditis there is extensive, widespread cell death that occurs over a relatively short time—days to weeks. By contrast, if a cardiomyopathy results, cell death is slow, patchy, and ongoing over months.

In this instance, drug toxicity is dose related and its effects are cumulative. The extent of cell damage then depends on the toxicity of the drug and the total dose administered. Cell damage also depends on drug absorption by the cell. The combination of these factors which determines both the extent and the speed of cell death.

Pathogenic Mechanisms

The mechanisms of direct drug toxicity are varied and depend on the drug. Drugs may interfere with or inhibit cell metabolism, block or alter cell transport, or cause hemodynamic alterations that result in cell ischemia. The mechanisms of action and resultant structural alterations caused by the cardiotoxic drugs emetine and cyclophosphamide have been characterized and serve as a model for other cardiotoxic drugs.

Emetine is an inhibitor of oxidative phosphorylation.[101] Structurally, its cardiotoxic effects are marked by mitochondrial swelling and widespread cell death.[104] By contrast, the cardiotoxic effects of cyclophosphamide appear to be secondary to capillary endothelial damage and thrombosis.[20,22] The result is multifocal cardiac necrosis characterized structurally by extensive contraction bands, myofibrillar lysis, and electron-dense intramitochondrial inclusions—structural findings similar to those described in ischemia.

Morphologically, the toxic effects of drugs on the heart produce an acute or a chronic myocarditis. The diagnosis of myocarditis is based on the finding of focal areas of cell death associated with an inflammatory infiltrate.

The type of myocarditis is determined histologically by the type and extent of the inflammatory infiltrate. Such myocarditis, directly induced by a drug, is best termed "toxic" myocarditis. On the other hand, the slow, patchy death of cells caused by a drug is usually referred to as a drug-induced cardiomyopathy.

Toxic Myocarditis

Pathology

Grossly, the heart in toxic myocarditis is not hypertrophied; cardiac chambers are frequently dilated and the myocardium is pale and soft.

Microscopically, there is usually extensive but patchy myocardial cell death and an extensive inflammatory infiltrate. Areas of acute cell death alternate with foci of recent and healing myocardial cell damage. The morphology could be confused with that of a myocardial infarction. In the areas of acute cell death, myocardial cells are hypereosinophilic and there is a predominant polymorphonuclear cell infiltrate (Fig. 32–3). Foci of myofiberlysis that represent areas of recent cell damage are associated with a mixed inflammatory infiltrate consisting of lymphocytes, plasma cells, and polymorphonuclear cells (Fig. 32–4). Eosinophils are notably absent. The lack of eosinophils, as well as the varying stages of cell damage, helps distinguishes a toxic from a hypersensitivity myocarditis. Healing areas of cell damage are characterized by proliferating fibroblasts and a sparse infiltrate of macrophages (Fig. 32–5). Patchy areas of fibrosis, indicative of healed cell damage, are uncommon. Frequently, there is moderate interstitial edema and a sparse nonspecific interstitial infiltrate

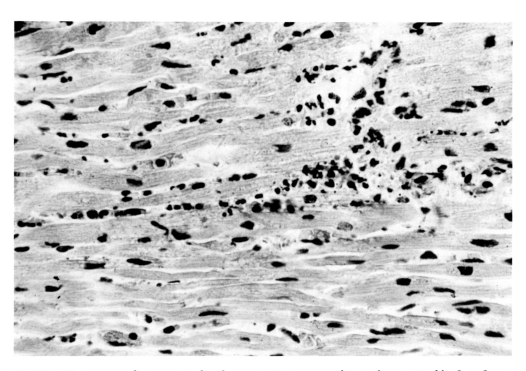

Fig. 32–3. Toxic myocarditis associated with arsenic. Toxic myocarditis is characterized by foci of acute cell death. Foci of cellular necrosis are usually prominent and marked by an inflammatory infiltrate rich in polymorphonuclear leucocytes. (H&E, × 240.)

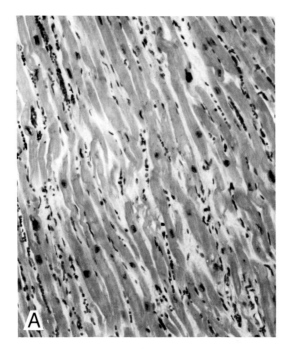 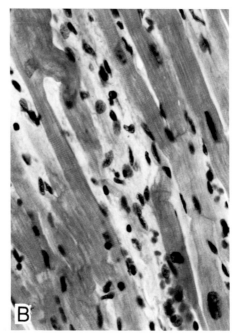

Fig. 32–4. Toxic myocarditis associated with emetine. In toxic myocarditis all stages of cell death are present and a diffuse interstitial inflammatory infiltrate is usually prominent. (**A**) Areas of recent cell damage are characterized by focal loss of myocytes and myocytolysis. (H&E, × 160.) (**B**) Areas of myocyte loss of the cellular infiltrate consist of lymphocytes, macrophages and polymorphonuclear leukocytes. (H&E, × 375.)

of lymphocytes, plasma cells, and macrophages. Endocardium and valves are usually not involved in these cases.

Endothelial damage and capillary microthrombosis may be prominent features, especially with cyclophosphamide cardiotoxicity. Although microthrombosis is best appreciated by electron microscopy, small arterial thrombi are occasionally seen by light microscopy. The microthrombi are thought to be secondary to drug-induced endothelial damage.[20] The larger vessels are normal, and a true vasculitis is rarely present.

Thus, a toxic myocarditis is characterized by multifocal areas of cell death of different ages. Areas of recent and healing cell damage are seen, but foci of acute cell death usually predominate and foci of fibrosis are usually not prominent.

The prevalence of recent and healing foci of cell death is an indicator of the drug toxicity and dosage. The prominence of foci of acute cell death is diagnostic of an acute toxic myocarditis, whereas the prominence of areas of healing and healed cell damage is diagnostic of a chronic drug-induced toxic myocarditis.

Clinical Features

The clinical findings are also useful in this differentiation. In acute toxic myocarditis, cardiac symptoms appear suddenly, over days to weeks, whereas in chronic toxicity their onset may be insidious, over months to years. Arrhythmias and ECG abnormalities are frequent in toxic myocarditis, usually in the absence of cardiomegaly.

Natural History

The natural history of toxic myocarditis is not well understood. Our knowledge of this entity is derived mainly from reports of fatal cases.

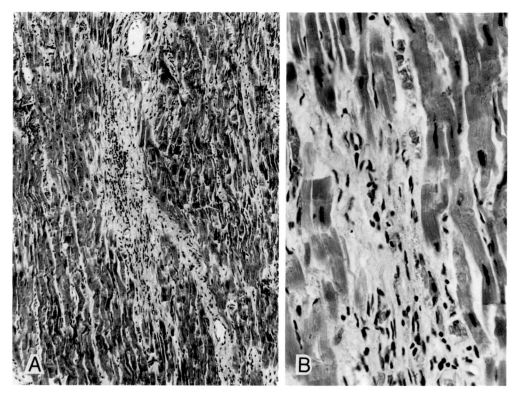

Fig. 32–5. Toxic myocarditis associated with arsenic. Healing areas of myocardial damage imply chronicity and are less prominent in toxic myocarditis than in drug-related cardiomyopathy. In (**A**) toxic myocarditis these foci are associated with an interstitial inflammatory infiltrate. (H&E, × 94.) (**B**) Areas of healing cell damage are marked by proliferation of fibroblasts and capillaries and scattered mononuclear cells and macrophages. (H&E, × 375.)

This probably explains why areas of healed cell damage are not described in toxic myocarditis. It seems logical to assume, however, that ongoing cell damage would cease if the toxin or drug were withdrawn. The residuum would be focal myocardial scars, but such scarring might not be of sufficient magnitude to impair cardiac function. We note that focal myocardial scars are a frequent autopsy finding. They are usually ascribed to subclinical ischemic heart disease, but this may not always be their cause.

Many drugs are suspected of being cardiotoxic. Toxic myocarditis, however, has only been histologically documented for a handful of drugs (Tables 20–3 and 32–2). Digitalis[60,81] and thyroid extract[36] can produce a toxic myocarditis experimentally, but there is no evidence that they do so in humans.

Table 32–2. Drugs Associated with Toxic Myocarditis

Adriamycin[18]
Antimony compounds[58]
Arsenicals[19]
Catecholamines[42,46,123]
Cyclophosphamide[4,47,71]
Daunorubicin[4]
Emetine hydrochloride[6,74,113]
Fluorouracil[84,107]
Lithium carbonate[87,98]
Phenothiazines[45,59,112]
Plasmocid[22]

Cocaine and the Heart

In recent years, abuse of cocaine and of "crack" cocaine (the latter made by adding ammonium and baking soda to an aqueous solution of cocaine hydrochloride to precipitate alkaloid cocaine, which is dried and smoked, allowing very high blood levels of the drug to be achieved very quickly) has increased alarmingly in some countries. With that have come more frequent reports of the drug's toxic effects, producing both morbidity and death. Karch[72] provides a brief history of cocaine abuse.

Clinical Features

The drug has both direct and indirect effects on the heart. Acute pulmonary edema, angina pectoris, myocardial infarction, coronary artery spasm, cardiac arrhythmias, and sudden death have all been reported, as well as a dilated cardiomyopathy with associated congestive cardiac failure.[29,82,95,126,132] (Endocarditis is also frequent among intravenous drug users; see Ch. 23.)

The cardiac consequences of cocaine abuse (1) are not unique to parenteral administration of the drug; (2) may occur in patients who do not, necessarily, have underlying heart disease; (3) may develop in those without seizure activity, a well-documented noncardiac complication of cocaine abuse; and (4) are not limited to massive doses of the drug.[63] Most cases have been reported among patients 20 to 40 years old, with a greater frequency among males.

Pathology

Endomyocardial biopsy reveals changes ranging from myocardial necrosis, which usually involves individual cells in a multifocal distribution, through a myocarditis, which may or may not accompany these changes, to myocyte hypertrophy and interstitial fibrosis.[63,64,105] Ultrastructurally, a striking feature is extensive loss of myofibrils with other myocells showing degenerative and necrotic changes. Remnants of Z bands are thickened and have an irregular arrangement. Mitochondria retain compact cristae but are often smaller than normal. Scavenger macrophages are seen and, in some patients, increased numbers of inflammatory cells.

Autopsy findings range from widespread contraction bands in myocytes to frank myocardial infarction in cases of sudden death to evidence of a toxic myocarditis. Morphologic findings include dilated cardiomyopathy and evidence of severe coronary artery obstructive lesions resulting from chronic intimal proliferation and/or coronary thrombosis.[63,73,120,126] Other authors have reported the adverse cerebrovascular effects of the drug[89] and amyloidosis occurring in addicts.[102]

Pathogenic Mechanisms

Here, because of the risk of contamination of cocaine with other substances during illegal manufacture and subsequent distribution, care must be observe in relating the drug and both observed clinical events and morphologic findings. Nevertheless, an association between cocaine and cardiac toxicity is certain.

Acute administration has two dose-related effects on the heart, a local anaesthetic one at low plasma concentrations and the prevention of norepinephrine reuptake by preganglionic sympathetic nerve endings at high plasma concentrations resulting in a local excess of norepinephrine at the synaptic cleft.[126] The latter mechanism could explain the frequency of contraction bands, a nonspecific finding in the hearts of cocaine abusers. Nevertheless, the lesion provides an anatomic substrate for cardiac arrhythmias and sudden death.[126] Coronary artery spasm with an indirect effect on myocardial cells may have a comparable explanation or result from direct adrenergic stimulation.[82]

Drug-related Cardiomyopathy

The sequel of chronic toxic myocardial damage is a cardiomyopathy (see also Ch. 20). The underlying process is identical to that in toxic myocarditis; however, cell death is gradual and progressive rather than acute.

Initial clinical findings are usually cardiomegaly and congestive heart failure rather than an arrhythmia. The term cardiomyopathy should be reserved for cases that present with cardiomegaly and congestive heart failure rather than being applied generally to all cases of drug-related heart disease.

Etiology

Drugs associated with the development of cardiomyopathy are listed in Tables 20–3 and 32–3. Many are implicated as a cause of toxic myocarditis (Tables 20–3 and 32–2). This relationship has been well established and documented in anthracycline-induced cardiomyopathy.

Anthracycline-Induced Cardiomyopathy

The anthracyclines daunorubicin and adriamycin are antitumor agents. Both are cardiotoxic and associated with the development of cardiomyopathy.[17,22,86] (See also Chs. 20 and 39.)

Clinical Features.   Symptoms usually appear weeks to months after treatment has con-

Table 32–3.   Drugs Associated with Cardiomyopathy

Adriamycin
Amphetamine[121]
Arsenicals[34,35]
Catecholamines (endogenous)[77]
Chloroquine[109]
Daunomycin[21]
Ephedrine[127]
Lithium[98,122]
Mitomycin C[23]
Rubidazone[8]

cluded. The clinical course is dominated by intractable congestive heart failure often preceded by progressive cardiomegaly. Adriamycin cardiotoxicity is dose related and occurs almost exclusively in patients receiving a total dose of more than 500 mg/m^2,[86] with as many as 30 percent of patients receiving more than this dose developing a cardiomyopathy. The mortality approaches 50 percent in this group. On the other hand, Buzdar and colleagues[24] report a 1 percent incidence of congestive cardiac failure in patients treated with up to 300 mg/m^2 and 4 percent in those treated with 450 mg/m^2 of doxorubicin. Available data does not suggest an increasing incidence with increasing dosage. Rather, the risk of developing a cardiomyopathy is roughly the same in patients receiving a total dosage of 600 mg/m^2 as in those receiving 1,000 mg/m^2.[86] This suggests a considerable individual variation in the degree of anthracycline cardiotoxicity.

Pathology.   As in other forms of congestive cardiomyopathy, the heart is enlarged (Fig. 32–6). All chambers are dilated, and mural thrombi are frequent in both ventricles (Fig. 32–7). Histologically there are multifocal areas of patchy fibrosis and myocardial degeneration throughout the heart (Fig. 32–8) (see also Figs. 39–3 and 39–4). Vacuolated myocardial cells are occasionally seen adjacent to areas of myocardial scarring (so-called Adra cells). As in toxic myocarditis, foci of healing cell damage are associated with fibroblast proliferation and a histiocytic infiltrate. Areas of acute damage are infrequent, and foci of fibrosis predominate.

Ultrastructurally, two types of cellular injury are seen: myofibrillar loss and vacuolar degeneration[14,21,66] (see also Ch. 39). Myofibrillar loss is characterized by either partial or total loss of myofibrils within the cell. Usually the nucleus is unaffected and mitochondria retain compact cristae. In vacuolar degeneration, the earliest change is distention of the sarcoplasmic reticulum and T-tubular system. The distended vacuoles swell

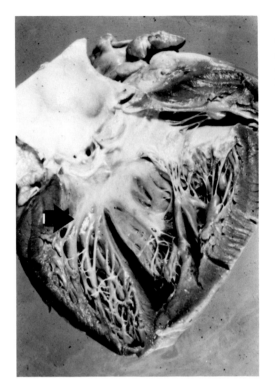

Fig. 32–6. In Adriamycin-related cardiomyopathy, is in other forms of dilated (congestive) cardiomyopathy, the ventricular chambers are dilated and the heart is hypertrophied. Left ventricular walls are not thickened despite a massive increase in heart weight (750 g). Mitral and aortic valves are normal but there is endocardial sclerosis, especially over the left ventricular outflow region (arrow).

These findings are not specific for anthracycline-induced or other drug-related cardiomyopathies. Nevertheless, they can be produced experimentally. Rabbits treated with both daunomycin and Adriamycin develop a cardiomyopathy similar clinically and morphologically to that observed in humans.[65] Morphologic changes are seen long before clinical signs and symptoms of cardiac disease are evident. The clear relationship of morphologic changes to Adriamycin administration and the lack of predictive clinical tests to identify patients at risk lead to the use of endomyocardial biopsy to monitor cardiotoxicity.[10,64] The myofibrillar and vacuolar changes are graded from the biopsy (see Ch. 39). By applying this scoring method it is possible to tailor treatment to a patient. Treatment can be stopped when morphologic evidence of cardiotoxicity is observed before the patient develops irreversible congestive heart failure. Druck and colleagues[33] reported their observations on radionucleotide imaging and endomyocardial biopsy in the assessment

and eventually coalesce, forming large, membrane-bound spaces. Frequently, there is loss of the outer mitochondrial membranes and cristae. The nuclei demonstrate variable degrees of chromatin disorganization and partial replacement of the chromatin by pale staining fibers and filaments. Myofibrillar loss and vacuolar degeneration can occur concomitantly in the same cell or in separate cells. These changes are progressive and lead to cell death; in severe cases of anthracycline cardiotoxicity, foci of frank cellular necrosis are apparent. As myocytes die they are replaced by fibrous tissue, which forms the patchy stellate scars observed in this cardiomyopathy.

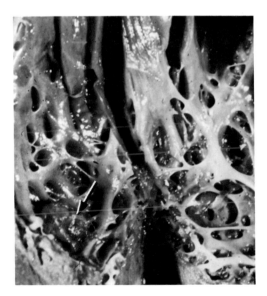

Fig. 32–7. Mural thrombus formation is common in Adriamycin-related cardiomyopathy. Thrombi may be present in any cardiac chamber. This small mural thrombus (arrow) was embedded between prominent trabeculae in the right ventricle.

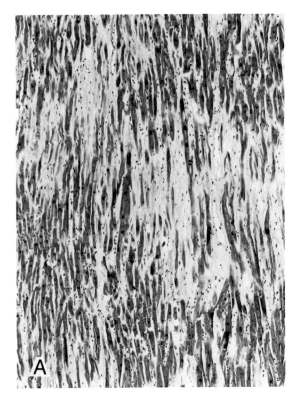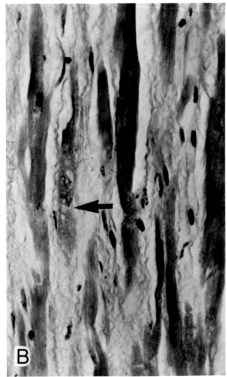

Fig. 32–8. Adriamycin-related cardiomyopathy is characterized, histologically, by (A) extensive patchy and interstitial fibrosis. Areas of healing cell damage are seen, but the predominant finding is myocardial scarring, which represents healed areas of cell damage. (H&E, × 63.) Adjacent to (B) areas of scarring, scattered myocytes are vacuolated (arrow), so-called Adria cells. In these areas, myocytes are being replaced by fibrous tissue. (H&E, × 375.)

of doxorubicin toxicity. This combination proved useful in diagnosis.

The cardiotoxicity of Adriamycin is enhanced by previous mediastinal irradiation.[13] In these patients there is more advanced myocyte degeneration as well as irradiation damage. Evidence of acute radiation effect, especially endothelial swelling, can also be found even when irradiation has preceded Adriamycin therapy by years. This is evidence that Adriamycin can activate a "recall" phenomenon. Adriamycin must be given cautiously in patients who have received previous mediastinal irradiation.

Pathogenic Mechanisms. Experimental and morphologic studies suggest several possible mechanisms of anthracycline-induced cardiotoxicity.[17,22] The nuclear changes indicate a possible disturbance of nucleic acid metabolism induced by the known binding of these drugs to DNA. Alterations in nucleic acid metabolism, especially RNA transcription, could impair protein synthesis with resultant myofiberlysis. The marked swelling of the sarcoplasmic reticulum suggests that cardiotoxicity is the result of generalized metabolic inhibition induced by the anthracyclines.

Catecholamine Cardiomyopathy

Catecholamines produce myocardial necrosis and a cardiomyopathy in experimental animals.[38,80] Epinephrine[42,46] and norepinephrine[123,124] are also cardiotoxic in humans. Both substances produce a toxic myocarditis after massive infusion and are associated with the development of cardiomyopathy in patients with pheochromocytoma.[77,128] The cardiotoxic effects of catecholamines illustrate the overlap between toxic myocarditis and drug-induced cardiomyopathy. Both disease states are produced by a single agent, depending on drug dosage.

Pathology.   The structural changes in catecholamine-induced cardiomyopathy are similar to those in Adriamycin-induced cardiomyopathy. Ultrastructurally, there is extensive myofiberlysis and swelling of the sarcoplasmic reticulum. The similarity of the structural changes suggests that cardiotoxic drugs may exert their effect by potentiating release of catecholamines either directly or via histamine release.[52]

Pathogenic Mechanism.   The mechanism of catecholamine cardiotoxicity may be multifactorial, including a direct toxic metabolic effect and ischemia secondary to an increased demand for oxygen caused by the inotropic stimulus of catecholamines.

Chloroquine Cardiomyopathy

Ratcliff and colleagues report endomyocardial biopsy findings in cases of chloroquine cardiomyopathy.[109]

FIBROTIC SYNDROMES

Fibrotic syndromes affecting the heart and blood vessels are known to occur during therapy with methysergide and ergotamine tartrate.

Cardiac Fibrosis

In cardiac fibrosis cardiac valves are most commonly involved.

Pathology

Grossly, the valves are thickened and distorted (Fig. 32–9; see also Fig. 24–10A & B). Microscopically, the thickening is secondary to a dense layer of fibrous tissue superimposed on the normal valve (Fig. 32–10; see also Fig. 24–10C). The underlying valve is neither fibrotic nor infiltrated by inflammatory cells. Aortic and mitral valves are most frequently involved. The tricuspid valve and endocardium of both ventricles are also affected. Interstitial myocardial fibrosis is reported,[94] but it is unclear whether this is an

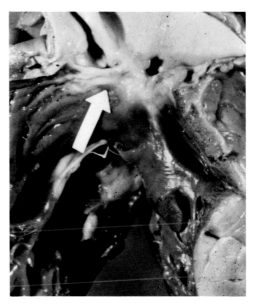

Fig. 32–9. Valvular fibrosis associated with methysergide is characterized by thickening and distortion of valve cusps (arrow) and leaflets. The mitral and aortic valves are most commonly involved. Tricuspid and pulmonary valve involvement (as in this photomicrograph) are rare but have been reported.[49]

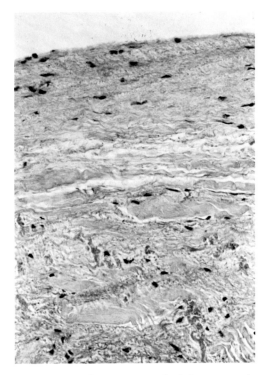

Fig. 32–10. Fibrous tissue is laid down over the normal endocardium in methysergide-induced fibrosis. A distinct cleavage plane is frequently seen between the underlying endocardium and the pannus of new fibrous tissue. This fibrosis is similar to that seen in carcinoid heart disease. (H&E, × 240.)

extension of endocardial fibrosis into the underlying myocardium or a generalized process.

Clinical Features

Clinically, patients with cardiac fibrosis present with cardiac murmurs that were not detected before the beginning of drug therapy.[5,50] The majority have murmurs of aortic insufficiency. However, murmurs of aortic stenosis, mitral stenosis, mitral insufficiency, and tricuspid insufficiency are also reported; many patients have multiple murmurs. When drug therapy is stopped, the murmurs regress partially or completely in 75 percent of cases. Approximately 25 percent

of patients with cardiac fibrosis have pleuropulmonary fibrosis and/or retroperitoneal fibrosis.

Etiology

Cardiac fibrosis is primarily associated with methysergide therapy, although similar cardiac changes are observed with prolonged ergotamine therapy.[5,50,79] Most patients are on long-term methysergide treatment (years) before symptoms develop. The appearance of cardiac symptoms is not, however, directly related to drug dosage or duration of therapy, rather to continuous, daily therapy. The incidence of cardiac fibrosis is approximately 3 percent in patients on continuous therapy and virtually nil in those on an interrupted therapeutic regimen.[79] Nevertheless, cardiac fibrosis can occur in patients on an interrupted regimen.[94]

Pathogenic Mechanisms

Methysergide-induced cardiac fibrosis closely resembles the cardiac lesions associated with the carcinoid syndrome[114] (see Ch. 31), and both states appear related to serotonin. Serotonin produces cardiac and valvular fibrosis in dogs[116] and stimulates fibroblast growth in tissue culture.[15] Methysergide is an antagonist of serotonin with a similar chemical structure. The exact mechanism of methysergide-induced fibrosis is unknown, but methysergide, like serotonin, may stimulate fibroblast growth directly or increase circulating serotonin levels by competing for serotonin binding sites.[9]

Vascular Fibrosis

Intimal fibroplasia and fibromuscular hyperplasia are reported in association with ergotamine[49,133,136] and methysergide[110,119] therapy. It is of interest that proliferative changes have also been described in the walls of blood vessels draining carcinoid tumors (See Ch. 31).

Pathology

The intima is thickened and replaced by loose myxomatous tissue in an intimal fibroplasia (Fig. 32–11). The internal elastic membrane is focally disrupted, but the media is not thickened. The myxomatous tissue consists of proliferating fibroblasts and smooth muscle cells. Large muscular and elastic arteries demonstrate intimal fibroplastic changes. Fibromuscular hyperplasia, by contrast, is more common in medium and small arteries. Here, the media is hypertrophied and there is intimal proliferation similar to that in intimal fibroplasia. Adventitial fibrosis is prominent in both entities. The vascular lesions are focal, and only selected vessels are involved. The intimal proliferation produces focal arterial narrowing and symptoms of ischemic disease.

Pathogenic Mechanisms

Ergotamine is a powerful vasoconstrictor. Clinical symptoms associated with ergotism, especially gangrene, may be secondary to vasoconstriction; however, the morphologic changes are not those of vasoconstriction. One theory proposes that the focal areas of intimal proliferation represent organized thrombi at sites of vasoconstriction.[136] This is not substantiated, and it is more likely that ergotamine, like methysergide, stimulates fibroblast proliferation (see also Ch. 10).

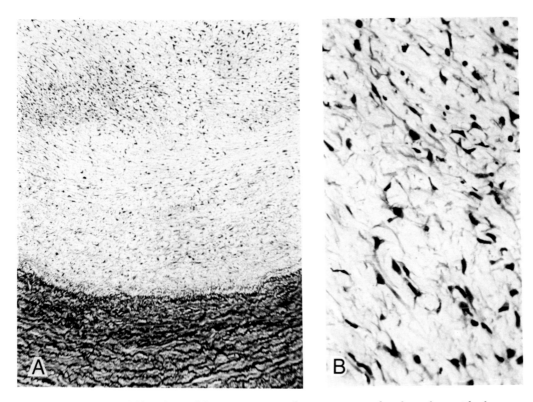

Fig. 32–11. (A) Intimal fibroplasia of the common carotid artery associated with methysergide therapy. This process is focal, and the vessel lumen is usually compromised. (H&E, × 90.) (B) The thickened intima is composed of fibroblasts and prominent myointimal cells in an acid mucopolysacharide matrix. The myointimal cells are branching and contain abundant myofilaments, similar to smooth muscle cells, although they lack a well-defined basement membrane. (H&E, × 275.)

DRUG-RELATED VASCULITIS

The association of drug therapy with development of a vasculitis is well recognized[43,100] (see also Ch. 12). Originally, drug-related vasculitis was considered analogous to panarteritis nodosa and was called "microscopic periarteritis nodosa." In the 1940s, Zeek and colleagues recognized that drug-related vascular lesions were not identical to classic panarteritis nodosa and proposed that they be classified as hypersensitivity angiitis.[137,138] Unfortunately, Zeek and subsequent authors grouped many other vasculitides together with drug-related vasculitis under the inclusive term "hypersensitivity angiitis."

Hypersensitivity angiitis commonly includes vascular lesions associated with serum sickness, systemic bacterial infections, protozoal infestations, reactions to influenza vaccines, as well as drug-related vasculitides. If the drug-related vasculitides are separated from the broad grouping of hypersensitivity angiitis, such vascular lesions can be divided into a nonnecrotizing and a necrotizing form. Most drug-related vasculitis, despite published reports to the contrary, is nonnecrotizing and secondary to delayed drug hypersensitivity.[100] Necrotizing drug-related vasculitis is uncommon and more frequently toxic in etiology.

Non-necrotizing (Hypersensitivity) Vasculitis

Pathology

Vascular lesions in this condition are monotonously alike and characterized by a predominantly mononuclear infiltrate with occasional eosinophils, in the absence of fibrinoid necrosis or necrotizing lesions of the vessel wall. Arterioles, capillaries, venules, small veins, and occasionally small arteries are affected; muscular and elastic arteries and large veins are spared. Capillaries and venous channels are most extensively involved (Figs. 32–12 and 32–13). The inflammatory infiltrate extends through the *full* thickness of the affected vessel wall, involving the media and intima, as well as the adventitia. The infiltrate consists of mononuclear cells, eosinophils, and scattered polymorphonuclear leukocytes. Eosinophils are prominent but comprise 10 percent or less of the cell population, and polymorphs are usually inconspicuous (Fig. 32–12). Foci of medial edema (inspissated plasma proteins) are occasionally seen in small arteries. These areas do not stain positively for fibrin with phosphotungstic acid-hematoxylin or the Movat stain. The endothelial lining of involved arterial and venous channels is intact, and thrombi are not found. The vascular lesions are uniformly bland appearing, and lesions in different stages of development are not seen. So-called pre-exudative lesions and healing lesions with periadventitial and medial fibrosis are not observed.[100]

Differential Diagnosis

The diagnosis of drug-related vasculitis must be based on both clinical information and the morphologic appearance of vascular lesions. Vascular lesions that resemble those seen in hypersensitivity vasculitis may be found in any of the "collagen diseases" (see Ch. 30). Other morphologic changes (periadventitial fibrosis, vessel wall scarring, fibrinoid necrosis, and focal necrotizing vasculitis) are usually present in collagen diseases and distinguish these vasculitides from drug-related vasculitis. The latter changes, however, are often focal and may not be present in small biopsy specimens. In drug-induced vasculitis, laboratory and clinical findings, such as positive serologic tests and drug history, are important; the diagnosis should not be made solely on the basis of morphology. Nevertheless, the finding of a bland vasculitis with prominent eosinophils, involving small arterial and venous channels, in the absence of necrotizing vascular lesions strongly suggests a drug-related hypersensitivity vasculitis.

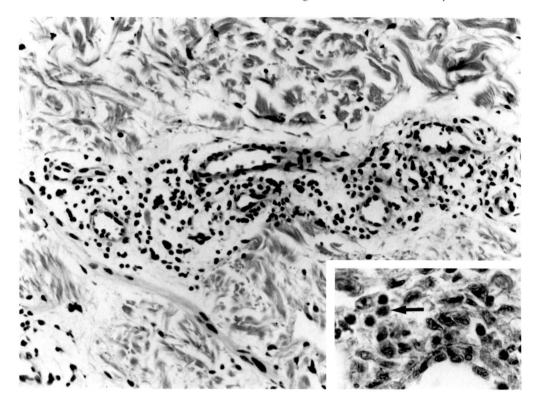

Fig. 32–12. Hypersensitivity vasculitis associated with ampicillin. The skin is a common site for vascular involvement in hypersensitivity drug reactions. The inflammatory infiltrate rings small vessels and extends through the vessel wall. Capillaries, arterioles, and small veins are all involved. The infiltrate (insert) consists of mononuclear cells and prominent eosinophils (arrow). (H&E, × 275; insert × 900.)

Clinical Features

Clinically, patients with drug-related vasculitis divide into two distinct groups.[100] One develops a localized skin reaction without other clinical signs or symptoms. In contrast, the second group develops a systemic vasculitis often with skin involvement. Clinical findings in these patients are often multiple and confusing. Malaise, shortness of breath, and findings of congestive heart failure are common, as are other symptoms secondary to specific organ involvement. The presence of a rash in association with eosinophilia or an unexplained fever is the most reliable clue to the possibility of a systemic drug-related vasculitis, irrespective of the organs involved. The most common sites of involvement are the skin and subcutaneous tissue, the heart, the liver, and the kidneys.

Treatment

Effective treatment depends on early diagnosis and prompt withdrawal of the offending medication followed by steroid administration. In patients with localized drug-related vasculitis, diagnosis is seldom a problem, and they respond dramatically to withdrawal of all medication, with or without steroid therapy. However, confusing and often conflicting symptoms tend to obscure the diagnosis of drug hypersensitivity. When all medications are withdrawn and steroid therapy is started early, symptoms promptly abate and the patients recover.

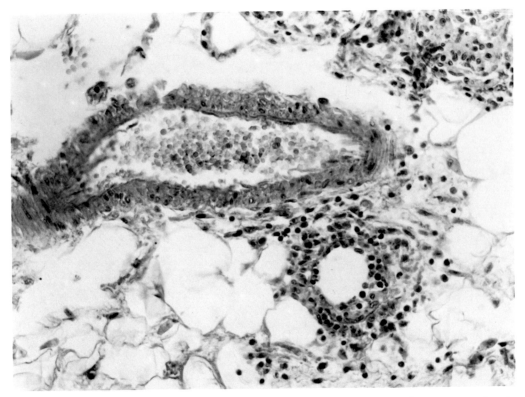

Fig. 32–13. Hypersensitivity vasculitis associated with allopurinol. Larger vessels, arteries, and veins are characteristically spared in hypersensitivity vasculitis. The arteriole, adjacent to the larger vein, is involved while the vein is spared in this photomicrograph. The inflammatory infiltrate extends through the entire thickness of the arteriole wall. (H&E, × 576.)

Pathogenic Mechanisms

The interval between first administration of a drug and development of vasculitis is extremely variable. The fact that a patient has been taking a drug for months or years, without side effects, does not exclude it as a possible etiologic agent. *Drug-induced vasculitis is neither dose-dependent nor time-dependent* and may occur at any time while the drug is being administered.

The lack of a dose-dependent response and clinical presentation suggest that this form of drug-related vasculitis is a delayed hypersensitivity phenomenon.[96] Experimental evidence also supports an immunologic mechanism. A non-necrotizing vasculitis has been reported in patients with previous drug-related vasculitis following rechallenge with nonpharmacologic doses of diphenhydramine[32] and levamisole.[92] In addition, deposits of IgG, IgA, and IgM were found in the involved vessels of a patient with propylthiouracil-induced vasculitis.[51] These reports suggest a specific antigen-antibody interaction as the cause of non-necrotizing drug-related vasculitis.

Drugs associated with hypersensitivity vasculitis are listed in Table 32–4. Many are also associated with hypersensitivity myocarditis.

Necrotizing Vasculitis (Toxic Vasculitis)

Unlike hypersensitivity vasculitis, necrotizing drug-related vasculitis may be indistinguishable from classic panarteritis nodosa.

Table 32–4. Drugs Associated with Nonnecrotizing Hypersensitivity Vasculitis

Allopurinol	Indocin
Ampicillin	Isoniazid
Bromide	Levamisole[92]
Carbamazepine	Methylthioruracil[57]
Chloramphenical	Oxyphenbutazone
Chlorothiazide	Penicillin
Chlorpropamide	Phenylbutazone
Chlortetracycline	Potassium iodine
Chlorthalidone	Procainamide[115]
Colchicine	Propylthiouracil[51]
Cromolyn sodium	Quinidine
Dextran	Spironolactone
Diphenylhydantoin	Sulfonamide
Diphenhydramine[32]	Tetracycline
Griseofulvin	Trimethadione

Table 32–5. Drugs Associated with Necrotizing Vasculitis

Arsenic[133]
Bismuth[133]
Gold[133]
Methamphetamine[26]
Sulfonamides[100]

Pathology

The involved vessels are usually medium-sized and small arteries. Capillaries, arterioles, and veins are spared. Acute as well as healing and healed lesions are present. Acute lesions are characterized by focal fibrinoid necrosis of the vessel wall. The associated inflammatory infiltrate is composed primarily of polymorphonuclear leukocytes, although eosinophils are occasionally prominent. Older lesions are distinguished by focal scarring of the media, adventitial fibrosis, and marked intimal proliferation with luminal narrowing. Occlusive thrombi are frequent in both acute and healing stages. Lesions are most often observed at sites of bifurcation, and in many instances there is aneurysmal dilation of the defective area of the vessel wall.

Etiology and Pathogenic Mechanisms

Only a few drugs are clearly associated with necrotizing vasculitis (Table 32–5). The etiology of this form of drug-related vasculitis is unclear. Precipitated drug or foreign material is occasionally found in the vessel wall, especially in areas of necrosis.[100] In these instances the necrotizing lesions are most probably toxic in etiology. In other cases, as in serum sickness in which a similar necro-tizing vasculitis has been reported,[28] the etiology appears to be antibody antigen related. The immunologic mechanism in these cases is more likely an immediate hypersensitivity reaction.

LUPUS-LIKE SYNDROMES

Syndromes indistinguishable from systemic lupus erythematosus (SLE) may follow the administration of a number of drugs.[1,46,53,85]

Clinical Features

As in "spontaneous" SLE, presenting complaints vary widely and include arthritis, fever, skin lesions, and renal involvement. Unlike spontaneous SLE, however, renal involvement is less frequent and usually less severe in drug-induced lupus.[53] In addition to clinical features of SLE, a high proportion of patients (75–100%) have antinuclear antibodies usually with positive LE cell tests. Antinuclear antibodies may also be present in the absence of other signs of the disease, especially in patients taking procainamide[85] (see also Ch. 30).

Most cases of drug-related lupus are completely reversible within weeks to months following withdrawal of the drug.

Pathology

Morphologic studies of drug-induced lupus are thus rare. Although morphologic changes similar to those in spontaneous SLE have been reported in lupus-like syndromes,[7,35,111] most cases studied have not substantiated these findings. The reports of morphologic changes are primarily in the early literature and probably represent cases of spontaneous SLE, rather than drug-induced lupus.

Etiology

Many drugs are associated with lupus-like syndromes.[52,85] Drugs in which this association is well documented are listed in Table 32–6. In addition, penicillin, sulfonamides, streptomyosin, tetracycline, and griseofulvin are reported to cause a lupus-like syndrome in occasional patients; however, the criteria for drug eligibility are not completely fulfilled in these reports.[85] Lupus-like syndromes usually occur only after months of therapy with large doses of drug and then only in 1 to 2 percent of the population exposed to the drug. As in spontaneous SLE, females are more frequently affected than males.

Pathogenic Mechanisms

Considerable epidemologic and experimental evidence now exists that drug-induced lupus occurs, not in a random population who de-

Table 32–6. Drugs Associated
with Lupus-like Syndromes

Carbamazepine
Chloropromazine
Diphenylhydantoin
D-Penicillamine
Isoniazid
Mephenytoin
Methyldopa
Methylthiouracil
Para-aminosalicylate
Phenylbutazone
Procainamide
Propylthiouracil
Reserpine
Trimethadione

velop drug hypersensitivity, but among individuals with an intrinsic tendency to the syndrome—a so-called lupus diathesis. The mechanism by which these drugs cause or unmask the lupus-like syndrome is unknown. The best evidence suggests that the drug either modifies nucleoprotein antigenicity or reinforces the antigenicity of circulating DNA, which is normally present in small amounts.

EFFECTS OF ESTROGENS

Epidemiologic investigations demonstrated modest risks of thromboembolic and vascular disorders associated with the use of oral contraceptives, and more specifically with the use of estrogens. These included deep vein phlebitis, pulmonary embolism, postoperative phlebitis, stroke, and myocardial infarction. The risk of thromboembolic disorders is greatest in premenopausal women. Studies in postmenopausal women on long-term estrogen therapy have not demonstrated a significant increase of thromboembolic disorders or myocardial infarction.[97,108]

The weight of evidence from both retrospective[117,129] and prospective[75,130] studies indicates that the risk of deep vein phlebitis and pulmonary embolism is fivefold, and that of stroke tenfold, in women taking oral contraceptives as compared to age-matched controls. The risk of thromboembolic disease is greatest in women under the age of 35 and does not correlate with smoking.[67] Evidence suggests that the population at greatest risk are women with prior thromboembolic disorders or with prominent risk factors for thromboembolic disorders, such as severe varicose veins, hypertension, or diabetes mellitus.[118] The incidence of thromboembolic disorders in women without these risk factors has diminished since the introduction, in the early 1970s, of newer oral contraceptives containing low-dose estrogens.

Retrospective epidemologic studies also

suggested an association between oral contractive use and myocardial infarction in premenopausal women.[67,93] The risk of myocardial infarction was increased fivefold in oral contraceptive users and was greatest in women over 35 years of age, heavy cigarette smokers, and women with pre-existing medical conditions, especially hypertension, diabetes mellitus, and a history of myocardial infarction.

Pathology/Pathogenic Mechanisms

Whether there is a morphologic basis for the thromboembolic disorders associated with estrogen use is not clear. Individual case reports document vascular changes in patients with phlebitis and pulmonary emboli,[62] stroke,[54] and myocardial infarction.[3] The vascular changes identical in all three reports. They consisted of intimal proliferation in veins and fibromuscular hyperplasia (intimal fibroplasia) in arteries. Medium and small vessels focally involved throughout the body, and thrombi frequent at sites of intimal narrowing. It is unclear whether the intimal proliferation was caused by the estrogens or sites of old organized thrombi. Other investigators have not found similar vascular lesions in women taking oral contraceptives. Evidence suggests that serum estrogen compounds in premenopausal women may alter lipids and accelerate the development of atherosclerosis.[70] Vascular lesions reported in oral contraceptive users are consistent with early atherosclerotic lesions.

REFERENCES

1. Alarcon-Segovia D, Wakim KG, Worthington JW, Ward LE: Clinical and experimental studies on the hydralazine syndrome and its relationship to systemic lupus erythematosus. Medicine 46:1, 1967
2. Alexander CS, Nino A: Cardiovascular complications in young patients taking psychotrophic drugs. A preliminary report. Am Heart J 78:757, 1969
3. Altshuler JH, McLaughlin RA, Neubuerger KT: Neurologic catastrophe related to oral contraceptives. Arch Neurol 19:264, 1968
4. Applebaum FR, Strauchen JA, Graw RG, Jr: Acute lethal carditis caused by high-dose combination chemotherapy. A unique clinical and patholgoic entity. Lancet 1:58, 1976
5. Bana DS, MacNeal PS, LeCompte PM, et al: Cardiac murmurs and endocardial fibrosis associated with methysergide therapy. Am Heart J 88:640, 1974
6. Banerjee D: Myocarditis in penicillin sensitivity. Indian Heart J 20:72, 1968
7. Bendersky G, Ramirez C: Hydralazine poisoning: review of the literature and autopsy study of persons with massive intestinal bleeding. JAMA 173:1789, 1960
8. Benjamin R, Billingham M, Mason J: Cardiotoxicity of adriamycin, DNA and rubidazone: Evaluation by ECG and endomyocardial biopsy. Cancer Treat Rep 62:935, 1978
9. Bianchine JR, Eade NR: Vasoactive substances and fibrosis. Res Clin Study Headache 2:60, 1969
10. Billingham ME: Some recent advances in cardiac pathology. Hum Pathol 10:367, 1979
11. Billingham ME: Morphologic changes in drug induced heart disease. p. 127. In Bristow MR (ed): Meyler and Peck's Drug Induced Heart Disease, vol. 5, Elsevier Science Publishers, Amsterdam, 1980
12. Billingham ME: Pharmacotoxic myocardial disease. An endomyocardial study. Heart Vessels. suppl. 1:278, 1985
13. Billingham ME, Bristow MR, Glatstein E, et al: Adriamycin cardiotoxicity: Endomyocardial biopsy evidence of enhancement by irradiation. Am J Surg Pathol 1:17, 1977
14. Billingham ME, Mason JW, Bristow MR, Daniels JR: Anthracycline cardiomyopathy monitored by morphologic changes. Cancer Treat Rep 62:865, 1978
15. Boucek RJ, Alvarez TR: 5-Hydroxytrytamine: A cytospecific growth stimulator of cultured fibroblasts. Science 167:898, 1970
16. Brem TH, Konwaler BE: Fatal myocarditis due to emetine hydrochloride. Am Heart J 80:476, 1980

17. Bristow MR, Mason JW, Billingham ME, Daniels JR: Doxorubicin cardiomyopathy: Evaluation by phonocardiography, endomyocardial biopsy, and cardiac catheterization. Ann Intern Med 88:168, 1978

18. Bristow MR, Thompson PD, Martin PR, et al: Early anthracycline cardiotoxicity. Am J Med 65:823, 1978

19. Brown CE, McNamara DH: Acute interstitial myocarditis following administration of arsphenamines. Arch Derm Syph 42:312, 1940

20. Buja LM, Ferrans VJ, Graw RG, Jr: Cardiac pathologic findings in patients treated with bone marrow transplantation. Hum Pathol 7:17, 1976

21. Buja LM, Ferrans VJ, Mayer RJ, et al: Cardiac ultrastructural changes induced by daunorubicin therapy. Cancer 32:771, 1973

22. Buja LM, Ferrans VJ, Roberts WC: Drug-induced cardiomyopathies. Adv Cardiol 13:330, 1974

23. Buzdar AU, Legha SS, Tashima CK, et al: Adriamycin and mitomycin C: Possible synergistic cardiotoxicity. Cancer Treat Rep 62:1005, 1978

24. Buzdar AU, Marcus C, Smith TL, Blumenschein GR: Early and delayed cardiotoxicity of doxorubicin. Cancer 55:2761, 1985

25. Chatterjee SS, Thakre MW: Fiedler's myocarditis: Report of a fatal case following intramuscular injection of streptomycin. Tubercle 39:240, 1958

26. Citron BP, Halpern M, McCarron M, et al: Necrotizing angiitis associated with drug abuse. N Engl J Med 283:1003, 1970

27. Clark E: Serum carditis: The morphologic cardiac alterations in man associated with serum disease. JAMA 110:1098, 1938

28. Clark E, Kaplan BI: Endocardial, arterial and other mesenchymal alterations associated with serum disease in man. Arch Pathol 24:458, 1937

29. Cregler LL, Mark H: Medical complications of cocaine abuse. N Engl J Med 315:1495, 1986

30. Contro S, Mond E: The electrocardiogram in hypersensitivity reactions. Am Heart J 52:510, 1956

31. Dalgaard JB: Fatal myocarditis following smallpox vaccination. Am Heart J 54:156, 1957

32. Davenport PM, Wilhelm RE: An unusual vasculitis due to diphenhydramine: Cutaneous and central nervous system involvement. Arch Dermatol 92:577, 1965

33. Druck MN, Gulenchyn KY, Evans WK, et al: Radionuclide angiography and endomyocardial biopsy in the assessment of doxorubicin cardiotoxicity. Cancer 53:1667, 1984

34. Dustan HP, Taylor RD, Corcoran AC, Page IH: Rheumatic and febrile syndrome during prolonged hydralazine treatment. JAMA 154:23, 1954

35. Edge JR: Myocardial fibrosis following arsenical therapy. Lancet 2:675, 1946

36. Farrant R: Myperthyroidism: Its experimental production in animals. Br Med J 2:1363, 1913

37. Fenoglio JJ Jr, McAllister HA Jr, Mullick FG: Drug-related myocarditis. I. Hypersensitivity myocarditis. Human Pathol 12:900, 1981

38. Ferrans VJ, Hibbs RG, Black WC, Weilbaecher DG: Isoproterenol-induced myocardial necrosis. A histochemical and electron microscopic study. Am Heart J 68:71, 1964

39. Field JB, Federman DD: Sudden death in a diabetic subject during treatment with BZ-55 (carbutamide). Diabetes 6:67, 1957

40. Findlay-Jones LR: Fatal myocarditis after vaccination against smallpox: Report of a case. N Engl J Med 270:41, 1964

41. Fleisher MS, Loeb L: Further investigations in experimental myocarditis. Arch Intern Med 6:427, 1910

42. Franz G: Eine seitene form von toxischer myocardschadigung. Virchows Arch (Pathol Anat) 298:743, 1937

43. French AJ: Hypersensitivity in the pathogenesis of the histopathologic changes associated with sulfonamide chemotherapy. Am J Pathol 22:679, 1946

44. French AJ, Weller CV: Interstitial myocarditis following the clinical and experimental use of sulfonamide drugs. Am J Pathol 18:109, 1942

45. Giles TD, Modlin RK: Death associated with ventricular arrhythmia and thioridazine hydrochloride. JAMA 205:108, 1968

46. Gormsen H: Om Dodelig Adrenalin Forgiftning. Ugeskrift For Laeger 101:242, 1939

47. Gottdiener JS, Appelbaum FR, Ferrans VJ, et al: Cardiotoxicity associated with high-dose

cyclophosphamide therapy. Arch Intern Med 141:758, 1981

48. Gotti EW: Adverse drug reactions and the autopsy. Arch Pathol 97:201, 1974

49. Gould SE, Price AE, Ginsberg HI: Gangrene and death following ergotamine tartrate (Gynergen) therapy. JAMA 106:1631, 1936

50. Graham JR: Cardiac and pulmonary fibrosis during methysergide therapy for headache. Am J Med Sci 254:1, 1967

51. Griswold WR, Mendoza SA, Johnston W, Nichols S: Vasculitis associated with propylthiouracil: Evidence for immune complex pathogenesis and response to therapy. Western J Med 128:543, 1978

52. Haft JI: Cardiovascular injury induced by sympathetic catecholamines. Prog Cardiovasc Dis 17:73, 1974

53. Harpey JP: Lupus-like syndromes induced by drugs. Ann Allergy 33:256, 1974

54. Hartman JD, Young I, Bank AA, Rosenblatt SA: Fibromuscular hyperplasia of internal carotid arteries: Stroke in a young adult complicated by oral contraceptives. Arch Neurol 25:295, 1971

55. Herman JE, Fleischmann P: Unusual evidence of myocardial involvement during a hypersensitivity reaction to oral penicillin. Israel J Med Sci 14:848, 1978

56. Herman JE, Schwartz Y, Bassan H: Primary cardiac involvement and painful salivary gland enlargement due to phenylbutazone. Harefuah 86:246, 1974

57. Hogewind F, Hadders HN, Meyler L: Arteriitis als gevolg van overgevoeligheid voor methylthiouracil. Nederland Tijd v. Geneesk 103:1009, 1959

58. Honey M: The effects of sodium antimony tartrate on the myocardium. Br Heart J 22:601, 1960

59. Horowitz JD: Drug therapy. Drugs that induce heart problems. Which agents? What effect? J Cardiovasc Med 8:308, 1983

60. Hueper WC, Ichniowski CT: Experimental studies in cardiovascular pathology. II. Pathologic lesions in organs of cats, guinea pigs and frogs produced by digitalis poisoning. J Lab Clin Med 26:1565, 1941

61. Irey NS: Tissue reactions to drugs. Am J Pathol 82:617, 1976

62. Irey NS, Manion WC, Taylor HB: Vascular lesions in women taking oral contraceptives. Arch Pathol 89:1, 1970

63. Isner JM, Estes NAM, Thompson PD, et al: Acute cardiac events temporally related to cocaine abuse. N Engl J Med 315:1438, 1986

64. Isner JM, Ferrans VJ, Cohen SR, et al: Clinical and morphologual cardiac findings after anthracycline chemotherapy. Analysis of 64 patients studied at necropsy. Am J Cardiol 51:1167, 1983

65. Jaenke RS: An anthracycline antibiotic-induced cardiomyopathy in rabbits. Lab Invest 30:292, 1974

66. Jaenke RS, Fajardo LF: Adriamycin-induced myocardial lesions: Report of a workshop. Am J Surg Pathol 1:55, 1977

67. Jick H, Dinan B, Herman R, Rothman KJ: Myocardial infarction and other vascular diseases in young women: Role of estrogens and other factors. JAMA 240:2548, 1978

68. Josue O: Hypertrophie cardiaque causee par l'adrénaline et la toxine typhique. Compt Rend Soc Biol 63:285, 1907

69. Kalikshtein DB, Odinokova VA, Paleev NR, Gurevich MA: Hypersensitivity of delayed type manifested during the development of allergic lesions of the myocardium. Bull Exp Biol Med 77:789, 1974

70. Kannel WB: Editorial: Possible hazards of oral contraceptive use. Circulation 60:490, 1979

71. Kantrowitz NE, Bristow MR: Cardiotoxicity of antitumor agents. Prog Cardiovasc Dis 27:195, 1984

72. Karch SB: The history of cocaine abuse. Hum Pathol 20:1037, 1989

73. Karch SB, Billingham ME: The pathology and etiology of cocaine-induced heart disease. Arch Pathol Lab Med 112:225, 1988

74. Kattwinkel EE: Death due to cardiac disease following the use of emetine hydrochloride in conditioned-reflex treatment of chronic alcoholism. N Engl J Med 240:995, 1949

75. Kay CK: Oral contraceptives and health. The Royal College of General Practitioners study. Am J Epidemiol 102:458, 1975

76. Kerwin AJ: Fatal myocarditis due to sensitivity to phenindione. Can Med Assoc J 90:1418, 1964

77. Kline IK: Myocardial alterations associated with pheochromocytomas. Am J Pathol 38:539, 1960

78. Kline IK, Kline TS, Saphir O: Myocarditis in senescence. Am Heart J 65:446, 1963

79. Kunkel RS: Fibrotic syndromes with chronic use of methysergide. Headache 11:1, 1971

80. Kutsuna F: Electron microscopic studies on isoproterenol-induced myocardial lesion in rats. Jpn Heart J 13:168, 1972

81. Kyser FA, Finsberg H, Gilbert NC: The effect of certain drugs upon the cardiotoxic lesions of digitalis in the dog. Am Heart J 31:451, 1946

82. Lange RA, Cigarrda RG, Yancy CW Jr, et al: Cocaine-induced coronary-artery vasoconstriction. N Engl J Med 321:1557, 1989

83. Langsjoen H, Stinson JC: Acute fatal allergic myocarditis: Report of a case. Dis Chest 48:440, 1965

84. Lang-Stevenson D, Mikhailidis DP, Gillett DS: Cardiotoxicity of 5-flourouracil. Lancet 2:406, 1977

85. Lee SL, Siegel M: Drug-induced systemic lupus erythematosus. p. 239. In Meyler L, Peck HM (eds): Drug-Induced Diseases, vol. 3. Excerpta Medica, New York, 1968

86. Lefrak EA, Pitha J, Rosenheim S, Gottlieb JA: A clinicopathologic analysis of adriamycin cardiotoxicity. Cancer 32:302, 1973

87. Len Tseng H: Interstitial myocarditis probably related to lithium carbonate intoxication. Arch Pathol 92:444, 1971

88. Levillain R: Myocardite experimentale: Étude anatomique de 210 coeurs de rats ayant ingéré du fluoro-uracile. Cir Soc Biol 166:340, 1972

89. Levine SE, Brust JCM, Futrell N, et al: Cerebrovascular complications of the use of the "crack" form of alkaloid cocaine. N Engl J Med 323:699, 1990

90. Lewitzky A: Ueber pathologisch-histologische Veranderungen des Herzens bei Digitalisvergiftungen. Zentralbl Allg Pathol 16:532, 1905

91. Lilienfeld A, Hochstein E, Weiss W: Acute myocarditis with bundle branch block due to sulfonamide sensitivity. Circulation 1:1060, 1950

92. Macfarlane DG, Bacon PA: Side effects of drugs. Levamisole-induced vasculitis due to circulating immune complexes Br Med J 2:407, 1978

93. Mann JI, Inman WHW: Oral contraceptives and death from myocardial infarction. Br Med J 2:245, 1975

94. Mason JW, Billingham ME, Friedman JP: Methysergide-induced heart disease. A case of multivalvular and myocardial fibrosis. Circulation 56:889, 1977

95. Mathias DW: Cocaine-associated myocardial ischemia. Review of clinical and angiographic findings. Am J Med 81:675, 1986

96. McCombs RP: Systemic "allergic" vasculitis: Clinical and pathological relationships. JAMA 194:1059, 1965

97. McKay Hart D, Lindsay R, Purdie D: Vascular complications of long-term estrogen therapy. Front Hormone Res 5:174, 1978

98. Mitchell JE, Mackenzie TB: Cardiac effects of lithium therapy in man: A review. J Clin Psychiatry 43:47, 1982

99. Mullick FG, McAllister HA: Myocarditis associated with methyldopa therapy. JAMA 237:1699, 1977

100. Mullick FG, McAllister HA, Wagner BM, Fenoglio JJ, Jr: Drug-related vasculitis: Clinicopatholgoic correlations in thirty patients. Hum Pathol 10:313, 1979

101. Murphy ML, Bullock RT, Pearce MB: The correlation of metabolic and ultrastructural changes in emetine myocardial toxicity. Am Heart J 87:105, 1974

102. Neugarten J, Gallo GR, Buxbaum J, et al: Amyloidosis in subcutaneous heroin abusers ("skin poppers amyloidosis"). Am J Med 81:635, 1986

103. Parker CW: Drug therapy: Drug allergy. N Engl J Med 292:511, 1975

104. Pearce MB, Bullock RT, Murphy ML: Selective damage of myocardial mitochondria to emetine hydrochloride. Arch Pathol 91:8, 1971

105. Peng SK, French WJ, Pelikan PCD: Direct cocaine cardiotoxicity demonstrated by endomyocardial biopsy. Arch Pathol Lab Med 113:842, 1989

106. Plafker J: Penicillin-related nephritis and myocarditis: A case report. South Med J 64:852, 1971

107. Pottage A, Holt S, Ludgate S, Langlands AO: Fluorouracil cardiotoxicity. Br Med J 1:547, 1978

108. Rakoff AE: Factors relating to morbidity and mortality of women on long-term estrogen therapy. Front Hormone Res 5:40, 1978

109 Ratcliff NB, Estes ML, Myles JL, et al: Diagnosis of chloroquine cardiomyopathy by endomyocardial biopsy. N Engl J Med 316:191, 1987

110. Regan JF, Poletti BJ: Vascular adventitial fibrosis in a patient taking methysergide maleate. JAMA 203:1069, 1968

111. Reinhardt DJ, Waldron JM: Lupus erythematosus-like syndrome complicating hydralazine (Apresoline) therapy. JAMA 155:1491, 1954

112. Richardson HL, Groupner KI, Richardson ME: Intramyocardial lesions in patients dying suddenly and unexpectedly. JAMA 195:254, 1966

113. Rinehart JF, Anderson HH: Effect of emetine on cardiac muscle. Arch Pathol 11:546, 1931

114. Roberts WC, Sjoerdsma A: The cardiac disease associated with the carcinoid syndrome (carcinoid heart disease). Am J Med 36:5, 1964

115. Rosin JM: Vasculitis following procaine amide therapy. Am J Med 42:625, 1965

116. Rossi P, Stevenson M, Khaksar P, Bellet S: Coronary arteriosclerosis induced in young dogs by prolonged intra-aortic infusions of serotonin. Circ Res 9:436, 1961

117. Sartwell PE, Masi AT, Arthes FG, et al: Thromboembolism and oral contraceptives: An epidemiologic case-control study. Am J Epidemiol 90:365, 1969

118. Sartwell PE, Stolley PD, Touascia JA, et al: Overview: Pulmonary embolism mortality in relation to oral contraceptive use. Preventive Med 5:15, 1976

119. Schwarts DT: Relation of superior mesenteric artery obstruction to renal hypertension. N Engl J Med 272:1318, 1965

120. Simpson RW, Edwards WD: Pathogenesis of cocaine-induced ischemic heart disease. Arch Pathol Lab Med 110:479, 1986

121. Smith HJ, Roche AHG, Jagusch MF, Herdson PB: Cardiomyopathy associated with amphetamine administration. Am Heart J 91:792, 1976

122. Swedberg K, Winblad B: Heart failure as complication of lithium treatment. Acta Med Scand 196:279, 1974

123. Szakacs JE, Cannon A: L-norepinephrine myocarditis. Am J Clin Pathol 30:425, 1958

124. Szakacs JE, Mehlman B: Pathologic changes induced by 1-norepinephrine. Am J Cardiol 5:619, 1960

125. Taliercio CP, Olney BA, Lie JT: Myocarditis related to drug hypersensitivity. Mayo Clin Proc 60:463, 1985

126. Tazelaar HD, Karch SB, Stephens BG, et al: Cocaine and the heart. Hum Pathol 18:195, 1987

127. van Mieghem W, Stevens E, Cosemans J: Ephedrine-induced cardiomyopathy. Br Med J 1:816, 1978

128. van Vliet PD, Burchell HB, Titus JL: Focal myocarditis associated with pheochromocytoma. N Engl J Med 274:1102, 1966

129. Vessey MP, Doll R: Investigation of relation between use of oral contraceptives and thrombo-embolic disease. A further report. Br Med J 2:651, 1969

130. Vessey M, Doll R, Peto R, et al: A long-term follow-up study of women using different methods of contraception—an interim report. J Biosoc Sci 8:873, 1976

131. Waugh D: Myocarditis, arteritis, and focal hepatic, splenic, and renal granulomas apparently due to penicillin sensitivity. Am J Pathol 28:437, 1952

132. Weiner RS, Lockhart JT, Schwartz RG: Dilated cardiomyopathy and cocaine abuse: Report of two cases. Am J Med 81:699, 1986

133. Wenzel DG: Drug-induced cardiomyopathies. J Pharm Sci 56:1209, 1967

134. Wynne J, Braunwald E: The cardiomyopathies and myocarditides. p. 1410. In Braunwald E (ed): Heart Disease. A Textbook of Cardiovascular Medicine, 3rd ed. WB Saunders, Philadelphia, 1988

135. Yater WM, Cahill JA: Bilateral gangrene of feet due to ergotamine tartrate used for pruritus of jaundice. JAMA 106:1625, 1936

136. Young JR, Humphries AW: Severe arteriospasm after use of ergotamine tartrate suppositories. JAMA 175:1141, 1961

137. Zeek PM: Periarteritis and other forms of necrotizing angiitis. N Engl J Med 248:764, 1953

138. Zeek PM, Smith CG, Weeter JC: Studies on periarteritis nodosa. III. The differentiation between the vascular lesions of periarteritis nodosa and hypersensitivity. Am J Pathol 24:889, 1948

33

Cardiovascular Diseases in the Tropics

B. N. Datta

The socioeconomic development of under-privileged peoples, most of whom live in the tropics, determines the pattern of disease prevalent in their countries. During the last 5 to 7 years, heart diseases in the tropics have become a focus of attention for cardiologists all over the world. The World Health Organization (WHO) and the International Society and Federation of Cardiology designated 1982 the "Year of Tropical Cardiology." Also, most developing Asian and African countries have now invested in cardiac investigative laboratories and cardiothoracic surgery centers. This has considerably enriched the literature on tropical cardiology. Despite these "advances," the basic pattern of cardiac morbidity and mortality in tropical countries has not changed for the better. For example, infective conditions such as rheumatic heart disease, infective endocarditis, and pericarditis continue to extract a heavy toll of life, especially among the young, while the rapid sophistication of life-style has made diseases such as hypertension and ischemic heart disease common (these are classified as "modern Western pattern dominated by degenerative diseases").[10] Recognition of cardiomyopathies has improved, but many still have not yielded their enigmatic cause. The hot, humid climate of the tropics by itself produces edema and heart failure.[260]

Extensive clinical and some postmortem data are available from the 1950s on the prevalence of cardiac diseases in the tropics. However, comparison of published data poses a problem, because of their variety. There are hospital statistics and population surveys—both clinical and autopsy—some expressed as a proportion of total hospital patients, others as cardiac diseases only. This chapter attempts to sift such data. Some data have been condensed in Table 33–1 (clinical information) and Table 33–2 (autopsy reports). My own experience, updated to 2,500 autopsies on cardiac diseases examined over 25 years, is shown in Table 33–3.

Both in India and Africa, the last two to three decades have seen a marked increase in the incidence of cardiac diseases and deaths.[144,277,314] A recent survey from China of more than 25,000 patients, spanning a 32-year period from 1948 to 1979, reported a decrease in rheumatic heart disease by 50 percent but showed an increase in the incidence of ischemic heart disease by a spectacular 500 percent.[305,306]

In general, in Asia and Africa, heart diseases account for 8 to 20 percent of all medical ad-

Table 33–1. Clinical Prevalence of Common Heart Diseases in the Tropics
(% of Hospital Admissions)

Country	Heart Disease				
	Rheumatic	Hyper-tensive	Ischemic	Cardio-myopathy	Cor Pulmonale
Africa					
East[74]	18.3–26.0	19.5–36.0	0.7–2.1	15.1–46.0	0.6–5.0
South[74]	23.6	19.6	0.4	37.5	10.9
Asia					
India[225]	22.7	11.2	10.0–21.0	2.0–3.0	10.0–18.0
Malaysia[18]	16.6	54.0	0.1	0.1	—
Hong Kong[55]	40.6	26.6	12.7	—	—
Philippines[231]	21.3	23.9	26.4[a]	—	—
Thailand[284]	38.4	10.6	—	—	—

[a] Also includes heart muscle disease.
(Data derived from references 18, 55, 74, 225, 231, and 284.)

Table 33–2. Autopsy Prevalance of Heart Disease (% of Cardiac Diseases)

Heart Disease	Total Cases				
	Uganda[135] 637	Johannesburg[145] 120	Philippines[141] 1,240	Southern India[247] 250	Northern India[a] 2,500
Rheumatic	19.7	20.8	23.3	30.0	21.4
Hypertensive	20.5	43.3	24.3	15.0	17.9
Cardiomyopathy	17.6	14.1	—	3.0	10.4
Myocardial infarct	0.5	11.7	35.3[b]	8.0	15.0
Cor pulmonale	7.7	—	5.0	—	8.1
Infective endocarditis	6.1	—	—	4.0	8.2
Pericarditis	8.5	—	—	—	10.4
Congenital	3.7	—	5.0	10.0	10.6

[a] Author's own data. See Table 33–3 for details.
[b] Cases listed as coronary atherosclerosis and not as infarcts.

missions to hospitals.[29,45,74,203,280] In some countries, the population is a mixture of ethnicities and races. Differences in the patterns of diseases noticed among ethnic groups have been based on economic and social differences; they are not attributable to racial differences.[280] For example, Indian migrants to various parts of Africa and the Far East show disease patterns similar to European settlers in these communities. The major factors, therefore, are ecologic and economic.

THE NORMAL HEART IN THE TROPICS

In Uganda, normal heart weight is 267 g for men and 226 g for women.[67] Nigerians have hearts of similar weight, which is lighter than the American average by a factor of 0.83 in men and 0.92 in women.[47] Some normal heart parameters among adults in northwest India

Table 33–3. Cardiac Diseases at Autopsy, Chandigarh, India 1964–1988[a]

Cardiac Disease	Number	Total Autopsy (%)	Cardiac Cases (%)
Rheumatic	536	4.8	21.4
Hypertensive	447	4.0	17.9
Infarction	373	3.4	15.0
Pericarditis	281	2.5	11.3
Congenital	261	2.3	10.4
Cardiomyopathies	261	2.3	10.4
Cor pulmonale	202	1.8	8.1
Infective endocarditis	201	1.8	8.1
Isolated aortic valve disease	130	1.2	5.2
Miscellaneous conditions (aortic aneurysm, Takayasu's arteritis, primary pulmonary hypertension, primary and secondary tumors, etc.)	154	1.4	6.1

[a] Total autopsies: 11,000.
Cardiac diseases: 2,500 (22.7%).

Table 33–4. Normal Heart Parameters in Northwest India

Parameter	Male		Female	
	Range	Average	Range	Average
Heart weight (g)	150–350	290.0	140–300	212.4
Orifice diameters (mm)				
Mitral	19–30	24.5	17–26	21.4
Tricuspid	20–36	28.9	21–34	26.6
Aortic	15–26	19.0	13–21	17.2
Pulmonic	14–26	18.3	14–21	17.0
Wall thickness (mm)				
Left ventricle (posterior)	11–18	14.2	10–17	13.2
Right ventricle (anterior)	2–5	3.7	2–3.5	2.9

(Data from Dewan, Indarjit and Sahni[93])

are shown in Table 33–4, as found at my center, in Chandigarh, India.

TROPICAL CARDIOMYOPATHIES AND CARDIOMEGALY

I am convinced that if nature had not inflicted on the African certain peculiar and obscure heart diseases, the "Dark Continent" would not have attracted such a trail of investigators as it did in the last three to four decades. Many of these investigators not only immortalized themselves in the annals of cardiology but, in the process, rendered invaluable service to tropical cardiology. The term *tropical heart disease* has become almost synonymous with the obscure conditions called *cardiomyopathies*.

WHO[339–342] and the International Society and Federation of Cardiology have been very active in the field of cardiomyopathies and have drawn up, in some detail, the definition, nomenclature, classification, and description (clinical and morphologic), as well as the etiopathogenesis, of these conditions. In 1986, WHO made recommendations for the early detection and prevention of cardiomyopathies.[339] Details of cardiomyopathies are described elsewhere in this book (see Ch. 20); here the relevance of tropical location with regard to the prevalence of cardiomyopathies and possible etiopathogenetic mechanisms will be presented. The classification and terminology is used according to the WHO definition.[339,342] Thus, we have three categories:

1. Dilated heart cardiomyopathy (DCM)
2. Restrictive cardiomyopathy (RCM), exemplified by endomyocardial fibrosis (EMF)
3. Hypertrophic cardiomyopathy (HCM)

Endomyocardial Fibrosis

Unlike DCM, which has a worldwide prevalence, EMF is almost exclusively a disease of the tropics, East Africa being its "homeland." EMF is also known as *Davies disease* after the detailed description of it given by J.N.P. Davies and his colleagues 40 years ago.[90] It has been reported from almost all tropical countries in Africa and from Arabian countries, South America, India, and China. Its major loci of occurrence are Uganda and Nigeria in Africa and Kerala in southern India—two sites with near identical rain-forest topography about 15 degrees north and south of the equator, respectively.[32,45,76,77,81,106,112,121,142,214,280] EMF or a condition similar to it has also been described in Switzerland[200] and England,[59] as well as in European residents in parts of Africa.[49]

The clinical expression of EMF depends on its morphologic location in the heart. It may affect both ventricles or predominantly one ventricle, being labeled as biventricular (BiV-EMF), right ventricular (RV-EMF), or left ventricular (LV-EMF). In two separate au-

topsy series from Uganda[40,278] the location was BiV-EMF in 56 and 51 percent, LV-EMF in 36 and 38 percent, and RV-EMF in 4 and 11 percent respectively. Indian data are similar. Postmortem data reflect, the poor outcome of BiV-EMF and LV-EMF and a comparatively better prognosis for RV-EMF, since in clinical studies RV-EMF is the most common presentation.[69,70,91,228,287] Clinically, in Kerala, among 150 cases, 52 percent were diagnosed as RV-EMF, 11 percent as LV-EMF, and 37 percent as BiV-EMF,[214] but, at autopsy, in the same area, RV-EMF was found rarely.[161]

Considerable clinical and investigative data have emerged over the last 5 years. In African cases, onset with fever, malaise, and at times with itching and urticaria, suggests an infective/inflammatory disease, albeit of a nonspecific nature,[106,122] features that are not noticed in cases from Kerala.[320] The patient then develops cardiac failure and, though this presentation may be predominantly one-sided, investigation will reveal biventricular disease in the majority. ECG features are rather nonspecific, except possibly in African children with RV-EMF.[150] Echocardiography (especially 2D and M-mode color-coded) is very helpful in demonstrating the thickened endocardium and obliteration of the ventricular apices. Infundibular dilation together with a crenelated cavity characterizes RV-EMF, whereas tethering of the posterior mitral leaflet and a greater amplitude of septal motion demonstrate LV-EMF.[88,95,112,242,316] The pathologic state of obliterated apex and infundibular dilation of RV-EMF is shown very well on angiography (see Figs. 33–7 and 33–8).[91,142,144,184] On the basis of clinical presentation, different varieties have been recognized:[340] (1) arrhythmic, with a very large right atrium, (2) pericardial type, with recurrent large pericardial effusion, (3) pseudocirrhotic with severe recurrent ascites and a fibrotic liver, (4) a calcified type with linear calcification of the right ventricular apex or outflow, and (5) a mitral regurgitant form.

At autopsy a variable amount of pericardial effusion is seen, particularly in children with

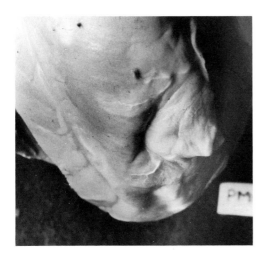

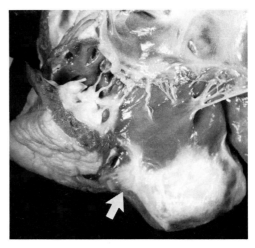

Fig. 33–1. EMF. External surface of heart. Note the dimple marking the right ventricular apex.

Fig. 33–3. EMF. Right ventricular cavity showing endocardial sclerosis over the papillary muscles. The cavity has been smoothed out and the apex drawn in (arrow).

RV-EMF. A characteristic feature in Ugandan cases is a notch or depression that externally marks the right apex and is caused by an indrawing of the obliterated ventricular cavity (Figs. 33–1 to 33–3). The heart is usually enlarged. On opening the left chambers in an established case, it appears as if a tenacious,

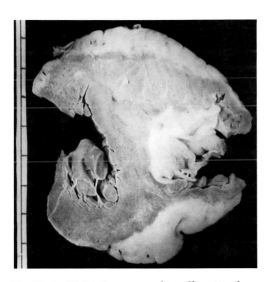

Fig. 33–2. EMF. Transverse slice of heart to show the near total obliteration of the right ventricular cavity.

thick white paint poured over the posterior mitral leaflet has trickled down into the inflow tract, tethering the leaflet and chordae tendinae to the underlying endocardium; flattened the posterior papillary muscle; and, in accumulating at the apex, traveled up the outflow tract for a little distance (Figs. 33–4 and 33–5). The insides of the chamber are thus smoothed. Hudson described the process as starting at the apex and "crawling up to involve the mitral apparatus."[32] A white ridge may form a little above the apex, at times it may calcify. The cut edges of the ventricle reveal an extension of the thickened endocardium into the inner one-third or one-half of the wall thickness (Fig. 33–6). Thrombi at various stages of organization may be seen. The distinction between inflow and outflow regions, so well demarcated in the left ventricle, is not maintained in the right ventricle, where the entire chamber may be incarcerated, forming a shallow cavity resembling a porcelain saucer. The thinner RV myocardium also permits the thickened endocardium to extend to the epicardium.

Histologically, the thickened endocardium is densely collagenous, almost cartilagenous, with a few fine strands of elastic fibers in the

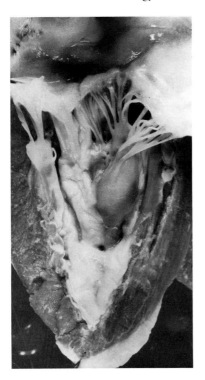

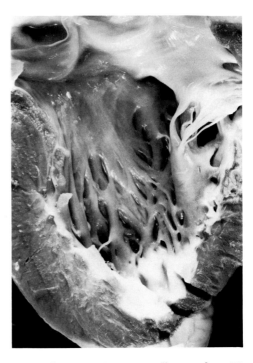

Fig. 33–4. EMF. Left ventricular inflow tract reveals a densely thickened endocardium coating the posterior leaflet of the mitral valve and its chordae tendineae and papillary muscles and filling the apex of the cavity.

Fig. 33–5. EMF. Specimen illustrated in Fig. 33–4, showing the left ventricular outflow region spared by the process, the apex is "frozen" and the endocardial sclerosis "crawls" a little distance up the outflow tract.

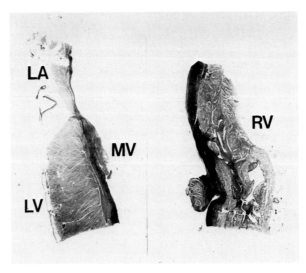

Fig. 33–6. EMF. Sections of the two ventricles. Left ventricle (LV) and atrium (LA) show the mitral valve leaflet left (MV) plastered to the thick mural endocardium. "Trapping" of the papillary muscles and extension of the thickened endocardium into the deeper myocardial are seen in the right ventricle (RV). (Masson's trichrome, × 4.) (From Datta and Aikat,[77] with permission.)

superficial and deeper layers. Three zones may be identified in the earlier stages of EMF. The inner (luminal surface) layer of dense collagen is followed by a layer of loose connective tissue and then a layer of "granulation tissue." In the last-named zone there is abundant vascularization and variable inflammatory cell exudate including lymphocytes, monocytes, plasma cells, and sometimes a few eosinophils and Anitschkow's myocytes.[69,70] The cellularity of this layer determines the "activity" of the disease. In fact, as will be discussed later, an acute endomyocarditis, rich in eosinophils, is claimed to represent the acute stage. In the outflow tract the sclerosis is fibroelastic and also lacks this inflammatory zone. An extension of the lesion (in the inflow tracts) into the myocardium produces a serrated infiltration by tongue-shaped processes. The trabeculae carnae and papillary muscles may appear embedded in dense collagenous scar. The trapped myofibers as well as the underlying myocardium show varying degrees of "degenerative" changes, including vacuolization, fragmentation, and enlarged and atypical nuclei. Medial and intimal proliferation of intramural arteries has been noticed[8]—a feature seen in DCM and HCM also.

The description just detailed applies to a fully developed ease; five sites or patterns of sclerotic patches have been described.[278] These vary from scattered, unconnected patches to a completely solidified base-to-apex sclerosis, involving the mitral apparatus. The earliest lesions appear as gelatinous gray-green endocardial swellings with increased glycosamineglycosides, at times with fibrinoid necrosis and inflammatory infiltration with or without eosinophils. This may correspond to the necrotic stage of eosinophilic endomyocarditis described by Olsen and Spry.[221]

Studies of endomyocardial biopsies by electron microscopy show endocardial endothelial cell proliferation, collagenization, and edema. Small vessels have endothelial swelling with clusters of polymorphs and eosinophils, at times with degranulation of the latter, as seen in one study[162] but not in another.[177]

Extracardiac lesions have been described in patients with EMF. Prominent among them is an immune complex glomerulonephritis.[75] Its occurrence has been used as evidence of an immune disturbance in EMF, but its frequency or clinical expression is not known.

Nature and Etiology of Endomyocardial Fibrosis

On clinical grounds generally, and on morphologic grounds rarely, EMF may be confused with rheumatic valvular disease and, still more rarely, with DCM.[111,280] Among 172 specimens of EMF and 188 of rheumatic heart disease, features of both were found in 21 cases.[280] Probably both diseases represent an altered immune response to one or more antigens in the particular geographic area.[280] In the face of diagnostic sophistication, these "overlaps" are only of academic/historic interest. In passing, it may be recorded that the entity *Becker's disease* (cardiovascular collagenosis) in South Africa has long since lost its separate identity from EMF.[91,195] Distinction of EMF from endocardial fibroelastosis, whether congenital or acquired, is not a problem.

In the past decade, the classification of Löffler's disease (Löffler's endocarditis fibroplastica or eosinophilic heart disease) and of EMF have been extensively discussed. Brockington and Olsen studied much material from both diseases and concluded that EMF represents the late stage of Löffler's disease.[48] A *unitarian theory* was proposed to show that EMF and Löffler's disease belong to the same disease spectrum, the origin of which can be traced to the eosinophil leukocyte, both on clinical and morphologic grounds. Accordingly,[48,88,89,220,222,340,342] eosinophilia, due to a wide variety of causes, may be associated with an endomyocardial disease that starts as an acute myocarditis and ends as EMF. The former, found in temperate climates, does not progress to the healed stage because of its severity. In tropical climates, the same condition with a milder eosinophilia is not seen in its acute stage, but insidiously leads to its fibrotic end-stage and presents as EMF. By this time the eosinophilia, both in the blood and in the myocardium, has disappeared or decreased. This disease spectrum has been regarded as *eosinophilic-endomyocardial disease*. Clinically, a patient may present with (1) a systemic arteritis involving brain, retina, lungs, gastrointestinal tract, kidneys, and heart, (2) congestive cardiac failure, or (3) an eosinophilia-associated disease that subsequently develops into heart disease. Morphologically, Olsen and coworkers[220,222] recognize three stages:

1. A *necrotic stage* developing, on an average, 5.5 weeks after the onset of symptoms. The heart shows intense myocarditis and arteritis with abundant eosinophil infiltration.
2. A *thrombotic stage* follows in about 10 months; the inflammation abates and thrombi develop over the endocardium.
3. In about 24.5 months a *fibrotic stage* develops with all features of an established EMF.

It is proposed that the eosinophil damages tissue in two ways. (1) There is active degranulation of eosinophils in circulation, and a cationic protein, released from the granules, is cytotoxic and thrombogenic. This occurs when there are $1 \times 10^9/L$ or 15-percent degranulated eosinophil cells in circulation. (2) There is an immune mechanism in which eosinophil granules and immunoglobulin E (IgE) are involved.

This unitarian hypothesis has clarified many issues, but it still fails to explain some aspects of both Löffler's disease and EMF. This is extensively discussed in publications by Olsen and colleagues.[48,220,222,288] Eosinophilia that is related to parasites is almost universal in the population living in geographic areas endemic for EMF (Filaria is possibly the most common), yet Löffler's disease, the presumed acute stage of EMF, is virtually nonexistent in these areas. Compared with the number of patients with eosinophilia, the incidence of

even classic EMF is rare. Spry, in a comprehensive review, concedes that the role of eosinophils in EMF in the tropics is not yet settled.[288]

Only two case reports of idiopathic hypereosinophilia with endomyocarditis, proved by endomyocardial biopsy, are available from India, one an autopsy finding and the other from the Postgraduate Institute at Chandigarh.[258] Even though eosinophilia is equally prevalent in EMF-nonendemic areas (northern or eastern India, parts of China, other Far Eastern countries, Arabian and Mideastern countries) cases of EMF are still rarer in these areas. The common entity, *tropical eosinophilia syndrome*, to my knowledge, has not been associated with endomyocardial disease. Conversely, the proposed end stage of Löffler's disease, EMF, is a curiosity in temperate zones. Reference has been made already to cases described in Switzerland and the United Kingdom. Two additional cases of EMF have been reported in the United Kingdom, one with the well-known association with daunorubicin therapy,[336] the other in a 4-year-old child with restrictive cardiomyopathy.[337] Neither had eosinophilia. In endomyocardial biopsies in southern India, an eosinophil infiltrate is rarely found, if at all.[89,161] EMF developed in mice infected with *Plasmodium berghei* but without eosinophilia in an experimental study.[101] The team in Kerala has, in elaborate studies, found no deposition of eosinophil protein in the diseased endocardial tissue.[282] Estimation of trace elements in their autopsy tissues show an excess of thorium in conjugation with a magnesium deficiency. High levels of thorium are found in the staple diet of the Kerala population.[311]

There is no doubt that eosinophil leukocytes—structurally and/or functionally abnormal ones—are cardiotoxic, but to consider all EMF due to the eosinophil seems a very restricted viewpoint of this restrictive cardiomyopathy. The relationship between classic EMF seen in the tropics and the eosinophil leukocyte is as yet an open question. In the serologic study at Kerala, evidence for involvement of coxsackievirus (B1) has been presented.[246]

Relationship to Parasitic Infestation

The tropical habitat is conducive to the co-existence of humans and parasites. In view of this geographic overlap, patients with EMF are likely to harbor one or more parasite(s). A cause-and-effect relationship is possible, mediated through either the eosinophilic leukocyte or immune mediation, or both. Filariasis heads the list of such parasites, but a critical analysis makes one concede that the association of EMF and filariasis is only topographic.[117,148,245,265] Other parasites that have been detected in cases with EMF include toxoplasmosis,[230] schistosomiasis,[152] and trichinosis.[9] By 1977 more than 32 cases of trichinosis with eosinophilic endocarditis had been recorded.[9] Eosinophil-associated myocarditis was shown, also, in the invasion of the heart by *Ascaris lumbricoides* larvae (see Ch. 34). EMF and African trypanosomiasis occur together in Uganda with pancarditis but notably without eosinophilia.[236] Malaria has also been implicated, including the experimental study referred to earlier.

Immune Mechanisms

Fibrin and IgG deposits are detected on myocardial sarcolemma in more than 40 percent of cases of EMF in Africa, but the same proportion of rheumatic disease and DCM cases show similar reactivity.[312] Elevated antimalarial, antiheart antibodies, and IgE (parasite-related) have also been reported.[153] A similar experience was recorded in one report from Kerala[319] but another investigation found no immune reactivity in EMF.[160]

Malnutrition

An unspecified "conditioning effect" of malnutrition in EMF has been considered.[279] A diet rich in plantains, a source of serotonin, is mentioned only for historic interest.[71] Experimentally, a 5HT-rich, protein-deficient diet produced lesions in rats but not in monkeys.[196] The possible role of tapioca in Kerala has been investigated without success. Reference has been made to thorium in the diet and tissues. EMF has been described in families, too.[185,229]

Finally, knowledge concerning the etiology of EMF has been summarized by Hudson: "Factors certainly include infection, infestation and malnutrition but there must be something else, otherwise the disease would be much more widespread among underprivileged people of all the countries. The part played by noxious herbs and other substances which may be consumed secretly is not known."[132]

It should be noted that surgery (decortication of the thickened endocardium with valve replacement) offered relief to many patients at a number of centers.[201] The preoperative, operative, and postoperative pictures of a case from Trivandrum are shown in Figures 33–7 and 33–8.

Dilated Cardiomyopathy

DCM, also known as idiopathic cardiomegaly (ICM), has a worldwide prevalence with a tropical and subtropical preponderance.[16,77,121,134,136] Ikeme's statement that DCM is an "amorphous area" in tropical cardiology,[136] in view of its lack of specific diagnostic, clinical, or pathologic features, is equally applicable to nontropical cases. DCM is best looked on as end-stage heart disease, resulting from processes that are yet undefined.

The detailed pathology of DCM is described in Chapter 20. The gross and microscopic features of DCM found in the tropics do not differ from those cases seen elsewhere.[251] An example from the author's collection is illustrated in Figures 33–9 and 33–10. In succeeding paragraphs special conditions applicable to the problem of etiopathogenesis of DCM in the tropics will be highlighted. DCM causes 2 to 25 percent of clinical

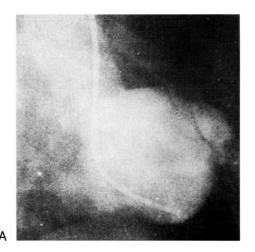 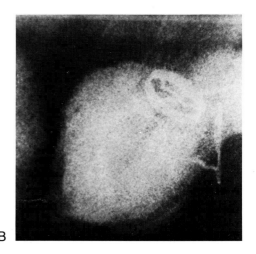

A   B

Fig. 33–7. (**A**) Pre- and (**B**) postoperative angiograms of left ventricle in a case of endomyocardial fibrosis subject to decortication and mitral valve replacement. Note prosthesis in place in Fig. B. (Courtesy of Professor M. S. Valiathan, Trivandrum, Kerala, India.)

cardiac disease in the tropics, and its frequency in adults in clinical practice in Africa is rated second only to hypertension.[108,136,158] The prevalence of DCM in Arab countries—Saudi Arabia, Egypt, and Libya—remains between 3 and 6 percent of hospitalized cases of cardiac diseases.[218]

The Heart and Nutrition

The vast population of most tropical, under-developed countries exist in a state of chronic under/malnutrition. There is certainly reason to believe that malnutrition contributes to the prevalence, severity, natural history, and

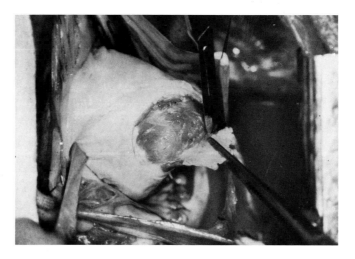

Fig. 33–8. Operative picture of case shown in Fig. 33–7, showing the decortication of the thickened mural endocardium. (Photograph courtesy of Professor M. S. Valiathan, Trivandrum, Kerala, India.)

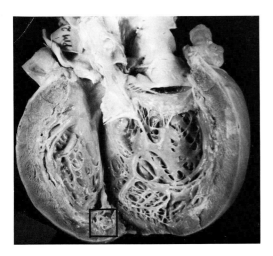

Fig. 33–9. Idiopathic cardiomegaly (heart weight, 850 g). The deep longitudinal furrow shows the extreme flabbiness of the specimen. Patches of endocardial sclerosis are seen. The boxed area includes the mural thrombus. (From Datta and Aikat,[77] with permission.)

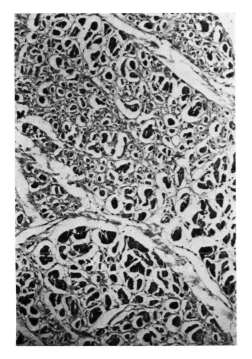

Fig. 33–10. Dilated cardiomyopathy. The photomicrograph shows the characteristic variation of fiber size and fine lacy fibrosis isolating individual fibers. (From Datta and Aikat,[77] with permission.)

prognosis of almost all diseases in these countries, yet only a few conditions, such as beriberi, kwashiorkor, and vitamin deficiencies are specific, well-defined, nutritional diseases.[203]

Attempts were made in the early 1950s to define "nutritional heart disease."[120] In the 12 cases in Higginson's report,[130] the gross and microscopic features were not different from those of DCM (cardiomegaly, flabby heart, myofiber atrophy, disarray, fibrosis, and mural thrombi). Furthermore, these cases had an excess of iron, which was not satisfactorily explained[6] in view of the known relationship between iron overload and heart disease. In the malnourished person, the heart is atrophic. In a group of starved children, 22.5 percent with kwashiorkor had atrophic hearts and 43 percent with marasmus had cardiomegaly.[235] Degenerative changes that included vacuolization, fatty change, edema, mitochondrial proliferation, and fragmentation of myofilaments were described in the hearts by both light and electron microscopy. Nuclear changes of the type seen in DCM (hyperchromatic, pyknotic, wrinkled, insect-like configuration) were not apparent in these cases.[235] Atrophy also characterizes the heart in famine conditions. McKinney claims to have produced a DCM-like heart in rats fed a tryptophan-deficient diet.[196] Monkeys on a protein/calorie-deficient diet develop an atrophic heart.[56]

Alcohol and the Heart

The details of alcohol-induced heart disease are discussed elsewhere (see Ch. 20); the relevance to underdeveloped tropical countries lies in the relationship of alcohol to beriberi heart disease in the African, as discussed below. Elevation of myocardial enzymes in biopsy has been considered a feature of alcoholic cardiomyopathy distinct from DCM.[250,342] Other than that, there is no morphologic distinction between the two.

Beriberi Heart Disease

The frequency of the pure nutritional variety of beriberi heart disease, an ancient disease of the Orient, is probably decreasing; however, the alcoholic variety is on the increase. A dietary deficiency of thiamine and an excessive alcohol consumption are considered important causes for intractable congestive heart failure in many tropical regions. Undernutrition or malnutrition frequently goes hand-in-hand with an overindulgence in alcohol, especially beer.[6,103,272,273]

Beriberi, which occurs in young adults endemically in Africa, Southeast Asia, and India, is characterized by edema, cardiovascular disturbances (cardiomegaly, tachycardia, systolic murmur, and hypotension), and peripheral neuritis. The disease occurs in four forms:

1. Classic or wet beriberi
2. Acute pernicious beriberi or Shoshin type
3. Classic or Shoshin beriberi with persistent cardiomegaly
4. Thiamine deficiency complicating other forms of heart disease

The clinical, high-output cardiac failure is associated with peripheral vasodilation and a peripheral arteriovenous shunting of blood. The heart is enlarged and flabby, with right-sided dilation and failure being more pronounced than effects on the left heart. Histologically, nonspecific degenerative changes with edema are seen. The Shoshin or pernicious form of beriberi is not different morphologically, but has a shorter course with biventricular failure and may end in sudden death. The response to thiamine is dramatic; cardiomegaly may disappear within hours or days. This dramatic therapeutic response is considered a point of distinction between beriberi and other forms of congestive heart failure, yet in the late stages with irreversible structural changes, therapy may fail. Such a chronic, nonspecific course is not a feature of nutritional beriberi but occurs more frequently in patients with chronic alcoholism.[272,273]

The difference between the oriental type of beriberi (thiamine deficiency due to eating polished rice) and the occidental type (deficiency in alcoholics not consuming thiamine) may be attributable to alcoholic cardiomyopathy.[7,139]

In studies from South Africa beriberi was distinguished from DCM by being more frequent in males (10 males per 1 female in beriberi and 3.3 to 1 in DCM).[272,273] Again, red cell thiamine levels were normal in DCM and, whereas patients with DCM did not respond to thiamine, those with nutritional beriberi did not develop chronic heart failure. The authors considered alcohol a potent link between beriberi and DCM. Apparently, beriberi and alcohol are a greater, unrecognized problem in South Africa, Japan, and New Zealand and must be kept in mind in cases of intractable cardiac failure.[139,165,211]

In Thailand, infants breast-fed by thiamine-deficient mothers develop beriberi with congestive heart failure that may prove rapidly fatal.[284] A peculiar feature of beriberi is the rapid response of peripheral vasodilation to thiamine therapy. This adds to the burden of an already incapacitated heart, and congestive failure worsens on initial thiamine treatment. The situation is similar in cases of kwashiorkor when they are treated (see below).

Kwashiorkor (Protein/Calorie Malnutrition in Children)

Unlike the situation in beriberi and DCM, in kwashiorkor the heart is atrophic, flabby, and rather pale brown (compare the "parboiled" appearance in DCM). Histologically, myofibers are small with indistinct striations, especially in papillary muscles and subendocardial regions.[333] Myocardial vacuolization, frequently due to fat, is present, and there may be minute areas of necrosis with an infiltration of mononuclear cells and Anitschkow's myocytes. Similar findings have been reported in an experimental model of kwashiorkor in the rhesus monkey.[56] Children with kwashiorkor may at times develop severe, even fatal, heart failure due to electrolyte disturbances when given therapy.[25,286,333]

During the famine of 1968 to 1969, 72.2 percent of 1,900 Biafran children evacuated had features of kwashiorkor,[301] and 538 had abnormalities such as heart murmurs, arrythmias, and cardiomegaly. The majority recovered with treatment, although heart failure worsened in some following an excess sodium intake. The authors believed that magnesium deficiency had an important role in cardiac damage in kwashiorkor. Usually, distinction between kwashiorkor and DCM is not a problem. Furthermore, there is no connection between childhood malnutrition and adult DCM.

Chronic Anemia

Enlargement of the heart occurs in chronic anemia irrespective of its cause. Congestive heart failure in such patients is common, but death purely due to anemia is rare. Clinical studies in India reveal severe cardiac dysfunction in anemic patients, most of whom suffered from hookworm infestation, malaria,

bleeding disorders, and/or nutritional deficiency.[255,264] Cardiac function usually recovers on restoration of a normal hematologic status. Morphologically, the heart is mildly enlarged and flabby, with loss of its epicardial fat; the valves appear rather edematous. Histologic investigation shows nonspecific anoxic damage in the form of fiber vacuolization, fatty infiltration, and stray foci of atrophy and replacement fibrosis, mostly in the subendocardial zone. An iron deficiency anemia is a comparatively easy experimental method of producing cardiomegaly in weanling rats.[80,82] Such animals show considerable cardiomegaly and all of the features recorded above. The gross and light microscopic changes are illustrated in Figures 33–11 through 33–14; one can appreciate their lack of specificity. Ultrastructurally, the heart shows proliferation of mitochondria with widespread degenerative changes but no increase in myofilaments; thus, there is no true hypertrophy.

As in humans, experimental animals recover rapidly when their diet is restored with iron supplements. Furthermore, there seem to be no aftereffects of the cardiac derangement once the animals have recovered. Deficiency of vitamin B12 and folate affect the

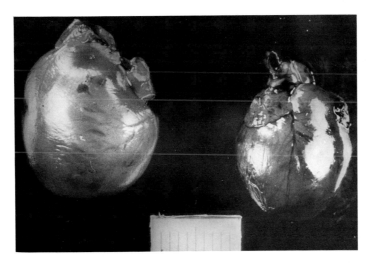

Fig. 33–11. Cardiomegaly in experimental chronic anemia in the rat. The pale globular and enlarged heart of an anemic animal (left) is compared to the heart from a weight-matched normal rat (right). (Scale indicated, 1 cm.)

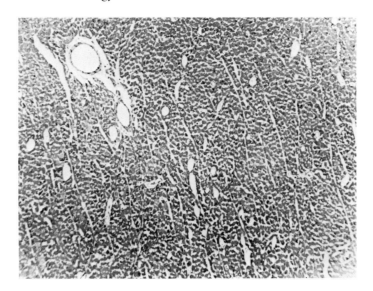

Fig. 33–12. Heart from an anemic rat, showing the wide dilation of vessels. (H&E, × 44.) (From Datta and Silver,[85] with permission.)

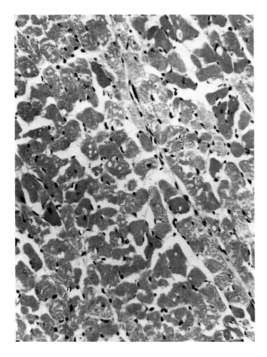

Fig. 33–13. Vacuolization, hyalinization, and general "moth-eaten" appearance of myocardium in an anemic rat. Note the shrunken nuclei. (H & E, × 440.)

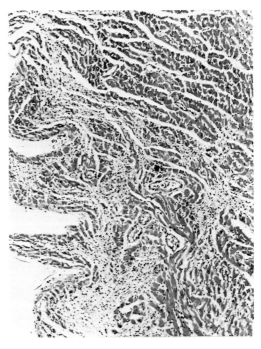

Fig. 33–14. Atrophy and fibrosis in the subendocardial zone ("watershed area") of an anemic rat heart. (H & E, × 68.) (From Datta and Silver,[85] with permission.)

heart similarly, but the cardiomegaly is not as appreciable. In fact, the heart is likely to be atrophic as this kind of deficiency seriously interferes with protein biosynthesis in the myocardium.

Hypertension and DCM in Africa

Statements that DCM could be "hypertension in disguise" or could represent a state of "truncated hypertension" or "failed hypertension" have been in print for some time.[94] Hypertension has been reported in more than 50 percent of patients with DCM in Africa.[13,104,137,249]

Generally diastolic blood pressure shows a transient elevation during periods of congestive failure that tends to return to normal on recovery,[104,105] but there is also evidence to the contrary. In some patients the pressure may become considerably elevated on recovery.[137] Radiologically, unfolding of the aorta may be seen in middle-aged and elderly African patients with DCM[46] in addition, arterial changes of hypertension in the ocular fundi are known in cases of DCM and persist even after cardiac failure has been controlled.[227] Other evidence linking DCM and hypertension is related to the role the latter has in the genesis of postpartum cardiac failure. All these aspects have been discussed in a debate.[94]

In addition to the clinical study from Ibadan[104] referred to above at autopsy, in patients dying of hypertension it is as common to find a large and flabby heart with dilated chambers indistinguishable from DCM as it is to find one with concentric left ventricular hypertrophy.[13] Furthermore, the authors found that a great many autopsy patients with large, flabby hearts had significant anemia in life. It has been argued that anemia contributed to early cardiac failure in the hypertensive, leading to the dilated heart. In my own autopsy cases of DCM,[38] evidence of hypertension, as observed in the renal arteries, was

found in only 7 percent of patients younger than 40 years of age. I would agree that such patients should be classified as "dilated heart in hypertension" and not DCM.[13] I am of the opinion that DCM is "end-stage heart disease" and that in some cases, at least at autopsy, there is evidence that "failed hypertension"—a failure to maintain blood pressure at hypertensive levels while the stimulus for hypertension persists—could lead to a DCM-like clinical picture.

An experimental model referred to earlier[80,82] provides some evidence that chronic anemia curtails cardiac hypertrophy in response to a work overload similar to that caused by hypertension. Anemic rats, when subjected to the additional burden of aortic constriction, demonstrated a true myofilament hyperplasia (proliferation of Z discs) in the heart but simultaneously, mitochondrial degeneration became more pronounced and accelerated. Such a heart does not develop concentric left ventricular hypertrophy.

Apart from chronic anemia, such factors as alcohol and malnutrition, including beriberi, might also introduce variation in the cardiac response to hypertension,[127,136,137] as "conditioning factors"[3401] with DCM as the end result.

Finally, to quote Ikeme et al., "it is suggested that hypertension is an important associated causative factor in DCM in the tropics and the extent of myocardial damage produced by nutritional factors may determine the levels of blood pressure, when presenting in heart failure."[137]

Myocardial Anoxia

Obliterative lesions of intramural coronary arteries have been described in cases of "heart muscle disease" and are favored to cause anoxic damage to the heart.[52,161] I have seen coronary arterioles showing marked medial and intimal hypertrophy in some cases of DCM and in hypertrophic obstructive cardiomyopathy. The occurrence of similar obliterative proliferative arterial changes has been noted by Brazilians in cases of EMF.[8] By their very sporadic and focal nature, these lesions are likely to be a result of organized thromboemboli in small arteries: I would not attach any etiologic significance to them.

Immunologic Mechanisms in DCM

From Cameroon, abnormal immunologic findings have been reported in cases of DCM.[41] Tissue autoantibodies against skeletal, cardiac, and smooth muscles have been demonstrated. The authors suggested they might be an expression of altered immune response to trypanosomal infection in the population. The finding of IgG and fibrin on sarcolemma and subsarcolemma in cases of EMF, DCM, and rheumatic heart disease was mentioned earlier. Endomyocardial biopsy studies in East African patients have shown a higher ratio of T helper/supressor cells, in support of a presumed viral myocarditis.[262] However, in a series of biopsies in New Delhi, no T-cell alterations were detected.[163]

Viral Infections

The possibility of a relationship between viral myocarditis and DCM is being investigated all over the world (see Chs. 19 and 20). Falase et al. from Nigeria found that the percentage of patients with DCM who had a fourfold rise (or fall) in antibody titer against at least one coxsackievirus B was greater than in normal controls.[109] Because infections by coxsackieviruses are common in Nigeria, the authors believed that a viral myocarditis could be a factor weakening the heart and leading to congestive failure in association with other influences. Madhavan et al. from Pondicherry (southern India) also found evidence for coxsackievirus infection in one case of DCM.[89] Similar evidence has come from many centers using endomyocardial biopsies; patients have

been treated with cytotoxic drugs as a result.

There has been no clear breakthrough in our understanding of the etiology of DCM in the tropics. It should be considered an end-stage disorder with many causes. The size of the clinical problem is likely to fluctuate with availability of better diagnostic facilities. Lowenthal sums up by stating, "Idiopathic heart disease of South African blacks may consist largely of undiagnosed examples of well recognized causes of heart disease."[186] Ikeme grouped DCM into four subclasses: (1) DCM affecting children and young adults, caused, possibly, by viral myocarditis; (2) DCM in elderly and middle-aged adults with unfolded aorta, being hypertensive in origin; (3) DCM in middle-aged and the elderly due to alcohol; and (4) postpartum congestive failure, DCM peculiar to parturient females and possibly related to hypertension.[136]

Peripartum or Postpartum Cardiac Failure

Unexplained heart failure developing during pregnancy or soon after childbirth has attracted attention as a separate form of congestive cardiomyopathy. This may be acceptable to a clinician because of the unique setting in which heart failure develops. However, a pathologist presented with a large, flabby, pale heart, with no valvular, coronary, or congenital lesion, cannot determine the sex or race of the patient, or whether the patient was a pregnant woman. Peri- or postpartum cardiac failure (PPCF) has no morphologic features distinct from DCM. PPCF (also known as *puerperal cardiomyopathy*) has been reported in white women, but the majority of patients are blacks "from widely separated areas, such as New Orleans, . . . South Africa, . . . Jamaica, and Arabia. . . ."[195] Cases have been reported from India and China. Incidence is difficult to assess, but one report from the United States recorded it as 1 in 1,300 deliveries and 1 in 4,000 pregnancies.[156] The incidence works out to be about 0.005 percent of deliveries in whites and 1 percent in Zarian women in Nigeria.[87] Among clinical studies in India, PPCF forms 13 to 18 percent of all cases of congestive cardiomyopathy (DCM).[119,296]

Clinically, at my center (the Postgraduate Institute at Chandigarh), 48 patients with PPCF accounted for 10 percent of all cardiomyopathies: 23 percent were hypertensive.[167] By contrast, hypertension exists in 11 percent of all cases of PPCF in the West and 81 percent in Africa.[86] A high prevalence of PPCF in the Hausa community of Zarie is noted, accounting for 306 cases.[315] In this community the pregnant and postpeurperal woman is subjected to a very high salt intake and restricted to heated and humid environments. In a study of 244 cases of PPCF in Zarian women, Davidson and Parry recognized a multiplicity of factors overloading the heart.[87] There is pressure load due to postpartum hypertension (which is common in this population) and a high salt intake. Also, there is volume overload due to the hot and humid climate, anemia, and splenomegaly (both common in the community) and an output overload due to heat and infection. The heart develops congestive failure under the multifactorial strain. Sanderson et al., reporting on the same area, concluded that PPCF is neither a serious heart muscle disorder nor a serious cardiomyopathy, but is the result of multiple factors.[261] However, the situation in Zaire is not duplicated elsewhere in the world. Among endomyocardial biopsies from 11 African women with PPCF in Nairobi, five showed "healing myocarditis" and 9 a high T helper/supressor cell ratio, suggesting an inappropriate immunologic reaction.[263]

Grossly, in PPCF the heart has the same features as in any example of DCM. Histologically, myocardial degenerative changes with endocardial sclerosis, inflammatory reaction, and mural thrombi are seen. The histochemical and electron microscopic features have been described but show no specificity.[50,330] Interestingly, two of my autopsied cases of endomyocardial fibrosis were diagnosed clinically as puerperal cardiomyopathy because of the patient's history. This illustrates the futility of maintaining PPCF as a distinct pathologic entity. However, it does not deny that pregnancy and its associated physiologic state may contribute to or precipitate progressive congestive cardiac failure in susceptible women.

Keshan Disease

Keshan disease (KSO) is a cardiomyopathy found mainly in China in a broad geographic belt running from northeast to southwest and also in Tibet, North Korea, and Japan. Selenium deficiency in the drinking water is possibly its cause. Dietary supplementation with sodium selenite has caused a considerable decline in its incidence,[124] but other factors such as infection (a number of viruses have been blamed as cofactors) and protein deficiency are also important. The disease, occurring mostly in children, may present in four forms:

1. Acute, with shock and arrhythmias
2. Subacute with shock and congestive failure
3. Chronic (the major form), in which the disease resembles dilated cardiomyopathy
4. Compensated

The heart at autopsy is grossly dilated, as in DCM, but, in addition has an appreciably thickened endocardium. Histologic investigation shows disseminated military foci and broad zones of necrosis/degeneration and inflammatory infiltration, especially in the subendocardial zone. Myofibers appear "juicy" due to numerous minute vesicles that, on ultrastructure analysis, are shown to be greatly distended sarcoplasmic tubules and mitochondria (Figures 33–15 to 33–17). Similar necrotic changes may occur in the conduction tract also. Scarring and fibrosis develop over time.

A case of Keshan disease has been detected in Long Island, New York, in a 2-year-old child with progressive cardiac failure.[68] The cardiac failure was traced to her poor dietary

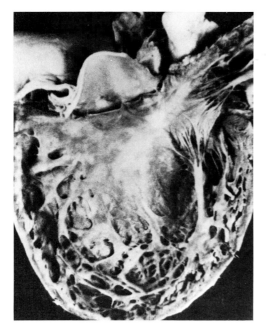

Fig. 33–15. Keshan disease. Dilation of the left ventricle is shown with marked thinning of its wall and papillary muscles in a 28-year-old man. (Heart weight, 519 g.) The right ventricle was similar. (From Gu and Cheng,[124] with permission.)

intake of dairy products and meat (the main source of selenium in the United States). The diagnosis of Keshan disease was suspected on detection of low levels of serum selenium and was confirmed when she recovered after selenium therapy.

HYPERTROPHIC CARDIOMYOPATHY

In the first edition of this book, HCM was presented as a rather rare condition in the tropics.[219] Within 5 years, that situation changed. The detection of HCM increased after installation of echocardiographic equipment centers in developing countries. Clinical case series of substantial number have been reported from India[226] and South Africa.[202] Autopsy experience, however, is limited to three cases in Africa[219] and slightly more in my own material in India.[77] From Groote-Schuur Hospital, Cape Town, Rose presented a critical analysis of the well-known histopathologic features of HCM.[252] Apart from minor variations in the incidence of various features, the basic clinical and morphologic aspects of different types of HCM are the same as in the West. They are described in Chapter 20.

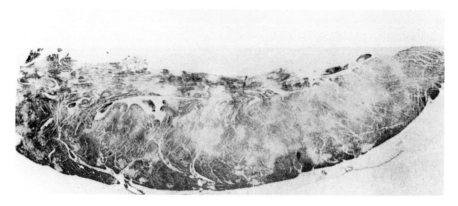

Fig. 33–16. Keshan disease. The blotchy appearance of a slice of left ventricle is caused by focal myocardial necrosis. (Phosphotungstic acid hematoxylin, × 1.5) (From Gu and Cheng,[124] with permission.)

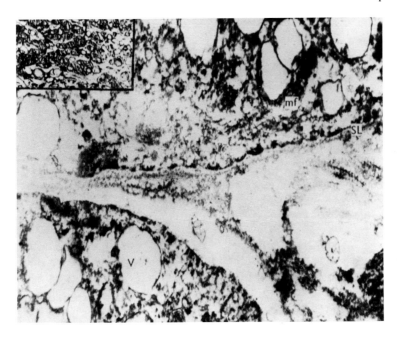

Fig. 33–17. Keshan disease. Two adjacent myocytes showing numerous dilated vesicles (V) with residual myofilaments (mf) between. (× 35,000.) **(Inset)** The semithin section with hydropic change and myocytolysis of fibers. (From Gu and Cheng,[124] with permission.)

VALVULAR HEART DISEASE

Rheumatic Heart Disease

Acute rheumatic fever (ARF) and rheumatic heart diseases (RHD) remain the most common heart diseases in children and young adults in the tropics.[28,29,203,292] WHO has recorded a decline in the prevalence of RHD in some countries.[151] For example, the incidence in Japan between 1968 and 1971 dropped from 4.6 to 0.1/1,000, and in Venezuela a twofold reduction occurred between 1950 and 1969. China has recorded a 50-percent decline between 1948 and 1976.[305,306] This, however, is not true for most tropical countries, where, despite occasional reports of decline, the disease has been static, if it did not actually increase between 1937 and 1975.[3]

Incidence

Hospital-based data indicate that RHD accounts for 20 to 50 percent of all heart diseases seen both clinically and at autopsy (see Tables 33–1 to 33–3). WHO estimates a population incidence of 100 to 200/100,000 in the young.[338] In school-aged children, the incidence figures in different countries are: India, 6 to 11 per 1000[194,215] and as low as 2.33 per 1000 (urban) and 1.66 (rural)[14]; Soweto, South Africa, 7/1,000[197]; Iran, 1/1,000[197]; Thailand, 1/1,000[239]; and Ivory Coast, 1/1,000.[30] It has been estimated that in India 88,000 new cases appear every year.[323] In comparison with the disease in western countries, several clinicopathologic differences have been highlighted in the pattern and presentation of RHD in the tropics (before the antibiotic era)[225,275,280]:

1. Early age of onset, with faster progression and early death

2. Severe degree of valvular stenosis
3. Severe degree and higher frequency of pulmonary hypertension
4. Higher rates of recurrence, even with antibiotic therapy
5. Differences in diagnostic criteria

Early Age of Onset

In clinical data available from India, Africa, Pakistan, and the Far East as well as the Middle East, up to 78 percent of patients are younger than 30 years of age and 45 percent are younger than 20.[5,15,34,79,118,140,147,197,203,224,275,280] In India, at autopsy, 80 to 98 percent are younger than the age of 40.[79,169,172,254] In Johannesburg, 61 percent are younger than 30 years old.[145] By contrast, in the United Kingdom and the United States, only 3 percent are younger than 20. In Israel, 8 percent are younger than 16. In Johannesburg the number of black children below 5 years of age affected are twice as many as for white children. The mortality rate is 4 percent in the former, 1 percent in the latter.[280]

Faster Progression Leading to Early Death

This has been a common clinical experience. In Jamaica 11 percent of school children with RHD die within a few weeks of onset, and another 11 percent within 1 to 3 years.[280] In India, 10 to 14 percent of patients had their first attack of ARF before their fifth birthday, in contrast to the rarity of the disease in children under 6 in temperate climes.[12,275] On follow-up, 26 percent of patients lost the murmur of mitral regurgitation and 17 percent the murmur of aortic regurgitation, which in contrasts with western figures of about 70 percent losing the murmur in the postantibiotic era.[12] Even with penicillin therapy the recurrence rate of streptococcal infection in patients with ARF in India is far higher (0.020/patient year) than in the West (0.004/patient year). The continued states of malnutrition, overcrowding, and dampness predispose to recurrent infection, and Indian patients show poor

bioavailability of penicillin.[285] In Nigeria, 50 percent of 20 children with ARF died within a year and 9 percent in 1 to 5 years, the former due to the carditis and the latter to complications such as pulmonary hypertension or infective endocarditis.[151] In Zimbabwe, chronic rheumatic valvular disease developed within 3 years of onset of RHD.[188]

Development of Valvular Lesions

Mitral regurgitation is the most common clinical dysfunction in Asian and African school-aged children.[172,183,194,225] That position is assumed by the evidence of mitral stenosis in autopsy data.[82,34,66,172,187] This process of transition has yet to be worked out; possibly serial ECG studies will provide an answer. Mitral stenosis develops at a faster pace if the initial attack of ARF starts early in life and is delayed if the onset is in adolescence.[3] A major contribution of tropical studies has been the recognition of juvenile mitral stenosis.[34,275] It is common to see 9- to 10-year old children with advanced mitral stenosis in need of surgery.[34] Seventy-five percent of juvenile cases have grade 3 to 4 stenosis,[28] and 30 percent of valvotomies in India are performed on patients younger than 20 years.[318]

Aortic valves also become significantly stenosed in the young. Whereas in the West up to 6.5 percent of cases of rheumatic aortic stenosis are younger than 30 years of age, in India 60 percent of such cases are younger than 30.[318] That RHD presents as anatomically isolated aortic valve disease (up to 1.5 percent) has been reported in autopsy studies both from India and Africa.[79,172]

Organic tricuspid valve stenosis is also more frequent and severe in the tropics (Fig. 33–18). Both clinically and at autopsy, 30 to 34 percent of cases have organic valvulitis of the tricuspid valve. In an occasional report these figures have gone as high as 41.4 percent in India[79,172,254,310] and 33 percent in Mexico.[1] These were autopsy figures, whereas on 2D echocardiography, only 8.6 percent had organic tricuspid stenosis in Delhi[192] and 1.2 to

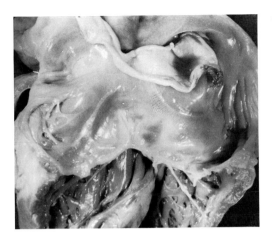

Fig. 33–18. Chronic rheumatic heart disease affecting tricuspid valve with severe fibrosis, commissural fusion, and almost total disappearance of chordae tendineae.

5 percent had organic tricuspid stenosis in the West.

A low prevalence of valvular calcification (lower than 10 percent) in clinical/surgical reports had been the common experience until the late 1970s.[28,318] At autopsy in Chandigarh, 32 percent of cases had valvular calcification.[82] With the recent use of cardiac fluoroscopy, however, 34.7 percent of 320 cases with valvular heart disease were detected to have calcified valves—a figure comparable to western data.[324]

Development of Pulmonary Hypertension

The prevalence of pulmonary hypertension in RHD in India is about 60 percent.[34,275] Severe grades (arteritis) have been reported in 4 percent of cases of mitral stenosis in lung biopsy studies.[298] In a recent assessment of 101 patients, suprasystolic pulmonary arterial pressures were noted in 40.[204] In Sudan, pulmonary hypertension seems uncommon.[147] An example of necrotizing lesions of pulmonary arteries, the forerunner of the plexiform lesion, is shown in Figure 33–19 from one of my cases.

Clinical Diagnosis

Indian studies continue to show a fairly low prevalence of subcutaneous nodules (1 to 6.2 percent) as compared to cases in the United Kingdom (21 percent) or the United States (7.5 percent). Erythema marginatum is also rare (0.4 percent, compared to 11 percent in Boston).[35,224,239,275,280,293] At autopsy, most cases are either burnt out and show acellular, collagenized, and badly deformed valves and myocardial scars or show some evidence of recurrence. Only 3 percent of 260 autopsies in Chandigarh showed acute rheumatic pancarditis with organizing fibrinoid vegetations on valves, numerous Aschoff bodies, and fine fibrinous pericarditis.[79] The frequency of detection of Aschoff bodies at autopsy is highly variable, depending on sampling and the individual pathologist's concept of a granuloma. In any case, the finding is usually of little relevance to the patient's clinicopathologic state. Among 260 autopsies reported from Chandigarh, Aschoff bodies were detected in 26.4 percent. Additional relevant data from this study include the development of infective endocarditis in 9.2 percent of cases and pericarditis in 46.1 percent, including an active fibrinous pericarditis in 30.1 percent.[79]

Other points of interest include differences in genetic markers in different populations. Whereas HLA-DR4 predisposes individuals to ARF and RHD in Saudi Arabia and the United States, patients in India show an association with HLA-DR 3.[244]

A histologic study of autopsy specimens suggests that medial hypertrophy and adventitial scarring of intramyocardial arteries in rheumatic mitral stenosis correlates with severity of left ventricular dysfunction.[294]

Infective Endocarditis

In earlier reports and some recent ones, from India and Africa, infective endocarditis in the tropics shows some notable differences from its pattern in the West.[53,85,110,199,267] These include the following:

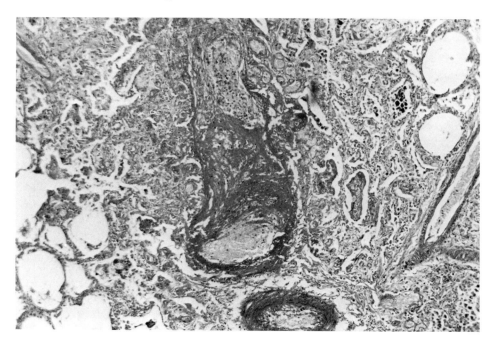

Fig. 33–19. Severe pulmonary arterial hypertension in chronic rheumatic mitral stenosis. Fibrinoid necrosis of arterioles, the forerunner of plexiform lesions, is shown. (H&E, × 200.)

1. The majority of patients are younger than 40. In my series of 120 autopsied cases, the average age was 28.[33,84,85]

2. There is a higher rate of infection of previously normal cardiac valves: about 40 percent in adult cases and a still higher frequency in children.[33,85] Among pre-existing valvular diseases favoring the development of infective endocarditis, rheumatic and congenital heart diseases are the majority. Association with atherosclerotic valvular and ischemic heart disease or cardiomyopathies is rare. Intravenous drug abusers have (so far) not been encountered with this complication; infection of prosthetic heart valves is becoming more common as more are inserted.

3. Low rates of positive blood cultures are obtained in life; up to 60 percent of cases remain "negative."[33,324] Nevertheless, *Staphylococcus aureus* and *Streptococcus viridans* are still common causative organisms. Recent reports from Saudi Arabia note that uncommon organisms such as brucella and salmonella may cause the disease.[155,302] Tuberculosis, too, is a cause.[325]

4. Failure to identify, even at autopsy, other predisposing conditions. In only about 15 percent of Nigerian and 25 percent of Indian cases could the cause be determined.[80,110] Prominent were pre-existing chest infections and puerperal sepsis.

Because of the continued sizable number of cases of infective endocarditis with underlying rheumatic valvular disease in tropical cases, there is a need to continue classifying cases into acute and subacute infective endocarditis, a trend long discontinued in the West. Acute and subacute cases can be differentiated on both clinical and morphologic grounds. The reports cited herein highlight a greater accuracy of clinical diagnosis in the subacute group (the majority of acute cases were diagnosed at autopsy only), a better survival of patients with subacute infection, and the dominance of peripheral manifestations.

Embolic manifestations from cardiac vegetations show the same pattern of distribution as is described in classic texts—namely, kidney and spleen affected more often, with a fair number of cases developing central nervous system manifestations.

Anatomically Isolated Aortic Valve Disease

The concept of anatomically isolated aortic valve disease has not proved well-liked with cardiologists and pathologists in Asia and Africa. Apparently, the condition continues to be included among cases of infective endocarditis or of congenital or rheumatic valvular disease.

Among 100 examples of isolated aortic stenosis observed in Chandigarh there were 52 bicuspid valves, 4 unicuspid unicommissural valves, and 43 tricuspid diseased aortic valves.[83] Calcification was noted in 42 percent, infective endocarditis in 39 percent, and fibrous sclerosis in 19 percent. The youngest patients, about 30 years of age, had infective lesions. Fibrous sclerosis was seen in those over 30 and calcification in patients older than 40. Four of the 100 cases were considered rheumatic in origin. In fact, in a study of rheumatic heart disease at Chandigarh, 1.5 percent of cases had isolated aortic valve lesion.[79]

In 64 autopsies recorded in western Nigeria 4 cases of isolated aortic valve disease (other than rheumatic), 2 cases with calcification, and 2 cases with minor lesions were found.[47] Cases of isolated aortic valve infective endocarditis were not defined separately, although the aortic valve was the seat of lesions in 33 of 64 cases.

Mitral Valve Prolapse Syndrome

Like hypertrophic cardiomyopathy the myxomatous degeneration of mitral valve in the tropics is proportional to the availability of an echocardiographic machine. From a virtual absence of reports from Africa and India some years ago, it has been suggested that mitral valve prolapse has now emerged as more common in the African black than in the African white because of an excessive reactivity and proliferation of connective tissue in blacks. The condition has been estimated to occur clinically in 15 percent of black Ugandans older than 60 years of age,[98] and at autopsy it was detected in 10 of 236 cases of rheumatic valve disease.[146] In India, 16 percent of healthy[72] and 18 percent of symptomatic[216] women had myxomatous degeneration of mitral valve.[11]

HYPERTENSIVE HEART DISEASE

In a review of hypertension in Africa, Koate showed that only after 1940 did hypertension among the African black populations south of the Sahara receive due attention.[176] The incidence of hypertension seen in overall heart disease has varied from 14 percent in Gambian hospitals to 44.4 percent in the Sudan. This has been the experience in Nigeria.[149] India and Far Eastern countries also provide a similar picture.[280] In the adult and middle-aged populations of India and the Far East hypertension is the most common cause of heart disease.[138] It is seen in 20.5 to 43.3 percent of cardiac autopsies, with the highest recorded incidence in Johannesburg.[145] In Durban, it is the second most common cause of death, next only to violence.[268] In addition, the incidence is steadily rising, due to westernization, and hypertension is therefore more common especially among urban dwellers. In clinical practice the incidence has varied between 16 and 36 percent of all common heart diseases (Table 33–1), the highest being found in Malaysia.[18] Walker found that hypertension is common among Indians and colored or mixed race adults in South Africa, yet in black school children blood pressure is far lower than in white school children.[329]

In Indian cities, the hospital-based incidence of hypertension is again 16 to 30 percent of the total for common heart diseases.[29,73,281] A population survey in Rohtak (northern India) showed an incidence of 64.3 /1,000 (59.9 males and 69.9 females per 1,000). The authors reported the incidence to be twice as much in the local rural population, making it about one-third the figures reported from the West.[126] In Johannesburg[269,270] and the Cape Peninsula,[291] the incidence among blacks is 25 percent and among Indians 19 percent—the same as in India. The effect of hypertension varies from place to place. Attention has been drawn to the frequency of cardiac complications compared with neurologic ones, but reports vary, due possibly to sample variations. In Senegal,[176] 75 percent of 1,177 clinical patients had cardiac, 21.7 percent renal, and 3.14 percent neurologic complications.[176] In Durban, of 343 autopsies on hypertensive black patients studied over 10 years (1965 to 1975), 41.9 percent had cardiovascular lesions.[268] In another study of 1,232 autopsies on South African blacks older than 50 years of age, 64 percent died of essential hypertension and 36 percent had underlying renal disease.[145] In an autopsy study in Lagos, of 266 patients with hypertension who died suddenly, 62 percent had intracerebral complications (hemorrhage in 58 percent and infarction in 4 percent), 23 percent had cardiac failure, and 15 percent had uremia.[206] This incidence of stroke is higher than in Europeans and Americans. A clinical survey from Senegal of 696 cases showed a similar distribution, namely, two-thirds had essential hypertension and one-third had secondary, mainly renal, hypertension.[176] A peculiar tendency of the African hypertensive to develop congestive heart failure despite the lack of coronary atherosclerosis has been commented on from Durban.[145,268] Only 2.2 percent of 434 cases in that series died of myocardial infarction. The Zambian study also showed

that left axis deviation on ECG, a usual clinical feature of the hypertensive white, is unusual in the hypertensive African black.[182] Another feature noted by the Durban group in hypertensive patients at autopsy was a large, flabby heart occurring in about half of the cases; the other half presented with classic concentric left ventricular hypertropy. The former feature, because of its relevance to DCM in Africa, is discussed earlier under the etiology of DCM, where evidence is presented that the natural history of hypertension in the tropics can be modified by a number of additional factors, especially dietary considerations.

ISCHEMIC HEART DISEASE

Myocardial infarction is traditionally a disease of affluence and therefore uncommon in the tropics, but its incidence there is increasing, parallel with an increasing westernization of those countries.[145,271] WHO has already voiced concern over this.[96] Among South African blacks, the incidence of ischemic heart disease (IHD) increased from 0.8 percent of cardiac deaths in 1969 to 11.7 percent in 1976,[145] although it is still regarded as a rare condition.[327] On the Ivory Coast, Bertrand et al. reported an increase in IHD incidence in blacks from 2.2 percent in 1965 to 5.3 percent in 1981.[31] The general figures in the few population surveys show an incidence of IHD of 8 percent in the north and 4 percent in southern Africa.[208] Among Hong Kong Chinese, deaths due to IHD registered an increase from 5.5 percent in 1971 to 8.4 percent in 1981.[59] In eastern India, deaths from IHD increased from 13.5 percent in 1970 to 14.6 percent in 1979.[180]

A study from Djibouti reports 431 cases of IHD over a period of 5 years (1972–76), representing 4.4 percent of all medical admissions.[116] Similarly low prevalence rates of myocardial infarction are seen in other parts of

Africa—namely East Africa.[74] In Johannesburg in 1970, 950 whites and 48 blacks died of myocardial infarction, the national figure for South Africa being 1,118 whites, 1,047 Asians, 941 mixed race, and 51 blacks.[271]

The mortality rates for all arteriosclerotic diseases (coronary, cerebral, hypertensive) in the different racial populations of South Africa per 100,000 is 1,156 for blacks, 2,166 for whites, 3,472 for Indians (highest), and 2,682 for races of color (higher than the black).[290] Another study in the South African black found 39 cases of myocardial infarction amongst 758 cases of sudden death.[313] In the Congo basin, between 1975 and 1980 only 25 cases of IHD were detected amongst 889 cases of cardiac diseases.[43] In Johannesburg, South African whites have almost the same mortality rate from coronary artery disease (885 per 10,000) as whites in the United States (906 per 10,000).[326] Chesler et al. found the overall incidence of myocardial infarction in South African blacks as 0.05 percent of all medical admissions, with no apparent increase over the last two decades.[57] The same trend was recorded for Indians in South Africa and Indians in India.[326] In Fiji there was increase of hospital incidence of IHD from 6.6 to 32 per thousand from 1960 to 1979.[307] The explosive increase in China has already been referred to.[305] IHD was the cause of death of 7 to 12 percent in Mozambique, Mauritius, and Malaysia.

In most centers in India, the incidence of coronary heart diseases is not as low as in Africa. In fact, in some reports it is as high as in the West.[212] Ten to twenty percent of cardiac diseases are due to coronary heart disease.[29] Deaths from coronary diseases have varied from about 5 to 35 percent. In Gujarat in western India, the hospital incidence for coronary artery disease rose from 16.3 to 23.5 percent between 1961 and 1965.[212] Population surveys (for IHD) have shown a figure of 5 to 6 percent for higher income groups and 0 to 1 percent for lower income groups.[29] In the urban population of Chandigarh, the incidence was 66 males and 63.7 females/1,000 population above the age of 30 years.[266] Other estimates are 45 to 65/1000 in males and 28 to 49 in females.[180] For myocardial infarction a population survey in Rohtak (northern India) revealed an incidence of 1.29 per 1,000.[125]

In a study of 1,000 hospitalized cases in Eastern India, 52 percent had myocardial infarction; 18 percent of the total were manual workers.[22] In the series from Gujarat of 1,105 cases of coronary disease, 62 percent had myocardial infarction and 4 percent were less than 30 years old.[212] The peak incidence of infarcts in India is between the ages of 40 and 60 years, with some reports finding more cases in the fifth or sixth decade. Roughly 8 percent of infarcts occur in those younger than 40 years.[22,276] The major change in the recognition of coronary artery disease in the last 5 to 7 years has been the application of angiographic and other sophisticated techniques to define the patterns of disease. Determination of risk factors has also been valuable.

Coronary Atherosclerosis

The pattern and severity of coronary and aortic atherosclerosis studied by intimal surface mapping technique in India and Africa revealed that, as far as the fatty streak is concerned, the extent of the lesion and age spread in the population affected is identical to that seen in the United States. Further progression to a fibrous plaque or a complicated lesion then slows, so that after the age of 20 years the extent of atherosclerosis in Indians and Africans lags behind that found in Americans, with the lag period being 10 to 20 years.[193,209,210] The Chinese, however, show some differences: mainland Chinese follow this pattern while the incidence of atherosclerosis in Hong Kong Chinese is similar to the western population.[59] Of 26 cases of myocardial infarction in Nigeria, nonatheromatous causes of coronary occlusion far outweighed atherosclerosis and included thromboemboli arising from the heart chambers or valves—in cases of infective endocarditis, EMF or ICM; in the remaining two-thirds predisposing causes included diabetes mellitus, hypertension, thyrotoxicosis, and aortic valve disease.[107]

Risk Factors

It has been stated that the urban black in Africa (Durban area) is exposed to all risk factors, including hypertension, cigarette smoking, obesity, and diabetes mellitus, listed for coronary heart disease in the Framingham, Massachusetts study, with the exception of hyperlipidemia, yet coronary atherosclerosis is hardly seen in African subjects.[268] Walker aptly summarized the situation by stating that in South Africa the population is in various stages of transition, from "primitiveness" to "sophistication" and that risk factors underlying coronary atherosclerosis do not have the same degree of noxiousness in different populations.[326] As is discussed later, these comments are applicable to most tropical countries, including China.

Lipids and Cholesterol

It is generally appreciated that in India, Sri Lanka, and parts of Africa little correlation exists between blood levels of lipids (including those of cholesterol) and the prevalence of coronary heart disease. Although hypercholesterolemia is as much a risk in India as it is in the United States, Indians frequently develop myocardial infarction at cholesterol levels well within the "normal" range, even when the prevalence of IHD in urban Indians is not very much lower than in Americans. In South Africa, 55 percent of whites and 45 percent of Indians have cholesterol levels above 6.0 IU (220 mg/100 ml)[326] whereas only 25 percent of urban and 10 percent of the rural blacks reach that level from youth to old age.[328] The black population of Transvaal does not show a fall in the levels of high-density lipoproteins (HDL) in the serum, as is seen in whites there.

Whites in the United States (Framingham, Massachusetts study) and Indians in Kampala and Durban have very similar cholesterol levels.[326] Conversely, nomadic tribes in Africa have high blood cholesterol levels (from a diet rich in animal fat and milk) yet an extremely low level of coronary heart disease.[280] The Masai tribe in Africa presents yet another peculiarity. Members consume a high cholesterol genic diet yet do not show hypercholesterolemia—possibly due to inborn differences in their cholesterol metabolism.[37] These observations suggest ethnic and racial differences in the interrelationship between diet, serum lipids, and atherosclerosis. However, a dominant role for life-style and physical activity as the determinants of the differences has been voiced.[273,280] In fact, Seftal believes that the rarity of coronary heart disease in the South African black is quite consistent with his lifestyle.[273] Applicable to such a discussion is the thesis, popularized by Trowell, Painter, and Burkitt,[304] of the anti-atherogenic properties of the high-fiber content diet consumed in the tropics.

In India, the situation is also different; the incidence of myocardial infarction is appreciably high, but its relationship with hypercholesterolemia is not a direct one. In a study of 85 cases of myocardial infarction in Chandigarh,[179] only 18 percent of patients and 15 percent of matched normal controls had cholesterol levels above 6.0 IU (250 mg), which is the usually accepted upper limit for the population (the normal average is around 200 mg). Normal lipid and cholesterol levels in Indian patients with IHD are recorded in 54 to 80 percent of the cases,[179,299,332] although the low-density lipoprotein (LDL)/HDL cholesterol hold the same status in Indians as in Western profiles. Among the young (under 40 years) the importance of cigarette smoking has been emphasized both in India[332] and Africa.[26,27] In 50 percent of cases only two or none of the nine recognized risk factors were applicable; 36 percent of young myocardial infarction victims showed no risk factors.[331]

Similarly, in a multicenter study in Africa, more than 26 percent of cases of IHD had no risk factors.[26,27] However, the situation is not consistent. A study of 54 cases of myocardial infarction in New Delhi, for example, showed hyperlipidemia and hypercholesterolemia in every case.[129]

Diabetes Mellitus

Diabetes mellitus and impaired glucose tolerance are highly significant factors in promoting atherosclerosis in a number of studies in the tropics, especially among Indians.[51,64,100,157,271,334]

An interesting pattern of vascular complications of diabetes among various groups in the tropics shows an unequal racial distribution of atherosclerotic vascular diseases.[157] Within India as well as among Indians living in Africa and Southeast Asian countries, diabetes is significant in the atherogenic profile.[51] In India the incidence of diabetes among hospitalized cases of IHD varies between 10 and 24 percent.[22] Diabetic blacks and whites on the Ivory Coast seem equally prone to IHD,[303] with the incidence in blacks as high as 22 percent.[31] In one Malaysian study, Chinese showed a higher prevalence of cerebral atherosclerosis, whereas Indians showed a higher prevalence of coronary atherosclerosis. Africans suffer far more from metabolic complications of diabetes than from vascular ones. It has been suggested that the etiopathology of diabetes in the African is different.[334] Among Indians in South Africa, both hypertension and diabetes have been regarded as possible expressions of a common biochemical disturbance.[270]

Hypertension

It has already been noted that hypertension has a high prevalence in the tropics, yet, unlike its significant atherogenic effect among the Western population, hypertension does not promote coronary atherosclerosis in the African black. In Durban among 434 cases

dying of hypertension, only 2.2 percent had a myocardial infarction; the corresponding figure for London was quoted as 27 percent and for New Zealand, 41.5 percent.[268] The Indian situation is similar to that in the West; 25 to 46.4 percent of cases of IHD have hypertension.[331,332]

Coagulation Factors

Increased fibrinolysis and lower platelet counts are a feature of the coagulation profile of the African population.[99] Venous thrombi and thromboembolism were reported in 2.4 percent of Africans and 52 percent of Americans in a comparative study. Interestingly, in my own analysis of records over an 18-year period, the incidence of pulmonary thromboembolism and infarction in 7,000 routine hospital autopsies was only 3.1 percent,[78] mostly in association with cardiac disease. The generally accepted figure in the United States and the United Kingdom range between 9 and 23 percent and in Africa, between 2 and 6 percent.

Smoking

Smoking is considered an important risk factor in India in myocardial infarcts occurring in those younger than 40 years.[331,332] Seventy-six percent of 100 young patients with myocardial infarction were smokers in a study from southern India.

Physical Activity and Socioeconomic Status

While earlier recording the incidence of coronary heart disease in India, it was mentioned that 15 to 20 percent of cases of myocardial infarction occur among manual laborers and those who are economically poor.[22,180,276]

Chronic anemia is another factor influencing coronary artery anatomy and physiology. It causes a compensatory vasodilation and opening up of anastomoses in the heart.

Morphology of Coronary Arteries and Myocardial Infarction

Anatomic Pattern of Coronary Arteries

The presence and incidence of a third primary division of the left coronary artery, demonstrated by postmortem coronary radiography, was reported to be higher in Bantu (74 percent) than in European hearts (38 percent).[44] This was not so among Nigerians.[99] In a study of 125 injected specimens at Chandigarh, I found more than two primary branches arising from the left coronary artery in 80 percent of hearts (unpublished). No difference in the existence and density of intercoronary anastomoses were found in various races by other workers.[232] The pattern of coronary artery dominance that favors the right artery in the western heart as well as the Indians heart[61] is reportedly balanced between the two coronary arteries among South Africans.[232] It is difficult to determine what contribution, if any, these anatomic variations make to the overall pattern of coronary artery disease: it is probably none, as the general pattern of coronary arterial disease is the same as in western studies.

Cardiac Findings

In 272 cases of myocardial infarction studied at autopsy in my department over the last 18 years,[39] most morphologic features are similar to those reported from the West. Males outnumbered females by 6.2 to 1 and had an average age of 58 and 47 years, respectively. The most common site of infarction was anteroseptal (43 percent), and the artery most commonly containing an occlusion was the left anterior descending. Thrombotic occlusion (recent or old) formed over atherosclerotic stenosis was seen in 46 percent of cases. Complications included cardiac aneurysm in 36.5 percent and rupture (of free wall, septum, or papillary muscles) in 0.7 percent of fresh in-farcts. The 35 postinfarction aneurysms were analyzed. These patients were, on an average, a decade older than those who died without aneurysms.[62]

INFECTIOUS DISEASES OF THE HEART

Infectious diseases of the heart, consisting of parasitic, bacterial, fungal, and viral diseases, are dealt with in part in Chapter 34. Parasitic and bacterial diseases are more common in the tropics. Three bacterial diseases that are rampant and often involve the heart are described here. They are tuberculosis, salmonellosis (including typhoid fever), and leprosy. Syphilis and viral myocarditis are also mentioned.

Tuberculosis

Tuberculosis is possibly the most common chronic bacterial disease in the world. Cardiac tuberculosis, however, is rare, except for pericarditis. In the preantibiotic era the incidence of tuberculoma was reported as 0.3 percent in all autopsies.[123] In recent years, reports from Bombay highlighted the tendency for tuberculosis to involve superficially located coronary arteries and the conduction fibers of the heart.[170] Among 14 cases, destruction of the sinuatrial node, atrial conduction tracts, and tuberculous arteritis were frequently noted. Only seven cases were found among 32,980 autopsies on patients over 46 years in this series. Another report from Bombay mentions nine cases among 9,333 autopsies over 10 years.[159] Pillay and Bhigjee describe myocardial tuberculosis from South Africa.[234] Tuberculoma with rupture/aneurysm formation have been described.[128,133] Tuberculous endocarditis and tuberculous aneurysms of the aorta are discussed elsewhere in the chapter.

Salmonellosis

Typhoid fever and other salmonella diseases are major public health problems in developing as well as developed countries. In cases of typhoid admitted to the hospital, it is not unusual to find ECG abnormalities, if looked for, and at autopsy stray foci of myocardial necrosis and degenerative lesions may be found (hydropic swelling, hyalinization of fibers, fatty infiltration), but cardiac involvement in typhoid rarely attracts attention. Radiologic enlargement of the heart in addition to ECG changes in typhoid in children have been noted in 15 percent of cases in Tunisia.[181] Apart from the myocarditis, salmonella may be responsible for purulent pericarditis, especially nonenteric salmonella-like S. *typhimurium*.[36] Endocarditis is a rare complication of typhoid; case reports are available from South Africa,[205] India,[178] and Saudi Arabia.[302]

Leprosy

There are no specific lesions in the heart in leprosy. In a clinical study from Chandigarh, a state of dysautonomia was described, in 3 of 15 leprosy patients studied. Both sympathetic and parasympathetic systems were involved.[166] Holla et al. described a case of "leproma of the heart" from western India and in the review mentioned the occurrence of rhythm disturbances, ventricular hypertrophy, raised serum enzyme levels, and congestive cardiac failure in patients with leprosy.[131]

Syphilis

A survey of the literature in India reveals that the incidence of cardiovascular syphilis in hospital data varies from 0.4 to 31.6 percent, with the condition being more prevalent in the south than the north.[247] The incidence is apparently declining. The lesions of cardiovascular syphilis in the tropics do not differ from those found in the West.

Viral Myocarditis

The belief that the coxsackievirus B group causes a variety of heart diseases has its followers in both Asia and Africa. Attempts have been made to relate DCM to viral infections. In a Nigerian study, of 44 patients with DCM a significant percentage showed a fourfold change in the antibody titers against one of the group of coxsackievirus B.[105] The findings were especially relevant to coxsackieviruses B2, B3, and B6. In a study of 50 patients with heart disease in Pondicherry, South India, viruses were implicated in 29.[189] The viruses included coxsackieviruses A9, B2, B3, B4, B5, influenza A, ECHO9, and cytomegalovirus, and the diseases included myocarditis, rheumatic heart disease, and DCM. Similarly, coxsackievirus B infection was related to valvular heart disease in children in Thailand.[240]

CHRONIC COR PULMONALE

Right ventricular hypertrophy secondary to chronic lung disease is another common cardiac problem in the tropics. In Africa, up to 10 percent of medical cases suffer from chronic cor pulmonale (Tables 33–1 and 33–2); in Sudan, this change is demonstrated in up to 12 percent of autopsies on cardiac patients.[100] In India, the situation has been reviewed by Wig in patients with chronic obstructive pulmonary disease.[335] Cor pulmonale is far more frequent in northern and central India (16 to 20 percent of cardiac diseases) than in southern India (4 percent). A high figure of 31 percent was encountered in Jaipur.[29] In Delhi, 5 percent of medical admissions and 10 percent of deaths in hospitalized patients are due to chronic cor pulmonale.[335] The usual causes in India are presented in a review[29] and include bronchiectasis (47.5 percent), chronic bronchitis (41.9 percent), bronchial asthma, and pulmonary tuberculosis (4.5 percent each).

The etiology of chronic obstructive pulmonary disease in the tropics is somewhat different from its etiology in the West. Industrial smog is replaced by different kinds of air pollution and respiratory infections caused by over-crowding. Thirty percent of villagers and 10 percent of the urban population suffer some form of chronic lung disease.[335] Factors contributing to this higher prevalence include smoking of cigarettes and bidies (cigarettes handmade by wrapping tobacco filling in a leaf), and the hookah (water pipe), the last named being more common in villages.[191,335] The villager is also exposed to the smoke of burning dried cow-dung cakes used as cooking fuel. The poverty and the cold climate of northern Indian villages results in overcrowding in single rooms that are poorly ventilated and frequently shared by cattle. The kitchen is in the same room, and exposure to cow-dung smoke is inevitable. This domestic air pollution is possibly one reason that chronic respiratory diseases are sometimes reported as more frequent in females. The closely packed dwellings also aid in the spread of infections. In Africa, exposure to mining dusts also promotes chronic obstructive pulmonary diseases.

CONGENITAL HEART DISEASE

The incidence of congenital heart disease in autopsy series from various countries is listed in Table 33–2. In an analysis of 222 autopsied cases in Bombay, a comparison of the patterns of various congenital lesions in Asian and Western countries was made.[168] Tetrology of Fallot was the most common congenital lesion in India and some Asian countries, whereas ventricular septal defect (VSD) is the most

common lesion in the West. In northern India, too, tetrology of Fallot was the most common lesion among 95 autopsies on patients in the pediatric age group.[190] However, cases between 1 month and 1 year of age showed a VSD more often. A similar analysis of 210 cases was presented from Ghana.[42] In northern India, 7.6 percent of neonates had congenital cardiac malformations.[21] A report from Sri Lanka showed a very high incidence of situs inversus and dextrocardia (1:2,500) especially in rural areas.[309]

In the late 1970s the incidence of congenital heart disease in Thailand was shown to be 2.7 per 1,000 births,[238] and in black school-aged children in Soweto, 3.9 per 1,000.[198] The figures do not differ very much from those of whites.

SENILE CARDIAC AMYLOIDOSIS

There is no mention of senile cardiac amyloidosis in reports from the tropics, except for the finding of senile amyloid in 10 percent of hearts of elderly Ugandans.[97]

CARDIAC LESIONS IN SCORPION BITES

Scorpion bites are a frequent event in tropical countries, especially those with deserts. For example, 50 children were admitted to a hospital in Patna in eastern India in 1 year alone. The majority were in shock, and 15 died. Echocardiographic and ECG features of "myocarditis" were recorded in 21.[4] Murthy and co-workers have done elaborate experimental studies on the pathophysiology of scorpion bite in dogs.[243] Acute myocarditis, hypokalemia, and hyperglycemia developed, which the author attributed to an autonomic storm and release of catecholamines. Enzyme studies pointed toward a cardiac sarcolemmal defect.

ACQUIRED IMMUNE DEFICIENCY SYNDROME

The ravages of acquired immune deficiency syndrome (AIDS) do not spare any organ; cardiac involvement in this disease is not specific. Because of its frequency, especially of seropositivity (against the human immunodeficiency virus [HIV]) in Africa, interest has been focused on the African states. I am not aware of any morphologic studies from Africa, but the cardiac pathology affecting the U.S. white possibly would be applicable to the black African. The lesions described include pericardial effusion and tamponade,[114] metastatic Kaposi's sarcoma,[283] a DCM-like cardiomyopathy, and myocarditis in the absence of Kaposi's sarcoma.[65] The myocarditis is presumably due to any of the viruses—cytomegalovirus, Epstein-Barr virus, or HIV, though in view of suppression of both T and B cells, a nonimmune mechanism could operate.[65]

Kaposi's sarcoma, until the early 1960s, was a curiosity known for its high frequency in blacks (estimated to be 200 times higher in the Congo than in Chicago) on the one hand, and a predeliction to affect East European Jews[253] on the other. The pattern of Kaposi's sarcoma in Africa has radically altered. Two forms are recognized: the endemic or typical African Kaposi's sarcoma and the atypical or AIDS-associated Kaposi's sarcoma.[23,24] The endemic lesion accounts for 4 to 12 percent of malignant tumors in blacks in the Congo, Zimbabwe, Malawi, Zambia, Uganda (East and central Africa).[213] With the identification of AIDS came the identification of AIDS-associated Kaposi's sarcoma in 1983 or so. In Zambia 24 percent and in Uganda 8 percent of patients with endemic Kaposi's sarcoma were seropositive to HIV; almost all cases of AIDS-associated Kaposi's sarcoma in Zambia and Uganda were seropositive.[24] The two forms also differ in their natural history. Endemic Kaposi's sarcoma in adults is an indolent disease presenting mainly with cutaneous nodular lesions of the skin, though visceral involvement does occur. The tumor responds to cytotoxic therapy, greatly extending patient life expectancy. Endemic Kaposi's sarcoma in children uncommonly involves the skin but appears as lymph node enlargement. It rapidly spreads to internal organs and has a poor prognosis. AIDS-associated Kaposi's sarcoma in adults has features similar to endemic Kaposi's sarcoma in children and is frequently associated with opportunistic infections of all kinds. Doubts as to whether this atypical AIDS-associated Kaposi's sarcoma is a true tumor have been voiced.[24] In South Africa, too, endemic Kaposi's sarcoma is 10 times more common in blacks, than in whites. Studies have not revealed any underlying immunodeficiency or viral infection in endemic Kaposi's sarcoma in the black population of Africa.[233]

HEAT INJURY

Exposure to high atmospheric temperature and hyperthermia associated with various infectious fevers in equatorial countries produces nonspecific cardiac damage, detectable by ECG recordings. Not only the temperature but also the duration of exposure to that temperature is important.[102] Nonspecific vacuolization and hyaline changes in myocardial fibers have been noted after an exposure to heat for more than 24 hours. Foci of contraction band necrosis and hemorrhage were found in the myocardium of 10 acute heat stroke victims.[54] Electron microscopic detected changes of malignant hyperthermia induced by anesthetic agents include damage to the myofilaments and to the intercalated discs.[113]

EPIDEMIC DROPSY

Epidemic dropsy is caused by the ingestion of sanguinine, a toxic alkaloid found in the seeds or oil of the Mexican poppy (*Argemone mexicana*). Sanguinine, consumed either as seeds contaminating wheat or as oil adulterating cooking oils, causes widespread capillary dilation and increased capillary permeability. It may cause the formation of small, tumorous angiomata in the skin. The heart is usually dilated and histologically shows intensely congested capillaries separating myofibers with edema. Epidemic dropsy is found in South Africa, Mauritius, the Fiji islands, India (especially its eastern parts), Burma, and other Far Eastern countries.[257]

SUBVALVULAR VENTRICULAR ANEURYSMS

Subvalvular ventricular aneurysm is a peculiar entity almost restricted to Africans. Rare cases occurring in blacks in other countries have been published. Reports are available from South Africa, Congo, Nigeria, and India.[47,63,99,237] The patients may be asymptomatic, with the aneurysm discovered as an incidental finding at autopsy. There may be features of mitral or aortic regurgitation, depending on the site and size of the aneurysm. The heart may be enlarged and its shape distorted. Usually a localized pericarditis covers the bulge. The aneurysm is actually a herniation or outpouching of the ventricular wall deep to the overhang of valve leaflets or cusps. It measures from a few millimeters to several centimeters in diameter. Endocardium lining the pouch is thick, and the thin aneurysm wall may contain very little or no muscle, which has been replaced by scar tissue that may, at times, calcify. A mixed inflammatory reaction is usually present in the wall. The lumen contains laminated thrombi.

In a review of 34 cases (38 aneurysms) reported up to 1973, 27 were submitral and 11 in subaortic locations.[237] Rare examples in the left atrium and the membranous septum are known.[47] The etiology of these aneurysms is unknown. A few patients had aortitis, but it was not related to the aneurysms. Herniation of the ventricle through a congenital weakness of the fibrous annulus has been suggested to cause these lesions.[99] This etiology would, in my opinion, put these aneurysms in the same class as congenital berry aneurysms of cerebral arteries.

PERICARDITIS

Pericarditis accounts for up to 5 percent of cardiac diseases in India[2] and 0.2 to 10.8 percent in Africa.[47] Tuberculosis continues as the major cause of both effusive and chronic constrictive pericarditis in Asian and African reports. The acute, benign form of pericarditis, which is not due to tuberculosis, is common in the West but rare in India.[2] In India in collective reviews,[2,17] 40 to 85 percent of cases of chronic constrictive pericarditis are due to tuberculosis. Indeed, tuberculosis is responsible for 40 to 60 percent of all kinds of pericarditis in India. Ten of 13 autopsied cases in Sudan were tuberculous.[100] Because rheumatic and hypertensive heart disease are so common in the tropics, rheumatic and uremic pericarditis are also frequent causes of pericarditis. In 107 cases from Uganda, 72 were a part of an overwhelming systemic infection whereas pericarditis was the main disease in 35 cases.[47] A review of 100 cases of tuberculous pericarditis from Durban showed that 82 percent presented with effusion and 18 percent with constriction. Fifteen percent of those with effusion developed constriction within 4 months.[92]

Among 140 cases examined in my department, uremic pericarditis was recorded in 31 percent, rheumatic pericarditis in 27 percent, and tuberculous (including chronic constrictive pericarditis) in 14 percent. Another 27 percent showed serofibrinous and purulent pericarditis as a part of congestive cardiac failure, septicemias, chest infections, or other miscellaneous causes. Rare forms of pericarditis due to parasites (amebic, filarial, guinea worm) are described in Chapter 34 (see also Ch. 22).

IDIOPATHIC AORTITIS: TAKAYASU'S DISEASE

Many centers worldwide have reported the existence of an idiopathic, granulomatous aortitis under a variety of names, including Takayasu's aortitis, young female arteritis, aortic arch syndrome, pulseless disease, and, lately, occlusive thrombotic aortopathy (OTAP).[256] (See Ch. 9 also.) Edington and Gilles included the conditions under the broad category of "arteritis of obscure etiology." Among etiologic mechanisms considered, tuberculosis and autoimmunity figure prominently.[259]

The disease affects any part of the aorta and/ or its branches as well as arteries. Clinical manifestations depend on its location, as some synonyms of the disease suggest (aortic arch syndrome, middle aortic syndrome, etc.). The most frequently involved arteries are the renal, the mesenteric, and those to the head and neck (Figs. 33–20 and 33–21). Coronary and pulmonary arteries have also shown arteritis in some cases. In Japan 44 to 100 percent, in Mexico 50 percent, and in India up to 26 percent of patients had pulmonary artery

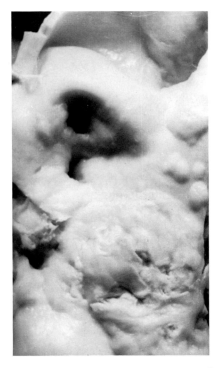

Fig. 33–20. Idiopathic aortoarteritis. Ascending arch of aorta showing buttonlike plaques of heaped intima and their extension into the neck arteries.

involvement.[308] Patients are young and include children. Females are affected 3 to 4 times more often than males.[343]

The appearance of the aorta is characteristic. Involvement may be restricted to a sin-

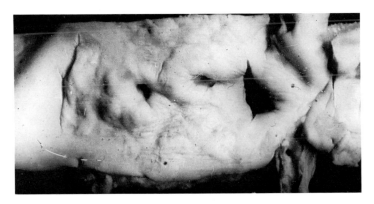

Fig. 33–21. Idiopathic aortoarteritis. Abdominal aorta showing intimal wrinkling and raised intimal plaques, especially around the major arterial ostia. The renal artery arises at the bottom right.

gle segment, or there may be more than one site affected with normal "skip areas" between. A diffuse involvement may occur. The intima is heaped up and markedly wrinkled, presenting with dense, gray plaques. The thickening extends to the periadventitial tissues. The result is the formation of one or more stenosed sites in the aorta interspersed with aneurysmal outpouchings. Multiple aneurysms are reported more commonly in Africans who are affected with the condition than in Indians who are; the first case of this kind from India was reported from New Delhi in 1985.[107] When the arch is involved, it usually affects the dome extending into the branches to the neck and upper limbs. The inferior intimal surface of the arch may be spared.

Histologic findings vary with the stage of the disease and may be active or quiescent. An initial inflammatory reaction appears at the medial-adventitial junction and consists of mononuclear cells, plasma cells, and sometimes a granulomatous reaction with disruption of the elastica and fibrosis.[171] Fibrinoid necrosis is not a feature. Inflammation spreads to the adventitia and periadventitia while the overlying intima undergoes fibrocollagenous thickening. The vasa vasora are thickened and have an onion skin appearance (see also Ch. 9). Among 197 cases from Japan,[343] lesions were most frequent in the aortic arch and its branches.

Although 22 percent had tuberculosis in the past, the authors of this Japanese study believe that the most likely cause is some postinfection allergy. In their opinion, classic Takayasu's disease features are not common. A report from Singapore of 48 cases of aortoarteritis emphasizes the greater prevalence of the disease in Japan, India, and Southeast Asia and records that 69 percent of cases had hypertension.[300] The incidence of hypertension in the European reports was quoted at 48 percent and in South Africa 42 percent. Kinare of Bombay, in her extensive experience with this disease, found no laboratory or clinical evidence of an autoimmune basis for this disease and believes tuberculosis plays an important role in its causation.[171,174] In some cases significant titers against streptococci and coxsackieviruses were also detected. In reports from Chandigarh, however, no evidence linking aortoarteritis to tuberculosis has been seen, with support for some kind of immune sensitization of aorta.[256]

ANEURYSMS OF THE AORTA

In two reports, one of 102 autopsied cases[175] and the other of 75 clinical cases,[274] both from western India, aneurysms of the aorta contributed to less than 1 percent of cardiac diseases. Causes for the aneurysms were syphilis (67.7 percent at autopsy and 42.2 percent in clinical cases) and atherosclerosis (16.8 and 49.3 percent, respectively). Dissecting aneurysms were rare in autopsy cases and accounted for 2.8 percent of clinical ones. Nonspecific aortitis was responsible for less than 5 percent at autopsy. Tuberculosis very rarely causes aneurysms of the aorta.[295]

OCCLUSIVE DISEASE OF PERIPHERAL ARTERIES

Arterio-occlusive disease in the tropics has not been adequately studied pathologically. As it is, a pathologist sees "end-stage" disease when all evidence of the etiologic development of the arterial occlusion has been overshadowed by scar tissue and gangrenous changes. Usually, three categories of arterio-occlusive disease are considered:

1. Thromboangiitis obliterans (TAO) or Buerger's disease
2. Arteriosclerotic or atherosclerotic occlusive disease (ASO)
3. Thromboembolic occlusion (TEO)

TAO is considered common in Asia. In a comprehensive pathologic study by Kinare,

89 limbs, amputated for arterial occlusions, were analyzed.[173] On a clinical basis there were 54 cases of ASO, 25 cases of TAO, and 10 of TEO. As expected, histologic differentiation between ASO and TAO proved difficult. In a similar study of 28 cases from Chandigarh,[217] it was concluded that TAO is a distinct disease; it is the most common peripheral arterio-occlusive disease in northern India. Venous involvement was found to be a significant feature. A recent clinical survey in Chandigarh spread over 7 years (1970 to 77) collected 122 cases of TAO and 32 cases of ASO.[321] The patients with TAO were exclusively men (barring a woman in whom tissue diagnosis was not available), mostly between the ages of 21 and 40 years, and generally of a low economic status; characteristically 98.3 percent were smokers, 55 percent being classed as heavy smokers. A significant number hailed from the hill districts. By contrast, patients with ASO were older, there were four men to one woman, and 60 percent were light to moderate smokers. Unlike the cases of Buerger's disease, the majority of patients with ASO had associated diabetes mellitus, ischemic heart disease, (IHD) or hypertension (Rose also discusses Buerger's disease in Ch. 10).

In the section on IHD it was mentioned that diabetes has a significant role in arterial atherosclerosis only in some races. Among Indians, peripheral and coronary arteries are significantly affected. The frequency of both diabetes and its vascular complications among Indian settlers abroad approaches that among European residents of those countries and is greater than that seen in indigenous inhabitants.[157] In a study of 200 cases of diabetes mellitus in northern India, the incidence of arterio-occlusive lesions was 9 percent.[297] The authors contrasted this finding with the reported incidence of 4.3 to 5 percent from the West and 2 to 5 percent in previous reports in India. It is interesting that an appreciably higher incidence of impaired glucose tolerance was found among cases of peripheral vaso-occlusive disorders in nondiabetics, es-

pecially those with arteriosclerotic occlusion, Buerger's disease, and in association with IHD in northern India.[51] This impairment was more marked during the acute occlusive episode.

PERIPHERAL VASCULAR DISEASE IN LEPROSY

Arteriographic and histologic abnormalities were detected in 50 percent of limb arteries and in more than 75 percent of smaller digital arteries in patients younger than 40 years suffering from various forms of leprosy in northern India.[164] Histologic lesions consisted of intimal thickening and organizing thrombi in the arteries and medial muscular and fibrotic proliferation in arterioles. Capillaries showed endothelial proliferation. It is likely that such occlusive vascular changes play a significant role in the development of mutilating deformities of fingers and toes in leprosy.

IDIOPATHIC SYMMETRIC GANGRENE OF THE LIMBS

Like annular subvalvular aneurysms, symmetric gangrene of the limbs is a peculiar, idiopathic cardiovascular lesion found among Africans (see also Ch. 10). Rare cases have been described from India also. It occurs in children and young adults and involves the upper or lower limbs, starting usually as edema of toes or hands. Gradually, gangrene sets in symmetrically in both limbs.[115] No cause is known, although an association with malnutrition and infections in the tropics is unavoidable. Coagulation abnormalities have been described. Steiner and Hutt, in a pathologic study, found mucoid swelling of the arterial walls with heaping of the intima into polyplike plaques, suggesting organized thrombi.[289] All sizes of arteries and even veins were involved; they suggested the name *peripheral mucoid arteriopathy*.

CEREBROVASCULAR DISEASE

The incidence of cerebrovascular disease (CVD) or stroke in the population under 40 years is higher in African-Asian countries than in the West.[329] In contrast with figures of 2.8 to 7 percent of strokes in the young from the United States, cerebrovascular disease accounts for 20 to 30 percent of such strokes in India.[60] In Africa, the incidence is about the same as it is in the West (3.5 percent of autopsies). CVD is becoming an increasingly prevalent cause of death and morbidity in the elderly urban African black. Hypertension and diabetes in the adult and sickle cell disease in children are the underlying causes.[223]

The main point of interest in Africa, particularly, is the complete dissociation between cerebral atherosclerosis and stroke. Although there is a low prevalence of atherosclerosis of coronary intracranial and peripheral limb vessels as well as a correspondingly low frequency of IHD and ischemic peripheral arterial disease, the rate of CVD is not low. This paradox has been discussed by others.[248] The major cause of CVD appears to be the higher prevalence of hypertension.[154]

From Uganda, James presented 207 autopsied cases of CVD and reviewed two other African reports.[154] James' work revealed the following:

Intracerebral hemorrhage: 11 to 36 percent
Subarachnoid hemorrhage: 13 to 17 percent
Cerebral infarction (nonembolic): 18 to 64 percent
Cerebral infarction (embolic): 5 to 23 percent
Arteriosclerotic occlusion: 1 percent

The cause of nonembolic occlusion included hypertension (33 to 64 percent), degenerative vascular disease (14 to 24 percent), miscellaneous (8 to 29 percent), and unknown (17 to 33 percent). The wide range shown in the data also matches general data in India.[60] Fourteen-year autopsy data from my institute of 362 cases show the incidence of CVD to be 7.6 percent of all autopsies, with the mean age being 43.3 years. Of the total, 36.8 percent were below the age of 40 years.[20] This contrasts with Western reports in which the incidence of CVD included hemorrhage in 38.1 percent and venous thrombosis in 9.3 percent.[60] Emboli arose in the heart in the majority; rheumatic heart disease in 51.6 percent, infective endocarditis in 19 percent, hypertension in 38.6 percent. Hemorrhage was caused by ruptured aneurysms in 11.6 percent of cases. The impression that intracranial aneurysms are rare in Asia is being disproved as more studies become available. In Chandigarh, 42 aneurysms were detected among 362 autopsies (11.6 percent) of CVD.[19] Of these, 33 were saccular and 9 myocotic, with the respective mean ages of patients at 43.3 years and 25.8 years. In clinical studies, on the other hand, much higher figures are detected. In a multicenter analysis of 661 cases of subarachnoid hemorrhage, there were 187 instances (36.7 percent) of aneurysms and 35 of arteriovenous malformation (7.1 percent).[20] These figures are similar to western data.

The incidence of cerebral arterial atherosclerosis here seems similar to western observations, but its severity is much less.[143,193]

The well-known "medial gap" or "medial discontinuity" found in cerebral arteries in the West is also equally prevalent in our material in Chandigarh, where such gaps were seen in 55 of the 56 sets of circle of Willis studied.[143]

In the Far East (specifically, Taiwan),[187] the situation is similar to that in Africa in that there is a higher incidence of CVD (25.4 to 30.1 percent) than of ischemic heart disease (7.4 to 17.2 percent) among atherosclerotic disease. Hypertension has been implicated as the main promotional factor. Data from the Phillipines followed a similar pattern. The incidence of myocardial infarction was one-third of CVD, although 67 percent of cases were coronary artery disease versus 29.9 percent CVD and 3.1 percent peripheral vascular diseases.[231]

Another important cause of CVD in India and parts of Africa is aseptic cerebral venous thrombosis (ACVT).[19,20,99] The Chandigarh data revealed 34 cases, which accounted for 9.3 percent of all CVD. There is higher frequency of ACVT in pregnancy and puerperium than in the West—21 of 34 cases.[19]

REFERENCES

1. Aceves S, Carrol R: The diagnosis of tricuspid valve disease. Br Heart J 19:211, 1957
2. Agarwal BL, Agarwal RK, Misra DN: Pericarditis: A clinical study of 77 cases. Indian Heart J 26:6, 1974
3. Agarwal BL, Prasad S: Rheumatic mitral stenosis: accelerated and delayed types. Indian Heart J 34:286, 1982
4. Agarwal RK, Singh DK, Shrinath M, Kumar R: Cardiovascular involvement in scorpion bite. Indian Heart J 40:311, 1988 (abst)
5. Al-Bahrani IR, Thamer MA, Al-Omeri MM: Rheumatic heart disease in the young in Iraq. Br Heart J 28:824, 1966
6. Alexander CS: Nutritional heart disease. Cardiovasc Clin 4:1972
7. Anderson SH, Charles TJ, Nicol AD: Thiamine deficiency at a district general hospital. Q J Med 55:15, 1985
8. Andrade ZA, Teixeira ARL: Changes in the coronary vasculature in endomyocardial fibrosis and their possible significance. Am Heart J 86:152, 1973
9. Andy JJ, O'Conell JP, Daddario RC, Roberts WC: Trichinosis causing extensive ventricular mural endocarditis with superimposed thrombosis. Am J Med 63:8214, 1977
10. Anonymous: The tropical heart. Editorial. S Afr Med J 62:463, 1982
11. Antani J, Rao MS, Biradar NS, et al: Incidence and clinical profile of click-murmur syndrome in Indian females. Indian Heart J 34:285, 1982
12. Arora R, Manoharan S, Sethi KK, Khaliullah

13. Attah EDB, Falase AO: Large flabby hearts in hypertension. Am Heart J 94:189, 1977
14. Avasthi G, Singh D, Singh C: Prevalence survey of rheumatic fever and rheumatic heart disease in urban and rural school children in Ludhiana. Indian Heart J 39:26, 1987
15. Ayuthya ASN, Ratanabanangkoon K, Pongpanich B: Juvenile rheumatic fever and rheumatic heart disease at Ramathibodi Hospital, Thailand. Southeast Asian J Trop Med Public Health 7:77, 1976
16. Babu SK, Khattri HN, Datta BN, et al: Cardiomyopathy in Northern India. Indian Heart J 29:35, 1977
17. Balasubramaniam V, Druiraji M, Basu SN, Ahuja IM: Etiology of chronic constrictive pericarditis. Indian Heart J 26:253, 1974
18. Balasundaram R: Cardiovascular disease in a West Malaysian town. Trans R Soc Trop Med Hyg 64:607, 1970
19. Banerjea AK, Varma M, Vasistha RK, Chopra JS: Cerebrovascular disease in northwest India. Study of autopsy material. J Neurol Neurosurg Psychiatry 52:512, 1989
20. Banerjee AK, Bansal AK: Aseptic cerebral venous thrombosis. Editorial. Bulletin PGI Chandigarh 23:116, 1989
21. Banerjee CK, Mahajan CM, Narang A, Bidwai PS: Congenital cardiac malformations in the new born. A clinico-pathologic study. Indian J Paediatrics 22:619, 1975
22. Banerjee JC, Mukherjea SK: Some observations on coronary heart disease. A study of 1000 cases. Indian Heart J 22:288, 1970
23. Bayley AC: Kaposi's sarcoma in Africa. Postgrad Doctor Mid East 10:248, 1987
24. Bayley AC, Downing RG, Cheingsong-Popov RG, et al: HTLV III serology distinguishes atypical and endemic Kaposi sarcoma in Africa. Lancet 1:359, 1985
25. Bayo S, Kuakavi N, Ndiaye P, Quenum: Les lésions du myocarde dans le kwashiorkor de sevrage à Dakar. À propos soixante quatre cas. Arch Anat Cytol Pathol 27:69, 1979
26. Ben Ismail JL: Coronary heart disease in Africa. A multicenteric prospective study I. Trop Cardiol 8:93, 1982
27. Ben Ismail JL: Coronary heart disease in Africa. A multicenteric prospective study II. Trop Cardiol 9:105, 1982

28. Berry JN: Prevalence of chronic rheumatic heart disease in an urban community. Indian Heart J 23:248, 1971

29. Berry JN: Epidemiology of heart disease in India. p. 86. In Ahuja MMS (ed): Progress in Clinical Medicine. Arnold Heinmann, New Delhi, 1976

30. Bertrand Ed Coly M, Chauvet, J, et al: A study of heart disease, particularly rheumatic disease in school children in the Ivory Coast. Bull WHO 57:471, 1979

31. Bertrand ED, Kacou GM, Mounkam Mbouende Y, N'Dori R: Maladie coronarie sous dévelopement et développement. Cardiol Trop (spécial numéro 51), 1984

32. Bertrand, ED, Renambot J, Chauvet J, et al: Study of 14 cases of endomyocardial fibrosis Bull WHO 51:417, 1974

33. Bhandari S, Kaul U, Shrivastva S, et al: Infective endocarditis in children. Indian J Pediatrics 51:529, 1986

34. Bhatia ML: Juvenile rheumatic disease in India. In Ahuja MMS (ed): Progress in Clinical Medicine. Arnold Heinmann, New Delhi, 1976

35. Bhattacharya SK, Jha BN, Somani PN: Carditis in acute rheumatic fever in Varanasi, India. Trop Geogr Med 26:271, 1976

36. Bhusnurmath B, Datta BN: Hypertension and dilated cardiomyopathy. An autopsy experience of 42 cases. Trop Cardiol 13:145, 1987

37. Bhusnurmath B, Datta BN, Khattri HN, et al: Myocardial infarction at autopsy. Morphological observations on 272 cases. Indian Heart J 37:353, 1985

38. Bijlsma A: The variety of endomyocardial fibrosis. Trop Geogr Med 28:199, 1975

39. Bird T: *Salmonella typhimurium* pericarditis. Br Heart J 31:659, 1969

40. Biss K, Taylor CB, Lewis LA, et al: Atherosclerosis and lipid metabolism in the Masai of East Africa. Afr J Med Sci 2:249, 1971

41. Blackett K, Ngu JL: Immunological studies in congestive cardiomyopathy. Br Heart J 38:605, 1976

42. Blankson JM, Christian EC: Congenital heart disease in Ghana. An analysis of 210 clinical and necropsy cases. Trop Cardiol 1:5, 1975

43. Bouramone C, Nkoua JL, Ekoba J: Les cardiopathies ischèmique en République populaire du Congo. Cardiol Trop 6:17, 1980

44. Brink AJ: Coronary arteries of Bantu hearts. S Afr Med J 33:407, 1959

45. Brockington IF: Heart diseases in tropical Africa. The last few years. Acta Cardiol 35:317, 1980

46. Brockington IF, Bohrer SP: Enlargement of the aortic shadow in Nigerian heart muscle disease. Acta Cardiol 25:346, 1970

47. Brockington IF, Edington GE: Adult heart disease in western Nigeria. A clinico-pathological synopsis. Am Heart J 83:27, 1972

48. Brockington IF, Olsen EGJ: Löffler's endocarditis and Davie's endomyocardial fibrosis. Am Heart J 85:308, 1973

49. Brockington IF, Olsen EGJ, Goodwin JF: Endomyocardial fibrosis in European residents in tropical Africa. Lancet 1:583, 1967

50. Burch GE, Gilles TD, Tsui C-Y: Epidemiology. In Burch GE (ed): Cardiomyopathy. Cardiovasc Clin 4:275, 1972

51. Burman SN, Rastogi GK, Wahi PL: Glucose tolerance in peripheral vaso-occlusive disorders. Indian Heart J 29:155, 1977

52. Campbell M, Summerell JM, Bras G, et al: Pathology of idiopathic cardiomegaly in Jamaica. Br Heart J 33:193, 1971

53. Cassel GA, Haitas B, Lakier JB, Barlow JB: Infective endocarditis at the Johannesberg Hospital. A retrospective analysis of 40 patients. S Afr Med J 55:624, 1979

54. Chao TC, Sinniah R, Pakiam JE: Acute heat stroke deaths. Pathology 13:145, 1981

55. Chau YN, Pan JYC, Barnes RJ: Epidemiological survey of cardiovascular disease in Hong Kong. p. 37. In Elia Kim M, Neufield HN (eds): Cardiology Current Topics and Progress. Academic Press, San Diego, 1970

56. Chauhan S, Nayak NC, Ramalingaswamy V: The heart and skeletal muscle in experimental protein malnutrition in rhesus monkey. J Pathol 90:301, 1965

57. Chesler E, Mitha AS, Weir EK, et al: Myocardial infarctions in the black population of South Africa. Coronary angiographic findings. Am Heart J 95:691, 1978

58. Cheung FMF, Pang SW, Loke SL, Lau SH: Coronary atherosclerosis among Hong Kong Chinese. Pathology 16:381, 1984

59. Chew CYC, Zaidy GM, Raphael MJ, et al: Primary restrictive cardiomyopathy. Br Heart J 39:399, 1977

60. Chopra JS, Prabhakar S, Das KC, et al: Stroke

in young. p. 217. In Greenhalg RM, Rose FC (eds): Progress in Stroke Research I. Pitman, London, 1979

61. Chopra P, Sethi U, Gupta PK, Tandon HP: Coronary arterial stenosis. An autopsy study. Acta Cardiol 38:183, 1983

62. Chopra VK, Bhusnurmath B, Datta BN: Ventricular aneurysms. Clinicopathological correlation. Indian J Chest Dis Allied Sci 22:9, 1980

63. Chugh VK, Sabharwal U: Subvalvular cardiac aneurysm. Indian Heart J 30:171, 1978

64. Cleave TL, Campbell GD: Diabetes, coronary thrombosis and the saccharine disease. 2nd Ed. John Wright, Bristol, England, 1969

65. Cohen IS, Anderson DW, Virmani R, et al: Congestive cardiomyopathy in association with acquired immunodeficiency syndrome. N Engl J Med 315:628, 1986

66. Cole TO: Problems of rheumatic fever in Nigerians. Trop Cardiol 6:181, 1980

67. Coles RM, Davies JNP: The heart weight in normal subjects in Uganda. E Afr Med J 36:76, 1959

68. Collipp PJ, Chen SY: Cardiomyopathy and selenium deficiency in a two-year-old girl. N Engl J Med 304:1304, 1981

69. Connors DH, Somers K, Hutt MJK, et al: Endomyocardial fibrosis in Uganda. Part I. Am Heart J 74:687, 1967

70. Connors DH, Somers K, Hutt MJK, et al: Endomyocardial fibrosis in Uganda. Part II. Am Heart J 75:107, 1967

71. Crawford MA: Endomyocardial fibrosis and carcinoidosis. A common denominator? Am Heart J 66:273, 1963

72. Dalal JJ, Vengsarkar AS, Nair KG: The click-murmur syndrome. Clinical and echocardiographic study of 51 cases. J Assoc Physicians India 26:665, 1978

73. Dalal PM, Shah KD, Jhaveri GC: Hypertension in India. International Congress on Hypertension. Bombay, October 1977

74. D'Arbela PG, Kanyerezi RB, Tulloch JA: A study of heart diseases in the Mulago Hospital, Kampala. Trans R Soc Trop Med Hyg 60:782, 1966

75. Datey A, Parameswaran A, Bhaktaviziam A: Renal lesions in obliterative cardiomyopathy. J Pathol 140:113, 1983

76. Datta BN: Heart diseases in the tropics and Parasitic heart diseases. p. 884. In Tsung CO (ed): International Textbook of Cardiology. Pergamon Press, Elmsford, NY, 1986

77. Datta BN, Aikat BK: Cardiomyopathy in North India. An autopsy study of 30 cases. Indian Heart J 26:219, 1974

78. Datta BN, Babu SK, Khattri HN, et al: Endomyocardial fibrosis in Chandigarh area. Trop Geogr Med 29:346, 1977

79. Datta BN, Bharti B, Khattri HN, et al: Anatomically isolated aortic valve disease. Autopsy study of 100 cases. Jpn Heart J 29:661, 1988

80. Datta BN, Khattri HN, Bidwai PS, et al: Infective endocarditis at autopsy in N India. Analysis of 120 cases. Jpn Heart J 23:330, 1982

81. Datta BN, Misra NP: Infective endocarditis. p. 213. In Misra NP (ed): Progress in Cardiology. Arnold Hemmann, New Delhi, 1981

82. Datta BN, Nagrani B, Khattri HN, et al: Rheumatic heart disease at autopsy. An analysis of 260 cases at Chandigarh. Indian Heart J 30:39, 1978

83. Datta BN, Ramesh K, Bhusnurmath B: Autopsy incidence of pulmonary vascular episodes. A study of 218 cases. Angiology 37:744, 1986

84. Datta BN, Silver MD: Cardiomegaly in chronic anemia in rats. An experimental study, including ultrastructural histomatic and stereological observations. Lab Invest 32:503, 1975

85. Datta BN, Silver MD: Cardiomegaly in chronic anaemia in rats: Gross and histologic features. Indian J Med Res 64:447, 1976

86. Davidson BMD, Parry EHO: Peripartum cardiac failure. Q J Med 47:431, 1978

87. Davidson NMD, Parry EOH: The etiology of peripartum cardiac failure. Am Heart J 97:535, 1979

88. Davies J, Spry CJF, Sapsford R, et al: Cardiovascular features of 11 patients with eosinophilic endomyocardial disease. Q J Med 52:23, 1983

89. Davies J, Spry CJF, Vijayaraghavan G, DeSouza JA: A comparison of the clinical and cardiological features of endomyocardial disease in temperate and tropical regions. Postgrad Med J 59:179, 1983

90. Davies JNP: Endocardial fibrosis in Africans. East Afr Med J 25:476, 1948

91. Davies JNP: African endomyocardial fibrosis. Cardiovasc Clin 4:275, 1972

92. Desai HN: Tuberculous pericarditis. A review of 100 cases. S Afr Med J 55:877, 1979

93. Dewan D, Indarjit D, Sahni D: Personal communication, 1989

94. Dickinson J: That congestive cardiomyopathy is really hypertension in disguise. Debate. Postgrad Med J 48:777, 1972

95. Disnot B, Ekra A, Bertrand E: Echocardiographic signs in 45 cases of endomyocardial fibrosis. Trop Cardiol 7:117, 1981

96. Dodu SRA: Coronary artery disease in developing countries: The threat can be averted. WHO Chron 38:3, 1984

97. Drury B: The cardiac pathology of elderly Ugandan Africans. E Afr Med J 50:566, 1973

98. Drury RAB: Myxomatous degeneration of cardiac valves in Uganda. E Afr Med J 50:566, 1978

99. Edington GM, Gilles HM: Pathology in the Tropics. 2nd Ed. Edward Arnold Publishers, London, 1976

100. El Hasan AM, Wasfi A: Cardiovascular diseases in Khartoum. Trop Geogr Med 24:118, 1972

101. Eling WMC, Jerusalem CR, Hermsen CC, et al: Role of macrophages in pathogenesis of endomyocardial fibrosis in murine malaria. Trans R Soc Trop Med Hyg 78:43, 1984

102. Ellis PF: Heat illness II. Pathogenesis. Trans R Soc Trop Med 70:412, 1976

103. Engbers JG, Molhoek GP, Arntzenius AC: Soshin beri beri, a rare diagnostic problem. Br Heart J 51:581, 1984

104. Falase AO: Cardiomyopathy of unknown origin among Nigerian adults: role of hypertension in etiology. Br Heart J 39:671, 1977

105. Falase AO: Four year follow-up of the blood pressure of adult Nigerians with cardiomegaly of unknown origin. Cardiol Trop 4:59, 1978

106. Falase AO: Endomyocardial fibrosis in Africa. Postgrad Med J 59:170, 1983

107. Falase AO, Cole TO, Osuntokun BO: Myocardial infarction in Nigeria. Trop Geogr Med 25:147, 1973

108. Falase AO, Fabiyi A, Odegbo-Olukoya OO: Coxsackie B virus and heart muscle disease in Nigerian adults. Trop Geogr Med 31:237, 1979

109. Falase AO, Fabiyi A, Ogimba EO: Heart muscle disease in Nigerian adults. Afr J Med 6:165, 1977

110. Falase AO, Jaiyesimi F, Iyun AO, Attah EB: Infective endocarditis. Experience in Nigeria. Trop Geogr Med 28:9, 1976

111. Falase AO, Kolawale TM, Lagundoye SB: Endomyocardial fibrosis. Problems in differential diagnosis. Br Heart J 38:369, 1976

112. Fawzy ME, Zaidy G, Halim M, et al: Endomyocardial fibrosis: A report of eight cases. J Am Coll Cardiol 5:983, 1985

113. Fenoglio JA, Irey N: Myocardial changes in malignant hyperthermia. Am J Pathol 89:51, 1977

114. Frink L, Reichek N, St. John Sutton MG: Cardiac abnormalities in acquired immune deficiency syndrome. Am J Cardiol 54:1161, 1984

115. Gelfland M: Symmetrical gangrene in the Africans. Br Med J 1:847, 1947

116. Gendron Y, Ardouin C, Sinol J: Les condiopathies ischèmiques de l'Africain à Djibouti. Éfinde de 431 observations en 5 ans. Bull Soc Pathol Exog 70:427, 1977

117. Gerbaux A, Dubost C, Maurice P, et al: Endomyocardite fibroseuse observée au cours la Filariose. À propos d'un cas traité chirurgicalement. Ann Med Inteme 124:471, 1973

118. Gharagozoloo RA, Daneshpajooh M, Ghavamian P: Rheumatic fever and rheumatic heart disease among 56,800 inhabitants of South East Tehran from 1972–74. Acta Trop 33:215, 1976

119. Ghosh JC, Neelakanthan MK, Chhetri MK: Peripartal cardiomyopathy. Indian Heart J 26:212, 1974

120. Gillanders AD: Nutritional heart disease. Br Heart J 113:177, 1951

121. Goodwin JF: Geographic distribution of cardiomyopathies. p. 31. In Bajusz E, Rona G, Brink AJ, Lochna A (eds): Cardiomyopathies. University Park Press, Baltimore, 1973

122. Goodwin JF: Endomyocardial disease—clinical features. Postgrad Med J 59:154, 1983

123. Gore I, Saphir O: Myocarditis: A classification of 1402 cases. Am Heart J 34:827, 1947

124. Gu B-Q, Cheng TO: Keshan disease. p. 752. In Cheng TO (ed): International Textbook of Cardiology. Pergamon Press, Elmsford, NY, 1986

125. Gupta SP, Khetrapaul NN: Incidence of acute myocardial infarction in Rhotak city, based on total population study. Indian Heart J 30:370, 1978 (abst)

126. Gupta SP, Siwach SB, Moda VK: Epidemi-

ology of hypertension. Indian Heart J 30:315, 1978

127. Gwata T: Cardiomyopathy in Rhodesia. Cent Afr J Med 23:247, 1977

128. Halim MA, Mercer EN, Guinn GA: Myocardial tuberculoma with rupture and pseudoaneurysm formation. Br Heart J 54:603, 1985

129. Harshwardhan JS, Gupta MP: Serum lipid patterns in acute and old myocardial infarction. Indian Heart J 32:75, 1980

130. Higginson J, Gillanders AD, Murray JF: The heart in chronic malnutrition. Br Heart J 14:213, 1952

131. Holla VV, Zawan PB, Deshmukh SD, Sardar SS: Leproma of heart. Indian Heart J 35:111, 1983

132. Hudson REB: Pathology of cardiomyopathies. In Burch GE (ed): Cardiomyopathy. Cardiovasc Clin 4:289 1972

133. Human DG, Rose A, Fraser CB: Tuberculous aneurysms of the left ventricle. S Afr Med J 64:26, 1983

134. Hutt MSR: Pathology of cardiomyopathies. Geographic aspects. Postgrad Med J 48:738, 1972

135. Hutt MSR: Cardiac pathology in the tropics. p. 511. In Pomerance A, Davies MJ (eds): The Pathology of the Heart. Blackwell Scientific Publications, London, 1975

136. Ikeme AC: Idiopathic cardiomegaly in Africa. Bull WHO 54:544, 1976

137. Ikeme AC, D'Arbella PG, and Somers K: The role of hypertension in the pathogenesis of idiopathic cardiomegaly. Trop Cardiol 1:135, 1975

138. Ikeme A, Pole JD, Larbi E, et al: The prevalence cardiovascular abnormality in a tropical urban population. The Mamprobi survey. Cardiol Trop 4:113, 1978

139. Ikram H, Maslowski AH, Smith BL, Nicholls MG: The hemodynamic, histopathologic and hormonal features of alcoholic cardiac beri beri. Q J Med 50:359, 1981

140. Ilyas M, Peracha MA, Ahmed R, et al: Prevalence and pattern of rheumatic heart disease in the frontier province of Pakistan. J Pak Med Assoc 29:165, 1979

141. Imperial ES, Felarca A: Autopsy study of heart disease in the Philippine General Hospital. Am Heart J 66:470, 1965

142. Indian Council of Medical Reserach: Pro-

ceedings of Workshop on Endomyocardial fibrosis in India. Trivandrum, 1981. Indian Council of Medical Research, New Delhi, 1983

143. Indian Council of Medical Research: Epidemiological study on subarachnoid hemorrhage in India (1972–75). Indian Council of Medical Research, New Delhi, 1983

144. International Society and Federation of Cardiology, Scientific Council on Cardiomyopathy: Workshop on multicentric research project on endomyocardial disease, London. Postgrad Med J 59:133, 1982

145. Isaacson C: The changing pattern of heart disease in South African blacks. S Afr Med J 52:793, 1977

146. Isaacson C: Myxomatous degeneration of heart valves in blacks. S Afr Med J 57:537, 1980

147. Ismail SA, Gabir MH: Observations on rheumatic heart disease in the Sudan. Trans R Soc Trop Med Hyg 64:772, 1970

148. Ives FA, Willis AJ, Ikeme AC, Brockington IF: Endomyocardial fibrosis and filariasis. Q J Med 36:495, 1967

149. Jain PS, Gera SC, Abergowe CQ: Incidence of hypertension in Ahmed Bellu Hospital, Nigeria. J Trop Med Hyg 80:90, 1977

150. Jaiyesimi F: Scalar electrocardiogram in children with endomyocardial fibrosis. A useful diagnostic tool. Trop Cardiol 7:107, 1981

151. Jaiyesimi F, Abiaye AA: Fatal rheumatic carditis in early life. Trop Cardiol 8:7, 1982

152. Jaiyesimi F, Onadeko M, Antia AU: Endomyocardial fibrosis, schistosomiasis and dermatosis: A new facet of an old problem. Cardiol Trop 5:27, 1979

153. Jaiyesimi F, Salimonu LS, Amtia AU: Serum immunoglobulins in children with cardiomyopathies. Trans R Soc Trop Med Hyg 78:127, 1984

154. James PD: Cerebrovascular disease in Uganda. Trop Geogr Med 27:125, 1975

155. Jeroudi MO, Halim MA, Harder EJ, et al: Brucella endocarditis. Report of 4 cases. Br Heart J 58:279, 1987

156. Johnson JB, Mir GH, Flores P, Manu M: Idiopathic heart disease associated with pregnancy and puerperium. Am Heart J 72:809, 1966

157. Jones JJ, Watkins PS, Owyong LY, et al: Di-

abetes and its vascular complications in Malaysia. Trop Geogr Med 30:439, 1978

158. Kalichurun S: The heart in cardiomyopathy. S Afr Med J 50:155, 1976

159. Kapoor OP, Mascrehans E, Ranawase MM, Gadgil RK: Tuberculoma of the heart. Report of 9 cases. Am Heart J 86:334, 1973

160. Kartha CC, Mathai A, Balakrishnan KG, Valiathan MS: Immunological studies in endomyocardial fibrosis. Indian Heart J 36:90, 1984

161. Kartha CC, Sandhyamani S: An autopsy study of tropical endomyocardial fibrosis. Indian J Med Res 82:439, 1985

162. Kartha CC, Valiathan MS: Cardiac ultrastructure in tropical endomyocardial fibrosis. Indian J Med 87:275, 1988

163. Kaul UA, Tatke MA, Khalilullah M: Immunologic studies in idiopathic congestive cardiomyopathy. Indian Heart J 40:325, 1985

164. Kaur S, Wahi PL, Chakravarti KN, et al: Peripheral vascular deficit in leprosy. Int J Leprosy 44:332, 1976

165. Kawai C, Wakabayashi A, Matsumura T, Yui Y: Reappearance of beri-beri heart disease in Japan. Am Med J 69:383, 1980

166. Khattri HN, Radhakrishnan K, Kaur S, et al: Cardiac dysautonomia in leprosy. Int J Leprosy 46:172, 1978

167. Khattri HN, Wander GS, Varma JS, et al: Peripartum cardiomyopathy. Indian Heart J 40:103, 1988

168. Kinare SG: Congenital heart disease. Cardiovasc Rev 11:46, 1971

169. Kinare SG: Chronic rheumatic valvular disease. Ann Indian Acad Med Sci 8:47, 1972

170. Kinare SG: Interesting facets of cardiovascular tuberculosis. Indian J Surg 37:144, 1975

171. Kinare SG: Non-specific aortitis (Takayasu's disease). Pathol Microbiol 43:134, 1975

172. Kinare SG: Rheumatic heart disease in the young. Pathologic aspects. Indian Heart J 35:135, 1983

173. Kinare SG, Iyer I, Murthy A, et al: Nonspecific aortitis—immunologic studies. Indian Heart J 35:337, 1987

174. Kinare SG, Kher YR, Rao G, Sen PK: Pattern of occlusive peripheral vascular disease in India. Angiology 27:165, 1976

175. Kinare SG, Pai AM: Aneurysms of aorta. Morbid anatomical study of 102 cases. Indian Heart J 15:241, 1963

176. Koate P: Arterial hypertension in black Africans. Bull Trop Dis 56:841, 1978

177. Krishnaswamy H, Datey A, Krishnaswamy S, Cherian G: Electron microscopic findings in endomyocardial fibrosis. Indian Heart J 34:276, 1982

178. Kulpati DDS, Bhargava SP, Gupta GD, Sharma ML: Salmonella endocarditis. J Assoc Phys India 16:535, 1968

179. Kumar M, Chakravarti RN, Singh A, Wahi PL: Serum lipid profiles in patients of myocardial infarction in the Chandigarh area. Atherosclerosis 24:355, 1976

180. Kundu SC, Bhattacharya TD, Banerjee D, et al: Profile of myocardial infarction among railroad workers in Eastern India. Indian Heart J 35:151, 1982

181. Latrous L, Mazhoud N, Mazigh R, et al: Complications cardiovasculaires de la fièvre typhoidide. Tunis Med 54:847, 1976

182. Levitt D: Hypertensive heart disease in the Zambian. E Afr Med J 54:174, 1977

183. Lewis BS, Gotman MS: Natural history of rheumatic heart disease in childhood. p. 63. In Borman JB, Gotman MS (eds): Rheumatic Valvular Disease in Children. Springer-Verlag, New York, 1980

184. Liu YQ, Wang ZL, Wei EY: Radiological study of four cases of endomyocardial fibrosis. Chin Med J 96:569, 1983

185. Lowenthal MN: Endomyocardial fibrosis: familial and other cases from North Zambia. Med J Zambia 12:2, 1978

186. Lowenthal MN: Hypertensive heart disease and cardiomyopathy in blacks. Diagnostic confusion. S Afr Med J 55:547, 1979

187. Lue HC, Tseng WP, Liu GJ, et al: Clinical and epidemiological features of rheumatic fever and rheumatic heart disease in Taiwan and Far East. Indian Heart J 35:339, 1983

188. Lutalo SM, Mbonga N: Experience on follow-up of registered rheumatic fever patients in Zimbabwean midlands. Trop Geogr Med 38:277, 1986

189. Madhavan HN, Agarwal SC, Badrinath S: Role of viruses in myocarditis during the years 1973–76 in Pondicherry area. Indian J Med Res 67:190, 1978

190. Mahajan CM, Banerjee CK, Bidwai PS, Datta BN: Congenital cardiac malformation in children. An autopsy study. Indian J Pediatr 13:759, 1976

191. Malik SK, Singh K: Smoking habits, chronic bronchitis and ventilatory function in rural males. Indian J Chest Dis Allied Sci 20:73, 1978

192. Manoharan S, Mohan JC, Arora R, et al: Organic tricuspid valve involvement in rheumatic heart disease. Indian Heart J 38:60, 1986

193. Mathur KS: Arterial disease. In Ahuja MMS (ed): Progress in Clinical Medicine in India. Arnold Heinmann, New Delhi, 1976

194. Mathur KS, Wahal PK: Epidemiology of rheumatic heart disease. Study of 29,922 school children. Indian Heart J 34:367, 1982

195. McKinney B: Pathology of Cardiomyopathies. Butterworth (Publishers), London, 1974

196. McKinney B: Endocardial changes produced in Patus monkey by ablation of cardiac lympatics and the administration of plantain diet. Am Heart J 91:484, 1976

197. McLaren MG, Hawkins DM, Koornhof HS, et al: Epidemiology of rheumatic heart disease in black school children of Soweto, Johannesburg. Br Med J 3:474, 1975

198. McLaren MJ, Lachman AS, Barlow JB: Prevalence of congenital heart disease in black school children of Soweto, Johannesburg. Br Med J 41:554, 1979

199. Mehta AP, Kalyani MD, Kinare SG: Infective endocarditis. J Postgrad Med 24:40, 1978

200. Mess OM, Turina M, Benning A, et al: Endomyocardial fibrosis in Switzerland. Br Heart J 40:406, 1978

201. Metras D, Coulibaly AO, Ouattara K: The surgical treatment of endomyocardial fibrosis: results in 55 patients. Circulation 72(suppl. 2):274, 1985

202. Meyer M, De Moor MMA, Human DG: Hypertrophic cardiomyopathy in infancy and childhood. S Afr Med J 71:490, 1987

203. Miall WE, Bras G: Heart disease in the tropics. Br Med J 28:79, 1972

204. Mohan JC, Reddy KS, Karloopia BD, et al: Extreme pulmonary hypertension in rheumatic heart disease in India. Indian Heart J 36:313, 1984

205. Mokhobo KP: Typhoid cardiac involvement. S Afr Med J 49:55, 728, 1975

206. Mordi VPN, Okuwobi BO: Sudden deaths in Lagos and their relation to hypertension. Cardiol Trop 4:27, 1978

207. Mukhopadyay AK, Chopra P: Diffuse nonspecific aortitis with multiple saccular aneurysms and aortoenteric fistula. Br Heart J 54:102, 1985

208. Multaf C: Enquête épidémiologique sur les coronaropathies en Afrique. Cardiol Trop 9:105, 1983

209. Murthy MSN, Datta BN, Ramalingaswamy V: Aortic atherosclerosis in N. India. J Pathol Bacteriol 83:135, 1962

210. Murthy MSN, Datta BN, Ramalingaswamy V: Coronary atherosclerosis in N. India. J Pathol Bacteriol 85:93, 1963

211. Naidoo DP: Beri beri heart disease in Durban. A retrospective study. S Afr Med J 72:241, 1987

212. Naik CH: Incidence and epidemiology of coronary artery disease in Gujarat. Indian Heart J 20:3, 1968

213. Naik KG: Kaposi's sarcoma in Zambia. A histopathologic study. Indian J Cancer 13:132, 1976

214. Nair DV: Endomyocardial fibrosis in Kerala state. Indian Heart J 34:412, 1982

215. Nair DV, Kabir HA, Thankum S: Epidemiological survey of rheumatic heart disease in school children at Allepey. Indian Heart J 32:65, 1980

216. Nambiar U, Alurkar VM, Druiraj M, et al: Mitral valve prolapse in apparently healthy Indian women. Indian Heart J 34:285, 1982

217. Narasimham P, Sodhi JS, Bhagwat AG: Pathologic pattern of peripheral arterio-occlusive disease in the young adult of North India. Bull PGI 12:25, 1978

218. Noah MS: Dilated cardiomyopathy in Saudi Arabia. A review of 55 cases. Trop Geogr Med 38:283, 1986

219. Ogunnowo PO, Odesanni WO, Andy JJ: Hypertrophic cardiomyopathy. Cardiol Trop 13:61, 1984

220. Olsen EGJ: Myocarditis—a case of mistaken identity? Br Heart J 50:303, 1983

221. Olsen EGJ, Spry JFC: The pathogenesis of Loffler's endomyocardial disease. p. 281. In Yu PN, Goodwin JF (eds): Progress in Cardiology. Lea & Febiger, Philadelphia, 1979

222. Olsen EGJ, Spry JCF: Relation between eosinophilia and endomyocardial disease. Prog Cardiovasc Dis 27:241, 1985

223. Osuntokun BO: Stroke in the African. Afr J Med Sci 6:39, 1977

224. Padmavati S: Rheumatic fever and rheumatic heart disease in developing countries. Bull WHO 56:543, 1979

225. Padmavafi S: The challenge of rheumatic fever and rheumatic heart disease in India. Indian Heart J 34:364, 1982

226. Panja M, Kar AK, Chetri M, Panja S: A profile of apical cardiomyopathy. Indian Heart J 40:92, 1985

227. Parry EHO: Idiopathic cardiomegaly. Clinical diagnosis. Cardiologia 52:36, 1968

228. Parry EHO, Abrahams DG: The natural history of endomyocardial fibrosis. Q Med J 34:383, 1965

229. Patel AK, Ziegler JL, D'Arbela PG, Somers K: Familial cases of endomyocardial fibrosis in Uganda. Br Med J 4:331, 1971

230. Pauley JW, Jones R, Green WPD: Myocardial toxoplasmosis. Lancet 2:624, 1954

231. Paulion-Abundo HP, Helen P: Epidemiology of cardiovascular disease in the Philippines. p. 39. In Eliakim M, Neufield HN (eds): Cardiology. Current Topics and Progress. Academic Press, San Diego, 1976

232. Pepler WJ, Meyer BJ: Interarterial coronary anastomoses and coronary arterial pattern. A comparative study of South African Bantu and European hearts. Circulation 22:14, 1960

233. Phillips JI, Sher R: Kaposi's sarcoma in different populations in South Africa. S Afr Med J 71:615, 1987

234. Pillay SU, Bhigjee AI: Myocardial tuberculosis and polycythaemia. S Afr Med J 54:453, 1978

235. Piza J, Troper L, Cespedes R, et al: Myocardial lesions and heart failure in infantile malnutrition. Am J Trop Med Hyg 20:343, 1971

236. Poltera AA: Pathology of African trypanosomiasis. Br Med Bull 41:169, 1985

237. Poltera AA, Jones AW: Subvalvular left ventricular aneurysm. A report of 5 Ugandan cases. Br Heart J 35:1085, 1973

238. Pongpanich B, Ayuthya PSN, Jayavasu J, Sankavibha N: Coxsackie group B virus and acquired valvular heart disease in children. J Med Assoc Thailand 59:452, 1976

239. Pongpanich B, Chesdavanijkul W, Chiemchanya S, et al: Congenital heart disease in children born at the Ramasthibodi Hospital. J Med Assoc Thailand 61:261, 1978

240. Pongpanich B, Dhanavaravibul S, Limsuvan A: Prevalence of heart disease in school children in Thailand. Southeast Asian J Trop Med Public Health 7:91, 1976

241. Pruthi PK, Sharma D, Kalil A, Prakash K: Clinical bacteriological and immunological correlationship of rheumatic activity. Indian Heart J 36:235, 1984

242. Puigbo JJ, Combellas I, Acquatella H, et al: Endomyocardial disease in South America. Report on 23 cases in Venezuela. Postgrad Med 59:162, 1983

243. Radhakrishna MK, Billimoria FR, Khopkar M, Dave KN: Acute hyperglycemia and hyperkalemia in acute myocarditis produced by scorpion venom injection in dogs. Indian Heart J 38:71, 1986

244. Rajapakse CNA, Kalim AO, Al-Nozha I, Al-Aska AK: A genetic marker for rheumatic heart disease. Br Med J 58:659, 1987

245. Rao CK, Kumar S: Role of filariasis in endomyocardial fibrosis. J Communic Dis 14:91, 1982

246. Raveendranath M, Shanmugam J, Valiathan MS, et al: Prevalence of Coxsackie group B infection in EMF. Indian Heart J 35:284, 1983 (abst)

247. Reddy DB, Chengalraju G, Parvathi G, Suvarnakumari G: Syphilitic heart disease. Autopsy study of 13 cases. Indian Heart J 26:61, 1974

248. Reef H, Issacson C: Cerebrovascular disease in Africa. Circulation 25:66, 1962

249. Rees PH, Rees MC, Fulton FM, Gichinga HN: Cardiomyopathy in Nairobi. E Afr Med J 51:863, 1974

250. Richardson J, Wodak AD, Atkinson L, et al: Relation between alcohol intake, myocardial enzyme activity and myocardial function in dilated cardiomyopathy. Br Heart J 56:165, 1986

251. Roberts WC, Ferrans VJ: Pathologic anatomy of cardiomyopathies. Hum Pathol 6:287, 1975

252. Rose AG: Evaluation of pathologic criteria for diagnosis of hypertrophic cardiomyopathy. Histopathology 8:395, 1984

253. Rothman C: Remarks on sex, age and racial distribution of Kaposi's sarcoma and on possible pathogenetic factors. Acta Union Internationale Cancer 18:322, 1962

254. Roy S, Tandon HD: Pathology of acute rheumatic fever. Ann Indian Acad Med Sci 8:99, 1972

255. Roy SB, Bhatia ML, Mathur VS, Virmani S:

Haemodynamic effects of chronic severe anaemia. Circulation 28:346, 1963

256. Sagar S, Marwah RK, Ganguly NK, Sharma BK: Immunopathology of occlusive thromboaortopathy. Indian Heart J 40:58, 1988

257. Sainani GS: Epidemic dropsy. p. 92. In Ahuja MMS (ed): Progress in Clinical Medicine in India. Arnold Heinmann, New Delhi, 1976

258. Sakhuja V, Manjunath S, Varma S, Anand IS: Idiopathic hyper-eosinophilic syndrome with restrictive cardiomyopathy. Indian Heart J 39:82, 1987

259. Samantray SK: Takayasu's arteritis. A study of 45 cases. Aust NZ J Med 8:68, 1978

260. Sanderson JE: Oedema and heart failure in the tropics. Lancet 2:1159, 1977

261. Sanderson JE, Adesanya CO, Anjorin FI, Parry EHO: Postpartum cardiac failure— Heart failure due to volume overload? Am Heart J 97:613, 1979

262. Sanderson JE, Koech D, David IHA, Ojaimbo HP: T-lymphocyte subsets in idiopathic cardiomegaly. Am J Cardiol 55:755, 1985

263. Sanderson JE, Olsen EGJ, Gate D: Peripartum heart disease. Br Heart J 56:285, 1986

264. Sanghvi LM, Misra SM, Banerjee K: Cardiac enlargement in chronic severe anaemia. Circulation 22:412, 1960

265. Sapru RP, Balakrishnan KG, Sasidharan K, et al: Clinical profile of endomyocardial fibrosis. p. 3. In Sapru RP (ed): Endomyocardial fibrosis in India. Indian Council of Medical Research, New Delhi, 1983

266. Sarvotham SG, Berry JN: Prevalence of coronary heart disease in an unknown population in N India. Circulation 37:939, 1968

267. Sasikumar M, Drurairaj M, Alurkar VM, et al: Infective endocarditis—a changing spectrum. Indian Heart J 35:282, 1983 (abst)

268. Seedat YK, Pillay N: Myocardial infarction in the African hypertensive patient. Am Heart J 95:388, 1977

269. Seedat YK, Seedat MA, Nkomo MN: The prevalence of hypertension in the urban Zulu. S Afr Med J 53:923, 1978

270. Seedat YK, Seedat MA, Reddy K: The prevalence of hypertension in Indian population of Durban. S Afr Med J 54:10, 1978

271. Seftal HC: The rarity of coronary heart disease in the South African blacks. S Afr Med J 54:99, 1978

272. Seftal HC, Metz J, Lakier JB: Cardiomyopathies in Johannesberg Bantu. I. Etiology and characteristics of beri beri heart. S Afr Med J 46:1707, 1972

273. Seftal HC, Metz J, Lakier JB: Cardiomyopathies in Johannesburg Bantu. II. Etiology of idiopathic cardiomyopathy. S Afr Med J 46:1823, 1972

274. Sepaha GL, Jain SR, Dixit VP, Chhabra MI: Aortic aneurysms. A study of 75 cases. Indian Heart J 20:116, 1968

275. Shah SL, Goyal BK, Sheth A, et al: Juvenile mitral stenosis in India. Indian Heart J 27:6, 1975

276. Shah VV: Coronary profile of Indian patients in a lower economic group. J Assoc Phys India 21:351, 1975

277. Shah VV: Prevalence and early detection of heart disease. J Assoc Phys India 25:407, 1977

278. Shaper AG, Bellhouse BJ: Localization of lesions in endomyocardial fibrosis. Br Heart J 35:962, 1973

279. Shaper AG, Coles RM: The tribal distribution of endomyocardial fibrosis. Br Heart J 27:121, 1965

280. Shaper AG, Hutt MSR, Fejfar Z (eds): Cardiovascular Diseases in the Tropics. British Medical Association, London, 1974

281. Sharma BK, Arora OP, Bansal BC, Khurana SK: Hypertension among the industrial workers and professional classes in Ludhiana. Indian Heart J 37:380, 1985

282. Shibu S, Kartha CC, Basu D, Appukuttan PS: Increase in extracellular matrix components and absence of eosinophil granule protein in heart tissue affected with endomyocardial fibrosis. Indian J Med Res 84:191, 1986

283. Silver MA, Macher AM, Reichert CM, et al: Cardiac involvement by Kaposi's sarcoma in acquired immune deficiency syndrome. Am J Cardiol 53:983, 1984

284. Sindhavananda K, Jumbala B, Sriwann C, et al: Heart disease in Thailand. p. 41. In Eliakim M, Neufield HN (eds): Cardiology. Current Topics and Progress. Academic Press, San Diego, 1970

285. Sinha N, Saran RK, Hasan M, Bhatia ML: Rheumatic fever prophylaxis in developing countries. Why are early injections needed? Indian Heart J 35:26, 1983

286. Smythe PM, Swanpoel A, Campbell JAH: The heart in kwashiorkor. Br Med J 1:67, 1962

287. Somers K, Brenton DP, Sood NK: Clinical

features of endomyocardial fibrosis of right ventricle. Br Heart J 30:309, 1968

288. Spry CJF: Eosinophils and endomyocardial fibrosis. A review of clinical and experimental studies. p. 293. In Kawai CH, Abelman WH (eds): Cardiomyopathy Update I. Pathogenesis of Myocarditis and Cardiomyopathy. University of Tokyo Press, Tokyo, 1987

289. Steiner IO, Hutt MSR: Vascular changes in idiopathic gangrene of the tropics. Trop Geogr Med 24:219, 1972

290. Steyer K, Jooste PL, Fourie JM, et al: Hypertension in the colored population of Cape Peninsula. S Afr Med J 69:165, 1988

291. Steyer K, Jooste PL, Langerhove ML, et al: Coronary risk factors in the coloured population of Cape Peninsula. S Afr Med J 67:619, 1985

292. Strasser T: Rheumatic fever and rheumatic heart disease in the 1970s. WHO Chron 32:18, 1978

293. Subramanyam G, Byotra SP, Arora S, Gupta MP: Clinical profile of rheumatic fever and rheumatic heart disease. A study of first 1500 cases. J Assoc Phys India 26:1072, 1978 (abst)

294. Subramanyam R, Kartha CC, Balakrishnan KG: Intramyocardial coronary arterial changes in rheumatic mitral valve disease. Indian Heart J 35:268, 1983 (abst)

295. Subramanyam K, Chittipuntulu G, Rama Chandra Rao S, et al: Tuberculous aneurysm of aorta. J Assoc Phys India 21:339, 1973

296. Talwalkar PG, Narula DV, Mistry GJ, Wagholikar UC: Peripartum cardiomyopathy—a clinico-pathologic study. J Assoc Phys India 26:793, 1978

297. Tandon DL, Wahi PL, Rastogi GK: Peripheral vascular disease in diabetes mellitus. Indian J Med Res 61:1187, 1973

298. Tandon HD, Kasturi J: Pulmonary vascular changes associated with isolated mitral stenosis in India. Br Heart J 37:26, 1975

299. Taskar SP, Iyyer IR, Neurkar SV, et al: Lipid profile in patients with myocardial infarction in the city of Bombay. Indian Heart J 35:169, 1983

300. Teoh PC, Tan LKK, Chia BL, et al: Nonspecific aorto-arteritis in Singapore with special reference to hypertension. Am Heart J 95:683, 1978

301. Thomas J, Josserand C, Chastel C, et al: The cardiovascular manifestation of protein calorie malnutrition. Med Trop 32:505, 1973

302. Tongia RK, Chowdhury MNH, Al-Nozha M: Infective endocarditis. Experience at the University Hospital, Riyadh. Saudi Med J 7:321, 1986

303. Touze JE, Sess D, Darracq R, et al: Silent coronary artery disease in black African diabetic patients. Trop J Med 39:144, 1987

304. Trowell H, Painter N, Burkitt D: Aspects of the epidemiology of diverticular disease and ischaemic heart disease. Am J Digest Dis 19:864, 1974

305. Tung CL, Chen WC, Liang SP, et al: A reappraisal of the changing proportions of various types of heart diseases in Shanghai and its relationship to serum cholestrol levels. Chin Med J 97:171, 1984

306. Tung CL, Cheng TO: The changing incidence of heart disease in modern China. p. 10. In Cheng TO (ed): International Textbook of Cardiology. Pergamon Press, Elmsford, NY, 1986

307. Tuomilheto J, Ram P, Eseroma R, et al: Cardiovascular disease and diabetes mellitus in Fiji Bull WHO 62:133, 1989

308. Tyagi S, Kaul UA, Gambhir DS, et al: Pulmonary artery involvement in aortoarteritis. Indian Heart J 39:46, 1987

309. Uragooda CG: Dextrocardia and situs inversus in Sri Lanka. Trop Geogr Med 29:14, 1977

310. Uthaman B, Parameshwaran A, Bakthaviziam A, et al: Tricuspid valve involvement in rheumatic heart disease. A necropsy study. Indian Heart J 30:359, 1978 (abst)

311. Valiathan MS, Kartha CC, Pandey VK, et al: A geochemical basis for endomyocardial fibrosis. Cardiovasc Res 20:679, 1986

312. Van der Geld H, Peetom P, Somers K, Kanyarezi BR: Immunological studies in endomyocardial fibrosis. Lancet 2:1210, 1966

313. Van Staden DA, Kloppers PL, Feherson JP: Ischemic heart disease in the South African black. S Afr Med J 58:271, 1980

314. Vaughan JP: A review of cardiovascular diseases in developing countries. Am J Trop Med Parasit 72:101, 1978

315. Veille JC: Peripartum cardiomyopathy—a review. Am J Obstet Gynecol 148:805, 1984

316. Vijayaraghawan G: Echocardiographic features of EMF. p. 134. In Sapru RP (ed): Endomyocardial Fibrosis in India. Indian Council of Medical Research, New Delhi. 1983

317. Vijayaraghawan G: p. 22. In Sapru RP (ed): Endomyocardial fibrosis in India. Indian

Council of Medical Research, New Delhi, 1983

318. Vijayaraghavan G, Cherian G, Krishnawamy S, Sukumar IP: Left ventricular endomyocardial fibrosis in India. Br Heart J 39:563, 1977

319. Vijayaraghavan G, Cherian G, Krishnaswamy S, et al: Rheumatic aortic stenosis in young patients presenting with combined aortic and mitral stenosis. Br Med J 39:294, 1977

320. Vijayaraghavan G, Sadanandan S: Immunological phenomena in tropical endomyocardial fibrosis. Indian Heart J 36:87, 1984

321. Wahi PL: Peripheral vascular disease in North India. Report of the Indian Council of Medical Research, New Delhi, 1979

322. Wahi PL, Ghosh PK, Wahi S, Katariya S: Valvular calcification in Indian patients. Indian Heart J 38:326, 1986

323. Wahi PL, Grover A: Rheumatic fever: A challenge. Editorial. Indian Heart J 39:1, 1987

324. Wahi PL, Kohli RS: Infective endocarditis: East and West. Indian Heart J 34:378, 1982

325. Wainwright J: Tuberculous endocarditis. Report of 2 cases. S Afr Med J 56:731, 1979

326. Walker ARP: Studies bearing on coronary heart disease in South African population. S Afr Med J 47:85, 1973

327. Walker ARP: Coronary disease in blacks in underdeveloped populations. Am Heart J 104:1410, 1984

328. Walker ARP, Walker BF: High density lipoprotein cholesterol in a population free of coronary heart disease. Br Med J 4:1336, 1978

329. Walker ARP, Walker BF, Wadvalla M, Dayal L: Blood pressure of Indian and colored children aged 10–12 years. S Afr Med J 54:315, 1978

330. Walsh JJ, Burch GE, Black WC, et al: Puerperal cardiomyopathy. In Burch GE (ed): Cardiomyopathy. Cardiovasc Clin 4:202, 1972

331. Wasir HS, Bahrani AK, Bhatia ML: Risk factor profile in patients with angiographically proven coronary artery disease. Indian Heart J 37:221, 1985

332. Wasir HS, Bhandari S, Kaushik VS, Bhatia ML: Critical evaluation of coronary risk factors in patients with myocardial infarction. Indian Heart J 37:366, 1985

333. Wharton BA, Balmer SE, Somers K, Templton AC: The myocardium in kwashiorkor. Q J Med 38:107, 1966

334. Wick ACB, Jones JJ: Diabetes mellitus in Rhodesia. A comparative study. Postgrad Med J 50:659, 1974

335. Wig KL: Some aspects of chronic obstructive lung disease. Indian J Chest Dis 15:331, 1973

336. Wilcox RG, James PD, Toghill PJ: Endomyocardial fibrosis associated with daunorubicin therapy. Br Heart J 38:860, 1976

337. Wiseman MN, Giles MS, Camm AJ: Unusual echocardiographic appearance of intracardiac thrombi in a patient with endomyocardial fibrosis. Br Heart J 57:179, 1986

338. World Health Organization: Community control of rheumatic heart disease in developing countries. WHO Chronicle 34:336, 1980

339. World Health Organization: Cardiomyopathies. WHO Technical Report Series 697, Geneva, 1984

340. World Health Organization: Approaches to prevention and early detection of cardiomyopathies. Bull WHO 64:365, 1986

341. World Health Organization and the International Society and Federation of Cardiology: Report of a task froce on definitions and classifications of cardiomyopathies. Br Heart J 44:672, 1980

342. World Health Organization Task Force on Primordial Prevention of Cardio-Vascular Disease in Developing Countries. WHO CVD, Geneva, 6 December 6, 1982

343. Yoshitoshi Y, Masuyama Y, Koide K: Nonspecific arteritis of aorta and its branches. p 318. In Eliakim M, Neufield HN (eds): Cardiology. Current Topics and Progress. Academic Press, San Diego, 1970

34

Parasitic Diseases of the Heart

B. N. Datta

The hot, humid climate of the tropics is most conducive to the biologic growth of both vectors and parasites; hence, the higher incidence of parasitic diseases in the tropics. Nevertheless, parasitic diseases still occur in temperate climates. Furthermore, with population migrations and travel by air, parasitic diseases must be considered in the differential diagnosis of some cardiologic disease in those geographic areas.

Parasitic diseases of the heart can be conveniently classified into four categories:

1. *Specific parasitic heart diseases*, in which the parasite regularly produces a specific clinicopathologic cardiac disorder overshadowing any other manifestation. Trypanosomiasis is the typical example; toxoplasmosis, trichinosis, and schistosomiasis may also be included.
2. *Significant parasitic heart diease.* Here, the cardiac involvement forms an important, but not specific or exclusive, component of an otherwise systemic parasitism. Examples are hydatid disease, cysticercosis, and amebiasis (pericardial).
3. *Incidental parasitic heart disease.* In these cases the heart is an incidental site of disseminated parasitic infestation with no specific clinicopathologic features. Any parasite, from malaria to guinea worm, may

involve the heart with or without symptoms and signs.
4. *Nonparasitic cardiac manifestation of systemic parasitic disease*, in which the heart is involved secondarily by conditions such as anemias (as in intestinal helminths), septicemia, or circulatory disturbances (filariasis, pulmonary schistosomiasis) or by immunologic or toxic disturbances (eosinophilia, immune disturbance).

The following descriptions of specific infestations are arranged according to the classical parasitic classification. The biology of parasites is not detailed here; two recent textbooks may be consulted for more information.[57,100]

PROTOZOAN PARASITES

Trypanosomiasis

Like leishmania, trypanosomes are unicellular flagellate protozoa living in the blood and tissues of humans and other animals. In humans, two forms of trypanosomial disease exist: African trypanosomiasis or African sleeping sickness caused by *Trypanosoma brucei*, and American trypanosomiasis caused by *Trypanosoma cruzi*. The parasite in the blood is 20 μm long (trypanosomal form), and in cells, in its leishmanial form, it is 4 μm × 1.5 μm. Unlike *T. cruzi*, *T. brucei* has the ability to change its antigenic structure with each cycle, a process called *variable antigenic type* (VAT).[100]

African Trypanosomiasis

African trypanosomiasis exists in two forms. One, caused by *T. brucei gambiense* is prevalent along the west coast of Africa between 20° N and 20° S of the equator and in the vicinity of lakes Victoria and Tanganyika. The other form, *T. brucei rhodesiense*, is prevalent in the eastern parts of the continent—for example, in Uganda, Kenya, Tanzania, Zambia, and Zimbabwe. *T. brucei rhodesiense* has a large reservoir in African bush game. On the other hand, Zambian trypanosome does not seem to thrive in animal hosts; humans are the main reservoir. A third form of *T. brucei*—*T. brucei brucei*—is not pathogenic to humans; it affects domestic animals only.

The two pathogens are spread by the bite of the tsetse fly (*Glossina* species) through its salivary ducts (cyclic transmission). After introduction into the skin, the parasites localize for a time in regional lymph nodes and the central nervous system (CNS). The latter possibly serves as a reservoir.[64] The patient develops fever, lymphadenitis, skin eruptions, and both physical and mental lethargy. Although cardiac lesions develop, the major morbidity, "sleeping sickness," is caused by CNS lesions.

The disease manifests a two-stage process.[75] Stage 1 is infection without CNS involvement. Stage 2 is the dominant CNS disease. In stage 1, there is pericarditis, and valves, conduction tissue, and autonomic nerves are involved. The heart may be normal in size or enlarged and dilated. There is often a pericardial effusion and a mild lymphocytic infiltration in the pericardium.[75] A focal or diffuse pancarditis is seen, including myocytolysis, necrosis, and inflammatory cell infiltration. The lesions are denser in epicardial and subepicardial zones and may leave small myocardial scars. Cardiac aneurysms may form, as in Chagas' disease. The clinical picture mimics that of a dilated heart cardiomyopathy. A mouse model of African trypanosomiasis shows pancarditis and valvulitis.[76]

American Trypanosomiasis

Also known as South American trypanosomiasis or Chagas' disease/syndrome, the American form of trypanosomiasis is a major public health and social problem in Latin America. Twenty-four million people are believed to be infected with *T. cruzi*, and 65 million live in the endemic area, which spans both Americas from Texas to Argentina and includes the Caribbean.[101] The population prevalence rates, based on complement fixation seropositivity, are 40 to 50 percent in Venezuela, and up to 70 percent in Brazil.[34] Autopsy records in Brazil show a 6-percent incidence, and in Trujillo a 1.16 percent incidence.[50] In another center in Brazil, Ribeirão Prêto, 20 percent of autopsies reveal evidence of Chagas' disease with 64.8 percent of the cases showing cardiac lesions alone, 2.2 percent lesions of hollow viscera alone, and 32.8 percent, both.[7] In Curaço, more than 76 percent of cardiomyopathies diagnosed at autopsy are due to Chagas' disease.[91] Isolated cases have been reported from California[70] and Guyana.[79]

T. cruzi is a hemoflagellate that alternates its life between an intermediate host, the winged reduviid bug, and a vertebrate host, humans or other animals, the latter both wild and domestic. It is these animal hosts, in the tropical forests, that form a vast reserve for the parasite. The bug defecates while biting, causing itching, and the trypanosomes are rubbed in or enter the skin through wounds and abrasions (stercoral spread)[77,102] or through intact membranes. The conjunctiva is a common portal of infection, with conjunctivitis and periorbital edema forming the well known *Romana sign*. The natural history of the disease extends over years. It starts as an acute illness (1 to 3 months), is followed by a latent phase, and then in symptomatic or asymptomatic form emerges after 10 to 20 years as chronic Chagas' disease.[77] Carditis and cardiac lesions dominate the clinical picture in both acute and chronic stages, especially in the latter.

Acute Phase

During the acute phase the parasite multiplies extensively by binary fission. Distended host cells (muscle, myocardium), form "pseudocysts." The parasite's intracellular habitat provides protection from host immune defenses and drugs and ensures a life-long infection. As these pseudocysts rupture, parasitemia develops. There is generalized lymphadenopathy, hepatosplenomegaly, and an acute myocarditis. About 10 percent of patients die due to either acute meningoen-

cephalitis or acute myocarditis.[77] At this stage the heart is either normal in size or slightly enlarged, flabby, and has a mottled appearance. Histologically, there are extensive areas of myocardial necrosis loaded with released parasites as well as pseudocysts (Fig. 34–1A). Inflammatory destruction of cardiac ganglia and nerve fibers may be demonstrated.

The acute phase represents a stage of anergy, and patients pass into a latent period for the next 10 to 20 years. Even if asymptomatic (as many are) electrocardiographic (ECG) recordings show abnormalities.[85] At autopsy, a granulomatous myocarditis has been detected in 38 percent of cases, together with necrosis of small vessels. Gangliolysis and neurolysis also may be seen, although cardiac conduction tissue is generally not affected.[85] Frequently, the acute phase passes unnoticed and the patient later presents a full-blown picture of Chagas' disease. The cardiologic diagnosis in such cases can be a problem in nonendemic areas, especially due to migration of carriers to other countries during the asymptomatic latent period. Pointed in-

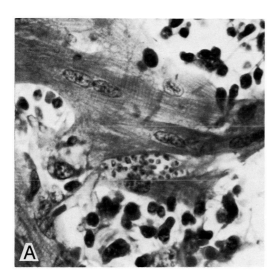 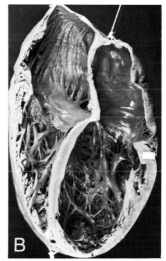

Fig. 34–1. Myocarditis in acute Chagas' disease. (**A**) Parasites forming pseudocysts in myocardial fiber are seen in the center of the photograph, with associated inflammatory reaction. (H&E × 160.) (Specimen courtesy of H. Miziara, M.D., Brazil.) (**B**) Chagasic cardiomyopathy showing marked cardiac dilation with wall thinning. The latter is especially marked at the apex of the left ventricle where a small aneurysm has a thrombus in its lumen. (Specimen courtesy of J. Keystone, M.D., Toronto.)

vestigations are essential (Holter ECG monitoring, for example) with a high degree of suspicion. The case of an Ecuadorian immigrant in New York is illustrative. The individual was treated for ischemic heart disease for some time before investigation revealed the diagnosis of chronic Chagas' cardiomyopathy.[27]

Chronic Phase

The dominant feature during the chronic phase is congestive cardiac failure due to *Chagasic cardiomyopathy*.[101,102] The ECG may reveal right bundle branch block, complete or incomplete left anterior hemiblock, nodal dysfunction, or QRS abnormalities. Sick sinus syndrome, requiring pacemaker implantation, has been detected in 6 percent of cases.[66] Two types of electrophysiologic dysfunction can be recognized: a myogenic form showing dominant myocardial involvement and a neurogenic form due to conduction tissue involvement.[73] The basic biventricular asynergy, dysfunction, and aneurysms are clearly defined by echocardiography and/or angiocardiography.[3] These investigations have been used in Brazil to distinguish Chagas' disease from dilated cardiomyopathy (DCM).[92] Furthermore, during this latent period, 60 percent of patients show histologic abnormalities in the myocardium on endomyocardial biopsy.[54] The condition develops in 90 percent of infected patients and is responsible for the death of up to 70 percent.[39,77]

There is some geographic variation in the "tissue tropism" of *T. cruzi*. Whereas cardiac disease is the principle lesion in Argentina and Venezuela, the gastrointestinal tract is the site favored by the parasite in Brazil. The latter leads to the characteristic "megas" of Chagas' disease, namely, megaesophagus, megastomach, and megacolon.[85] The heart is enlarged and dilated, weighing 500 to 600 g. The gross morphology is best seen in coronal base to apex section (Fig. 34–1**B**). Chambers are dilated, especially on the right side of the heart and are thin-walled. A characteristic feature is the formation of a thin-walled aneurysm, usually at the left ventricular apex. Its lumen is frequently packed with thrombus. The aneurysm is apical in 47 percent of cases;

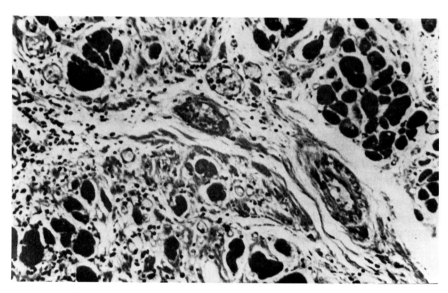

Fig. 34–2. Chronic chagasic cardiopathy. The myocardium shows degenerative changes, hypertrophy, and atrophy, with interstitial inflammation and fibrosis. Stain and magnification not available. (Courtesy of Paulo Becker, M.D., Ribeirão Prêto, Brazil. From Amorim,[7] with permission.)

in another 27 percent, it is located in the posterior wall, deep to the posterior leaflet of the mitral valve.[77] This feature is helpful in distinguishing Chagas' cardiomyopathy from DCM. Cardiac valves are normal, and the coronary arteries are considerably dilated. Microscopically, there is myocardial atrophy, patchy scars, and interstitial fibrosis. In the aneurysm, the endocardium nearly approximates the pericardium.

In contrast to the acute phase, parasites are difficult to find, although an occasional granuloma may still be seen. Focal arteritis has been observed. Destruction of cardiac ganglia, nerves, and the conduction nodes and fibers is noted[10] (Figs. 34–2 through 34–4). Preferential involvement of the right bundle and anterior fascicular branches of the left bundle occurs. The cardiac lesions have been likened to the piecemeal necrosis of (viral) hepatitis.[85]

A congenital form of Chagas' disease (acute) also exists, due to transplacental migration of the trypanosomes. Generally, this happens in asymptomatic mothers with a placenta that is either deficient or impaired. Acute myocarditis as well as other systemic lesions are present and the infant dies by the fourth day.[62]

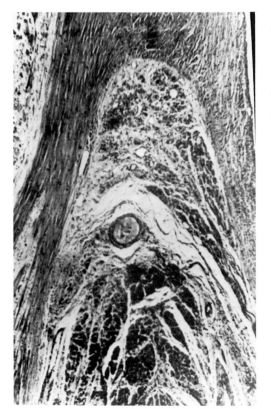

Fig. 34–3. Chronic chagasic cardiopathy showing fibrosis, atrophy, and fragmentation of conduction tissue fibers including the inferior one-third of the atrioventricular (AV) node and right half of the main bundle. Stain and magnification not available. (Courtesy of J. A. Mello de Oliveira, M.D., Ribeirão Prêto, Brazil. From Amorim,[7] with permission.)

Pathogenesis of Chagas' Disease

Infection and Disease. It has been aptly stated that "in South American trypanosomiasis and Chagas' disease, the distinction between infection and disease extends beyond that of intellectual convenience. The degree of infection is a good indication of the severity of the disease but once a state of chronic infection has been gained, anecdotal evidence suggests there may be a negative correlation between the level of persistent infection and eventual disease outcome."[38]

Many authors have emphasized the observed destruction of ganglia, nerve fibers, and conduction tracts of the heart and nerves in the cardiac valves.[45] In Koberle's[38] opinion, the result is a "denervated" heart, incapable of reacting to normal demands so that, with time, it dilates and fails.

This denervation, based on destruction of ganglia, has been confirmed in humans and experimental animals over the years,[7,53,80] and is used to explain the alimentary tract "megas" of Chagas' disease. In the rat experimental model, gangliolysis is accompanied by reduced cardiac norepinephrine levels, which recover subsequently. Recovery is impeded in the protein-deficient rat.[53] This neurogenic theory, however, is not satisfactory. The lesion is inconsistent both in its existence and in quantitation in humans, the dog,[7,90] and the "Peru strain" of rhesus monkey.[60]

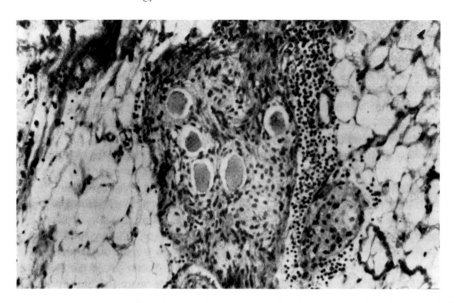

Fig. 34–4. Chronic chagasic cardiopathy. Cardiac neuroganglia show neuronal depletion and chronic inflammation. Stain and magnification not available. (From Amorin,[7] with permission.)

Similar neuroganglion atrophy occurs even in rheumatic and hypertensive hearts without Chagas' type dilation.[52] Ganglion reduction has recently been found in DCM also[8] (see Ch. 33).

Finally, the mechanism of ganglion destruction is not clear; it does not seem to be direct parasitic destruction. Alternative pathogenetic mechanisms such as toxic, enzymatic, and immune lysis have been suggested as the cause of the perpetual cardiac derangement.[7,77,85,92] The autoimmune hypothesis suggests that an immune reactivity to *T. cruzi* is initiated during the acute phase, matures during the latent phase, and causes progressive cardiac damage.[85,92] This reaction is also expressed in circulating antibodies used for serologic tests, including agglutination, complement fixation, enzyme-linked immunosorbent assay (ELISA), biotin H3-Avidin, as well as *T. cruzi* specific monoclonal antibodies.[17,28,49,94,101] Endomycardial biopsy has provided other, more direct evidence. The endocardial-vascular-interstitial (EVI) antibody, although detected in 93 percent of patients and in 96 percent of asymptomatic cases, has been considered nonspecific.[98,102] In mice, the progressive loss of cardiac ganglia precedes development of the anti *T. cruzi* immune response.[80] This suggests that the immune injury is a result of cardiac damage. Use of BALB/C mice in another set of experiments,[2] on the other hand, supports a direct role of autoimmune injury, elicited by cross-reacting sarcoplasmic reticulum-adenosine triphosphate (SRA) antigens shared by striated muscle and *T. cruzi*. Thus, there is considerable debate on the pathogenesis of chronic chagasic cardiopathy. A detailed review on the subject may be consulted elsewhere.[38]

Kala-azar: Leishmaniasis

Three varieties of Leishmaniasis affect humans: the cutaneous form (*Leishmania tropica*), the generalized form or Kala-azar or visceral leishmaniasis (*L. donovani*), and the mucocutaneous form or espundia (*L. brasi-*

liensis). The causative organisms, although named differently, cannot be distinguished from each other morphologically. The insect vector responsible for the spread of the disease is also the same (sandfly, *Phlebotomus* species), although the animal reservoir differs. Involvement of the heart is extremely rare and is described only in the visceral form of Kala-azar, a myocarditis, with necrotic foci containing Leishman-Donovan (L-D) bodies in phagocytic cells. The heart, however, may show secondary atrophy due to the severe anemia and debilitation associated with the disease and may also show L-D bodies within macrophages incidentally.

Malaria

Among the sporozoa, members of the genus *Plasmodium* are the most widespread human parasites. Four species infect human beings: *P. falciparum*, which causes malignant tertian malaria; *P. vivax*, which causes benign tertian malaria; *P. malariae*, which causes quartan malaria; and *P. ovale*, the cause of ovale tertian malaria. Malaria, which, together with viral hepatitis, has played a decisive though latent part in several wars, including both world wars, was under fair control but has re-emerged as a major health problem during the last ten years, especially in India.

Malaria does not cause a specific cardiac lesion. The heart may show changes secondary to toxemia or hyperthermia. In fatal cases, especially of falciparum malaria, parasitized red cells suffuse myocardial capillaries (Fig. 34–5). This is believed to produce focal ischemic change.[58] Myofibers show malarial pigment (hemozoin) and may demonstrate such nonspecific changes as hyalinization with loss of striations, vacuolization, and fatty acid change.[55] In chronic malaria, the severe anemia adds to nonspecific cardiac incapacitation. The possible role of malaria in initiating an abnormal immune state in the African-Asian population relevant to dilated cardiomyopathy and endomyocardial fibrosis has already been mentioned (Ch. 33).

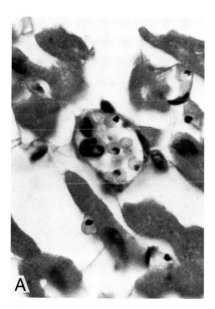
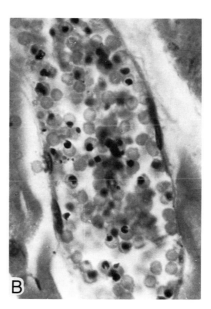

Fig. 34–5. (**A,B**) Heart in malaria. Sections showing capillaries stuffed with red cells, many of which contain malarial parasites. (H&E, × 660.)

Toxoplasmosis

The sporozoon protozoa important to humans and animals is *Toxoplasma gondii*. This organism is a crescentic or pyriform nucleated structure, 4- to 6-μm long and 2- to 3-μm wide, with a conoid tip on one end to penetrate the host. Cats harbor the oocysts and pass them in their feces. Infected soil and animals such as flies, snails, cockroaches, and earthworms help pass the infection to cattle and other domestic animals, which then act as intermediate hosts. Ingestion of uncooked or partially cooked meat, unpasteurized milk, and close contact with pets, including kissing, passes the infection to humans. Infection has also been transmitted by renal transplants and during the handling of infected material by laboratory staff.[48]

The parasite has a worldwide distribution. Surveys based on allergic skin tests place the prevalence rates to 100 percent in Tahiti, 30 percent in South Africa, up to 21 percent in India,[30,74] and 15 to 42 percent in England.[81] Infection occurs at any age, including in utero, and can occur by transplacental congenital infection. Immune suppressed patients and those with organ transplants or AIDS are susceptible. In the tissues, the parasite multiplies in macrophages, forming a "pseudocyst" packed with the protozoa (Fig. 34–6), although a true cyst may be detected.

In the adult, infection may occur in one of three forms: acute, glandular, or localized. The acute form[48] produces a miliary infection with a severe course. The glandular form involves lymph nodes and follows a course similar to that of infectious mononucleosis. The localized form affects one or two organs only. There may be a myocarditis, hepatitis, glomerulonephritis, meningoencephalitis, or chorioretinitis. Infection in the neonate is usually severe, and death occurs as a result of meningoencephalitis or myocarditis.[35,37]

In utero infection can be a cause of abortion (up to 6 percent of all abortions in Costa

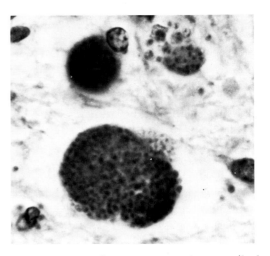

Fig. 34–6. Toxoplasmosis, a pseudocyst packed with sporozoa. The section is from the brain of a case of generalized toxoplasmosis. (H&E, × 1,100.)

Rica).[74] Myocarditis occurs in infants in 50 percent of cases but is uncommon or rare in adults. In the adult, trophozoites mature into the encysted state and may remain dormant in the tissues throughout life. One or more granulomas or cysts without inflammatory reaction may be detected incidentally in an otherwise normal heart. Clinically, myocarditis appears usually in chronic infection when an appreciable degree of myocardial fibrosis has occurred in the heart. Leak et al. observed 18 patients with a variety of cardiac diseases with no apparent cause other than a serologic one and other evidences of toxoplasmosis. Clinical manifestations of the disease include rhythm disturbances, chest pain, pericarditis, and cardiac failure. The authors recommended certain diagnostic aids in suspected cases: detection of IgM immunofluorescent antibodies in early cases, cell wall antibodies in intermediate states, and antibodies to soluble internal antigens in late states. *T. gondii* has been implicated as a possible cause of endomyocardial fibrosis.[69]

Sarcocystis

Sarcocystis, another genus of the sporozoa group allied to toxoplasmosis, is found in many mammals. *Sarcocystis lindemanni* is infective to humans under the name of sarcosporidosis. This fusiform, minute protozoan exists as round or crescentic cysts (Miescher's tubes), within myocardial fibers. Each cyst contains hundreds of trophozoites. Three cases showing cardiac sarcocystis were referred to by Lui and Roberts[51] in addition to an earlier report.[31] Faust et al.[24] cite positive identification of a parasite in a heart forwarded by Gadgil from Bombay.[24] The parasite secretes a toxic by-product, sarcocystin, which dissolves muscle fibers. Infection in humans is usually silent and of no clinical significance, although myocardial scars may result from destroyed areas.[41,42]

Amebiasis

The ameba is a protozoan of worldwide distribution that affects the heart by producing a specific suppurative pericarditis. *Entameba histolytica*, from its habitat in the colon, spreads to produce an amebic liver abscess and then crosses the diaphragm into the pericardium. The event, however, is rare (0.2 to 2.8 percent of liver abscesses)[5] and occurs usually in cases of left lobe abscess; which is less common than right lobe abscess. Two types of pericardial effusion are known: definitive amebic suppurative pericarditis, and reactive or sympathetic serous or serosanguinous effusion. Until 1976, 132 cases of amebic pericarditis had been reported. Of these, 109 were suppurative and 23 were nonsuppurative.[46] *E. histolytica* was found in the pericardial plus in only 9 instances. Twenty-five cases were recorded in Natal during 3 years.[39] In 12, the aspirate was typical "anchovy sauce" pus, and, in 3, it was a serous "reactive" or presuppurative effusion, with an incidence of 2 percent of amebic liver abscesses. Cases secondary to right lobe abscess and lung abscess have rarely been recorded. In the department of pathology at Chandigarh, among 80 cases of amebic liver abscess examined at autopsy, pericardial invasion was seen twice. Reports of 6 cases from Bombay,[40] 2 from South India,[93] and 4 from Sri Lanka[29] are available up to 1976. A very interesting case was reported from Vietnam[96] of a young man who developed massive hematogenous spread of amebiasis from a liver abscess that caused amebic valvular endocarditis. At autopsy, apart from pericarditis, the tricuspid valve and right ventricular mural endocardium showed nodular vegetations. Trophozoites of *E. histolytica* were found in them.

Balantidiasis

The ciliated protozoan *Balantidium coli* is a large, single-cell parasite whose normal habitat is the intestine of animals and humans. Like the ameba, it exists in a trophozoite or cyst form and is similarly responsible for dysentery in endemic, sporadic, or epidemic form. Unlike *E. histolytica*, *B. coli* rarely invades the intestine. I am aware of only one published case of myocarditis caused by this parasite.[87] Foci of myocardial necrosis with foreign body giant cell reaction were noted, and the parasite was seen in arterioles and the myocardium.

HELMINTHIC PARASITES

Tapeworms

Cestode or tapeworm infestation in humans produces two sets of clinical features: (1) those due to the adult form of the parasite, which include toxic reactions, allergic reactions, physical obstruction of gut, etc.; and (2) those due to tissue invasion by larvae, which are far more serious. Some tapeworms (e.g., *Taenia solium, T. saginata, Diphylobothrium latum,* and *Hymenolepis nana*) depend on humans for their existence, whereas for others (e.g., *Echinococcus granulosus*) humans are incidental hosts.

Cysticercosis

The tapeworm of genus *T. solium* lays eggs in the pig or human small intestine. The eggs hatch and pass into the circulation to migrate all over the body as cysticerci. No tissue or organ in the body is spared, and the brain is particularly a favored site. Infection is passed to humans and animals by consumption of infected flesh or by ingestion of food contaminated by human or pig feces. Cysticercosis is a worldwide problem and is one of considerable magnitude in Latin America and the Indian subcontinent. It is uncommon, however, in Muslim, mid-Asian countries. In Guatemala[1] 4 instances were found among 118 cases of cysticercosis over 10 years. A report of 6 cases seen at autopsy and accounting for 46.1 percent of generalized cysticerosis comes from western India.[23] One case actually caused fatal occlusion of a coronary artery by external pressure. The Medical Re-

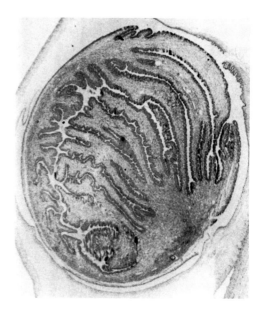

Fig. 34–8. Cysticercosis heart. Higher-power photograph of the larva in Figure 34–7. (H&E, × 60.)

search Council in Britain collected nine cases of cardiac cysticercosis.[22] A cardiac infestation may be an unsuspected finding at autopsy[86] (Figs. 34–7 and 34–8).

Echinococcus Granulosus: Hydatid Disease

Hydatid disease of humans and animals is a parasitic problem world-wide but even more so in tropical areas and in sheep- and cattle-breeding countries. The adult *T. echinococcus* is a small (3- to 6-mm) worm that lives in the dog intestine. The eggs, passed in feces, are ingested by other animals as well as by humans. The oncospheres pass through the intestinal wall and lodge in capillaries of various organs. The heart is involved in 0.5 to 2 percent of human infestations. An extensive, collective review by Dighiero et al.[21] of 300 cases of cardiac hydatid disease is most informative. The cardiac cyst is always primary and the hexacanth embryo passes from the liver (and rarely via the subclavian vein from the thoracic duct lymph) into the right heart,

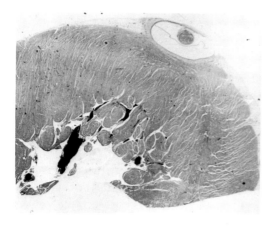

Fig. 34–7. Cysticercosis heart. A larval cyst is embedded in the epicardium, an incidental finding at autopsy. (H&E, × 4.)

escaping the pulmonary filter and entering the coronary circulation. Because of the greater vascularity of the left ventricle, the majority of larvae lodge in the wall of this chamber.[36] One survey found 43 to 77 percent of cysts in the left ventricle and 7 to 20 percent[36] in the septum. Cardiac hydatid cysts do not enlarge much and they rupture early due to the kinetic action of the heart. A cyst within the heart may present in at least five different ways.[72]

1. As a dead cyst with marked fibrosis and calcification around it (this is usually clinically silent)
2. As a living, intact cyst
3. As cyst rupturing into the pericardium
4. As pediculated cyst projecting into a heart cavity
5. As a cyst rupturing into a chamber

The clinical presentation depends on the actual location of the cyst. It may remain entirely in the heart wall, cause valvular obstruction, or lead to pericardial involvement, either as acute pericarditis or as a secondary pericardial cyst.[71]

A ruptured cyst produces at least two manifestations: (1) an immediate and at times paroxysmal hypersensitivity state due to leakage

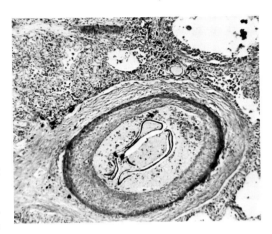

Fig. 34–10. Hydatid cyst embolism including fragments of daughter cysts and hydatid sand in a pulmonary artery. (Same case as in Fig. 34–9.) (H&E, × 160.)

of protein-rich hydatid fluid into the circulation or (2) metastatic hydatid disease in either pulmonary or systemic circulation. Rupture into the right ventricle is more common (88 percent of cases)[72] because of its thinner wall. In another review,[83] up to 27 percent of cysts were incidental findings at autopsy; 16 percent in cases of sudden death, presumably owing to cardiac arrhythmia induced by the location of the cyst. In another 25 percent the rupture was the primary cause of death. Among a total of 269 cases of hydatid cysts up to 1963,[20] 104 had ruptured. Ninety-four were located in the left ventricle, of which 35 (37 percent) had ruptured, 34 were in the right ventricle, of which 30 (80 percent) had ruptured. Twenty-four of the latter 30 colonized the lung and are included among a total of 43 cases of pulmonary hydatid embolization reported up to 1976.[67] The specimen illustrated in Figures 34–9 and 34–10 came from a case of sudden death due to embolization of the pulmonary artery from a ruptured hydatid cyst in the right ventricle. In recent years,[56] echocardiography has helped the clinical diagnosis of cardiac hydatid disease. Successful surgical removal of cardiac cysts has been achieved.[36,68,83] Involvement of the heart by *E. multilocularis* (alveolar hydatid

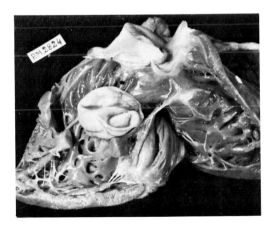

Fig. 34–9. Hydatid cyst of the heart. The right ventricle is opened to show the cyst located in the crista supraventricularis.

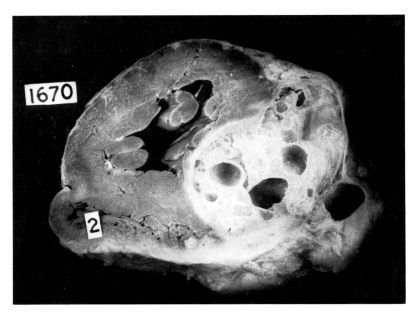

Fig. 34–11. Echinococcus multilocularis. An incidental finding in a man dying in an automobile accident. The entire heart was riddled with parasitic cysts. (Photograph courtesy of Professor Inderjit, Chandigarh.)

disease) was encountered in an unrelated accidental death at autopsy by Indarjit at Chandigarh (Fig. 34–11).

Flatworms

Schistosomiasis

Trematodes are flatworms that pass through a mollusk habitation at one stage of their natural history. *Schistosoma* or blood flukes that pose a health threat to humans include S. *haematobium* (*Bilharzia*), S. *mansoni*, and S. *japonicum*. S. *haematobium* is endemic all over Africa; the Nile Valley has been its traditional home even in the days of the pharaohs. S. *mansoni* is actively present in South America, and S. *japonicum* in the Far East, including China. A pocket of S. *haematobium* infestation is known in western India near Bombay,[89] as well as in central India.

Adult worms normally live in the pelvic venous plexuses and, rarely, in portal vein radicals, where the eggs are laid. These escape from the blood vessels and through the bladder or rectal mucosa and pass into urine or feces. On contact with water the eggs hatch into miracidia, infect an appropriate snail species, mature into fork-tailed cercariae, and escape into the water. They penetrate human skin on contact and change to young worms (schistomules), enter capillaries, and are transported to the lungs, from which they pass to the left heart, the systemic circulation, the mesenteric artery, and the portal circulation. After growth in the liver, larvae swim to the rectal veins and the pelvic and vesicle plexuses. By this time they are mature and restart the life cycle.

The effects of *Schistosoma* in the human body are due mainly to the eggs, apart from an occasional hypersensitivity reaction to the presence of adult worms or their products in the bloodstream.[99] Involvement of the heart occurs rarely. It is either by direct infiltration by the adult worm or, more commonly, as a reaction to extensive pulmonary schistosomiasis that leads to pulmonary hypertension. This usually follows establishment of portocaval shunting and collateral circulation[19] and therefore, is more frequent in the presence of cirrhosis of the liver. Bertrand et al.[13] believe that direct involvement of the heart has rarely been proved and that cardiac deficiency might in fact be due to anemia and the specific therapy given to patients. Van der Horst[97] records a case of pericarditis caused by *S. haematobium* and refers to earlier publications describing adult worms in the myocardium and coronary artery. The eggs may be arrested in the myocardium and produce a granulomatous reaction. As in liver or bladder, this focus becomes fibrotic.

The frequency of corpulmonale has varied from place to place. Infection with *S. haematobium* rarely causes pulmonary hypertension, despite the high concentration of its ova in the lungs.[9] Pulmonary hypertension is most frequent with *S. mansoni.*[82] Bertrand et al.[13] estimate that 21.6 percent of cases develop pulmonary hypertension. Variable figures (2.1 to 13 percent) have been reported from Brazil also.[19] The pulmonary lesions may be in the form of localized necrotizing arteriolitis and obliterative endarteritis due to the impaction of the ova of *S. haematobium* or the migrating larvae of *S. mansoni.*[15] In addition to arteritis, there is a widespread thrombosis. Organization of the thrombi produces the usual angiomatoid and plexiform lesions and severe pulmonary hypertension.[82] Associated with the ova or without their physical presence, an obliterative arteritis may occur as a result of hypersensitivity. A detailed account of the pathology of schistosomiasis based on 400 autopsies in Egypt is presented in a series of articles by Cheever et al.[18]

Heterophydiasis

Besides schistosomiasis, cardiac involvement by some other trematodes of the family Heterophyidae or flukes has been known. These parasites are endemic in Africa (Egypt), the Far East, and India. Infection is possibly acquired by eating raw fish.

Heterophyes heterophyes lays eggs in the intestine, from which they pass into lymphatics and veins. The eggs become trapped between myocardial fibers, leading to capillary congestion and rupture with hemorrhages. The heart is enlarged and flabby and the clinical presentation of the patient and the gross appearance of the heart are similar to those found in beriberi.[6] Kean and Breslau[41] estimate that more than 14 percent of fatal cardiac cases in the Philippines are due to heterophyid myocarditis. Another member of the same family that causes similar myocarditis is Yokogawa's fluke or *Metagonimus yogogawai*, found in the Sino-Japanese areas of the USSR. Humans and other animals are infected from eating uncooked freshwater trout. Cardiac lesions have also been recorded in infection by *Haplorchis yogogawai*, *H. pumilio*, *H. taichui*, and *Diorchitrema pseudocirratum.*[6] From Canada, Fernandes et al.[25] reported a fatal case of systemic infestation with mesocerceria of *Alaria americanus*, presumably obtained by the patient eating inadequately cooked frog's legs. In their passage through organs, including the heart, the parasites left necrotic tracks while parasites, and granulomata devoid of parasites, were obvious in some tissues. A hypersensitivity vasculitis and bleeding diathesis due to disseminated intravascular coagulation and a circulatory anticoagulant killed the man 8 days after onset of his illness.

Roundworms

Filariasis

Parasites of the plasmid nematode family frequently invade humans. Among the most important are filarial worms, including *Wuchereria bancrofti* (Bancroft's filaria), *Loaloa*, *Brugia malayi* (Malaysian filaria), and *Onchocerca volvulus* (convoluted filaria). Filaria are known more for causing elephantiasis of limbs and scrotum, and rarely produce cardiac manifestations. Most of the northern and central regions of Africa, coastal regions of India, and southeast Asian countries are the habitat of this mosquito-borne scourge.

Bancroft's larvae have been found in 6 hearts.[63] Although massive lymphedema of lower limbs and, at times, ascites and pleural effusion, result from lymphatic blockage by the microfilariae, curiously, the pericardial space is rarely involved. Only 4 cases of filarial pericardial effusion have been reported in India.[84] The often mentioned relationship of filaria to endomyocardial fibrosis in Africa and also in Kerala is based more on the geographic concurrence of the two conditions than on sound etiologic grounds. The fact that filariasis is associated with eosinophilia, which in turn is a possible cause of endocarditis and its thickening, has been advocated as evidence for associating the two diseases (see the discussion of endomyocardial fibrosis in Ch. 33).

Two other plasmid nematodes infect the heart. *Dirofilaria immitis* or the dog heartworm is a natural parasite of dogs the world over. On rare occasions it infects the heart and lungs of humans, as well, but without much clinical disease.[33]

Dracunculus medinensis or the guinea worm is a third member of the group. This parasite is very commonly found in Egypt and India, especially in central and western India. Humans are the definitive host, and adult worms live in the soft tissues. The male guinea worm is short, whereas the female is about 100 cm in length. The gravid female migrates to a subcutaneous location, usually the lower limb, and protrudes its gravid uterus through a blister on the skin. The larvae are then passed out into water, usually ponds and step wells. The rhabditoid larvae quickly invade the intermediate host, the cyclops. Humans are infected by drinking contaminated water; in about a 1 year, the larvae grow into adults in tissues. Kinare et al. of Bombay detected a 53.5-cm dead gravid female in a pericardial abscess in a 35-year-old man.[44] Another similar instance was recorded in a patient with chronic constrictive pericarditis.[12]

Ascariasis

The roundworm *Ascaris lumbricoides* is the most common human intestinal helminth in the world with prevalence rates of up to 90 percent in certain Asian countries.[88] The infection is acquired by swallowing eggs, which germinate in the duodenum and ileum and enter lymphatics and capillaries. After passage through pulmonary capillaries and alveoli, they enter the air passages and reach the small intestine, where they mature to adults. The entire cycle takes 25 to 30 days and some larvae may pass into the systemic circulation from the lungs. The heart is rarely invaded. Case reports record the occurrence of larvae in the hearts of children, with an active, eosinophil-dominated myocarditis.[4] Adult worms have been reported in the right ventricular cavity.[14,78]

Strongyloidiasis

Strongyloides stercoralis or the threadworm is a parasite of the tropics and other warm climates, including the Pacific Islands and parts of North America. It usually parallels hookworm in its geographic distribution, but unlike hookworm, strongyloides has not only an animal parasitic form larva but also a free-living, soil form (filariform) larva. Fecal-contaminated soil infects humans through the intact skin. The maturation of the larvae again involves migration through lungs, bronchi, and trachea. Arrest of the larvae, while wandering in the cardiac vasculature, is a rare event. Kyle et al.[47] described finding filariform larvae in the myocardium with a mild mononuclear reaction around them. The patient had nonspecific ECG changes. Larvae have also been found in pericardial fluids.

Trichinosis

The parasite *Trichinella spiralis* belongs to the roundworm family and is known to involve skeletal and cardiac muscle during its larval stage. It is far more common in Europe, the USSR, North America, and Iceland than in the tropics. Spencer[88] believes that 50 percent of the population in endemic areas of Europe and North America might harbor the infection. In the United States, however, the incidence dropped from 16.1 percent in 1943 to 4.2 percent in 1968.[103]

Infestation is conveyed to humans by consumption of raw or undercooked flesh (sausage is a common mode) containing larval cysts. Pork is the most common source, but other animals, including bears, foxes, cats, rats, and dogs, also harbor the infestation. The minute adult worms develop in the duodenum and jejunum and deposit larvae, which gain entry into mesenteric vessels and disseminate widely. Larvae prefer to lodge in muscle poor in glycogen.[32] An inflammatory reaction develops that contributes a "cyst" wall around the larvae and is associated with blood eosinophilia. In the myocardium, however, larvae do not encyst; they either escape or are destroyed by the inflammatory reaction.[32] In addition to such foci of myocarditis, nonspecific fatty change and vacuolization are seen. During early parasitization, the myocarditis may prove fatal.[43] Diagnosis is made by muscle biopsy; at autopsy a section of diaphragm is the usual site used to establish the intensity of infestation in terms of the number of cysts/g of muscle.

Cases of trichinosis with eosinophilia, mural endocarditis, and thrombosis similar to Löffler's fibroplastic endocarditis have been reported.[11] A report from the Soviet Union[65] mentions that massive infection (4,400 to 22,500 larvae/g of muscle tissue) favors development of myocarditis. Toroyan[95] from the USSR reports a case of trichinella myocarditis in a 43-year-old woman who had been treated for rheumatic heart disease. The larvae were detected at autopsy.[95]

Toxocara canis

Toxocara canis, an ascarid, is a dog parasite found all over the world. It resembles *Ascaris lumbricoides* in its life cycle and shares the condition of "visceral larva migrans" in which larvae wander through the body tissues undergoing stages of maturation. During migration, the larvae incite granulomatous inflammatory reaction wherever they are caught in the tissues, including the myocardium. A peripheral eosinophilia is associated with it.[16]

Mikhael and colleagues[61] discuss a fatal case in a boy of 18 months. The visceral larva migrans had induced granulomatous lesions in many organs, including the heart, although cerebral involvement and symptoms predominated. The authors' paper includes a table showing the prevalence of *T. canis* infestations among dogs and puppies at specific locations in different countries.

Ancylostomiasis

Also known as hookworm, ancylostomiasis is not known to produce direct cardiac lesions. The severe anemia of ancylostoma infestation, however, is usually associated with cardiomegaly and nonspecific degenerative changes.

REFERENCES

1. Acha PN, Aguilar FG: Studies on cysticerosis in Central America and Panama. Am J Trop Med Hyg 13:48, 1964
2. Acosta AM, Santos-Buch CA: Autoimmune myocarditis induced by *Trypanosoma cruzi*. Circulation 71:1255, 1985
3. Acquatella H, Schiller NB, Puigbo JJ, et al: M-Mode and two dimensional echocardiography in chronic Chagas' heart disease. Circulation 62:787, 1980
4. Adelson L: Larval myocardial ascariasis. Ohio Med J 48:723, 1952
5. Adeyemo AO, Aderoumu A: Intrathoracic complication of amebic liver abscess. J R Soc Trop Med Hyg 77:17, 1984
6. Africa CM, Garcia EY, DeLeon W: Heterophydiasis with cardiac involvement. Philip J Publ Hlth 2:1, 1935
7. Amorim DS: Chagasic cardiomyopathy. p. 191. In Kawai C, Abelmann WH (eds): Pathogenesis of Myocarditis and Cardiomy-

opathy. Update I. University of Tokyo Press, Tokyo, 1987

8. Amorim DS, Olsen EGJ: Assessment of heart neurones in dilated (congestive) cardiomyopathy. Br Heart J 47:11, 1982

9. Andrade ZA, Andrade SG: Pathogenesis of schistosomal pulmonary arteritis. Am J Trop Med Hyg 19:305, 1970

10. Andrade ZA, Andrade SG, Oliviera GB, Alonso DR: Histopathology of the conducting tissue of the heart in Chagas' myocarditis. Am Heart J 95:316, 1978

11. Andy JJ, O'Connel JP, Daddario RC, Williams RC: Trichinosis causing extensive ventricular mural endocarditis with superimposed thrombosis. Am J Med 63:824, 1977

12. Balasubramaniam V, Druiraj M, Basu SN, Ahuja IM: Etiology of chronic constrictive pericarditis. Indian Heart J 26:253, 1974

13. Bertrand ED, Charles D, Burdin CD, et al: Cardiac symptomatology in schistosomiasis. Trop Cardiol 6:167, 1980

14. Boetliger C, Werne J: *Ascaris lumbricoides* found in the cavity of the human heart. JAMA 93:312, 1929

15. Briers PJ: Schistostomiasis with particular reference to pulmonary and abdominal lesions. Proc R Soc Med 67:861, 1974

16. Brill R, Churg J, Beaver PC: Allergic granulomatosis associated with visceral larva migrans. Am J Clin Pathol 23:1208, 1953

17. Camargo ME, Takeda GKF: Diagnostico de labortorio. p. 175. In Brener Z, Andrade Z (eds): *Trypanosoma cruzi* e doenca de Chagas. Guanabara, Rio de Janeiro, 1979

18. Cheever AW, Kamal IA, Elwi AM et al: *Schistostoma mansoni* and *Schistosoma hematobium* infection in Egypt. III. Extrahepatic pathology. Am J Trop Med Hyg 27:55, 1978

19. Chen MG, Mott KE: Progress in assessment of morbidity due to *Schistosoma mansoni* infection. A review of literature. Trop Dis Bull 85:R2, 1988

20. DiBello R, Menondez H: Intracardiac rupture of hydatid cysts of heart. Circulation 27:366, 1963

21. Dighiero J, Canabal EJ, Aguire CV, et al: Echinococcus disease of the heart. Circulation 17:127, 1958

22. Dixon HBF, Lipscomb FM: Cysticercosis. An analysis and follow up of 450 cases. MRC Special Rep Sci 299:41, 1961

23. Dutta SK, Banerjee AK, Pal A: Cysticercosis with involvement of the heart. Report of six cases. Indian Heart J 34:329, 1982

24. Faust EC, Russel PF, Jung RC (eds): Craig and Faust's Clinical Parasitology. 8th Ed. Lea & Febiger, Philadelphia, 1970

25. Fernandes BJ, Cooper JD, Cullen JB, et al: Systemic infection with *Alaria americanus* (Trematoda). Can Med Assoc J 115:1111, 1976

26. Ferriera A, Rossi MA: (1971) A desnervação na cardiopátia chagásica. Rev Inst Med Trop São Paulo 13:391, 1971

27. Fiet A, El-Sharif N, Korostoff S: Chagas' disease masquerading as coronary artery disease. Arch Intern Med 143:144, 1983

28. Fife EVH: Serodiagnosis of trypanosomiasis. p. 395. In Saduri S, Cohen S (eds): Immunology of Parasitic Infection. Blackwell Scientific Publications, Oxford, 1976

29. Ganeshanathan N, Maridason AD, Dharamaratne DAI: Amoebic pericarditis. Ceylon Med J 21:39, 1976

30. Gautam OP, Chabbra MB, Bhardwaj RM, et al: Current status of toxoplasmosis research in India. Haryana Agriculture University. Hissar, India, April 1979

31. Gilmore HR Jr, Kean BH, Posey FM Jr: A case of sarcosporidiosis with parasites found in human heart. Am J Trop Med 22:121, 1942

32. Goldberg E: The glycolytic pathway in *Trichinella spiralis* larvae. J Parasitol 44:363, 1958

33. Gould SE: Pathology of the Heart. Charles C Thomas, Springfield, IL, 1960

34. Guimaraes AG, de Abreu NN, Santofillio AA, et al: Haemodynamics in chronic Chagas' myocarditis and its differential diagnosis with endomyocardial fibrosis. Trop Cardiol 3:87, 1977

35. Hakkila J, Frick HM, Halonen PI: Pericarditis and myocarditis caused by toxoplasma. Report of a case and review of the literature. Am Heart J 55:758, 1985

36. Heyat J, Mokhtari H, Hajaliloo J, Shahibi JG: Surgical treatment of echinococcal cyst of the heart. J Thorac Cardiovasc Surg 61:755, 1971

37. Hocherein M quoted by Stryker WA: Parasitic disease of the heart. p. 824. In Gould SE (ed): Pathology of the Heart. 2nd Ed. Charles C Thomas, Springfield, IL, 1960

38. Hudson L, Britten V: Immune response to

South American trypanosomiasis and its relation to Chages' disease. Br Med Bull 41:175, 1985

39. Hutt MSR, Köberle F, Salfelder K: Leishmaniasis and Trypanosomiasis. p. 351. In Spencer H (ed): Tropical Pathology. Springer-Verlag, Heidelberg, 1973

40. Kapoor OP, Shah NA: Pericardial amoebiasis following amoebic liver abscess of left lobe. J Trop Med Hyg 75:7, 1972

41. Kean BH, Breslau RC: Parasites of the Human Heart. Ch. 10. Grune & Stratton, Orlando, FL, 1964

42. Kean BH, Grocott RG: Sarcosporidiosis and toxoplasmosis in man and guinea pig. Am J Pathol 21:467, 1945

43. Kershaw WE, St. Hill CA, Semple AB, Davis JBH: The distribution of larvae of *Trichinella spiralis* in cases of trichinosis at Liverpool in 1953. Ann Trop Med Parasitol 50:355, 1956

44. Kinare SG, Parulkar GB, Sen PK: Constrictive pericarditis resulting from Dracunculosis. Br Med J 1:845, 1962

45. Köberle F: Chagas' disease and Chagas' syndrome. The pathology of American trypanosomiasis. Adv Parasitol. 6:63, 1968

46. Kulpati DD, Venkatachulum CG, Saha NC: Amoebic pericarditis. J Assoc Phys India 24:119, 1976

47. Kyle LH, McKay DG, Sparling JH Jr: Strongyloidosis. Annals Intern Med 29:1014, 1984

48. Leak D, Meghji M: Toxoplasmic infection in cardiac disease. Am J Cardiol 43:841, 1979

49. Lemesre JL, Archain D, Orozoco O, et al: Specific and sensitive immunological diagnosis of Chagas' disease by competitive enzyme immunoassay using a *T. cruzi* specific monoclonal antibody. Am J Trop Med Hyg 34:86, 1986

50. León A: Morfología de la miocarditis Chagásica. Kasmera 3:299, 1977

51. Liu CT, Roberts LM: Sarcosporidiosis in a Bantu woman. Am J Clin Pathol 44:639, 1965

52. Lopez ER: Comparative study of intracardiac ganglia in rheumatic, hypertensive and Chagas' disease. Rev Med Trop São Paulo 12:365, 1970

53. Machado CRS, Moraes-Santos T, Machado ABM: Cardiac noradrenalin in relation to protein malnutrition in chronic experimental Chagas' disease in the rat. Am J Trop Med Hyg 33:835, 1984

54. Mady C, Pereira Bersetto AC, Stoff N, et al:

55. Maegraith BC: Malaria. p. 319. In Spencer H (ed): Tropical Pathology. Springer-Verlag, Heidelberg, 1973

56. Malouf J, Saksouk FA, Alam S, et al: Hydatid cyst of the heart. Diagnosis by two dimensional echocardiography and computed tomography. Am Heart J 109:605, 1985

57. Manson-Bahr PEC, Apted FIC: Manson's Tropical Diseases. 18th Ed. Ballière-Tindall, London, 1983

58. Markel WC: *Plasmodium falciparum* malaria. The coronary and myocardial lesions observed at autopsy. Arch Pathol 41:290, 1964

59. McLeod IN, Wilmot AJ, Powel SJ: Amebic pericarditis. Q J Med 35:293, 1966

60. Mikhael NZ, Montpetit VJA, Orizaga M, et al: *Toxocara canis* infestation with encephalitis Can J Neurol Sci 1:114, 1974

61. Miles MA, Marsden PD, Pelitt LE, et al: Experimental *Trypanosoma cruzi* infection in rhesus monkeys III. E.C.G. and histopathological findings. Trans R Soc Trop Med Hyg 73:528, 1979

62. Nadia N, Coura JR: American trypanosomiasis. p. 235. In Warren KS, Mahmoud AAF (eds): Tropical and Geographical Medicine. McGraw-Hill, New York, 1984

63. Nagasawa, 1927. Quoted in Gould SE: Pathology of the Heart. Charles C Thomas, Springfield, IL, 1960

64. Ormerod WE, Venkatesan S: An amastigote phase of sleeping sickness. Trans R Soc Trop Med Hyg 65:736, 1971

65. Ozeratskovskaya NN, Tumolskaya NA, Vikhert AM, et al: Pathogenesis of organic and systemic lesions in trichiniasis. R Medskaya Parazit 38:521, 1969

66. Palmero HA, Caeiro TF, Losa D: Prevalence of slow heart rates in chronic Chagas' disease. Am J Trop Med Hyg 30:1179, 1981

67. Palant A, Deutsch V, Kishon Y, et al: Pulmonary hydatid emolisation. Br Heart J 38:1086, 1976

68. Papo I, Ginsberg E, Albreht M, et al: Surgical treatment of cardiac echinococcosis. Report of nine cases. Texas Heart Inst J. 9:3, 1982

69. Pauley JW, Jones R, Green WPD: Myocardial toxoplasmosis. Lancet 2:624, 1954

70. Pearlman JD: Chagas' disease in northern

California. No longer an endemic diagnosis. Am J Med 75:1057, 1983

71. Perez-Gomez F, Duramn H, Tamames S, et al: Cardiac echinococcosis. Br Heart J 35:1326, 1973

72. Peters JM, Dexter L, Weiss S: Clinical and theoretical consideration of involvement of left side of the heart with echinococcal cysts. Am Heart J 29:143, 1945

73. Pimenta J, Miranda M, Periera CB: Electrophysiologic findings in long-term asymptomatic Chagasic individuals. Am Heart J 106:374, 1983

74. Piza G quoted by Spencer H: Other protozoal diseases gaining entry through the bowel. p. 299. In Spencer H (ed): Tropical Pathology. Springer-Verlag, Heidelberg. 1973

75. Poltera AA: Pathology of African trypanosomiasis. Br Med Bull 41:169, 1985

76. Poltera AA, Hochmann A, Lambert PH: A model for cardiopathy induced by *Trypanosoma brucei* in mice. Am J Pathol 99:325, 1980

77. Puigbo JJ, Hirschhaut E, Boccalandro I, et al: Diagnosis of Chagas' cardiomyopathy. Postgrad Med J 53:527, 1977

78. Rabinovich JJ: A rare case of metastatic ascariasis in the heart and large vessels. Soviet Med 21:117, 1957

79. Rambajan I: The first autochthonous case of Chagas' disease. With notes on possible vectors in Guyana. Trop Geog Med 36:73, 1984

80. Ribiero DR, Hudson L: Denervation and immune response in mice infected with *Trypanosoma cruzi*. Clin Exp Immunol 44:349, 1981

81. Rose CF, Bourne GL: Incidence of toxoplasmosis at a London Hospital. J Clin Pathol 22:649, 1969

82. Sadigursky M, Andrade ZA: Pulmonary changes in schistosomal cor pulmonale. Am J Trop Med Hyg 31:779, 1982

83. Saidi F: Surgery of hydatid disease. WB Saunders, London, 1976

84. Samantray SK, Pulimood BM: Pericardial effusion due to filariasis. J Assoc Phys India 23:349, 1975

85. Santos-Buch CA: American trypanosomiasis. Int Rev Exp Pathol 19:63, 1979

86. Saxena H, Samuel KC, Singh B: Cysticercosis of the heart. Indian Heart J 24:313, 1972

87. Sidorow P: Quoted in Gould SE: p. 29. Pathology of the Heart. Charles C Thomas, Springfield, IL 1960

88. Spencer H: Tropical Pathology. Springer-Verlag, Heidelberg, p. 469, 1973

89. Srivastava KK, Arora MM: *Schistosoma haematobium* infection in Raipur district of Madhya Pradesh. Indian J Med Res 57:2016, 1969

90. Suarez, JA: The intracardiac neurovegetative ganglia and the pathogenesis of Chagas' myocarditis. Gaz Med Bahia 69:73, 1969

91. Suarez JA, Puigbo JJ, Rhode N, et al: Cardiomyopathy in Venezuela. Morbid Anatomy of 210 cases. Acta Med Venez 15:320, 1968

92. Suarez JA, Puigbo JJ, Valecillos RI: Estúdio clinicopátálogical de la miocárdiopátia cronicá Chagásica y de las micocárdiopatiás de etiologia des conocida. Acta Med Venez 17:25, 1970

93. Suryanarayan K, Chittipantulu G, Venkataramana G: Amoebic pericarditis. Indian Heart J 26:241, 1974

94. Tarleton RL, Schulz CL, Grogl M, Kuhn RE: Diagnosis of Chagas' disease in humans using a Biotin 3H-Avidin radioimmunoassay. Am J Trop Med Hyg 33:34, 1984

95. Toroyan IA: Trichinella myocarditis. Arch Patol 40:66, 1978

96. Trinz P: A case of tricuspid valvular and right parietal endocarditis due to *E. histolytica* in the course of fatal systemic amebiasis. Bull Soc Pathol Exot 67:359, 1974

97. Van der Horst R: Schistosomiasis of the pericardium. Trans R Soc Trop Med Hyg 73:243, 1979

98. Vieira LMM, Vieira ARM, Albanesi Filho FM, et al. Determinacáo do auticórpo EVI na cardiopátiá Chagásica crônica. Arg Bras Cardiol 45:413, 1985

99. von Lichtenberg F: Immunologic aspects of parasitic infection. Pan Am Hlth Org WHO Sci Publ 150:107, 1967

100. Warren KS, Mahmoud AAF: Tropical and Geographic Medicine. McGraw-Hill, New York, 1984

101. World Health Organization: Recent developments in the field of Chagas' disease. Bull WHO 60:463, 1982

102. World Health Organization: Cardiomyopathies. WHO Technical Report Series 697, Geneva, 1984

103. Zimmerman WJ, Steele JH, Kagan IG: The changing status of trichiniasis in the U.S. population. Publ Hlth Rep 83:857, 1968

35

Tumors of the Heart and Pericardium

Hugh A. McAllister, Jr.

METASTATIC NEOPLASMS

Metastatic cardiac tumors are 16 to 40 times more common than primary cardiac tumors, and carcinomatous invasion is more common than sarcomatous invasion.[6,35] Nevertheless, attention should be focused on the detection of primary cardiac tumors, as resection is more likely to result in cure of the heart disease.

The heart is involved in approximately 10 percent of patients with malignant neoplasms; of these, 85 percent have tumor in the pericardium.[63] Approximately 10 percent of patients with secondary neoplasms of the heart have clinical evidence of cardiac disease; in 90 percent of these, the clinical dysfunction is the result of pericardial involvement, usually a pericardial effusion or neoplastic thickening of the pericardium or both.[63] Although pericardial effusion, usually hemorrhagic, is frequent in patients with cardiac metastases, pericardial effusion, which is usually serous, is also common in patients who have malignant neoplasms without cardiac metastases. These "nonmetastatic" serous pericardial effusions are most commonly secondary to hypoalbuminemia. Pericardial injury secondary to chemotherapy or radiation therapy, as well as infective pericarditis in an immunologically compromised host, must also be considered.[55]

Nearly every type of malignant tumor from any organ and tissue has been reported to metastasize to the heart, with the sole exception of tumors primary to the central nervous system. In absolute numbers the most common neoplasms with cardiac metastases are lung, in males, and breast, in females, followed by leukemia and lymphoma, especially reticulum cell sarcoma. Approximately 10 percent of patients with carcinoma of the lung or breast will have cardiac metastases.[63] Among specific malignant neoplasms, those with the highest percentage of metastases to the heart are melanoma (70 percent), leukemia, and lymphoma.[63]

Forms of metastatic growth in the heart somewhat depend on the mode of spread and origin of the tumor. Some malignant neoplasms, especially carcinoma of the lung, breast, and esophagus, frequently involve the heart and pericardium by direct extension from contiguous structures. However, the primary tumor is far removed from the heart in approximately 50 percent of patients with carcinoma of the lung and breast with cardiac metastasis. In this latter case, there is no evidence of direct extension of the primary tumor to involve the heart; rather frequently, however, there is evidence of retrograde lymphatic spread of the tumor. Indeed, most carcinomas appear to reach the heart by retrograde lymphatic spread; if so, multiple small nodules, many of microscopic size, are found throughout the myocardium and epicardium.

Besides direct extension from contiguous structures and lymphatic spread, carcinoma may occasionally reach the heart by direct venous extension. This is especially true for renal cell carcinoma and hepatoma, which may extend along the inferior vena cava into the right atrium. Hematogenous spread, although unusual for carcinoma, is the main route of metastasis for sarcoma, lymphoma, and leukemia, as well as melanoma involving the heart.

Carcinomatous metastases are usually grossly visible, multiple, discrete, small, firm nodules; microscopically, they resemble the

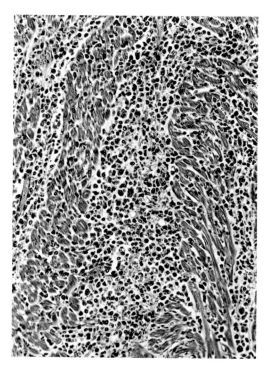

Fig. 35–2. Sarcomatous involvement of the heart is usually diffuse as is the case in this patient with malignant lymphoma infiltrating the myocardium. (H&E, × 165.)

primary tumor and metastases in other organs (Fig. 35–1). Diffuse infiltration is characteristic of sarcomatous metastases (Fig. 35–2). In either case tumor necrosis is uncommon.

PRIMARY TUMORS OF THE HEART AND PERICARDIUM

Although primary tumors of the heart and pericardium are rare, with an incidence of 0.001 to 0.28 percent in reported or collected autopsy series, many of these tumors or cysts that, in the past, would have caused the patient's demise are now amenable to surgical removal. Therefore, it has become important to enhance our knowledge of their distribution, histologic identification, and biologic behavior.

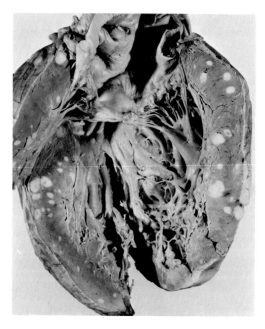

Fig. 35–1. Multiple nodules of malignant cells throughout the pericardium and myocardium are often found when the heart is involved by metastatic carcinoma. Nodules of metastatic papillary carcinoma of the thyroid were apparent microscopically in this heart. Cardiac metastases from carcinoma are usually well circumscribed both macroscopically and microscopically.

At the Armed Forces Institute of Pathology (AFIP), we reviewed 533 primary tumors and cysts of the heart and pericardium; their relative incidence is summarized in Table 35–1.[54] Considering all age groups, the most common cardiac tumor is the myxoma. Forty percent of all benign cardiac tumors are myxomas, and 25 percent of all tumors and cysts of the heart and pericardium are myxomas.[52] In adults, almost one-half of the benign tumors are cardiac myxomas[54] (Table 35–2). Approximately one-fourth of all tumors and cysts of the heart and pericardium are malignant. Of these, one-

Table 35–1.   Tumors and Cysts of the Heart and Pericardium

Type	N	%
Benign		
Myxoma	130	24.4
Lipoma	45	8.4
Papillary fibroelastoma	42	7.9
Rhabdomyoma	36	6.8
Fibroma	17	3.2
Hemangioma	15	2.8
Teratoma	14	2.6
Mesothelioma of the AV node	12	2.3
Granular cell tumor	3	—
Neurofibroma	3	—
Lymphangioma	2	—
Subtotal	319	59.8
Pericardial cyst	82	15.4
Bronchogenic cyst	7	1.3
Subtotal	89	16.7
Malignant		
Angiosarcoma	39	7.3
Rhabdomyosarcoma	26	4.9
Mesothelioma	19	3.6
Fibrosarcoma	14	2.6
Malignant lymphoma	7	1.3
Extraskeletal osteosarcoma	5	—
Neurogenic sarcoma	4	—
Malignant teratoma	4	—
Thymoma	4	—
Leiomyosarcoma	1	—
Liposarcoma	1	—
Synovial sarcoma	1	—
Subtotal	125	23.5
Total	533	100.0

(From McAllister and Fenoglio,[54] with permission.)

Table 35–2.   Tumors and Cysts of the Heart and Pericardium in Adults

Type	N	%
Benign		
Myxoma	118	26.6
Lipoma	45	10.1
Papillary fibroelastoma	42	9.5
Hemangioma	11	2.5
Mesothelioma of the AV node	9	1.1
Fibroma	5	—
Teratoma	3	—
Granular cell tumor	3	—
Neurofibroma	2	—
Lymphangioma	2	—
Rhabdomyoma	1	—
Subtotal	241	54.3
Pericardial cyst	80	18.0
Bronchogenic cyst	6	1.4
Subtotal	86	19.4
Malignant		
Angiosarcoma	39	8.8
Rhabdomyosarcoma	24	5.4
Mesothelioma	19	4.3
Fibrosarcoma	13	2.9
Malignant lymphoma	7	1.6
Extraskeletal osteosarcoma	5	1.1
Thymoma	4	—
Neurogenic sarcoma	3	—
Leiomyosarcoma	1	—
Liposarcoma	1	—
Synovial sarcoma	1	—
Subtotal	117	26.3
Total	444	100.0

(From McAllister and Fenoglio,[54] with permission.)

third are angiosarcomas, 20 percent are rhabdomyosarcomas, 15 percent are mesotheliomas, and 10 percent are fibrosarcomas.

In infants and children, the most common cardiac tumor is the rhabdomyoma[51] (Tables 35–3 and 35–4). In infants (under 1 year of age) more than 75 percent of these tumors and cysts are rhabdomyomas or teratomas. Rhabdomyomas, fibromas, and myxomas are the most common cardiac tumors in children aged 1 to 15 years, accounting for 80 percent of benign tumors and 60 percent of all tumors and cysts in this age group. Malignant tumors are rare in the pediatric age group and com-

Table 35–3.   Tumors and Cysts of the Heart and Pericardium in Infants

Type	N	%
Benign		
Rhabdomyoma	28[a]	58.3
Teratoma	9	18.8
Fibroma	6	12.5
Hemangioma	1	2.1
Mesothelioma of the AV node	1	2.1
Subtotal	45	93.7
Bronchogenic cyst	1	2.1
Subtotal	1	2.1
Malignant		
Fibrosarcoma	1	2.1
Rhabdomyosarcoma	1	2.1
Subtotal	2	4.2
Total	48	100.0

[a] Includes three stillborn infants.
(From McAllister and Fenoglio,[54] with permission.)

Table 35–4.   Tumors and Cysts of the Heart and Pericardium in Children

Type	N	%
Benign		
Rhabdomyoma	35	39.3
Fibroma	12	13.5
Myxoma	12	13.5
Teratoma	11	12.4
Hemangioma	4	4.5
Mesothelioma of the AV node	3	3.4
Neurofibroma	1	1.1
Subtotal	78	87.6
Pericardial cyst	2	2.2
Bronchogenic cyst	1	1.1
Subtotal	3	3.4
Malignant		
Malignant teratoma	4	4.5
Rhabdomyosarcoma	2	2.2
Neurogenic sarcoma	1	1.1
Fibrosarcoma	1	1.1
Subtotal	8	9.0
Total	89	100.0

(From McAllister and Fenoglio,[54] with permission.)

prise less than 10 percent of all tumors and cysts of the heart and pericardium.

Pericardial Tumors

Pericardial Cysts

Most patients with pericardial cysts are asymptomatic; the cysts are first noted either on a chest radiograph or as an incidental finding at autopsy. However, slightly more than one-third of the 82 patients with pericardial cysts in the AFIP series were symptomatic.[54] Chest pain, usually precordial or substernal, was the most frequent symptom. These patients ranged from 4 to 82 years of age, although 62 percent were in their twenties or thirties at the time the cyst was discovered. Most series in the literature indicate a nearly equal incidence in males and females (see also Ch. 22).

Sites of pericardial cysts in this series are summarized in Table 35–5. Pericardial cysts are most commonly located at the right heart border, and a small but significant number (8 percent) project into either the anterosuperior or posterior mediastinum.[19] They range in size from 1 to 15 cm or more in diameter. Commonly they appear multilobulated externally; however, although the cyst lining is frequently trabeculated, most are unilocular. They contain clear yellow fluid and occasionally communicate with the pericardial sac. The wall of the cyst is composed mainly of

Table 35–5.   Pericardial Cyst: Location in 82 Patients

Site	N	%
Right costophrenic angle	57	70
Left costophrenic angle	18	22
Anterior and superior mediastinum	4	4
Posterior mediastinum	3	4
Total	82	100

(From McAllister and Fenoglio,[54] with permission.)

collagen with scattered elastic fibers and is lined by mesothelial cells. Although these mesothelial cells usually form a single layer, foci of hyperplastic mesothelial cells are occasionally encountered. Rarely, foci of calcification and accumulations of lymphocytes and plasma cells are present.

The pericardial cyst and the pericardial diverticulum are microscopically identical, and both probably originate as persistent blind-ending parietal pericardial recesses.[56]

The pericardial cysts were successfully excised from 78 patients in this series, and the 30 symptomatic patients experienced prompt relief of all symptoms. All 78 patients were alive and well without evidence of recurrence or symptoms at least 2 years following surgery. The four remaining pericardial cysts were incidental findings at autopsy.

Some tumors of the pericardium may simulate the clinical and radiologic picture of a pericardial cyst.[77] Ultrasonic diagnosis, computed tomography (CT), and magnetic resonance imaging (MRI) may help differentiate pericardial cysts from these solid pericardial tumors.[74,76,78]

Solid tumors of the pericardium include lipoma, hemangioma, lymphangioma, leiomyoma, neurofibroma, heterotropic tissue, benign and malignant teratomas, mesothelioma, thymoma, liposarcoma, angiosarcoma, and synovial sarcoma.

Lipomas

Lipomas, exclusive of lipomatous hypertrophy of the atrial septum (see later discussion), occur throughout the heart, including the pericardium. They are less frequent than interatrial lipomas and are usually not associated with symptoms unless they are situated in the visceral or parietal pericardium and protrude into the pericardial sac. Parietal pericardial lipomas are often mistaken clinically for pericardial cysts, and visceral pericardial lipomas are frequently associated with a pericardial effusion. Relief of symptoms follows surgical excision of visceral or parietal pericardial li-

pomas. In contrast to interatrial lipomas, these tumors are encapsulated masses of adult adipose tissue. The pericardial lipomas are frequently bosselated and may be 10 cm or more in diameter. Grossly, these lipomas are identical to adult fat or lipomas elsewhere in the body. Microscopically, they consist of mature fat cells with varying amounts of fibrous tissue, myxoid matrix, and blood vessels. Rarely, fetal fat cells are present.

Leiomyoma

In the AFIP series, there are no examples of a leiomyoma arising in the heart, and a search of the literature has not yielded any report of one. There is, however, one report of a leiomyoma arising in the parietal pericardium.[10]

Heterotopic Tissue

Heterotopic islands of thymic tissue and thyroid have been described in the parietal pericardium.[78] Thyroid rests in the heart have also been reported.[65]

Mesothelioma

Mesotheliomas are malignant tumors of either visceral or parietal pericardium and are derived from mesothelial cells. They represent the third most common primary malignant neoplasm of the heart and pericardium. The clinical and pathologic findings of 19 patients dying of mesothelioma of the pericardium were available in the AFIP series. Dyspnea, usually with cough and signs of pericardial effusion, is the most common clinical finding. Frequently, pericardial effusion is recurrent, and cytologic examination of the aspirated fluid may be of diagnostic value. Many patients have symptoms of pericarditis and nonspecific ST-segment and T-wave changes on electrocardiogram (ECG). Clinical findings of pericarditis and pericardial effusion frequently are present without a history or accompanying signs of an inflammatory disease. Other patients have signs and symptoms of constrictive pericarditis, often with severe

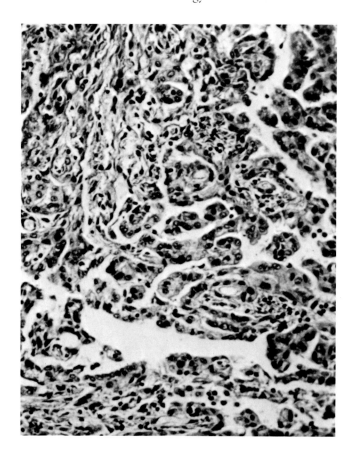

Fig. 35–3. Tubular and tubulopapillary areas are characteristic of the mesothelioma. Usually solid, papillary, and tubular areas are admixed within a single tumor. (H&E, × 180.)

right-sided congestive heart failure.[69] Occasionally, the only clinical findings are fever, malaise, and weight loss. Cardiomegaly may be present on chest radiograph.

The patients in the AFIP series ranged in age from 17 to 83 years. Although there were no children in this series, mesotheliomas have been reported in the pediatric age group. Most series indicate a male-to-female ratio of nearly 2:1 in frequency.

The majority of pericardial mesotheliomas diffusely cover the parietal and visceral pericardium, encasing the heart. Solitary or localized pericardial mesotheliomas exist but are distinctly rare. Histologically, a localized mesothelioma is identical to a diffuse mesothelioma and may be an epithelioid or fibrous type.

Microscopically, mesotheliomas are characterized by cellular irregularity and histo-logic variability. The tumor may consist of tubules or solid cords of malignant cells (tubular or tubulopapillary pattern) or spindle-shaped cells with a connective tissue stroma (fibrous pattern) (Figs. 35–3 and 35–4). Frequently, both patterns are present in the same tumor. In either histologic pattern, the cells are usually strikingly irregular in appearance, and the nuclei most frequently are large, rounded, and vesicular, with prominent nucleoli. Cellular pleomorphism and anaplasia are unusual, and atypical mitoses may be seen. Fibrous or mixed fibrous and epithelioid mesotheliomas predominate in the pericardium, as is the circumstance with pleural mesotheliomas. Involvement of asbestos in the induction of some pericardial mesotheliomas has been suggested.[42]

The mesothelioma, whether nodular or sheetlike, invades contiguous structures, in-

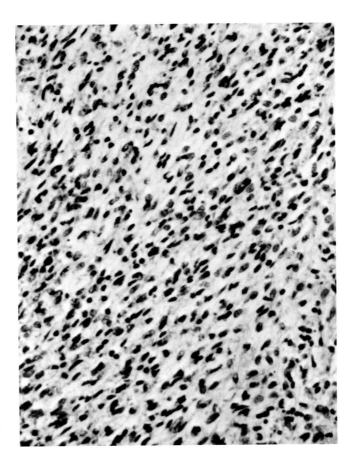

Fig. 35–4. Most pericardial mesotheliomas are composed, at least in part, of spindle-shaped cells that imitate fibroblasts; hence, the designation fibrous mesotheliomas. Although the cells are spindle-shaped, the nuclei are usually rounded and vesicular with prominent nucleoli, unlike the elongated, blunt-ended nuclei of fibroblasts. (H&E, × 225.)

cluding the heart, only superficially (Fig. 35–5). This is an important differential diagnostic point in that other primary sarcomas, most notably angiosarcoma, can diffusely involve the pericardium but, unlike mesotheliomas, almost invariably have a significant intramyocardial or intracavitary component.

Pericardial mesotheliomas frequently spread to the adjacent pleura and mediastinum and may involve mediastinal lymph nodes. Occasionally, pericardial mesotheliomas spread through the diaphragm and involve the peritoneum. Distant metastases are extremely unusual. Cytologic examination of the pericardial fluid may aid diagnosis. The distinction between hyperplastic and malignant mesothelial cells is, however, extremely difficult. Indeed, differentiation of mesothelial hyperplasia and mesothelioma on a

pericardial biopsy poses a major diagnostic problem to the pathologist. Exfoliative cytology is usually helpful in establishing the diagnosis of metastatic carcinoma of the pericardium. Most metastatic carcinomas that are likely to be confused with mesothelial hyperplasia can be identified by differential histochemical staining of a pericardial biopsy. However, mesothelial hyperplasia may be a complication of treatment by radiotherapy, or be secondary to pericarditis following the spread of carcinoma to the pericardium. Finding only mesothelial hyperplasia in a patient suspected of having metastatic pericardial carcinoma, therefore, does not exclude the diagnosis of metastatic carcinoma involving the pericardium.

There is no specific treatment for pericardial mesothelioma. Surgical excision is usually

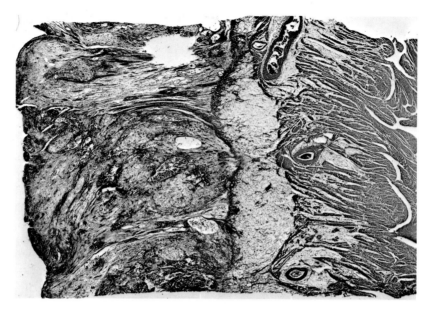

Fig. 35–5. Mesothelioma tends to obliterate the pericardial space and may actually constrict the heart causing symptoms of constrictive pericarditis. Occasionally the parietal pericardium is not invaded. The tumor may extend along blood vessels from the epicardium into the heart, although the myocardium is usually not directly invaded. (H&E, × 5.)

not possible. Although chemotherapy and radiotherapy may produce temporary improvement, there is no well-established correlation between this treatment and the course of the disease. Prognosis is generally poor, with as many as 60 percent of patients dying within 6 months of diagnosis; survivals of 5 and 6 years were reported in an AFIP series.[54]

Thymoma

Thymomas are primarily tumors of the anterior mediastinum; however, they are occasionally primary within the pericardium. Presumably, they are derived from thymic rests, which, incidentally, are not infrequently encountered in the parietal pericardium. The pericardium can be accepted as the primary sight of origin only in those tumors in which there is no evidence of anterior mediastinal involvement.

Four thymomas originating in the parietal pericardium were in the AFIP series. Three of the four patients were women. In one, thymoma was an unexpected finding at autopsy. The remaining three patients had clinical findings of intractible congestive heart failure, pericardial effusion, and a mediastinal or pericardial mass by chest radiograph. At operation, each patient had an intrapericardial thymoma attached to the pericardium, either at the base of the heart or over its anterior aspect. No patient had myasthenia gravis.

Liposarcoma

Although lipomas of the heart are relatively frequent, liposarcomas of the heart and pericardium are distinctly rare. Only six primary in the heart or pericardium have been reported in the literature.[54] The only such tumor in the AFIP series was in a 30-year-old woman with severe congestive heart failure, believed, clinically, to stem from chronic rheumatic heart disease. At autopsy, however, a large tumor replaced the right atrium and extended to the pericardium, constricting the superior and inferior vena cavae. No metastases were found. The neoplasm presumably originated in the epicardial fat.

Microscopically, the tumor resembled embryonal adipose tissue containing signet ring and stellate cells, with numerous tiny vacuoles. Myxoid areas were frequent. The vacuoles and intracellular spaces stained intensively with Oil-red O stain.

Synovial Sarcoma

The only reported case of primary synovial sarcoma in the heart was that of a 30-year-old man who had progressive dyspnea, syncopal episodes, and a systolic ejection murmur that was believed to represent pulmonic stenosis.[54] At autopsy, a 15 × 10 cm tumor was found at the base of the heart involving the pericardium and invading the outflow tract of the right ventricle and pulmonary artery. It extended into the right ventricle, obstructing the pulmonary valve. No metastases were found. Microscopically, the tumor had the classic biphasic pattern and staining properties characteristic of synovial sarcoma.

Other Tumors

Benign and malignant teratomas are most commonly extracardiac, but intrapericardial examples occur. Because these tumors are usually attached to the base of the heart and derive their blood supply from the vasa vasorum of the aorta and pulmonary artery, they are discussed under the section on primary tumors of the heart. Hemangiomas, lymphangiomas, and angiosarcomas may primarily involve the pericardium, myocardium, or both. They are discussed under primary tumors of the heart. Serosal papillomas are discussed as part of the differential diagnosis of papillary fibroelastomas of the endocardium or cardiac valves.

Primary Cardiac Tumors

Myxoma

Before 1960, cardiac myxomas were generally misdiagnosed as chronic rheumatic heart disease. Since that time, clinicians have become increasingly aware of the ability of cardiac myxomas to imitate mitral valve disease. As newer diagnostic methods of cardiology have become available, these tumors have been correctly diagnosed and surgically excised in most cases. The clinical presentation of a cardiac myxoma mostly depends on the cardiac chamber involved by the tumor. The presentations of 130 patients in the AFIP series are summarized in Table 35–6.[54] Of the 57 patients with clinical signs and symptoms of mitral valve disease in this series, 56 had a myxoma in the left atrium; the other had a myxoma in the right atrium. Signs and symptoms included dyspnea, progressive or refractory congestive heart failure, systolic and diastolic murmurs, and atrial arrhythmias. Although the distinction between those patients with cardiac myxoma and those with intrinsic mitral valve disease may be difficult by physical examination, diagnosis may be aided by murmurs of changing intensity and laboratory findings such as an elevated erythrocyte sedimentation rate or increased gamma globulin levels. Either anemia or polycythemia may be present in these patients. Evidence has been

Table 35–6. Cardiac Myxoma: Clinical Presentation

Clinical Presentation	N
Signs and symptoms of mitral valve disease	57
Embolic phenomena	36
No cardiac symptoms—incidental finding	16
Signs and symptoms of tricuspid valve disease	6
Sudden unexpected death	5
Pericarditis	4
Myocardial infarction	3
Signs and symptoms of pulmonary valve disease	2
Fever of undetermined origin	2

[a] One patient with multiple myxomas had signs and symptoms of mitral and tricuspid valve disease.
(From McAllister and Fenoglio,[54] with permission.)

presented that myxomas may produce erythropoietin.[17]

The second most common clinical presentation of patients with cardiac myxoma is with embolic phenomena. In 36 patients in the AFIP series, the initial event was embolic and occurred in patients with myxomas arising in either the left or right side of the heart. Diagnosis was difficult in the six patients with pulmonary emboli from right atrial myxoma. Each had persistent fever, changing murmurs, and progressive congestive heart failure. Slightly more than one-third of patients with a myxoma located in the left ventricle or the left atrium died of a cerebrovascular accident, and an embolic myxoma was found at autopsy. Symptoms or signs in the remaining 18 patients were sudden hemiparesis, sudden diplopia, or sudden loss of blood supply to an extremity. The common denominator in these patients was sudden onset of symptoms or signs suggesting arterial occlusion. Many of these tumors were diagnosed following arterial embolectomy. Occasionally, the myxoma was not identified microscopically, and some patients had repeated episodes of peripheral embolization before a cardiac myxoma was suspected. All but one of the patients with a myxoma in the left ventricle presented with signs or symptoms of emboli. An additional 18 had episodes of arterial embolic occlusion during the course of their disease or evidence of myxoma emboli at autopsy. Three patients who presented with signs or symptoms of myocardial infarction had a myxoma embolus in at least one coronary artery at autopsy. Thus, patients with a myxoma in the left side of the heart most frequently have symptoms of mitral valve disease or of embolic phenomena. These were the presenting symptoms in 86 of 108 patients with myxomas of the left atrium or left ventricle in the AFIP series.

By contrast, myxomas arising in the right side of the heart may mimic any number of clinical entities. In addition to pulmonary emboli, patients with myxomas in the right atrium or ventricle may have signs or symptoms of tricuspid valve disease or pulmonary stenosis. Occasionally, patients with a myxoma in the right atrium or ventricle may present with pericarditis or with fever of undetermined origin. Rhythm disturbances are frequently present, especially right bundle branch block and atrial flutter or fibrillation. As with myxomas on the left side of the heart, advances in diagnostic cardiology have greatly aided the diagnosis of right atrial and ventricular myxomas.

More than 50 percent of patients with cardiac myxoma are in their fourth, fifth, and sixth decades; however, myxomas occur in all age groups. Twelve percent of patients in the AFIP series were over age 70 years, and 9 percent were in the pediatric age group (15 years or under). Most published series indicated a nearly equal sex distribution. It appears, however, that nonfamilial cardiac myxoma is mainly a disorder of middle-aged women (mean age: 51 years), usually occurs in the left atrium, presents as a single tumor, and is not associated with any particular lesions elsewhere.

By contrast, familial cardiac myxoma is mainly a disorder of young men (mean age: 24 years), is less commonly found in the left atrium, often multicentric, and occasionally associated with unusual or rare conditions.[13] These include skin pigmentation, such as lentigo and several types of nevi, which commonly affect the lips and oral cavity, cutaneous myxomas, pigmented nodular adrenocortical disease (with or without Cushing syndrome), myxoid mammary fibroadenomas, pituitary adenomas, and testicular tumors. This familial myxoma syndrome appears to follow a pattern of mendelian dominant inheritance.[14]

The locations of the myxomas in this series are summarized in Table 35–7.[54] The myxomas were multiple in 5 percent of the patients, and in one patient a myxoma was present in each of the four cardiac chambers. The majority of myxomas arising in the atria, either left or right, are attached to the atrial septum, usually in the region of the limbus of the fossa ovalis; however, 10 percent originate in sites

Table 35–7. Cardiac Myxoma: Location of 138 Myxomas in 130 Patients[a]

Site	N	%
Left atrium	103	74.5
Right atrium	25	18.1
Right ventricle	5	3.7
Left ventricle	5	3.7

[a] Multiple myxomas were present in six patients. (From McAllister and Fenoglio,[54] with permission.)

in the atria other than the septum. After the atrial septum, the most common site is the posterior atrial wall, followed by the anterior wall and the atrial appendage. By contrast, only one of the 10 ventricular myxomas originated from the ventricular septum. Although myxoma imitators such as papillary fibroelastomas, sarcomas, and, rarely, metastatic carcinomas, have been localized to valves, I am not aware of a documented example of a true myxoma arising from a cardiac valve.

Although cardiac myxomas differ in clinical presentation, depending on the chamber in which they are located, they are similar in gross and microscopic appearance, irrespective of their location. Grossly, most have a short, broad-based attachment and are pedunculated, gelatinous, and polypoid (Fig. 35–6), although some tumors have a rounded, smooth surface (Fig. 35–7). True sessile myxomas are distinctly rare. The majority of so-called sessile myxomas have previously embolized, leaving only the broad base of the polypoid tumor attached to the endocardium. Characteristically, myxomas are soft and gelatinous and frequently contain areas of hemorrhage. Their size varies from 1 to 15 cm in diameter, although most myxomas are 5 to 6 cm in diameter.

Microscopically, myxomas have a myxoid matrix composed of acid mucopolysaccharide within which are polygonal cells with scant eosinophilic cytoplasm (Fig. 35–8). These cells are arranged singly, often assuming a

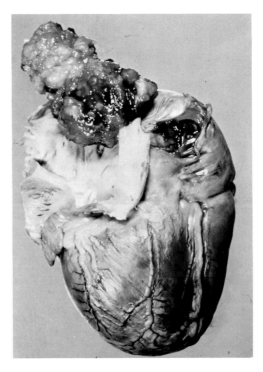

Fig. 35–6. Most cardiac myxomas consist of multiple, friable, polypoid fronds and have a distinctive mucoid or gelatinous appearance. Approximately 75 percent of cardiac myxomas arise in the left atrium, as shown here, and 18 percent arise in the right atrium.

stellate shape, and in small nests; they are occasionally multinuclear.[28] The surface of the myxoma is covered by the polygonal cells, usually in a monolayer with focal clustering in crevasses (Fig. 35–9). These cells also form vascular-like channels throughout the myxoid stroma, simulating primitive capillaries (Fig. 35–10). Ultrastructurally, the polygonal cells closely resemble multipotential mesenchymal cells.[24,70,73] Occasionally, glandular elements are present within myxomas. These usually stain positively with both mucicarmine and periodic acid-Schiff (PAS) reagent with diastase pretreatment. Immunoperoxidase studies demonstrate positivity of the glandular cells for carcinoembryonic antigen (CEA), epithelial membrane antigen (EMA), and keratin.[1,32] Factor VIII-related antigen (FVIIIAg)

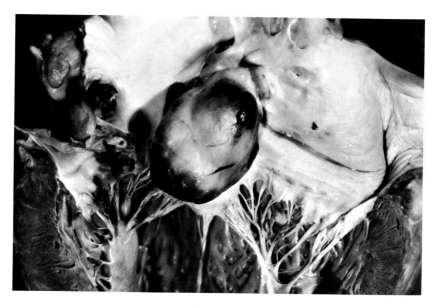

Fig. 35–7. Although most cardiac myxomas are polypoid and friable, a significant percentage are rounded and solid. Their surface is smooth, glistening and gelatinous, and foci of hemorrhage and thrombus are frequently present.

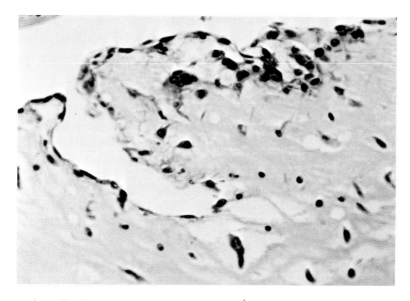

Fig. 35–8. Histologically, the cardiac myxoma consists of an acid mucopolysaccharide matrix within which are embedded polygonal cells and occasional blood vessels. The surface of the fronds of the myxoma is covered by cells similar to those embedded in the matrix. (H&E, × 305.)

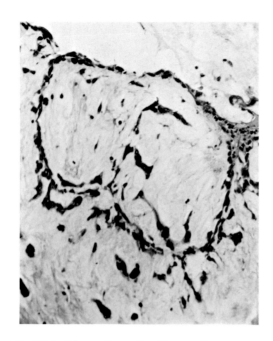

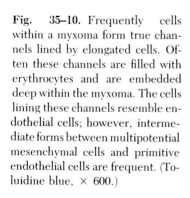

Fig. 35–9. The surface cells of the cardiac myxoma are usually arranged in a monolayer; however, foci of multilayered hyperplastic cells are frequent. In these areas, the surface cells extend in crypts into the myxoma and appear to merge with the multipotential mesenchymal cells of the matrix. (H&E, × 150.)

is identified only in cells lining vascular spaces. An electron microscopy study of one tumor revealed well-formed glands having basement membranes, junctional complexes, and apical secretory granules.[32] The stroma contains variable amounts of reticular fibers, collagen, elastic fibers, and smooth muscle cells. Large arteries and veins are commonly present at the base of the tumor and communicate with the subendocardium. Lymphocytes and plasma cells are not infrequent, especially at the site of attachment to the subendocardium, and foci of extramedullary hematopoiesis are commonly found throughout the tumor. Foci of microscopic calcification are present in approximately 10 percent of myxomas, and areas of metaplastic bone occasionally occur. Rarely, a cardiac myxoma infarcts or undergoes degenerative changes to produce the so-called Gamna body of the heart.[15,75]

Although arguments supporting a thrombotic origin of cardiac myxomas have appeared in the literature,[67] they do not account for the following points:

1. True thrombi, even in the atria, organize into fibrous tissue; myxomas do not.

Fig. 35–10. Frequently cells within a myxoma form true channels lined by elongated cells. Often these channels are filled with erythrocytes and are embedded deep within the myxoma. The cells lining these channels resemble endothelial cells; however, intermediate forms between multipotential mesenchymal cells and primitive endothelial cells are frequent. (Toluidine blue, × 600.)

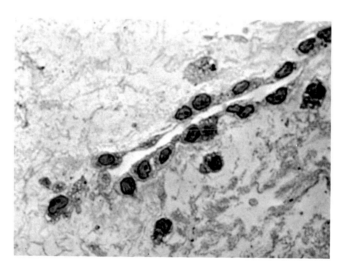

2. Fluid influx into the lesion in the low-pressure system of the atria cannot explain the myxomatous appearance of myxomas arising in the ventricles.

3. True thrombi are most frequent in patients with underlying cardiac disease and occur most frequently in the right atrium and right atrial appendage, whereas underlying cardiac disease is infrequent in patients with myxomas, and most myxomas arise in the left atrium, usually from the atrial septum. Myxomas arising from the atrial appendage of either atrium are a distinct rarity, whereas this is the most common location for atrial thrombi. The most compelling argument against the thrombotic origin of the cardiac myxoma is based on tissue culture work.[31] When thrombi are placed in tissue culture, fibroblasts overgrow the culture, as is true of cultured granulation tissue, whereas the cells obtained from cardiac myxomas grown in tissue culture are mononuclear and polygonal or multinuclear, and collagen formation does not occur. These tissue cultured cells closely resemble the primitive multipotential mesenchymal cells characteristic of the cardiac myxoma.

Embryonal rests have been reported in the heart in the region of the limbus of the fossa ovalis, and many investigators have speculated that these tissue rests contain the cells of origin of the cardiac myxoma.[50] Although embryonal rests may occur in this region, more frequently clusters of "cardiac reserve" cells (multipotential mesenchymal cells) are found. In either case, the cardiac myxoma is most likely derived from these multipotential mesenchymal cells of the subendocardium. Although an occasional report has suggested that myxoma originates from endothelial or endocardial cells,[58] the overwhelming evidence gathered from immunoperoxidase,[9,33,57,68] ultrastructural,[70,73] and cytogenetic[18] studies supports the theory (originally proposed in the AFIP fascicle) that cardiac myxomas arise from subendocardial mesenchymal cells.

Complete surgical excision of a myxoma and its base along with a small rim of unaffected endocardium and myocardium is the treatment of choice. Surgical excision should not be unduly delayed because of the high incidence of embolization. As is now well recognized, special care must be taken during the operation to avoid embolization, and all cardiac chambers should be explored for the occasional multicentric tumor. If not completely excised, the cardiac myxoma can recur although, in many cases, recurrence is probably caused by multiple foci of tumor growth.[34] Despite this tendency for recurrence, the existence of a true malignant cardiac myxoma remains in doubt. The malignant cardiac myxomas reported in the literature that we reviewed have either been malignant tumors of other types that had extensive areas of myxoid degeneration, or multiple myxomas that were benign.[54] Follow-up information was available in 33 patients in the AFIP series who had surgical excision of a cardiac myxoma. Twenty-nine patients were alive and well at least 2 years after surgery, and nine had been followed for more than 10 years without evidence of recurrence or metastases. Two patients were dead, 4 and 6 years postoperatively, of causes unrelated to their hearts. In both patients, no residual myxoma was detected at autopsy. A third patient died of a myocardial infarction 2 years after excision of a cardiac myxoma; an autopsy was not performed.

Papillary Fibroelastoma

Forty-two patients with fibroelastomas were identified in the AFIP series. They ranged in age from 25 to 86 years, although 55 percent were older than 60 years. The tumors are incidental findings at autopsy, or on surgically excised valves, and are not associated with cardiac dysfunction in the majority of patients. However, in at least three reported cases, these tumors were associated with paroxysmal angina pectoris, or sudden unexpected death.[54] In these three patients, the papillary tumor was located on the aortic side of the aortic valve and partially obstructed the ostium of a coronary artery.

Although they most frequently arise from the valvular endocardium, papillary fibroelastomas may arise anywhere in the heart, and occasionally are multiple. When these tumors occur on the atrioventricular (AV) valves they usually project into the atria. Although they may arise from the free edge of the valve, more commonly they arise from its midportion (Fig. 35–11). On the semilunar valves, these tumors arise with nearly equal frequency on the ventricular and arterial side and may be situated anywhere on the valve.[54]

Grossly, the tumors resemble a sea anemone, with multiple papillary fronds attached to the endocardium by a short pedicle. Histologically and ultrastructurally, the papillary fronds consist of a central core of dense connective tissue surrounded by a layer of loose connective tissue and covered by endothelial cells, which are frequently hyperplastic (Figs. 35–12 and 35–13). The mantle of loose connective tissue consists of an acid mucopolysaccharide matrix, within which are embedded collagen fibrils, elastic fibers, scattered smooth muscle cells, and occasional mononuclear cells. Usually a fine meshwork of elastic fibers surrounds a central collagen core.[29] Occasionally, however, the entire central core appears to consist of elastic fibers. The central core of the papillary fibroelastoma is continuous with the connective tissue of the endocardium and merges imperceptibly with it. Similarly, the endothelial cells covering the papillary fronds are contiguous with the normal endothelial cells covering the endocardium or the cardiac valve.

The papillary fronds of these tumors are microscopically similar in structure to normal chordae tendineae, and the tumors replicate all components of normal endocardium. These observations suggest that the papillary fibroelastoma is a hamartoma; however, the fact that the tumors are rarely found in children and are more frequent in older patients, many

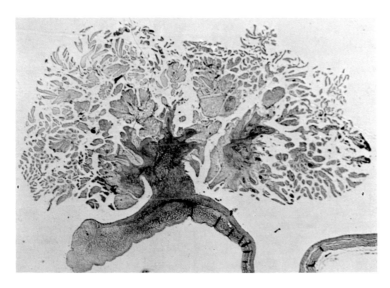

Fig. 35–11. Papillary fibroelastomas are most frequently located on the cardiac valves. These tumors consist of multiple papillary fronds arranged on a stalk that merges imperceptibly with the valve substance. (H&E, × 12.)

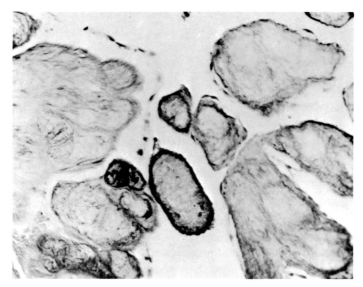

Fig. 35–12. The fronds of the papillary fibroelastoma consist of a collagen core surrounded by elastic and loose connective tissue. They are covered by endothelial cells that bear no resemblance to the cardiac myxoma. (Elastic van Gieson, × 70.)

of whom have had long-standing cardiac disease, has suggested to some authors that the tumors are secondary to mechanical damage and represent a degenerative process.[39]

The frequent occurrence of papillary fibroelastomas on the atrial surface of the AV valves, and on the ventricular surface of the semilunar valves, parallels the location of Lambl's excrescences; however, Lambl's excrescences do not usually occur on the arterial side of the semilunar valves or on the mural endocardium, whereas the papillary fibroelastomas do. Lambl's excrescences are most frequently located along the line of closure of the valves, whereas papillary fibroelastomas are located more frequently on the midportion or body of the valve, away from the contact surface. Lambl's excrescences have been reported in 70 to 80 percent of adult heart valves, whereas papillary fibroelastomas are

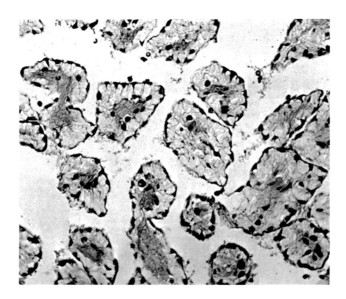

Fig. 35–13. The endothelial cells covering the papillary fronds are in continuity with the endothelial cells covering the normal adjacent endocardium or valve and are structurally identical to these adjacent cells. Focally, especially at the tips of the papillary fronds, the endothelial cells are multilayered and hyperplastic. The loose connective tissue, mainly acid mucopolysaccharide, is clearly visible between the collagen core and the covering endothelial cells. (H&E, × 195.)

rare. Lambl's excrescences are multiple in more than 90 percent of affected hearts, whereas papillary fibroelastomas are rarely multiple. Finally, Lambl's excrescences, unlike papillary fibroelastomas, contain deposits of fibrin, lack an abundant acid mucopolysaccharide matrix, and do not contain smooth muscle cells as a significant component[49,62] (see also Ch. 5).

Papillary fibroelastomas are not to be confused with polypoid myxomatous valvular lesions of childhood (incompletely differentiated or dysplastic valves).[54] Nor should the papillary fibroelastoma of the endocardial surface be confused with papillary projections from the epicardium. The fronds of the serosal papilloma are composed of loose connective tissue, covered by mesothelial cells, often with a central blood vessel. Unlike the papillary fibroelastoma, they lack a collagen core surrounded by an elastic tissue mantle. The epicardial papillomas are occasionally complex structures with multiple papillary fronds; however, they more frequently consist of only one or two fibrous tissue stalks. Histologically, the epicardial papilloma resembles a fibrous pericardial adhesion. Surgical excision would appear to be indicated in those patients with symptoms of angina pectoris secondary to obstruction of a coronary ostium by the fronds of a papillary fibroelastoma.

Rhabdomyoma

The most common primary cardiac tumor in infancy and childhood is the rhabdomyoma. In the AFIP series of 36 patients, 78 percent were under 1 year of age, and only one patient was over age 15 years. Ninety percent of rhabdomyomas were multiple and occurred with nearly equal frequency in the right or left ventricles, including the ventricular septum. Although reportedly infrequent in the atria, rhabdomyomas involved either one or both atria in 30 percent of these patients. In no case did a rhabdomyoma originate in a cardiac valve. In 50 percent of patients, at least one of the tumor masses was intracavitary and obstructed 50 percent or more of one of the cardiac chambers or valve orifices (Fig. 35–14). Symptoms referable to obstruction of intracardiac blood flow were present in nine patients—none of whom had tuberous sclerosis and all of whom would appear to have been good surgical candidates. The incidence of tuberous sclerosis associated with rhabdomyomas in the 30 patients whose brain was examined was 37 percent.

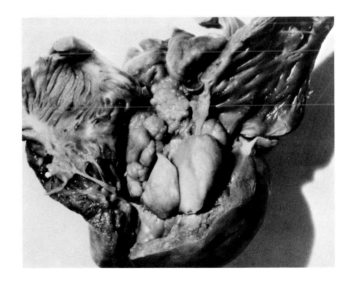

Fig. 35–14. This rhabdomyoma fills the right ventricle of a newborn infant and clearly obstructs the tricuspid valve. In approximately 50 percent of children with rhabdomyomas, at least one of the tumors is intracavitary and partially obstructs at least one valve orifice.

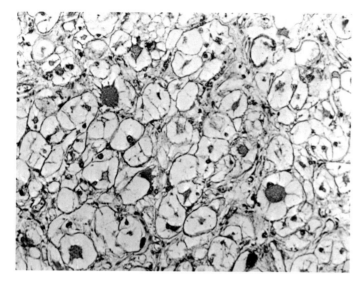

Fig. 35–15. Rhabdomyomas are composed of vacuolated, large, ovoid cells. Islands and strands of cytoplasm are present against the cell membrane and occasionally in the center of the cell. If the tissue is fixed in methyl alcohol, the vacuolated areas seen in the formaldehyde-fixed tissue are easily demonstrated to contain abundant glycogen. (H&E, × 125.)

Grossly, these tumors are white to yellow-tan and vary in diameter from millimeters to centimeters. Microscopically, they are circumscribed but not encapsulated and are easily distinguished from the surrounding myocardium. The rhabdomyoma cells are large, up to 80 μm in diameter, and contain abundant glycogen. The histologic demonstration of glycogen in their cytoplasm depends on the speed and type of fixation. Glycogen is best demonstrated with the PAS reaction, or with Best's carmine stain on frozen sections from unfixed tissue, or following methanol or nonaqueous fixation. Classic "spider cells" with centrally placed cytoplasmic masses containing the nucleus and elongated projections of slender myofibrils extending to the periphery of these cells are present in each tumor (Figs. 35–15 and 35–16). More frequently, however, the cytoplasmic mass is eccentrically placed, usually against the cell wall, and the cytoplasmic projections traverse the vacuolated cells. Rarely, microscopic calcification is found within rhabdomyoma cells. Many of the rhabdomyomas in newborns contain collections of nucleated red cells, myelocytic precursor cells, and occasional megakaryocytes, consistent with extramedullary hematopoiesis.

Ultrastructurally, cellular junctions resembling intercalated discs are located around the total periphery of the rhabdomyoma cells interconnecting them. This ultrastructural feature is unlike that seen in normal myocardial cells or Purkinje cells where intercalated discs are located at the poles of the cell, but is suggestive of embryonic cardiac myoblasts.[20] Thus, rhabdomyomas are probably not abnormal proliferations of specialized Purkinje cells, or of nonspecialized myocardium. Nor is the rhabdomyoma a localized form of glycogen storage disease. In glycogen storage disease (types II, III, and IV), the contractile elements are compressed around the periphery of the cardiac muscle cells by the accumulated glycogen. The cell, however, maintains its cylindrical shape, and intercalated discs are located at the two poles of the cell. The preservation of a relatively normal cell shape distinguishes glycogen-laden cardiac muscle cells in glycogen storage disease from rhabdomyoma cells. The preponderance of multiple, as opposed to solitary, cardiac rhabdomyomas, and their most frequent occurrence in infants, suggests that the cardiac rhabdomyoma is a hamartoma or malformation rather than a true neoplasm. The clinical behavior and microscopic appearance of these

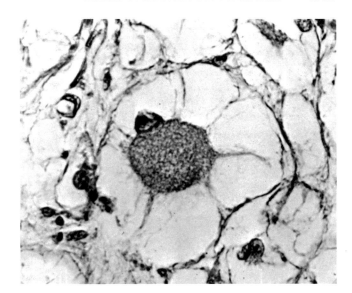

Fig. 35–16. The spider cell with a central cytoplasmic mass and strands of cytoplasm that extend to the cell membrane is pathognomonic of the cardiac rhabdomyoma. The nucleus is usually centrally located, but may be eccentrically placed, as in this cell. (H&E, × 525.)

tumors suggests that rhabdomyoma cells eventually lose their ability to divide. A similar loss of mitotic activity occurs in normally differentiated human cardiac muscle cells soon after birth. The rhabdomyoma cells appear to undergo arrest of development and to lose the ability to differentiate fully. The ovoid shape and the peripheral location of cellular junctions of intercalated disc type in rhabdomyoma cells are reminiscent of cardiac myoblasts and suggest that the tumor is a fetal hamartoma derived from embryonic cardiac myoblasts.

Although the cardiac rhabdomyoma has been described repeatedly in the literature as a nonsurgical lesion because of its tendency for multiplicity, cardiac rhabdomyomas have been excised successfully.[54] Surgical management is only necessary in patients presenting with symptoms related to obstruction of intracardiac blood flow or with arrhythmias that are resistant to conventional medical treatment.[60] Since there is no evidence to suggest that rhabdomyoma cells are capable of mitotic division after birth,[23] and, indeed, regression of the tumor has been demonstrated in infancy by two-dimensional echocardiography,[2] these patients should be considered for surgical treatment.

Fibroma

Cardiac fibromas are almost always solitary and located in the ventricular myocardium, frequently in the ventricular septum. The clinical findings in 17 patients with cardiac fibromas in the AFIP series depended on the location of the tumor. Ten fibromas of the ventricular septum were inoperable, and the patients either died suddenly or developed intractable congestive heart failure. Most of these tumors encroached on, or invaded, the conduction system, usually the left and right bundle branches, and the patients either developed ventricular fibrillation or died suddenly and unexpectedly. Seven patients with fibromas located in the left ventricular free wall or atrium presented with cardiomegaly, often as an incidental finding on a chest radiograph. In five patients, the mass lesion was identified by cardiac catheterization, and surgical excision was attempted. One of these patients died postoperatively, but four were alive and well, without evidence of recurrence, at least 2 years after surgery.

Cardiac fibromas occur at all ages and in both sexes; however, they are more frequent in children and, as such, are the second most common primary cardiac tumor in the pedi-

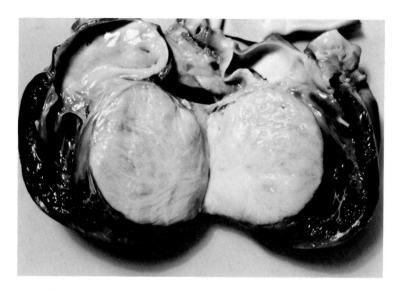

Fig. 35–17. Cardiac fibromas are most commonly solitary and located in the ventricular septum. This fibroma virtually replaces the ventricular septum and encroaches on the left ventricular chamber.

atric age group.[54] These firm gray-white tumors are often large and sometimes exceed 10 cm in diameter[38] (Fig. 35–17). Grossly, they appear sharply demarcated, but microscopically they interdigitate with the adjacent myocardium (Fig. 35–18). There may be an impression of satellite nodules, but, when traced, these nodules connect to the main tumor mass in a different plane. The central portion of the tumor is composed of hyalinized fibrous tissue, often with multiple foci of calcification and cystic degeneration, probably secondary to a poor blood supply. This central calcification may often be seen on chest radiographs. Elastic tissue may also be prominent, as in many of the fibromatoses of the superficial soft tissues.[54] Indeed, fibromas of the heart are connective tissue tumors derived from fibroblasts and have the same spectrum of appearance and behavior as the soft tissue fibromatoses in other areas of the body. These definable masses of proliferating connective tissue should not be confused with reactive fibrous tissue proliferation in the endocardial or epicardial layers of the heart. Areas of cellular fibrous tissue are present in each tumor, usually at the periphery. Mitotic figures are rare in the areas of cellular fibrous tissue, and, as in the extracardiac fibromatoses, cellularity is not an indication of malignancy. Because of the invasive growth of these tumors, normal cardiac muscle cells are frequently entrapped in the growing fibrous tissue and are left intact deep within the tumor, occasionally in central locations. The myocardial cells eventually degenerate and become vacuolated as they are separated from the syncytium of the contracting myocardium; this observation led pathologists to speculate that the fibroma is a "healing rhabdomyoma" or a "mesoblastic tumor."[54] Rather, by both light and electron microscopy, these are degenerating cardiac muscle cells, not embryonic (rhabdomyoma) muscle cells, and are not an intrinsic, developing part of the fibroma. True "spider cells," diagnostic of the rhabdomyoma, are not found in the cardiac fibroma.

Cardiac fibromas located outside the ventricular septum are amenable to surgical excision, and patients usually do well after surgery. Surgical resection of ventricular septal fibromas may not be possible, especially if the tumor is close to the conduction system; such patients often succumb to ventricular arrhyth-

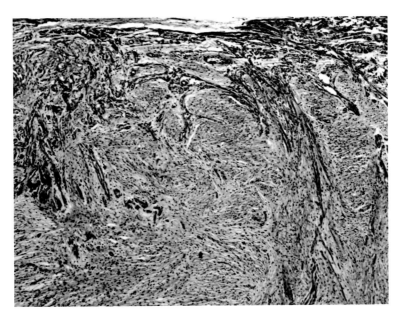

Fig. 35–18. Fibromas commonly contain foci of cellular fibrous tissue, usually at the periphery of the tumor. Individual myofibers and bundles of myofibers are entrapped by the expanding fibrous tissue. These are normal, although degenerating myofibers, not rhabdomyoblasts, and do not arise from the replicating cells of the fibroma. (H&E, × 50.)

mias.[44] The efficacy of permanent cardiac pacing in patients with large ventricular septal fibromas has not been adequately evaluated.

Lipomatous Hypertrophy of the Atrial Septum and Lipoma

Lipomatous hypertrophy (interatrial lipoma) is a nonencapsulated mass of adipose tissue in the atrial septum that is in continuity with the epicardial fat. Most probably, it represents atypical hyperplasia of primordial fat rather than a true neoplasm. The clinical significance of the lesion has been debated in the literature[61]; however, we believe that it may be associated with cardiac symptoms, especially cardiac arrhythmias.

The clinical and pathologic findings in 45 patients with abnormal accumulations of adipose tissue in the heart and pericardium were reviewed at the AFIP.[54] Thirty-two of the 45 patients had lipomatous hypertrophy of the atrial septum. In 28 percent of these 32 pa-

tients, the cause of death appeared directly related to the atrial tumor. The patients died either suddenly or following prolonged episodes of atrial or ventricular arrhythmia, or of intractable congestive heart failure. The etiology of the cardiac symptomatology was clinically uncertain in each case, and at autopsy no abnormality or cardiac disease other than lipomatous hypertrophy of the atrial septum was found. Of the remaining patients, approximately 50 percent had either conduction disturbances or evidence of congestive heart failure; however, in each case the relationship of these findings to coexistent cardiopulmonary disease was unclear. In only 10 of the 32 patients was lipomatous hypertrophy an incidental finding at autopsy.

Ten patients in this series had chronic or debilitating diseases; however, this did not correlate with the size of the interatrial lipoma or with the presence of rhythm disturbance. Similarly, the body habitus of the patient and the amount of epicardial fat did not correlate with the interatrial lipoma or with the rhythm disturbances.

Although most patients with lipomatous hypertrophy of the atrial septum are over 60 years of age, approximately 25 percent of the patients in this series were younger, with one dying at age 22 years.

In lipomatous hypertrophy of the atrial septum, the mass of accumulated fat frequently causes the atrial septal endocardium to bulge, most frequently into the right atrium (Fig. 35–19). This may be detected by either two-dimensional echocardiography[30] or MRI.[46] Rarely an interatrial lipoma protrudes so far into the atrium that this entity must be considered in the angiographic differential diagnosis of intracavitary masses. Interatrial lipomas vary in size from 1 or 2 cm up to 7 or 8 cm in maximum diameter. They may extend into the region of the AV node, but most often they are located anterior to the foramen ovale. The interatrial lipoma is situated in the area of at least two proposed interatrial conduction pathways. The inter-

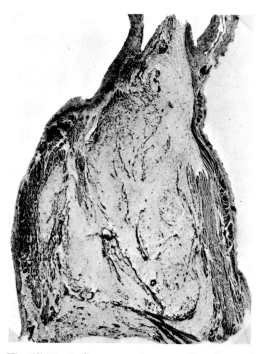

Fig. 35–20. In lipomatous hypertrophy, the atrial septum is thickened by adipose tissue and the myofibers are compressed against the endocardium. Islands of atrial myofibers are trapped in the lipoma and often do not appear to be in contact with the myofibers compressed against the endocardium. Blood vessels and fibrous tissue septae are abundant. (H&E, × 8.)

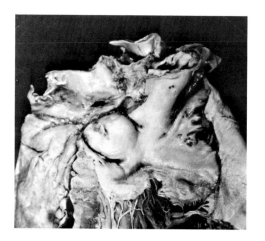

Fig. 35–19. Occasionally, a portion of the tumor in lipomatous hypertrophy of the atrial septum projects into the atrial cavity, usually the right atrium. The intracavitary portion of the tumor may be large enough to be detected by angiography and mistakenly interpreted as a myxoma. The intracavitary portion of this tumor is situated just proximal to the region of the AV node.

ruption of these pathways could be the major reason for rhythm disturbances in these patients.

Microscopically, there are varying proportions of mature adipose tissue and granular or vacuolated cells.[61] Fat droplets can usually be detected both in the mature fat cells and in the granular cells with Oil-red O stain. By both light and electron microscopy, the granular cells are identical to fetal fat cells.[41] The presence of fetal fat is a hallmark of lipomatous hypertrophy of the atrial septum; occasionally, these interatrial masses consist almost entirely of fetal fat. Myocardial cells are invariably entrapped in the mass, especially at the periphery (Fig. 35–20). Many of the entrapped myocardial cells demonstrate bizarre, hypertrophic, atrophic, or degenerative changes. Often the muscle nuclei are large, hyperchromatic, and pleomorphic. Neither classic "spider cells" nor neoplastic muscle cells are found in the interatrial lipoma. Varying amounts of fibrosis and foci of chronic inflammatory cells, predominantly lymphocytes and plasma cells, are frequently present. When located within the myocardium, lipomas are usually small and irregular in contour and have a barely definable, but definite capsule; varying numbers of myocardial cells are entrapped in the tumor. Like the cardiac fibroma in which cardiac myofibers may be entrapped, "spider cells," characteristic of rhabdomyoma, are not identified in true lipomas. An association of cardiac lipoma and tuberous sclerosis has been reported, however, and lipomas may be present in the heart and other viscera of patients with tuberous sclerosis in the absence of cardiac rhabdomyoma.

Hemangioma

Hemangiomas are composed of benign proliferations of endothelial cells, usually forming channels containing blood. They may occur at any site in the heart or pericardium and may be mainly intramural or mainly intracavitary. The clinical and pathologic findings in 15 patients with cardiac hemangioma have been reviewed at the AFIP.[54] In greater than 50 percent of these patients, who ranged in age from 7 months to 80 years, the tumors were incidental findings at autopsy. Signs and symptoms in the remaining patients depended on the location of the tumor. In three patients, the tumors were intracavitary and mimicked the symptoms of patients with myxomas. Two patients had a mass discovered on routine chest radiograph and underwent surgery with the probable diagnosis of pericardial cyst. A hemangioma was present in both patients. The final two patients presented with cardiomegaly and recurrent pericardial effusion. In both, the cardiac enlargement suggested a mass lesion and, in both, an intra-myocardial hemangioma was discovered at surgery.

Grossly, hemangiomas are red and hemorrhagic. Microscopically, they are classified according to the morphologic pattern and interrelationship of the vascular channels, endothelial cells, and supporting stroma. This microscopic classification (capillary, cavernous, intramuscular, hemangioendothelioma) is descriptive of varying growth patterns and does not necessarily imply differences in prognosis.[5]

When the tumors produce symptoms, the treatment of choice is surgical excision. The varied presentation of hemangiomas underscores the importance of a complete clinical evaluation in all patients with cardiac symptoms.

Varix

Varices are dilated blood vessels in the subendocardium that are frequently mistaken for hemangiomas. They may occur at any site in the heart but are most common in the subendocardium of either the atrial or ventricular septum. Varices are microscopically different from hemangiomas and consist of either a single or cluster of normally formed vascular channels, usually veins, which are dilated and frequently thrombosed, resembling hemorrhoids. The exact frequency of varices is unknown; however, they are usually incidental findings.[40]

Blood Cysts

Blood cysts are found on the endocardium, particularly the valvular endocardium, in newborns and infants (see Fig. 35–12). These cysts are usually lined by normal-appearing endothelial cells that are not delimited by a basement membrane. Occasionally, the lining cells are absent in the intravalvular portion of the blood cyst, in which case the cyst wall consists of endocardial stroma.[7] They contain blood, probably derived from the cavitary blood of the heart. These cysts are not true blood vessels or hemangiomas; they have no clinical significance.

Mesothelioma of the Atrioventricular Node

Mesotheliomas are always located in the region of the AV node and are composed of nests of mesothelial cells. They most likely originate in mesothelial rests, similar to adenomatoid tumors of the ovary and testis, and are always benign. Most patients with mesotheliomas have partial or complete heart block, usually of long duration, and often die of either complete heart block or ventricular fibrillation. This tumor has appropriately been referred to as the smallest tumor capable of causing sudden death. The 12 patients studied at the AFIP ranged in age from 11 months to 71 years, a distribution similar to that reported in the literature.

Grossly, the tumors are usually poorly circumscribed, slightly elevated nodules, located in the atrial septum immediately cephalad to the junction of the septal and anterior leaflets of the tricuspid valve in the region of the AV node (Fig. 35–21). On cross section, they are usually multicystic. Microscopically, the cysts are lined by uniform polygonal cells, frequently multilayered, with a suggestion of a "brush border" (Fig. 35–22). Interspersed with these cysts are multiple nests of cells of markedly varying size. The small nests appear solid, whereas the large nests frequently have a central lumen. The cells in the nests are often squamoid (Fig. 35–23). The nuclei are usually ovoid, and many have a cleftlike longitudinal indentation resembling so-called "coffee bean" nuclei. Foci of positive staining are present intracellularly and in the lumens of the cyst with the PAS reaction and with alcian blue. The intracellular PAS positivity is partially abolished by prior diastase digestion, whereas the extracellular PAS positivity is usually unaffected. Both the intracellular and extracellular positivities with alcian blue are abolished by prior hyaluronidase digestion. Occasionally, the amorphous material in

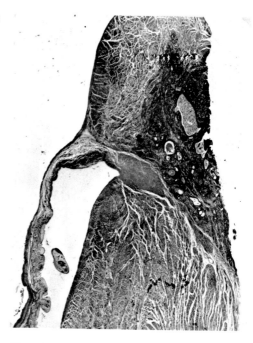

Fig. 35–21. Mesotheliomas of the AV node are located in the atrial septum at or close to the region of the AV node and are delineated from the ventricular myocardium by the fibrous annulus. The tumor is primarily subendocardial and only rarely replaces the full thickness of the atrial septum. This tumor completely replaced the AV node. (H&E, × 6.)

the cyst lumen will stain weakly positive with Best's mucicarmine.[26] The cellular nests and cystic structures are set in a dense connective tissue stroma. Within this stroma, collagen and elastic fibers are abundant and mast cells are frequent. The tumor usually replaces part or all of the AV node, and may extend proximally into the atrial septum and distally into the AV bundle.

Ultrastructurally, these tumors are strikingly similar to adenomatoid tumors of the ovary and testis. The luminal surface of the polygonal cells lining the cysts have numerous, widely spaced microvilli. These cells are multilayered, and there are numerous intercellular spaces bound on all sides by tight junctions and desmosomes. These are features of mesothelial cells and present further ev-

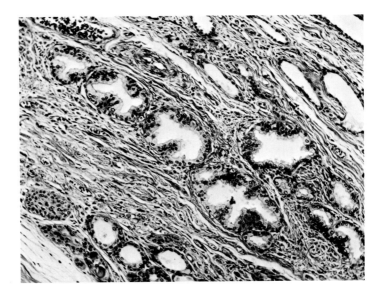

Fig. 35–22. The cells lining the smaller channels and spaces in the mesothelioma of the atrioventricular node vary widely in appearance. Occasionally, the lining cells are plump, cuboidal, or columnar, and there is a suggestion of cilia or a brush border by light microscopy. (H&E, × 150.)

idence that the tumors are of mesothelial origin with focal metaplasia.[22] Although some immunohistochemical studies have been interpreted to indicate that the tumors have an endodermal origin,[27,47] these findings have not been correlated with ultrastructural observations, so such a conclusion seems premature.

Since AV block, both complete and partial, is the major clinical manifestation of this tumor, the use of a pacemaker to maintain normal ventricular function appears indicated. However, even with cardiac pacing, two patients in our series developed ventricular fibrillation. Cardiac pacing, coupled with drug therapy to suppress residual AV nodal activity and possible accessory AV pathways, is probably indicated. (See also Ch. 37.)

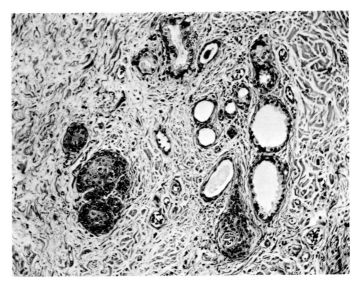

Fig. 35–23. In other areas of the same tumor illustrated in Fig. 35–22, small nests of cells which vary markedly in size are interspersed with the cysts. The small nests appear solid, whereas the large nests frequently have a central lumen. The cells in the nest are often squamoid. (H&E, × 115.)

Teratomas

Most true teratomas of the heart and pericardium are extracardiac but intrapericardial and arise from the base of the heart. They are usually attached to the root of the pulmonary artery and aorta and receive their blood supply from the vasa vasorum of these vessels (Fig. 35–24). Although intracardiac teratomas have been reported, most of the reports describe cysts that do not include all three germ layers. Teratomas may occur in adults, but the majority present in the pediatric age group. Females are affected much more commonly than males.[54]

The clinical and pathologic findings in 14 patients with intrapericardial teratomas were available for study at the AFIP. The patients ranged in age from less than 1 day to 42 years; however, 11 were in the pediatric age group. All were female, with one exception—a 10-week-old boy. Two patients in this series died suddenly and unexpectedly; the remaining 12 all presented with signs and symptoms relating to the heart. Dyspnea and cardiomegaly were among the presenting symptoms and signs in each patient. The infants were usually cyanotic and occasionally had cardiac murmurs. With the aid of newer diagnostic techniques in cardiology, a diagnosis of an extracardiac mass was established in each case since 1960. The teratoma was excised in eight patients; six were alive and well without evidence of recurrence at least 2 years after surgery, and two died during the postoperative period.

Intrapericardial teratomas may assume massive proportions, measuring up to 15 cm in diameter. They are pear shaped, usually smoothed surfaced, and lobulated. On section, the teratoma contains numerous multiloculated cysts and intervening solid areas (Fig. 35–25). Microscopically, intrapericardial teratomas resemble teratomas elsewhere in the body, and derivatives of all three germ layers are present. Like all teratomas, intrapericardial teratomas have a malignant potential, although this is decidedly unusual. Nevertheless, all teratomas should be adequately sampled in order to avoid overlooking the rare malignant example.

Surgical excision following diagnosis is the only effective therapy. Since these tumors usually receive their blood supply from the vasa vasorum of the aorta and pulmonary artery, effective removal must include a careful dissection of the root of these great arteries.

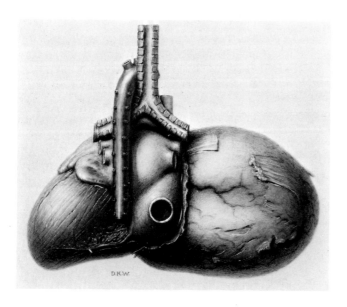

Fig. 35–24. Cardiac teratomas are usually intrapericardial and attached to the root of a pulmonary artery and aorta. These tumors may reach massive proportions.

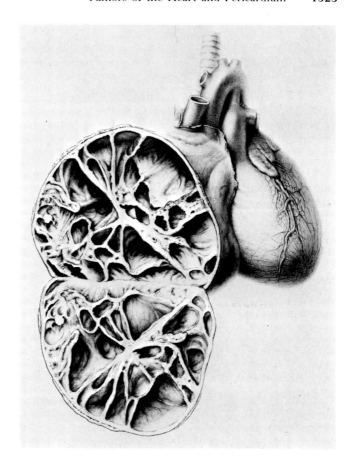

Fig. 35–25. On section the teratoma contains numerous multi-loculated cysts and intervening solid areas similar to teratomas occurring elsewhere in the body.

Bronchogenic Cysts

Bronchogenic cysts are usually contained within the myocardium, especially the ventricular myocardium, although occasionally they may project into a cardiac chamber or into the pericardial space. They rarely exceed 1 to 2 cm in diameter. Bronchogenic cysts are misplaced elements of the respiratory tract, and, unlike teratomas, contain only elements derived from mesoderm and ectoderm, arranged in an orderly manner resembling a bronchus.

Of the seven patients with cardiac bronchogenic cysts in the AFIP collection, five were male and two female—a sex distribution similar to that of bronchogenic cysts in the skin and subcutaneous tissues. In six of the seven patients, the cyst was an incidental find-ing at autopsy. These six patients ranged in age from 36 to 75 years. The other patient, a 6-month-old infant, presented with cardiomegaly and a loud systolic murmur. At autopsy, a large cyst protruded from the ventricular septum into the right ventricle displacing the tricuspid valve into the right atrium.

Intracardiac bronchogenic cysts are, with rare exception, incidental findings of no clinical significance. In the unusual exception, surgical excision would be indicated for relief of symptoms.[25]

Granular Cell Tumor

The granular cell tumor is a rare and apparently incidental finding in the heart that occurred in only three patients in the AFIP series.[20] All were adults, and none had cardiac symptoms. The tumors are frequently multiple.[53] Histologically, they are identical to granular cell tumors elsewhere in the body. The granular tumor comprises individual cells that are rounded or elongated and filled with cytoplasmic granules. These granules stain red with Masson's trichrome stain and exhibit a positive reaction with PAS that is unaffected with prior diastase digestion.[53]

Lymphangiomas and Hamartomas

Lymphangiomas are proliferations of lymphatic channels without proliferations of blood-carrying channels. They are uncommon in the heart but, as elsewhere in the body, are frequently diffuse proliferations rather than distinct tumors. Therefore, total excision is often not practical.[71,72] Cardiac transplantation may be considered an alternative treatment in these cases.[37] There were two cardiac lymphangiomas in the AFIP collection; one was found in the parietal pericardium and the other in the left ventricular myocardium. Lymphatic ectasia, which may occur in the heart, must be distinguished from lymphangioma.

Approximately 12 primary cardiac tumors composed of more than one type of mesenchymal tissue have been reported. Anbe and Fine[3] reviewed these tumors and concluded that all but two were, in fact, lymphangiomas of the heart. The two exceptions were considered best classified as arterial or venous malformations (vascular hamartomas). So-called lymphangioendotheliomas of the AV node are discussed under Mesothelioma of the Atrioventricular Node.

Intrapericardial Paraganglioma

Paragangliomas, such as pheochromocytomas and chemodectomas, may rarely be localized within the pericardium. Although these tumors may be found overlying or within any cardiac chamber, they most commonly occur over the base of the heart in the major region of vagus nerve distribution.[43] Detection and localization have been provided by iodine-131 metaiodobenzylguanidine (^{131}I-MIBG) nuclear scanning. Magnetic resonance imaging can further localize cardiac paragangliomas without the need for contrast material and may provide detailed information for better guidance of surgical excision. Although definitive diagnosis can only be made histologically, benign pathologic characteristics do not necessarily predict a favorable outcome, as these tumors are highly vascular, adherent, and difficult to resect. Human cardiac explantation and autotransplantation have been applied in a case involving a large cardiac paraganglioma.[17]

Neurofibroma

Although exceedingly rare, neurofibromas have been reported in the heart, especially as a complication of von Recklinghausen's disease. In the AFIP collection, three neurofibromas involved the heart. One was present in the parietal pericardium, and two in the left ventricular myocardium. Two of the patients had von Recklinghausen's disease, whereas, during childhood, the third had a neuroblastoma treated with radiation. Neurofibromas have also been reported in the right ventricle.[66] Neurofibromas occurring in the heart are identical grossly and microscopically to those occurring elsewhere in the body.

Angiosarcoma

Angiosarcoma is the most frequently occurring primary cardiac sarcoma and is two to three times more common in men than in women. The site of origin is most frequently the right side of the heart, especially the right atrium, followed by the pericardium. Eighty percent of the primary cardiac angiosarcomas in the 39 patients in the AFIP series originated in the right atrium or pericardium.[54] In approximately 25 percent of these patients, a portion of the angiosarcoma was intracavitary and obstructed a valve orifice. The tricuspid valve was most frequently obstructed by a right atrial tumor mass (seven patients), although the pulmonary valve was obstructed in two patients and the mitral valve in one. All 39 patients ranged in age from 15 to 76 years, although 70 percent were between 20 and 50 years. Seventy-seven percent of patients had clinical findings of right-sided heart failure or of pericardial disease. These findings included congestive heart failure, pericardial effusion, dyspnea, and pleuritic chest pain. However, a significant number of patients (10 percent) had symptoms suggestive of malignancy (fever, weight loss, and malaise) without cardiac findings or before cardiac findings were noted. Systolic murmurs and atrial arrhythmias were present in six patients, each of whom also had evidence of right-sided heart failure. All patients presented with cardiomegaly by chest radiograph and with ECG abnormalities, such as nonspecific ST-segment and T-wave changes and/or low voltage. Only 11 patients had distant metastases; in three they were confined to the nervous system. Five additional patients had local spread of the tumor either to the adjacent pleura or mediastinum, or both.

Microscopically, angiosarcomas are composed of malignant cells forming vascular channels; however, there is usually considerable variation in histology, even within the same tumor. Most angiosarcomas contain foci of solid areas of spindle cells; occasionally, they are composed almost entirely of sheets of rounded anaplastic cells or spindle cells. Even in these cellular, solid-appearing angiosarcomas, a reticulum stain will usually demonstrate a vascular pattern in at least part of the tumor. The vascular channels vary markedly in size and configuration, but there are usually multiple anastomosing channels lined by rounded or elongated, often multilayered, endothelial cells. Occasionally these proliferating endothelial cells fill the vascular channels, thus giving the tumor a solid appearance. Pleomorphism and anaplasia may be marked, and mitoses are usually frequent, as are intraluminal tufting projections of multilayered endothelial cells without an intervening stroma. Spindle cell areas commonly merge imperceptibly with vascular and solid areas.

Anastomosing vascular channels, foci of endothelial tufting, and spindle cell areas are the most reliable indicators of angiosarcoma. In combination with these features, pleomorphism, anaplasia, and mitoses are adjunctive diagnostic aids; alone, however, they are not reliable indicators of malignancy in an endothelial tumor.

These tumors are often subclassified on the basis of their microscopic appearance; however, since their clinical course and prognosis appear to be identical, irrespective of the subclassification, the all-inclusive term, angiosarcoma, is preferable. Without treatment, prognosis is poor; most patients die within a year of the onset of symptoms. In the future, newer pathologic techniques for the identification of sarcomas, aggressive surgical resection, and advanced chemotherapy and radiotherapy may contribute to better survival for patients with these tumors.

Kaposi Sarcoma

Metastatic Kaposi sarcoma to the epicardium and myocardium has been described in autopsy studies of patients with acquired immune deficiency syndrome (AIDS),[12] and primary Kaposi sarcoma has also been reported in this group of patients.[4]

Rhabdomyosarcoma

Rhabdomyosarcoma, the second most common primary sarcoma of the heart, is a neoplasm composed of malignant cells with features of striated muscle. Rhabdomyosarcomas have been reported in patients ranging in age from 3 months to 80 years but, like other primary sarcomas, they are rare in the pediatric age group. In the AFIP collection of 26 rhabdomyosarcomas primary in the heart, the ages range from 1 to 66 years, with only two patients in the pediatric age group. The incidence of cardiac rhabdomyosarcoma in the adult population is nearly equal in all decades. A slightly increased incidence in men over women has been reported.[54]

The majority of patients in the AFIP collection had nonspecific symptoms, characterized by fever, anorexia, malaise, and weight loss—symptoms more indicative of malignancy than of cardiac disease. However, findings of pericardial disease, pleuritic chest pain, pleural effusion, dyspnea, and embolic phenomena—both pulmonary and cerebral—were common in patients with rhabdomyosarcoma. A common denominator in all patients was cardiomegaly by chest radiograph and nonspecific electrocardiographic changes, such as ST-segment and T-wave changes, low voltage, and/or varying degrees of bundle branch block. Most frequently the heart borders were irregular and the contour of the heart was distorted. In addition, 50 percent of patients had unexplained murmurs, usually systolic and of recent onset and/ or intractable atrial or ventricular arrhythmias. Findings of obstruction to blood flow, such as congestive heart failure, were common. In each patient in which a cardiac murmur was noted, a large portion of the rhabdomyosarcoma was intracavitary, and there was significant obstruction of at least one valve orifice. Approximately 50 percent of the patients in this series had partial obstruction of at least one valve orifice, the mitral and pulmonic orifices being the most frequently obstructed. Unlike benign intracavitary tumors, the cardiac valves are often invaded, occasionally with extensive valve replacement by adjacent intracavitary rhabdomyosarcoma.[54]

Unlike angiosarcoma, rhabdomyosarcoma does not have a propensity for arising in a particular cardiac chamber. These tumors originate with equal frequency in the left and right heart; in approximately 60 percent of patients, the tumor involves multiple sites within the heart at autopsy. The pericardium is involved in 50 percent of these patients, usually by direct extension of the tumor from the myocardium. However, diffuse pericardial involvement characteristic of mesothelioma or angiosarcoma is not a feature of rhabdomyosarcoma. Occasionally, the tumor extends beyond the parietal pericardium to the contiguous mediastinum or pleural cavity. Microscopically, both juvenile forms (embryonal or alveolar) and adult forms occur. However, the adult form is much more common. The diagnosis of rhabdomyosarcoma is made by identifying convincing rhabdomyoblasts. This is often extremely difficult in that the tumors usually exhibit marked pleomorphism and anaplasia. The nuclei vary widely in size, shape, and chromaticity. Pyknotic nuclei are rare, but giant forms and abnormal mitoses are frequent; the nuclei are often large and vesicular (Fig. 35–26). Spindle cell foci as well as solid, cellular, and loose myxoid areas are frequently present within the same tumor. Microscopic foci of necrosis and hemorrhage are common. This marked variation in the microscopic appearance of rhabdomyosarcoma is one indicator to its diagnosis and should precipitate the search for rhabdomyoblasts. Cross-striations may be identified by light microscopy using the phosphotunsic acid hematoxylin stain; the appropriate area of the paraffin block is then excised and processed for electron microscopy. Ultrastructurally, both thick and thin filaments (actin and myosin) as well as a Z-band material must be identified. Only rarely will these elements be organized into the characteristic sarcomere of striated muscle; more commonly they are arranged haphazardly throughout the cytoplasm.[59] Immunohistochemical analysis of these neoplasms is also helpful. Monoclonal antidesmin and monoclonal antimyoglobin antibodies, as well as immunoperoxidase detection of intracellular Z-protein, aid in identifying myoblastic differentiation.

Excision of the main tumor mass, followed by combined radiation therapy and chemotherapy, is recommended. In spite of therapy, prognosis is generally poor, although 3-year survivals following treatment have been reported. Most patients, however, die within 1 year of diagnosis.

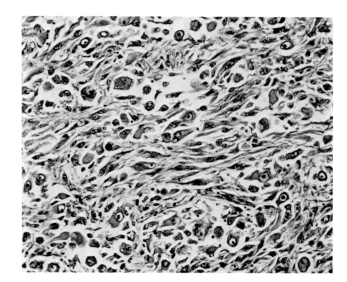

Fig. 35–26. Marked cellular pleomorphism and nuclear atypia are characteristic of rhabdomyosarcoma. Multinucleated cells and abnormal, often bizarre, mitoses are frequent. Strap-shaped and racquet-shaped cells are highly suggestive but not diagnostic of rhabdomyosarcoma. (H&E, × 195.)

Fibrosarcoma and Malignant Fibrous Histiocytoma

Fibrosarcoma and malignant fibrous histiocytoma are malignant mesenchymal tumors that are primarily fibroblastic in their differentiation. The clinical and pathologic findings of 14 patients with malignant cardiac fibroblastic tumors were available at the AFIP. The clinical findings associated with these tumors are often multiple and confusing. The most common findings in patients with fibrosarcoma of the heart include systolic murmurs, often of changing intensity and recent onset; nonspecific ECG changes including ST-segment and T-wave changes, low voltage, and bundle branch block; arrhythmias, especially atrial arrhythmias; and findings of pericardial disease including chest pain, fever, and dyspnea. Eight percent of the patients in this series had one or more of these signs or symptoms. In addition, two patients had symptoms usually suggestive of malignancy, including weight loss, fever, and malaise.

Five of the 14 patients had distant metastases involving other viscera, and in two additional patients there was a direct spread of the tumor to involve adjacent structures. The patients in this series ranged in age from less than 1 year to 87 years.

These tumors arise with equal frequency on the left and right sides of the heart, with no predilection for any single site. They may be nodular or infiltrative, and are firm and gray-white. In slightly more than one-half of the patients, they involve multiple sites within the heart at autopsy. The pericardium is invaded in approximately one-third, and a portion of the tumor protrudes into a cardiac chamber causing significant obstruction of a valve orifice, or invasion of a valve leaflet in 50 percent of patients. The mitral valve was involved in four patients, the pulmonary valve in two, and the tricuspid valve in one.

Microscopically, fibrosarcomas consist of spindle-shaped cells with elongated blunt-ended nuclei and tapering cytoplasm. Although mitoses are usually frequent, pleomorphism and anaplasia are generally minimal. Nucleoli are not prominent. The spindle cells are arranged haphazardly, occasionally in broad bundles or fascicles that may course at acute angles to one another; however, palisading nuclei and interlacing cords of cells are not features of fibrosarcoma. Tumor necrosis is rare, but foci of myxoid change are common. Metaplastic cartilage and bone are often present but do not provide sufficient reason to classify these tumors as malignant mesenchymomas.

Malignant fibrous histiocytoma has fibrosarcomatous areas, but it is differentiated from fibrosarcoma in that the former has a whorled pattern of the spindle cells and the presence of giant cells, often with multiple nuclei. Immunohistochemical studies may aid in establishing the fibroblastic origin of these sarcomas.

Ultrastructurally, both fibrosarcoma and malignant fibrous histiocytoma consist primarily of fibroblastic cells. The nuclei are usually multilobed, and the elongated cell body contains multiple cytoplasmic processes. The cells lack a basement membrane and collagen fibrils are present in cellular bays, closely associated with the cell membrane. In addition, malignant fibrous histiocytomas contain so-called pale cells which are ovoid with few cytoplasmic processes and sparse, rough-surfaced endoplasmic reticulum. Like fibroblastic cells, however, they lack a basement membrane.[54]

Although radiation and chemotherapy have been tried with minimal success, no therapy has been especially effective for treating malignant fibroblastic tumors of the heart; however, in the future, aggressive surgical resection with advanced chemotherapy and radiotherapy may contribute to better survival.

Cardiac transplantation may also have a therapeutic role for patients with localized disease.

Lymphoma

By definition, a primary lymphoma of the heart must involve only the heart and pericardium. Lymphomas primary in the heart have been found in patients from 14 months to 84 years of age.

The AFIP series included seven examples. The patients ranged in age from 18 to 77 years, with a nearly equal incidence among men and women. In three of these patients, lymphoma was an incidental finding at autopsy. In the remaining four, the most common findings were congestive heart failure, cardiomegaly, and pericardial effusion. All four patients died of intractable congestive heart failure without clinical suspicion of malignant disease.[54] An increased incidence of lymphoma, including cardiac lymphoma, has been noted in patients with AIDS,[16,36] and in transplant patients receiving immunosuppresive therapy.[64] Most of these cardiac lymphomas have been of B-cell lineage.

In the AFIP series, all sites in the heart were involved without apparent predilection for any specific site. In two patients, the lymphoma diffusely involved the pericardium (both visceral and parietal) and the myocardium. Both patients had cardiomegaly by chest radiograph and died of intractable congestive heart failure. In the remaining five patients, the lymphoma was localized, although there were multiple sites of involvement in three patients. A portion of the lymphoma was intracavitary in two patients and partially obstructed the pulmonary valve in another.

Surgical excision followed by radiation therapy or chemotherapy is the treatment of choice. In none of the patients in the AFIP series was the tumor diagnosed antemortem, and all died within a year of the onset of the symptoms.

Extraskeletal Osteosarcoma

When extraskeletal osteosarcoma is primary in the heart, it most commonly arises in the left atrium, usually from the posterior wall, near the entrance of the pulmonary veins (Fig. 35–27). Of the five tumors in the AFIP series, three were primary in the left atrium, one was in the right atrium, and one in the right ventricle. The five patients in this series—four men and one woman—ranged in age from 16 to 58 years.[54] Their clinical findings were similar to those associated with other sarcomas of the heart: progressive congestive heart failure, dyspnea, and cardiac murmurs of recent onset. Systolic murmurs were present in three of the patients; in all three, an intracavitary tumor was diagnosed with the aid of angiography, and the intracavitary portion of the tumor was excised surgically.

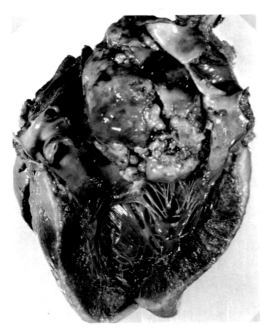

Fig. 35–27. This osteosarcoma originated in the posterior wall of the left atrium. A large portion of the tumor is intracavitary and has partially replaced the mitral valve, obstructing the valve orifice.

A portion of the tumor was intracavitary in four of the five patients; the mitral valve was obstructed in two, the tricuspid valve in one, and the pulmonary in another. In the fifth patient, both the mitral and aortic valves were invaded by the tumor, although neither valve orifice was obstructed.

Microscopically, these tumors have fibrosarcomatous areas in close association with areas of osteoid and malignant osteoblasts. Foci of apparent chondrosarcoma are not uncommon. Many tumors, especially fibrosarcomas, contain foci of metaplastic bone or cartilage and should not be confused with extraskeletal osteosarcoma. Pure extraskeletal chondrosarcomas primary in the heart are rarely encountered.

In three patients, metastases were to the lungs, adjacent soft tissues, or liver. Metastases and secondary sites of involvement within the heart contained foci of osteoid and were composed entirely of osteoid and malignant osteoblasts in two tumors.

Four patients in the series died within 2 years in spite of surgery, radiation therapy, and/or chemotherapy. The remaining patient, who lived 4 years after onset of symptoms, was treated with radiation therapy and chemotherapy following excision of the intracavitary portion of the tumor.

Malignant Nerve Sheath Tumors

All four patients with malignant nerve sheath tumors in the AFIP series were male, and ranged in age from 9 to 52 years. All presented with pleuritic chest pain, dyspnea, and pericardial effusion. Two patients had nonspecific ECG findings of low voltage and left ventricle strain. A systolic murmur was present in one patient. In three of these patients, a diagnosis of pericardial tumor was made antemortem with the aid of echocardiography and angiocardiography. Surgical excision was attempted in each patient.[54]

All four tumors involved the visceral pericardium over the base of the heart. In three patients, primary involvement was over the outflow tract of the right ventricle and pulmonary artery. In the fourth, the bulk of the tumor was situated over the right atrium. In each patient, the underlying myocardium was invaded; in two, the parietal pericardium was involved. The main mass of the tumor was intrapericardial in all four patients. In one, the adjacent mediastinum was involved, and there were metastases to the lungs in two patients.

These tumors presumably are derived from the cells of nerve sheaths. In all probability, when they involve the heart primarily, they originate in the cardiac plexus or the vagus nerve innervation of the heart.

All reported malignant nerve sheath tumors, as well as the four tumors in this series, were located on the visceral pericardium at the base of the heart on the right side—the precise location of the vagus nerve innervation of the heart.

Three of the patients in this series were diagnosed antemortem. Of these, two died within a year despite radiation and chemotherapy following surgical excision of the main intrapericardial mass. The third patient had evidence of recurrent disease 1 year after surgery.

Malignant Teratoma

Malignant teratomas, unlike most primary cardiac sarcomas, occur most commonly in children. Like their benign counterparts, they are primarily intrapericardial, attached to the base of the heart, and more common in females. A malignant teratoma is a teratoma in which one of the elements has undergone a malignant change, either metastasizing to or invading adjacent structures. The malignant portion may be a carcinoma or a sarcoma. When the malignant portion of the tumor is embryonal carcinoma, the tumor is termed teratocarcinoma. The most common malignancy is embryonal carcinoma, but examples of choriocarcinoma and squamous cell carcinoma have also been recognized.[8]

All four malignant teratomas in the AFIP collection occurred in children—three girls and one boy—ranging in age from 1 to 4 years. Each child in this series had congestive heart failure, usually associated with anorexia and vomiting. All four had cardiomegaly by chest radiograph; two had arrhythmias and nonspecific electrocardiographic findings, and one had a systolic murmur. Three of the tumors were primarily intrapericardial, attached to the root of the aorta and pulmonary artery. In each, elements derived from all three germ layers were identified. Two patients had metastases to the lungs and mediastinum, and another patient had extensive invasion of the myocardium of the left and right ventricles. In the fourth patient, the tumor was situated over the anterior surface of the heart and had invaded the ventricular septum and right ventricle. A large portion of the tumor was intracavitary within the right ventricle, but it did not appear to obstruct either the tricuspid or pulmonary valve. The main mass of this tumor and the pulmonary metastases were both embryonal carcinoma and choriocarcinoma.

Surgical excision of the pericardial mass was attempted in one patient; however, the tumor had invaded the heart so extensively that excision was impossible. All four children died within 3 months of the onset of symptoms.

Leiomyosarcoma

Malignant tumors derived from smooth muscle are extremely rare in the heart and pericardium. Approximately eight leiomyosarcomas of the heart have been reported; however, in at least half of the cases the heart was not unequivocally the primary site of the tumor.[54]

Microscopically, leiomyosarcomas in the heart are recognized by their elongated cells with blunt-ended nuclei. These cells grow in interlacing cords, and the suggestion of nuclear palisading is often present. The nuclei may be large and vesicular or hyperchromatic, and mitoses are often, but not always, numerous. In poorly differentiated examples of this neoplasm, immunohistochemistry and electron microscopy may help distinguish leiomyosarcomas from fibrosarcomas and neurogenic sarcomas. Ultrastructurally, these cells contain haphazardly oriented bundles of myofibrils with characteristic spindle-shaped densities, presumably tropomyosin. The cell membrane is distinct, and there is a well-defined basement membrane. Marginal dense bodies similar to the spindle-shaped densities of the myofibrils are frequently found against the cell membrane.

TUMORS OF THE MAJOR BLOOD VESSELS

Tumors arising in major blood vessels are distinctly uncommon. The majority are of smooth muscle origin; leiomyomas and leiomyosarcomas account for 70 percent of all reported cases and for more than 90 percent of tumors arising in large veins.[54]

Approximately 65 percent of all primary tumors of major blood vessels arise in large veins. Most smooth muscle tumors of large veins are malignant; indeed, slightly more than 75 percent of all benign and malignant tumors arising in large veins are leiomyosarcomas.[45] Approximately half of leiomyosarcomas of the large veins arise in the inferior vena cava; they are much more common in women, outnumbering men by 8:1. Veins of the lower extremity are the next most frequently involved (60 percent), followed by veins of the torso (25 percent) and the upper extremities and head and neck (15 percent).[45] Approximately 16 percent of smooth muscle tumors of veins are benign. They have the microscopic appearance of leiomyomas elsewhere in the body.

Primary neoplasms of large arteries are extremely unusual, and with few exceptions all of those reported have been malignant. Histologically, approximately one-fourth of the sarcomas of the pulmonary artery are leiomyosarcomas.[45] These tumors appear to arise in the main pulmonary artery and may grow in a retrograde fashion, involving the pulmonary valve, or extend along branches of the pulmonary artery into the lung. Less commonly, fibrosarcoma, angiosarcoma, rhabdomyosarcoma, osteosarcoma, chondrosarcoma, and malignant mesenchymoma primary in the pulmonary artery have been reported.

In the aorta, sarcomas are equally divided between the thoracic and abdominal regions. The sarcomas of the aorta and its major tributaries appear to arise in the wall of the vessel affected. They rarely occlude the vessel lumen, but, rather, grow along the intimal surface. Many of these tumors are confined to the intimal layer of the artery without evidence of invasion of the muscular wall. The two most common types of sarcoma involving major arteries are leiomyosarcoma and fibrosarcoma. Intimal fibroplasia involving the large arteries must not be confused with sarcoma.[54]

REFERENCES

1. Abenoza P, Sibley RK: Cardiac myxoma with glandlike structures. An immunohistochemical study. Arch Pathol Lab Med 110:736, 1986
2. Allenlay AL, Ferry DA, Lin B, et al: Spontaneous regression of cardiac rhabdomyoma in tuberous sclerosis. Clin Pediatr 26:532, 1987
3. Anbe DT, Fine G: Cardiac lymphangioma and lipoma. Report of a case of simultaneous occurrence in association with lipomatous infiltration of the myocardium and cardiac arrhythmia. Am Heart J 86:227, 1973
4. Autran B, Garlin I, Leibowitch M: AIDS in a Haitian woman with cardiac Kaposi sarcoma and Whipple disease. Lancet 1:767, 1983
5. Baroldi G, Colombo F, Manion WC: Benign primary hemangioma of the right atrium of the heart. Report of a case. Med Ann DC 36:287, 1967
6. Bearman RM: Primary leiomyosarcoma of the heart: Report of a case and review of the literature. Arch Pathol 98:62, 1974
7. Begg JG: Blood-filled cysts in the cardiac valve cusps in foetal life and infancy. J Pathol 87:177, 1964
8. Berry CL, Keeling J, Hilton C: Teratoma in infancy and childhood. A review of 91 cases. J Pathol 98:241, 1969
9. Boxer ME: Cardiac myxoma: An immunoperoxidase study of histogenesis. Histopathology 8:861, 1984
10. Brandes WW, Gray JAC, MacLeod NW: Leiomyoma of the pericardium. Report of a case. Am Heart J 23:426, 1942
11. Burns ER, Schulman IC, Murphy MJ Jr: Hematologic manifestations and etiology of atrial myxoma. Am J Med Sci 284:17, 1982
12. Cammarosano C, Lewis W: Cardiac lesions in acquired immune deficiency syndrome (AIDS). J Am Coll Cardiol 5:703, 1985
13. Carney JA: Differences between nonfamilial and familial cardiac myxoma. Am J Surg Pathol 9:53, 1985
14. Carney JA, Hruska LS, Beauchamp GD, Gordon H: Dominant inheritance of the complex of myxomas, spotty pigmentation, and endo-

crine overactivity. Mayo Clin Proc 61:165, 1986

15. Coard KC, Silver MD: Gamna body of the heart. Pathology 16:459, 1984

16. Constantino A, West TE, Gupta M, Loghmanee F: Primary cardiac lymphoma in a patient with acquired immune deficiency syndrome. Cancer 60:2801, 1987

17. Cooley DA, Reardon MJ, Frazier OH: Human cardiac explantation and autotransplantation: Application in a patient with a large cardiac pheochromocytoma. Texas Heart Institute Journal 12:171, 1985

18. Dewald GW, Dahl RJ, Sparbeck JL, et al: Chromosomally abnormal clones and nonrandom telomeric translocations in cardiac myxomas. Mayo Clin Proc 62:558, 1987

19. Feigin DS, Fenoglio JJ, McAllister HA Jr, Madewell JE: Pericardial cysts: A radiologic-pathologic correlation and review. Radiology 125:15, 1977

20. Fenoglio JJ, McAllister HA Jr: Granular cell tumors of the heart. Arch Pathol 100:276, 1976

21. Fenoglio JJ, Diana DJ, Bowen TE, et al: Ultrastructure of a cardiac rhabdomyoma. Hum Pathol 8:700, 1977

22. Fenoglio JJ, Jacobs DW, McAllister HA Jr: Ultrastructure of the mesothelioma of the atrioventricular node. Cancer 40:721, 1977

23. Fenoglio JJ, McAllister HA Jr, Ferrans VJ: Cardiac rhabdomyoma: A clinicopathologic and electron microscopic study. Am J Cardiol 38:241, 1976

24. Ferrans VJ, Roberts WC: Structural features of cardiac myxomas. Hum Pathol 4:111, 1973

25. Fine G: Neoplasms of the pericardium and heart. p. 868. In Gould SE (ed): Pathology of the Heart and Blood Vessels. Charles C Thomas, Springfield, IL, 1968

26. Fine G, Morales AR: Mesothelioma of the atrioventricular node. Arch Pathol 92:402, 1971

27. Fine G, Raju U: Congenital polycystic tumor of the atrioventricular node: A histogenetic appraisal with evidence for its endodermal origin. Hum Pathol 18:791, 1987

28. Fine G, Morales A, Horn RC: Cardiac myxoma. A morphologic and histogenetic appraisal. Cancer 22:1156, 1968

29. Fishbein MC, Ferrans VJ, Roberts WC: Endocardial papillary elastofibromas. Histologic,

histochemical, and electron microscopic findings. Arch Pathol 99:335, 1975

30. Fyke FE, Tajik AJ, Edwards WD, Seward JB: Diagnosis of lipomatous hypertrophy of the atrial septum by two-dimensional echocardiography. J Am Coll Cardiol 1:1352, 1983

31. Glasser SP, Bedynek JL, Hall RJ, et al: Left atrial myxoma. Report of a case including hemodynamic, surgical, histologic and histochemical characteristics. Am J Med 50:113, 1971

32. Goldman BI, Frydman C, Harpaz N, et al: Glandular cardiac myxomas. Histologic, immunohistochemical and ultrastructural evidence of epithelial differentiation. Cancer 59:1767, 1987

33. Govani E, Severi B, Cenacchi G, et al: Ultrastructural and immunohistochemical contribution to the histogenesis of human cardiac myxoma. Ultrastruct Pathol 12:221, 233, 1988

34. Gray IR, Williams WG: Recurring cardiac myxoma. Br Heart J 53:645, 1985

35. Griffiths GC: A review of primary tumors of the heart. Prog Cardiovasc Dis 7:465, 1965

36. Guarner J, Brynes RK, Chan WC, et al: Primary non-Hodgkin's lymphoma of the heart in two patients with the acquired immunodeficiency syndrome. Arch Pathol Lab Med 111:254, 1987

37. Hall RJ, Cooley DA, McAllister HA Jr, et al: Neoplastic diseases of the heart. p. 1382. In Hurst JW (ed): The Heart. 7th Ed. McGraw-Hill, New York, 1989

38. Heath D: Cardiac fibroma. Br Heart J 31:656, 1969

39. Heath D, Best PV, Davis BT: Papilliferous tumours of the heart valves. Br Heart J 23:20, 1961

40. Heggtveit HA: Thrombosed varices of the heart. Am J Pathol 48:50a, 1966

41. Heggtveit HA, Fenoglio JJ, McAllister HA Jr: Lipomatous hypertrophy of the interatrial septum: An assessment of 41 cases. Lab Invest 34:318, 1976

42. Hoch-Ligeti C, Restrepo C, Stewart HL: Comparative pathology of cardiac neoplasms in humans and in laboratory rodents: A review. J Natl Cancer Inst 1:127, 1986

43. Hui G, McAllister HA Jr, Angelini P: Left atrial paraganglioma: Report of a case and review of the literature. Am Heart J 113:1230, 1987

44. James TN, Carson DJ, Marshall TK: De subitaneis morbitus. 1. Fibroma compressing His bundle. Circulation 48:428, 1973

45. Kerorkian J, Cento DP: Leiomyosarcoma of large arteries and veins. Surgery 73:390, 1973

46. Levine RA, Weyman AE, Dinsmore RE, et al: Noninvasive tissue characterization: Diagnosis of lipomatous hypertrophy at the atrial septum by nuclear magnetic resonance imaging. J Am Coll Cardiol 7:688, 1986

47. Linder J, Shelburne JD, Surge JP, et al: Congenital endodermal heterotopia of the atrioventricular node: Evidence for the endodermal origin of so-called mesotheliomas at the atrioventricular node. Hum Pathol 15:1093, 1984

48. Lund JT, Ehman RL, Julsrud PR, et al: Cardiac masses: Assessment by MR imaging. AJR 152:469, 1989

49. Magarey FR: On the mode of formation of Lambl's excrescences and their relation to chronic thickening of the mitral valve. J Pathol 61:203, 1949

50. Mahaim I: Les tumeurs et les polypes du coeur. Masson et Cie, Paris, 1945

51. McAllister HA Jr: Primary tumors of the heart and pericardium. p. 1. In Harvey WP (ed): Current Problems in Cardiology. Year Book Medical Publishers, Chicago, 1979

52. McAllister HA Jr: Primary tumors of the heart and pericardium. p. 325. In Sommers SC and Rosen PP (eds): Pathology Annual. Appleton-Century-Crofts, East Norwalk, CT, 1979

53. McAllister HA Jr, Fenoglio JJ: Granular cell tumor of the heart: A report of three cases. Arch Pathol 100:276, 1976

54. McAllister HA Jr, Fenoglio JJ Jr: Tumors of the Cardiovascular System. Fascicle 15, Second Series. Atlas of Tumor Pathology. Armed Forces Institute of Pathology, Washington, DC, 1978

55. McAllister HA Jr, Hall RJ: Iatrogenic heart disease. p. 871. In Cheng TO (ed): The International Textbook of Cardiology. Pergamon Press, New York, 1986

56. McAllister HA Jr, Hall RJ, Cooley DA: Surgical pathology of tumors and cysts of the heart and pericardium. p. 343. In Waller BF (ed): Contemporary Issues in Surgical Pathology. Churchill Livingstone, New York, 1988

57. McComb RD: Heterogeneous expression of factor VIII/Von Willebrand factor by cardiac myxoma cells. Am J Surg Pathol 8:539, 1984

58. Morales AR, Fine G, Casto A, Nadji M: Cardiac myxoma (endocardioma): An immunocytochemical assessment of histogenesis. Hum Pathol 12:896, 1981

59. Morales AR, Fine G, Horn RC: Rhabdomyosarcoma: An ultrastructural appraisal. Pathol Annu 7:81, 1972

60. Ott DA, Garson A, Cooley DA, McNamara DG: Definitive operation for refractory cardiac tachyarrhythmias in children. J Thorac Cardiovasc Surg 90:681, 1985

61. Page DL: Lipomatous hypertrophy of the cardiac interatrial septum: Its development and probable clinical significance. Hum Pathol 1:151, 1970

62. Pomerance A: Papillary "tumours" of the heart valves. J Pathol 81:135, 1961

63. Roberts WC, Spray TL: Pericardial heart disease. Curr Probl Cardiol 2:1, 1977

64. Rodenburg CJ, Kluin P, Maes A, Paul LC: Malignant lymphoma confined to the heart, 13 years after cadaver kidney transplant. N Engl J Med 313:122, 1985

65. Rogers AM, Kesten HD: A thyroid mass in the ventricular septum obstructing the right ventricular outflow tract and producing a murmur. J Cardiovasc Surg 4:175, 1963

66. Rosenquist GC, Krovetz LJ, Haller JA, et al: Acquired right ventricular outflow obstruction in a child with neurofibromatosis. Am Heart J 79:103, 1970

67. Salyer WR, Page DL, Hutchins GM: The development of cardiac myxomas and papillary endocardial lesions from mural thrombus. Am Heart J 89:4, 1975

68. Schuger L, Ron N, Rosenmann E: Cardiac myxoma. A retrospective immunohistochemical study. Pathol Res Pract 182:63, 1987

69. Sytman AL, MacAlpin RN: Primary pericardial mesothelioma: Report of two cases and review of the literature. Am Heart J 81:760, 1971

70. Tanimara A, Kitazono M, Nagayama K, et al: Cardiac myxoma: Morphologic, histochemical, and tissue culture studies. Hum Pathol 19:316, 1988

71. Trout HH, McAllister HA Jr: Treatment of vascular anomalies in infancy and childhood. p. 380. In Ernst CB, Stanley JC (eds): Current

Therapy in Vascular Surgery. BC Decker, Philadelphia, 1987

72. Trout HH, McAllister HA Jr, Giordano JM, Rich NM: Vascular malformations. Surgery 97:36, 1985

73. Valente M: Structural profile of cardiac myxoma. Appl Pathol 1:251, 1983

74. Vasile N, Nicoleau F, Mathieu D: CT features of cardio-pericardial masses. Eur J Radiol 1:21, 1986

75. Wang S-C, Dirkman SH, Goldberg SL, Depisch LM: Gamna-Gandy body in a cardiac myxoma. Mt Sinai J Med 41:524, 1974

76. Williamson BR, Sturtevant NV, Black WC, et al: Epicardial lipoma: A CT diagnosis. Comput Radiol 9:169, 1985

77. Wychulis AR, Connolly DC, McGoon DC: Pericardial cysts, tumors, and fat necrosis. J Thorac Cardiovasc Surg 62:294, 1971

78. Zanca P, Chuang TH, DeAvila R: True congenital mediastinal thymic cyst. Pediatrics 36:615, 1965

36

Cardiovascular Trauma

H. Alexander Heggtveit

Cardiovascular trauma ranks second only to craniocerebral injury as a major cause of morbidity and mortality in both civilian and military spheres. Mechanical injuries of the heart and blood vessels are increasingly the basis for accident insurance or worker's compensation claims. Cardiac surgery and invasive cardiologic procedures have widened the range of iatrogenic lesions of the cardiovascular system. Rich and Spencer[86] and Symbas[108–110] have addressed the current status and management of cardiovascular trauma. The pathologic findings and older literature have been assessed in books by Gould[34] and Hudson.[45] In this chapter, the basic types and mechanisms of heart and blood vessel injuries are reviewed with emphasis on iatrogenic vascular trauma. While some of the consequences may be the same, it is convenient to consider separately the effects of penetrating and nonpenetrating injury.

PENETRATING INJURIES

Common in military casualties,[86] penetrating wounds of the heart and great vessels are becoming much more frequent in the civilian population as urban violence escalates.[6,85] Penetrating wounds are usually the result of a bullet (Fig. 36–1) or knife (Fig. 36–2) wound to the chest or neck and less often are caused by puncture wounds from other sharp objects

such as ice picks, metal shrapnel, pins, or arrows (Fig. 36–3). Multiple penetrating wounds of the heart can result from indriven fragments of fractured ribs in falls from great height or other severe crushing injuries of the chest (Fig. 36–4). The nature of an injury inflicted on the vascular structures is related to the physical properties of a missile as well as to its velocity and force. High-velocity projectiles such as rivets or bullets possess great kinetic energy. Thus, even a small-caliber bullet can inflict extensive injury, out of proportion to its size. More massive wounds result from larger-caliber slugs or shotgun injuries (Figs. 36–5 and 36–6). Generally speaking, the closer the range, the greater the destructive force released; in the case of very close range or contact gunshot wounds, the destructive force is compounded by the effect of the muzzle blast of hot gases. Gunshot wounds tend not only to penetrate but also to perforate the heart or great vessels. The associated massive tissue destruction often leads to exsanguinating hemorrhage.

By contrast, knife wounds are of low velocity and are more likely to produce localized penetrating injuries, which, although transmural, do not necessarily perforate a chamber. Such wounds may seal or close spontaneously, especially when confined to the thicker left ventricle. Despite lower intracavity pressures in the atria and right ventricle, these thin-walled chambers are more likely to bleed when punctured. Thus, the site of a

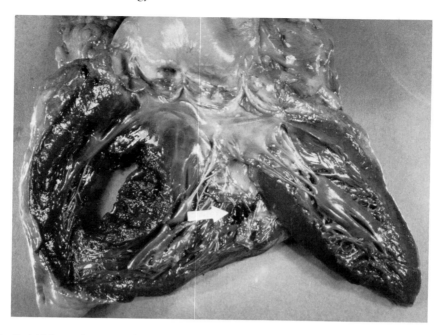

Fig. 36–1. Suicidal gunshot wound of heart (0.22-caliber handgun). The bullet produced a small entry wound in the anterior free wall of the right ventricle (not shown), a large ventricular septal defect, and a small exit wound in the posterobasal wall of the left ventricle beneath the mitral valve (arrow).

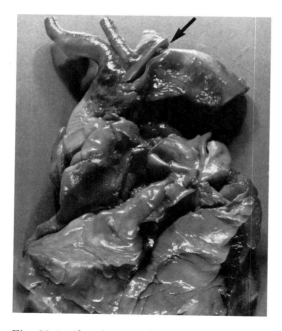

Fig. 36–2. Sharply incised stab wound of aortic arch (arrow) resulting from a single downward thrust of a broad kitchen knife in the left supraclavicular region.

wound is important in determining the outcome of the injury. Hemopericardium with cardiac tamponade is a common sequel of major penetrating wounds of the heart and aortic root. Rapid accumulation of 150 to 200 ml of blood in the pericardial sac will increase intrapericardial pressure and decrease the systolic ejection of the ventricles, leading to a decline in central aortic pressure and diminution of coronary blood flow with ultimate cessation of cardiac function. If the associated pericardial wound communicates with the pleural cavity, fatal hemothorax may result.

Table 36–1 lists the location and types of lesions seen in penetrating wounds of the heart. Arrhythmias and conduction defects may occur as well as structural damage to any of the cardiac tissues. Intracardiac shunts[7,84] or fistulas[3,80] may develop as well as valvular and coronary artery lacerations. Coronary artery injuries, depending on the size of the injured vessels, result in cardiac tamponade and varying degrees of myocardial ischemia or even infarction.[109]

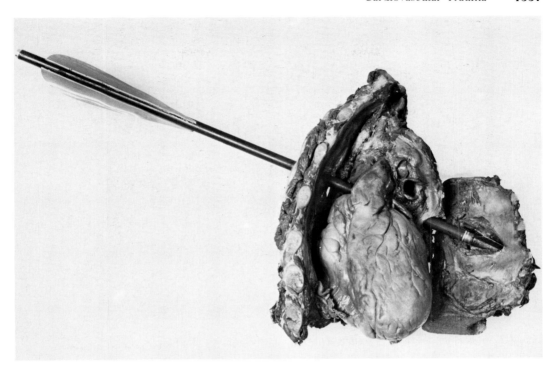

Fig. 36–3. Suicidal crossbow wound of aorta in a 21-year-old man. The thoracic structures are viewed from the left side. The bolt penetrated the ascending aorta (behind the pulmonary artery in the photograph) and then passed through the descending aorta before lodging in the thoracic spine. The hunting tip went through 6 cm of bone. Death resulted from massive left-sided hemothorax.

The resorption of hematomas produced by penetrating wounds is slow; healing begins at the epicardial and endocardial portions of the wound and extends gradually into the transmural segment.[34] The end result is focal endocardial fibrosis and localized fibrous pericardial adhesions with a connecting, often ill-defined path of myocardial scarring between. Constrictive pericarditis does not usually result unless there has been organization of an associated hemopericardium. Post-traumatic aneurysm of the left ventricle may be an early or late consequence of penetrating or nonpenetrating wounds.[50]

Infection, leading to suppurative pericarditis, myocardial abscess, or bacterial endocarditis, is always a risk with penetrating wounds of the pericardium and heart. One of the unique features of missile injury to the heart and blood vessels is the possibility of intracardiac retention or embolization of a bullet or other foreign object.[3,98,116] In persons surviving the acute injury, the surgical treatment of penetrating wounds of the heart, aorta, and peripheral vessels has produced generally good results.[6,17,86,87,110]

NONPENETRATING INJURIES

Nonpenetrating chest trauma with injury to the heart and aorta has become increasingly common, particularly as a result of rapid deceleration in high-speed automobile accidents.[62,93] Airplane crashes, falls from great height, and other severe crushing injuries of the thorax and lower body may lead to non-

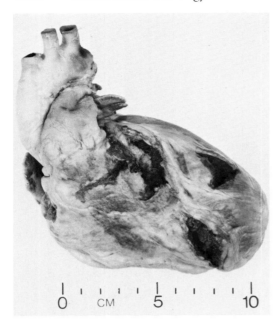

Fig. 36–4. Specimen from a 19-year-old youth who fell from the twenty-second floor of an apartment block, sustaining multiple traumatic injuries. Several irregular penetrating wounds of the atria and ventricles resulted from indriven ends of broken ribs, most of which were fractured anteriorly and posteriorly. This is an example of nonpenetrating thoracic trauma causing penetrating cardiac wounds.

Table 36–1.   Cardiac Lesions Produced by Penetrating Wounds

I. Pericardial injury
   A. Laceration
   B. Hemopericardium
      1. With cardiac tamponade
      2. Without cardiac tamponade
   C. Effusion with fibrinous pericarditis
   D. Recurrent pericarditis with effusion
   E. Pneumopericardium
   F. Suppurative pericarditis
   G. Constrictive pericarditis

II. Myocardial injury
   A. Laceration
   B. Penetration or perforation
   C. Rupture
   D. Retained foreign body
      1. Infected (abscess)
      2. Sterile
   E. Structural defects
      1. Aneurysm formation
      2. Septal defects
      3. Aortocardiac fistula

III. Valvular injury
   A. Leaflet injury
   B. Papillary muscle or chordae tendineae laceration or rupture

IV. Coronary artery injury
   A. Thrombosis or laceration
      1. With myocardial infarction
      2. Without myocardial infarction
   B. Arteriovenous fistula
   C. Aneurysm

V. Embolism
   A. Foreign body
   B. Thrombus
      1. Septic
      2. Sterile

VI. Bacterial endocarditis

VII. Rhythm or conduction disturbances

(Adapted from Hurst,[45a] with permission.)

penetrating cardioaortic injuries. Damage to the heart and great vessels from blunt trauma is often masked by associated major visceral or musculoskeletal injury or by lack of external evidence of chest injury.[62] The effects of blunt force injuries are governed by the site and extent of injury and by the phase of the respiratory and cardiac cycles when the trauma was sustained. Physical forces acting externally on the body to produce major cardiovascular lesions do so through any one or more of the following six mechanisms[110]:

1. Unidirectional force against the chest
2. Bidirectional or compressive force against the thorax
3. Indirect forces (i.e., compression of the abdomen and lower extremities resulting in marked increase in intravascular pressure)
4. Decelerative forces, particularly when imparting differential deceleration to the heart and great vessels
5. Blast forces of great magnitude
6. Concussive force, indicating a jarring force that interferes with cardiac rhythm but is

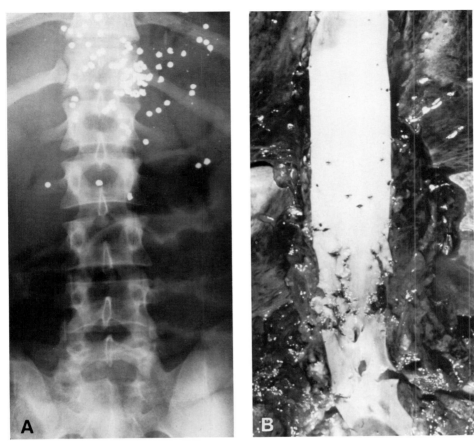

Fig. 36–5. Close range homicidal shotgun wound (0.20-gauge, No. 5 shot) in a young man. (**A**) Radiograph showing clustering of lead pellets in lower chest and upper abdomen. (**B**) Aorta with multiple perforating wounds above level of celiac artery.

not of sufficient magnitude to produce a significant lesion

The major sequelae of nonpenetrating trauma to the heart and great vessels are listed in Table 36–2.

Pericardial Lesions

Pericardial tears from blunt trauma are usually transverse across the base of the heart near the reflexion of the visceral and parietal pericardium, at a site that represents an area of relative fixation or suspension.[62] Such rents carry a potential danger of herniation or luxation of the heart.[70] When myocardial tears coexist, the integrity of the parietal pericardium may prevent exsanguination by inducing tamponade to control bleeding long enough to permit surgical treatment. Larger pericardial defects may allow excessive bleeding from smaller myocardial lacerations that might otherwise have sealed, with some relative increase in intrapericardial pressure. Traumatic pericarditis is a common accompaniment of closed cardiac injuries and is usually characterized by simple serous or sanguinous effu-

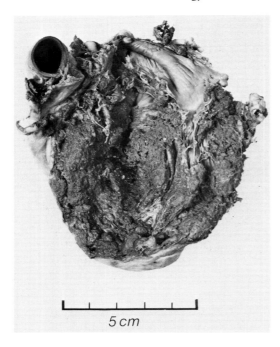

Fig. 36–6. Homicidal shotgun wound of heart in an 8-year-old boy. Major portions of the atrial and ventricular walls have been carried away and the chambers laid open by the charge of large-sized buckshot at close range.

sions and fibrinous exudate. Such reactions are probably secondary to pericardial and underlying myocardial contusions. Delayed or recurrent pericarditis with effusion following trauma is a poorly understood clinical entity that may have an autoimmune basis. Chronic constrictive pericarditis with calcification may be late sequel of recurrent post-traumatic pericarditis or result from organization of blood in the pericardial sac (see Ch. 22).

Cardiac Commotion

Cardiac commotion (commotio cordis) is an old term denoting a disturbance of cardiac function, induced by impact or agitation of the heart, which is out of proportion to the

Table 36–2.   Nonpenetrating Trauma of Heart and Great Vessels

I. Pericardial injury
  A. Hemopericardium
  B. Rupture or laceration
  C. Serofibrinous or suppurative pericarditis
  D. Constrictive pericarditis
  E. Recurrent pericarditis with effusion

II. Myocardial injury
  A. Contusion
    1. Anginal syndrome
    2. Aneurysm
    3. Delayed rupture
    4. Thromboembolism
    5. Myocarditis with or without failure
  B. Laceration
  C. Rupture, including septal rupture

III. Coronary artery injury
  A. Laceration with or without myocardial infarction
  B. Thrombosis with or without myocardial infarction
  C. Arteriovenous fistula

IV. Valvular injury
  A. Laceration, rupture, contusion
  B. Papillary muscle or chordae tendineae injury

V. Disturbances of rhythm or conduction

VI. Great vessel injury
  A. Laceration, rupture
  B. Aneurysm formation
  C. Thrombotic occlusion

(Adapted from Hurst,[45a] with permission.)

degree of observed anatomical alterations.[34] As such, it is roughly analogous to so-called cerebral concussion. Nonfatal transient disturbances of cardiac activity may occur after chest trama, but pathologic documentation of damage is obviously impossible in survivors. Occasional instances of nonpenetrating chest trauma leading to heart failure and death have had neither gross nor microscopic evidence of cardiac injury at autopsy. Traumatic arrhythmias and disturbances of conduction may be manifestations of cardiac commotion; however, underlying myocardial contusions are probably responsible for most clinical cases of this syndrome.

Myocardial Contusions

Cardiac damage caused by blunt chest trauma presents a spectrum of injury ranging from cardiac rupture to arrhythmias or heart failure without morphologic evidence of injury.[62,93] Somewhere in the middle of the spectrum is myocardial contusion, an entity with its own range of variable and transient clinical signs or functional consequences. Myocardial contusion (Fig. 36–7) may occur with or without external signs of trauma or fractures of the bony structures of the chest wall. The most common cause of this injury is steering wheel impact, compressing the heart between the sternum and vertebrae. Sudden accelerations or decelerations may cause the heart to be thrust against the sternum or vertebrae, injuring the myocardium. Also, sudden increase in intrathoracic or intra-abdominal pressure may result in subendocardial and myocardial hemorrhages.[109,110]

Precordial pain, which clinically simulates angina pectoris or acute myocardial infarction,[49] is the most common symptom of myocardial contusion and may be associated with rhythm or conduction disturbances. When extensive damage is present throughout the myocardium, early death is the rule, although later deaths have been reported. Causes of death include ventricular fibrillation, prolonged cardiac standstill, myocardial rupture, and/or heart failure.[62] Pathologically, there may be subepicardial, intramyocardial, or subendocardial extravasation of blood with focal, microscopic fractures of the muscle bundles of the heart. Varying degrees of myocardial necrosis (often of the contraction band type) are usually present in contusions[49] but this may be minimal, the dominant feature being interstitial hemorrhage. Healing takes place rapidly with infiltration of leukocytes and resorption of blood and necrotic tissue, followed by replacement fibrosis. Extensive transmural contusions may, with healing, give rise to true post-traumatic aneurysms of the ventricular wall.[62,93]

While subendocardial hemorrhages may be

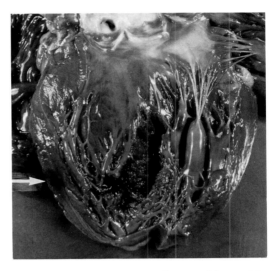

Fig. 36–7. Traumatic ventricular septal laceration caused by blunt thoracic injury in a young man struck by an automobile. The left ventricular free wall was contused (arrow) but not ruptured.

contusive in origin (Fig 36–8), very similar extravasations, although usually smaller, may be seen in hypoxic or asphyxial states.[34] Larger subendocardial hemorrhages are often found in patients with circulatory or hypovolemic shock or hemorrhagic diatheses. It is not as widely appreciated that subendocardial hemorrhage, myocytolysis, and myocardial necrosis may develop in the left ventricle secondary to isolated spontaneous or traumatic intracranial hemorrhage[40,55a] (Fig. 36–9). These cardiac alterations are most likely the result of a pressor sympathetic effect mediated by a neurohormonal mechanism. Catecholamine release, primarily norepinephrine from the terminal nerve endings in the myocardium, may induce a state of relative anoxia due to augmented myocardial oxygen consumption.[55b] Altered hemodynamic patterns, mechanical factors, or excessive production of adrenal corticosteroids may also contribute to the pathogenesis of such secondary myocardial lesions.[40] These lesions are not uncommon in early endomyocardial biopsies recovered from transplanted hearts. Both

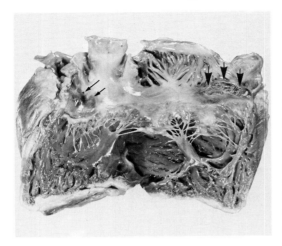

Fig. 36–8. Specimen from victim of a motor vehicle accident, showing multiple injuries. Focal subendocardial hemorrhage is seen in the atrioventricular node region just above the septal cusp of the tricuspid valve (small arrows). An incomplete transverse endomyocardial tear is present in the right atrium immediately proximal to the posterior leaflet of the tricuspid valve (large arrows).

acute and healing lesions of this type must be distinguished from a rejection reaction.

Rupture of the Heart

Myocardial laceration and rupture may be produced by the same forces that cause contusion and are the lesions most often found at autopsy in fatalities attributable to non-penetrating chest trauma.[62] Rupture of the right ventricle occurs most frequently (Fig. 36–10), followed in diminishing order by rupture of the left ventricle (Fig. 36–7), right atrium, and left atrium (Fig. 36–11). Massive compression of the chest may result in explosive ruptures of the roof of the atria and/or apex of the ventricles (Fig. 36–12). Rupture of the heart may occur immediately or within the first 2 weeks of injury, following softening and necrosis in a contused segment of the wall

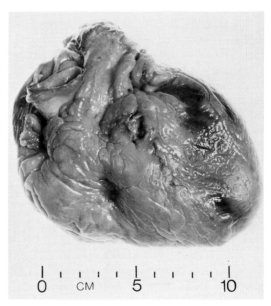

Fig. 36–10. Linear vertical tear over outflow tract of right ventricle with larger defect on inner surface of chamber. Compression injury of chest with fatal hemopericardium. The defect, adjacent to the ventricular septum, exposed the left anterior descending coronary artery, which, however, remained intact.

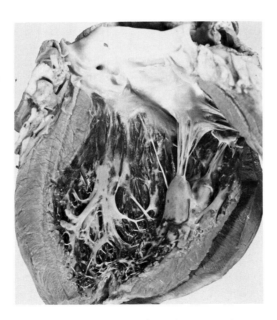

Fig. 36–9. Massive subendocardial hemorrhage in dilated left ventricle of patient dying after severe craniocerebral trauma with swelling and herniation of the brain.

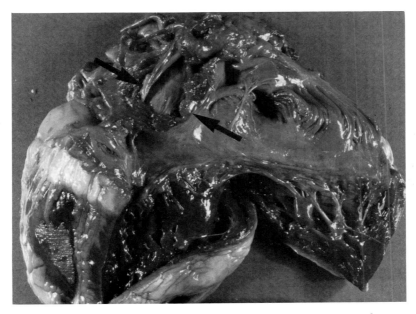

Fig. 36–11. Traumatic atrial septal defect (arrows) resulting from nonpenetrating thoracic trauma sustained in a motor vehicle accident.

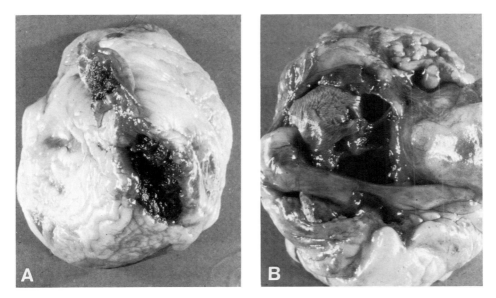

Fig. 36–12. Blowout lacerations of (**A**) apex of right ventricle and (**B**) dome of right atrium. The victim had been run over, the wheels of the automobile traversing his chest.

before healing occurs. The heart is usually ruptured when the anterior chest wall is driven in by an external force, or it may be ruptured by forceful compression against the vertebral column.[110] The ventricles are most vulnerable in late diastole or early systole when the ventricular chambers are full and the valves closed. The atria are at risk during ventricular systole because of maximum venous return. A sudden increase in hydrostatic pressure within the heart chambers causes tearing of atrial or ventricular walls from within outward, beginning with the endocardium. As a result, partial or incomplete endomyocardial lacerations (Fig. 36–8) or complete full-thickness tears (Fig. 36–10) may be found. The size of a rupture tends to be larger on the endocardial aspect and smaller on the epicardial surface of the heart. Ventricular ruptures from blunt trauma usually have a vertical orientation while those in the atria are most often horizontal. With larger ventricular free-wall lacerations, death from cardiac tamponade is commonly a swift sequence. Smaller tears may be compatible with survival long enough to permit surgical correction.[62,110] Rarely, a false or pseudoaneurysm of the left ventricle may develop when bleeding from a rupture is contained by pericardial adhesions and organizing blood clot[50,62,110] (see Ch. 22). The interventricular septum appears acutely susceptible to injury secondary to nonpenetrating chest trauma (Fig. 36–7). Isolated traumatic ventricular septal defects may occur as the major cardiac lesion[12,62] or be associated with valvular damage[104] or ventricular aneurysm.[106] Although small ventricular defects may close spontaneously, the treatment of choice is surgical closure, particularly in the presence of cardiac failure.[62] Other less common types of intracardiac or cardioaortic shunt may develop secondary to nonpenetrating chest trauma.[28]

Coronary and Valvular Injuries

The question of whether nonpenetrating chest trauma can cause direct injury to the coronary arteries has been strongly debated in the literature.[49,62,93] Cumulative evidence from clinical cases with angiographic documentation now supports such a relationship,[55,82,83,117] although documented pathologic observations are still few (Fig. 36–13). Invariably, the left anterior descending coronary artery is the traumatized vessel, usually resulting in myocardial infarction. Intimomedial tears and intramural dissections with superimposed thrombosis appear to be the major mechanisms involved. Nonpenetrating traumatic injuries of the atrioventricular or semilunar valves may induce clinically significant valvular incompetence.[62,93] The aortic valve is most commonly involved, followed by the mitral and, rarely, the tricuspid. The bodies of the aortic cusps may be torn or the cusps avulsed along their basal attachments. Injuries of the mitral valve may result in tears of the anterior or posterior leaflets but more commonly cause ruptures of the chordae tendineae or papillary muscles. Early operation with prosthetic valve replacement affords the best chance of survival.[62,93] Bacterial endocarditis may develop on traumatically ruptured valves.[71]

Laceration and Rupture of Aorta

An unusual occurrence until well into this century, traumatic laceration and rupture of the aorta now occurs with alarming frequency and is seen in 1 of every 6 or 10 automobile fatalities.[109,110] The types of injury leading to aortic rupture are similar to those causing rupture of the heart and include direct blunt force to the chest, vertical deceleration, horizontal deceleration with or without chest compression, or crushing injuries involving some flexion mechanism to the spine. More than 95 percent of traumatic aortic injuries involve the thoracic aorta; the usual site of tearing is the aortic isthmus at the level of the ligamentum arteriosum, 2 to 3 cm beyond the origin of the left subclavian artery (Fig. 36–14). This represents a point of relative fixation or suspension of the descending thoracic aorta by the ligamentum, intercostal arteries, and pa-

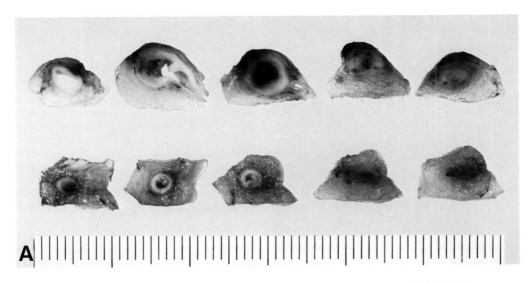

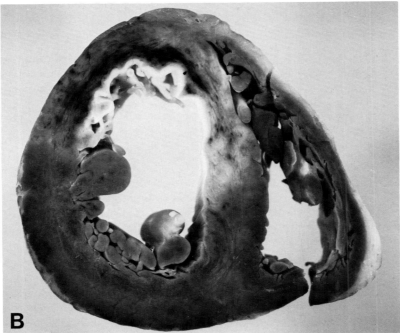

Fig. 36–13. Post-traumatic coronary occlusion and myocardial infarction in a 17-year-old boy who sustained a severe concussion and bilateral fractured clavicles in a motorbike accident. An aortogram was normal, but cardiac investigations were not done. He died suddenly 3 months later while playing basketball. (**A**) Serial slices of left main coronary artery and left anterior descending (LAD) branch clockwise from upper left. Slight aneurysmal dilation and recent retrograde extension of thrombus are seen at the LAD origin (slices 2 and 3) followed by organized occlusion (slices 4 to 7) and, further along, distal prolapse and LAD occlusion by a torn intimomedial flap. (**B**) Transverse midventricular slice of heart showing late healing anteroseptal infarct with richly vascularized scar and secondary endocardial fibrosis.

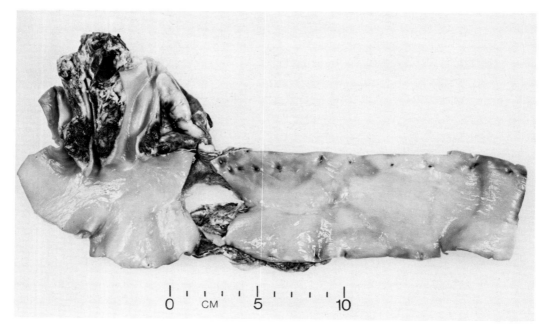

Fig. 36–14. Same case illustrated in Figure 36–4. Complete transection of the aorta just beyond the attachment of the ligamentum arteriosum. Mediastinal hemorrhage surrounds the branches of the aortic arch. Thus, while the heart in this case suffered penetrating trauma, the aorta manifested the classic effects of blunt trauma.

rietal pleura, rendering it relatively immobile compared with the aortic arch and heart. The different rate of deceleration of the mobile arch and the relatively fixed descending aorta place unusual stresses on the aortic isthmus in deceleration accidents. The second most frequent site of rupture is in the ascending aorta proximal to the innominate artery (Fig. 36–15). This too is a point of relative fixation by the pericardial reflexion and partial suspension of the heart by bronchi and mediastinal structures.[4]

Four main mechanical stresses appear to contribute to acute traumatic rupture of the aorta.[110] Shearing stress and bending stress are more likely to cause rupture at the isthmus. Shearing stress is related to differential deceleration and relative fixation, while bending stress is caused by chest compression with flexion of the aortic arch over the left main stem bronchus and left pulmonary artery. During sudden compression or direct blunt force to the chest, the heart may be displaced into the left posterior chest and the aorta rotated. The ascending aorta bears the brunt of this torsion stress. In addition, horizontal linear impact trauma to the sternum produces an acute lengthening of the aorta, creating an intra-aortic pressure wave or "waterhammer" stress that is greatest in the ascending aorta.[110]

Traumatic rupture of the ascending aorta is often associated with other cardiac injuries. Combined rupture of the aortic valve and ascending aorta have been reported after blunt chest trauma[20] including one patient with prior aortic dissection.[22] Charles and colleagues[20] suggested that depression of a fractured sternum contacting the forward moving heart in diastole resulted in injuries in the aortic root following a steering wheel injury. Aronson[4] reported rupture of the ascending aorta after a minor fall in a patient with extreme cardiomegaly. It was postulated that the unusually heavy heart exerted a se-

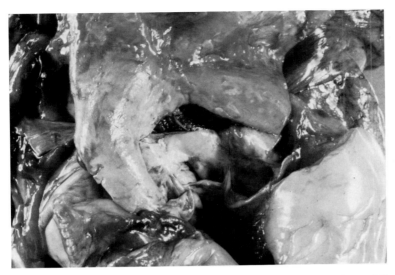

Fig. 36–15. Transverse laceration of ascending aorta just above aortic valve. The middle-aged female victim was driving a snowmobile on a country road and was struck by a car. Death was caused by hemopericardium with cardiac tamponade.

vere downward force as a result of its mass and the inertia concomitant with the fall. The aorta ripped at the proximal site of maximum stress. This type of rupture is usually seen in falls from great height or in air crash victims.

The aorta exhibits less tensile strength to longitudinal than to transverse stress; thus the majority of aortic lacerations are horizontal. Tears in the aorta range from small lacerations to circumferential transections with separation of the proximal and distal aortic segments. As in the heart, aortic lacerations develop from within outward and may involve the intima only, the intima and a varying amount of media, or the full thickness of the aorta. In the latter situation, the parietal pleura will tear and fatal hemothorax will ensue. Nevertheless, a patient may survive a complete transection of the aorta. The adventitia may remain intact because it is the toughest layer of the aortic wall and has the greatest tensile strength. Patients retaining a largely intact adventitia and pleura may survive the initial injury with bleeding limited to the mediastinal tissues. Such cases are amenable to successful surgery if a diagnosis can be estab-

lished.[2] Major aortic rupture may be accompanied by multiple intimal contusions and minor intimomedial lacerations (Fig. 36–16). When minor lacerations alone are produced by chest trauma, they are of no great consequence and probably resolve leaving small fibrous intimal plaques. However, serious lacerations will require graft replacement of the lacerated aorta, if an accident victim survives, and carries the risk of additional cross-clamp injury (Fig. 36–17).

Major dissection is not a feature of traumatic rupture of the aorta since there is usually no underlying medial disease. However, limited "dissection" or undermining of the torn edges may lift an intimal or intimomedial flap[37]; this can cause obstruction by prolapse or thrombosis or simulate coarctation in the thoracic[57] or abdominal[24,99] aorta. Although abdominal aortic injury is more commonly caused by penetrating wounds,[73] when lacerations from blunt force do occur, they are often associated with intimal flap prolapse and stenosis.[24,34,99] Occlusive thrombi, frank rupture, intramural hematomas, simple contusions, false aneurysms, and atheroemboli may also result from

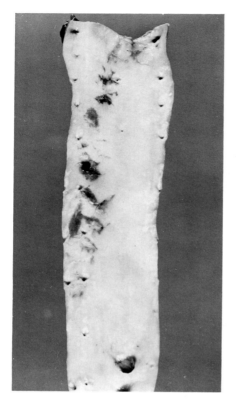

Fig. 36–16. Distal portion of completely transected aorta of driver killed in motor vehicle accident. A number of intimal contusions and shallow transverse intimal tears are present in the descending thoracic aorta.

blunt trauma to the abdominal aorta.[78] Most cases of abdominal aortic injury present with signs of leg ischemia or of an "acute abdomen," or of both.[78]

Post-traumatic Aortic Aneurysm

The ability of the adventitia to withstand great mechanical forces and remain intact, after tearing of the inner layers of the aortic wall, facilitates development of post-traumatic aneurysms. The parietal pleura and organization of periaortic mediastinal hematoma may give support to the weakened aorta and limit bleeding until healing occurs. Such aneu-

rysms are usually found in the upper thoracic aorta some time after the injury (Fig. 36–18). They may be discovered by chance or, since they continue to expand, cause pressure on an adjacent structure or late rupture may occur. Swanson and Gaffey[107] reported a case of traumatically induced false aneurysm with secondary bacterial aortitis of the descending aorta and fistula formation between the aorta and esophagus. When diagnosed, the affected

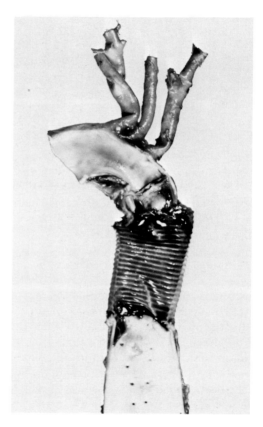

Fig. 36–17. Transverse laceration of descending limb of aortic arch at the classic location, surgically repaired with insertion of Dacron graft. The patient, a passenger in a motor vehicle accident, died in the early postoperative period with recurrent bleeding from another transverse laceration between the left subclavian artery and the proximal graft anastomosis. While this second laceration may have been initiated during the accident, it may well have resulted from aortic cross-clamping during surgery.

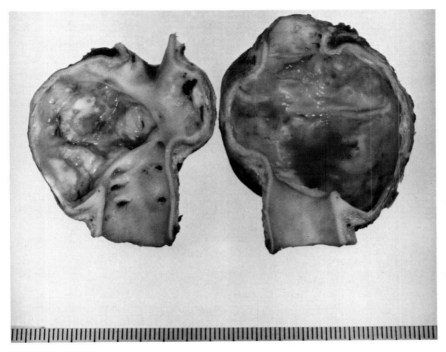

Fig. 36–18. Surgically resected post-traumatic aneurysm of descending thoracic aorta in 23-year-old automobile driver involved in a head-on collision 9 months previously. The aortic injury escaped notice at the time of the accident, and a mediastinal mass was detected on routine chest x-ray when the patient returned for treatment of a nonunited fracture of the tibia and fibula. The specimen has been hemisected in the coronal plane. This is a true aneurysm with the adventitia holding intact after almost complete circumferential laceration of the full thickness of intima and media.

patient requires early operation; surgical results are good.[66] The inner margins of post-traumatic aneurysms are formed by the edges of the original laceration. The undermined edges may produce an intimal flap or rolled-in cuff of intima and media, which can present as a coarctation.[51] False aneurysm of the abdominal aorta due to total rupture and peri-aortic hematoma formation has been reported after a fall causing blunt abdominal trauma.[94]

Blunt Injuries to Branches of the Aortic Arch

Nonpenetrating chest trauma may involve branches of the aortic arch, causing early laceration or avulsion of the innominate, common carotid, or subclavian arteries and lead to massive mediastinal hemorrhage.[110] Incomplete lacerations result in post-traumatic aneurysms which most often involve the innominate artery.[19,41] My colleagues and I[41] reported two cases of innominate arterial aneurysm following steering wheel injuries in young men (Fig. 36–19). One also involved the proximal portions of the right subclavian and common carotid arteries. Both were associated with partially obstructing intimomedial flaps or shelf like stenoses caused by limited dissection with lifting of the torn edges; in both cases, the adventitia had remained intact, containing major bleeding. Resection and graft replacement of the aneurysms was performed four and eleven months after the injuries and produced excellent long-term results.

Blunt Injuries of Peripheral Arteries

Although less frequently seen than penetrating injuries, blunt trauma of the peripheral arteries may result in lacerations, transections, avulsions, contusions, secondary thrombosis, and arteriovenous fistulas.[17,85] The intimal flap mechanism may play an important role in vascular stenosis[37]; occasionally, false aneurysms develop.[86] The development of post-traumatic-pseudoaneurysms of the superficial temporal artery is a hazard of hockey puck injuries in the absence of protective head gear.[18]

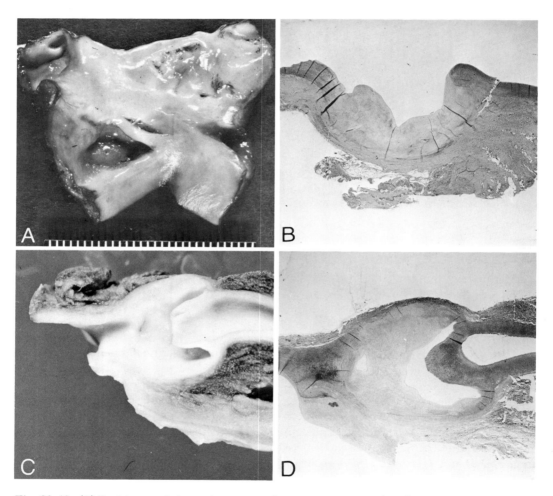

Fig. 36–19. (**A**) Post-traumatic innominate arterial aneurysm associated with transverse intimomedial tears resulting from steering wheel injury of chest 10 months previously. (**B**) Longitudinal histologic section through aneurysm showing intact adventitia and myointimal repair tissue partially filling the defect ($\times$ 6). (**C**) Post-traumatic aneurysm involving innominate bifurcation and proximal common carotid artery discovered 4 months after steering wheel injury. The projecting intimal flap or shelf, due to limited dissection, may cause obstruction to blood flow and secondary thrombosis. (**D**) Low-power histologic section of aneurysm showing the dark intimomedial flap of original vessel wall and the lightly textured myointimal repair tissue partially filling the sac ($\times$ 6). (*Figure continues.*)

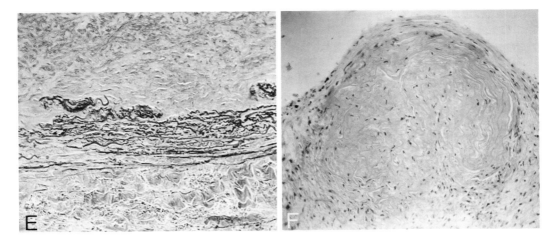

Fig. 36–19 *(Continued).* **(E)** Myointimal repair tissue in the wall of the aneurysm (above) is separated from the adventitia (below) by a few residual elastic fibers in the outer media. (Elastic tissue stain, × 185.) **(F)** Subintimal knot of retracted elastic fibers near the edge of innominate aneurysm. (Hematoxylin, phloxine, and saffron stain, × 185.) (From Heggtveit et al.,[41] with permission.)

IATROGENIC INJURY

Operative Injury

Operative injury to blood vessels is, fortunately, uncommon during general surgical procedures and is usually encountered during particularly difficult or complicated operations (Fig. 36–20). Cardiovascular surgery, however, carries an inherent risk of damage when the heart and vascular structures are approached and manipulated directly (see Ch. 40). Penetrating wounds or vascular cross-clamp injuries may manifest as early or delayed bleeding or show up later as aneurysmal dilations. Black and colleagues[11] described 50 vascular injuries in 45 patients following cardiac valve replacement over a 10-year period. Lesions of the aorta were most common, and coronary and femoral arteries were damaged less frequently. The injuries included stenosis or occlusion (17 patients), laceration or perforation (16 patients), dissecting aneurysm (13 patients), and false aneurysm (4 patients). Nine patients suffered injuries caused by surgical clamps; 12 injuries were caused by sutures. Tearing of the aortic root from the base

of the heart occurred in 5 patients. Inadvertent coronary ligation is apt to occur during emergency attempts to control major intraoperative bleeding and the left circumflex coronary artery is at special risk during mitral valve replacement. We have seen transverse lacerations, dissections, and small saccular aneurysm develop in the proximal aorta at the site where clamps were applied to create coronary bypass graft ostia (Fig. 36–21). Although such clamps are applied parallel to the long axis of the aorta, the intimomedial tears tend to be horizontal, as are lacerations caused by aortic cross-clamping (Figs. 36–18 and 36–20). Coronary ostial obstruction, resulting from intimal proliferation, may be a late result of coronary cannulation[21] or high perfusion pressures distending the proximal coronary arteries during surgery.[97] The turbulence from lateral-flow aortic valve prostheses may be a contributing factor to such narrowings of the coronary orifices[21] as well as to the fibromuscular intimal thickening observed in the ascending aorta.[97]

Ventriculotomy sites represent penetrating wounds with the additional factor of ischemic necrosis at their margins as a consequence of

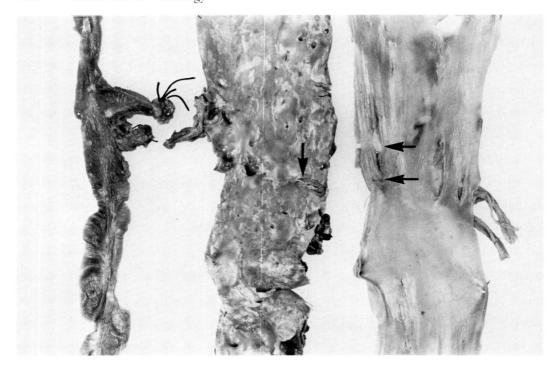

Fig. 36–20. Operative vascular injuries in a 64-year-old woman undergoing left nephrectomy for a large renal cell carcinoma. Massive hemorrhage occurred during the operation, and the patient died 2 days later from continued bleeding and ischemic infarction of liver, spleen, and stomach. The celiac artery was clipped and ligated (at left, with silk ligature), several small transverse intimomedial cross-clamp tears were present in the aorta (center, arrow) and a vertical, partially sutured 2-cm laceration was found in the inferior vena cava (right, arrows).

incision or suture obliteration of subtending blood vessels.[56] False aneurysms may develop at such points of injury.[88,93] Damage to components of the cardiac conduction system is a special hazard in surgical correction of congenital heart defects[56] (see Ch. 37). As increasing numbers of patients undergo a second or third cardiac operation, it is apparent that repeat median sternotomy may be an especially hazardous procedure.[5,65] If the pericardial sac has been left open after open heart surgery, the heart becomes closely bound to the posterior surface of the sternum. Penetrating wounds of the great vessels, right atrium, or right ventricle may occur on reopening the sternum or on subsequent blunt dissection to free the heart from encasing adhesions (Fig. 36–22). Although the closed

pericardial sac may become largely obliterated by fibrous adhesions, it serves as a cleavage plane that facilitates separation from the sternum. Thus, the complications of pericardial tamponade or constriction from postoperative closure of the pericardium are probably less than the risks of repeat sternotomy where the pericardium has been left open at initial operation.[5]

Cardiac Massage

A wide range of cardiac injuries may occur secondary to open- or closed-chest cardiac massage. Adelson documented the anatomic changes in the hearts of 60 patients who died during or after open-chest cardiac massage.[1]

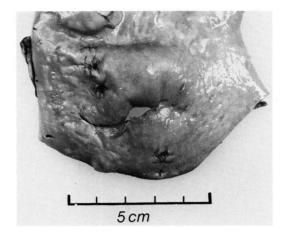

Fig. 36–21. Transverse intimal tear of ascending aorta between bypass graft ostia. This laceration was probably related to the application of an occluder clamp during creation of the proximal graft anastomoses. The laceration was associated with localized intramural dissection followed by external rupture into the pericardial sac and death at the end of the operative procedure.

Manual massage can injure any and all portions of the cardiac tissues and gross laceration of the ventricles in more than 10 percent of cases (Fig. 36–23). Closed-chest resuscitation, in addition to cardiac contusions, may produce traumatic rupture of the aorta or right ventricular structures from sternal compression.[15,33,75]

In a series of 705 autopsies on persons undergoing prehospital cardiac resuscitation, 42.7 percent had thoracic complications (rib and sternal fractures, mediastinal hematomas), 30.8 had percent abdominal visceral complications, 13 percent had pulmonary complications, and only 0.5 percent displayed heart and great vessel trauma.[58] Among 130 hospitalized patients dying after cardiopulmonary resuscitation, 27 (21 percent) had major complications, including 11 cases (8 percent) with cardiac laceration or hemorrhage[10]; all of the latter had pericardiocentesis or placement of a transvenous pacemaker during

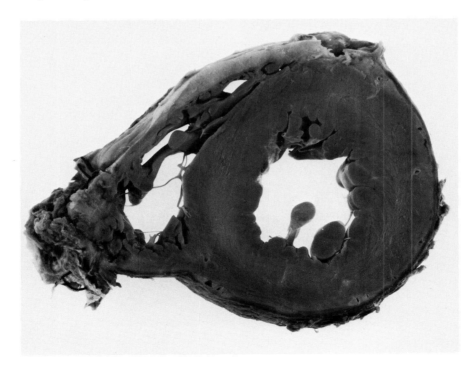

Fig. 36–22. Intraoperative right ventricular lacerations sustained when freeing the heart from adhesions during reoperation for coronary artery disease. Attempts were made to repair the wound, but the patient died on the operating table.

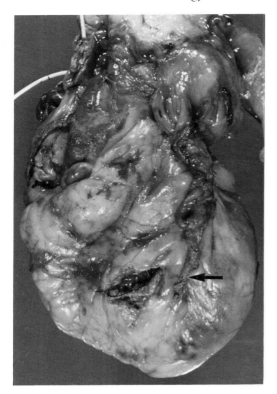

Fig. 36–23. Laceration of anterior free wall of right ventricle caused by manual open-chest cardiac massage. Patient had sustained a myocardial infarct during coronary bypass surgery, and resuscitation failed. Arrow indicates distal end of left internal mammary artery graft to left anterior descending branch.

the attempted cardiopulmonary resuscitation. Subepicardial contraction band necrosis of myofibers in the anterior or posterior myocardial wall is a common finding in patients who had cardiac massage before death.

Catheters and Cannulas

The use of a wide range of intravascular catheters, cannulas, and other invasive instruments for diagnosis and therapy is a routine occurrence in medical and surgical wards. All vascular cannulations involve a penetrating wound of the vessel at the point of insertion

and the possibility of further trauma as the catheter is advanced within the lumen (Fig. 36–24). Complications include local bleeding and mural tears or contusions with endothelial injury or intimal flaps. The latter may induce intraluminal thrombosis, remote embolization, or intramural dissection. Emboli may derive from thrombi or disrupted atheroma or be of extraneous foreign material. On reaching the heart, catheters may contuse, tear, penetrate, or become tangled in cardiac structures. Wound infections, bacterial endocarditis, or false aneurysms may also complicate angioinvasive techniques.

Polyethylene Catheters

Catheter embolization to the heart or pulmonary arteries is a well-recognized complication of intravenous fluid therapy using polyethylene tubing. This may result from disengagement of the catheter from the needle during administration of fluid or severing of the tubing by the needle through which the catheter has been introduced.[103] While much less common with current methods, catheter loss into the venous circulation may sometimes occur as a result of faulty bonding of the catheter shaft to the hub.[102] Embolization of polyethylene catheter fragments[48] or silicone

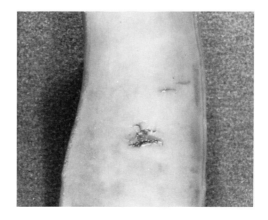

Fig. 36–24. Carotid angiogram puncture site in a young adult. Note two small nonperforating intimal tears on opposite wall just above point of entry.

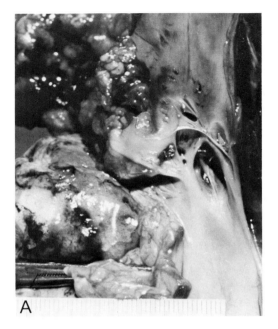 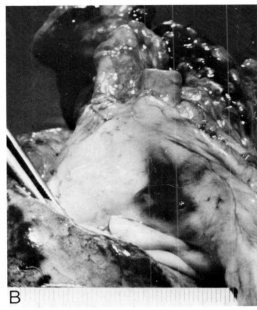

Fig. 36–25. (A) Multiple perforations of right internal jugular vein induced during attempted insertion of a CVP line. (B) Hematoma and puncture wounds at dome of right pleural cavity due to malpositioned CVP catheter. Death resulted from massive hemothorax.

rubber ventriculoatrial shunt tubing[30] has caused myocardial perforation and cardiac tamponade. Even intact indwelling polyethylene catheters of various types may perforate the right atrium or ventricle, causing fatal cardiac tamponade from hemopericardium[25,46,52] or intrapericardial infusion of intravenous fluid.[32,60,112]

Central Venous Lines

The ubiquitous insertion of central venous pressure (CVP) lines via subclavian and internal jugular veins is fraught with hazards ranging from simple knotting[68] and thrombosis to perforation of the heart and lethal tamponade.[25,31,52,112] In a prospective study of 141 autopsies on patients with indwelling right heart catheters,[29] three deaths were attributable to catheter use, two to perforation. Twelve (29 percent) of 42 patients with central venous catheters exhibited mural thrombi in the right side of the heart. Perforation of the

dome of the right pleural cavity with resultant hemothorax or hydrothorax has been seen on a number of occasions (Fig. 36–25). It is not generally appreciated that the large veins of the neck are thin-walled, delicate structures with a network of venous valves at the junction of subclavian and jugular veins, which may snare or misdirect a CVP line or guide leading to perforation of the vessel wall (Fig. 36–25A).

Swan-Ganz Catheters

Balloon-tipped, flow-directed, Swan-Ganz catheters have been associated with cardiac arrhythmias[64,76] and may become snared or entangled in the heart.[13] Tricuspid and pulmonary valve injury with insufficiency have been reported,[81,100] as well as perforation of the pulmonary artery[27]; minor pulmonary valve contusion is more frequent (Fig. 36–26). Other complications of these commonly employed devices include pulmonary thromboembolism and infarction, balloon rupture,

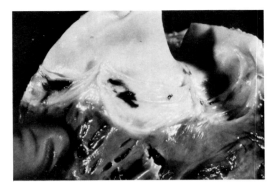

Fig. 36–26. Contusions of pulmonary valve following passage of a Swan-Ganz catheter. Thrombus forming in a pulmonary artery branch at the wedged tip of the catheter resulted in segmental infarction of the lung.

catheter knotting, and infection.[76] In one study, 33 percent of 99 patients with indwelling pulmonary arterial catheters had mural thrombi in the right side of the heart

at autopsy.[29] We found a high incidence of mural or occlusive thrombi due to endothelial damage along the course of veins traversed by these catheters (Fig. 36–27). The incidence and severity of such venous thrombosis are directly proportional to the number of catheters passed, the degree of right heart failure and the duration of catheterization. The inferior vena cava virtually always exhibits mural thrombi when catheters have been inserted via the femoral veins in patients with congestive cardiac failure (Fig. 36–28). Intimal injury and stasis both play a major role in the pathogenesis of these thrombi. In a critical assessment of the procedure, Robin[89] suggested that as many as 8 percent of patients with acute myocardial infarction may die as a result of complications from pulmonary arterial catheterization; he called for a moratorium on their use. He believes the information gained from the procedure does not justify the associated high morbidity and mortality.

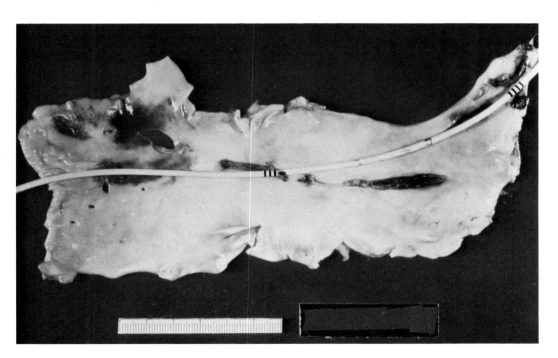

Fig. 36–27. Intimal contusions and linear thrombi of inferior vena cava secondary to insertion of Swan-Ganz catheter.

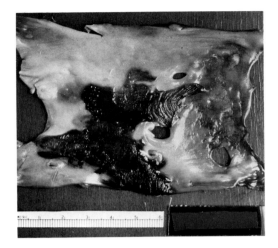

Fig. 36–28. Extensive mural thrombus of inferior vena cava at level of hepatic vein secondary to passage of several venous catheters in patient with marked right heart failure.

Cardiac Pacemakers

Transthoracic implantation of epicardial or myocardial pacemaker electrodes is associated with early and continuing local myocardial injury[39] (see Ch. 38). Initial changes are related to the trauma of electrode insertion and movement before proliferation of fibrous tissue anchors the electrode securely in place. Subsequent damage is the result of tissue reaction to the implanted metal and progressive electrical injury induced by chronic artificial stimulation.[90] The myocardium around and between implanted electrodes undergoes focal continuing necrosis and replacement fibrosis resulting in increasing electrical threshold and ultimate "exit block" with pacemaker failure.[90] Pervenous endocardial pacemakers are associated with a different set of pathological reactions related to their route of insertion.[39,44] Before becoming anchored, the tip of the electrode catheter traumatizes the right ventricular endocardium. Subsequent mural thrombosis and endomyocardial fibrosis may impede electrical activation of the heart muscle and invoke the risk of pulmonary embolization.[39,44,96] Electrode catheters become encased in an endothelialized sheath of fibrous tissue or "neo-endocardium," which is often incomplete. Usual points of encasement and attachment of the catheter by organized and endothelialized mural thrombi are in the superior vena cava, at the sinoatrial junction, at the level of the triscuspid valve, and at the catheter tip in the apex of the right ventricle (Fig. 36–29). Surprisingly, tricuspid valve dysfunction is not often found with pacemakers in place, but valve injury may occur if attempts are made to remove a well-secured unit.[44] Pacemaker electrodes can become knotted together in the heart.[14] Perforation of the ventricular septum can occur,[105] and sometimes right ventricular free wall perforation with lethal cardiac tamponade ensues[8,43] (Fig. 36–30). Perforation of the

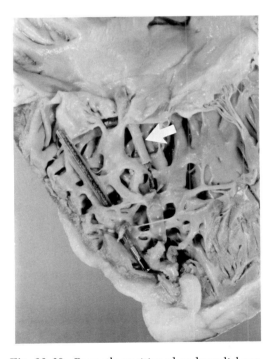

Fig. 36–29. Recently positioned endocardial pacing catheter in right ventricle of elderly patient with complete heart block. The partial fibrous sheath, which encased a previously failed and removed pervenous pacer, is seen passing through the commissure between the septal and posterior leaflets of the tricuspid valve (arrow).

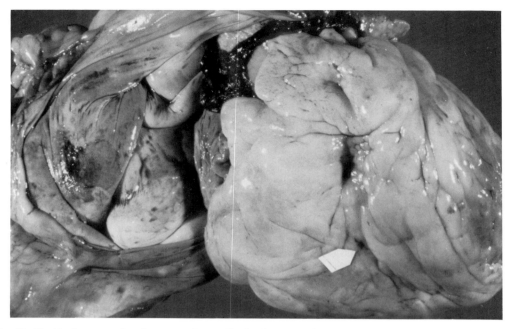

Fig. 36–30. Perforation of mid anterior free wall of right ventricle (arrow) with hemopericardium, caused by a temporary pervenous pacing wire. There was excessive epicardial fat and fatty infiltration of the myocardium.

right ventricle is more likely to occur with stiffer and hard-tipped catheters than with more flexible or soft-tipped ones.[43] Infection along the course of a pacemaker wire is uncommon.

Aortography and Angiography

Arterial trauma secondary to diagnostic procedures frequently involves a vessel at the point of vascular invasion or cannulation.[87] Lacerations, stenoses, thromboses, false aneurysms, or arteriovenous fistulas occur locally and are amenable to surgical correction.[87] Aortographic injection of contrast material may result in vasospasm with depression of renal function,[9] and intramural aortic dissection is a known hazard of transfemoral or translumbar aortography.[118] Nunn[79] cites the following complications of peripheral angiography:

1. Reactions to contrast media (much less likely with non-ionic media)
2. Vasovagal response to arterial puncture
3. Local hemorrhage
4. Vein and nerve injuries in the area
5. Subintimal injection of contrast material
6. Arterial thromboembolism
7. Intravascular injection of foreign material
8. Problems with catheters and guidewires such as breakage, knots, kinks, and creation of false channels

Intra-aortic Balloons

Intra-aortic balloon counterpulsation employed in the treatment of cardiogenic shock may be associated with a higher frequency of complications than that predicted from purely clinical studies.[47] Most necropsy patients with counterpulsation devices inserted exhibit major or minor evidence of vascular injury. Dam-

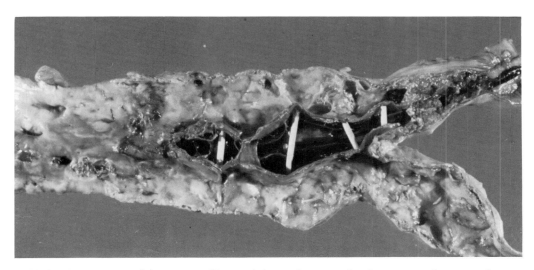

Fig. 36–31. Laceration and disruption of lower abdominal aorta and right common iliac artery by intra-aortic balloon inserted via right femoral artery in a patient with left ventricular failure at the end of coronary bypass surgery.

age ranges from small intimal contusions, tears, and mural thrombi in the aorta to extensive aorto iliac lacerations, dissections and occlusive thrombi in the iliac and femoral arteries (Figs. 36–31 to 36–33). Intramural dissection usually begins in the common iliac artery as it curves over the pelvic brim. Usually the balloon catheter re-enters the true lumen of the aorta before reaching the upper abdominal segment. Soft atheromatous plaques also serve to divert the balloon intramurally and initiate dissection. Such retrograde re-entry dissections are more likely to occur during intraoperative insertion of balloon pumps without fluoroscopic guidance. Secondary ischemic changes in the lower extremities and spinal cord are not uncommon. Dissections have been encountered with both surgically installed and percutaneously inserted devices. Intraoperative insertion of balloon pumps through the ascending aorta has led to balloon tip occlusion of the superior mesenteric artery with ischemic necrosis of the bowel and stroke following occlusion of the carotid arteries.

Coronary Angiography

The complication rate of coronary angiography is generally low in institutions studying a large volume of case material[16,36,101] and higher in those where smaller groups of patients are investigated.[16,72,77,111] As is the case with other angioinvasive procedures, thrombosis and distal thromboembolism may result from injury at the entry sites.[16,86] Sones,[101] reviewing his vast experience, found 39 deaths (0.07 percent). The commonest complications were brachial artery occlusion, which occurred in 2.8 percent and ventricular arrhythmias, which were seen in 0.82 percent. Other less common sequelae included acute myocardial infarction, coronary artery dissection, coronary or cerebral emboli, and left ventricular perforation. Guss and co-workers[36] found 12 coronary dissections or embolizations in 2,981 patients. They found significantly fewer coronary occlusions following the Sones brachial artery approach (0.19 percent) as compared with the Judkins transfemoral technique (0.88 percent). In a study

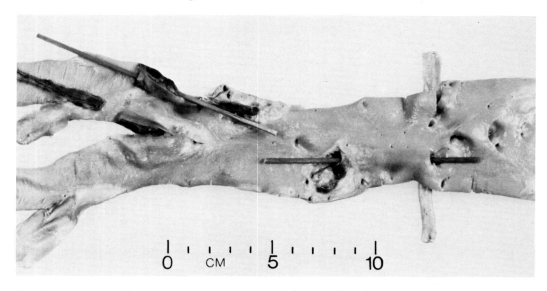

Fig. 36–32. Aorta and iliac arteries opened to show intraluminal thrombus and two intramural dissections caused by insertion of an intra-aortic balloon pump. The first dissection in the left common iliac artery (probe) re-entered the true lumen just above the bifurcation. The balloon tip then burrowed into an atheromatous plaque and returned to the aortic lumen just proximal to the right renal artery ostium. This 68-year-old man with perioperative myocardial infarction and left ventricular failure developed ischemic changes in his left leg.

of 3,044 coronary angiograms from 18 cooperating hospitals, Takaro and colleagues[111] reported 66 deaths (2.1 percent), the greater proportion with the transfemoral route. In a small series of patients, de la Torre et al.[26] found a relatively high incidence of coronary thromboemboli (4 percent) after switching from the transbrachial to the transfemoral approach; their six cases involving the left main coronary artery or one of its branches. It has been our experience, and that of others,[38] that the left coronary system is the site of predeliction for coronary thromboemboli occurring during transfemoral coronary arteriography (Fig. 36–34). This may be due to the thrombogenic properties of the left coronary catheter or to the procedure in which introduction of a second catheter is required.[26] Thrombus forming on a catheter may be wiped off on the vessel wall during removal and picked up on the tip of the second catheter when inserted over the retained guidewire.[111] Also, we believe that there is a greater risk of picking up fragments of damaged endothelium, atheromatous debris, or mural thrombi from the aorta or iliofemoral vessels when catheters are introduced from below (Fig. 36–34). Skeletal muscle coronary embolism is a less common complication of coronary angiography[67]; we have seen a case of adipose tissue embolism to the coronary circulation induced during the procedure. Coronary ostial stenosis due to intimal proliferation and atherosclerosis has been reported as a long-term complication of coronary angiography[53]; presumably, it represents a reparative response to endothelial injury incurred during the procedure.

Angiocardiography

The passage of catheters through the left and right sides of the heart during angiocardiography may also induce perforating wounds.[59,61,112] The wounds may, in turn,

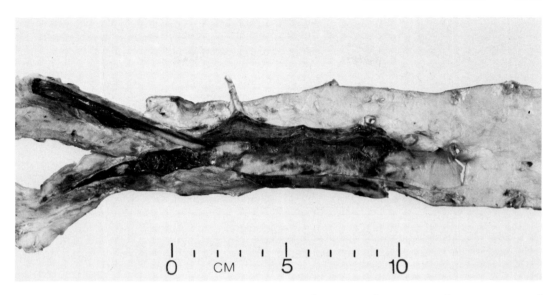

Fig. 36–33. External view of lower abdominal aorta and common iliac arteries showing intramural dissection resulting from pervenous transfemoral insertion of an intra-aortic balloon pump. The dissection started at the distal end of the right common iliac artery (above left) and re-entered the aortic lumen at the level of the celiac artery. The dissection propagated down the left common iliac artery and extended into both mesenteric arteries as well as the left renal artery. This 62-year-old man developed myocardial infarction one hour after cardiac catheterization studies. The intra-aortic balloon pump was inserted before emergency coronary artery bypass surgery. He died two days after operation with gangrene of both lower extremities.

cause hemopericardium or transmyocardial extravasation of contrast material, which may result in cardiac tamponade.[74] Exploration of the heart with semirigid catheters is more likely to cause intracardiac perforation, particularly in infants and children.[59] When this procedure was instituted in the 1960s, we observed three instances of fatal cardiac tamponade due to right atrial perforation during angiocardiography in newborn infants. Atrial perforations are more serious because there may be a tendency to tear the chamber wall in comparison with a "clean" ventricular penetration.[61] Where myocardium is sparse or virtually absent, such as between pectinate muscles of the right atrium or in areas of fatty infiltration of the right ventricular wall or wherever the chamber is abnormally thin, there would be a greater tendency for continued bleeding with development of tamponade. The heart is probably perforated

more frequently than is generally recognized, but seldom does this cause serious complication.[61] Bacterial endocarditis is a rare complication of right and left heart catherization.[69]

Balloon Angioplasty

Percutaneous balloon angioplasty has become increasingly useful and common in the treatment of obstructive coronary artery disease,[54,114,115] avoiding, or at least postponing, the greater morbidity associated with coronary bypass surgery. The technique inflicts calculated trauma by balloon expansion across the stenotic vascular segment (see Ch. 44). Intimal or intimomedial tears and plaque fractures appear mainly responsible for successful dilation of the narrow lumen.[114] Stretching of the vessel or compression of plaque components do not account for significant luminal

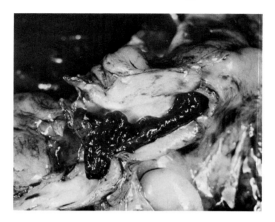

Fig. 36–34. Fatal coronary thromboembolism occurring during selective coronary angiography by the Judkins technique. The embolus lies in the left main coronary artery and straddles the bifurcation into the anterior descending and circumflex branches. Histologically, the fibrin-platelet mass of the thrombus contained a central coiled strip of endothelial and foam cells that were probably picked up by the catheter tip as it was advanced along the aorta from below. The thrombus was likely dislodged from the catheter tip when it was flushed, immediately before injection of the dye.

expansion. Since the extent of induced trauma is difficult to control, the procedure is associated with a wide range of complications, including coronary arterial dissection, thrombosis, distal embolization, rupture, and aneurysm formation.[42,92,115] Thus, early acute closure of coronary arteries postangioplasty, with or without myocardial infarction, continues to be a major concern and may require emergency coronary artery bypass grafting. A later problem is restenosis, which develops 2 to 4 months after balloon dilation. Restenosis is mediated primarily by endothelial denudation and vascular disruption, leading to superimposed thrombotic and reparative processes with myointimal hyperplasia the major mechanism.[23,35,63] Balloon angioplasty has also been applied to atherosclerotic aorto-coronary saphenous vein bypass grafts, where extensive plaque disruption, luminal thrombosis, and atheroembolism are major hazards.[91]

Restenosis in vein grafts may be caused by accelerated vein graft atherosclerosis as well as myointimal hyperplasia.

Interventional Cardiology

Balloon dilation is now employed to reopen stenotic valves and expand coarcted aortas. New invasive technologies are being introduced into the cardiologic arena at a rapid pace. Atherectomy devices, various laser systems, balloon pyroplasty (thermal balloon angioplasty), intravascular ultrasound (diagnostic and therapeutic), and intravascular stents already in clinical use or being evaluated can be expected to broaden the range of iatrogenic cardiovascular lesions. Waller[114] provided a detailed clinicomorphologic assessment of the current status and future treatment of atherosclerotic coronary artery disease by evolving interventional approaches (see Ch. 44). Any invasive vascular procedure has the potential of causing significant morbidity and mortality. The risks attendant to these techniques should not be overlooked or underestimated.

REFERENCES

1. Adelson L: A clinicopathological study of the anatomic changes in the heart resulting from cardiac massage. Surg Gynecol Obstet, 104:513, 1957

2. Allmendinger PD, Low HB, Takata H, et al: Deceleration injury: Laceration of the thoracic aorta. Am J Surg 133:490, 1977

3. Alter BR, Whelling JR, Martin HA, et al: Traumatic right coronary artery-right ventricular fistula with retained intramyocardial bullet. Am J Cardiol 40:815, 1977

4. Aronson W: Aortic rupture after a minor fall in a patient with extreme cardiomegaly. JAMA 186:729, 1963

5. Asanza L, Rao G, Voleti C, et al: Should the pericardium be closed after an open-heart operation? Ann Thorac Surg 22:532, 1976

6. Asfaw I, Arbulu A: Penetrating wounds of the pericardium and heart. Surg Clin North Am 57:37, 1977

7. Asfaw I, Thoms NW, Arbulu A: Interventricular septal defects from penetrating injuries of the heart. J Thorac Cardiovasc Surg 69:450, 1975

8. Bassan MM, Merin G: Pericardial tamponade due to perforation with a permanent endocardial pacing catheter. J Thorac Cardiovasc Surg 74:51, 1977

9. Beall AC, Crawford ES, Couves CM, et al: Complications of aortography. Surgery 43:364, 1958

10. Bedell SE, Fulton EJ: Unexpected findings and complications at autopsy after cardiopulmonary resuscitation (CPR). Arch Intern Med 146:1725, 1986

11. Black LL, McComb RJ, Silver MD: Vascular injury following heart valve replacement. Ann Thorac Surg 16:19, 1973

12. Bloch B, Meir J: Isolated traumatic tears of the intraventricular septum. Forensic Sci 9:81, 1977

13. Block PC: Snaring of a Swan-Ganz catheter. J Thorac Cardiovasc Surg 71:917, 1976

14. Boal BH, Keller BD, Ascheim RJ, Kaltman AJ: Complication of intracardiac electrical pacing—Knotting together of temporary and permanent electrodes. N Engl J Med 280:650, 1969

15. Bodily K, Fischer RP: Aortic rupture and right ventricular rupture induced by closed chest cardiac massage. Minn Med 62:225, 1979

16. Bourassa MB, Noble J: Complication rate of coronary arteriography. A review of 5250 cases studied by a percutaneous femoral technique. Circulation 53:106, 1976

17. Burnett HF, Parnell CL, Williams GD, Campbell GJ: Peripheral arterial injuries: A reassessment. Ann Surg 183:701, 1976

18. Campbell JJ, Fournier P, Hill DP: Puck aneurysm. Can Med Assoc J 81:922, 1959

19. Castagna J, Nelson RJ: Blunt injuries to branches of the aortic arch. J Thorac Cardiovasc Surg 69:521, 1975

20. Charles KP, Davidson KG, Miller H, Caves PK: Traumatic rupture of the ascending aorta and aortic valve following blunt chest trauma. J Thorac Cardiovasc Surg 73:208, 1977

21. Chawla SK, Najaki H, Javid H, Serry C: Coronary obstruction secondary to direct cannulation. Ann Thorac Surg 23:135, 1977

22. Cleveland JC, Cleveland RJ: Successful repair of aortic root and aortic valve injury caused by blunt chest trauma in a patient with prior aortic dissection. Chest 66:447, 1974

23. Cox JL, Gotlieb AI: Restenosis following percutaneous transluminal angioplasty: Clinical, physiologic and pathological features. Can Med Assoc J 134:1129, 1986

24. Dajee H, Richardson IW, Iype MO: Seat belt aorta: Acute dissection and thrombosis of the abdominal aorta. Surgery 85:263, 1979

25. Dane TEB, King EG: Fatal cardiac tamponade and other mechanical complications of central venous catheters. Br J Surg 62:6, 1975

26. de la Torre A, Jacobs D, Aleman J, Anderson GA: Embolic coronary artery occlusion in percutaneous transfemoral coronary angiography. Am Heart J 86:467, 1973

27. Deren MM, Barash PG, Hammond GL, Saieh T: Perforation of the pulmonary artery requiring pneumonectomy after the use of a flow-directed (Swan-Ganz) catheter. Thorax 34:550, 1979

28. DeSa'Neto A, Padnick MB, Desser KB, Steinhoff NG: Right sinus of Valsalva-right atrial fistula secondary to nonpenetrating chest trauma: A case report with description of noninvasive diagnostic features. Circulation 60:205, 1979

29. Ducatman BS, McMichan JC, Edwards WD: Catheter-induced lesions of the right side of the heart. A one-year prospective study of 141 autopsies. JAMA 253:791, 1985

30. Dzenitis AJ, Mealey J, Waddell JR: Myocardial perforation by ventriculoatrial-shunt tubing. JAMA 194:1251, 1965

31. Fraser RS: Catheter-induced pulmonary artery perforation: Pathologic and pathogenic features. Hum Pathol 18:1246, 1987

32. Friedman BA, Jurgelett HC: Perforation of atrium by polyethylene CV catheter. (Letter.) JAMA 203:1141, 1968

33. Gerry JL Jr, Bulkley BH, Hutchins GM: Rupture of the papillary muscle of the tricuspid valve. A complication of cardiopulmonary resuscitation and a rare cause of tricuspid insufficiency. Am J Cardiol 40:825, 1977

34. Gould SE (ed): Pathology of the Heart and Blood Vessels. 3rd Ed. Charles C Thomas, Springfield, IL, 1968, p. 834

35. Gravanis MB, Roubin GS: Histopathologic phenomena at the site of percutaneous transluminal coronary angioplasty: The problem of restenosis. Hum Pathol 20:477, 1989

36. Guss SB, Zir LM, Garrison HB, et al: Coronary occlusion during coronary angiography. Circulation 52:1063, 1975

37. Hare RR, Gaspar MR: The intimal flap. Arch Surg 102:552, 1971

38. Hartveit F, Andersen KS, Maehle BO, Kalager T: Fatal coronary embolism due to thrombus detached from a coronary catheter. A case report. Acta Pathol Microbiol Immunol Scand [A] 248 (Suppl):95, 1974

39. Heggtveit HA: Pathological considerations of artificial cardiac pacemakers in man and dog. Lab Invest 16:652, 1967

40. Heggtveit HA: The donor heart: Brain death and pathological changes in the heart. Laval Med 41:178, 1970

41. Heggtveit HA, Campbell JS, Hooper GD: Innominate arterial aneurysms occurring after blunt trauma. Am J Clin Pathol 42:69, 1964

42. Hill JA, Margolis JR, Feldman RL, et al: Coronary arterial aneurysm formation after balloon angioplasty. Am J Cardiol 52:261, 1983

43. Hirose T, Vera CA, Bailey CP, Edberg SH: Perforation of right ventricular wall by the endocardial pacing catheter. Dis Chest 54:510, 1968

44. Huang T, Baba N: Cardiac pathology of transvenous pacemakers. Am Heart J 83:469, 1972

45. Hudson RE: Cardiovascular Pathology. Vol. 2. Edward Arnold, London, 1965, p. 1604

45a. Hurst JW (ed): The Heart. 4th ed. McGraw Hill, New York, 1978

46. Iglesias A, Rufilanchas JJ, Maronas JM, Figuera D: Perforation of the right ventricle and cardiac tamponade caused by a venous catheter. Postgrad Med J 53:225, 1977

47. Isner JM, Cohen SR, Virmani R, et al: Complications of the intraaortic balloon counterpulsation device: Clinical and morphologic observations in 45 necropsy patients. Am J Cardiol 45:260, 1980

48. Johnson CE: Perforation of right atrium by a polyethylene catheter. JAMA 195:584, 1966

49. Jones FL: Transmural myocardial necrosis after nonpenetrating cardiac trauma. Am J Cardiol 26:419, 1970

50. Killen DA, Gobbel WG, France R, Vix VA: Post-traumatic aneurysm of the left ventricle. Circulation 39:101, 1969

51. Kinley CE, Chandler BM: Traumatic aneurysm of thoracic aorta: A case presenting as a coarctation. Can Med Assoc J 96:279, 1967

52. Kline IK, Hofman WI: Cardiac tamponade from CVP catheter perforation. JAMA 206:1794, 1968

53. Knutson EL, Smith JC: Coronary ostial stenosis complicating coronary arteriography. Arch Pathol Lab Med 100:113, 1976

54. Kohchi K, Takebayashi S, Block PC, et al: Arterial changes after percutaneous transluminal coronary angioplasty: Results at autopsy. J Am Coll Cardiol 10:592, 1987

55. Kohli S, Saperia GM, Waksmonski CA, et al: Coronary artery dissection secondary to blunt chest trauma. Cath Cardiovasc Diagn 15:179, 1978

55a. Kolin A, Norris JW: Myocardial damage from acute cerebral lesions. Stroke 15:990, 1984

55b. Kolin A, Breziwa A, Lewis AJ, Norris JW: Quantitative evaluation of myocardial injury induced by acute cerebral ischemia and its prevention by β-adrenergic blockage. An ultrastructural morphometry study. Br J Exp Path 70:659, 1989

56. Korns ME, Schwartz CJ, Edwards JE, Lillehei CW: Pathologic sequelae and complications of ventriculotomy. I. With special reference to the myocardium. Arch Pathol 88:269, 1969

57. Koroxenidis GT, Moschos, CB, Landy ED, et al: Traumatic rupture of the thoracic aorta simulating coarctation. Am J Cardiol 16:605, 1965

58. Krischer JP, Fine EG, Davis JH, Nagel EL: Complications of cardiac resuscitation. Chest 92:287, 1987

59. Krovetz LJ, Shanklin DR, Schiebler GL: Serious and fatal complications of catheterization and angiocardiography in infants and children. Am Heart J 76:39, 1968

60. Lamberti, JJ: Serious complication of intracardiac catheters. (Letter.) JAMA 231:463, 1975

61. Lawton RL, Rossi NP, Funk DC: Intracardiac perforation. Arch Surg 98:213, 1969

62. Liedtke AJ, DeMuth WE: Nonpenetrating

cardiac injuries: A collective review. Am Heart J 86:687, 1973

63. Liu MW, Roubin GS, King SB III: Restenosis after coronary angioplasty. Potential biologic determinants and the role of intimal hyperplasia. Circulation 79:1374, 1989

64. Luck JC, Engel TR: Transient right bundle branch block with "Swan-Ganz" catheterization. Am Heart J 92:263, 1976

65. MacManus Q, Okies JE, Phillips SJ: Surgical considerations in patients undergoing repeat median sternotomy. J Thorac Cardiovasc Surg 69:138, 1975

66. McCollum CH, Graham JM, Noon GP, DeBakey ME: Chronic traumatic aneurysms of the thoracic aorta: An analysis of 50 patients. J Trauma 19:248, 1979

67. McHenry MM, Lee J: Skeletal muscle coronary embolism: A complication of coronary angiography. Circulation 59:189, 1979

68. McMichan JC, Michel L: Knotting of central venous catheters: Nonsurgical correction. Chest 74:572, 1978

69. Mason JW, Rossen RM, Colby T, Harrison DC: Bacterial endocarditis after cardiac catheterization. Chest 70:293, 1976

70. Matila S, Silvola H, Ketonen P: Traumatic rupture of the pericardium with luxation of the heart. Case report and review of the literature. J Thorac Cardiovasc Surg 70:495, 1975

71. Morgan MG, Glasser SP, Sanusi ID: Bacterial endocarditis. Occurrence on a traumatically ruptured aortic valve. JAMA 233:810, 1975

72. Morton BC, Beanlands DS: Complications of cardiac catheterization: One centre's experience. Can Med Assoc J 131:889, 1984

73. Myles RA, Yellin AE: Traumatic injuries of the abdominal aorta. Am J Surg 138:273, 1979

74. Nadimi M, Anagnostopoulos LD, Frank MJ: Cardiac tamponade after transmyocardial extravasation of contrast material. Am Heart J 72:369, 1966

75. Nelson DA, Ashley PF: Rupture of the aorta during closed-chest cardiac massage. JAMA 193:681, 1965

76. Nicholas WW, Nichols MA, Barbour H: Complications associated with balloon-tipped, flow-directed catheters. Heart Lung 8:503, 1979

77. Nitter-Hauge S, Enge I: Complication rates of selective percutaneous transfemoral coronary arteriography. A review of 1094 consecutive examinations. Acta Med Scand 200:123, 1976

78. Nizzero A, Miles JT: Blunt trauma to the abdominal aorta. Can Med Assoc J 135:219, 1986

79. Nunn DB: Complications of peripheral arteriography. Am J Surg 44:664, 1978

80. Orlick AE, Hultgren HN, Stoner JD, et al: Traumatic pulmonary artery—Left atrial fistula: An unusual case of cyanosis in an adult. Am Heart J 98:366, 1979

81. O'Toole JD, Wurtzbacher JJ, Wearner NE, Jain AC: Pulmonary-valve injury and insufficiency during pulmonary-artery catheterization. N Engl J Med 301:1167, 1979

82. Pifarre R, Grieco J, Garibaldi A, et al: Acute coronary occlusion secondary to blunt chest trauma. J Thorac Cardiovasc Surg 83:122, 1982

83. Pringle SD, Davidson KG: Myocardial infarction caused by coronary artery damage from blunt chest injury. Br Heart J 57:375, 1987

84. Rayner AV, Fulton RL, Hess PJ, Daicoff GR: Post-traumatic intracardiac shunts. Report of two cases and review of the literature. J Thorac Cardiovasc Surg 73:728, 1977

85. Rich NM: Vascular trauma. Surg Clin North Am 53:1367, 1973

86. Rich NM, Spencer FC: Vascular Trauma. WB Saunders, Philadelphia, 1978

87. Rich NM, Hobson RW, Fedde CW: Vascular trauma secondary to diagnostic and therapeutic procedures. Am J Surg 128:715, 1974

88. Rittenhouse EA, Sauvage LR, Mansfield PB, et al: False aneurysm of the left ventricle. Report of four cases and review of surgical management. Ann Surg 189:409, 1979

89. Robin ED: Death by pulmonary artery flow-directed catheter. (Editorial.) Time for a moratorium? Chest 92:727, 1987

90. Roy OZ, Heggtveit HA, Waddell WG. Canine myocardial thresholds and tissue responses to chronic pacing. Med Biol Eng 7:501, 1969

91. Saber RS, Edwards WD, Holmes DR Jr, et al: Balloon angioplasty of aortocoronary saphenous vein bypass grafts: A histopathologic study of six grafts from five patients, with emphasis on restenosis and embolic compli-

cations. J Am Coll Cardiol 12:1501, 1988

92. Saffitz JE, Rose TE, Roberts WC: Coronary arterial rupture during coronary angioplasty. Am J Cardiol 53:902, 1983

93. Saunders CR, Doty DB: Myocardial contusion. Surg Gynecol Obstet 144:595, 1977

94. Sethi GK, Scott SM, Takaro T: False aneurysm of the abdominal aorta due to blunt trauma. Ann Surg 182:33, 1975

95. Sharratt GP, Ross JK, Monro JS, Johnson AM: Intraoperative left ventricular perforation with false aneurysm formation. Br Heart J 38:1154, 1976

96. Sidd JJ, Stellar LI, Gryska PF, O'Dea AE: Thrombus formation on a transvenous pacemaker electrode. N Engl J Med 280:877, 1969

97. Silver MD, Wigle ED, Trimble AJ, Bigelow WG: Iatrogenic coronary ostial stenosis. Arch Pathol 88:73, 1969

98. Silverman EM, Littler ER: Bullet in the left ventricle from a remote gunshot wound to the heart. Chest 71:234, 1977

99. Sloop RD, Robertson KA: Nonpenetrating trauma of the abdominal aorta with partial vessel occlusion: Report of two cases. Am Surg 41:555, 1975

100. Smith WR, Glauser FL, Jemison P: Ruptured chordae of the tricuspid valve. The consequences of flow-directed Swan-Ganz catheterization. Chest 70:790, 1976

101. Sones FM Jr: Complications of coronary arteriography and left heart catheterization. Cleve Clin Q 45:21, 1978

102. Sprague DH, Sarwar H: Catheter embolization due to faulty bonding of catheter shaft to hub. Anaesthesiology 49:285, 1978

103. Steiner ML, Bartley TD, Byers FM and Krovetz, LJ: Polyethylene catheter in the heart. JAMA, 193:1054, 1965

104. Stephenson LW, MacVaugh H, Kastor JA: Tricuspid valvular incompetence and rupture of the ventricular septum caused by nonpenetrating trauma. J Thorac Cardiovasc Surg 77:768, 1979

105. Stillman MT, Richards AM: Perforation of the interventricular septum by transvenous pace-maker catheter. Am J Cardiol 24:269, 1969

106. Stinson EB, Rowles DF, Shumway NE: Repair of right ventricular aneurysm and ventricular septal defect caused by nonpenetrating cardiac trauma. Surgery 64:1022, 1968

107. Swanson SA, Gaffey MA: Traumatic false aneurysm of descending aorta with aortoesophageal fistula. J Forensic Sci 33:816, 1988

108. Symbas PN: Cardiac trauma. Am Heart J 92:387, 1976

109. Symbas PN: Great vessels injury. Am Heart J 93:518, 1977

110. Symbas PN: Cardiothoracic Trauma. WB Saunders, Philadelphia, 1989

111. Takaro T, Hultgren HN, Littman D, Wright EC: An analysis of deaths occurring in association with coronary angiography. Am Heart J 86:587, 1973

112. Thomas CS, Carter JW, Lowder SC: Pericardial tamponade from central venous catheters. Arch Surg 98:217, 1969

113. Wagner GR, Keates PG: Perforation of the heart during cardiac catheterization and selective angiocardiography. Circulation 28:585, 1963

114. Waller BF: "Crackers, breakers, stretchers, drillers, scrapers, shavers, burners, welders and melters"—The future treatment of atherosclerotic coronary artery disease? A clinical-morphologic assessment. J Am Coll Cardiol 13:969, 1989

115. Walley VM, Higginson LAJ, Marquis J-F, et al: Local morphologic effects of coronary artery balloon angioplasty. Can J Cardiol 4:17, 1988

116. Ward PA, Suzuki A: Gunshot wound of the heart with peripheral embolization. J Thorac Cardiovasc Surg 68:440, 1974

117. Watt AH, Stephens MR: Myocardial infarction after blunt chest trauma incurred during rugby football that later required cardiac transplantation. Br Heart J 55:408, 1986

118. Wolfman EF, Boblitt DE: Intramural aortic dissection as a complication of translumbar aortography. Arch Surg 78:629, 1959

37

The Conducting System: Anatomy, Histology, and Pathology in Acquired Heart Disease

Reginald E. B. Hudson

DEFINITION

The conducting system is the means by which the heart beat is initiated and propagated quickly into the myocardium 100,000 times a day, in a regular, orderly fashion, resulting in the most effective contraction expelling the heart's blood into the great arteries. The system (Fig. 37–1), which is neuromyocardial, comprises two main parts: (1) the *sinuatrial node* (sinoatrial node, SA node, sinoauricular node, sinus node, the pacemaker), and (2) the *atrioventricular* (AV) system of AV node extending as the atrioventricular (AV) bundle (of His), which terminates in left and right branches, to ramify in the subendocardium of the corresponding ventricles. The speed of impulse conduction in the AV system (4 m/ sec) is about 10 times that of ordinary myocardium.

The sinuatrial node may be likened to a generating station, producing a regular impulse that radiates through the atrial walls to reach the relay station (atrioventricular node), main cable (bundle of His) and its distributing network (bundle branches and their termination). Should the main station break down, other parts of the system are capable of taking over. Some authorities claim that the SA and AV nodes are connected by definitive tracts in the atrial walls; also, in some people, additional AV connections (e.g., Kent bundles) have been defined. These matters are discussed later.

The conducting system is under autonomic nervous control, but it can function when denervated, as evidenced by the surviving recipients of heart transplants.

HISTORY

Most of our current knowledge of the specific conducting system was established during that golden era of discovery between 1885 and 1915. The story begins in 1887 with the pioneer work of Augustus Desiré Waller in the physiology department of my alma mater, St.

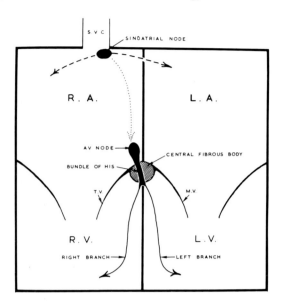

Fig. 37–1. Diagram of the conducting system of the heart. Note the possible connections of the sinuatrial node to the atria and to the AV node (arrows); also, how the bundle of His penetrates the central fibrous body of the heart to reach the top of the interventricular septum. (Modified from Hudson,[166] with permission.)

Mary's Hospital in London. Waller was the first to record body surface electromotive changes with each heart beat in man,[408] using Lippman's capillary electrometer in circuit with the extremities immersed in jars of saline; his "electrogram" was made on a photographic plate carried on a toy train, the image being that of a light beam focused on the plate and intercepted by the vertical fluctuation of the mercury column with each heart beat. Later, he called the tracing a "cardiogram." Waller demonstrated to learned societies electric activity of the heart in a variety of animals, dogs, horse, and two chimpanzees (from the variety stage). It is to be expected that the Animals Rights Lobby of those days accused Waller of cruelty, especially to his pet bulldog Jimmie, the matter being questioned in the British House of Commons on July 8, 1909, besides reports and letters to the press (e.g., from "Indignant").[389] It seems incredible that such brilliant fundamental research about the life force in all of us should have been resented. Waller also demonstrated his work to Einthoven, who later devised the string galvanometer, a faster and more sensitive instrument, to make electrocardiograms (ECG). Even the true inventor of the string galvanometer has been questioned, but Burchell's scholarly research established Einthoven's right to the credit.[53] Einthoven was awarded the Nobel Prize for Medicine in 1924, and it is possible that Waller, had he not died in 1922, might have shared the honor. Waller also became a physician at my other hospital, the National Heart Hospital in London, where he used the string galvanometer. The Waller Memorabilia are preserved in the Cardio-Pulmonary Unit at St. Mary's Hospital.[32] (His father, Augustus Volney Waller, is also renowned, for his study of nerve damage, "Wallerian degeneration.")

About that time, contraction of the heart was considered to be wholly neurogenic in origin,[266] or simply a myogenic peristaltic wave[133]—rather like that of the gut—but very regular and much faster. These ideas were held until 1893 because nobody knew the atria were actually connected to the ventricles by muscular bridges across the fibrous atrioventricular fibrous valve rings. In that year, Kent[213] described such connections in the mammalian heart; in numerous subsequent articles, he located the main connection spanning the lateral walls of the right atrium and ventricle. (These connections are currently, and perhaps rather loosely, referred to as bundles of Kent—a very belated tribute to a much-neglected pioneer.[418])

In the same year, 1893, Dr. Wilhelm His, Jr., announced, "I have succeeded in finding a muscle bundle which unites the auricular and ventricular walls . . . in a grown mouse, a newborn dog, and one adult (30 years old) human."[158] (William His, Sr., was Professor of Anatomy at Leipzig and obviously had taught his son well.) His's original article is preserved in the Library of the College of Physicians of Philadelphia.[226] William His, Jr., is sometimes confused with His, Sr. (just as Waller, Jr., is with Waller, Sr.).

The AV bundle of His was not the first part of the classic conducting system described. Many years before, in 1845, Purkyně (Purkinje), Professor of Anatomy in Breslau (Wroclaw) in Poland had described large, rather empty-looking cells in the subendocardium of ungulate hearts; he hypothesized that they belonged to the "apparatus of motion."[320] Then, in 1886, Schmaltz,[274,305] a German veterinary surgeon, suggested that these Purkinje fibers were the terminal elements of the musculomotor system, the viewpoint held generally today; that is, that they are the ultimate endings of branches of the Bundle of His. In an ungulate heart such as that of the sheep, Purkinje cells are prominent throughout the conducting system, but in the human heart, Purkinje cells are mainly in the subendocardial terminal network of the left branch. However, some writers still refer to the conducting system as the "Purkinje system," which is not quite accurate; in the human heart, the system is not so well differentiated as in ungulate hearts.

Although it seems certain that earlier workers must have noticed that the bundle of His emanated from a definite AV node near the ostium of the coronary sinus, credit for its discovery goes to Tawara, a research worker at Aschoff's Institute, who published his findings in 1906[390]; this fine work contains many hand-colored drawings of the AV system, often referred to nowadays as the His-Tawara system.

Thus, a definite muscular pathway between atria and ventricles was established, capable of rapid transmission of the impulse for contraction. But whence did this impulse originate? The answer came in a most remarkable manner from Keith and Flack.[210,211] Martin Flack was a medical student at the London Hospital Medical College, where Keith was a lecturer. One summer afternoon in 1906,

Flack called on the Keiths at their farmhouse, "Mann's Place," at Bredgar in Kent, where Keith had a laboratory. Flack was persuaded to cut serial sections of the heart of a mole while the Keiths went for a bicycle ride in the nearby countryside. When Keith returned, he and Flack examined the sections and noted a distinct compact mass of cells at the junction of the superior vena cava and right atrium, reminding Keith of Tawara's node, just described. In their 1907 paper, they wrote: "There is a remarkable remnant of primitive fibres persisting at the sinuatrial junction in all mammalian hearts. These fibres are in close connection with the vagus and sympathetic nerves, and have a special arterial blood supply; in them the dominating rhythm of the heart is believed to normally arise." This prophetic statement was amply confirmed by the brilliant work of Lewis and the Oppenheimers at the Royal College of Surgeons in London, where Keith was now a professor. In 1910,[250] they reported that electric exploration of the exposed dog heart had located the point of primary activity: this area was sectioned by the Oppenheimers, and it proved to correspond with Keith and Flack's node. Thus it was that the sinuatrial node became established as the "pacemaker" of the heart.

The main facts about the human conducting system were confirmed by numerous observers during the next 30 years. Waning interest was revived by the Glomsets in 1940[143] in startling fashion. They considered that the impulse for contraction was initiated and transmitted solely by nerve pathways (indeed, this seems the case in the pig heart[38]), and not by the classic muscular system; however, their work coincided with the development of intracardiac surgery, which soon demonstrated the arrhythmias could result from operative trauma in the area of the classic conducting system. It is now known that the transplanted human heart can function without autonomic monitoring at all. Nevertheless, the Glomsets' studies served to remind us of the importance of the nerve elements of the system, as noted by numerous earlier workers; it is now agreed by all experts that the system is neuromyocardial. Moreover, there is consensus confirming the classic descriptions of the conducting system.[11]

Anomalous AV connections outside or additional to the His-Tawara system would provide a convenient explanation for disorders of rhythm, the pre-excitation syndromes (e.g., the Wolff-Parkinson-White syndrome[424] of paroxysmal tachycardia, short PR and corresponding long QRS intervals of the ECG). The extra pathway provides a shortcut, as it were, for pre-excitation of the ventricles; sometimes more than one such tract is postulated. The impulse may travel in an antegrade or retrograde fashion. Such pathways were described by Kent; others have been reported by Mahaim,[264] James,[170] Lev,[243] and Brechenmacher.[44] In the last-named author's two cases, the anomalous path was from the AV node or AV bundle to the tracts of Paladino, which normally skirt the right aspects of the AV node to reach the tricuspid valve orifice. In a few patients, the extra pathway has been pinpointed electrically and interrupted surgically, curing the arrhythmia; it would not be unfair to state that such attempts have proved unsuccessful in many other patients.

Electrical exploration of the endocardial surface of the heart is now practiced commonly, using special catheter or balloon electrodes introduced percutaneously into veins or arteries.[5] Tracings can be made with the tip of an electrode in contact with the area of the SA node,[328] AV node, bundle of His, and its branches; abnormalities of conduction can be registered and analyzed[338]; from these "His-bundle" tracings, experts may be able to locate a lesion as being proximal or distal to the bundle itself, although histologic correlation may be poor.[339] Sometimes extravagant interpretations are deduced from such investigations by workers who have never seen the conducting system; those of us who have seen it have done so only in dead macroscopic or microscopic sections of the heart.

Ingenious apparatus is now available to help the cardiac surgeon locate the conducting system in the exposed field of operation; this is valuable especially in hearts with congenital anomalies.[151,254,329]

ANATOMY AND HISTOLOGY

Sinuatrial Node (Pacemaker)

The pacemaker is a distinctive crescentic collection of neuromyocardial cells wrapped around the anteromedial quarter of the arterial circle that lies at the junction of the superior vena cava with the right atrium. At its widest and in mature hearts it is about 3 mm in diameter; this part commonly lies just below the highest part of the crest of the right

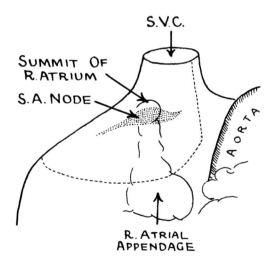

ANTERIOR   **A**SPECT

Fig. 37–2. Diagram showing the usual relationship of the sinuatrial node to the "summit" of the right atrial appendage. (From Hudson,[164] with permission.)

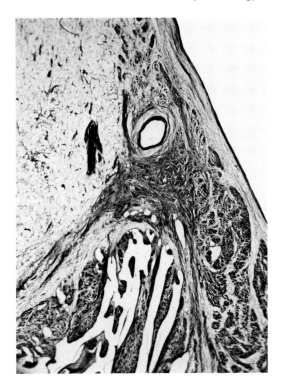

Fig. 37–3. Sinuatrial node with its artery in vertical section. It lies just deep to the fatty surface epicardium and adjacent to the endocardium, and sends strands upward into the superior vena cava and downward into the right atrial myocardium. (Holmes silver, × 20.) (From Hudson,[165] with permission.)

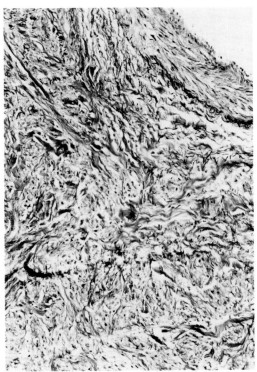

Fig. 37–4. Sinuatrial node—muscular, elastic and fibrous components: at top right is a portion of the node artery wall. (Elastic van Gieson, × 95.) (From Hudson,[165] with permission.)

atrial appendage, which I named the "summit" (Fig. 37–2); most often it lies to the right of this surgical landmark, but it may lie more medially. The summit is a constant feature of the heart, almost without exception.[163,164] In 25 hearts from infants under 1 year of age, Anderson et al. located the node in 22 at the lateral junction of the superior vena cava and right atrium; only 3 were sited more medially.[9]

The general histology of a node from an adult heart and seen in vertical section is shown in Figure 37–3; in this example, there is a single large artery, but sometimes there are several smaller arteries. The densely stain-

ing node extends into the superior vena cava and downward into the right atrium. Its outer surface is in direct contact with the epicardial fat, and its inner surface is near the endocardium. Figure 37–4 shows a portion of the node in greater detail; it comprises muscle, fibrous, and elastic fibers. A high-power view demonstrates the striations of the muscle fibers (Fig. 37–5).

Blood Supply

Arteries

The sinuatrial node receives a rich blood supply from the arterial circle, which it partly embraces. This circle is fed by an artery that arises from the proximal few millimeters of

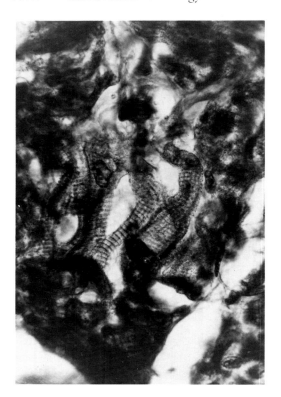

Fig. 37–5. Striated myocardium of the sinuatrial node. (Holmes silver, × 770.) (Modified from Hudson,[165] with permission.)

either the right (in 55 percent of hearts) or the circumflex (45 percent) coronary artery,[169] entering the node from either the front or back; this applies in both the infant and adult heart. In cross section, the artery provides a valuable marker for the node; its medial coat is often disposed in two or three layers (Fig. 37–6). Injection techniques have demonstrated free anastomoses with other atrial arteries.

Veins

In an injection-radiographic study of 25 hearts, Eliška and Elišková[99] found that veins from the upper SA node drain into the superior vena cava at its entry into the right atrium; veins from the lower part drain di-

rectly into the right atrium; the midpart of the node drains in both directions.

Lymphatics

The lymphatics are numerous in the epicardium adjacent to the node.

Nerves

Pioneer workers were well aware of the numerous nerves in the sinuatrial node; this has since been confirmed amply by many observers, including Rossi.[344,350] One can usually find parasympathetic ganglia in the nearby epicardium, and a fortunate section may show a ganglion cell in the node or a nerve entering the node (Fig. 37–7); terminal filaments ramify on the surface of each muscle cell.[385]

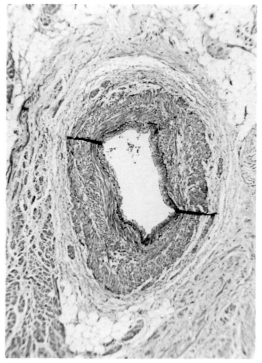

Fig. 37–6. Sinuatrial node artery showing muscle layers of its media. (Elastic van Gieson, × 80.) (Modified from Hudson,[165] with permission.)

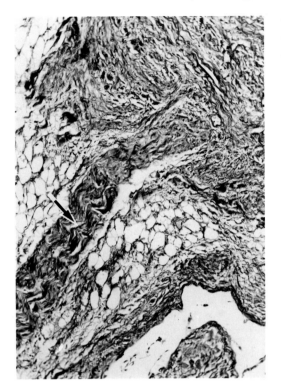

Fig. 37–7. Autonomic nerve (arrow) entering the sinuatrial node. (Elastic van Gieson, × 93.) (From Hudson,[165] with permission.)

Atrioventricular System of His-Tawara

The AV system of His-Tawara comprises the AV node of Tawara, the AV bundle of His, its right and left branches, and their termination in the subendocardium of the ventricles.

The general anatomy is shown in Figures 37–8A,B. The AV node lies just deep to the right atrial endocardium between the orifice of the coronary sinus and the membranous septum (pars membranacea). To paraphrase the description of its location given by Davies and colleagues[80] the node landmarks were clearly defined by Koch,[221] who described the anatomic triangle that bears his name, that is, the continuation of the eustachian valve and the annulus of the tricuspid valve (Fig. 37–8A and Fig. 1–15). This triangle has its apex at the central fibrous body and its base at the coronary sinus. The atrial component of the node is entirely contained within the triangle. The eustachian valve, having guarded the entrance of the inferior vena cava, fuses with the thebesian valve. The commissure of the two valves buries itself in the substance of the sinus septum as the tendon of Todaro,[395] a structure that may be defined by dissection (Fig. 1–15) in most hearts and is a recognized landmark in histologic section.

The AV node is about 8 × 4 × 1 mm in the adult heart. From its anterior end emerges the compact bundle of His, up to 4 mm thick, which penetrates the central fibrous body (which unites the annuli of the tricuspid, mitral, and aortic valves) to course along the summit of the muscular interventricular septum. Soon after its formation, the bundle starts to give off a thin sheet of fibers that fans down the left side of the septum, deep to the unstriated muscle of the endocardium; this is the left branch. There is, therefore, no bifurcation into the two equal divisions so commonly illustrated by physiologists. When the last left-sided fibers have emanated, what remains of the AV bundle continues as the right branch: a thin cord, coursing down the right side to run in the moderator band, which unites the ventricular septum to the base of the main papillary muscle of the tricuspid valve. Figure 37–8B shows the anatomy from the left side of the heart; the AV bundle runs in the base of the pars membranacea, which fills the gap between the muscular septum and the aortic attachments of the right and noncoronary cusps of the aortic valve. Some workers[106] suggest that connections may span the cavity of the left ventricle in "false tendons" extending from the muscular septum to the papillary muscles of the mitral valve. I have found striated muscle in the ends of such tendons but not in their middle portions in the adult heart. Such false tendons are a normal feature of human and animal hearts;

AV-SYSTEM — ANATOMICAL RELATIONS

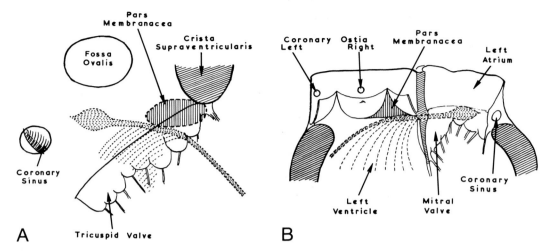

Fig. 37–8. Diagram of the AV system of His-Tawara (**A**) From right side, showing its relationships to the coronary sinus ostium and the pars membranacea. The left fascicles are represented by the dotted lines. (**B**) From left side, showing how the bundle of His lies in the base of the pars membranacea, sending a fan of left fascicles down the left side of the interventricular septum. (From Hudson,[166] with permission.)

they were detected by cross-sectional echocardiography in 21.7 percent of children and in 0.4 percent of adults; as well as in 48 percent of 686 postmortem hearts of different ages by Gerlis et al.[136] Malouf et al.[267] found them in 25 percent of 488 normal, diseased, or congenitally malformed hearts; Gerlis et al. suggested that they were a possible source of innocent murmurs. Beattie et al.[21] considered them to be Purkinje fibers, traversing the cavity of the left ventricle. They were present in 29 of 167 autopsied hearts and therefore subject to tension.

The Atrioventricular Node of Tawara

The AV node of Tawara (Fig. 37–9) comprises a collection of special myocardial fibers. Its deep surface lies against the central fibrous body; its superficial surface lies just deep to the endocardium of the right atrium. The muscle fibers present a distinctive, more delicate, lacy appearance than nearby ordinary myocardium (Fig. 37–10).

Traced forward from the coronary sinus end, the AV node condenses somewhat and penetrates deeply into the central fibrous body (Fig. 37–11) as it must do to reach the ventricle, where it lies on the summit of the muscular interventricular septum as the AV bundle of His; sometimes there is obvious cartilage in the central fibrous body of the infant's heart,[119] much less commonly, cartilage is also found here in the adult.

Meijlen[279] considered that the AV node had the dual role of delaying the rate of impulse conduction to the ventricles, while protecting them from rapid atrial arrhythmias. Delay lessened, but protection increased, as the size of a mammal increased, with humans somewhere between the rat and the whale heart (100,000 times its weight).

The Atrioventricular Bundle of His

The AV bundle of His is a compact cord, rounded or roughly triangular in cross section, up to 4 mm in diameter and 20 mm in length

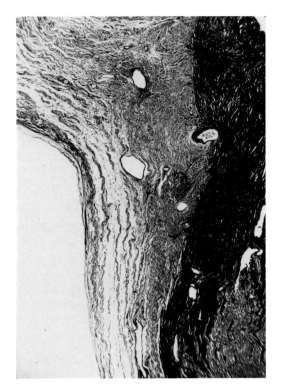

Fig. 37–9. AV node in vertical section, lying against the central body (the dark-staining tissue on the right) and covered by right atrial endocardium on the left. (Elastic van Gieson, × 16.) (From Hudson,[166] with permission.)

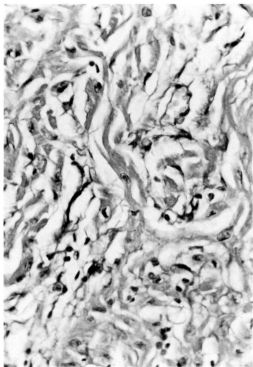

Fig. 37–10. Delicate myocardium of the AV node. (Elastic van Gieson, × 400.) (From Hudson,[165] with permission.)

(Fig. 37–12). It resembles ordinary myocardium (Fig. 37–13). Serial sections often reveal direct connections to the adjacent interventricular septum, called Mahaim fibers (Fig. 37–14).

The Bundle Branches

Bifurcation of the bundle of His is a misnomer; the bundle gives off left fascicles almost as soon as it is formed; it continues to do so throughout its length, thus forming a thin sheet called the left branch (Figs. 37–15 and 37–16). What remains of the bundle then descends the right side of the interventricular septum as the right branch, a thread up to 1 mm in diameter (Fig. 37–17), emerging gradually toward the surface endocardium.

The Left Branch

The left branch is a thin sheet of fibers, fanning out down the left side of the ventricular septum, from their origin in the bundle of His in the base of the membranous septum (see Fig. 37–8B). At some point in their descent, individual fibers give way to the large, rather empty-looking Purkinje cells (Fig. 37–18), considered the termination of the AV system.

An important normal variation in left bundle branch anatomy occurs in about 15 percent of normal human hearts, in which the His bundle courses to the right side of the crest of the interventricular septum and gives rise to the left bundle branch by a narrow stem only 1 mm or so in maximal dimension.[272] This stem then courses over the ridge of the septum and widens abruptly upon reaching the left

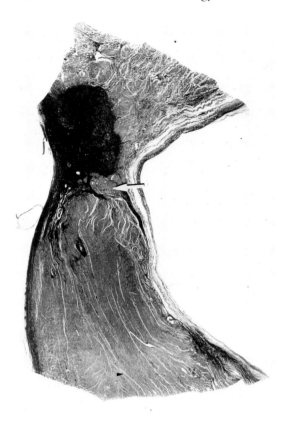

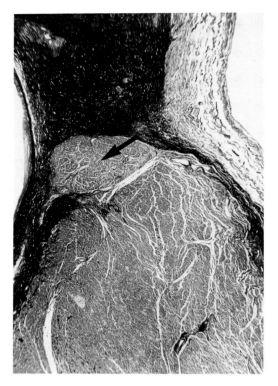

Fig. 37–11. AV node (arrow) penetrating the dark-staining central fibrous body to reach the summit of the muscular interventricular septum. (Elastic van Gieson, × 5.) (From Hudson,[165] with permission.)

Fig. 37–12. Bundle of His (arrow) on the summit of the interventricular septum. (Elastic van Gieson, × 17.) (From Hudson,[165] with permission.)

side of the septum. In this unusual anatomic configuration the left bundle branch may be uniquely vulnerable to small lesions.

The Right Branch

The right branch is the continuation of the main bundle after emergence of the left fascicles. It courses through the muscular interventricular septum as a thread about 1 mm thick, reaching the subendocardial surface of the ventricle at some point (Fig. 37–19). From there, it passes into the moderator band to traverse the apex of the right ventricular cavity and reaches the main papillary muscle of the tricuspid valve. Then it is thought to ramify over the lining of the chamber. Its appearance is that of the surrounding myocardium, but it may stain a little paler and often contains an obvious vessel (Fig. 37–20). Sometimes it can be identified in a random section.

Great interest was aroused by Rosenbaum's "hemiblock" theory[341]; he reasoned that there are *three* main pathways from the bundle of His, that is, the whole right branch and the anterior and posterior divisions of the left branch. The left anterior division courses toward the anterior papillary muscles; the posterior division, toward the posterior papillary muscles of the mitral valve. Moreover, Ro-

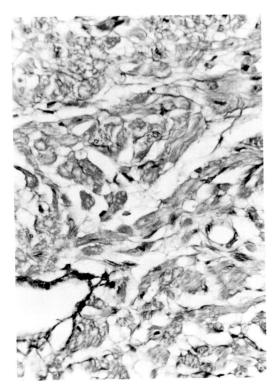

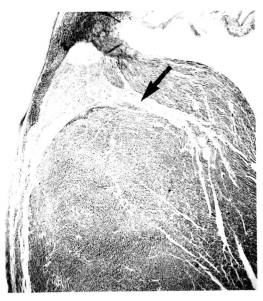

Fig. 37–14. Mahaim fiber (arrow) from the bundle of His entering directly into the interventricular septum. (Elastic van Gieson, × 13.) (From Hudson,[165] with permission.)

Fig. 37–13. Myocardium of the bundle of His. (Elastic van Gieson, × 430.) (From Hudson,[165] with permission.)

senbaum was able to interpret ECGs accordingly into 11 types of heart block, the chief three being left anterior hemiblock alone, left anterior hemiblock with right bundle branch block, and left posterior hemiblock with right bundle branch block (RBBB). Rosenbaum's view has been much argued about; the consensus of most observers, including me, does not support such a clear-cut anatomic division of the left branch, which is now regarded as an interlacing sheet of ribbonlike bands, forming random patterns, often with a third main division to the central area of the ventricular septum. Such anatomy can be verified only by horizontal, instead of the usually vertical, serial sectioning, that is, along the bundle of His instead of across it.[85,272]

Blood Supply of the Atrioventricular System

Arteries

The AV system is nourished by perforating septal arteries from either or both main coronary arteries (Fig. 37–21). The particular coronary artery which crosses the posterior crus of the heart (the common junction of the atria and ventricles) makes a U bend into the septum around the middle cardiac vein, which is ascending to join the coronary sinus. From the apex of the bend, one or more septal branches penetrate the septum.[147] This was demonstrated further by the elegant injection-corrosion studies of James and Burch[179]; the branch crossing the crus was the right coronary artery in 83 percent of normal hearts, the left circumflex artery in 7 percent, and both arteries in 10 percent. The right coronary

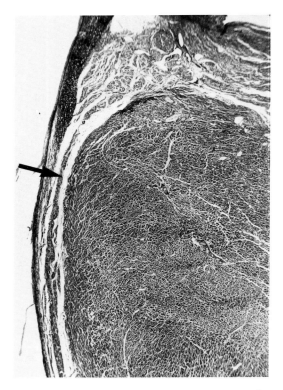

Fig. 37–15. Bundle of His yielding a left fascicle (arrow). (Elastic van Gieson, × 43.) (From Hudson,[165] with permission.)

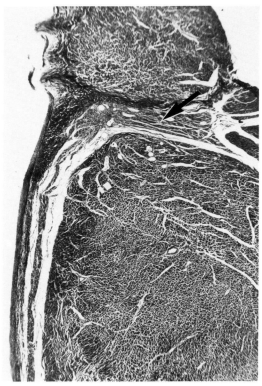

Fig. 37–16. Termination of bundle of His (arrow), which is about to divide into separate branches. (Elastic van Gieson, × 400.) (From Hudson,[165] with permission.)

artery supplied the AV node in 90 percent, and the SA node in 55 percent of normal hearts.

The main branches of the bundle and their terminal arborizations (as well as most of the septum) are nourished by perforating arteries derived from the anterior descending branch of the left coronary artery; the orifice of the largest of these arteries can be seen easily as one opens the proximal 2 to 3 cm of the descending artery in the autopsied heart. Frink and James,[123] in a differential injection study of all three main coronary arteries in 10 normal hearts, showed that the blood supply to most parts of the AV system was dual, that is, from both sets of perforating arteries. Somewhat different results came from an injection study

of 10 normal necropsy hearts done by Van der Hauwert et al.,[403] who found that only the proximal part of the AV node received an adequate blood supply from the ramus septi fibrosi of Gross, which derived in all 10 hearts from the right coronary artery; it mainly turned back within the node with only a small twig continuing into the bundle of His. Moreover, no anastomoses were demonstrated with the anterior penetrating arteries. This means that the bundle and distal part of the AV node had a poor blood supply and were, therefore, more vulnerable to hypoxia. It is possible that discrepancies between these two studies arose from differences in the techniques of injection—a notorious snag in such work.

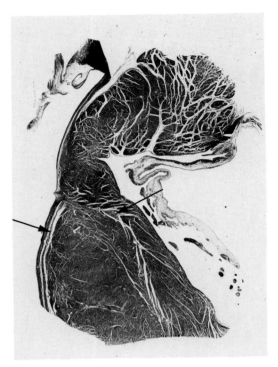

Fig. 37–17. Separated right and left branches (arrows); the left branch is the thin subendocardial fascicle, and the right branch is a compact cord. (Elastic van Gieson, × 5.) (From Hudson,[165] with permission.)

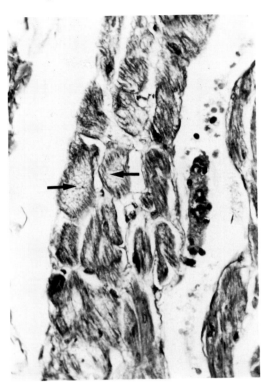

Fig. 37–18. Purkinje cells of the left branch (arrows). (Elastic van Gieson, × 400.) (From Hudson,[165] with permission.)

Veins

In their injection-radiographic study of 50 hearts, Eliška and Elišková[99] found that the AV node and bundle of His drained mainly into a thebesian vein which entered the right atrium near the coronary sinus; some blood drained into the middle and the great cardiac veins. The bundle branches drained into oblique septal veins. Truex and Schwartz[399] suggested that blood from myocardial sinusoids and venous channels coursed through sinusoids in the bundle of His and this might be a way in which noxious substances affected the rhythm of the heart.

Lymphatics

Lymphatic vessels are plentiful in the AV system; this may become obvious if they carry metastases from cancer of the lung or elsewhere.

Nerves

The AV node lies near the origin of the left horn of the sinus venosus (coronary sinus), and the SA node is near the origin of the right horn (superior vena cava). Lewis stated that the AV node was supplied by the left, and the SA node by the right sympathetic and parasympathetic nerves.

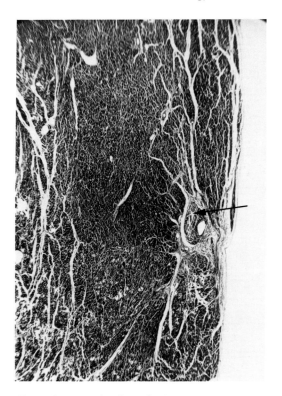

Fig. 37–19. Right branch (arrow) approaching endocardium of the right ventricle. (Elastic van Gieson, × 16.) (From Hudson,[165] with permission.)

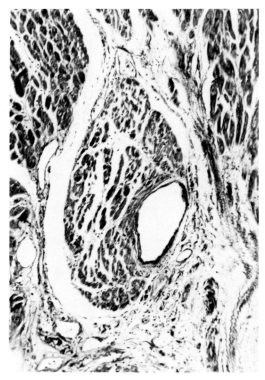

Fig. 37–20. Right branch detail. (Elastic van Gieson, × 102.) (From Hudson,[165] with permission.)

Many workers since Tawara have studied the nerves of the AV system, including Blair and Davies[41] and Rossi.[344] It is agreed that the AV system is well supplied with nerves, but they are not so conspicuous as those of the SA node. Indeed, Stotler and McMahon[385] could not trace nerves from the AV node further than the bundle of His; this rather countered Glomset's view that any system in the heart is entirely nervous. James and Spence[197] demonstrated that cholinesterase activity of frozen sections of the area was strongest in the conducting system, especially in the SA node (confirming one's histologic experience that parasympathetic ganglia are abundant near the pacemaker, and their nerves inside it). Kent et al.[214] also showed cholinesterase activity to be strongest in the nodes and atrial

myocardium of the human and the canine heart, and considered, from their dog experiments, that vagal stimulation enhanced the stability of the AV conducting system.

Myocardium

All observers agree that the muscle of the conducting system is specialized myocardium, that of the AV node being most distinguishable from ordinary myocardium (often referred to as "working" myocardium). A special feature of muscle cells of the bundle and its branches is their content of clumps of periodic acid-Schiff (PAS) positive glycoprotein, first reported by Gee,[134] in more than 70 percent of hearts at necropsy from patients of all ages (Fig. 37–22). In general, however, the muscle of the conducting system does not stain differentially with routine stains.

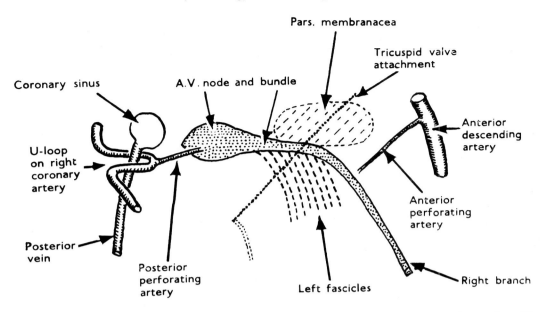

Fig. 37–21. Diagram of the blood supply to the AV system from the perforating arteries. (From Hudson,[165] with permission.)

Ultrastructure of the Conducting System

Investigation of the ultrastructure of the conducting system of the human heart must be done on the dead specimen with tiny blocks of tissue. Identification and correct sampling require a highly skilled investigator. It is thus not surprising that few studies have been reported, although there are several concerning the animal heart in which terminal "circulatory" fixation and immediate postmortem sampling are possible, for example, the steer[331] and dog.[203,367]

Nevertheless, studies came from James and colleagues about the human heart. The SA node[195] was examined from a child of 2 years and from two adults of 38 and 45 years, as well as from three dogs (in one dog terminal fixation with circulating glutaraldehyde was done). The human and canine nodes were similar. Three types of cells were distinguished; ordinary working myocardium, node cells (principal or P cells), and transitional cells

(Fig. 37–23). The P cells appeared like primitive myocardial cells, in clusters, and empty looking, with large nuclei, sparse striated myofibrils, and scattered mitochondria; the cells contacted each other and transitional cells, which in turn contacted working myocardial cells. P cells were thought to be the site of pacing. The AV node[193] was examined in hearts from two patients aged 2 and 38 years. Transitional cells, with structure between that of P cells and working myocardium, were the main cells seen (Fig. 37–23); P cells like those in the SA node were also found. The bundle of His[194] from one human and two dog hearts was composed mainly of Purkinje cells with few myofibrils, shorter and broader than working myocardium, with a large perinuclear clear zone, and with oblique junctions and more nexus formations. Fine collagen septa separated the strands of the bundle. (In light microscopic studies I found that the bundle resembles closely ordinary myocardium.) The bundle branches[196] showed similar structure in human and canine

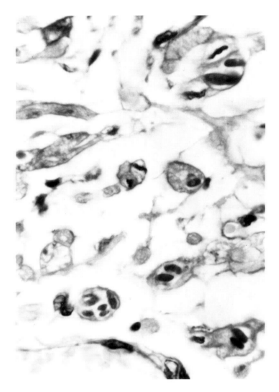

Fig. 37–22. Dark-staining masses of glycoprotein in the muscle cells of the bundle of His. (PAS, × 970.) (From Hudson,[166a] with permission.)

hearts. The left branch comprised Purkinje cells and working myocardial cells, but the right branch was almost all working myocardial cells.

Internodal Pathways

It is much disputed whether the impulse from the SA node travels to the AV node through the atrial wall in random fashion or via special pathways. The early workers Wenckebach, Thorel, and Bachman each described a different pathway, but the matter was not pursued seriously until James thoroughly restudied the problem in 1963.[172] James's findings from histology of 76 hearts and dissection of 42 are illustrated in Figure 37–24. James confirmed the pioneer studies and de-

scribed the three internodal pathways as follows:

Anterior: Connecting the SA node to the left atrium in front of the superior vena cava (corresponding to Bachman's bundle) and sending a strand to the AV node
Middle: Running behind the superior vena cava and corresponding to Wenckebach's bundle
Posterior: Traversing the crista terminalis of the right atrium, and corresponding to Thorel's bundle

A confirmatory report came from Meredith and Titus,[272] who studied seven human hearts from patients aged 5 to 81 years. However, some workers[10,95] do not agree with James. It is obvious that such analyses are extremely difficult technically; large blocks of tissue are required, and meticulous close-serial sectioning is essential—a formidable combination of obstacles to anyone working on the histological anatomy of the conducting system.

The matter is not entirely academic; acquired lesions of the pathways have been invoked to explain some ECG abnormalities. Cardiac surgeons often operate in the area concerned, especially, for example, in Mustard's operation for transposition of the great vessels. Although such procedures may interfere with one or more of the supposed tracts, surgeons plan to keep any such damage to the minimum—which, on first principles, is a good thing. By contrast, Gillette et al.[141] concluded on clinical evidence that arrhythmias following Mustard's operation were more likely the result of damage to the SA node than to internodal pathways. Hollman[161] noted that Lewis was the first to describe a patient with mitral stenosis and a nonbeating left atrium (presumably fibrotic) and a beating right atrium, a phenomenon detected by jugular pulse tracing. Atrial standstill, with absent P waves, was described by Pierard et al.[309] in familial Ebstein's anomaly in a father aged 56 who died of cardiac infarction (and had fibrofatty changes in the AV system) and in his son of 18 years who received permanent pacing.

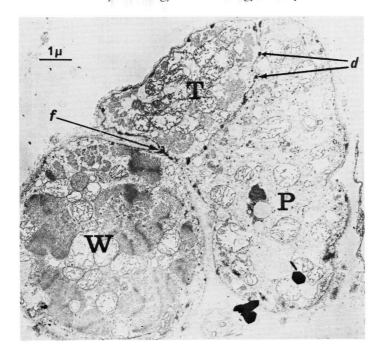

Fig. 37–23. Electron micrograph of the human sinuatrial node showing P cell (P), working myocardial cell (W), and transitional cell (T). (From James et al.,[196] with permission.)

PRACTICAL METHODS OF STUDYING THE CONDUCTING SYSTEM

Sinuatrial Node

Figure 37–25 shows a reliable way to examine the sinuatrial node. The superior vena cava is fixed intact by gentle packing, and vertical strips cut as shown. Each strip is lettered separately, and this is noted on a ground plan for reference; it is sectioned lengthwise. Verhoeff-van Gieson staining is excellent for routine study. In tiny hearts, the whole area may be excised, embedded, and cut in part-serial section, either horizontally or vertically.

Atrioventricular System

It should be emphasized that, in my view, there is no better method than serial histologic sectioning of a single block of tissue from the requisite area; the closeness of the serial cutting depends on the block size and on one's facilities and enthusiasm. Under ideal conditions, a small specimen may yield several hundreds, or a large one, several thousands of sections, each about 8 μm thick. Most workers have to compromise by "picking up," for

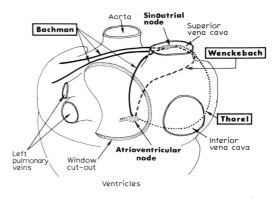

Fig. 37–24. Suggested internodal tracts; posterior view of the atria. (From James,[172] with permission.)

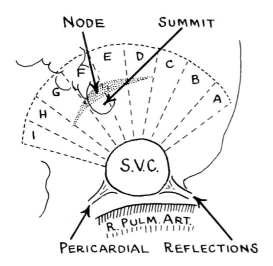

Fig. 37–25. Diagram of overhead view of the right atrium showing the strips, A to I, to be taken for histology of the sinuatrial node. (From Hudson,[164] with permission.)

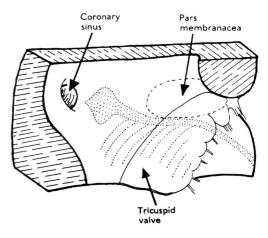

Fig. 37–26. Tissue block for histology of the AV system. Note the "corner off" the lower left border. (From Hudson,[165] with permission.)

example, every thirtieth section for staining and study, in the meantime retaining the "in-between" ribbons of sections should any of the series be spoiled or indicate a need for closer study of an area. Macroscopic dissection of the AV node and bundle of His was practiced by pioneer workers and by a few later experts,[419] but only as an exercise in highly skilled anatomic display; pathology needs histologic methods, and the results are proportional to the trouble taken.

The requisite block of tissue from the heart is shown in Figure 37–26. First, the membranous septum is identified by holding the opened heart against a light shining into its left-sided cavities. Next, the septum is excised boldly to include the coronary sinus orifice and the membranous septum, trimming extraneous tissue freely. The block is refixed in 10 percent formal-saline and, if necessary, decalcified and washed. It is then taken through alcohols, either manually or mechanically (50, 70, 90, and 4 × 100 percent strengths), leaving it in each fluid 24 to 48 hours. Next it is immersed in alcohol-chloroform, chloroform, and four successive paraffin-wax

baths. Vacuum is applied in the last two paraffin-wax baths, and finally the block is embedded face down in fresh wax. The "face down" is a matter of choice; I favor the membranous septum end. With very large blocks that are too tall for the microtome, the block may be taken through, *almost* bisected vertically at its middle, until the final embedding, when the "hinge" may be severed and the opposing faces embedded face downward (Fig. 37–27). This method ensures that the first sections from either half-block will show a recognizable part of the AV system, often the AV bundle itself; this encourages further exploration.

For orientation and identification, it is a good idea to remove the lower corner along the left side of the block at the last alcohol or the chloroform stage; all subsequent sections will show this "corner off" and can be taken up onto the glass slides all in the same way, making microscopy easier as one passes from one slide to the next. It is also good practice at this stage of dehydration to make a rough sketch of the block from both sides, inserting cotton thread "markers" to facilitate any later measurements and to pinpoint the origin of a particular section.

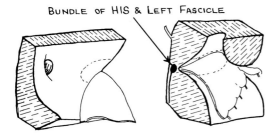

BUNDLE OF HIS & LEFT FASCICLE

Fig. 37–27. Tissue block transected; the opposing faces will show an obvious part of the AV system. (From Hudson,[165] with permission.)

The wax ribbons of sections are laid in order on sheets of cardboard in a stack; the cards can be kept separated by pieces of cork glued to each corner. At every thirtieth section, two (or three) sections are taken onto slides for staining and study. I found that hematoxylin and eosin (H&E) provides a satisfactory routine stain because the section usually survives intact and gives a general picture of the tissues present. The second method of staining is a matter of choice; I like trichrome stains best because the conducting system stands out clearly against the blue or green background. Unfortunately, the system cannot be stained differentially by routine methods.

Sections are cut starting from the anterior surface of the block, working backward toward the coronary sinus end; the early sections will soon encounter some left fascicles and the end of the right branch, and the series is continued until the AV node is passed. Once the series has been selected, the final set can be numbered boldly 1, 2, 3, and so on, from the AV node to the end of the right branch in the block.

The trays of spare ribbons are preserved until the investigation is complete. Additional "fill-in" sections may be required; also, further stains may be needed such as silver to help identify nervous tissue, or PAS to demonstrate glycoprotein masses in the muscle cells of the AV bundle.

Vertical sections, as just described, are not the best way of studying the left branch origin

and distribution because of its interlacing pattern. For this reason, some workers prefer to cut along the system horizontally, that is, parallel to the AV bundle, from above downward. This method, however, yields very few sections containing the AV bundle, the sections are somewhat unwieldly. A compromise is to cut the upper two-thirds or so of the block vertically and the remaining lower one-third horizontally, as suggested by Davies.[79]

Although it may be difficult to interpret results, a good series of sections will provide for discussion with experienced colleagues. No histopathologist faced with the task need be daunted, provided embedding is thorough and the microtome-knife sharp. The field is ever open to further exploration.

PATHOLOGY OF THE CONDUCTING SYSTEM

It must be admitted that, however carefully done, clinical findings and postmortem histology do not always correlate well. Established arrhythmias may remain inexplicable by microscopic study; or apparent pathology may be found in the heart of a patient who never displayed clinical evidence of abnormal conduction. This is not cause for dismay but testifies to the difficulties of such studies and to our incomplete knowledge of cardiac conduction.

General Remarks

The conducting system is not free of those pathologic processes that affect the rest of the heart, nor should this be expected. The general pathology which follows concentrates on the SA node (pacemaker), but much the same description applies to the AV system.

In a study of the SA nodes from 65 human hearts with congenital or acquired diseases, I found 15 nodes that were obviously abnormal; these came from patients who had

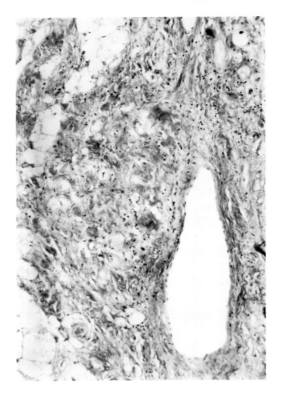

Fig. 37–28. Damaged sinuatrial node; note fibrofatty replacement of node muscle. From a woman of 49 years with chronic atrial fibrillation from cardiomyopathy. (Elastic van Gieson, × 100.) (From Hudson,[165] with permission.)

chronic arrhythmias, especially atrial fibrillation. The most striking abnormality was the depletion of the myocardium of the node and its replacement by fibrous and fatty tissue; an example is shown in Figure 37-28 (compare with Fig. 37-4). The dilated right atrium usually showed similar pathology. These findings were confirmed by Davies and Pomerance[81]; in acute fibrillation cases, however, they found no lesion of the node itself, but there was often associated acute pericarditis or pulmonary embolism.

When interpreting the histology of the SA node, it should be remembered that depletion of myocardium with increased fibrofatty elastic tissue has been reported as an aging change by some observers, for example, Lev[238] and Davies and Pomerance[82]; I have not been quite so convinced of this, nor was Rossi[345] in his study of the nerve components of the system.

In my experience, the most common lesion of the conducting system is focal hemorrhage, in the SA node, the AV system, or in both. Ferris[118] found focal hemorrhage in the area of the node and "internodal path ways" of 11 of 50 infants dying suddenly, and considered it to be hypoxic. Similar findings came from a study of 15 infant "cot deaths"(crib deaths) by Anderson et al.,[13] who reported similar hemorrhages in 15 control specimens; in addition, the crib death babies' hearts showed specialized tissue related to the AV orifices. Lie et al.[252] also found hemorrhages in the conducting system of 27 percent of 26 hearts from newborn to 2-year-old babies with the sudden infant death syndrome (SIDS) and in 29 percent of control hearts from explained deaths; the authors discussed the "moulding" of the AV system in the myxoid central fibrous body as a possible cause.

Arterial lesions in the SA node artery are seen occasionally. Focal stenosis of the artery is shown in Figure 37-29, but in general I found the vascular supply of the conducting system remarkably free from complete obstructions. Engel et al.[101] found that only 21 percent of 80 hearts in patients with coronary artery disease showed some angiographic obstruction of the SA node artery, but this was not considered clinically important. By contrast, James and colleagues stressed the significance of arterial lesions of the conducting system in the demise of patients suffering from various diseases. For example, James and Marshall[187] reported two patients, a boy of 7 years and a man of 64 years, whose deaths were associated with multifocal stenoses of the SA node artery due to fibromuscular dysplasia.

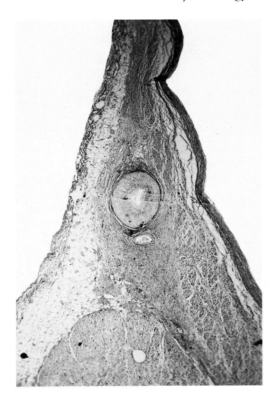

Fig. 37–29. Local stenosis of the artery of the sinuatrial node from a woman of 47 years with mitral stenosis and atrial fibrillation. There is much fibrofatty replacement of node muscle. (Elastic van Gieson, × 14.) (From Hudson,[165] with permission.)

Pathology in Arrhythmias

Bradycardias

Sick Sinus Syndrome

This form of sinuatrial heart block, also known as bradycardia-tachycardia syndrome, lazy sinus syndrome, and sinuatrial disease, was reviewed by Short.[374] It was given the colorful title of "sick sinus syndrome" by Ferrer,[116] who has now contributed a monograph about it[117]; for a change, Shaw and Eraut[369] have called the condition "lazy sinus syndrome";

other names are being coined, and the clinical literature is now extensive since the original description by Lown in 1967.

Victims complain of palpitations (often due to atrial fibrillation), breathlessness, dizziness, even of fainting attacks, and may suffer angina pectoris or heart failure after a number of years. The only reliable treatment in those with severe bradycardia is the insertion of a demand pacemaker. By contrast, some patients have no complaint[370] apart from attacks of palpitations from "lone fibrillation."

The syndrome has been associated with many diseases—hypertension, coronary artery disease, rheumatic heart disease, cardiomyopathy, pericarditis, congenital heart anomalies, surdocardiac syndrome—and with aging (it is commoner in the elderly).[72] Familial incidence, with autosomal dominance in three generations, is recorded.[233] It has also been reported in a man of 41 who had no right superior vena cava.[56]

Comparatively few pathology studies of the conducting system have been made in this condition. Evans and Shaw[111] (following their preliminary report with Brownlee to the British Cardiac Society) published findings about 8 necropsy hearts; the SA node was atrophic in 4, fibrotic in 3 (one showing amyloidosis, too); 7 of the 8 hearts also showed lesions in the AV system. Only one of 5 hearts specially injected showed some coronary artery narrowing, and this was reflected in the normality of the sinus node artery in all 8 hearts. The etiology was multifactorial and not coronary artery atheroma. Demoulin and Kulbertus,[86] in a Belgian study of the SA nodes from six necropsy hearts from patients aged 28 to 75 years, also reported damage (hemorrhage and fibrosis, as well as amyloidosis in one case) in all cases, accompanied by damage to the atria and to the AV system in six.

Lev et al.[245] studied two fatal cases of the syndrome; both in life had prolonged sinus recovery times. In one, aged 16, the approaches to the SA and AV nodes, and the "preferential atrial pathways," were fibrotic; in the other patient, aged 17, these areas were fatty. The etiology of the condition was unknown.

It is possible that some of the 15 hearts with grossly abnormal pacemakers that I described in a study[163] were examples of the syndrome, not then defined as such; several different diseases were represented.

From a postmortem injection study of 69 hearts, Shaw et al.[372] concluded that coronary artery disease was not the main cause of the sick sinus syndrome. Crossen and Cain[74] recommended pacing in severe symptomatic cases, as did Chung[65] in an extensive review of the condition, in which sudden death could occur.[101] A Belgian study of five childhood cases included one diagnosed before birth; the syndrome is a dangerous disorder in young children.[98]

Heart Block

Blockage of the impulse for contraction of the heart may occur anywhere in the conducting system and be attributable to congenital or acquired causes.

Sinuatrial Block.   A whole heart beat is dropped, no PQRST is written in the ECG, occasionally or at regular intervals. Sinuatrial block may occur in health but is often associated with intrathoracic invasion involving the vagus,[83] such as by lymphomas, or carcinoma of the bronchus, esophagus, breast, or stomach.

Atrioventricular Block.   There is delay or loss of the impulse on its way from the SA node to the AV system; however, P-waves continue to be written in the ECG. The block may be in the AV node, the AV bundle, or the bundle branches.

Three degrees of AV block are recognized. *First-degree block* is prolongation of the PR (PQ) interval; Campbell[60] considered that it was not always benign, as was thought formerly. *Second-degree block* is the periodical dropped beat, which may be preceded by progressive lengthening of the PR interval in preceding beats (known as the Wenckebach phenomenon or as Mobitz type I conduction); or the beat may simply be dropped, with constant PR-intervals (Mobitz type II conduction). Both second-degree blocks were known to Wenckebach,[417] who observed the a-c intervals of the jugular pulse; later, Mobitz[284] used the corresponding ECG PR interval. Shaw et al.[371] considered that all those with second-degree AV block should be paced to improve survival. In *third-degree (complete) heart block*, the atria and ventricles beat independently at their own intrinsic rates—the latter usually at 30 to 50 beats/min.

As with all readily observed human abnormalities, the slow pulse of heart block has a long history, dating from Galen's "rare pulse" in the second century, AD, and its first proper description by Vesalius in 1555; accurate timing awaited the invention of Harrison's watch with a seconds hand in 1760. A fascinating historic account of the matter came from Liebowitz and Ullmann.[253]

Congenital AV block may be partial or complete and be detected at any age from gestation onward; the prelabor heart rate is below 80/min.[313] Surprisingly, the abnormality may cause little disability in adults in whom the heart rate is usually over 40 beats/min, faster than in acquired heart block. Asymptomatic cases may have a lesion in the AV system, nevertheless, and may require future treatment.[231] By contrast, Seda et al.[368] reported a truck driver of 52 who suffered symptomatic second-degree heart block only when standing; the ECG evidence disappeared when he lay down. Congenital AV block may be familial; this was known to Morquio,[287] who reported slow pulse and sudden death in 5 of 8 children of a family, and who is credited with the first description of the disease. An affected mother and her two boys were reported by Veracochea et al.[404] Often, the heart has some structural anomaly, especially ventricular septal defect, alone, or as part of a more complex malformation, such as pulmonary atresia, transposition (simple or cor-

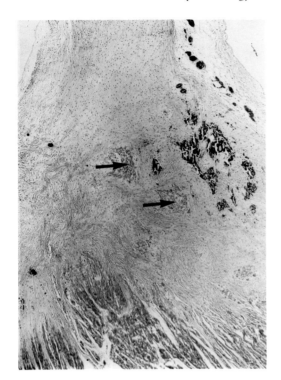

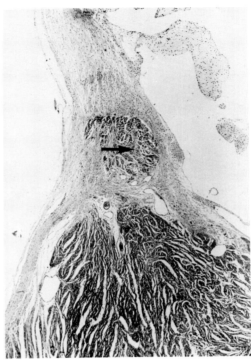

Fig. 37–30. Congenital heart block in a neonate. The AV node (arrows) is fragmented in the large central fibrous body, which also contains much dark-staining pigment. (H&E, × 49.) (From Hudson,[165] with permission.)

Fig. 37–31. Bundle of His (arrow) from the same heart as seen in Fig. 45–30; it is virtually normal. (H&E, × 49.) (From Hudson,[165] with permission.)

rected) of the great vessels, or aneurysm of the membranous septum.[392]

Figure 37-30 shows the histopathology in a neonate of 2 days; the AV node is fragmented by the extensive central fibrous body; more distally, however, the bundle of His looks virtually normal (Fig. 37-31). The fetal heart rate was 40/min, and the electrocardiogram (ECG) at birth was typical of complete heart block; at autopsy, all heart chambers showed mild fibroelastosis.

Many similar cases of congenital AV block have been reported; in 1926, Wilson and Grant[422] described a female baby of 14 months; Lev et al.[241] reported two babies, ages 3 days and 2½ years. James and colleagues have contributed several studies; in 1975[188] they reported their findings in the

heart of a female neonate, whose brother also had complete heart block but had survived by pacemaking to 6 years. In 1976,[185] they described the condition in the heart of a boy of 11 and a youth of 20 years, and in the same year,[198] histopathologic details were given about a black man of 30 years, whose family had suffered sudden deaths. Anderson et al. reported several cases; in 1975[12] they described three cases, and in the same year[135] recorded the findings in a 39-year-old mother of three children who had never sought treatment for her slow heart rate (34 to 54 beats/min); at autopsy, no nodal tissue could be identified around the SA node artery. In 1977,[14] the findings were reported at necropsy in three neonates of 2, 2, and 18 days.

The relatively benign nature of other cases of congenital heart block is well illustrated by the remarkable natural history reported by the late Maurice Campbell, M.D., with a succession of colleagues over the years—Suzman, Thorne, and Emanuel. The last-named paper[59] concerned the current state of six patients followed up to 40 years, survivors of the nine first reported in 1934. Four lived normal lives, and only one suffered a Strokes-Adams attack since several attacks in babyhood; one patient had corrected transposition. Reid et al.[326] reviewed 35 patients ages 12 days to 85 years: 21 (including three neonates) required permanent pacemakers; the sole death involved an unpaced 5-year-old.

Recently, attention has been directed to the presence of some connective tissue disease, especially systemic lupus erythematosus (SLE) in the mothers of neonates with congenital heart block. SLE is a multisystem disease in which numerous circulating autoantibodies react against blood cells and coagulation factors and cause hemolytic anemia, leukopenia, thrombocytopenia, clotting defects, renal disease, and other manifestations. Chameides et al.[62] reported eight children with complete heart block; at least five of their mothers had SLE. Histology in one infant at autopsy revealed fibrotic damage to the AV node, the bundle of His, and its branches. It was suggested that these lesions were postinflammatory, due to transplacental antibodies. McCue et al.[275] described 20 neonatal cases; 14 came from 11 mothers; seven mothers had definite evidence of SLE and four had laboratory evidence (antinuclear factor, rheumatoid factor, and low complement levels). Winkler et al.[423] tabulated data about 13 families with congenital heart block, and added details of a family in which the mother had SLE and her two infants, her husband, and his father had congenital heart block. Winkler et al.[423] postulated that there was interaction between genetic heart block and environmental SLE. Also, the prognosis in such cases was worse than in the sporadic type. In a European cooperative study, Esscher and Scott[108] added, in their second report,[109] 27 personal cases to 40 in the literature. In 24, the heart block was detected before birth, and seven of the nine infant necropsies disclosed endocardial fibroelastosis. However, many babies had grown up free of symptoms; the oldest was 40 years old at the time of the second report. An immunodiffusion study by the team of the sera of 25 to 47 mothers demonstrated antibodies to Ro (SSA), as did the sera of their infants up to 6 months of age.[262] Stephensen et al.[383] reported the additional complication of persistent ductus arteriosus.

Acquired AV block is one of the commonest conduction abnormalities. *Partial* block, in which the patient notices occasional missed beats by the thumping beats which follow (palpitations), is experienced at times by every healthy person and some who have a low tolerance for tea or coffee. Missed beats are common in infections, in digitalis overdosage and in chronic heart disease (ischemic, hypertensive, myocardial), when they may become established and progress to complete block.[57] The heart rate in acquired *complete* AV block (usually 40 or fewer beats per minute) is slower than in the congenital form. Campbell[58] found that the usual sufferer was a man over 60 years of age with myocardial disease from ischemia, hypertension, and cardiomegaly; less common were rheumatism or syphilis. Over half of Campbell's 67 patients suffered Stokes-Adams fainting attacks—often the first evidence of heart block, and of serious import. Other excellent clinical accounts came from Kay[204] concerning 80 cases; he related the form of the ventricular complexes to the probable site of the lesion in the AV system. Penton et al.[307] described 251 cases, aged 10 to 85 years; the heart block was permanent in 176, transient in 29, and paroxysmal in 19. One patient had clinical heart block for 47 years (presumably of the congenital type); by contrast, Gilchrist[140] reported that 11 of 25 patients with cardiac infarction died within 5 hours of the onset of heart block.

Besides those conditions mentioned above, heart block may be caused by the trauma of investigations or surgery, or by chemicals, cardiac infarction, local calcification (e.g., aortic valve), amyloidosis, myocarditis (of all varieties including sarcoidosis and tuberculosis), infective endocarditis,[165,223] by autoimmune diseases (vitiligo, hypothyroidism, SLE, pernicious anemia), by primary or secondary tumors and leukemias. It is a regular feature of certain congenital heart anomalies (e.g., corrected transposition), and has been reported in chloroquine overdosage.[96]

Clinicopathologic correlation is far from perfect; lesions of the AV system may be found when there is no block—and vice versa. The tedious nature of the histologic investigation usually ensures that only clinically proven cases will be studied, and this introduces the bias of inadequate control; there will be a tendency to attribute the block to a lesion that may in fact be only an artifact. Despite this, many authentic studies have accumulated, including those of Kries,[223] Mahaim,[263] Yater et al.,[431] Gertz et al.,[138] Di Gregorio et al.,[89] Castoldi,[161] Merron and Rao,[281] Harrison and Lennox,[153] Lenègre and Chevalier,[237] Zanchi and Lenègre,[432] Lev et al.,[240] Rossi,[344] and James and Reynolds.[191]

Good reports have come from St. George's Hospital in London; by 1969[152] their series had grown to 65 patients, ages 10 to 82 years (25 female, 40 male); 60 needed pacemaking. The commonest pathology was *bilateral bundle-branch fibrosis* in 26 patients; this group of primary chronic block was described separately[78] and subdivided into three subgroups according to the main distribution of the fibrosis in the bundle or branches. The cause of this fibrosis in the elderly is obscure. An example I studied is shown in Figure 37-32; it came from a man of 85 years. The condition has been called "Lenègre's disease"[235] (specific fibrosis of the AV system) and "Lev's disease"[239] (degenerative aging fibrosis of the cardiac skeleton in the area). Other reports came from Rossi[344] (who found nerve lesions in 2 of 4 cases) and from Zoob and Smith,[437] concerning 51 clinical cases. I studied the necropsy hearts from two of the Zoob and Smith's series, and suggested that the fibrosis might

be postinflammatory. James et al.[192] found scattered fibrosis in the necropsy hearts from two younger patients, a youth of 16 and a woman of 36 years, both of whom died suddenly. Fairfax[113] stated that "Purkinje tissue antibodies" occurred in 8.6 percent of patients with idiopathic chronic heart block compared with 4.2 percent of normal controls.

From a historic viewpoint, the classic studies of Eppinger, Rothberger, and their colleagues[103,104,356] about the electrocardiographic results of injury to the septum (and thereby to the AV bundle and its branches), were followed by much confusion among experts. This took several years to resolve and resulted in the reversal of the original electrical distinctions between right and left bundle branch block. Many authorities took part in this "change-about," Lewis[249] being a pioneer. Histologic studies are difficult because of the extensive areas to be studied. Early papers came from Yater,[430] Mahaim,[265] Lenègre and Chevalier,[236] Zanchi and Lenègre,[432] Unger et al.,[400] and Lev et al.[246] By contrast, some workers (e.g., Sanabria[359] and Rossi, alone[346] and with Lévy[352]) were less successful, suggesting that the electrical changes were less specific of damage than thought hitherto. Indeed, Ostrander[302] thought that right or left bundle branch block may not be of itself or serious import, especially in older people who are overweight, hypertensive, hyperglycemic, or hypercholesterolemic.

Stokes-Adams Disease. Huchard[162] in 1899 proposed this name for the combination of slow pulse with syncopal attacks. Noted by Morgagni[286] in 1761 and by several other writers, the definitive account came from Stokes of Dublin in 1846.[384] Nearly 20 years earlier, Adams,[1] a fellow Dubliner, described his case: a man of 68 whose pulse was 30 beats/min 3 days after the syncopal attack, and who suffered over 20 attacks in 7 years, falling completely insensible, with an even slower pulse rate, but recovering without paralysis. Some writers still use the reverse, historically correct eponym (Adams-Stokes disease).

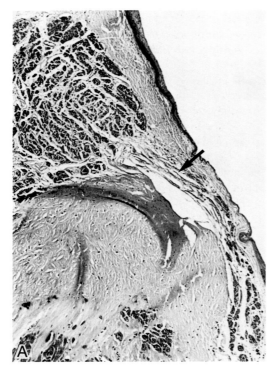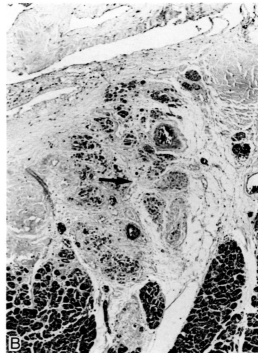

Fig. 37–32. Complete heart block in a man of 85 years, due to bilateral branch damage. **(A)** Fibrotic interruption (arrow) of the left branch as it leaves the well-preserved bundle of His. **(B)** Severe fibrofatty replacement of the right branch (arrow). (Both H&E, × 85.) (From Hudson,[166a] with permission.)

Parkinson et al.[306] analyzed the electrocardiograms during the syncope of 8 cases plus 56 recorded in the literature and subdivided them into (1) ventricular standstill alone, (2) ventricular tachycardia or fibrillation alone, (3) following standstill, and (4) extreme bradycardia of heart block, which accounted for the remaining few cases.

Stokes-Adams attacks have been reported complicating partial or complete heart block of acute rheumatic carditis and diphtheria, cholecystitis, ischemic heart disease, and other illnesses. Stokes-Adams attacks must be distinguished from neurogenic cardiac syncope, including an ordinary faint; ventricular standstill from vagal or carotid sinus origin; or myogenic syncope without heart block (e.g., nodal bradycardia or ventricular tachycardia). Some faints have acquired special names (e.g., swallowing faint). Sapru et al.[362] reported a woman of 20 years with this peculiarity, caused by dropped beats, who was cured only by surgical division of all autonomic nerves to the lower part of the esophagus. Rarely, swallowing causes paroxysmal atrial tachycardia as reported in a man aged 52 years, described by Bexton et al.[34] The symptom could also be provoked by inflation of a balloon in the esophagus probably from autonomic sympathetic stimulation. Weight-lifter's black-out[67] is caused by the warming up hyperventilation, tachycardia, and the very high intrathoracic pressure during lifting (160 to 260 mmHg), leading to reduced cardiac output and fall of cerebral blood flow with the Valsalva maneuver as occurs in the "mess trick" or "fainting lark." "Micturition fainting"[227] may happen when one leaps from a warm bed and stands to pass water.

Kearns-Sayre Syndrome. In 1958, Kearns and Sayre[208] described patients with complete heart block, retinal pigmentation and external ophthalmoplegia often presenting with ptosis and slow pulse. The weakened ocular and skeletal muscles may show abnormal mitochondria with excess glycogen granules. Uppal[401] recorded a boy aged 12 years, suffering ptosis and blackouts; at age 19, he had syncope on walking, with a heart rate of 44 to 72 beats/min; a pacemaker was inserted to combat the bilateral bundle branch block (BBB) and Stokes-Adams attacks successfully. A man aged 32 years with ptosis and divergent squint reported by McCornish et al.[276] had first-degree heart block with left BBB and HV prolongation. Endomyocardial biopsy disclosed hypertrophy with increased mitochondria. A demand pacemaker was inserted to combat the risk of complete heart block and sudden death. Two further sporadic cases, a man aged 30 and a woman aged 26 were reported by Charles et al.[64]; both suffered syncopes, held in check by permanent pacing. In the man, electron microscopy (EM) of an AV biopsy revealed proliferation of mitochondria with glycogen accumulations; left anterior hemiblock developed in the woman, at 19, which progressed to complete block. A youth aged 21, in whom intractable heart failure necessitating transplant surgery developed was described by Channer et al.[63]; his excised heart (less its atria), weighed 500 g. Histology showed diffuse foci of fibrosis and myocardial degeneration; EM study revealed vacuolated mitochondria of greatly varied sizes.

Right Bundle Branch Block

Right bundle branch block (RBBB) may be familial, as reported by Esscher et al.[107] in two families descended from an emigrant glassblower in Sweden, eight generations back in 1761; it occurred in 20 of 91 members. Right ventriculotomy is a common cause of RBBB, if it disrupts a lesser fascicle.[225] Dancy et al.,[77] from an echocardiographic study, reported that symptoms occurred in 10 of 24 patients with more distal lesions, showing pro-

longation of the isovolumic right ventricle and therefore the more distal lesions.

Left Bundle Branch Block

Left bundle branch block is not always benign. In an extensive survey of 3,983 males, aged 15 to 64 years, observed for more than 30 years, Rabkin et al.[321] detected 29 cases, five of which died in 5 years. Left ventricular hypertrophy is commonly present; Zymslinski et al.[438] found autopsy confirmation of this in 41 of 43 cases.

The danger of converting branch block to complete heart block during cardiac catheterization was pointed out by Wood;[428] this has been amply confirmed, and extended, by Rosenbaum's[341] "trifascicular" hemiblock view that there are three main branches of the AV bundle, that is, right, left anterior, and left posterior hemidivisions. In his tribute to Sir Thomas Lewis, Rosenbaum[342] confessed to using Fig. 4 of Sir Thomas's 1925 third edition of *The Mechanism and Graphic Registration of the Heart Beat* as a basis for his theory; it shows the bifurcating left branch of the His bundle of the walrus heart (the specimen itself is in the London Museum of the Royal College of Surgeons). *Bifascicular block* involves the right branch (RBB), with either left anterior hemiblock (LAH) or left posterior hemiblock (LPH). This may occur alone in 10 to 15 percent of those with Lev's or Lenègre's disease and may be harmless, but it may be associated with heart disease, with syncopal attacks, or even with sudden death, especially if deteriorization to trifascicular block occurs.[70,88] This event is more reliably indicated by clinical worsening than by sophisticated intracardiac ECG; Surawitz reached this conclusion from a survey of 1,242 patients from six studies.[387]

In a joint study with colleagues,[378] I found histologic damage to right and left main branches in the necropsy heart from a man of 62 years who had permanent LAHB with intermittent RBBB and LPHB, and who developed trifascicular block. Histologically, it was not possible to distinguish LAH and LPH. Rossi[349] found distinct left *anterior* lesions in only 2 of 8 patients with bifascicular block although all 8 had left, and 7 had right main branch lesions; he defined *three* interconnecting left branch divisions in most hearts.

Tachycardias

Paroxysmal Tachycardia

The sudden onset of rapid ectopic beats arising from the atrium, AV node, or ventricle, up to 240 beats/min and lasting seconds to weeks, may occur in health; this is the atrial variety of paroxysmal tachycardia. The ventricular type is much more serious and occurs in a heart damaged by ischemia, hypertension, aortic valve disease, or digitalis overdosage; it can complicate infectious diseases of infancy and childhood. A distressing accompaniment of all forms of paroxysmal tachycardia is *polyuria;* it starts about an hour after the start of the attack.[42] Wood[427] suggested that polyuria was due to inhibition of antidiuretic hormone; Kinney et al.[218] attributed it to decreased reabsorption of sodium.

In recent years, certain forms of tachycardia associated with pre-excitation along rapid "extra" pathways have received much attention; these are discussed separately below.

Methods of Treatment. Intractable tachycardia may be life-threatening; numerous "tricks" may be resorted to in an attempt to bring relief, such as breath-holding; applying pressure on the eyeballs (the oculocardiac reflex of Aschner)[17]; plunging the face under cold water with breath held (the "diving" reflex), causing vagal slowing of the heart[420]; carotid sinus pressure; and drugs (e.g., atropine, amyl nitrite, prostigmine, digitalis). In his AHA International Lecture, Krikler[224] surveyed European medical practice from the classic use of quinidine and digitalis; then β-blockers, verapamil, diltiazem, calcium antagonists, somatostatin, and amiodarone. Josephson[201] considered amiodarone to be the best drug at that time. A review by Di Marco[90] added encainamide, flecainide, and ATP. Ward and Camm[409] considered that

ventricular tachycardia could herald dangerous fibrillation; direct electrical stimulation could stop it, followed by drugs (e.g., disopyramide, tocainide, amiodarone, or sotalol). McGovern and Ruskin[277] recommended Holter monitoring during drug therapy.

Somatostatin is a 14-amino acid peptide isolated from ovine hypothalamus by Brazeau et al.[43] as an inhibitor of the secretion of immunoreactive pituitary growth hormone. Later, a 28-aminopeptide was found. It occurs in sympathetic and sensory nerves of mammals. Infusion into a human subject causes bradycardia and a drop in cardiac output. Using radioimmunoassay, Day et al.[84] found it in seven fresh necropsy hearts, especially in the right atrium and AV node. Webb et al.[413,414] reported that its presence in the SA and AV nodes suggested their control by it; it could, like the calcium channel blocker verapamil, terminate ventricular tachycardia,[413] but less actively, given as infusion of 12.5 μg/min to six of seven patients.[414] However, these may all fail to give relief, and so may electric shock therapy (introduced by Zoll and Linenthal[435]). Ward and Davies[411] reported using high-energy electric shock (210 to 375 W/sec) through a transvenous pacing wire to terminate intractable tachycardia in a man aged 55 years; he died 5 months later. Autopsy revealed extensive coronary artery disease and healed anteroseptal infarction, but no AV node was found, nor were any signs of endocardial injury at its site. The His bundle and bifurcation were intact. For these reasons, surgical means have been resorted to, often successfully, if a causative site for "re-entry" of the impulse can be defined before operation. For example, Spurrell et al.[382] explored four such cases by isochrone mapping, then cured the ventricular tachycardia by appropriate incision in ventricle or septum. Denes et al.[87] cured chronic tachycardia in a man of 44, whose heart contained a bundle of Kent, by severing the bundle of His. Aneurysm resection may relieve a left ventricular cause. In ischemic cases, encircling endocardial incision may sever a re-entry pathway;

precise mapping and incision is better.[228] A full review followed, by Morady and Scheinman.[285] Nathan et al.[293] described their surgical experience since 1977 of 54 patients with ventricular tachycardia or fibrillation; several techniques were used. Mortality was 22 percent; the surviving 40 were brought under control.

Cryosurgery (i.e., freezing the AV system) has been successful too; it was used by the team at Duke University in Durham. Reversible heart block occurs at 0°C and permanent block at −60°C; 5 patients with preexcitation[129] and 2 without it[154] were so treated. Bentall et al.[30] treated 7 patients suffering intractable Wolff-Parkinson-White tachycardia by cryosurgery, curing 6 and relieving the symptoms in 1, after endocardial mapping had located the accessory pathway(s); the method was also applied to the bundle of His in 2 patients with atrial arrhythmias. Bennet[29] discussed surgical management and concluded that accurate localization with cryotherapy of the pathways was the method of choice, as recommended by the Duke University team's report on two patients in 1980; it succeeded in 17.[220]

Torsade de Pointes

A special variety of ventricular tachycardia is *torsade de pointes* described by MacWilliam[261]; the QRS polarity oscillates in runs of 3 to 20 beats; it can complicate many heart diseases and drug treatments. Rossi and Matturri[353] reported the histopathology in 2 cases: a man aged 55 dying of cardiac infarction and a man aged 87 with pulmonary tuberculosis, dying of syncope. The former showed infarction of the atrium and ventricle at autopsy involving the bundle branches; the latter showed fibrosis of the AV system, as in Lev-Lenègre disease.

In experiments on isolated perfused pig hearts, the arrhythmia could be produced by stimulating both ventricles together, suggesting an interaction of two ectopic foci.[294] Fontaine et al.[121] credited Dessertene with naming the condition in 1966. The attack

might necessitate cardiac massage, pacing, or even DC shock, but intravenous isoproterenol was valuable therapy.

Wolff-Parkinson-White (WPW) and Other Preexcitation Syndromes

Parkinson in England and White in the United States were the doyens of cardiology in their time. They would be gratified at the enormous interest now shown in their classic 1930 paper with Wolff[424] about healthy young people getting attacks of tachycardia associated with an ECG short PR interval and corresponding widened QRS, simulating bundle branch block.

As mentioned, the phenomenon has been attributed to some pathway of more rapid conduction inside or outside the AV system, "writing" the first part of the QRS wave of the ECG; the normal slower conducted impulse writes the rest, so that this part of the wave is slurred. Two forms are described: type A, with the slurred Δ wave upward, and a right bundle branch pattern; and type B, with the Δ wave downward in leads V_1 and V_2 and left bundle branch pattern.[340] Type A indicates a left-sided posterior or septal, and type B a right-sided anomalous AV connection.

The syndrome may occur in the neonate,[206] in children,[139] or in adults, in apparent health, or in a variety of heart diseases. It may also accompany congenital heart anomalies such as Ebstein's anomaly[242,397] or Fallot's tetrad.[271] It may lead to other arrhythmias, such as dangerously rapid atrial fibrillation,[75] to fatal ventricular fibrillation,[92] or to complete heart block.[243]

The arrhythmias occur if the impulse travels retrogradely from ventricle to atrium, through either the normal or the anomalous pathway, setting up a "circus" movement.[95] What triggers an attack is not known, although various factors have been blamed; usually the attack comes "out of the blue" and may go away as mysteriously.

Most of our current knowledge and extensive literature derives from sophisticated exploration of electric impulses from the epi-

and endocardial surfaces of the heart during the cardiac cycle to locate accessory pathways for fast conduction.[94] Sometimes surgical ablation of such tracts, or even of the AV node and bundle of His by injection (procaine, formalin), freezing, cautery, ligation, or transection may succeed in abolishing the arrhythmia. When all such treatment fails, the insertion of an artificial pacemaker may be required.

Large series of WPW cases were described by Giardina et al.[139] (62 infants and children), Miller et al.[283] (13 cases), and Gallagher et al.[126] (92 cases).

Three main ECG pre-excitation syndromes are now distinguishable.[73]

1. *Classic WPW syndrome:* The PR interval is short, QRS wider, with slurred Δ wave either upward (type A) or downward (type B). A Kent or other bundle may be defined (e.g., that of Lev et al.[243])

2. *Lown-Ganong-Levine syndrome*[259]: PR interval is short, but QRS is normal. The abnormality has been attributed to the tract described by James,[170] normally connecting the atria to the high interventricular septum via part of the AV node and AV bundle. Bundle of His recordings in three cases by Mandel et al.[268] suggested partial bypass of the AV node or accelerated conduction distal to it. Benditt et al.[28] studied 12 patients, ages 12 to 59 years, and defined three subgroups: 6 patients had regular tachycardia, 2 had atrial fibrillation, and 4 had ventricular tachycardia.

3. *Normal PR-interval but wider QRS, with Δ wave:* This is attributed to Mahaim fibers from the AV node or bundle direct into the interventricular septum. Such fibers are common in the normal heart; indeed, they were the only accessory pathways found by Lev and Lerner[244] in 22 fetal and neonatal hearts and 5 adult hearts. Sometimes more than one tract is defined in the same heart[130]; this may frustrate surgical ablation. When no accessory pathway for pre-excitation can be defined, it has been proposed that it lies within the AV system

itself[317,373]; another view suggests that there are hyperexcitable foci in the heart.[379] Pritchett et al.[317] reported a man aged 50 whose intractable chronic, supraventricular attacks of tachycardia were cured by excision of the AV node without causing expected heart block; it was postulated that re-entry was in the AV node itself and that the operation had changed both antegrade and retrograde conduction.

When one considers that histologic confirmation may require expert preparation and scrutiny of thousands of serial sections from the correct part of the heart, searching for a mere wisp of muscle fibers making an accessory AV connection, it is no surprise that pathology lags far behind clinical studies; indeed, up to 1975, Rossi[348] reckoned that fewer than 20 reliable cases were available in the literature. Moreover, it is almost impossible at autopsy to verify that an abnormal tract was present in the scar of surgical ablation.

Despite these formidable obstacles, some good histologic studies have been done since Wood et al.[426] in 1943 found an anomalous right-sided bundle of Kent, and Öhnell[299] a left-sided one in 1944. Truex et al.[398] cut 11,500 sections to find a right atrial-septal connection in their case; Lev et al.[243] cut 14,662 sections to find, as well as Mahaim and James tracts, another one from the atrium to the bundle of His. In a study of two cases, Lunel[405] found numerous tunnels for anomalous septal and parietal pathways in the annulus fibrosus. James and Puech[190] studied 14,165 slides from their case, a woman aged 22 years who died of a stroke after a long history of type A WPW syndrome. These workers found several lesions, and an AV connection in the mitral valve annulus.

In a truly international study, Brechenmacher et al.[45] studied 16,000 slides from the heart of a policeman of 42 who suffered type A WPW syndrome. Epicardial mapping supported the view that there was a left-sided connection, but left atrial incisions missed it; there were also fibers from the interatrial septum to the bundle of His. Another international study was by Becker et al.[24] of 53 normal hearts at autopsy; 8 came from patients who had proven pre-excitation, and 6 of these contained 7 accessory connections; in 4, tracts skirted the mitral valve annulus, and one each was found in the septum, the tricuspid valve annulus, and anteriorly. The same team, in another clinicopathologic report[22] of 7 patients, 2 with Ebstein's anomaly of the tricuspid valve, got good correlation in at least 4 cases; the entire AV junction was studied (but in separate blocks of tissue—always a disadvantage when searching for tenuous accessory connections).

Rossi of Milan has contributed many expert and thoughtful studies. With Knippel and Taccardi,[351] Rossi studied the case of a woman of 41 who had type A WPW syndrome that became so intractable that the AV bundle was severed surgically; a tiny, left-sided bundle of Kent was found posterolaterally in the mitral valve annulus of the heart. In a later study[348] of 9 autopsy hearts (8 human and 1 dog) which had shown various arrhythmias, including WPW syndrome, Rossi found James's fibers from the atrium to the distal part of the AV node in the heart of a man aged 70 who had *not* suffered pre-excitation; in the heart of a woman of 41 who had had WPW syndrome, he found Mahaim fibers, a left-sided Kent bundle, and also "ring tissue"—islets of tiny pale interlacing myocardial fibers in the atrial wall near the valve ring. Rossi concluded that only Kent bundles were of proven importance in pre-excitation syndromes, other connections not having proved as responsible. In another case, a woman of 47 years with type B WPW syndrome underwent aortic valve replacement and two surgical attempts to sever suspected accessory AV connections; one effort succeeded, but she died 7 weeks later from infective endocarditis. Rossi et al.[355] found fibrosis of the SA node and of the left bundle branch origin; it was not possible to identify the bundle of Kent presumed to be in the posterolateral scar. Mahaim and James fibers were present, however.

The pre-excitation syndromes have continued to excite interest; numerous clinical reports, especially concerning management have appeared. A definitive review concerning 68 patients in 5 years, 30 of whom needed surgical relief (18 successful) came from the team at Duke University, who acknowledged the pioneer epicardial mapping procedure of Durrer and Roos in 1967 in Amsterdam; their series had then grown to 92.[128] The team also reported five patients with dual antegrade pathways[318] and a man aged 60 who died of cardiac infarction 18 months after studies that suggested impaired antegrade conduction; three AV pathways were confirmed at autopsy, one fibrotic and the other two partly so.[219] A full account of the diagnosis and treatment of WPW patients came from Wellens[415] (a colleague of Durrer). Robinson et al.[336] reported that the syndrome often presented with atrial fibrillation, which was not a cause for worry. Gerlis et al.[137] described an unusual cause of pre-excitation in a youth aged 18 and a girl aged 11 who died; at autopsy, the hearts showed aneurysms of the coronary sinus in the muscular walls of which the accessory pathway was found on meticulous histological search.

Most accounts of pre-excitation include methods of treating patients with intractable medical response by a variety of physical means, as in other tachycardias. Invasive techniques include cryoablation of the AV system followed by pacemaking as by the Duke University team[220] and also by the team at Hammersmith Hospital in London, who treated 20 adults since 1977, under bypass conditions, after endo- and epicardial mapping; 17 of the 20 patients were relieved, some after a repeat procedure[357] and by transvenous electric ablation of the accessory pathways when located, as in three patients by Ward and Camm[410] by three shocks of 50 to 100 joules (J) to the defibrillator electrode sited as near to the pathways as possible.

Fibrillation

Fibrillation is a very rapid flickering movement of a heart chamber instead of a proper contraction. Atrial fibrillation impairs filling of the ventricles, but ventricular fibrillation halts the circulation and, unless it is remedied, life itself.

Most of our knowledge about fibrillation comes from clinical and experimental observation. Several theories in turn have been advanced to explain the abnormality, e.g., Lewis's[248] "circus" movement of the wave of contraction traveling continuously round the base of the great veins because the tissue ahead is always excitable; Prinzmetal's[315,316] ectopic focus in the atrium; Burn's[54] shortening of the normally protective refractory period of cardiac muscle with its fibers out of phase for some reason.

Atrial (Auricular) Fibrillation

This may occur without apparent heart disease (lone fibrillation),[112] the only complaints being palpitations and polyuria; sometimes it is familial.[425] More often, the arrhythmia complicates mitral stenosis especially if the valve annulus is calcified[291]; thyrotoxicosis, ischemic heart disease, constrictive pericarditis, hypertension, or an infection; it is rare in congenital heart anomalies (excepting atrial septal defect) and in infective endocarditis. It is more common with advancing age; Rossi,[345] in a study of necropsy hearts from 37 patients aged 60 to 90 years, found degenerative changes in ganglia and nerves of the heart but little wrong with the conducting system.

In a histologic study[163] of the human pacemaker of 65 hearts, I found 15 nodes obviously diseased from fibrofatty replacement of the node myocardium; 14 of the 15 nodes came from those with established atrial fibrillation; in 8 of the remaining 49 nodes without apparent lesions, paroxysmal atrial fibrillation had occurred.

If the fibrillation is too fast, it may be slowed by drugs such as digitalis or quinidine (which carries a risk of dangerous syncope[330]) or abolished, sometimes permanently in suitable cases by intravenous pirmenol,[396] by direct current electric shock, as introduced by Lown et al.[258]

McMichael[278] in his account of the history of atrial fibrillation between 1628 and 1819, said that Harvey was the first to realize that the pulse was caused by the heartbeat, which started in the atria, the right one fibrillating at death. Other pioneers added to this fundamental knowledge—Lower, deSenac, and Laennec. The precise nature of the pulse was studied by Rawles and Rowland[324] in 76 patients, 36 having digitalis therapy; it was concluded that the pulse is not always "irregularly irregular" as is usually taught; 34 had pulsus alternans, a regular rhythm.[280] (Anyone recording arm blood pressure in such patients will have noticed the large variation in the loudness of the beats.) A study of 15 patients at open heart surgery showed that the onset of atrial fibrillation occurred when an atrial premature beat came during (11 patients) or after (4 patients) the atrial vulnerable period.[314] Whereas insurance records indicate that paroxysmal cases have no increased mortality,[125] Kowey et al.[124] reported that they suffered more serious symptoms and were better if converted to sustained fibrillation with digoxin or with propranolol if necessary. Ambulatory 24-hour ECGs of 66 patients showed pauses of 1.5 to 4 seconds and several other abnormalities (e.g., coupling, bigeminy, and ventricular tachycardia[310]). DC electrical conversion succeeded in 14 of 20 patients, but improved treadmill capacity was delayed.[255]

Ventricular Fibrillation

Ventricular fibrillation is the most serious and dreaded of the arrhythmias and the presumed ultimate event at life's end. It was described by Hoffa and Ludwig[160] in 1850. The circulation halts at once, and the ventricles gradually cease to beat. ECG monitoring—which every lay "televiewer" of medical drama will have seen repeatedly—has demonstrated the agonal tracings. Monitoring has also shown that ventricular arrest for periods of 2 to 11 seconds or more is not uncommon in patients being monitored for 24 hours; this may be due to sinus arrest, heart block, or atrial fibrillation, but only occasionally is it fatal.[312]

Verrier et al.[406] produced ventricular fibrillation in 60 percent of dogs by stimulating the ventricle and stellate ganglion at the same time; reserpine inhibited this sympathetic reaction. Human counterparts were reported by Coumel et al.[69] in four children (two boys aged 7 and 10 years and two girls aged 9 and 12 years), in whom severe ventricular tachycardia developed up to 380 beats/min with syncope from emotion or exertion, inducible by infusion of isoprenalin; 10 more examples had been recorded, all dying before 20 years and often suddenly. At autopsy, no lesion was found either in the heart or in its conducting system.

Immersion in seawater may cause ventricular fibrillation; Harries et al.[150] described two children, a boy aged 13 years immersed for 20 minutes at 15°C who died, and a girl aged 11 years for 6 minutes who survived resuscitation. The Scottish physiologist Mac-Williams[260] said that in 1889 sudden death in apparent health was caused by "fibrillar mode of contraction (delirium)," and Halsey[148] in 1915 secured ECG proof of this. Although atheromatous coronary disease is the most common cause, there are many others, including cardiac, pulmonary asphyxia (café coronary), extracardiac, and miscellaneous.[91] In acute myocardial infarction, ventricular arrhythmias range from premature beats to tachycardia to fibrillation, the last-named often coming without warning; lignocaine was a useful prophylactic at that time,[71] but β-blockers were much preferred by Kert and Hunt.[217]

Endocardial resection of any visible scar (ectopic focus) plus coronary bypass surgery was applied to 21 survivors of fibrillation in-hospital, 15 becoming free of tachycardia or fibrillation for up to 42 months.[209] The team at St. Bartholomew's Hospital in London[293] applied various procedures of surgery to 54 patients in 10 years (ventriculotomies, cryoablation, and bypass grafting); 52 survived, 28 relieved without, and 12 with medical treatment—a remarkable record, requiring good mapping.

The ideal treatment of heart attack arrhythmias (especially tachycardia and fibrillation) is started within minutes. This has been achieved by Pantridge in Belfast and by Chamberlain in Brighton,[298] who established highly trained mobile teams able to diagnose and apply any necessary electric shock therapy in the patient's home and maintain it during transit to the nearest cardiac coronary care unit; the former team even made *transtelephone defibrillation* possible by a bedside attendant (e.g., spouse), with 18 of 20 such cardioversions successful.[76] Kerber and Sarnat[215] treated 52 patients during 1974 to 1976, 38 successfully; however, but 14 failed because of delay (over 7 to 14 minutes), acidosis, or hypoxia. In the meantime it is worth remembering the first-aid value of the precordial thump, now banned in the United States, but defended in Britain by the Brighton team,[55] from wide experience.

Sudden Death in Sports

The sudden death of Pheidippides in 490 BC after his 22-mile run from the battlefield of Marathon to Athens with the good news of the Greek victory over invading Persians has not discouraged the thousands of today's would-be marathoners in their even longer run of more than 26 miles. Northcote and Ballantyne[297] of Scotland reported six cardiac deaths and reviewed the literature recording 80 coronary, 15 hypertrophic obstructive cardiopathy (HOCM), 8 coronary artery anomalies, 3 myocarditis, 2 conduction disorder, and 1 ruptured aortic valve; these investigators warned of the danger signs of angina, extreme fatigue, or fever. In America, Maron et al.[270] reported 29 patients aged 13 to 30 years who died "on the field" in a variety of sports, 22 of whom came to autopsy. Coronary atheroma was uncommon, and there was always a good autopsy explanation for the death; only seven had suspected heart disease in life. In Cape Town, Opie[301] reported on 21 men (mean age 25) in whom known ischemic heart disease was present in at least nine and possibly nine others. Bad coronary artery family history, smoking, and psychological factors were concerned as well. Aging referees were to take warning. (See Ch. 21 for further discussion.)

Arrhythmias and Sudden Death in Infants

Southall et al.[380] studied the 24-hour ECGs of 134 healthy neonates up to 10 days of age; heart rates ranged from 82 ± 12 to 175 ± 9 beats/min. There were various "abnormalities," including sinus bradycardia, variation in P waves and PR intervals, atrial premature beats, sinus pauses, and sinoatrial and Wenckebach block. Nathan et al.[292] made His-bundle ECGs in 25 of 27 normal neonates up to 4 days of age, using a high-resolution filtered 6-lead system; PH measured 60 to 105 and HV 10 to 25 msec. Bharati et al.[39] studied the conducting systems of 15 infants dying suddenly (plus those of 8 controls); the main finding was a left-sided His bundle and some inflammatory cells in and near the SA nodes of a heart with myocarditis, but no respiratory cause such as was found in 7 of the 8 controls.

Congenital Cardiac Arrhythmias with Prolonged QT Interval

The QT interval is measured from the onset of QRS to the end of the T wave; QT_c is corrected for heart rate, the upper limit being 440 msec. A prolonged QT interval may be congenital or acquired from numerous carriers and lead to attacks of syncope, even to sudden death.[36] Bharati et al.[37] studied the hearts from six patients, aged 9 months to 19 years, suffering seizures, one suddenly fatal in a girl 16 years. All showed fatty infiltration of the pathways to the AV node, as well as fibrosis and chronic inflammatory lesions in the left ventricle especially. The prolonged QT interval does not play a major role in SIDS.[212]

Isolated (Romano-Ward Syndrome)[337,412]

The familial syndrome described by Romano and Ward is now widely recognized as a cause of syncope, even of sudden death from ventricular fibrillation, afflicting infants,[269] children, or adults, and precipitated by emotion or exertion. Several members of a family may be involved. Inheritance is by autosomal dominance. Variants are described with AV dissociation,[216] electrical alternans of the TU wave,[157] or with torsade de pointes.[102]

I studied the conducting system in the heart from the second fatal case in the family described by Professor Ward; it came from a girl of 14 years. The formalin-fixed heart weighed 280 g and showed no macroscopic abnormality. Histology revealed no lesion of the SA node, AV node, or bundle of His, but both bundle branches were attenuated and poorly defined although no definitive lesion was found.

Philips and Ichinose[308] reported vascular changes and diffuse extensive fibrosis of the conducting system in the heart of a 3-year-old boy who died suddenly at play; he belonged to an affected family. Wellens et al.[416] investigated an epileptic girl of 18 years. Her fainting attacks, which started at age 14, were first precipitated by a clap of thunder and then regularly by an awakening alarm clock. The attacks, which lasted up to about 2 minutes, started with prolonged QT intervals and progressed to ventricular fibrillation from which she recovered, fortunately, each time.

The syndrome may present with epilepsy, as in the girl aged 16 years in the tragic family reported by Ballardie et al.[19] Her two sisters died after convulsions; one of them, aged 20 years, as well as their father, all had prolonged QT intervals. Vincent and Abildskov,[407] surveyed a family of 57 members, ages 3 hours to 70 years, in three generations. Six died suddenly and 29 had syncope, as had 14 of 23 survivors; 28 were symptomless. None of the infants died.

Congenital Nerve Deafness (Syndrome of Jervell and Lange-Nielsen; Surdocardiac Syndrome)

Surdus means deaf. In 1957, Jervell and Lange-Nielsen[199] described a Norwegian family of 6 siblings, 4 of whom were born deaf and suffered fainting attacks in childhood.

Three died suddenly—a boy aged 9 and his two sisters, aged 4 and 5 years; one autopsy provided no cause for this. Fraser et al.[122] collected 9 such cases from schools for the deaf; a necropsy showed only some hemorrhage in the SA node and some change in Purkinje fibers. Many more reports have appeared concerning this recessive syndrome, affecting people from birth[229] to 61 years.[124] Little more has been learned of the histopathology.

An important cooperative clinicopathologic study of 8 patients with the long-QT syndrome, ages $1\frac{1}{2}$ to 18 years, came from James et al.[183]; 3 were deaf. All had focal lymphocytic neuritis and neural degeneration, possibly viral, affecting the conducting system and myocardium. James and co-workers suggested, therefore, that the condition might not be congenital after all. They stressed (rightly) that few workers, apart from Rossi, paid sufficient attention to the state of nerve components of the conducting system.

It may be mentioned here that "crash" dieting can cause attacks of prolonged QT interval with low-voltage ventricular tachycardia, syncope, and even sudden death. Isner et al.[167] reported 17 such fatalities, 16 in women aged 23 to 51 losing an average of 45 percent of body weight in 5 months on a liquid protein diet. Heart histology revealed the lesions of cachexia—namely, attenuated muscle fibers with increased lipofuscin (see Ch. 21).

Conducting System in Various Diseases

Cardiac Infarction

Despite ECG evidence of abnormal conduction, the SA node, AV node, and bundle of His seem relatively immune to permanent visible structural damage in acute cardiac infarction.[97] However the bundle branches may be involved in massive septal infarction, which of itself is more dangerous anyway, so that a victim may not survive to develop permanent block.[388] It is presumed that temporary heart block is more likely due to ischemic hypoxia or to a reversible lesion such as hydropic change or hemorrhage. In a large series, bilateral bundle branch block carried a mortality of 59 percent, and complete block a mortality of 85 percent.[144] Mullins and Atkins[289] considered that patients in whom trifascicular block develops should have an artificial pacemaker inserted permanently.

Lie[251] agreed that the conducting system rarely showed overt lesions in acute infarction; lethal arrhythmias were probably due, therefore, to electrical instability of the ischemic myocardium. Corr and Sobel[68] considered that lack of oxygen with production of noxious substances in an ischemic area of myocardium led to its depression, allowing a re-entry pathway for the production of premature ventricular contraction and arrhythmia. Becker et al.[23] related the degree of bundle branch disturbance, found in 23 of 38 cases, to the amount of infarct damage. Particularly dangerous are premature beats, which may lead to fatal ventricular tachycardia or fibrillation without warning. Rizzon et al.[333] obtained good clinicopathologic correlation in their study of 8 hearts from 15 patients with left posterior hemiblock, 10 of whom also had RBBB; the left branch divided into three interlacing bands—anterior, middle, and posterior.

Pericarditis

Spontaneous pericarditis, or that following the trauma of cardiac surgery or mediastinal irradiation, can damage the SA node and its related nerves and ganglia directly; it can possibly set up in inflammatory ectopic pacemakers in the atrial walls. James[171] found the pacemaker involved in all of 38 patients dying with pericarditis present; 26 had atrial arrhythmias in life.

Aortic Valve Disease

The bundle of His lies in the base of the membranous septum between the right and noncoronary aortic valve cusps (see Fig. 38–8B); it may therefore be liable to damage by any disease of the valve, including fibrosis, calcification, and infection. An infected sinus of Valsalva aneurysm I studied involved the AV node and bundle in the heart of a young man who died suddenly of complete heart block in the outpatient department of our hospital. Jones and Roberts[200] studied the histology of the hearts of 12 patients who had aortic stenosis. Three had suffered complete heart block, the cause being obvious fibrocalcific destruction of the bundle of His, but only two of the nine with left bundle branch block had visible lesions of this branch on microscopy.

Rheumatoid Arthritis

Rheumatoid nodules and arteritis in the heart may involve the AV system; Figure 37–33

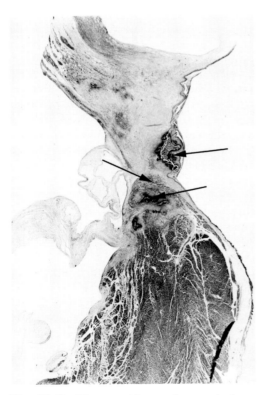

Fig. 37–33. Rheumatoid granulomata (right arrows) near the bundle of His (left arrow); from a woman of 70 with first-degree heart block. (H&E, × 7.) (From Hudson,[166a] with permission.)

shows several such nodules near the system, one being directly beneath the bundle of His. The patient, a woman aged 70 years, had first-degree heart block. The SA node can be involved in rheumatoid fibrous or constrictive pericarditis. James[175] studied the conducting system in the hearts of two cases of rheumatoid arthritis and one of ankylosing spondylitis; all three showed focal degeneration in the nodes and bundle of His; narrowing of arteries and inflammation were also found.

Systemic Lupus Erythematosus

For a discussion of systemic lupus erythematosus (SLE), see the earlier section on congenital heart block.

Marfan Syndrome

Medial hyperplasia and some degeneration were reported by James et al.[182] in the arteries of the SA node and AV system in the heart of a youth aged 20 years who died of syncope following atrial fibrillation. A second youth who died of ruptured aortic dissection had hemorrhagic damage of the nodes with intimal proliferation and medial degeneration in his arteries.

Polyarteritis Nodosa

Supraventricular arrhythmias, especially atrial flutter, may occur if the heart is involved. James and Birk[178] studied the hearts from six men, aged 47 to 73, and found arteritis with infarction and scarring in the SA node and some fibrosis also in the AV node; all six cases had pericarditis.

Wegener's Granulomatosis

Allen et al.[8] reported two women, aged 53 and 67, who died of renal failure due to severe necrotizing granulomatosis involving the kidneys, lungs, spleen, heart, systemic vessels, and skin; abnormal P waves were found in the ECG of one, attributable to atrial involvement. Histology of the conducting system was studied by serial section; previously, only four such studies had been published.

Polymyositis

Reid and Murdoch[327] described a man aged 37 who had polymyositis with pain and wasting of the thighs; 4 years later, the patient had complete heart block and syncope, necessitating artificial pacemaking and continuous steroid therapy. Serum creatine kinase level was 644 IU/I (normal = 50); muscle biopsy confirmed the myositis.

Dermatomyositis

Behan et al.[27] described a woman aged 59 with dermatomyositis who died 12 days after admission, with muscle pain, rash, and weakness; creatine kinase level was 2,248 IU (normal = 100), and the ECG showed RBBB and right axis deviation. Autopsy revealed a pale, flabby heart weighing 380 g. Histologic examination showed myocarditis, with severe infiltration of the SA and AV nodes, right branch fibrosis, but no involvement of the His bundle and left branch. She also had bronchopneumonia and evidence of right breast surgery (for cancer) 7 years previously. Behan et al. stated that the heart was involved in 70 percent of those with this disease, with one-third having conduction system involvement. In infants, the histologic lesions were associated with maternal Anti-RO antibodies, which cross the placenta to produce heart block.

Diphtheria

Myocarditis and conduction disturbances are well-known to occur in diphtheria (as in many other acute infectious diseases, especially in children). An early report in 1915 from Parkinson[305] concerned a man of 22 with complete heart block on the twenty-second day, followed by atrial fibrillation which lasted 6 months. A reminder of the danger of death in 10 percent of diphtheria cases came from Matisonn et al.,[273] who described how a black boy of 8 years, with severe disease, complete heart block, and Stokes-Adams attacks, required lifesaving artificial pacemaking and respiration.

Mumps

The first report of an infant dying of mumps affected a girl aged 8 months who died of crib death. At autopsy, the dilated heart showed diffuse myocarditis. Foci of lymphocytes and plasma cells were found in the submandibular glands and in the submucosa of the larynx, trachea, nasopharynx, and skeletal muscles. Mumps virus was isolated from the myocardium, which also contained the antigen.[52]

Arita et al.[15] described a man aged 32 who caught mumps from his two sons; on August 5 he developed swollen parotids and fever; on August 30 he became dizzy with a pulse of 40 beats/min. His mumps CFT measured 1:64, but it fell to 1:4 during the sixth week. Temporary pacing became displaced on the eighth day, causing Stokes-Adams attacks; permanent pacing was inserted. Arita et al. noted that Pujol was first to report myocarditis in mumps, in a French paper published in 1918.

Sarcoid Heart Disease

Arrhythmias, heart block, heart failure, or sudden death may occur in cardiac sarcoidosis. In the United Kingdom, Fleming has for several years conducted a valuable continuous survey, and by 1974[120] had records of 128 adult cases; 71 had survived with rhythm upsets (12 requiring artificial pacemaking for heart block), or heart failure. Sudden death occurred in 23 of the 57 fatal cases; and 45 autopsies were made, disclosing the correct diagnosis in 22. Rossi[347] found a sarcoid nodule destroying the AV node in the heart of a woman of 67 years who died in complete heart block. Fawcett and Goldberg[115] reported a similar finding in the heart of a man aged 60. James[176] found sarcoid foci and also focal fibromuscular dysplasia of the arteries of the SA and AV nodes in the heart of a black woman aged 30 who died suddenly in syncope. Roberts et al.,[334] in an autopsy study of 8 adults (5 of whom had died suddenly), found 3 with granulomas in the bundle of His; all 3 had suffered complete heart block. A further report[335] concerned 35 necropsy cases, 26 of whom had shown clinical evidence of the massive sarcoidosis of the heart found at autopsy; 6 had died suddenly, 12 after a short period of arrhythmias or of heart block.

Silverman et al.[375] reported about 84 sarcoidosis autopsies; 23 involved the heart. Only 4 had macroscopic lesions there, and these patients had died suddenly; in the remaining 19 cases, the heart lesions were microscopic. An interesting case report from Papoulos et al.[304] showed that attacks of hypercalcemia in summer, suffered by a man aged 36, coincided with rises of his serum vitamin D.

Trypanosomiasis

In an autopsy study of 10 African males ages 13 to 45, Poltera et al.[311] found myocarditis in all and lesions of the conducting system in 2; the autopsy diagnosis of this disease depended on the finding of diffuse mononuclear meningoencephalitis, since the organism, *T. gambiense*, was not seen in human histology. Conducting system lesions may also occur in Chagas disease (see Ch. 34).

Thrombotic Thrombocytopenic Purpura, Moschowitz Disease, Disseminated Intravascular Coagulation

Thrombotic thrombocytopenic purpura (TTP), Moschowitz disease, and a disseminated intravascular coagulation (DIC) are a group of generalized diseases that may involve the conducting system with platelet-fibrin thrombosis of small vessels, focal hemorrhages, and infarcts. James and Monto[189] described such lesions in the hearts from 3 patients, ages 26, 28, and 55. In the 26-year-old patient, a woman who suffered Stokes-Adams attacks, an infarct had interrupted the bundle of His. A similar case[186] concerned a pregnant woman of 19 who died in the second trimester of DIC; she also had paroxysmal tachycardia.

Amyloidosis

Hobbs[159] wrote that amyloidosis was attributable to one of three possible causes:

1. Production of homogeneous A proteins from a deranged lymphoreticular system
2. Production of monoclonal B proteins (mainly V portions of immunoglobulins) by immunocytomata
3. Local production of ?C-proteins from deranged cells of neuroembryonic origin

Amyloidosis is widespread in aging humans and animals as an eosinophilic hyaline protein that is fibrillar on electron microscopy. It can be demonstrated in sections by staining with Congo red, by sodium sulfate-Alcian blue (of Lendrum et al.[234]) and by thioflavine-T (frozen sections in UV light). It develops in hamsters with leishmaniasis and, if immunized with diphtheria-pertussis-tetanus vaccine,[436] as well as by feeding mice with casein; this reaction can be inhibited by thymosine hormone or by colchicine.[366]

Primary amyloidosis is idiopathic or caused by multiple myeloma in 10 percent of patients; it comprises light chains of immunoglobulin, including Bence Jones proteins.

Secondary amyloidosis, A/AA from many proteins, is associated with caseating tuberculosis, tertiary syphilis with suppuration, lepromatous leprosy, rheumatoid arthritis, bedsores, pyelonephritis, renal carcinoma, and Hodgkin's disease. Traces of serum AA is a normal precursor.[49] There is a *third* type associated with medullary carcinoma of the thyroid. In so-called senile amyloidosis, deposition occurs in the atria or whole heart and great vessels, the material being unique; or it may involve the pancreatic islets; or the brain (in the plaques of Alzheimer's disease, vessels, and meninges[51]).

Arrhythmias such as atrial fibrillation and heart block are common in cardiac amyloidosis. James,[174] in a study of 5 such hearts from patients aged 58 to 79, found deposition in all parts of the conducting system, the pacemaker being especially damaged in 4 hearts. By contrast, Ridolfi et al.[332] studied 23 hearts from patients aged 44 to 88 and found only 3 with amyloid in the conducting system; however, 9 showed fibrosis of the SA node and the bundle branches. The amyloidosis was attributable to senility in 18 and to plasma cell dyscrasia in 3; it was familial in one and primary in another.

During the past 10 years, more reports of heart involvement have been published. In Japan, Sawayama[363] found clinical cardiac abnormalities in 12 of 19 adult patients with familial amyloid polyneuropathy; two required pacemakers. From Sweden, Ericksson et al.[105] in 1964 reported 16 patients with familial amyloidosis and polyneuropathy whose ECGs were monitored for 24 hours and then for up to 15 months; five needed pacemakers. Allen and Doherty[7] described a man aged 54 with bilateral bronchiectasis in whom generalized amyloidosis developed, who died suddenly in cardiac arrest. Autopsy confirmed his widespread amyloidosis and a large heart (580 g) with deposition in the interstitium and endocardium, SA and AV nodes, and left bundle branch, explaining ECG findings of long PR and incomplete LBBB. Primary amyloidosis causing angina pectoris in a man aged 32 with nephrotic syndrome (excessive proteinuria) was reported by Saltissi et al.[358] In a study of 25 right atrial appendices, the team at St. Bartholomew's hospital, in London[205] demonstrated fibrils of amyloid in 10 specimens, with six also reacting for human atrial natriuretic peptide.

Friedreich's Ataxia

Common occurrences in this familial disease include ischemic lesions of the heart, atrial arrhythmias, heart block, Stokes-Adams attacks, and lung arteriopathy. These were attributed by James and Frisch[181] to widespread lesions of the small arteries, 100 to 300 μm in diameter. Cystic degeneration of the media, intimal hyperplasia, and endothelial deposits were also found.

Hypertrophic obstructive cardiopathy may occur. Van der Hauwaert and Dumoulin[402] reported it in two male siblings aged 16 and 21 years. More than 90 percent of sufferers have ECG abnormalities; three of the six original patients of Friedreich had "fatty" hearts at autopsy.[48] Gottdeiner et al.[145] found symmetric HOCM in 13 of 24 patients by echocardiography. However, a major study of 71 patients (35 females, 36 males, aged 11 to 58) by Bach et al.[18] found numerous ECG abnormalities, but HOCM was infrequent. From Milan,[303] a biventricular radionuclide angiographic study of 21 patients suggested hypokinesis of the right ventricle as the cause of heart failure in this disease. A multicenter study by James et al.[180a] of three young men ages 20, 22, and 20 coming to autopsy from heart failure and atrial arrhythmias, reported pleomorphic nuclei and focal fibrous lesions of the hearts, including the conducting systems, coronary artery lesions, and focal degeneration of nerves and ganglia.

Dystrophia Myotonica

Thomson[393] reported vacuolar degeneration, fibrosis, and fatty replacement in the myocardium, with cystic medial degeneration of the arteries, as occurs in the skeletal muscles. This could cause the atrial flutter and heart block in his case, a woman aged 69.

Severe active myocarditis in a mother aged 59 and her son aged 32 was found at autopsy, suggesting that an infective agent (? virus) was responsible; her other affected son was still alive at 31 years.[323]

The Becker X-linked type of muscular dystrophy[26] starts later and is milder; heart involvement may appear much later, or not at all. Emery and Skinner[100] studied 29 males out of 67, from 10 families, ages 2½ to 21 years.

Wyatt and Cox[429] detected "characteristic inclusion bodies" in an EM study of fibroblasts cultured from the skin biopsies of four patients with Duchenne dystrophy. But a later EM study of the autopsied hearts and skeletal muscles from two boys aged 10 and 12 years who died disclosed no virus particles, but extensive cell damage, producing a "motheaten" look, with total loss of thick and thin myofilaments, and other lesions, adequate reason for the several ECG abnormalities found in 64 of 75 patients with Duchenne's myopathy, ages 5 to 18 years.[361]

Myoglobinemia was detected in 14 of 18 Duchenne patients and in 10 of 16 carriers (plus 9 of 27 possible carriers by Adornato et al.[3])—an adjunct to raised CPK levels in carrier detection. Mitral valve prolapse was detected in 6 of 22 Duchenne patients and in seven carriers by Biddison et al., but it has also been reported in up to 17 percent in normal females.

A team at Duke University[319] carried out serial electrophysiologic studies of the conduction system at 3-year intervals, of nine patients with dystrophia myotonica. They found that seven had HV prolongation and seven had first-degree heart block with HV over 55 msec in three cases; if symptoms warranted, permanent pacing might be needed. AV block and arrhythmias were found in 12 males of 101 family members with the X-linked milder scapuloperoneal form of dystrophy; even so, pacemaking might prove essential and life saving.[155] Komajda et al.[222] studied the electrophysiology of conduction in 12 cases of dystrophia myotonica in Paris; seven had syncope. His-bundle recordings showed diffuse lesions in all; two had AV node lesions and three had His-bundle lesions; pacing was recommended if sudden death threatened. Sanyal et al.[360] suggested that mitral valve prolapse in the hearts of three Duchenne children at autopsy was caused by their disease process in the posterior papillary muscle and base of ventricle, that is, loss of actin and myosin myofilaments in the myofibrinolysis and fibrosis.

Although two-thirds of mothers of Duchenne dystrophy infants are carriers with some increase in their serum CPK levels, one-third are not, and therefore cannot be so identified,[93] but additional DNA analysis may permit much more accurate identification of the carrier state. Also, the probable responsible gene seems to be in the center of the short arm of X at the breakpoint.[149]

The only certain preventive against this distressing disease lies in counseling all family members and relatives to identify female carriers early, before possible conception can occur.[132]

In northern Sweden, where myotonic dystrophy is prevalent, Oloffsson et al.[300] found that the severity could be graded by the ECG changes of first-degree AV block and left anterior hemiblock in mild cases to atrial fibrillation, flutter, abnormal Q, and repolarization abnormalities in the most severely affected.

Hemochromatosis

In a study of five hearts from patients aged 66 to 83, with hemochromatosis, James[173] found iron deposition in the myocardium and AV node but not in the SA node; all five patients had suffered rhythm disorders—atrial flutter or fibrillation, sinus tachycardia, heart block, or syncope. Schellhammer et al.[364] studied the hearts of six patients dying with the acquired form of the disease and, although the myocardium and conducting system (but not nerves or ganglia) showed iron deposition and fibrosis, there was no correlation between the arrhythmias (present in three of the six patients) and the amount of iron deposition or the scarring.

Skinner and Kenmuir[377] reported a man of 32 with congestive cardiomyopathy due to primary hemochromatosis. He had sparse hair and testicular atrophy but no obvious skin pigmentation or diabetes mellitus. He responded to venesection. His serum iron measured 305 μ/dl, (normal = 75 to 175 μ/dl). Injection of iron-chelating disferrioxamine caused excess iron excretion in the urine.

Repeated blood transfusion is lifesaving for victims of incurable thalassaemia major; this may lead to heart failure from hemosiderosis by the second decade, treatable by chelation. Kaye and Owen[207] did this for 28 patients aged 7 to 23 years on transfusion treatment, by intramuscular disferrioxamine, 500 mg/day. None had heart failure, but three had ECG abnormalities of ventricular ectopic beats. In seven adequately chelated patients no such changes developed, possibly because it limited the deposition of iron in the myocardium.

Kwashiorkor

In a study of seven hearts from children aged 1 to 3 years in Uganda, dying of protein malnutrition, Sims[376] found that the myocardial atrophy and myocytolysis involved the conducting system, which also showed interstitial edema. These lesions could account for sudden death in Kwashiorkor, a disease of starvation. The dire effects of "crash" dieting were mentioned earlier in the section on congenital nerve deafness.

Tumors of the Conducting System

Primary or secondary tumors of the heart may involve the conducting system, and may be benign or malignant (see also Ch. 35).

Primary Tumors

Intrinsic tumors of the conducting system itself are few and rare; only two or three may be mentioned.

Rhabdomyoma

Rhabdomyoma may be single or multiple; it may occur alone, or it may be one of the manifestations of tuberous sclerosis. Figure 37–34 shows an example of a tumor nodule adjacent to the SA node in the heart of an infant; the heart of this child contained literally hundreds of such nodules, some being quite massive. Another example that I studied was a

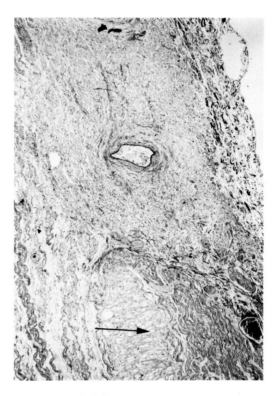

Fig. 37–34. Rhabdomyoma nodule (arrow) abutting the sinuatrial node. From an infant of 13 days whose heart contained numerous such tumors of all sizes. (Elastic van Gieson, × 39.) (From Hudson,[165] with permission.)

solitary tumor that the late Lord Brock excised from the interatrial septum of a female patient of the late Paul Wood, M.D. In doing so, Brock cured the patient's bizarre arrhythmia, which Wood had diagnosed as being caused by the tumor. James et al.[177] reported "multifocal Purkinje cell tumors causing arrhythmias in a black woman of 9 months; there was no tuberous sclerosis. The tumors were not considered typical rhabdomyomata. (Their illustrations reminded me of the cardiac lipidosis of Ross and Belton.[343])

Developmental Heterotopia

Developmental heterotypia is an inclusion cyst of the interatrial septum resulting from dislocation of foregut endoderm into the dorsal mesocardium.[421] It has a glandular epithelial cystic structure and no capsule and may cause heart block.[288] The cysts are lined with cuboidal, columnar, or squamous epithelium. James and Galakhov,[184] in reporting two examples, stated that the tumor was confined to the AV node area. Ariza et al.[16] reported fatal obstruction of the superior vena cava by such a tumor in the heart of an infant aged 6 months.

Mesothelioma

Several further examples of these heterotopic inclusion cysts have been reported as "mesothelioma of the AV node." Garcia et al.[131] described 10 cases, confirmed at autopsy (6 females, 4 males, aged 43 to 96); one patient had had atrial fibrillation, six had first-degree block and two complete heart block, and one was normal. From Tokyo, Nishida et al.[296] reported a man of 31 who suffered alcoholic cirrhosis and Mobitz type 2 heart block; a pacemaker was inserted but he died at 33 from subarachnoid hemorrhage from a ruptured aneurysm. At autopsy, the 340 g heart had a 1 cm tumor of the AV node. Fatal complete heart block, with rates down to 35 per minute, was diagnosed as congenital from the age of 10 in a man aged 23 who died with angina pectoris after loading bales of straw on to a lorry. At postmortem examination, the heart weighed 560 g and contained a mesothelioma of the AV node and His bundle.[110]

Other Tumors

These may invade or compress the septum. For example, James et al.[180] found a tiny fibroma pressing on the AV bundle in the heart of a man aged 40 years who died suddenly. Lenègre's view that senile fibrosis of the AV system is a specific disease has been already mentioned.

Secondary Tumors

Involvement of the conducting system directly or indirectly is quite common when metastases invade the heart; almost any tumor

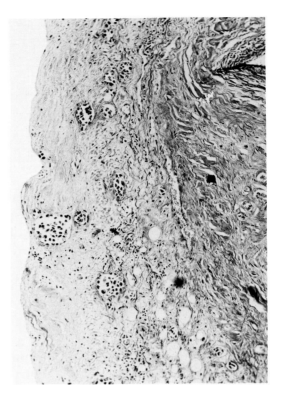

Fig. 37–35. Metastases from carcinoma of the bronchus in epicardial lymphatics adjacent to the sinuatrial node on right of picture. (Elastic van Gieson, × 114.) (From Hudson,[165] with permission.)

may do so, producing arrhythmias and heart block. Examples are shown in Figures 37–35 and 37–36, both of which are from patients with bronchial carcinoma.

Trauma to the Conducting System

Cardiac Catheterization and Surgery

Cardiac catheterization and surgery[166] are the chief causes of trauma to the conducting system. Hypothermia, when used to aid cardiac surgery, can lead to the cessation of all elec-

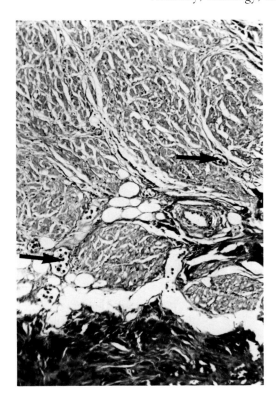

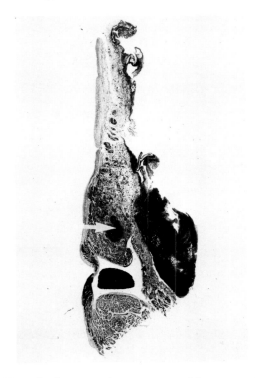

Fig. 37–37. Hemorrhagic necrosis of the sinuatrial node (arrow); surgical repair of Fallot's tetralogy in a girl aged 6 years. (H&E, × 7.5.) (From Hudson,[166] with permission.)

Fig. 37–36. Metastases (arrows) of carcinoma of the bronchus in lymphatics of the bundle of His. (Elastic van Gieson, × 98.) (From Hudson,[165] with permission.)

trical activity of the heart[386] and must be monitored most carefully.

The SA node is especially vulnerable to damage during intubation of the superior vena cava for bypass surgery; it may be pinched, incised, sutured, or otherwise damaged. Figure 37–37 shows an example of traumatic hemorrhagic necrosis.

The AV system is vulnerable to exploratory catheterization, especially in bundle of His electrocardiography; to deliberate interatrial septal rupture (Rashkind[322] procedure) or excision (Mustard[290] operation) for transposition of the great arteries. It is also liable to damage all operations to repair ventricular septal defects (AV cushion defects, "membranous" septal defects); and at valve surgery, especially

of the aortic valve (Fig. 37–38). In cushion and membranous ventricular septal defects, the AV node and proximal part of the bundle of His nearly always lie in the posteroinferior rim of the defect, nearest to the coronary sinus ostium.

There is no doubt that injury to the conducting system adds to the risks of patients undergoing cardiac surgery; fortunately, any such injury is often transitory. Reid et al.[325] reported a remarkable recovery to normal rhythm 11 years after cardiac surgery had caused complete heart block.

Deliberate injury to the bundle of His by injection, freezing, cautery, or incision in the management of intractable dangerous tachycardias has been described earlier.

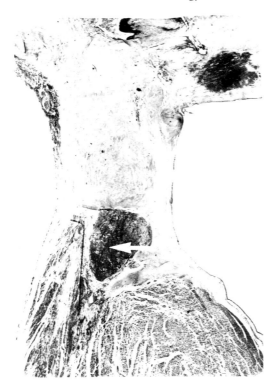

Fig. 37–38. Hemorrhagic necrosis of the bundle of His (arrow); surgical replacement of the mitral and aortic valves, in a man aged 44 years. (H&E, × 10.) (From Hudson,[166] with permission.)

Transplantation Surgery

In December 1967, the South African surgeon, Christiaan Barnard boldly defied all then existing ethics by removing the viable heart from 18-year-old Louise Darrell, recently dead from a traffic accident, and orthotransplanting it without delay into a grocer Louis Washkansky, age 53, suffering terminal heart failure; it continued to function for 18 days.

The heroic procedure was copied worldwide; no hospital, properly equipped or not, that valued public and official support could afford to ignore the challenge. In 10 years, the Chicago Registry reported 333 transplants in 325 patients. Monitoring the implant be-

haviour for signs of rejection, and for its physiologic properties has become a specialized branch of cardiology. Determining donor death became a subject of fierce controversy until 1975, when the British Transplantation Society defined it as "the irreversible cessation of brain function, incapable of spontaneous respiration."

Soon after the death of Washkansky, world media focused on the life story of his successor, a dentist, Dr. Blaiberg, who proved all critics wrong by surviving 19½ months. At autopsy, Thompson[394] found severe coronary atheroma, and commented: "It is a sad irony that a brave pioneer should produce in the coronary arteries of his transplanted heart the same disease that determined the dysfunction of his original heart."

Undismayed, Barnard resumed cardiac surgery and research; his next procedure was a heterotopic heart transplant in two men alongside their own hearts, using its two ventricles to augment the beat of the host's hearts by connecting the paired aortas and pulmonary trunks and ligating the graft's venae cavae—the so-called "piggyback" transplant.[20,47] The host now had a mixture of pulses to tide over a crisis. The Yacoub team[6] found that the donor heart suffers fewer arrhythmias than does the host's diseased heart. The miracle is that the excised, denervated donor heart can continue to beat when suitably nourished by the host; its careful removal and reinsertion can ensure that its conducting system remains intact and able to regulate physiologic beating in the host, although atrial arrhythmias and increased sinus node recovery time[35] and ventricular premature beats soon manifest, together with other evidence of graft rejection.[31] In 1980, the Barnard team[67a] reported that during the first 6 years, two of their 11 orthotopic transplant patients had survived 9 and 11 years; during the second 6 years, three of 30 heterotopic transplant patients were still alive after more than 4 years.

In the absence of nervous control by the host, the transplant has a high resting rate that responds slowly to exercise by host catecholamines. The stroke volume reacts to increased stretch on the Frank-Starling principle.

Crush Injuries

These can involve the areas of the conducting system, but any such damage is overshadowed by that of the major injury to the coronary arteries and myocardium. Several examples are recorded of heart block resulting from crush injury of the chest; in one case, the block continued for 18 years.[66] Hyperextension of the neck by traffic accident can rupture the superior vena cava and damage the SA node, producing aberrant pacemaker activity.[256]

Manual Resuscitation

The conducting system is not likely to be damaged directly by the various techniques of manual resuscitation—chest thumping, internal or external cardiac massage.[202] In any case, such damage is not so important relatively when life is at stake; reported lesions include fractured ribs or sternum, fat embolism, laceration of the liver or spleen, and gastroesophageal laceration. However, His bundle and left branch hemorrhage was found at necropsy in a man of 35 who died after external cardiac massage for arrest, by Rossi and Matturi.[354] It was attributed to hammering of the crest of the interventricular septum against the central fibrous body.

Irradiation Injury

Injudicious irradiation of the mediastinum for cancers (e.g., lung, breast, thymus, lymphomas) may cause ischemic fibrosis of the pericardium, epicardium, myocardium, and even the papillary muscles, months to years later, due to loss of capillaries.[114,146] The SA node may become involved in this process because of its position in the epicardium.

Lightning and Electric Shock Injury

Among five adults (including three physicians) and three children sheltered under a tree struck by lightning, three adults were injured; two so seriously that they had to be rushed to hospital within 30 minutes; a man aged 41 had temporary paralysis of legs and right arm, was gasping for breath, and had first-degree burns of the right shoulder, singed hair on the chest and left leg, and loss of the right eardrum. The heart suffered inferior infarction. A man aged 43 had total paralysis with ECG changes, severe central chest pain, and singe and exit burns. Surprisingly, both men recovered completely.

Lewin et al.[247] reported a youth aged 19 who was unconscious from contact with a home generator (220 V AC and 50 Hz); his cardiac arrest was remedied at hospital, where he had ECG evidence of myocardial injury, with raised serum enzymes and echocardiographic changes of left ventricular hypokinesis. All resolved in a few days and remained normal 1 year later.

Complications of Therapy by Shock and Pacemaking

Electroconversion

It has been known since 1794[295] that an electric shock could restart a recently stilled heart. The method has been refined for human therapy, using alternating[435] or direct current. The dramatic possibilities have become a cliché in the cinema and on television. Direct current is now preferred, as pioneered by Lown et al.[258] The shock is applied up to a safe maximum now generally recommended at 400 W-sec,[2] too little may mean fatal delay, and too much may damage the myocardium or induce further arrhythmias. The shock depolarizes the whole heart, extinguishing ectopic foci and allowing the SA node to resume pacemaking in selected patients with uncontrollable arrhythmias (atrial flutter, fibrillation, or tachycardia; ventricular tachycardia and standstill). In cardiac surgery, it is used to restart the heart stilled for operation, and to deal with postoperative arrhythmias. The somewhat dramatic procedure (known variously as cardioversion, defibrillation, countershock, conversion, electroreversion, or electroconversion) is not without complications, for example, relapse (the most common) embolism from the atrium, further arrhythmias, pulmonary edema, hypotension; also, previous digitalis dosage may suddenly become excessive and toxic.

Pacemaking

The detection of natural electric activity during the cardiac cycle was bound to result in the development of artificial pacemakers by which the tiny stimulus for contraction could be applied to the heart when the natural means was disordered—as in heart block, cardiac arrest, and cardiac surgery. Since the practice of electrical stimulation was introduced in 1952 by Zoll[434] and colleagues, the actual apparatus used has gone through highly sophisticated refinement in function, durability, and size (see Ch. 38). Although they cannot match nature's exquisite built-in pacemaker, models are now available that can operate for years "on demand," that is, when stimulation is required to maintain the circulation. The whole apparatus may be implanted in the body at operation; with the pacing electrode entering the heart via a vein (e.g., jugular or axillary). Ingenious electrodes have been devised both to sense heartbeats and to ensure endocardial attachment.

The intravenous electrode may invoke mass thrombosis in the right atrium,[257] become enveloped by the formation of a fibrous tunnel around it,[25] or break off and embolize (e.g., to the lung).[391] Pacemaker leads may become displaced,[46] in one case recorded, the lead moved to the level of L4 and stimulated the

nerves to the right adductor muscles, causing the leg to jerk in time with the heartbeat.[33]

It is possible, in dire necessity, to pace the right ventricle for a short while through the annulus of a tricuspid valve prosthesis.[230]

Other difficulties to be encountered include failure of the impulse from the lead from high threshold or poor insulation or its extrusion from the entrance wound.

In expert hands, artificial pacemaking is invaluable; initial overenthusiasm has been tempered by experience. The pioneer team at St. George's Hospital in London consider that artificial pacemaking improves survival in heart failure from chronic heart block, especially with syncope.[156] Of 839 patients followed for 14 years, 288 died, the worst mortality ($\times 4.5$ standard) being among those with ischemic heart disease. The prognosis was not influenced by the persistence of the heart block, the heart rate, and the duration of the QRS complex of the ECG.[142]

In a review of the "pacing industry," the British Medical Journal[50] estimated that one-third of a million were in use worldwide, for conditions such as sick sinus syndrome, complete and bilateral bundle branch block, refractory tachycardia, and carotid sinus syndrome. In 1978, there were 66,723 new implants and 30,025 generator replacements in the United States; corrresponding figures in the United Kingdom were 4,200 and 3,300.

Sowton,[381] from unique experience, reviewed the multitude of possible hazards threatening pacemaker wearers, in hospital and in everyday life; even a store's burglar alarm has been set off. The manufacturer's careful instructions to wearers has minimized such dangers. But endocardial pacing itself carries the risk of endocarditis,[232] and prolonged pacemaking may cause a syndrome of dizzy spells, syncope, shortness of breath, decreased exercise tolerance, and postural hypotension. It is caused by the paced ventricular beat coinciding with the atrial contraction, producing "cannon waves" in the jugular pulse, and liver pulsation[212a]; the syndrome may be avoided by the use of dual-chamber pacing systems, the most sophisticated of which are ventricular demand (VVI) and universal atrioventricular (DDD); the original fixed-rate asynchronous mode is known as AOO VOO DOO, as assigned by the International Commission for Heart Disease (ICHD) code.[4]

ACKNOWLEDGMENTS

My warmest thanks are due to Barry Richards, Director of Medical Illustrations, National Heart Hospital and Institute of Cardiology, London, for his expert help with the illustrations, and to my wife, Dorothy, for helping me with the typing and for encouraging my often flagging efforts at all times.

REFERENCES

1. Adams R: Cases of diseases of the heart, accompanied with pathological observations. Dubl Hosp Rep 4:353, 1827

2. Adgey AAJ: Electrical energy requirements for ventricular defibrillation. Br Heart J 40:1197, 1978

3. Adornato BT, Kagen LJ, Engel WK: Myoglobinaemia in Duchenne muscular dystrophy patients and carriers. A new adjunct to carrier detection. Lancet 2:499, 1978

4. AHA Council Clin Cardiol Newsletter: Dual chamber cardiac pacing systems. 10:1, 1984

5. Alanis J, González H, López E: The electrical activity of the bundle of His. J Physiol (Lond), 142:127, 1958

6. Alexopoulos D, Yusuf S, Bostock J, et al: Ventricular arrhythmias in long term survivors of orthotopic and heterotopic cardiac transplantation. Br Heart J 59:648, 1988

7. Allen DC, Doherty CC: Sudden death in a patient with amyloidosis of the cardiac conduction system. Br Heart J 51:233, 1984

8. Allen DC, Doherty CC, O'Reilly DPJ: Pathology of the heart and the cardiac conduction system in Wegener's granulomatosis. Br Heart J 52:674, 1984

9. Anderson KR, Yen Ho S, Anderson RH: Location and vascular supply of sinus node in human heart. Br Heart J 41:28, 1979

10. Anderson RH, Becker AE: Anatomy of conducting tissues revisited. Br Heart J 40(suppl):2, 1978

11. Anderson RH, Becker AE: Anatomy of conducting tissue revisited. Br Heart J 40(suppl):2, 1978

12. Anderson RH, Becker AE, Gerlis L: The morphogenesis of congenital heart block. Pathological Society of Great Britain and Ireland, Proceedings of Meeting January 9–11, 1975 (abst 13)

13. Anderson RH, Bouton J, Burrow CT, Smith A: Sudden death in infancy: A study of cardiac specialized tissue. Br Med J 2:135, 1974

14. Anderson RH, Wernick ACG, Losekot TG, Becker AE: Congenitally complete heart block. Developmental aspects. Circulation 56:82, 1977

15. Arita M, Ueno Y, Masuyama Y: Complete heart block in mumps myocarditis. Br Heart J 46:342, 1981

16. Ariza S, Rafel E, Castillo JA, Garcia-Canton JA: Intracardiac heterotopia-mesenchymal and endodermal. Br Heart J 40:325, 1978

17. Aschner B: Wiener klinische wochenshrift, 21, 1529, cited by Dewar KMS, Wishart HY: The oculocardiac reflex. Proc R Soc Med 69:373, 1908

18. Bach PM, Child JS, Perloff JK, et al: Cardiac involvement in Friedreich's ataxia. Circulation 68 (4, pt 2), III-334, 1983 (abst 1334)

19. Ballardie FW, Murphy RP, Davis J: Epilepsy: A presentation of the Romano-Ward syndrome. Br M J 287:896, 1983

20. Barnard CN, Losman JG: Left ventricular bypass. S Afr Med J 49:303, 1975

21. Beattie JM, Gaffney FA, Buja LM, Blomqvist CG: Left ventricular false tendons in man: Identification of clinically significant morphological variants. Proceedings of the British Cardiac Society, York, Apr. 2–3, 1986

22. Becker AE, Anderson RH, Durrer D, Wellens HJJ: The anatomical substrates of Wolff-Parkinson-White syndrome. A clinico-pathologic correlation in seven patients. Circulation 57:870, 1978

23. Becker AE, Anderson RH, Lie KI: Acute anteroseptal myocardial infarction; a clinicopathologic correlation of the conduction disturbance. In Proceedings of the Pathological Society of Great Britain and Ireland, One hundred thirty-fourth Meeting, 1977 (abst 6)

24. Becker AE, Anderson RH, Wellens HJJ, Durrer D: The anatomy of ventricular pre-excitation. p. 24. In Proceedings of British Cardiac Society, Fifty-fifth Annual General Meeting, Edinburgh, March 31–April 1, 1976 (abst)

25. Becker AE, Becker MJ, Clandon DG, Edwards JE: Surface thrombosis and fibrous encapsulation of intravenous pacemaker catheter electrode. Circulation 46:409, 1972

26. Becker PE: Zur Genetik der Myopathien. Dtsch Z Nervenheilkd 173:482, 1955

27. Behan WMH, Aitchison M, Behan PO: Pathogenesis of heart block in a fatal case of dermatomyositis. Br Heart J 56:479, 1986

28. Benditt DG, Pritchett ELC, Smith WM, et al: Characteristics of atrioventricular conduction and the spectrum of arrhythmias in Lown-Ganong-Levine syndrome. Circulation 57:454, 1978

29. Bennett JG: Surgery for cardiac arrhythmias. Br Med J 296:1687, 1988

30. Bentall, HH, Rowland E, Krickler, DM: Endocardial mapping and cryosurgery for arrhythmias. Br Heart J 41:371, 1979 (abst)

31. Berke DK, Graham AF, Schroeder JS, Harrison DC: Arrhythmias in the denervated transplanted heart. Circulation 48(suppl 3):112, 1973

32. Besterman E, Greese R: Waller—pioneer of electrocardiography. Br Heart J 42:61, 1979

33. Bettencourt-Gomes SG: Displacement of a pacemaker. Br Med J 1 397, 1975

34. Bexton RS, Nathan AW, Hellestrand KJ, Camm AJ: Paroxysmal atrial tachycardia provoked by swallowing. Br Med J 282:952, 1981

35. Bexton RS, Nathan AW, Hellestrand KJ, et al: Electrophysiological abnormalities in the transplanted human heart. Br Heart J 50:555, 1983

36. Bhandari AK, Scheinman M: The long QT syndrome. Mod Concepts Cardiovasc Dis 54:45, 1985

37. Bharati S, Dreifus L, Bucheleres G, et al: The anatomic base of prolonged QT interval. Circulation 70(4, pt 2):II–371, 1984 (abst 1483)

38. Bharati S, Handler B, Parr G, et al: The conduction system of the pig heart. Circulation 66(4, pt 2):II–342, 1982 (abst 1369)

39. Bharati S, Krongrad E, Lev M: Sudden infant death syndrome: Conduction system study. Circulation 68(4, pt 2):III–268, 1983 (abst 1073)

40. Biddison JH, Dembo DH, Spalt H, et al: Familial occurence of mitral valve prolapse in X-linked muscular dystrophy. Circulation 59:1299, 1979

41. Blair DM, Davies F: Observations on the conducting system of the heart. J Anat 69:303, 1934–35

42. Borst JG: The maintenance of an adequate cardiac output by regulation of urinary excretion of water and sodium chloride; an essential factor in the genesis of edema. Acta Med Scand 130(suppl 207):1, 1948

43. Brazeau P, Vale W, Burgus R: Hypothalamic polypeptide that inhibits the secretion of immunoreactive pituitary growth hormone. Science 179:77, 1973

44. Brechenmacher C: Atrio-His bundle tracts. Br Heart J 37:853, 1975

45. Brechenmacher C, Cowmel P, Fanchier J-P, Cachera, J-P, James, TN: De subitaneis mortibus. XXII. Intractable paroxymal tachycardias which proved fatal in Type A Wolff-Parkinson-White syndrome. Circulation 55:408, 1977

46. Brewster, GM, Evans AL: Displacement of pacemaker leads—A 10 year survey. Br Heart J 42:266, 1979

47. British Medical Journal: Cardiac implantation. Br Med J 2:707, 1975

48. British Medical Journal: Cardiac involvement in Friedreich's ataxia. Br Med J 1:261, 1978

49. British Medical Journal: Pathogenesis of amyloid disease. Br Med J 1:216, 1979

50. British Medical Journal: The pacing industry. Br Med J 282:2, 1981

51. British Medical Journal: The senile amyloidoses. Br Med J 282:846, 1981

52. Brown NJ, Richmond SJ: Fatal mumps myocarditis in an 8-month-old child. Br Med J 281:356, 1980

53. Burchell HB: Did Einthoven invent a string galvanometer? Br Heart J 57:190, 1987

54. Burn, JH: The cause of fibrillation. Br Med J 1:1379, 1960

55. Caldwell G, Millar G, Quinn E, et al: Simple mechanical methods for cardioversion: Defence of the precordial thump and cough version. Br Med J 291:627, 1985

56. Camm AJ, Dymond D, and Spurrell RAJ: Sinus node dysfunction associated with absence of right superior vena cava. Br Heart J 41:504, 1979

57. Campbell M: Partial heart block with dropped beats. Br Heart J 5:55, 1943

58. Campbell M: Complete heart block. Br Heart J 6:70, 1944

59. Campbell M, Emanual R: Six cases of congenital complete heart block followed for 34–40 years. Br Heart J 29:577, 1967

60. Campbell RWF: Chronic Mobitz type 1 second degree atrioventricular block. Has its importance been underestimated? Br Heart J 53:585, 1985

61. Castoldi P, Clinica Med Ital 73:5–8, 1942, cited by Rossi L: Atrioventricular conduction system and nerves in the human heart. Sci Med Ital 3:514, 1955

62. Chameides L, Truex R, Vetter V, et al: The association of maternal systemic lupus erythematosus with congenital heart block. Circulation 53/54(suppl II):228, 1976

63. Channer KS, Channer JL, Campbell MJ, Rees JR: Cardiomyopathy in the Kearns-Sayre syndrome. Br Heart J 59:486, 1988

64. Charles R, Holt S, Kay JM, et al: Myocardial ultrastructure and the development of atrioventricular block in Kearns-Sayre syndrome. Circulation 63:214, 1981

65. Chung EK: Sick sinus syndrome: Current views. Mod Concepts Cardiovasc Dis 49:67, 1980

66. Coffen TH, Rush HP, Miller RF: Traumatic complete heart block of 18 years duration; with review of the literature. North Med (Seattle) 40:195, 1941

67. Compton D, Hill PMcN, Sinclair JD: Weight-lifters' blackout. Lancet 2:1234, 1973

67a. Cooper DKC, Charles RG, Fraser RC, et al: Long-term survival after orthotopic and heterotopic cardiac transplantation. Br Med J 281:1093, 1980

68. Corr PB, Sobel BE: The importance of metabolites in the genesis of ventricular dysrhythmia induced by ischemia. Mod Concepts Cardiovasc Dis 48:43, 1979

69. Coumel P, Fidelle J, Lucet V, et al: Catecholamine-induced severe ventricular arrhythmias with Adam-Stokes syndrome in children; report of four cases. Br Heart J 40(suppl):28, 1978

70. Council on Clinical Cardiology of the American Heart Association: The Management of Patient with Bifascicular Block. Donoso E (ed). Council on Clinical Cardiology Newsletter. Vol. 1. AHA, Dallas, May 1974

71. Council on Clinical Cardiology of the American Heart Association: Ventricular Dysrhythmias in Acute Myocardial Infarction. Donoso E (ed). Council on Clinical Cardiology Newsletter. Vol. 2, No. 1. AHA, Dallas, August 1977

72. Council on Clinical Cardiology of the American Heart Association: The Sick Sinus Syndrome. Donoso E (ed). Council on Clinical Cardiology Newsletter. Vol. 3, No. 1. AHA, Dallas, February 1978

73. Council on Clinical Cardiology of the American Heart Association: Dysrhythmias in the Pre-excitation Syndrome. Donoso E (ed). Council on Clinical Cardiology Newsletter. Vol. 4. AHA, Dallas, May 1–4, 1979

74. Crossen KJ, Cain ME: Assessment and management of sinus node dysfunction. Mod Concepts Cardiovasc Dis 55:43, 1986

75. Curry PVL, Krickler DM: Atrial fibrillation in the Wolff-Parkinson-White syndrome. Br Heart J 37:779, 1975 (abst)

76. Dalzell GWN, Cunningham SR, Wilson CM, et al: Ventricular fibrillation: The Belfast experience. Br Heart J 58:441, 1987

77. Dancy M, Leech G, Leatham A: Prognosis in complete right bundle branch block: An echocardiographic study. Circulation 62(4 pt 2):III–200, 1980 (abst 760)

78. Davies M, Harris A: Pathological basis of primary heart block. Br Heart J 31:219, 1969

79. Davies MJ: Pathology of Conducting Tissue of the Heart. Butterworth (London), 1971, pp. 34–37

80. Davies MJ, Anderson RH, Becker AE: The Conduction System of the Heart. Butterworths (Publishers) London, 1983, p. 25

81. Davies MJ, Pomerance A: Pathology of atrial fibrillation in man. Br Heart J 34:520, 1972

82. Davies MJ, Pomerance A: Quantitative study of ageing changes in the human sinuatrial node and internodal tracts. Br Heart J 34:150, 1972

83. Davies P: Sino-auricular block associated with intrathoracic new growths. Br Heart J 19:431, 1957

84. Day SM, Gu J, Polak JM, Bloom SR: Somatostatin in the human heart and comparison with guinea pig and rat heart. Br Heart J 53:153, 1985

85. Demoulin JC, Kulbertus HE: Histopathological examination of concept of left hemiblock. Br Heart J 34:807, 1972

86. Demoulin J-C, Kulbertus HE: Histopathological correlates in sinoatrial disease. Br Heart J 40:1384, 1978

87. Denes P, Wyndham CRC, Rosen, KM: Intractable paroxysmal tachycardia caused by a concealed retrogradely conducting Kent bundle. Demonstration by epicardial mapping and cure of tachycardias by surgical interruption of the His bundle. Br Heart J 38:758, 1976

88. Dhingra RC, Wyndham C, Bauernfeind R, et al: Significance of chronic bifascicular block without apparent organic heart disease. Circulation 60:33, 1979

89. Di Gregorio NJ, Crawford JH: Auricular flutter and complete heart block. Am Heart J 17:114, 1939

90. Di Marco JP: Investigational antiarrhythmic drugs for treating supraventricular arrhythmias. Clin Cardiol Newsl 11:Aug., 1985

91. Doyle JT: Mechanisms and prevention of sudden death. Mod Concepts Cardiovasc Dis 45:111, 1976

92. Dreifus LS, Hriat R, Watanabe Y, et al: Ventricular fibrillation. A possible mechanism of sudden death in patients with Wolff-Parkinson-White syndrome. Circulation 43:520, 1971

93. Dubowitz V: The female carrier of Duchenne muscular dystrophy. Br Med J 284:1423, 1982

94. Durrer D, Schoo L, Schwilenburg RM, Welens HJJ: The role of premature beats in the initiation and the termination of supraventricular tachycardia in the Wolff-Parkinson-White syndrome. Circulation 36:644, 1967

95. Durrer D, Van Dam RTh, Freud GE, et al: Total excitation of the isolated human heart. Circulation 41:1970, 1970

96. Edwards AC, Meredith TJ, Sowton E: Complete heart block due to chronic chloroquine toxicity managed with a permanent pacemaker. Br Med J 1:1109, 1978

97. Ekelund L-G, Moberg A, Olsson AG, Orö L: Recent myocardial infarction and the conduction system. A clinicopathological correlation. Br Heart J 34:774, 1972

98. Ektor H, Van der Hauwaert LG: Sick sinus syndrome in childhood. Br Heart J 44:684, 1980

99. Eliška O, Elišková M: Venous circulation of the human conduction system. Br Heart J 42:508, 1979

100. Emery AEH, Skinner R: Clinical studies in benign (Becker type) X-linked muscular dystrophy. Clin Genet 10:189, 1976

101. Engel TR, Meister SG, Feitosa GS, et al: Appraisal of sinus node artery disease. Circulation 52:286, 1975

102. Enrico JF, Essinger S, Poli S, Perret Cl: Syndrome de Romano-Ward et "torsades de pointe." Schweiz Med Wochenschr 103:301, 1973

103. Eppinger H, Rothberger JC: Zur Analyse des Elektrokardiogramms. Wien Klin Wochenschr 22:1091, 1909

104. Eppinger H, Stoerk O: Zur Klinic des Elektrokardiogramms. Z Klin Med 71:157, 1910

105. Eriksson P, Karp K, Bjerle P, Olofsson BO: Disturbances of cardiac rhythm and conduction in familial amyloidosis with polyneuropathy. Br Heart J 51:658, 1984

106. Esmond WG, Moulton GA, Cowley RA, et al: Peripheral ramifications of the cardiac conducting system. Circulation 27:732, 1963

107. Esscher E, Hardell L-I, Michaelsson M: Familial, isolated, complete right bundle-branch block. Br Heart J 37:745, 1975

108. Esscher E, Scott JS: Congenital heart block and maternal connective tissue disease. Br Heart J 40: 457, 1978

109. Esscher E, Scott JS: Congenital heart block and maternal systemic lupus erythematosus. Br Med J 1:1235, 1979

110. Evans D, Stovin PGI: Fatal heart block due to mesothelioma of the atrioventricular node. Br Heart J 56:572, 1986

111. Evans R, Shaw DB: Pathological studies in sinotrial disorder (Sick sinus syndrome). Br Heart J 39:778, 1977

112. Evans W, Swann P: Lone auricular fibrillation. Br Heart J 16:189, 1954
113. Fairfax AJ: Immunological aspects of chronic heart block: A review. Proc R Soc Med 70:327, 1977
114. Fajardo LF, Stewart JR: Pathogenesis of radiation-induced myocardial fibrosis. Lab Invest 29:244, 1973
115. Fawcett FJ, Goldberg MJ: Heart block resulting from myocardial sarcoidosis. Br Heart J 36:220, 1974
116. Ferrer MI: The sick sinus syndrome in atrial disease. J Amer Med Assoc 206:645, 1968
117. Ferrer MI: The Sick Sinus Syndrome. Futura, Mount Kisco, NY, 1974
118. Ferris JAJ: Hypoxic changes in conducting tissue of the heart in sudden death in infancy syndrome. Br Med J 2:23, 1973
119. Ferris JAJ, Aherne WA: Cartilage in relation to the conducting tissue of the heart. Lancet 1:64, 1971
120. Fleming H: Sarcoid heart disease in the United Kingdom. Br Heart J 41:379, 1979
121. Fontaine G, Frank R, Grosgogeat Y: Torsades de pointes: Definition and management. Mod Concepts Cardiovasc Dis 51:103, 1982
122. Fraser GR, Froggatt P, James TN: Congenital deafness associated with electrocardiographic abnormalities, fainting attacks and sudden death. A recessive syndrome. Q J Med (new series) 33:361, 1964
123. Frink RJ, James TN: Normal blood supply to the human His bundle and proximal bundle branches. Circulation 47:8, 1973
124. Furlanello F, Maccà F, Dal Palù C: Observation on a case of Jervell and Lange-Nielsen syndrome in an adult. Br Heart J 34:648, 1972
125. Gajewski J, Singer RB: Mortality in atrial fibrillation. Circulation 60(4 pt 2):II-52, 1979 (abst 195)
126. Gallagher JJ, Cassell J, Sealy WC, et al: Epicardial mapping in the Wolff-Parkinson-White syndrome. Circulation 57: 854, 1978
127. Gallagher JJ, Gilbert M, Svenson RH, et al: Wolff-Parkinson-White syndrome. The problem, evaluation and surgical corrections. (Special article.) Circulation 51:767, 1975
128. Gallagher JJ, Kasell J, Sealy WC, et al: Epicardial mapping in the Wolff-Parkinson-White syndrome. Circulation 57:854, 1978
129. Gallagher JJ, Sealy WC, Anderson RW, et al: Cryosurgical ablation of accessory atrio-

ventricular connections. A method for correction of the pre-excitation syndrome. Circulation 55:471, 1977
130. Gallagher JJ, Sealy WC, Kassell J, Wallace AG: Multiple accessory pathways in patients with the preexcitation syndrome. Circulation 54:571, 1976
131. Garcia R, Breneman GM, Fine G: "Mesothelioma" of the atrioventricular node. Incidence of heart block in ten cases. Circulation 68(4 pt 2):III-12, 1983 (abst 46)
132. Gardner-Medwin D. Recognising and preventing Duchenne muscular dystrophy. Br Med J 287:1083, 1983
133. Gaskell WH: On the innervation of the heart. J Physiol (Lond) 4:43, 1883
134. Gee DJ: A glycoprotein in cardiac conducting tissue. Br Heart J 31:588, 1969
135. Gerlis LM, Anderson RH, Becker AE: Complete heart block as a consequence of atrionodal discontinuity. Br Heart J 37:345, 1975
136. Gerlis LM, Davies MJ, Boyle R, et al: Preexcitation due to accessory sinoventricular connections associated with coronary sinus aneurysms. A report of two cases. Br Heart J 53:314, 1985
137. Gerlis LM, Wright HM, Wilson N, et al: Left ventricular bands. A normal anatomical feature. Br Heart J 52:641, 1984
138. Gertz G, Kaplan HA, Kaplan L, Weinstein W: Cardiac syncope due to paroxysms of ventricular flutter, fibrillation, and asystole in a patient with varying degrees of A-V Block and intraventricular block. Am Heart J 16:225, 1938
139. Giardina ACV, Ehlers KH, Engle MA: Wolff-Parkinson-White syndrome in infants and children. A long term follow-up study. Br Heart J 34:839, 1972
140. Gilchrist AR: Clinical aspects of high-grade heart block. Scott Med J 3:53, 1958
141. Gillette PC, Duff D, Mullins CE, McNamara DG: Sinus node function VS internodal conduction as the mechanism of post Mustard dysrhythmias. Circulation 54(4 pt 2): II-184, 1976 (abst 0720)
142. Ginks W, Leatham A, Siddons H: Prognosis for patients paced for chronic atrioventricular block. Br Heart J 41:633, 1979
143. Glomset DJ, Glomset AJA: A morphologic study of the cardiac conduction system in ungulates, dog, and man. I. The sinuatrial node.

II. The Purkinje system. Am Heart J 20:389, 677, 1940

144. Godman MJ, Alpert BA, Julian DG: Bilateral bundle-branch block complicating acute myocardial infarction. Lancet 2:345, 1971

145. Gottdiener JS, Hawley RJ, Maron BJ, et al: Hypertrophic cardiomyopathy in Friedreich's ataxia. Circulation 60(4 pt 2):II–242, 1979 (abst 947)

146. Greenwood RG, Rosenthal A, Cassady R, et al: Constrictive pericarditis in childhood due to mediastinal irradiation. Circulation 50:1033, 1974

147. Gross L: The Blood Supply to the Heart. Hoeber, New York, 1921

148. Halsey RH: A case of ventricular fibrillation. Heart 6:67, 1915

149. Harper PS: Isolating the gene for Duchenne muscular dystrophy. Br Med J 293:773, 1986

150. Harries MG, Golden FS, Fowler M: Ventricular-fibrillation as a complication of saltwater immersion. Br Med J 283:347, 1981

151. Harriman RJ, Krongrad E, Boxer RA, et al: Methods for recording electrograms of the sinoatrial node during cardiac surgery in man. Circulation 61:1024, 1980

152. Harris A, Davies M, Redwood D, Leatham A, Siddons H: Aetiology of chronic heart block. A clinicopathological correlation of 65 cases. Br Heart J 31:206, 1969

153. Harrison CV, Lennox B: Heart block in osteitis deformans. Br Heart J 10:167, 1948

154. Harrison L, Gallagher JJ, Kassell J, et al: Cryosurgical ablation of the A-V node-His bundle. A new method for producing A-V block. Circulation 55:463, 1977

155. Hassan ZU, Fastabend CP, Mohanty PK, Isaacs ER: Atrioventricular block and supraventricular arrhythmias with X-linked muscular dystrophy. Circulation 60:1365, 1979

156. Hetzel, MR, Ginks WR, Pickersgill AJ, Leatham A: Value of pacing in cardiac failure associated with chronic atrioventricular block. Br Heart J 40:864, 1978

157. Hiejima K, Sano T: Electrical alternans of TU wave in Romano-Ward syndrome. Br Heart J 38:767, 1976

158. His WJr: Die Thätigkeit des embryonalen Herzens und deren Bedeutung für Lehre von der Herzbewegung beim Erswachsenen. Arbeit Med Klin Lpz 14–49, 1893

159. Hobbs Jr: An ABC of amyloid. Proc R Soc Med 66:705, 1973

160. Hoffa M, Ludwig CFW: Einige newe Versuche über Herzbewegung. Z Rat Med 9:107, 1850

161. Hollman A: Thomas Lewis—The early years. Br Heart J 46:233, 1981

162. Huchard H: Traité clinique des maladies du coeur et de l'aorte. 3rd Ed. Vol 1. Doin, Paris, 1905

163. Hudson, REB: The human pacemaker and its pathology. Br Heart J 22:153, 1960

164. Hudson REB: The human conducting system and its examination. J Clin Pathol 16:492, 1963

165. Hudson REB: Cardiovascular Pathology. Vol. 2. Edward Arnold, London, p. 1971, 1965

166. Hudson REB: Surgical pathology of the conducting system of the heart. Br Heart J 29:646, 1967

166a. Hudson REB: Cardiovascular Pathology. Vol. 3. Edward Arnold, London, 1970

167. Isner JM, Sours HE, Paris AL, et al: Sudden unexpected death in avid dieters using the liquid-protein-modified-fast diet. Observation in 17 patients and the role of the prolonged QT interval. Circulation 60:1401, 1979

168. Jackson SHD, Parry DJ: Lightning and the heart. Br Heart J 43:454, 1980

169. James TM: Anatomy of the human sinus node. Anat Rec 141:109, 1961

170. James TN: Morphology of the human atrioventricular node, with remarks pertinent to its electrophysiology. Am Heart J 62:756, 1961

171. James TN: Pericarditis and the sinus node. Arch Intern Med 110:305, 1962

172. James TN: The connecting pathways between the sinus node and A-V node and between the right and left atrium in the human heart. Am Heart J 66:498, 1963

173. James TN: Pathology of the cardiac conduction system in haemochromatosis. N Eng J Med 271:92, 1964

174. James TN: Pathology of the cardiac conduction system in amyloidosis. Ann Intern Med 65:28, 1966

175. James TN: De subitaneis mortibus. XXIII Rheumatoid arthritis and ankylosing spondylitis. Circulation 55:669, 1977

176. James TN: De subitaneis mortibus. XXV. Sarcoid heart disease. Circulation 56:320, 1977

177. James TN, Beeson CWII, Sherman EB, Mowry RW: De subitaneis mortibus. XIII. Multifocal Purkinje cell tumours of the heart. Circulation 52:333, 1975

178. James TN, Birk RE: Pathology of the cardiac conduction system in polyarteritis nodosa. Arch Intern Med 117:561, 1966

179. James TN, Burch GE: Blood supply of the human atrioventricular system. Circulation 17:391, 1958

180. James TN, Carson DJL, Marshall TK: Fibroma compressing His bundle. Circulation 48:428, 1973

180a. James TN, Cobbs BW, Coghlam HC, et al: Coronary disease, cardioneuropathy, and conduction system abnormalities in the cardiomyopathy of Friedreich's ataxia. Br Heart J 57:446, 1987

181. James TN, Fisch C: Observations on the cardiovascular involvement in Friedreich's ataxia. Am Heart J 66:164, 1963

182. James TN, Frame B, Schatz, IJ: Pathology of the cardiac conduction system in Marfan's syndrome. Arch Intern Med 114:339, 1964

183. James TN, Froggatt P, Atkinson WJ Jr, et al: De subitaneis mortibus XXX. Observations on the pathophysiology of the long QT syndrome with special reference to the neuropathology of the heart. Circulation 57:1221, 1978

184. James TN, Galakhov I: De subitaneis mortibus. XXVI. Fatal electrical instability of the heart associated with benign congenital polycystic tumor of the atrioventricular node. Circulation 56:667, 1977

185. James TN, Marshall TK: De subitaneis mortibus. XVIII. Persistent foetal dispersion of the atrioventricular node and His bundle within the central fibrous body. Circulation 53:1026, 1976

186. James TN, Marshall M, Craig MW: De subitaneis mortibus. VII. Disseminated intravascular coagulation and paroxysmal atrial tachycardia. Circulation 50:395, 1974

187. James TN, Marshall TK: Multifocal stenoses due to fibromuscular dysplasia of the sinus node artery. Circulation 53:736, 1976

188. James TN, McKone RC, Hudspeth AS: De subitaneis mortibus. X. Familial congenital heart block. Circulation 51:379, 1975

189. James TN, Monto RW: Pathology of the cardiac conduction system in thrombotic thrombocytopenic purpura. Ann Intern Med 65:37, 1966

190. James TN, Puech P: De subitaneis mortibus. IX. Type A Wolff-Parkinson-White syndrome. Circulation 50:1264, 1974

191. James TN, Reynolds EW: Pathology of the cardiac conduction system in a case of diphtheria associated with atrial arrhythmias and heart block. Circulation 28:263, 1963

192. James TN, Schlant RC, Marshall TK: De subitaneis mortibus. XXIX. Randomly distributed focal myocardial lesions causing destruction of the His bundle or a narrow-origin left bundle branch. Circulation 57:816, 1978

193. James TN, Sherf L: Ultrastructure of the human atrioventricular node. Circulation 37:1049, 1968

194. James TN, Sherf L: Fine structure of the His bundle. Circulation 44:9, 1971

195. James TN, Sherf L, Fine G, Morales AR: Comparative ultrastructure of the sinus node in man and dog. Circulation 34:139, 1966

196. James TN, Sherf L, Urthaler F: Fine structure of the bundle-branches. Br Heart J 36:1, 1974

197. James TN, Spence CA: Distribution of cholinesterase within the sinus node and AV node of the human heart. Anat Rec 155:151, 1966

198. James TN, Spencer MS, Kloepfer JC: De subitaneis mortibus. XXI. Adult onset syncope, with comments on the nature of congenital heart block and the morphogenesis of the human atrioventricular septal junction. Circulation 54:1001, 1976

199. Jervell A, Lange-Nielsen F: Congenital deaf-mutism, functional heart disease with prolongation of Q-T interval, and sudden death. Am Heart J 54:59, 1957

200. Jones AA, Roberts WC: Complete heart block and left bundle branch block in aortic stenosis; an analysis of its cause from a study of serial sections in 12 patients. Circulation 58(suppl II):239, 1978 (abst 932)

201. Josephson ME: Electrophysiologic approach to recurrent ventricular tachycardia. Clin Cardiol Newsl 10:Apr., 1984

202. Jude JR, Kouwenhoven WB, Knickerbocker GG: External cardiac resuscitation. Monog Surg Sci 1:59, 1964

203. Kawamura K: Electron microscope studies on the conduction system of the dog. I. The Pur-

kinje fibres II. The sinoatrial and atrioventricular nodes. Jpn Circ J 25:594, 773, 1961

204. Kay HB: Ventricular complexes in heart block. Br Heart J 10:177, 1948

205. Kaye GC, Butler MG, d'Ardenne AJ, et al: Isolated atrial amyloid contains atrial natriuretic peptide: A report of six cases. Br Heart J 56:317, 1986

206. Kaye HH, Reid DS, Tynan M: Studies on a newborn infant with supraventricular tachycardia and Wolff-Parkinson-White syndrome. Br Heart J 37:332, 1975

207. Kaye SB, Owen M: Cardiac arrhythmias in thalassaemia major: Evaluation of chelation treatment using ambulatory monitoring. Br Med J 1:342, 1978

208. Kearns TP, Sayre GP: Retinitis pigmentosa, external ophthalmoplegia and complete heart block. Arch Ophthalmol 60:280, 1958

209. Kehoe RF, Moran JM, Loeb JM, et al: Extended endocardial resection for treatment of survivors of out-of-hospital ventricular fibrillation. Circulation 66(4 pt 2):II–344, 1982 (abst 1375)

210. Keith A: The sino-auricular node: A historical note. Br Heart J 4:77, 1942

211. Keith A, Flack MW: The form and nature of the muscular connections between the primary divisions of the vertebrate heart. J Anat Physiol 41:172, 1907

212. Kelly DH, Shannon DC, Libertson RR: The role of the QT interval in the sudden infant death syndrome. Circulation 55:633, 1977

212a. Kenny RA, Sutton R: Pacemaker syndrome. Br Med J 293:902, 1986

213. Kent AFS: Researches on the structure and function of the mammalian heart. J Physiol (Lond) 14:233, 1893

214. Kent KM, Epstein SE, Cooper T, Jacobowitz DM: Cholinergic innervation of the canine and human ventricular conducting system: Anatomic and electrophysiologic correlation. Circulation 50:948, 1974

215. Kerber RE, Sarnat W: Factors influencing the success of ventricular defibrillation in man. Circulation 60:226, 1979

216. Kernoham, RJ, Froggatt, P: Atrioventricular dissociation with prolonged QT interval and synopal attacks in a 10-year-old boy. Br Heart J 36:516, 1974

217. Kertes P, Hunt D: Prophylaxis of primary ventricular fibrillation in acute myocardial infarction. The case against lignocaine. Br Heart J 52:241, 1984

218. Kinney, MJ, Stein RM, Di Scala VA: The polyuria of paroxysmal atrial tachycardia. Circulation 50:429, 1974

219. Klein GJ, Hackel DB, Gallagher JJ: Anatomic substrate of impaired antegrade conduction over an accessory atrioventricular pathway in the Wolff-Parkinson-White syndrome. Circulation 61:1249, 1980

220. Klein GJ, Sealy WC, Pritchett ELC, et al: Cryosurgical ablation of the atrioventricular node-His bundle: Long term follow-up and properties of the junctional pacemaker. Circulation 61:8, 1980

221. Koch W: Weitene mitteilungen über den Sinusknoten des Herzens. Verh. Dtsch Ges Pathol 13:85, 1909

222. Komajda M, Frank R, Vedel J, et al: Intracardiac conduction defects in dystrophia myotonica. Electrophysiological study of 12 cases. Br Heart J 43:315, 1980

223. Kries J Von: Über die Bedeutung der Bahnreite fur die Reizleitung im Herzen. Skand Arch Physiol 29:84

223a. Klein GJ, Hackel DB, Gallagher JJ: Anatomic substrate of impaired antegrade conduction over an atrioventricular pathway in the Wolff-Parkinson-White syndrome. Circulation 61:1249, 1980

224. Krikler DM: Supraventricular arrhythmias: A European view of medical management. Circulation 70(4 pt 2):II-A-II-B, 1984 (abst)

225. Krongrad E, Hefler SE, Bowman FO Jr, et al: Further observations on the etiology of the right bundle branch block pattern following right ventriculatomy. Circulation 50:1105, 1974

226. Krumbhaar, EB: History of the Pathology of the Heart. p. 22. In Gould SE (ed): Pathology of the Heart. 2nd Ed. Charles C Thomas, Springfield, IL, 1960

227. Lancet: Fainting on micturition. Lancet 2:286, 1962

228. Lancet: Surgery for ventricular tachycardia. (Editorial.) 1:579, 1980

229. Langslett, A. and Sørland SJ: Surdocardiac syndrome of Jervell and Lange-Nielsen at birth. Br Heart J 37:830, 1975

230. Layton C, Boyle R: Transvenous pacing after tricuspid valve replacement with a Starr-Edwards prosthesis. Br Heart J 35:666, 1973

231. Leading Article: Asymptomatic complete heart block. Br Med J 2:1245, 1979

232. Leatham A, Davies JG, Parker DJ, Siddons AHM: Lessons from early days of pacing. Proc of the British Cardiac Society. Wembley, Nov. 21–22; Br Heart J 51:116, 1984 (abst)

233. Lehmann H, Klein UE: Familial sinus node dysfunction with autosomal dominant inheritance. Br Heart J 40:1216, 1978

234. Lendrum AC, Slidders W, Fraser DS: Renal hyalin: A study of amyloidosis and diabetic fibrinous vasculosis with new staining methods. J Clin Pathol 25:373, 1972

235. Lenègre J: Etiology and pathology of bilateral bundle branch block in relation to complete heart block. Prog Cardiovasc Dis 6:409, 1964

236. Lenègre J, Chevalier H: Étude anatomo-clinique et histologique d'un nouveau cas de bloc typique-de la branche gauche. Arch Mal Coeur 42:197, 1949

237. Lenègre J, Chevalier H: Correlation of electrocardiograms with lesions of the Tawara-His system of A-V block, bundle branch block and ventricular hypertrophy. (Lond) p. 15, 1952 (abst)

238. Lev M: Ageing changes in the human sino-atrial node. J Gerontol 9:1, 1954

239. Lev M: Anatomic basis for atrioventricular block. Am J Med 37:742, 1964

240. Lev M, Benjamin JE, White PD: A histopathologic study of the conduction system in a case of complete heart block of 42 years' duration. Am Heart J 55:198, 1958

241. Lev M, Cuadros H, Paul MH: Interruption of the atrioventricular bundle with congenital atrioventricular block. Circulation 43:703, 1971

242. Lev M, Gibson S, Miller RA: Ebstein's disease with Wolff-Parkinson-White syndrome. Report of a case with a histopathologic study of possible conduction pathways. Am Heart J 49:724, 1955

243. Lev M, Leffler WB, Langendorf R, Pick A: Anatomic findings in a case of ventricular pre-excitation (WPW) terminating in complete atrioventricular block. Circulation 34:718, 1966

244. Lev M, Lerner R: The theory of Kent. A histological study of the normal atrioventricular communications of the human heart. Circulation 12:176, 1955

245. Lev M, Nordenberg A, Bharati S, et al: The anatomic substrate for the sick sinus syndrome in adolescence. Circulation 59/60(suppl II):113, 1979 (abst 437)

246. Lev M, Unger PN, Rosen KM, Bharati S: The anatomic substrate of complete left bundle branch block. Circulation 50:479, 1974

247. Lewin RF, Arditti A, Sclarovsky S: Non-invasive evaluation of electrical cardiac injury. Br Heart J 49:190, 1983

248. Lewis T: Observations upon flutter and fibrillation. IV. Impure flutter; theory of circus movement. Heart 7:293, 1920

249. Lewis T: The Mechanism and Graphic Registration of the Heart-Beat. 3rd Ed. Shaw and Sons, London, 1925

250. Lewis T, Oppenheimer BS, Oppenheimer A: The site of the mammalian heart beat: The pacemaker in the dog. Heart 2:147, 1910

251. Lie JT: Histopathology of the conduction system in sudden death from coronary heart disease. Circulation 51:446, 1975

252. Lie J, Rosenburg HS, Erickson EE: Histopathology of the conduction system in the sudden infant death syndrome. Circulation 53:3, 1976

253. Liebowitz JO, Ullmann DTh: Early references to heart block. J His Med Allied Sci 20:43, 1965

254. Lincoln C, Butler P, Logan-Sinclair R, Anderson RH: A cardiac conduction monitor and probe for intra-operative identification of conduction tissue. Br Heart J 42:339, 1979

255. Lipkin DP, Frenneaux M, Stewart R, et al: Delayed improvement in exercise capacity after cardioversion of atrial fibrillation to sinus rhythm. Br Heart J 59:572, 1988

256. Livesley B, Oram S: Trauma to the sinuatrial node. Lancet 2:426, 1971

257. London AR, Runge PT, Balsam RF, et al: Large right atrial thrombi surrounding permanent transvenous pacemakers. Circulation 40:661, 1969

258. Lown B, Amarasingham R, Newman J: New method for terminating cardiac arrhythmias. JAMA 182:548, 1962

259. Lown B, Ganong WF, Levine SA: The syndrome of short P-R interval, normal QRS

complex and paroxysmal rapid heart action. Circulation 5:693, 1952

260. McWilliam JA: Cardiac failure and sudden death. Br Med J 1:6, 1889

261. MacWilliam JA: Some applications of physiology to medicine. II. Ventricular fibrillation and sudden death. Br Med J 2:215, 1923

262. Maddison PJ, Skinner RP, Taylor PV, et al: Serological studies in congenital heart block. Br Heart J 49:301, 1983

263. Mahaim I: Les maladies organiques du faisceau de His-Tawara. Masson, Paris, 1931

264. Mahaim I: Kent's fibers and the A-V paraspecific conduction through the upper connections of the bundle of His-Tawara. Am Heart J 33:651, 1947

265. Mahaim I: Electrocardiographie. In Lemierre A, et al (eds): Traite de Médecine. Vol. 10, Masson, Paris, 1948

266. Mahaim I: Traité de Médecine. Vol. 10, Masson, Paris, 1948

267. Malouf J, Gharzuddine W, Kutayli F: A reappraisal of the prevalence and clinical importance of left ventricular false tendons in children and adults. Br Heart J 55:587, 1986

268. Mandel WJ, Danzig R, Hayakawa H: Lown-Ganong-Levine syndrome. A study using His bundle electrograms. Circulation 44:696, 1971

269. Maron BJ, Clark CE, Goldstein RE, Epstein SE: Potential role of QT interval prolongation in sudden infant death syndrome. Circulation 54:423, 1976

270. Maron BJ, Roberts WC, McAllister HA, et al: Sudden death in young athletes. Circulation 62:218, 1980

271. Martins de Oliveira J, Mendeljohn D, Nogueira C, Zimmerman HA: Wolff-Parkinson-White syndrome and tetralogy of Fallot. Report of a case. Am J Cardiol 2:111, 1958

272. Massing GG, James TN: Anatomical configuration of the His bundle and bundle branches in the human heart. Circulation 53:609, 1976

273. Matisonn RE, Mitha AS, Chesler E: Successful electrical pacing for complete heart block complicating diphtheritic myocarditis. Br Heart J 38:423, 1976

274. Matovšek M, Posner E: Purkyně's (Purkinje's) muscle fibres in the heart. Br Heart J 31:718, 1969

275. McCue CM, Mantakes ME, Tinglestad JB, Ruddy S: Congenital heart block in newborns of mothers with connective tissue disease. Circulation 56:82, 1977

276. McComish M, Compston A, Jewitt D: Cardiac abnormalities in chronic progressive external ophthalmoplegia. Br Heart J 38:526, 1976

277. McGovern BA, Ruskin JN: Ventricular tachycardia: Initial assessment and approach to treatment. Mod Concepts Cardiovasc Dis 56:13, 1987

278. McMichael J: History of atrial fibrillation 1628–1819. Harvey-deSenac-Laennec. Br Heart J 48:193, 1982

279. Meijler FL: Comparative aspects of the dual role of the human atrioventricular node. Br Heart J 55:286, 1986

280. Meijler FL: The pulse in atrial fibrillation. Br Heart J 56:1, 1986

281. Menon TB, Rao CKP: Tuberculosis of the myocardium causing complete heart block. Am J Pathol 21:1193, 1945

282. Meredith J, Titus JA: The anatomic atrial connections between sinus and A-V node. Circulation 37:566, 1968

283. Miller HC, Svenson RH, Gallagher JJ, Wallace AG: Preoperative assessment of patients with Wolff-Parkinson-White syndrome. Br Heart J 37:558, 1975

284. Mobitz, W: Über die unvollständige Störung der Erregungsüberleitung zwischen Vorhof und Kammer des menschlichen Herzens. Z Ges Esp Med 41:180, 1924

285. Morady F, Scheinman MM: Paroxysmal supraventricular tachycardia. Mod Concepts Cardiovasc Dis 51:Part I: Diagnosis, 107: Part II: Treatment, 113, 1982

286. Morgagni, GB: De Sedibus et Causis Morborum, Venetiis, ex. Typog. Remondiniana. Ep 26, 1761

287. Morquio L: Sur une maladie infantile et familiale; çaractérisée par des modifications permanentes du pouls, des attaques syncopales et epileptiformes et la mort subite. Arch Med Enfants 4:467, 1901

288. Morris AW, Johnson IM: Epithelial inclusion cysts of the heart. Arch Pathol 77:36, 1964

289. Mullins CB, Atkins JM: Prognosis and management of ventricular conduction blocks in acute myocardial infarction. Mod Concepts Cardiovasc Dis 45:129, 1975

290. Mustard WT: Successful two-stage correction

of transposition of the great vessels. Surgery 55:469, 1964

291. Nair CK, Runco V, Everson GT, et al: Conduction defects and mitral annulus calcification. Br Heart J 44:162, 1980

292. Nathan AW, Bexton RS, Levy AM, Camm AJ: Noninvasive recording of the His bundle electrograms in neonates. Circulation 68(4 pt 2):III–329, 1983 (abst 1314)

293. Nathan AW, Large SR, Davies DW, et al: Results from surgical treatment for ventricular tachycardia and fibrillation. Proceedings of the British Cardiac Society, Wembley. Br Heart J 57:62, 1987 (abst)

294. Naumann-D'Alnoncourt C, Zierhut W, Blüderitz B: "Torsade de pointes" tachycardia. Re-entry or focal activity? Br Heart J 48:213, 1982

295. Nichols, Trans. Royal Humane Society, London, 1774, Cited by Perman E: Succesful cardiac resuscitation with electricity in the eighteenth century. Br Med J 2:1770, 1978

296. Nishida K, Kamijima G, Nagayama T: Mesothelioma of the atrioventricular node. Br Heart J 53:468, 1985

297. Northcote RJ, Ballantyne D: Sudden cardiac death in sport. Br Med J 287:1357, 1983

298. O'Doherty M, Tayler DI, Quinn E, et al: Five hundred patients with myocardial infarction monitored within one hour of symptoms. Br Med J 286:1405, 1983

299. Ohnell RF: Pre-excitation. A cardiac abnormality. Pathophysiological, pathoanatomical and clinical studies of an excitatory spread phenomenon. Acta Med Scand Suppl 152, 1944

300. Olofsson B-O, Forsberg H, Andersson S, et al: Electrocardiographic findings in myotonic dystrophy. Br Heart J 59:47, 1988

301. Opie LH: Sudden death and sport. Lancet 1:263, 1975

302. Ostrander LD Jr: Bundle-branch block. An epidemiologic study. Circulation 30:872, 1964

303. Palagi B, Picozzi R, Casazza F, et al: Biventricular function in Friedreich's ataxia: A radionuclide angiographic study. Br Heart J 59:692, 1988

304. Papapoulos SE, Clemens TL, Fraher LJ, et al: 1,25-Dihydroxycholecalciferol in the pathogenesis of the hypercalcaemia of sarcoidosis. Lancet 1:627, 1979

305. Parkinson J: Auricular fibrillation following complete heart-block in diphtheria. Heart 6:13, 1915–17

306. Parkinson J, Papp C, Evans W: The electrocardiogram of the Stokes-Adams attack. Br Heart J 3:171, 1941

307. Penton GB, Miller H, Levine SA: Some clinical features of complete block. Circulation 13:801, 1956

308. Philips J, Ichinose H: Clinical and pathologic studies in the hereditary syndrome of a long QT interval, syncopal spells and sudden death. Chest 58:236, 1970

309. Piérard LA, Henrard L, Demoulin JC: Persistent atrial standstill in familial Ebstein's anomaly. Br Heart J 53:594, 1985

310. Pitcher DW, Papouchado M, James MA, Rees JR: What is "controlled atrial fibrillation"? Br Heart J 53:97, 1985 (abst)

311. Poltera AA, Cox JN, Owor R: Pancarditis affecting the conducting system and all valves in African trypanosomiasis. Br Heart J 38:827, 1976

312. Pool J, Roodenburg A, Glaser B, Lubsen J: Ventricular arrest: A possible mechanism of sudden death. Br Heart J 40(suppl):24, 1978

313. Potter EL: Pathology of the Fetus and Newborn. Yearbook Medical Publishers, Chicago, 1952

314. Priest MF, Cooper TB, MacLean WAH, et al: Nature of onset of atrial fibrillation in man. Circulation 60(4 pt 2):II–254, 1979, (abst 990)

315. Prinzmetal M, Corday E, Brill IC, et al: Mechanism of the auricular arrhythmias. Circulation 1:241, 1950

316. Prinzmetal M, Corday E, Brill IC, et al: The Auricular Arrhythmias. Charles C Thomas, Springfield, IL, 1952

317. Pritchett ELC, Anderson RW, Benditt DG: Re-entry within the atrioventricular node; surgical cure with preservation of atrioventricular conduction. Circulation 60:440, 1979

318. Pritchett ELC, Prystowsky EN, Benditt DJ, Gallagher JJ: Dual atrioventricular nodal pathways in patients with Wolff-Parkinson-White syndrome. Br Heart J 43:7, 1980

319. Prystowsky EN, Pritchett ELC, Roses AD, Gallagher J: The natural history of conduction system disease in myotonic muscular dystrophy as determined by serial electrophysiologic studies. Circulation 60:1360, 1979

320. Purkyně JE: Mikroskopisch-neurologische

Beobachtungen. Arch Anat Wissensch Physiol 12:281, 1845

321. Rabkin SW, Mathewson FAL, Tate RB: Natural history of left bundle-branch block. Br Heart J 43:164, 1980

322. Rashkind WJ, Miller WW: Creation of an atrial septal defect without thoracotomy. A palliative approach to complete transposition of the great arteries. JAMA 196:991, 1966

323. Rausing A: Focal myocarditis in familial dystrophic myotonica. Br Heart J 34:1292, 1972

324. Rawles JM, Rowland E: Is the pulse in atrial fibrillation irregularly irregular? Br Heart J 56:4, 1986

325. Reid JM, Coleman EN, Doig W: Reversion to sinus rhythm 11 years after surgically induced heart block. Br Heart J 38:1217, 1976

326. Reid JM, Coleman EN, Doig W: Complete congenital heart block. Report of 35 cases. Br Heart J 48:236, 1982

327. Reid JM, Murdoch R: Polymyositis and complete heart block. Br Heart J 41:613, 1979

328. Reiffel JA, Gang E, Gliklich J, et al: The human sinus node electrogram: A transvenous catheter technique and a comparison of directly measured and indirectly estimated sinoatrial conduction time in adults. Circulation 62:1324, 1980

329. Reiffel J, Gliklich J, Gang E, et al: Human sinus node electrograms. Transvenous, catheter recorded technique and normal sinoatrial conduction times in adults. Circulation 59/60(suppl II):63, 1979 (abst 238)

330. Reynolds EW, Vander Ark CR: Quinidine syncope and the delayed repolarisation syndromes. Mod Concepts Cardiovasc Dis 45:117, 1976

331. Rhodin JAG, Del Missier P, Reid LC: The structure of the specialized impulse conducting system of the steer heart. Circulation 24:349, 1961

332. Ridolfi RL, Bulkley B, Hutchins GM: The conduction system in cardiac amyloidosis: Clinical and pathological features of 23 patients. Circulation 54(suppl II):135, 1976 (abst 0533)

333. Rizzon P, Rossi L, Baissus C, et al: Left posterior hemiblock in acute myocardial infarction. Br Heart J 37:711, 1975

334. Roberts WC, Ferrans VJ, Bulkley B, et al: Sarcoidosis of the heart; a study of 8 necropsy patients. Circulation 49/50(suppl III):129, 1974, (abst 508)

335. Roberts WC, McAllister HA Jr, Ferrans VJ: Sarcoidosis of the heart: A clinicopathologic study of 35 necropsy patients and review of 78 previously reported necropsy patients. Am J Med 63:86, 1977

336. Robinson K, Rowland E, Krikler DM: Wolff-Parkinson-White syndrome: Atrial fibrillation as the presenting arrhythmia. Br Heart J 59:578, 1988

337. Romamo G, Gemme G, Pongiglione R: Aritme cardiache rare dell'eta' pediatrica II. Accessi sincopali per fibrillazione. ventricalare parossitica. Clin Pediatr 45:656, 1963

338. Rosen KM: Catheter recording of His bundle electrograms. Mod Concepts Cardiovasc Dis 42:23, 1973

339. Rosen KM, Rahimtoola SH, Gunnar RM, Lev M: Site of heart block as defined by His bundle recording. Pathologic correlations in three cases. Circulation 45:965, 1972

340. Rosenbaum FF, Hecht HH, Wilson FM, Johnston FD: The potential variations in the thorax and the oesophagus, in anomalous atrioventricular excitation (Wolff-Parkinson-White syndrome). Am Heart J 29:281, 1945

341. Rosenbaum MB: The hemiblocks: Diagnostic criteria and clinical significance. Mod Concepts Cardiovasc Dis 39:141, 1970

342. Rosenbaum MB: Sir Thomas Lewis; a view from the south. Br Heart J 46:349, 1981

343. Ross CF, Belton EM: A case of cardiac lipidosis. Br Heart J 30:726, 1968

344. Rossi L: Atrioventricular conduction system and nerves in the human heart. Sci Med Ital 3:514, 1955

345. Rossi L: Sistema nervoso e di conduczione nel cuore senile. G Gerontol 23(suppl):75, 1960

346. Rossi L: Discordant features in pathology of the bundle branches. Acta Cardiol 19:286, 1964

347. Rossi L: Sarcoid heart disease. Br Heart J 1:546, 1973

348. Rossi L: A histological survey of pre-excitation syndrome and related arrhythmias. G Ital Cardiol 5:816, 1975

349. Rossi L: Histopathology of conducting system in left anterior hemiblock. Br Heart J 38:1304, 1976

350. Rossi L: Personal observations on the conduction system and nerves of the heart in patients dying with arrhythmias. (Interna-

tional Lecture, Miami, Fla.) Circulation 62(4 pt 2):III–4–III–5, 1980 (abst 11)

351. Rossi L, Knippel M, Taccardi B: Histological findings, His bundle recordings and body-surface potential mappings in a case of Wolff-Parkinson-White syndrome. Cardiology 60:265, 1975

352. Rossi L, Lévy A: Anomalies morphologiques et topographiques de la branche droite du faisceau de His au cours de l'hypertrophie cardiaque. Arch Mal Coeur 53:154, 1960

353. Rossi L, Matturri L: Histopathological findings in two cases of torsade de pointes with conduction disturbances. Br Heart J 38:1312, 1976

354. Rossi L, Matturri L: His bundle haemorrhage and external cardiac massage. Br Heart J 59:586, 1988

355. Rossi L, Thiene G, Knippel M: A case of surgically corrected Wolff-Parkinson-White syndrome. Clinical and histological data. Br Heart J 40:581, 1978

356. Rothberger CJ, Winterberg H: Experimentelle Beitrage zur Kenntnis der Reizleitungsstörung in den Kammern des Säugetierherzens. Z Ges Exp Med 5:264, 1917

357. Rowland E, Robinson K, Edmondson S, et al: Cryoablation of the accessory pathway in Wolff-Parkinson-White syndrome: Initial results and longterm follow up. Br Heart J 59:453, 1988

358. Saltissi S, Kertes PJ, Julian DG: Primary cardiac amyloidosis in a young man presenting with angina pectoris. Br Heart J 52:233, 1984

359. Sanabria T: Étude anatomo-pathologique du bloc de branche. Rapports entre l'image electrocardiographique et l'aspect microscopique du systeme de His-Tawara. Acta Cardiol 8:145, 1953

360. Sanyal SK, Johnson WW, Dische MR, et al: Dystrophic degeneration of papillary muscle and ventricular myocardium. A basis for mitral valve prolapse in Duchenne's muscular dystrophy. Circulation 62:430, 1980

361. Sanyal SK, Johnson WW, Thapar MK, Pitner SE: An ultrastructural basis for electrocardiographic alterations associated with Duchenne's progressive muscular dystrophy. Circulation 57:1122, 1978

362. Sapru RP, Griffiths PH, Guz A, Eisele J: Syncope on swallowing. Br Heart J 33:617, 1971

363. Sawayama T, Kurihara T, Araki S: Noninvasive cardiovascular findings in familial am-

yloid polyneuropathy. Br Heart J 40:1288, 1978

364. Schellhammer PF, Engle MA, Hagstrom JWC: Histological Studies of the myocardium and conducting system in acquired iron-storage disease. Circulation 35:631, 1967

365. Scheinberg MA, Cathcart ES: New concepts in the pathogenesis of primary and secondary amyloid disease. Clin Exp Immunol 33:185, 1978

366. Scherf L, Woods WT, James TN: Cellular structure and function of the canine AV node. Circulation 66(4 pt 2):II–379, 1982 (abst 1518)

367. Seda PE, McAnulty JH, Anderson CJ: Postural heart block Br Heart J 44:221, 1980

368. Schmaltz R: Die Purkinje'schen Fäden im Herzen der Haussäugethiere. Arch Wiss Prakt Thierheilk 12:161, 1886

369. Shaw DB, Eraut D: Atrial bradycardia or the lazy sinus syndrome. Bristol Med Chir J 84:213, 1969

370. Shaw DB, Holman RR, Gowers JI: Survival in sinoatrial disorder (Sick sinus syndrome). Br Med J 1:139, 1980

371. Shaw DB, Kekwick CA, Veale D, et al: Survival in second degree atrioventricular block. Br Heart J 53:587, 1985

372. Shaw DB, Linker NJ, Heaver PA: Chronic sinoatrial disorder (sick sinus syndrome): A possible result of cardiac ischaemia. Br Heart J 58:598, 1987

373. Sherf L, James TN: A new look at some old questions in clinical electrocardiography. Henry Ford Hosp Med Bull 14:265, 1966

374. Short DS: The syndrome of alternating bradycardia and tachycardia. Br Heart J 16:208, 1954

375. Silverman KJ, Hutchins SGM, Bulkley BH: Cardiac sarcoid: A clinicopathologic study of 84 unselected patients with systemic sarcoidosis. Circulation 58:1204, 1978

376. Sims BA: Conducting tissue of the heart in Kwashiorkor. Br Heart J 34:828, 1972

377. Skinner C, Kenmure ACF: Haemochromatosis presenting as congestive cardiomyopathy and responding to venesection. Br Heart J 35:466, 1973

378. Smithen CS, Bennett D, Hudson REB, Sowton E: Trifascicular block—An electrocardiographic hemodynamic and pathological correlation. J Electrocardiol 4(2):145, 1971

379. Sodi-Pallares D: New Basis of Electrocardiography. Kimpton, London, 1956

380. Southall DP, Richards J, Mitchell P, et al: Study of cardiac rhythm in healthy newborn infants. Br Heart J 43:14, 1980

381. Sowton E: Environmental hazards for pacemaker patients. J R Coll Physicians Lond 16:159, 1982

382. Spurrell RAJ, Yates AK, Thorburn CW, Sowton GE, Deuchar DC: Surgical treatment of ventricular tachycardia after epicardial mapping studies. Br Heart J 37: 115, 1975

383. Stephensen O, Cleland WP, Hallidie-Smith K: Congenital complete heart block and persistent ductus arteriosus associated with maternal systemic lupus erythematosus. Br Heart J 46:104, 1981

384. Stokes W: Observations on some cases of permanently slow pulse. Dublin Q J Med Sci 2:73, 1846

385. Stotler WA, McMahon RA: The innervation and structure of the conductive system of the human heart. J Comp Neurol 87:57, 1947

386. Stuckey JH, Hoffman BF, Bagdonas AA, Piera J, Venerose RS: Direct studies of the specialized conducting system during hypothermia. Circulation 22:819, 1960

387. Surawicz B: Prognosis of patients with chronic bifascicular block. Circulation 60:40, 1979

388. Sutton R, Davies M: The conduction system in acute myocardial infarction complicated by heart block. Circulation 38:987, 1968

389. Sykes AH: A.D. Waller and Jimmie; a centenary contribution. St Mary's Hosp Gaz 93:23, 1987

390. Tawara S: Das Reizleitungssystem des Säugetierherzens. Eine anatomischhistologische Studie uber das Atrioventrikularbündel und die Purkinjeschen Fäden. Fischer, Jena

391. Theiss W, Wirtzfeld A: Pulmonary embolisation of retained transvenous pacemaker electrode. Br Heart J 38:326, 1977

392. Thery Cl, Lekieffre J, Dupuis Cl: Atrioventricular block secondary to a congenital aneurysm of the membranous septum. Histological examination of conduction system. Br Heart J 37: 1097, 1975

393. Thomson, AMP: Dystrophia cordis myotonica studied by serial histology of the pacemaker and conducting system. J Pathol 96:285, 1968

394. Thomson JG: Production of severe atheroma in a transplanted human heart. Lancet 2:1088, 1969

395. Todaro F: Novelle ricerche sopra la struttura muscolare delle orecchiette del cuore umano e sopra la valvola d'Eustachio. Sperimentale 16:217, 1865

396. Toivonen LK, Nieminen MS, Manninen V, Frick MH: Conversion of paroxysmal atrial fibrillation to sinus rhythm by intravenous pirmenol. A placebo controlled trial. Br Heart J 55:176, 1986

397. Tonkin AM, Dugan FA, Svenson RH, et al: Co-existence of functional Kent and Mahaim-type traits in the pre-excitation syndrome: Demonstration by catheter technique and epicardial mapping. Circulation 52:193, 1975

398. Truex RC, Bishof JK, Downing DF: Accessory atrioventricular muscle bundles, II Cardiac conduction system in a human specimen with Wolff-Parkinson-White syndrome. Anat Rec 137:417, 1960

399. Truex RC, Schwartz MJ: Venous system of the myocardium with special reference to the conduction system. Circulation 4:881, 1951

400. Unger PN, Greenblatt M, Lev M: Anatomic basis of the electrocardiographic pattern in incomplete left bundle-branch block in coronary disease. Circulation 35/36(suppl II):254, 1967

401. Uppal SC: Kearn's syndrome, a new form of cardiomyopathy. Br Heart J 35:766, 1973

402. Van der Hauwaert LG, Dumoulin M: Hypertrophic cardiomyopathy in Friedreich's ataxia. Br Heart J 38:1291, 1976

403. Van der Hauwert LG, Stroobandt R, Verhaeghe L: Arterial blood supply to the atrioventricular node and main bundle. Br Heart J 34:1045, 1972

404. Veracochea O, Zerpa F, Morales J, et al: Pacemaker implantation in a familial congenital A-V block complicated by Adams-Stokes attacks. Br Heart J 29:810, 1967

405. Verduyn Lunel AA: Significance of annulus fibrosus of heart in relation to AV conduction and ventricular activation in cases of Wolff-Parkinson-White syndrome. Br Heart J 34:1263, 1972

406. Verrier RL, Thompson PL, Lown B: Ventricular vulnerability during sympathetic stimulation: Role of heart rate and blood pressure. Cardiovasc Res 8:602, 1974

407. Vincent GM, Abildskov JA: The Romano-Ward (prolonged QT) syndrome. Circulation 55/56(4 pt 2):II–156, 1977 (abst 598)

408. Waller Ad: A demonstration on man of electromotive changes accompanying the heart's beat. J Physiol (Lond) 8:229, 1887

409. Ward DE, Camm J: Recurrent ventricular tachycardia. Br Med J 290:1926, 1985

410. Ward DE, Camm AJ: Treatment of tachycardias associated with the Wolff-Parkinson-White syndrome by transvenous electrical ablation of accessory pathways. Br Heart J 53:64, 1985

411. Ward DE, Davies M: Transvenous high energy shock for ablating atrioventricular conduction in man. Observations on the histological effects. Br Heart J 51:175, 1984

412. Ward OC: A new familial cardiac syndrome in children. J Irish Med Assoc 54:103, 1964

413. Webb SC, Hendry WG, Bloom SR, Krikler DM: Somatostatin: A neuroregulatory peptide with electrophysiological activity. Proceedings of the British Cardiac Society of York, April 2–3, 1986. Br Heart J 55:513, 1986 (abst)

414. Webb SC, Krikler DM, Hendry WG, et al: Electrophysiological actions of somatostatin on the atrioventricular junction in sinus rhythm and reentry tachycardia. Br Heart J 56:236, 1986

415. Wellens HJJ: Wolff-Parkinson-White syndrome. Mod Concepts Cardiovasc Dis 52:53, 57, 1983

416. Wellens HJJ, Vermeulen A, Durrer D: Ventricular fibrillation occurring on arousal from sleep by auditory stimuli. Circulation 46:661, 1972

417. Wenckebach KF: Zur Analyse des unregelmässigen Pulses. II Ueber den regelmässig intermitterenden Puls. Z Klin Med 37:475, 1899

418. Wenckebach KF: Beiträge zur Kenntnis der menschlichen Herztätigkeit. .rch Anat Physiol Lpz Physiol Abt p. 297, 1906

419. Widran J, Lev M: The dissection of the atrioventricular node, bundle and bundle branches in the human heart. Circulation 4:863, 1951

420. Wildenthal K, Leshin SJ, Atkins JM, Skelton CL: The diving reflex used to treat paroxysmal atrial tachycardia. Lancet 1:12, 1975

421. Willis RA: Some unusual developmental heterotopias. Br Heart J 3:267, 1968

422. Wilson J, Grant RT: A case of congenital malformation of the heart in an infant associated with partial heart block. Heart 12:295, 1926

423. Winkler RB, Nova AH, Nova JJ: Familial congenital complete block and maternal systemic lupus erythematosus. Circulation 56:1103, 1977

424. Wolff L, Parkinson J, White PD: Bundle branch block with short P-R internal in healthy young people prone to paroxysmal tachycardia. Am Heart J 5:685, 1930

425. Wolff L: Familial auricular fibrillation. N Engl J Med 229:396, 1943

426. Wood FC, Wolferth CC, Geckeler GD: Histologic demonstration of accessory muscle connections between auricle and ventricle in a case of short P-R interval and prolonged QRS complex. Am Heart J 25:454, 1943

427. Wood P: Polyuria in paroxysmal tachycardia and paroxysmal atrial flutter and fibrillation. Br Heart J 25:273, 1963

428. Wood PH: Diseases of the Heart and Circulation. 2nd Ed. Eyre and Spottiswoode. JB Lippincott, London 1956, p. 187

429. Wyatt PR, Cox DM: Duchenne's muscular dystrophy: Studies in cultured fibroblasts. Lancet 1:172, 1977

430. Yater WM: Pathogenesis of bundle branch block. Arch Intern Med 62:1, 1938

431. Yater WM, Cornell VH, Claytor T: Auriculoventricular heart block due to bilateral bundle branch lesions. Arch Intern Med 57:132, 1936

432. Zanchi M, Lenègre J: Les lesions histologiques du système de Tawara His et de ses branches. Cardiologia 27:1, 1955

433. Zipes DP: Second-degree atrioventricular block. Circulation 60:465, 1979

434. Zoll PM: Resuscitation of the heart in ventricular standstill by external electrical stimulation. N Engl J Med 247:768, 1952

435. Zoll PM, Linenthal AJ: Termination of refractory tachycardia by external countershock. Circulation 25:596, 1962

436. Zoltowska A, Wrzolkowa T: Experimental amyloidosis in hamsters. J Pathol 109:93, 1973

437. Zoob M, Smith KS: The aetiology of complete heart block. Br Med J 1:1149, 1963

438. Zmyslinski RW, Richeson JF, Akiyama T: Left ventricular hypertrophy in presence of complete left bundle-branch block. Br Heart J 43:170, 1980

38

The Pathology of Cardiac Pacing

Gregory J. Wilson

INTRODUCTION AND HISTORIC BACKGROUND

Cardiac pacing is an important therapeutic modality that can be lifesaving. The classic indication for its use is atrioventricular (AV) node disease that produces complete heart block. Current indications for permanent cardiac pacing are much more extensive, however, and include sinus node dysfunction, intermittent and incomplete AV block, and bundle branch block. (For the pathology of the cardiac conduction system, see Ch. 37.) In addition, cardiac pacing technology is now applied to convert tachyarrhythmias and in the form of implantable defibrillator systems to protect patients from sudden cardiac death.

Although it had been known since the days of Galvani that electric currents have an effect on the heart, A. S. Hyman was the first investigator to grasp the principles inherent in modern cardiac pacing and to demonstrate their use. In 1932, he reported his work on producing contractions in the asystolic heart of a dog by a needle electrode placed percutaneously and directly into the atrial myocardium.[68] He labeled the apparatus used to supply repetitive small electric impulses to the heart an "artificial pacemaker," the first use of the term. Such impulses depolarize only the adjacent myocardial muscle fibers. The remainder of the myocardium is then activated by a propagated action potential, causing the entire heart to contract.

The construction of temporary, nonimplantable cardiac pacemakers would have been feasible with the electronics technology of the 1930s but did not occur until more than 20 years later, in association with the rapid development of cardiac surgery. In 1951, Callaghan and Bigelow[16] reported effective pacing of the sinoatrial node of the dog by means of intravenous electrodes. These investigators demonstrated the important principle that the heart's rhythm is "captured" by an extrinsic stimulus with a faster rate than the heart's spontaneous mechanism. In 1952, Zoll[170] showed that the arrested heart in patients with Stokes-Adams attacks could be restarted by the transthoracic application of an electrical stimulus, but it was not until 1957 that Weirick et al.[160] reported cardiac pacing in man using a percutaneous epicardial wire electrode and an external artificial pacemaker. In 1959, Furman and Schwedel[47] introduced the now dominant technique of endocardial pacing with long-term stimulation of the right ventricular endocardium achieved by an externally powered electrode on the end of a catheter inserted through the jugular vein. The first self-contained transistorized implantable pacemaker containing a long-lasting battery designed by Greatbatch and inserted clinically by Chardack,[19] was reported in 1960. This marked the birth of long-term cardiac pacing and of the pacemaker industry.

Over the past three decades, cardiac pacing has become a well-established therapeutic tool. More than 250,000 new and replacement permanent pacemakers are implanted worldwide each year. The indications for pacing are broad, so that a few pacemakers are implanted for complete heart block and the most common single indication is bradycardia related to sick sinus node syndromes. Most cardiac pacemakers are implanted in patients older than 60 years but they are also used in children, including infants. There are also interesting geographic variations in their use reflecting different patterns of heart disease. For example, in Bolivia and Brazil many implants are in patients who are under 40 years of age and are used to treat the effects of Chagas' disease.

Fortunately, only a very small proportion of patients undergoing cardiac pacing die directly as a result of pacemaker-related complications. However, a variety of complications may bring a patient to reoperation, and potentially lethal complications do exist. Pathologists should be aware of them. Also, the pathologist requires some understanding of the artificial components involved in cardiac pacing. This involves assimilating background information, including definitions and terminology relating to the technology involved.

TECHNOLOGY OF CARDIAC PACING

Pacemaker Systems

Cardiac pacing is achieved by a system of interconnected components consisting of (1) a pulse generator (which includes a power source and electric circuitry not only to initiate the electric stimulus but also to perform other functions); (2) one or more electrically insulated conductors leading from the pulse generator to the heart; (3) an electrode at the distal end of each of the one or more conductors; and (4) a tissue, or blood and tissue, interface between electrode and adjacent stimulatable myocardial cells. The pulse generator is commonly referred to as the pacemaker, which is permissible provided one keeps in mind the system concept mentioned above. The combination of one or more insulated conductors and electrodes into a single device to connect pulse generator and heart produces the pacing lead. In more complicated pacing systems, two leads may be used. Both pathologists and clinicians must appreciate that the function of the pacing system (pulse generator-pacing lead-myocardial tissue interface) is as vulnerable as its weakest link.

Temporary vs. Permanent Pacing and Route of Lead Insertion

Cardiac pacing may be performed on either a temporary or a permanent basis. Most temporary pacing is done on patients with acute myocardial infarction complicated by cardiac conduction system disturbances that have progressed, or are at risk of progressing, to life-threatening complete heart block. In this context, a single pacing lead is usually placed transvenously into the right ventricle, usually from the femoral vein, and the pulse generator is located outside the body. Much less common with transvenous placement is dual-chamber temporary cardiac pacing involving an additional atrial electrode either to sense atrial depolarization or to pace the atria, or both. In the context of cardiac surgery, temporary pacing is achieved by suturing insulated wires with bare ends contacting the surface of the atria or ventricles to the epicardial surface of the heart. Also, separate atrial and ventricular connections are commonly used. A temporary pacemaker is replaced by an implanted permanent one or its use is discontinued within a few days.

Permanent cardiac pacing involves long-term implantation of the pulse generator. If the route is transvenous, the pacing lead is placed with the electrode at its tip positioned against the endocardium of the right atrium (usually the atrial appendage) or right ventricle. The lead passes from there transvenously to the cephalic vein in the deltopectoral groove. If the cephalic vein is not suitable, the subclavian vein, external jugular vein, or even the internal jugular vein may be used. The lead is then tunneled from the vein to a subcutaneous position, usually in the right or left deltopectoral regions of the superior thorax, where it is connected to a pulse generator. The pulse generator may or may not be wrapped in a polyester fabric sac (commonly referred to as a Parsonnet's pouch after its originator[111]) to assist fixation to the pectoral fascia. If the transthoracic route is used, the pulse generator is usually placed in a similar location, and the electrode is inserted directly into the myocardium of the ventricles or atria or attached to their epicardial surfaces. The pacing lead is brought to the heart by an intercostal, subcostal-subxiphoid, or transmediastinal route. In some cases, particularly in infants and young children, in whom the soft tissues of the chest wall are thin, the pulse generator may be placed in an abdominal location. Rarely, the lead is placed transvenously into the inferior vena cava (e.g., through a lumbar vein), while the pulse generator is positioned in the retroperitoneal space; alternatively, the lead may be tunneled through the soft tissues of the abdominal wall and enter the thorax, either transdiaphragmatically or through an intercostal space above the diaphragm. The pulse generator may then occupy an anterior abdominal location subcutaneously deep to the rectus sheath or rectus muscle or, a lateral position at the subcutaneous, intermuscular, or retroperitoneal level. These are the most common

surgical approaches to both temporary and permanent cardiac pacing, and most are described in more detail, together with other variations, by Meere and Lesperance.[97]

A transthoracic pacemaker insertion is generally more invasive than a transvenous one and, in addition, usually involves the risk of a general anesthetic; this may be a significant problem in the elderly, who are the more likely recipients of pacemakers. Thus, in most centers, more than 90 percent of pacemaker implants are transvenous. This emphasis will be reflected in this presentation of pacing systems and their related pathology.

Ventricular vs. Atrial Pacing and Pacing Modes

In cardiac pacing, the pulse generator stimulates the heart by sending through the pacing lead a repetitive electrical pulse, which can be characterized by its amplitude, measured as either electromotive force (volts) or current (milliamperes), its duration (milliseconds) and its repetition rate (pulses/minute). Pacing may be at a fixed repetition rate, referred to as asynchronous, the asynchrony being between the stimuluting pulse and the spontaneous pattern of atrial and ventricular electromechanical activity. This may have serious implications. If the atria are contracting purposefully, the imposed asynchrony between atrial and ventricular contraction will eliminate the atrial booster pump effect on ventricular filling; this accounts for up to 50 percent of the cardiac output in the abnormal heart,[9,62,141] about 10 percent of the output under normal conditions. In addition, competition with a patient's spontaneous idioventricular rhythm can induce ventricular fibrillation if a pacing stimulus arrives during the vulnerable period (T wave) in myocardial repolarization. Despite these disadvantages, asynchronous ventricular pacing has been used for years, and with good results, in many patients with complete heart block. Nevertheless, the asynchronous mode is now obsolete, having been replaced by various types of noncompetitive pacing. Of these, the ventricular inhibited mode, commonly called "demand," is the most widely used with stimulation being interrupted by any spontaneous cardiac activity. The electric activity of myocardial depolarization associated with spontaneous contraction of the ventricles is sensed by the same lead used for pacing and is amplified by circuitry in the pulse generator to inhibit generation of the stimulation pulses. In this fashion, artificial pacing occurs only when necessary. This is a valuable feature, particularly when a patient has an intermittent conduction disorder or sinus node dysfunction and may be pacer-independent much of the time.

Another much less common mode of noncompetitive pacing is called "ventricular triggered." In this instance, the normal ventricular QRS complex is sensed through the pacing lead and the pacing stimulus is immediately emitted into the QRS complex. This mode is less popular because it increases battery drain, but its advantage is that inhibition of the pacemaker by spurious signals, termed electromagnetic interference, cannot occur. Such interference can arise from external sources, ranging from permanent magnets through alternating current motors to sources in the microwave frequency range[71] or, more commonly from internal myopotentials associated with skeletal muscle activity.[3,106,110,117]

Atrial synchronous pacing enables patients with total heart block to have a completely normal cardiac rhythm that is responsive to changes in atrial rate and involves atrial assistance to ventricular filling. It requires an additional pacing lead connected to the atrium. The atrial electrogram is sensed and, following a suitable delay to allow for atrial contraction, ventricular stimulation occurs. This form of pacing has a disadvantage in that it requires a reasonably stable atrial rhythm and will not work in the presence of atrial flutter or fibrillation. By contrast, with AV sequential pacing, the pulse generator emits both atrial and ventricular stimuli with a suitable delay. If a spontaneous ventricular contraction occurs, the pacemaker is inhibited and recycled for both atrial and ventricular stimuli. This permits appropriately timed atrial contractions under most circumstances although it does not represent an ideal in physiologic pacing in that there is no response to change in the spontaneous atrial rate.

For the majority of patients, some form of atrial pacing is the best choice physiologically, although adequate results can usually be achieved with simpler, less expensive, ventricular inhibited pacemakers.

There are more complex techniques for regulating the output of pacing stimuli, but they represent only variations on the themes presented above.

The Pacemaker Code

A three-letter (three-position) code is used to describe different configurations of pacing systems. The first letter refers to the chamber paced: V for ventricle, A for atrium, D for both atrium and ventricle. The second letter indicates the chamber sensed: V for ventricle, A for atrium, D for both atrium and ventricle, and O for no sensing. The third letter refers to the response of the pacemaker to a sensed beat: T for triggered, I for inhibited, and D for double, indicating atrial triggered and ventricular inhibited or, alternatively, atrial inhibited and ventricular inhibited. The most common pacing mode has been simple ventricular demand (VVI) with one unipolar or bipolar lead attached to a pacemaker, which paces the ventricle and is inhibited by the spontaneous electrical activation of the ventricle. The atrial demand pacemaker (AAI) is analogous to the VVI pacemaker, except that the lead is attached to the atrium, where sensing and pacing occur; this system maintains sequential AV contraction, provided there is no heart block. With the P-wave synchronous pacemaker (VAT), the atrial depolarization is sensed and, after an appropriate delay, the pacemaker fires into the ventricle. This mode is not used clinically because, as no sensing occurs in the ventricle, a pacing spike can fall on the T wave of a spontaneous ventricular beat and could provoke ventricular tachycardia or ventricular fibrillation. An AV sequential pacemaker (DVI) paces both the atria and ventricles sequentially. A disadvantage of this mode is that the rate of firing into the ventricles is not increased as atrial rate increases. Also, the atrial spike may rarely induce atrial arrhythmias by occurring shortly after the P wave. In fact, while a wide variety of pacing modes are available, almost all pacemakers are now of either the simpler VVI type or, increasingly are DDD also referred to as fully automatic, universal, or physiologic. DDD pacing combines the advantages of P-wave synchronous and AV sequential pacing without the disadvantages of either. DDD pacing has brought with it two special problems: "cross-talk" and pacemaker-induced endless loop tachycardia. With atrial and ventricular pacing and ventricular sensing, the atrial pacing spiker or its depolarizing effect on the atrial myocardium (afterpotential) might be sensed through the ventricular electrode and inhibit ventricular firing. This is cross-talk and its risk is greatly reduced by using a bipolar atrial lead. Cross-talk can be eliminated by designing the pacemaker so that it is committed to firing into the ventricles once the atrial lead has fired. In a noncommitted dual-chamber pacemaker cross-talk can still be eliminated, using a blanking period. For several milliseconds during and after firing through the atrial electrode, the ventricular system does not sense, thereby avoiding inappropriate inhibition during this blanking period. Pacemaker-mediated tachycardia can occur with a DDD pacemaker when retrograde AV conduction occurs in response to ventricular pacing. This causes atrial contraction. Sensing the P wave stimulates the ventricle, completing the endless loop. One approach to stop pacemaker-induced tachycardia is to block retrograde AV conduction with carotid sinus massage, but more practical is extending the atrial refractory period or reprogramming to the VVI mode.

Unipolar vs. Bipolar Pacing

The terms unipolar and bipolar refer to the number and polarity of electrodes in or on the heart. The electric discharge that stimulates the heart always takes place between two electrodes, an anode $(+)$ and a cathode $(-)$. It will be equally effective in terms of current threshold, no matter whether both electrodes are within the heart or one is located elsewhere in the body. With a unipolar system, the metal case of the pulse generator forms the anode and a single electrode at the end of the pacing lead, the cathode. In a bipolar system, two electrodes are positioned near the end of the lead to form the anode and cathode. Generally, the cathode is positioned to contact the heart because the threshold for inducing ventricular fibrillation is higher for cathodal than anodal stimulation.[20]

Neither bipolar nor unipolar pacing is superior in all circumstances. Unipolar pacing has the advantage that electrocardiographic (ECG) detection is easier; this is important in the analysis of pacemaker function by the ECG, either at the bedside or by transtelephone monitoring. However, unipolar systems are much more sensitive to electromagnetic interference produced by muscle movement, especially in the region of the pulse generator.[3,106,110,117] Such myopotentials may produce false sensing and so dangerously inhibit pacemaker output. Bipolar pacing may also cause sensing problems because the signal can be markedly attenuated if the two lead electrodes are oriented nearly at right angles to the depolarization wave passing through the heart[45] and, if the proximal intracardiac electrode is near the atrium, it may falsely sense and cycle from a P wave. Furthermore, bipolar stimulation has been implicated in some cases of pacemaker-induced ventricular fibrillation.[120]

Almost all temporary pacing is bipolar because the pulse generator is external to the body, whereas permanently implantable pacing systems use either bipolar or unipolar modalities. With the development of programmability (described below), some pacemakers can switch between unipolar and bipolar pacing.

Pacing Thresholds

The pacing threshold is the strength of the pacing stimulus needed to initiate a wave of depolarization through the myocardium, thus allowing the pacemaker to initiate contraction of the chamber being paced. The threshold may be measured as a current (milliamperes) or as an electromotive force (volts), or it may be stated as one of two derived functions: charge (the product of current and time) or energy (the product of voltage, current, and time). Charge is the most practical function as it describes threshold in the same terms by which chemical battery capacity is measured (milliampere hours); its consumption is inversely related to battery longevity.[46] Usually, the pacing threshold is stated in volts because most pacing circuitry acts as a voltage source producing pulses of a particular voltage with the amount of current that flows determined by the impedance of the lead, electrode, and tissue in concert.

Threshold varies with pulse duration in that a shorter pulse requires higher voltage and current levels. Thus, threshold measurements cannot be interpreted without knowing pulse duration. The calculated energy and charge thresholds, by contrast, are quite insensitive to pulse duration over the range of 0.25 to 1.0 msec within which most pulse generators are set.

Threshold levels (at any given pulse duration) are affected by a variety of factors (Table 38–1). Most important, from the pathologist's perspective, are the position of the electrode relative to stimulatable tissue and the maturity of the tissue response to the elec-

Table 38–1. Determinants of Stimulation Threshold at a Given Pulse Duration

Electrode surface area and shape

Position of the electrode relative to stimulatable tissue

Maturity of the tissue response to the electrode

Acute ischemia

Drugs and electrolyte balance

Anodal versus cathodal stimulation

Unipolar versus bipolar electrode configuration

The metal of which the electrode is fabricated

trode. To depolarize cardiac muscle cells a critical electrical field strength must exist across the cell membranes and this, in turn, is a function of the current density (mA/cm^2) achieved in the region of the stimulating electrode.[70,126] If an electrode is separated from myocytes by tissue that cannot be stimulated, the current density reaching the myocytes must be reduced. In this way, the stimulus threshold is determined by the distance between the electrode and excitable tissue through nonexcitable tissue. Note that this explanation does not rely on the misconception that fibrous tissue acts as an electric insulator. In fact, it has about the same conductivity as myocardium. A larger electrode has a higher surface area and a lower current density at its boundaries, for the same stimulus current. Thus, one may think of the electrode surrounded by nonexcitable tissue as functioning in an equivalent manner, regarding threshold as an imaginary electrode of larger dimensions (Fig. 38–1). This idea is known as the *virtual electrode hypothesis.* The effects of electrode shape on current density make the picture more complex, but there is no doubt that the virtual electrode captures the essence of the situation.

Nonstimulatable tissue separating an electrode from myocytes may be fibrosis induced by the electrode itself or myocardial scarring from some other cause, most commonly a healed myocardial infarction. If separation of the electrode and myocardial cells causes a

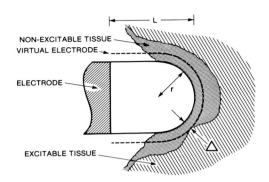

Fig. 38–1. The stimulation threshold for cardiac pacing is determined by the distance (Δ) between the electrode (tip radius [r]) and excitable tissue through nonexcitable tissue. The effect of the non-excitable tissue is similar to having an electrode of larger dimensions (r + Δ) called the virtual electrode.

stimulation threshold exceeding the capability of the pulse generator, *exit block* occurs. The threshold several weeks to months after electrode implantation may be two to three times that of the threshold of implantation although with improved lead designs, including the use of slow, local release of cortico-steroids, this is being reduced. This is explained by fibrous tissue, which forms around the electrode tip. The threshold may peak at its highest level, as much as 4 times that of implantation threshold, about 1 week after implantation. An inflammatory cell infiltrate (polymorphonuclear leukocytes and lympho-cytes) with associated edema can be seen in the endocardium and adjacent myocardium in the region of the electrode at this time. Presumably, the transient peaking of thresh-old is a response to injury, but it has received little study. More recent electrode designs have reduced this effect. The practical point is that, if pulse generator output is not set sufficiently high in the early postoperative phase, threshold peaking can cause a loss of pacing with potentially fatal consequences. By contrast, maintaining output at such high lev-els once thresholds have stabilized greatly shortens battery life. This dilemma has been

a stimulus for the development of pacemakers with adjustable ("programmable") variations in output.

Another factor that affects threshold is acute myocardial ischemia. In experimental stud-ies, this causes both an increased stimulation threshold and a decreased threshold for in-ducing ventricular fibrillation.[20] Normally, fibrillation threshold is far in excess of the maximum stimulus intensity available from any clinical pacemaker, but under ischemic conditions it may be one-tenth of normal or less, just as stimulation threshold in the same ischemic zone increases by 10 times or more. If a pacemaker electrode is located in or at the periphery of a zone of ischemic myocar-dium, the risk to a patient may be serious. Determination of early ischemic changes in the myocardium is difficult at autopsy but should be searched for carefully around the tip of an electrode in any patient with a pace-maker who dies suddenly.

Drugs and the electrolyte balance may also affect the threshold for stimulation[121,158] and can be clinically significant if that stimulation exceeds the threshold by less than 50 percent. In general, hypokalemia, hypernatremia, mineralocorticoids, meals, and sleep tend to elevate the threshold.

During diastole, the myocardium is more sensitive to cathodal than to anodal stimuli of constant current. However, cardiac sensitiv-ity to anodal stimulation is much greater dur-ing and immediately after the QRS complex during the relative refractory period.[98] This phenomenon explains instances of pace-maker-induced ventricular fibrillation related to stimulation of the myocardium from contact with the anode of a bipolar pacing lead. It is also one reason why, in all unipolar systems, the electrode in direct contact with the heart is the cathode. A bipolar electrode configu-ration also influences voltage (but not current) thresholds but only to the extent that the an-ode cannot be as large as in a unipolar system. This effect is small in practice. Finally, the material from which an electrode is made in-fluences threshold as a result of "polarization losses" related to electrochemical processes at the electrode-tissue fluid interface.[102] Platinum iridium electrodes which are most widely used are better than Elgiloy (a cobalt, iron, chromium, molybdenum, nickel, and manganese alloy) in regard to threshold. Elgiloy must be used only as a cathode in unipolar pacing due to its low resistance to electrolytic destruction as an anode.

Sensing the Cardiac Electrogram

Almost all permanent cardiac pacemakers sense the atrial or ventricular electrogram to inhibit the pacemaker if there is conduction through the AV node. Such sensing is achieved through the same electrode pair used for stimulation. Thus, output terminals for the pulse generator are also input terminals for sensing circuitry. The latter amplifies the cardiac electrogram and, when the wave of depolarization is sensed, inhibits the pulse generator from pacing the ventricles or, alternatively, triggers pacing of the ventricles after a suitable delay to allow added ventricular filling by atrial contraction. The sensing circuitry must distinguish a true cardiac depolarization wave from extraneous signals, and a unipolar electrode system in particular may have problems in this regard. Sensing the atrial electrogram can be especially difficult, as the peak signal strength of the P wave is typically only a few millivolts as compared with 10 to 20 mV for the R wave detected in the ventricles.

It must be realized that failure to sense the cardiac electrogram causes a pacemaker to function in the fixed-rate, competitive mode with a small but real risk of inducing ventricular fibrillation, particularly with bipolar pacing. Moreover, if in a demand pacemaker the sensing circuitry responds to spurious signals, the pulse generator may be inappropriately inhibited, placing the life of the patient with complete heart block in imminent danger.

For the pathologist, the sensing function is a source of frustration because there is no effective way of evaluating it at autopsy, except in the unusual circumstances of electronic component failure in the sensing circuitry.

Programmability

One of the most significant developments in cardiac pacing technology is programmability of pulse generator parameters. The circuitry within the pacemaker is designed to respond to electromagnetic impulses delivered from a hand-held programming tool positioned over the implant site of the pulse generator. In this fashion, the rate and output (both pulse width and amplitude) of the stimulating pulse can be modified; the internal logic of the pacemaker changed to different pacing modes; and the sensitivity of the sensing circuitry adjusted.

In addition to altering function in response to command, some pacemakers can signal information concerning the state of internal current consumption and battery drain to provide a guide to the timing of replacement. Given the ongoing revolution in microelectronics, the limitations on building "intelligence" into pacemakers are only those imposed by human imagination or, more importantly, by what is seen to be clinically useful.

Programmability is not without problems. Although rare, spontaneous and unwanted programming by electromagnetic interference termed "phantom" programming[17,39] can occur and, depending on the parameter(s) involved, may be potentially fatal. For this reason and others, the pathologist may need to determine the settings of a programmed pacemaker coming to autopsy and compare them with those in the clinical records.

Power Sources

Although a variety of power sources have been used in cardiac pacemakers, including batteries of mercury/zinc, nickel/cadmium (rechargeable), and even nuclear power, with the latter converting the heat from the radioactive decay of plutonium 238 to electric energy,[112] for practical purposes all current pacemaker batteries are based on lithium. Five types of lithium batteries are determined by the cathodal material: organic iodide, lead sulfide, thionyl chloride, cupric sulfide, and silver chromate with lithium iodide batteries predominating. These reliable batteries work routinely for 10 years and, theoretically, for 20 years.

With regard to the power source, only two issues are important, from the pathologist's perspective: (1) whether the source has completely discharged resulting in a failure to pace, and (2) the appropriate means of disposing of a pacemaker at autopsy, particularly of those with nuclear batteries. These questions are addressed in a later section dealing with the method of examining a pacemaker at autopsy.

With improvements in electronic circuitry and lithium battery technology in recent years, the modern pacemaker (Fig. 38–2) is ·

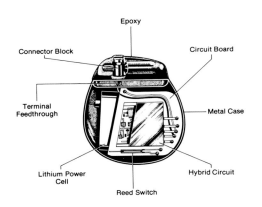

Epoxy

Connector Block

Circuit Board

Terminal Feedthrough

Metal Case

Lithium Power Cell

Hybrid Circuit

Reed Switch

Fig. 38–2. Cutaway view of a typical modern pacemaker shows its miniaturized electronics, lithium battery, and hermetically sealed feedthrough to the lead connector socket needed to eliminate any fluid intrusion. The outer metal shell, made of either stainless steel or titanium, serves as the anode for unipolar pacing and, if used as such, may be partially covered with an insulating polymer to reduce the area exposed.

a remarkably compact and highly reliable device. It represents the most successful implantable "organ" yet manufactured.

Sensor-Driven Rate-Responsive Pacing

The most sophisticated DDD pacemaker can only drive the ventricles as fast as the intrinsic atrial rate or at some rate set the last time the pacemaker was programmed. Many patients have disturbed sinuatrial function at the time of pacemaker implant (sick sinus syndrome is the leading indication for permanent implantable pacemakers) or within a few years thereafter; for these patients, the pacemaker does not increase rate with exercise, so that cardiac output can only increase, according to Starling's law of increased ventricular filling. The use of a physiologic sensing mechanism to supply information on metabolic demand for increased cardiac output can solve this problem.

Several sensing mechanisms have been developed. A simple and successful approach is based on a small piezoelectric sensor within the pacemaker designed to detect body motion. Another approach is to monitor respiration rate and tidal volume through transthoracic impedance measurement. This measurement can be made between the tip of the pacing lead and the pacemaker housing. Central venous temperature, oxygen saturation in mixed venous blood, stroke volume estimation through changes in intracardiac impedance that occur because blood is more conductive than tissue, and rate of pressure rise in the right ventricle are other possibilities, but all require special electrodes. Evoked depolarization offers an alternative approach. By sensing the depolarization response of the underlying myocardium from the pacing electrode, changes in neurally released and circulating catecholamines can be inferred. It is possible to develop an algorithm for the pacemaker microprocessor, to adjust the pacing rate. Such evoked response measurement imposes extraordinary demands on the ventricular electrode in regard to polarization phenomena. This electrode must be able to sense the myocardial evoked response; it is much smaller than the pacing spike (millivolts versus volts) and will be lost if there is not an almost instantaneous reversion to zero potential of the electrode after the pacing stimulus. It is attainable, using platinized-platinum microporous-surfaced electrodes. A description of how this is achieved is beyond the scope of this presentation.

During the 1990s, one can expect sensor-driven rate-responsive pacing to achieve its potential. The result will be that many patients paced only from the ventricle will enjoy the rate responsiveness achieved ideally with dual-chamber pacing, and DDD pacemakers will achieve their full potential in many patients with sinuatrial node disease.

Pacing Leads/Electrodes

Because the success or failure of a pacemaker is largely determined by the tissue response to a lead, and to the electrode in particular, the pathologist is in a key position to describe problems with pacing lead/electrode configurations in clinical use and, in this way, to point to future improvements. Pacing leads may be connected to the heart from either its endocardial or epicardial aspect and may involve quite different designs.

Endocardial Leads

An ideal endocardial pacing lead should provide stable fixation immediately from the time of implantation, achieve and maintain a minimal threshold for stimulation, maximize the amplitude of the cardiac electrogram to facilitate sensing, and function reliably for many years. So many new designs have been produced that it is possible to discuss only a representative sample, to emphasize the principles involved.

Early pacemakers had a cylindrical electrode, with either a flat or rounded tip, or a

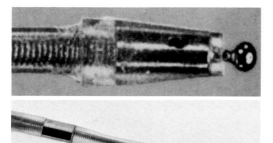

Fig. 38–3. Early endocardial leads had either a ball-shaped electrode at the distal end of the lead (Cordis ball-tip) or a cylindrical electrode with a flat or slightly rounded tip (Medtronic 6901). The latter example has been made bipolar by the addition of a cylindrical electrode on the body of the lead.

ball-shaped electrode in contact with the endocardium (Fig. 38–3). Electrode surface area has been reduced to achieve lower stimulation thresholds, and various means of achieving reliable fixation have been developed. Electrode fixation may be active or passive. In active fixation, the electrode is designed to

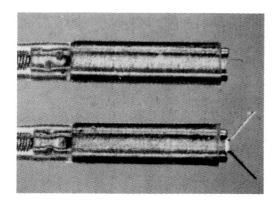

Fig. 38–4. Early "active" fixation endocardial lead (Biotronick IE-65-I) shown with and without deployment of its two projecting wires. The latter penetrate the endocardium and underlying myocardium.

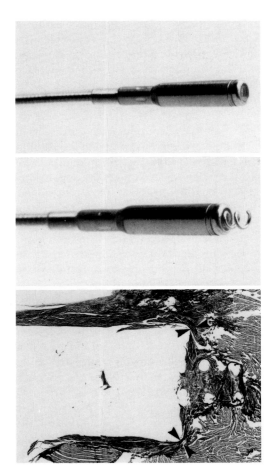

Fig. 38–5. A more recent "active" fixation endo-cardial lead (Medtronic 4016) with a ring shaped electrode is an extendable/retractable helix (top, center). The myocardial scarring that results at the site of penetration by the helix is thus divorced from the ring electrode which itself is separated from myocardium by only a thin fibrous tissue cap-sule (bottom, arrowhead).

grasp the endocardial surface to achieve pos-itive immediate fixation at implantation. One early positive fixation design[11] had metal wires held on a piston within a cylinder at the elec-trode tip (Fig. 38–4). When the appropriate implantation position was found, the wires were forced from the electrode tip through the endocardium and into the underlying myocardium.

Another design achieves positive fixation by an extendable/retractable helix positioned in the center of a ring-shaped electrode (Fig. 38–5) so that myocardial scarring at the site of penetration by the helix is separated from the tissue reaction to the ring electrode and, therefore, does not adversely affect stimula-tion threshold performance.[94] Retractability of the positive fixation mechanism can be a feature of critical importance if the lead re-quires subsequent removal—for example, in infective endocarditis.

Another approach to endocardial fixation, also employing the geometry of a helix, is shown in Figure 38–6. In this case, the elec-trode is formed as a double-wound helical coil that can be rotated around a trabeculum.[31] This approach is at the border-line between active and passive fixation.

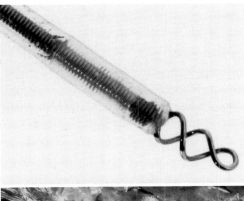

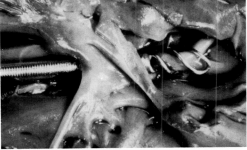

Fig. 38–6. Endocardial electrode formed from a double-wound helical coil of platinum iridium wire (Vitatron Helifix). This design is on the borderline between active and passive fixation.

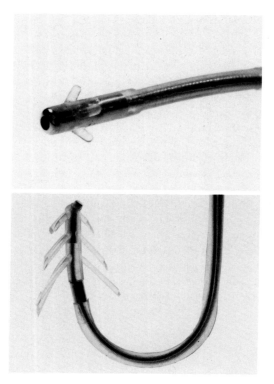

Fig. 38–7. Projections (tines) of silicone rubber added in the region of the electrode tip aid passive endocardial fixation. They have been used on both ventricular (Medtronic 6961, with ring electrode) and atrial leads (Medtronic 6990, bipolar J-shaped lead for positioning in right atrial appendage).

A very effective aid to passive fixation is the addition of projecting tines, or fins, in the region of the electrode tip.[65] This design has been used successfully for both ventricular and atrial endocardial leads (Fig. 38–7).

A quite different approach to improving fixation has been the development of electrodes with porous metal surfaces.[1,2,95,165] In one example, porous metal surfaces are created by coating a solid substrate with a metal powder of controlled particle size range.[95,165] The coating and substrate are sintered at high temperatures, so that the metal particles bond to each other and to the metal substrate by solid-state fusion. The particle-particle and particle-substrate bonds result in an interconnected network of pores uniformly distributed throughout the coating and allows tissue ingrowth (Fig. 38–8). There are other means of achieving porosity. For example, the electrode may consist of a random meshwork of platinum-iridium wires surrounded by an outer wire screen of the same material[2] (Fig. 38–9). Without passive or active fixation devices, porous electrodes are superior to smooth electrodes with regard to the stability of endocardial fixation and chronic stimulation thresholds. These advantages are achieved by the firm bonding of the electrode to the endocardium through tissue ingrowth into the electrode, with only a minimum of non-stimulatable fibrous tissue intervening between the electrode surface and underlying myocytes. Improved performance in sensing the cardiac electrogram has also been achieved with porosity. For sensing, a larger surface area is more effective.[45] This advance may be understood, in part, if the electrode is thought to have two different effective surface areas—a small area for stimulation and a much larger (three to five times) area for sensing.

An endocardial pacemaker lead may require a special design if it is implanted at a particular site. One example is the J-shaped atrial lead (see Fig. 38–7), which is curved to facilitate placing the electrode tip in the right atrial appendage, inherently the most stable site for fixation. Another example is the flexible distal tip lead with a cylindrical electrode (Fig. 38–10) adapted especially for pacing from the coronary sinus.[56] The flexible tip lies deep in the great coronary vein and prevents the electrode from being dislodged from the coronary sinus when the pacemaker is retracted by respiratory movement. A more common use of a cylindrical electrode is as an addition to the electrode at the lead tip to make any lead bipolar (see Fig. 38–3).

Epicardial Leads

Clinical use of epicardial leads is far less popular because of the entailed need for a thoracotomy. The predominant design is a "corkscrew" electrode (Fig. 38–11) in which the

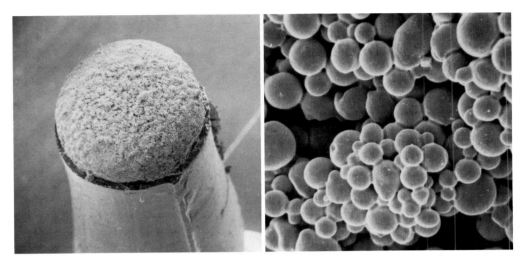

Fig. 38–8. Scanning electron micrographs showing low- ($\times$ 25) and high- ($\times$ 600) power views of a powder metal surfaced endocardial electrode (Cordis Telectronics porous). The metal particles (5 to 20 μm in diameter) bond to form an interconnected network of pores and provide a scaffolding for tissue ingrowth to anchor the electrode to the endocardium.

helical electrode is insulated over most of its length so that the stimulating surface area at its tip is small. The electrode is screwed into the myocardium; no sutures are needed for its attachment. This is a significant advantage

in that the electrode can be placed on the epicardium and fixed in place through a very limited incision, making possible a subxyphoid thoracotomy under local anesthesia. However, the lead is virtually impossible to

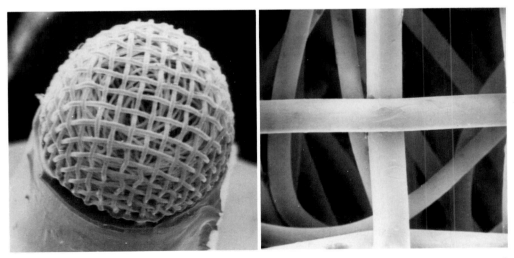

Fig. 38–9. Scanning electron micrographs showing low- ($\times$ 25) and high- ($\times$ 400) power views of an endocardial electrode (CPI porous) in which porosity is achieved by construction of a random meshwork of platinum-iridium wires (25-μm diameter) surrounded by an outer wire screen (40-μm diameter wire) of the same material.

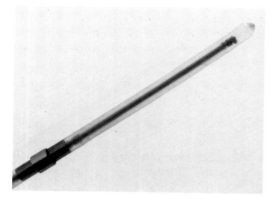

Fig. 38–10. Unipolar lead for coronary sinus pacing, incorporating a cylindrical electrode and a long, flexible tip. The latter lies deep in the great coronary vein to prevent electrode dislodgment.

remove at a later date, except by further surgery. The site of implantation in the myocardium depends on the type of thoracotomy used, which alters exposure. One further guiding principle as to the site of electrode location is to avoid scarred areas of those regions, such as the free wall of the right ventricle or apex, where the heart wall is thin and a corkscrew electrode could penetrate the right or left ventricular cavity with subsequent hemorrhage. To overcome the latter problem, a "two-turn" corkscrew electrode has been developed in addition to the "three-turn" electrode.

The Automatic Implantable Cardioverter-Defibrillator

The syndrome of sudden cardiac death is a major cause of mortality. It claims more than 400,000 victims each year in the United States alone. Many of these deaths occur in the context of a developing myocardial infarction. However, improvements in emergency and intensive medical care have saved many patients who previously would have died from ventricular tachycardia and ventricular fibrillation not associated with the onset of myo-

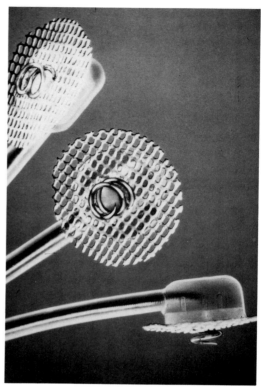

Fig. 38–11. The most commonly used epicardial lead is this "corkscrew" sutureless helical electrode (Medtronic 6917A), shown rotated through three different views. The electrode helix is insulated, except for about one-half turn at its tip, so that the exposed electrode surface area is small.

cardial infarction. These patients, who are at high risk of recurrent fatal ventricular arrhythmias, face an annual sudden cardiac death rate estimated in the range of 17 to 43.6 percent.[55,60,148] There are a variety of approaches to treatment. Antiarrhythmic drugs have their place but are variably effective and toxic. Surgical management includes isolated myocardial revascularization, if acute ischemia is the main problem, and simple ventricular aneurysmectomy, which may be curative in a small group with well-defined aneurysms. Unfortunately, endocardial resection operations have high associated mortality and failure rates of 20 to 30 percent, even in highly selected patients.[119] These shortcomings in medical and surgical management have contributed to the recent acceptance of the automatic implantable cardioverter defibrillator. Clinical experience in the United States with the available prototype devices from one manufacturer has been very positive with more than 5,000 implants and a 1-year arrhythmic mortality of only about 2 percent.[49,77,113,119] Pathologists will see increasing numbers of such devices at autopsy in the future.

The history of the implantable defibrillator centers around two tenacious individuals, Michel Mirowski and Morton Mower,[76] who fibrillated a dog's heart and then successfully defibrillated it with their first shock of 20 joules (J) from a crude prototype device, proving that when electrodes were placed directly on the heart, the energy requirement was a small fraction of the 400 J typically used with bulky external defibrillators. There is a limit to the miniaturization of batteries to provide the energy and of capacitors to hold the charge to be suddenly released, but this relatively low requirement made it possible to build an implantable device capable of more than 100 discharges. Such devices had dropped in size from 250 ml and 225 g to 100 ml and 180 g by the late 1980s. Mirowski and Mower developed their prototypes throughout the 1970s, facing skepticism about both the need for these devices and their practicality. The first patient was not treated until February 1980, nearly 11 years after initial success in the laboratory.

The automatic implantable cardioverter-defibrillator system developed by Mirowski and colleagues used a patch electrode sewn epicardially to the apex of the heart and a transvenous electrode positioned in the superior vena cava; the cardioverting shock was applied between the two electrodes, and the transvenous electrode was used for sensing. The system evolved through various design changes, so that stimulation is now performed through a pair of patch electrodes on the surface of the heart (anterioposterior orientation)

with a pair of screw-in epicardial electrodes performing the sensing function. The criteria for shocking the heart consist of the sensing of either a heart rate above a preset level (rate cutoff from 120 to 200 beats/min) or of an electrical signal that satisfies a probability density function consistent with fibrillation. In sinus rhythm and a wide variety of arrhythmias, the ECG signal is at or near the baseline most of the time. During ventricular fibrillation, the signal is always away from the baseline. The probability density function approach makes use of this difference.

The implantable cardioverter-defibrillator is subject to most of the complications described above for implantable pacing systems, but there have been several specific problems. One has been false-positive discharges, usually initiated by sinus or supraventricular tachycardia above the preset rate cutoff. Nonsustained ventricular arrhythmias that spontaneously terminate can also initiate undesired discharges because once the capacitors are fully charged, they are committed to discharge, regardless of the underlying rhythm. Thus, there was some truth to jocular descriptions of this device as a "bomb" inside the body[76] made during its early development. Another special problem has been interaction with pacemaker systems[32] often needed in these patients to treat underlying symptomatic bradycardia, severe bradycardia after defibrillation, or to provide a rate floor to minimize bradycardia related ventricular arrhythmias. Because the implantable cardioverter-defibrillator has automatic gain control activity that detects the largest amplitude signal and ignores smaller signals, ventricular electrograms, and pacing stimuli, if of similar strength, may be counted by the sensing circuitry. Such double counting of pacemaker stimuli and ventricular electrical activity may exceed the cutoff rate and produce false-positive shock delivery. Triple counting may occur if both the pacer stimulus and the local ventricular electrogram resulting from each pacing spike are counted. This can happen if the conduction time between the pacing stimulus and the rate counting electrodes exceeds the cardioverter-defibrillator sensing refractory period of 150 msec. By contrast, if the pacer spikes are sensed consistently at higher amplitude than the underlying cardiac rhythm, intrinsic ventricular arrhythmias, both ventricular tachycardia and fibrillation, may go undetected and cause death. These problems are greatly reduced with bipolar pacing and by implanting the bipolar rate sensing electrodes (epicardial screw-in leads) of the cardioverter-defibrillator on the lateral left ventricle, as far away from the right ventricular apex (where a pacing lead could be implanted) as possible.

Autopsy examination of the automatic implantable cardioverter-defibrillator[140] revealed foci of contraction band necrosis under the ventricular epicardial patch simulating electrode in some cases and vacuolar cytoplasmic clearing and loss of myocytes in the same location in five patients who had multiple defibrillations. These pathologic changes were confined to less than 2 percent of the total myocardial mass. Thrombus formation was associated with the superior vena cava electrode; in one patient defibrillated 59 times, there was destruction of the wall of the cava around the electrode which had been used both to deliver the shocks and for sensing.

Future generations of implantable cardioverter-defibrillators will be expected to have greater versatility in providing programmability and pacing capabilities, including antitachycardia and ventricular demand pacing with increasingly sophisticated sensing algorithms to avoid false-positive discharges. Both pacing and rate sensing will be possible from the transvenous lead. Also, intravenous and subcutaneous lead/electrode systems are being developed so that cardioversion and defibrillation can be accomplished without the need for epicardial patch placement. No doubt there will be new complications, some unanticipated, to be observed by alert pathologists. Nevertheless, these hybrid pacing-cardioverter-defibrillator devices can be ex-

pected to become increasingly common during the 1990s.

COMPLICATIONS OF CARDIAC PACING

Classification

A wide variety of complications may occur in cardiac pacing. Most are potentially life-threatening and should be considered as one attempts to establish the cause of death in any case of sudden death of a patient with a pacemaker. Not all complications involve specific pathologic findings, but when they do they are diagnostic.

In classifying complications, two approaches are possible. The first is temporal, dividing complications into those that are early and those that are late. The second is anatomic and divides complications into those affecting the portion of the pacing system involved, that is, the pacemaker pack (which houses the pulse generator and its controlling circuitry, power source, and lead connector socket[s]); the lead, exclusive of electrode(s); or the electrode(s). The first approach has the disadvantage that certain complications may occur either early or late but is needed to include a variety of problems that may occur operatively and cannot be readily linked to a specific portion of the implanted hardware. Therefore, a hybrid of these classifications is used here (Table 38–2).

Intraoperative Complications

Intraoperative complications are rare. They result largely from the route of insertion of a pacing lead.

Epicardial pacing involves the risk of com-

Table 38–2.   Complications of Cardiac Pacing

Intraoperative Complications
  Endocardial Approach
    Injury at the site of venous insertion
    Air embolism from the site of venous insertion
    Tricuspid valve perforation
    Perforation of the right ventricle or atrium
  Epicardial Approach
    Complications of thoracotomy and general anesthesia
    Perforation of the left ventricle
Complications related to the pacemaker pack and its site of implantation
  Battery depletion
  Electronic component failure
  "Phantom" programming
  Electromagnetic interference from
    Exogenous sources at home, in the workplace, or in the hospital
    Endogenous myopotentials
  Skin erosion due to pressure necrosis with secondary wound infection
  Infection of the pacemaker "pocket" with
    Septicemia
    Endocarditis from infection tracking along the lead
  Rotation of the pacemaker pack (packmaker twiddler syndrome) with
    Electrode dislodgment
    Lead fracture
Complications related to the pacing lead(s)
  Lead fracture
  Venous thrombosis and pulmonary thromboembolism
  Infection
  Lead failure
  Migration of epicardial leads
Complications related to the pacing electrode[a]
  Malposition
  Dislodgment
  Myocardial penetration and perforation
  Electrode corrosion and insulation failure
  Exit block

[a] All electrode complications may be considered lead complications because the electrode is part of the lead.

plications inherent in a thoracotomy and, in most patients, the associated use of a general anesthetic. In addition, specific complications relating to electrode placement are possible. Perforation of the corkscrew type of sutureless epicardial electrode through either the right or left ventricular wall may occur with a fatal outcome, as has been reported in one case of insertion into the apex of the left ventricle.[156]

The transvenous insertion of a pacemaker lead involves different risks such as air embolism, which may occur when fluctuation in intrathoracic pressures during respiration is transmitted to the neck veins and produces a sucking force during inspiration. Acute right heart failure results when large numbers of air bubbles impact in the pulmonary arterioles and capillaries.[72,125,169] Pneumothorax has occurred with subclavian vein introducer devices for pacing leads when the vein was perforated within the chest. Other complications include perforation of the tricuspid valve[54,115] or of the right ventricle.[41,53,67,81,100,103,127,162] Perforation through the right ventricular wall is most common during electrode positioning but may be delayed days or months after insertion. The stiff metal stilette passed into the pacing lead is one important mechanical factor; another is the thickness of the right ventricular wall at the site of electrode lodgment. Pacing of the diaphragm or chest wall muscles, chest pain, and/or a pericardial friction rub may result. Such perforation may be asymptomatic[41] but usually causes a loss of pacing. It can also result in a clinically evident cardiac tamponade[75,105] requiring thoracotomy, and death from either failure to pace[74] or tamponade.[48]

With either the transvenous or epicardial approach, the induction of ventricular fibrillation at implantation is a theoretical possibility, if the pacing stimulus competes with intrinsic cardiac electric activity and occurs in the vulnerable period of repolarization corresponding to the upswing of the T wave on the ECG. One case report exists of fibrillation induced by turning on a demand pacemaker during the temporary pacing of a patient with an acute myocardial infarction and who had a slow idioventricular rhythm.[131] This case suggests that the fibrillation threshold lowering effect of myocardial ischemia[20] is probably a requirement for this phenomenon. Also, it illustrates the point that a demand pacemaker, in which the pulse generator is inhibited when the intrinsic ventricular depolarization signal is sensed, can still produce ventricular fibrillation because the sensing inhibition does not operate at the moment the pulse generator is initially activated. Fortunately, this problem has been corrected in the newer external pacemakers.

Use of the femoral vein as the site of insertion of most temporary pacing leads is associated with several possible acute local complications. These include double puncture of the femoral artery and vein,[36,37] invited by the close anatomic relationship between the vessels in the femoral triangle, and femoral vein thrombosis.[24] The latter may be caused by local injury or compression by a large hematoma secondary to inadvertent arterial puncture. The thrombosis can cause pulmonary emboli. Arteriovenous fistulae may occur in association with cardiac catheterization by both the femoral artery and vein,[154] often performed in association with temporary pacing. Tearing of the femoral vein, with retroperitoneal hemorrhage, is another complication and infection a risk.

Use of unipolar electrocautery when a permanent pacemaker is implanted may be dangerous. Modern pacemakers employ microprocessors, and the software in memory may be "blown" by electrocautery. Also, a considerable electric current may pass down the lead and damage the myocardium through the electrode tip. Bipolar electrocautery avoids this problem, when the surgical field is near the pulse generator or lead. The nearby availability of both a noninvasive programming device for the pacemaker and an external pacemaker for backup protection, are wise precautions.

Complications Related to the Pacemaker Pack and Its Site of Implantation

Battery Depletion and Electronics-Related Failure, Including Electromagnetic Interference

Perhaps the most obvious complication related to the pacemaker is loss of the stimulus for pacing attributable either to failure of an electronic component or, more commonly, to battery depletion. In either event, the patient is at the mercy of intrinsic cardiac electrical activity, and the outcome may be fatal. A particularly interesting mode of electronic failure is the so-called "runaway pacemaker," in which very high stimulation rates exceeding 150 to 200 beats/min can be achieved, with catastrophic results.[107] This complication should have been eliminated by the increasing sophistication in design of pacemaker circuitry, yet occasional cases have been reported with "modern generation" pacemakers.[89,101,109] Another unusual cause for pulse generator-related loss of pacing is phantom programming, in which the output of the pacemaker is inappropriately reset to a level below the stimulation threshold by electromagnetic interference from a spurious signal, or by faulty signals from the programmer circuitry, or by misuse of the device by an uninformed operator.[39,77]

Electromagnetic radiation in the environment can also cripple demand-type pacemakers, used in most patients, by interfering with the sensing of the cardiac electrogram, a small signal often only a few millivolts in amplitude. Such interference may be thought of as an electrode-related problem in that the bipolar electrode configuration greatly reduces its effect. However, because the sensing circuitry is involved and can be protected by other means, it is usually regarded as a problem related to the pacemaker pack.

In the past, many reports appeared on interference with pacemaker function by devices ranging from electric razors, toothbrushes, and microwave ovens at home to electrosurgical and diathermy apparatus in hospital. Fortunately, recent generations of cardiac pacemakers have been greatly improved with regard to their resistance to electromagnetic interference.[38,69] Also, manufacturers of home appliances and such items as antitheft devices[29] in stores and libraries have been urged to use designs compatible with the degree of electromagnetic interference protection in existing pacemakers. Nevertheless, potentially fatal electromagnetic interference still occurs occasionally in the workplace and home environments. Arc welding remains the most common problem in industry. Experts in the field of pacer electromagnetic interference have a store of fascinating anecdotes relating close brushes with death of pacemaker recipients. Many of the current major risks of electromagnetic interference occur in the hospital environment. In addition to interference from electrocoagulation (especially unipolar units) and external cardiac defibrillation, therapeutic irradiation and magnetic resonance imaging (MRI) present risks. With therapeutic irradiation of malignancies, a pacemaker in the treatment field is not shielded with lead the semiconductor circuitry is likely to be damaged. The newer multiprogrammable pacers introduced during the 1980s frequently contain complementary metal oxide (CMOS) semiconductor "chips" that are particularly susceptible to damage from ionizing radiation.[13,89,90,157] The damage may be subtle and not appear as a life-threatening malfunction until long after radiotherapy. With MRI scanners, there are two problems. Asynchronous pacing tends to be provoked by the high magnetic field, but electronic circuitry damage does not occur; this is not a major problem. However, the radiofrequency signal from the scanner frequently causes rapid atrial pacing (up to 800 beats/min) or even total inhibition of atrial and ventricular output of dual-chamber DDD pacemakers.[34,63]

Pacemaker function usually reverts to normal when removed from the source of electric interference but, sometimes the pacemaker is permanently damaged. For example, the use of an electrocoagulator in a patient with a pacemaker may shorten battery life if the output capacitor of the pacemaker pulse generator is destroyed.[71] Furthermore, during cardiac defibrillation, in which potentials of thousands of volts may be generated, the output stage of a pacemaker can be destroyed, especially if one of the defibrillation electrodes is placed directly over the pacemaker pack of a unipolar pacing system.

Skeletal muscle potentials represent a source of electromagnetic interference from the patient's own body.[3,106,110,117] They can be as crippling to a demand pacemaker as electromagnetic fields of external origin. The extent of muscle contact with the anode is a key factor. Thus newer totally metal-encased pulse generators, which are implanted in a subpectoral (rather than subcutaneous) position totally surrounded by muscle, invite electromagnetic interference because they operate in the unipolar electrode configuration, whereby the metal case forms the anode. Solutions to this problem include the use of a bipolar electrode configuration, subcutaneous implantation, or the electric insulation of that portion of the pulse generator case in contact with muscle.

For the pathologist dealing with sudden death in a pacemaker patient, the problem with electromagnetic interference is that it is temporary and that no evidence of it may be found at autopsy. This emphasizes the importance of knowing the circumstances surrounding the sudden death. The situation is different with battery depletion, electronic component failure, and even "phantom" programming, which can be detected by a detailed electric examination of the pacemaker.

Surgical Complications

Surgical complications relating to implantation of the pulse generator are not unusual. Most common are erosion due to pressure necrosis, infection of the pacemaker pocket, and either migration or rotation of the pacemaker pack. Pressure necrosis of the skin overlying the pulse generator tends to occur in thin, elderly patients receiving bulky pacemakers and is less of a problem with newer, smaller designs. When the skin has broken, local infection, usually with some strain of *Staphylococcus*, is inevitable; under extreme circumstances, the entire pacemaker pack may extrude from the wound causing a loss of pacing (Fig. 38–12).

Infection of the pacemaker "pocket" may also occur by implantation of bacteria at operation and represents the most common source of pacemaker-related infection. *Staphylococcus epidermidis* is most frequently cultured and, although not normally regarded as pathogenic appears to be so in the presence of a foreign body. A local pacemaker pocket

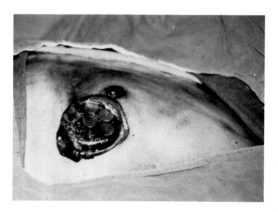

Fig. 38–12. This patient, shown with the left hemithorax draped for surgery, had a severe pacemaker pocket infection with complete erosion of the overlying skin and extrusion of the pacemaker. When he leaned forward, the anode, formed by the metal case of this unipolar pacemaker, lost contact with subcutaneous tissue; pacing ceased and syncope occurred.

infection may lead to the further complication of septicemia[73,134,139] or endocarditis, the latter caused by propagation of the local infection at the pulse generator site along the pacing lead and into the heart. With epicardial electrodes, a pacemaker pocket infection can spread to involve the mediastinum; two cases of resulting bronchocutaneous fistula have been reported.[23,153] Other complications of epicardial leads have been recurrent pericarditis with cardiac constriction[114] and even a case of cardiac strangulation.[12]

The guiding principle in the management of infected pacemakers has been to remove all foreign material, including the pulse generator and pacing leads.[40,92] Although some success has been reported with conservative therapy involving local debridement, antibiotics, and continuous closed irrigation with antiseptic solution,[52] this approach is probably only realistic when *S. epidermidis* is the offender.[94] Complete removal of the pacing system[129] may be necessary with infections caused by this microorganism.

Movement of the pulse generator either within a capacious tissue implant pocket or through fascial planes to a distant site can cause serious problems, the most common of which is electrode dislodgment. The placing of pulse generators in the abdominal wall has previously been associated with some bizarre symptoms: back pain caused by retroperitoneal migration with the formation of a large retroperitoneal hematoma,[8] chronic diarrhea,[21] and even small bowel infarction resulting from migration into the peritoneal cavity.[96] With the usual location of the pacemaker pocket in the anterior chest wall, downward migration of a heavy pulse generator has been reported,[78] but much more common has been the problem of rotation of the pulse generator within an enlarged pocket. Nowadays, pacemakers are quite compact, and one sees few migration problems.

Rotation may occur spontaneously but usually results when a patient habitually twists the generator within a capacious tissue pocket. This is referred to as *pacemaker twiddler syndrome*, after its initial description by Bayliss et al.[5] in 1968. Occasional cases are still reported.[161] Dislodgment of the electrode with resulting loss of pacing may be caused by one of two mechanisms:

1. The pacing lead may be reeled onto the pulse generator like fishing line.
2. The lead may coil when the pulse generator is rotated on its axis, causing the lead both to twist and pull back on the electrode. In this case, the lead may fracture before the electrode dislodges.

Such rotational movement of the pacemaker, of whatever cause, may be readily diagnosed radiographically.[152] The pacemaker twiddler syndrome has also occurred with abdominal implantation of pulse generators.[57] The important predisposing factor, whether the implant site is in the chest or abdominal wall, is an excessively spacious pulse generator pocket containing a pool of fluid, a seroma. Several means of preventing this complication have been discussed by Guharay et al.[57]; a synthetic fiber mesh pouch is used to closely surround the pacemaker and encourage tissue anchoring.[111]

The interface between a pacing lead and the pulse generator occurs at the connector socket in a pacemaker pack and is a weak link in pacing systems. If the connector seal fails, either fluid or tissue, or both, may enter the socket and cause current leakage with a resultant failure to pace.[25,138] A most unusual complication occurs when gas causes the uninsulated portion of the metal case of a pacemaker, which forms the anode in unipolar systems, to separate from the surrounding tissue pocket.[86] The gas is presumably generated as the result of infection. This complication might be regarded as an electrode failure but is better considered as a complication of the pacemaker pack. Air entrapment within a pulse generator pocket caused by subcutaneous emphysema as a complication of sub-

clavian venipuncture has also been described.[64]

Association with Neoplasia

Finally, neoplasia may occur in the tissues forming the pacemaker pocket. A carcinoma of the breast developed around a pulse generator[168] and a plasmacytoma, representing a manifestation of myelomatosis, arose in a pacemaker pocket.[59] Whether the presence of the pacemaker played some role in the pathogenesis of these tumors is unknown. However, given the large numbers of implanted pacemakers and the paucity of case reports of tumors arising from adjacent tissues, there is no reason to consider the association as anything more than coincidental.

Complications Related to Pacing Lead(s)

Although the pacing lead includes either one (unipolar) or two (bipolar) electrodes, it is convenient, conceptually, to separate complications into those related to the body of the lead, as distinct from the lead-pacemaker pack interface and the electrode(s). Some complications in which such distinctions blur are electrode malposition, dislodgment, and penetration, all of which might be considered lead problems. However, for this discussion, they will all be treated arbitrarily as electrode-related complications.

Fracture

During the course of a year, the heart contracts 30 to 40 million times. This, together with respiratory movement, exposes a lead to considerable stress due mainly to flexion, but also to torsion and elongation. Early lead designs involved conductors composed of numerous fine-stranded stainless steel wires. These had poor flexibility and frequently fractured. The subsequent winding of the lead into helical coils was a significant advance, with multistranded platinum tinsel wire replacing stainless steel. A further advance has been multifilar conductors made of composites of metal alloys, such as stainless steel, in a matrix of brazing material, such as silver. The composites provide very low resistance and have a flexibility more than 10 times that of earlier designs. However, some lead fractures will, no doubt, continue to occur. The handling of leads at implantation is a critical factor. Any sharp angulation results in increased stress at one point and premature fracture. Because introduction through the subclavian vein is common, the most frequent site of fracture is at the angulation point between clavicle and first rib. Leaving the introducing stilet in the lead will greatly accelerate fracture by this mechanism, sometimes producing it within a year. Lead fracture may cause intermittent or complete pacing failure. A complete break can usually be demonstrated radiographically; highly overpenetrated films are often required. More subtle losses of continuity can be discovered at autopsy by measuring the lead resistance. Lead fracture may also occur with epicardial implants and, interestingly, has been reported following multiple trauma[82]; in such cases, damage to the integrity of a pacing system may be as important as injury to a vital natural organ.

Alternatively, a lead may fail if the insulation layer, usually made of silicone rubber or polyurethane surrounding the conductor(s) is breached. In this unusual circumstance, a "short circuit" is created, with current leaking into the surrounding blood or tissue fluid instead of exiting from the electrode tip.

Polyurethane Biodegradation

Silicone rubber leads usually fail because of damage at implantation or explantation. Insulation may be cut by scalpels or ligatures or perforated by stilets, or joints may be pulled apart by forceps. Some segmented polyether polyurethane leads have failed as a result of biodegradation of the polymer. After months in the body, pits and microfissures may form in the polyurethane surface, particularly in the softer, more compliant, lower durometer grades of polyurethane. At this stage, the fissures may be only 10 to 20 μm deep; to the naked eye, the lead surface has a frosted or crazed appearance. It is when cracks extend through the full thickness of the insulation that lead failure occurs.

The basis for this biodegradation is not completely understood,[14] but it is placed in the category of a classic polymer failure mechanism known as environmental stress cracking. This requires a sensitive material, reactive chemical media, and tensile stresses.[116] The sensitive point is probably oxidation of the carbon-oxygen bond in the polyether soft segment with oxygen free radicals generated in vivo the likely oxidizing agent. Stress, built into the polymer through extrusion in tube form, definitely plays a role. Medtronic, affected by many more insulation failures than other companies, rapidly changed their manufacturing processes to reduce built in stress, when the problem was discovered in 1981.[145] While it is true that most polyurethane pacing leads have functioned without causing pacemaker failure, biodegradation places a cloud of uncertainty around use of this material, even though it is stronger and has a lower coefficient of friction than silicone; these properties are vital in making the thin, easily passed leads that have contributed so much to the clinical success of dual-chamber cardiac pacing. This problem must, and almost certainly will, be solved during the 1990s by new generations of polyurethane leads. Nevertheless, large cohorts of patients now carry affected leads. They should be examined carefully at autopsy. Scanning electron microscopy of suspicious lead surfaces will confirm the characteristic cracking, if it exists.[4]

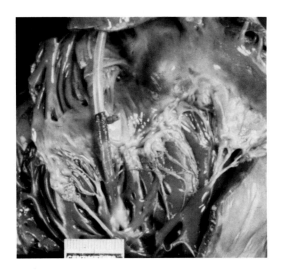

Fig. 38–13. Typical sheath of an endocardial lead shown extending back from the site of electrode contact with the endocardium of the right ventricle to the tricuspid valve apparatus to which it adheres. (Courtesy of M. D. Silver, M.D.)

Thrombosis and Thromboembolism

An endocardial pacing lead presents a foreign surface to the bloodstream. Some thrombus formation is inevitable with conventional silicone rubber lead coatings and even with the newer polyurethane ones.[146] The thrombi that form along the lead produce a sheath covering 30 to 80 percent of its length. The sheath is well formed within 12 hours[85] and then undergoes organization over several months, forming a fibrous sheath around the lead. This may extend from the site of electrode contact with the endocardium (usually at the right ventricular apex) back across the chordae tendineae and tricuspid valve, to which it may fuse, and into the right atrium,[66,123] as shown in Figure 38–13. Such lead ensheathment with adhesions to the endocardium and tricuspid valve apparatus usually causes no valve dysfunction and, in this sense, is a "normal" finding. However,

if a lead is to be removed, avulsion of part of the tricuspid valve is a possible complication.[88] Also, some cases of tricuspid valve stenosis have been reported.[87]

Major vein thrombosis and pulmonary thromboembolism may complicate endocardial pacing but are surprisingly infrequent. Subclavian vein obstruction demonstrated by venography does occur in a high proportion of patients with transvenous pacemakers,[147] but only infrequently causes symptoms.[28] The venous thrombosis may produce swelling of an arm[28,42,143] or the superior vena cava syndrome.[58,80,83,108,149,167] Pulmonary thromboemboli arising from transvenous pacing lead may lead to death.[79] However, asymptomatic pulmonary thromboembolism is more frequent.[135] The common factor in these cases appears to be congestive heart failure in the patient. It is highly questionable whether the risk of long-term anticoagulation for thousands of pacemaker patients with congestive heart failure would be outweighed by its benefit.

Infection

Infection is another major and not uncommon complication of pacing leads, whether they are endocardial or epicardial.[40] The infection may originate in the pacemaker pocket and track along the lead, which acts as a contaminated foreign body; alternatively, it may occur by implantation of bacteria on traumatized endocardium or thrombus contiguous with the lead.[15] The latter is much less common than the former, probably reflecting the organization of most pacemaker-induced endocardial lesions into dense layers of fibrous tissue with good endothelialization. In either event, the term endocarditis is appropriate and serves to emphasize the intracardiac location of the disease. Septicemia may develop,[43,130,133] and septic pulmonary emboli have occurred.[131,155] These complications are often fatal.[43,61,132,133] While an isolated infection of the pacemaker pocket may yield to conservative therapy with antibiotics and closed drainage,[52] the fundamental therapeutic principle in pacemaker-related endocarditis is removal of at least the lead and, when the pacemaker pocket is involved, the entire pacing system. Most leads can be removed by prolonged gentle traction,[10] but recourse to cardiotomy with cardiopulmonary bypass may be needed if the lead is incarcerated in fibrous tissue,[22,50,166] or if it is of such a design that it has an increased diameter, due to a flange or shoulder, near its tip. Rare cases have been reported in which the lead fragmented within the heart on traction, leaving its tip behind, or in which it came out with a large portion of avulsed right ventricular myocardium attached.[44]

Problems Particular to Epicardial Leads

Leads placed by the epicardial route are also subject to infection. The source is usually the pacemaker pocket, with the infection tracking along the lead to the myocardium producing an associated mediastinitis and the risk of bronchocutaneous fistula.[23,153] An unusual complication peculiar to epicardial leads is migration away from the original site of implantation.[159] This may occur subsequent to lead fracture or with an intact lead if its subcutaneous course is unusually slack.

Complications Related to Pacing Electrode(s)

A variety of complications are directly related to the interface between electrode and adjacent stimulatable cardiac cells. In transvenous pacing, electrode malposition or perforation through the myocardium may each result in a failure to pace, which can be fatal.

Malposition

An electrode may be malpositioned in the coronary sinus (Fig. 38–14) at insertion[100,142]; the problem will be missed on radiographs or flu-

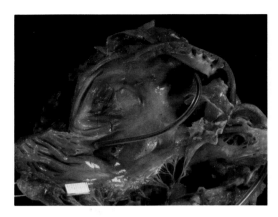

Fig. 38–14. Endocardial lead malpositioned in the coronary sinus at insertion. In this case, the electrode tip had been advanced so far that it lay in the posterior interventricular sulcus. (Courtesy of M. D. Silver, M.D.)

oroscopy performed in the frontal plane only. The result may be failure to pace due to a high stimulation threshold, which often occurs a few days to a week postimplantation. It must be appreciated, however, that a transvenous lead may be intentionally implanted in the coronary sinus for atrial pacing[56,104]; indeed, leads have been designed specifically for this purpose (see Fig. 38–10).

Dislodgment

Electrode dislodgment was once a very common complication of endocardial pacing, the prevalence varying with the technical skill of the physician implanting the lead. The availability of tined leads (see Fig. 38–7) for improved passive fixation and various positive fixation designs (see Figs. 38–4 and 38–5) has greatly reduced this complication. Projections from the body of the lead or the electrode at its tip may cause increased problems with lead incarceration. Dislodgment generally occurs within the first few days or weeks of electrode insertion. Late displacement is unusual because of fibrous tissue sheath formation around the electrode and body of the lead. Electrode dislodgment may occur as a result of either migration of the pacemaker pack or in the pacemaker twiddler syndrome. When dislocation of an electrode occurs, the tip of the lead most commonly flips into the right ventricular outflow tract or even into the pulmonary artery. Other possibilities include its looping within the body of the right ventricle or swinging back into the right atrium. If the electrode is dislodged into the superior vena cava, it may stimulate the phrenic nerve and cause diaphragmatic contractions.

Special problems with endocardial electrode dislodgment may occur in the presence of an anomalous venous return. The most common is a persistent left superior vena cava, which occurs in about 0.5 percent of the population[128] and results from failure of involution of the left cardinal vein. In this condition, the anomalous vein drains into the coronary sinus; a lead must take a tortuous course through a dilated coronary sinus into the right atrium and then loop in the atrium to cross the tricuspid valve. Thus, passage of the electrode may be very difficult[124] or impossible.[84]

Myocardial Penetration and Perforation

Perforation of the myocardium by endocardial electrodes has been discussed as an intraoperative complication. Delayed perforation can also occur, resulting from gradual penetration of electrode through the myocardium. The major predisposing factor is a stiff lead that is too long and exerts excessive pressure through the electrode tip on the underlying myocardium. With the widespread use of soft polyurethane leads this complication has become less common. In rare cases it has occurred when the metal stylet has been left in the lead at implant. Perforation can cause a failure to sense or pace, either of which can be fatal. The perforating electrode may also stimulate adjacent structures with twitching of intercostal, diaphragmatic, or abdominal muscles, and, sometimes, pain on stimulation. A pericardial friction rub may be another sign of late perforation. Hemopericardium with cardiac tamponade has not been de-

scribed in late perforation. Radiologic diagnosis of myocardial perforation is usually possible,[151] and both penetration and perforation are obvious at autopsy.

Exit Block

A much more common electrode-related complication is exit block, which is characterized by an increased chronic stimulation threshold that exceeds the maximum output capacity of the pulse generator in the absence of electrode displacement. In some cases, exit block can be readily explained by myocardial infarction with subsequent replacement fibrosis in the region of the electrode. Endocardial electrodes are usually placed in the apex of the right ventricle and positioned against the septum; thus, they are subject to this effect in a septal infarct. Another cause of fibrosis close to an electrode may be exceptionally high currents passing through the electrode. For example, if a patient is subjected to cardiac defibrillation after electrode placement, the very high defibrillation currents may be shunted through the zener diode placed at the output of the pulse generator in order to protect it from just such clinical events and pass along the lead, causing myocardial injury at the site of electrode placement.[150] Alternatively, induced currents to 160 mA and potentials to 140 V, more than 20 times the highest output of pacemakers, may be induced in pacemaker leads by electrocautery; this could be the cause of chronically elevated thresholds observed in some pacemaker patients subsequent to cardiac surgery when extensive electrocoagulation is performed.[137] Autopsy studies are needed to provide clinicopathologic correlations, to confirm these contentions.

Most cases of exit block, however, are not well explained. Increased fibrosis around the electrode tip is probably the cause, but no autopsy study has been performed to test this hypothesis.

Mechanical factors, specifically micromovements of the electrode tip, are responsible for much of the variability in occurrence of exit block. The electric stimulation from the electrode probably causes no injury, as reported in unipolar pacing in experimental animals by Contine and colleagues.[27] Bipolar endocardial pacing has a theoretically greater risk of causing myocardial injury because of the close spacing of the electrodes but in practice has not proved a problem.

Most pacemaker patients have long-term stimulation threshold stability, but about 20 percent develop a progressive increase in threshold, which, in some cases, is sufficient to produce exit block.[93] According to Conklin et al.,[26] this complication does not recur after repositioning of the electrode. Another therapeutic approach has been the use of prednisone, which has resulted in long-term decreases in threshold after discontinuation of the drug.[6] Corticosteroid elution has been incorporated into the design of both endocardial[118,122] and epicardial electrodes.[144]

CARDIAC PACING IN INFANTS AND YOUNG CHILDREN

Implantation of cardiac pacemakers in children is not frequent. Almost all cases have been for the treatment of heart block after repair of congenital heart defects or for congenital heart block with symptoms of congestive heart failure or syncope.[7,33,51,136,163,164] This group of young patients is subject to any of the complications of pacing described in the adult but, because so few children are paced, many of the complications have not yet been reported. In addition, special technical problems are related to the small size of the patient and to body growth.

In the infant, there is little space for a pacemaker pack. Innovative approaches to overcome the problem include implantation in the retroperitoneal,[91] pleural,[35] and properitoneal abdominal spaces[30] and, as smaller pacemakers have become available, within the planes of the anterior abdominal musculature.[164] Using the last approach, successful pacemaker placement has been achieved in a 2.2-kg infant. With abdominal placement, the pacing lead is brought into the thorax through a subcutaneous tunnel. The availability of smaller pacers in recent years (Fig. 38–15) has made the size problem less of an issue.

The use of epicardially placed leads in children is more popular because, historically, pacemakers were too large to safely implant in the pectoral area in most children. Silicone-coated leads were too bulky to insert easily into the cephalic vein and were considered likely to interfere with the tricuspid value. Also, transvenous lead dislodgment was more likely than in the adult because of many instances of dilated, poorly trabeculated ventricular chambers accessible from the right atrium in complex congenital heart disease. In addition, there was concern that growth of the child would place considerable traction on transvenous leads. However, in children weighing more than 15 kg and over 7 years of age transvenous pacemakers have been shown to be highly effective.[51] Pacemaker miniaturization and thinner, less stiff polyurethane-insulated pacing leads have contributed to this success. The endocardial approach offers a major advantage in that stimulation thresholds are generally lower than with epicardial leads. Also, physiologic dual-chamber pacing requiring an atrial electrode for sensing and pacing can be easily accommodated by placing two thin leads through the same vein. The postpericardiotomy syndrome is a frequent, and occasionally serious, complication of epicardial implantation; this risk is avoided with endocardial pacing. The older child often has adhesions from previous surgery which make a transthoracic approach difficult, again favoring an endocardial route. Traction of endocardial leads has not proved a major problem with growth. In the infant, however, small size continues to dictate the use of the epicardial leads, and, in many cases, the subxiphoid positioning of the pacemaker.

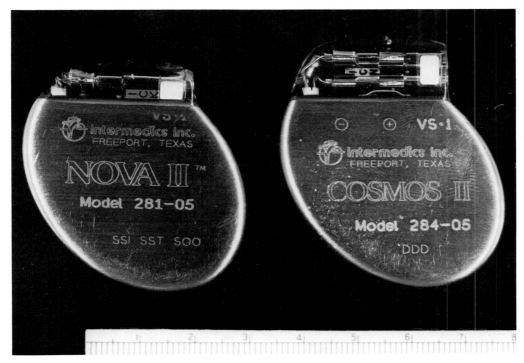

Fig. 38–15. Two examples of the very small implantable pacemakers now available from manufacturers, with one- and two-lead connectors typically for VVI and DDD pacing, respectively. Rule is marked in centimeters.

Because of the small size of pediatric patients, both skin erosion over the pacemaker pack, with infection and pacemaker extrusion, and lead fracture have been much more frequent complications than in the adult population.

EXAMINATION OF CARDIAC PACEMAKERS AT AUTOPSY

In examining cardiac pacemakers at autopsy, particularly in a case of sudden death, a pathologist must question whether a malfunction of the implanted hardware, or some host reaction to it, was responsible for death. This question may be impossible to resolve, but a detailed examination of the pacing system may provide an answer.

First, it is essential to document electrical continuity from the pulse generator through the lead(s) to the electrode tip(s). Radiographs (preferably at least two views with one at right angles to another), either taken shortly before death or prior to commencing the autopsy, can both indicate any lead fractures, and locate the position of electrodes,[151] thereby indicating the likelihood of electrode dislodgment before there is any interference with the body. If this cannot be done, it is still possible to establish electrical continuity during the autopsy.

On opening the body, special care should be exercised to not transect the lead. This is likely to occur near the entrance of the lead into the thoracic cavity, whether that is through the subclavian vein, as in most transvenous systems, or via an intercostal or perixiphoid substernal approach in a transthoracic system. The pulse generator and lead, including the electrode tip, should be exposed in situ by careful dissection. It is desirable to minimize traction or bending of the lead during this procedure. A search should be made for evidence indicating infection of the pulse generator pouch or of thrombosis along the course of the lead (in the case of transvenous placement), and appropriate photographs taken.

Often, a transvenous lead becomes included in a connective tissue sheath along the course of a vein. If thrombi are present along the lead(s), a careful search should be made for pulmonary thromboemboli and the possibility of an infection excluded. The lead(s) and pulse generator can then be separated by removing the lead terminal pin(s) from its (their) socket(s) in the pulse generator. This usually requires use of a screwdriver to loosen a set screw. The terminal pin and socket should be carefully examined for evidence of fluid intrusion, which can cause corrosion. Tissue ingrowth into the lead socket is another telltale sign of an electrode seal defect. These may be critical observations, as such fluid intrusion can form a parallel low-resistance path between cathode and anode (especially in unipolar systems) and cause loss of pacing. If the lead cannot be readily separated from the pulse generator (possibly as a result of corrosion), then it may be transected close to the body of the pulse generator. With the lead and pulse generator separated, the heart can be removed and photographs taken of the lead(s) in situ.[15] With a transvenous lead, special attention is paid to the course of the lead through the heart, the location of insertion of the electrode, and the relationship of the lead and the tricuspid valve.

After removal of the lead(s), sections are taken of unusual lesions along the course of the lead and at the site of contact of electrode and heart, the latter oriented to permit measurement of the minimum thickness of the nonstimulatable tissue (thrombus and/or fibrous tissue) separating the electrode from underlying myocytes. If there appears to be either a recent or old myocardial infarct in the vicinity of the electrode tip, more extensive sections to include this region should be taken. Examination of the conducting system may also be appropriate, but it is important to realize that many pacemakers are not inserted for complete heart block.

After its removal, the lead is tested for electrical continuity by measuring the resistance between the electrode tip and the proximal end of the lead with an ohm-meter. If the lead is bipolar (two electrodes near the distal end of the lead), the resistance of the conductor from each electrode must be determined. This must also be done if a second lead connected to the atrium is present. The measured resistance should be in the range of 5 to 50 ohms. If a lead is fractured, resistance should be too high to register on the meter. The lead should be put under tension when measuring resistance, to detect any "make/break" fracture, which is only apparent when the lead is stretched. An intermediate value can be recorded if fluid has penetrated into the conductor coil of the lead providing a high, but finite, resistance path across a fracture site.

The lead(s) should be examined with the distal portion photographed to record the appearance of the electrode, which may not be evident in situ in the heart because of buildup of thrombus or fibrous tissue (in the case of an endocardial lead) or simply because of the electrode of an epicardially placed lead was buried in the myocardium. So many electrode designs are available that specific identification as to manufacturer may be difficult. Furthermore, one cannot necessarily rely on the lead being from the same manufacturer as the pulse generator, as there is cross-compatibility of leads and pulse generators. The key features in description are the shape and size of the electrode, the absence or presence and type of devices on or about the electrode for active fixation, the presence or absence of tines for passive fixation, and the location of the electrode on the lead.

Fortunately, pulse generator identification is no problem. Unlike our colleagues in radiology, who have had to devise elaborate schemes for the radiographic identification of pulse generators, pathologists need only read the label. A more difficult task is to assess whether a pulse generator has failed. This may be attributable to a variety of causes, the most likely of which is battery depletion. Electronic component failure or phantom programming by electromagnetic interference, in the case of a programmable unit, are also possible but unlikely, given the current level of sophistication and reliability in pacemaker design. Most pathologists do not have at their disposal the electronic equipment necessary for such testing. What is required is to determine the amplitude (volts or milliamperes), duration, and repetition rate of the stimulating pulses by means of an oscilloscope with the pulse generator terminated by a 500-ohm resistor to the tissue load. Pacer manufacturers provide "pacer system analyzers"—test equipment used in the operating room at implantation—which can be used for this purpose. Some of the more sophisticated programmable pulse generators being implanted use telemetry to provide this information as well as data on internal current consumption and battery drain, and future designs can be expected to be even more sophisticated. Therefore, the most practical approach for the pathologist is to turn the unit over to an expert physician who implants pacemakers, a biomedical engineer, or the manufacturer for pulse generator testing. A pitfall in such testing used to be fluid intrusion into the epoxy case of the older generation of pacemakers with mercury/zinc batteries. With such a pacemaker, testing had to be done quickly to avoid uncertainty related to the possibility of the unit's "drying out" with resultant loss of evidence concerning the mode of failure. The modern lithium battery-powered pulse generator is hermetically sealed in a metal case, and, therefore, this problem occurs no longer.

An important limitation to testing pacemakers at autopsy remains that, if unrecognized, can result in the cause of death being incorrectly ascribed to pacemaker failure. As a body cools after death, battery voltage naturally falls somewhat particularly if the body is left in a refrigerated cold room prior to autopsy, as is normal practice in most hospitals. This can trigger an "end of battery life" indicator, in the memory of the pacemaker's microprocessor, one function of which is to monitor battery drain continuously by measuring its voltage output. Even if the body or explanted pacemaker is rewarmed the end of life indicator remains as a signal when the pulse generator is interrogated. A pathologist should not report battery failure unless battery function is directly tested on rewarming.

A practical, alternative approach to the above detailed examination in the hospital environment is to send the pulse generator and lead (preferably without separating them) to the manufacturer for examination. Manufacturers employ engineers with considerable expertise in this field, from whom an unbiased report can be expected. This approach is the most practical one for pathologists who do not have access to testing facilities. It is important to provide relevant clinical and autopsy information when pacer hardware is sent to the manufacturer and to pack it so that there is no danger of disease transmission to those who must test it but who may not have medical training, in handling the explant. At the very least, an explicit warning of danger should be placed on the package.

The presence of a nuclear-powered pulse generator posed special problems, but only in an administrative sense. Fortunately, there are almost no nuclear units in current clinical use. The electrical energy in nuclear pacers is generated by direct thermoelectric conversion from heat produced by α-emission from plutonium 238 (half-life: 86.4 years). A pathologist should contact both the local nuclear energy regulatory agency and the manufacturer to arrange for disposal of such units.

Because pacemakers are expensive and the current state of the art provides a battery life of 10 to 20 years, which may exceed the life expectancy of the elderly patients in whom most pacemakers are implanted, the reimplantation of used, refurbished pacemakers has been performed.

This practice has generated controversy—one important medicolegal issue being ownership of the pacemaker after the patient's death, another being the possible transmission of diseases between patients. A pathologist should be aware of the implications of complying with a request to remove a pacemaker for this purpose.

A pathologist may also be questioned by a mortician about disposal problems with pacemakers. It is useful to know that, on cremation, lithium batteries may explode. Interestingly, plutonium dioxide cannot be volatilized even at crematory temperatures but, in any event, special steps must be taken to retrieve any nuclear pacemakers before burial or cremation because safety in this field is such a sensitive public issue.

REFERENCES

1. Admundson D, McArthur W, MacCarter D, Mosharrafa M: Porous electrode-tissue interface. In Meere C (ed): Proceedings of the Sixth World Symposium on Cardiac Pacing, Montreal. Laplante and Langevin, Montreal, 1979
2. Admundson DC, McArthur W, Mosharrafa M: The porous endocardial electrode. PACE 2:40, 1979
3. Anderson ST, Pitt A, Whitford JA, Davis BB: Interference with function of unipolar pacemaker due to muscle potentials. J Thorac Cardiovasc Surg 71:698, 1976
4. Barbaro V, Bosi C, Caiazza S, et al: Implant effects on polyurethane and silicone cardiac pacing leads in humans: Insulation measurements and SEM observations. Biomaterials 6:28, 1985
5. Bayliss CE, Beanlands DS, Baird RJ: The pacemaker-twiddler's syndrome: A new complication of implantable transvenous pacemakers. Can Med Assoc J 99:371, 1968
6. Beanlands DS, Akyurekli Y, Keon WJ: Prednisone in the management of exit block. In Meere C (ed): Proceedings of the Sixth World Symposium on Cardiac Pacing, Montreal. Laplante and Langevin, Montreal, 1979
7. Beder SD, Hanisch DG, Cohen MH, et al: Cardiac pacing in children: A 15-year experience. Am Heart J 109:152, 1985
8. Bello A, Gilles Yepez CG, Barcelo JE: Retroperitoneal migration of a pacemaker generator: An unusual complication. J Cardiovasc Surg 15:256, 1974
9. Benchimol A, Ellis JG, Dimond EG: Hemodynamic consequences of atrial and ventricular pacing in patients with normal and abnormal hearts. Am J Med 39:911, 1965
10. Bilgutay AM, Jensen NK, Schmidt WR, et al: Incarceration of transvenous pacemaker electrode. Removal by traction. Am Heart J 77:377, 1969
11. Bleifeld W, Irnich W, Effert S: A new transvenous electrode with myocardial fixation for permanent pacing. Med Biol Eng 10:643, 1972
12. Brenner JI, Gaines S, Cordier J, et al: Cardiac strangulation: Two dimensional echo recognition of a rare complication of epicardial pacemaker therapy. Am J Cardiol 61:654, 1988
13. Brooks C, Mutter M: Pacemaker failure associated with therapeutic radiation. Am J Emerg Med 6:591, 1988
14. Bruck SD, Mueller EP: Materials aspects of implantable cardiac pacemaker leads. Med Prog Technol 13:149, 1988
15. Bryan CS, Sutton JP, Saunders DE, et al: Endocarditis related to transvenous pacemakers: Syndromes and surgical implications. J Thorac Cardiovasc Surg 75:758, 1978
16. Callaghan JC, Bigelow WG: An electrical artificial pacemaker for stand-still of the heart. Ann Surg 134:8, 1951
17. Cameron JR, Chisholme AW, Froggart GM, Harrison AW: "Phantom" programming. In Meere C (ed): Proceedings of the Sixth World Symposium on Cardiac Pacing. Montreal, 1979
18. Chandra MS, Patel MR, Laughlin DE, Rossie NP: False inhibition of demand pacemaker due to leakage of fluid into the pacemaker lead socket. J Thorac Cardiovasc Surg 75:765, 1975

19. Chardack WM, Gage AA, Greatbatch W: A transistorized self-contained implantable pacemaker for long-term correction of complete heart block. Surgery 48:643, 1960

20. Chardack WM, Ishikawa H, Fochler FJ, et al: Pacing and ventricular fibrillation. Ann NY Acad Sci 167:919, 1969

21. Charles R, Turner WL: Diarrhea induced by migration of a pacemaker generator. Br Heart J 40:425, 1978

22. Chavez CM, Conn JH: Septicemia secondary to impacted infected pacemaker wire: Successful treatment by removal with cardiopulmonary bypass. J Thorac Cardiovasc Surg 73:796, 1977

23. Chua FS, Leininger BJ, Hamouda AA, Pifarre RF: Bronchopleural cutaneous fistula from infected pacemaker electrodes. Chest 63:284, 1973

24. Cohen SI, Smith CK: Transfemoral cardiac pacing and phlebitis. Circulation 49:1018, 1974

25. Cohn JD, Santhanam R, Rosenblood MA, Thorson RF: Delayed pacemaker erosion due to electrode seal defects. Ann Thorac Surg 28:445, 1979

26. Conklin EF, Gianelli S Jr, Nealon TF Jr: Four hundred consecutive patients with permanent cardiac pacemakers. J Thorac Cardiovasc Surg 65:315, 1973

27. Contini C, Papi Pesola A, et al: Tissue reaction to intracavitary electrodes: Effect on duration and efficiency of unipolar pacing in patients with A-V block. J Cardiovasc Surg 14:282, 1973

28. Crook BRM, Gishen P, Robinson CR, Oram S: Occlusion of the subclavian vein associated with cephalic vein pacemaker electrodes. Br J Surg 64:329, 1977

29. Cueni T, Shenase M, Kappenberger L, Sowton E: The effect of electromagnetic interference from antitheft devices upon demand pacemakers. In Meere C (ed): Proceedings of the Sixth World Symposium on Cardiac Pacing. Montreal. Laplante and Langevin, Montreal, 1979

30. Donahoo JS, Haller JA, Zonnebelts S, et al: Permanent cardiac pacemakers in children. Technical considerations. Ann Thorac Surg 22:584, 1976

31. El Gamal M, Van Gelder B: Preliminary experience with the Helifix electrode for trans-venous atrial implantation. PACE 2:444, 1979

32. Epstein AE, Kay N, Plumb VJ, et al: Combined automatic implantable cardioverter-defibrillator and pacemaker systems: Implantation techniques and follow-up. J Am Coll Cardiol 13:121, 1989

33. Epstein ML, Knauf DG, Alexander JA: Long-term follow-up of transvenous cardiac pacing in children. Am J Cardiol 57:889, 1986

34. Erlebacher JA, Cahill PT, Pannizzo F, Knowles RJ: Effect of magnetic resonance imaging on DDD pacemakers. Am J Cardiol 57:437, 1986

35. Escano FB Jr, Berroya RB, Gianfrancesco H, et al: Intrapleural pacemaker generator in children. J Thorac Cardiovasc Surg 62:454, 1971

36. Escher DJW, Furman S, Solomon N: Transvenous emergency cardiac pacing. Ann NY Acad Sci 167:582, 1969

37. Falkoff M, Heinle RA, Ong LS, Barold SS: Inapparent double puncture of the femoral artery and vein: An important complication of temporary cardiac pacing by the transfemoral approach. PACE 1:49, 1978

38. Fetter J, Aram G, Holmes, DR, et al: The effects of nuclear magnetic resonance imagers on external and implantable pulse generators. PACE 7:720, 1984

39. Fieldman A, Dobrow RJ: Phantom pacemaker programming. PACE 1:166, 1978

40. Firor WB, Lopez JF, Manson EM, Mori M: Clinical management of infected pacemaker. Ann Thorac Surg 6:431, 1968

41. Fort ML, Sharp JT: Perforation of the right ventricle by pacing catheter electrode. Am J Cardiol 16:610, 1965

42. Friedman SA, Berger N, Carruti MM, Kosmoski J: Venous thrombosis and permanent cardiac pacing. Am Heart J 85:531, 1973

43. Furman S: Complications of pacemaker therapy for heart block. Am J Cardiol 17:439, 1966

44. Furman S: Removal of myocardial fragment containing a pacemaker electrode. Ann Thorac Surg 19:716, 1975

45. Furman S, Hurzeler, P, DeCaprio V: Cardiac pacing and pacemakers. III. Sensing the cardiac electrogram. Am Heart J 93:794, 1977

46. Furman S, Hurzeler P, Mehra R: Cardiac pacing and pacemakers. IV. Threshold of cardiac stimulation. Am Heart J 94:115, 1977

47. Furman S, Schwedel JB: An intracardiac

pacemaker for Stokes-Adams seizures. N Engl J Med 261:943, 1959

48. Furman S, Schwedel JB, Robinson G, Hurwitt ES: Use of an intracardiac pacemaker in control of heart block. Surgery 49:98, 1961

49. Gabry MD, Brodman R, Johnston D, et al: Automatic implantable cardioverter-defibrillator: Patient survival, battery longevity and shock delivery analysis. J Am Coll Cardiol 9:1349, 1987

50. Garcia R, Hakimi-Naini M: Bacterial endocarditis and incarceration of a transvenous pacemaker: Removal under cardiopulmonary by-pass after prolonged traction proved ineffective. Henry Ford Hosp Med J 23:135, 1975

51. Gillette PC, Shannon C, Blair H, et al: Transvenous pacing in pediatric patients. Am Heart J 105:843, 1983

52. Golden JT, Lovett WL, Harah JD, et al: The treatment of extruded and infected permanent cardiac pulse generators: Complication of a technique of closed irrigation. Surgery 74:575, 1973

53. Goswami M, Gould L, Gomprecht RF, Imperiale A: Perforation of the heart by flexible transvenous pacemaker. JAMA 216:2013, 1971

54. Gould L, Ramana Reddy CV, Yacob U, et al: Perforation of the tricuspid valve by a transvenous pacemaker. JAMA 230:86, 1974

55. Graboys TB, Lown B, Podrid PJ, DeSilva R: Long term survival of patients with malignant ventricular arrhythmias treated with antiarrhythmic drugs. Am J Cardiol 50:437, 1982

56. Greenberg P, Castellanet M, Messenger J, Ellestad MH: Coronary sinus pacing: Clinical follow-up. Circulation 57:98, 1978

57. Guharay BN, Gohse JC, Majum dar H, Basu AK: The pacemaker twiddler's syndrome: Another disadvantage of abdominal implantation of pulse generators. Br J Surg 64:655, 1977

58. Gundersen T, Abrahamson AM, Jorgensen I: Thrombosis of superior vena cava as a complication of transvenous pacemaker treatment. Acta Med Scand 212:85, 1982

59. Hamaker WR, Lindell ME, Gomez AC: Plasmacytoma arising in a pacemaker pocket. Ann Thorac Surg 21:354, 1976

60. Hamer A, Vohra J, Hunt D, Sloman G: Prediction of sudden death by electrophysiological studies in high risk patients surviving acute myocardial infarction. Am J Cardiol 50:223, 1982

61. Harris A, Redwood D, Davis M, Davis G: Causes of death in patients with complete heart block and artificial pacemakers. Br Heart J 30:495, 1969

62. Hartzler GD, Maloney JD, Curtis JJ, Barnhorst DA: Hemodynamic benefits of atrioventricular sequential pacing after cardiac surgery. Am J Cardiol 40:232, 1977

63. Hayes DL, Holmes DR Jr, Gray JE: Effect of 1.5 tesla nuclear magnetic resonance imaging scanner on implanted permanent pacemakers. J Am Coll Cardiol 10:782, 1987

64. Hearne SF, Maloney D: Pacemaker system failure secondary to air entrapment within the pulse generator pocket—A complication of subclavian venipuncture for lead placement. Chest 82:651, 1982

65. Holmes DR, Nissen RG, Maloney JD, et al: Transvenous tined electrode systems: An approach to acute dislodgement. Mayo Clin Proc 54:219, 1979

66. Huang TY, Baba N: Cardiac pathology of transvenous pacemakers. Am Heart J 83:469, 1972

67. Hurwitz BJ, Zion MM, Promud Obel IW: Myocardial perforation by flexible Elema endocardial pacing catheters. Thorax 29:678, 1974

68. Hyman AS: Resuscitation of the stopped heart by intracardiac therapy. Arch Intern Med 50:283, 1932

69. Irnich W: Interference with pacemakers. PACE 7:1021, 1984

70. Irnich W: Engineering concepts of pacemaker electrodes. p. 241. In Schaldach M, Furman S (eds): Advances in Pacemaker Technology. Springer-Verlag, New York, 1975

71. Irnich W, de Bakker JMT, Bisping HJ: Electromagnetic interference in implantable pacemakers. PACE 1:52, 1978

72. James TN: Air embolism. Am Heart J 61:423, 1966

73. Jara FM, Toled-Pereyra MD, Lewis JW Jr, Magilligan DJ Jr: The infected pacemaker pocket. J Thorac Cardiovasc Surg 78:298, 1979

74. Jensen NK, Schmidt WR, Garavella JJ, Lynch MF, Peterson CA: Intracavitary cardiac pacing. JAMA 195:916, 1966

75. Kalloor GJ: Cardiac tamponade: Report after insertion of a transvenous endocardial electrode. Am Heart J 88:88, 1974

76. Kastor JA: Michel Mirowski and the automatic implantable defibrillator. Am J Cardiol 63:1121, 1989

77. Kelly PA, Cannom DS, Garan H, et al: The automatic implantable cardioverter-defibrillator: Efficacy, complications and survival in patients with malignant ventricular arrhythmias. J Am Coll Cardiol 11:1278, 1988

78. Kim GE, Haverson S, Imparato AM: Late displacement of cardiac pacemaker electrode due to heavy weight pulse generator. JAMA 228:74, 1974

79. Kinney EL, Allen RP, Weidner WA, et al: Recurrent pulmonary emboli secondary to right atrial thrombus around a permanent pacing catheter: A case report and review of the literature. PACE 2:196, 1979

80. Koike R, Sasaki M, Kuroda K: Total venous obstruction—A possible complication of transvenous dual-chamber pacing. Jpn Circ J 52:1293, 1988

81. Kosowsky BD, Barr J: Complications and malfunctions of electrical cardiac pacemakers. Prog Cardiovasc Dis 14:501, 1972

82. Kromzon I, Mehta SS: Broken pacemaker wire in multiple trauma: A case report. J Trauma 14:82, 1974

83. Krug H, Zerbe F: Major venous thrombosis: A complication of transvenous pacemaker electrodes. Br Heart J 44:158, 1980

84. Kukral JC: Transvenous pacemaker failure due to anomalous venous return to the heart. Chest 59:458, 1971

85. Lagergren H, Dahlgren S, Nordenstam H: Cardiovascular tissue response to intracardiac pacing. Acta Chir Scand 132:696, 1966

86. Lasala AF, Fieldman A, Diana DJ, Humphrey CB: Gas pocket causing pacemaker malfunction. PACE 2:183, 1979

87. Lee ME, Chaux A: Unusual complications of endocardial pacing. J Thorac Cardiovasc Surg 80:934, 1980

88. Lee ME, Chau A, Matloff JM: Avulsion of a tricuspid valve leaflet during traction on an infected, entrapped endocardial pacemaker electrode. J Thorac Cardiovasc Surg 74:433, 1977

89. Lee RW, Huang SK, Mechling E, Bazgan I: Runaway atrioventricular sequential pace-

90. maker after radiation therapy. Am J Med 81:883, 1986

90. Lewin AA, Serago CF, Schwade JG, et al: Radiation induced failures of complementary metal oxide semiconductor containing pacemakers: A potentially lethal complication. Int J Radiat Oncol Biol Phys 10:1967, 1984

91. Lindesmith GG, Stiles QR, Meyer BW, et al: Experience with an implantable synchronous pacemaker in children. Ann Thorac Surg 6:358, 1968

92. Loffler S, Kasper J, Postulka J, et al: Septic complications in patients with permanent pacemakers. Cor Vasa 30:400, 1988

93. Luceri RM, Furman S, Hurzeler P, Escher DJW: Threshold behaviour in long-term ventricular pacing. Circulation 54(suppl II):32, 1976

94. MacGregor DC, Wilson GJ, Dutcher RG, et al: A new positive fixation endocardial pacemaker lead using an extendable/retractable helix. In Meere C, (ed): Proceedings of the Sixth World Symposium on Cardiac Pacing, Montreal. Laplante and Langevin, Montreal, 1979

95. MacGregor DC, Wilson GJ, Lixfeld W, et al: The porous-surfaced electrode: A new concept in pacemaker lead design. J Thorac Cardiovasc Surg 78:281, 1979

96. Matern WE, Jaffe MS, Towbin R: Unusual complication from a cardiac pacemaker. JAMA 238:969, 1977

97. Meere D, Lesperance J: Surgical techniques in cardiac pacing. p. 127. In Thalen HJ, Meere C (eds): Developments in Cardiovascular Medicine. Vol. 3: Fundamentals of Cardiac Pacing. Martinus Nijhoff, Boston, 1979

98. Mehra R, Furman S: A comparison of cathodal, anodal and bipolar strength-interval curves with temporary and permanent electrodes. Br Heart J 41:468, 1979

99. Meyer JA, Miller K: Perforation of the right ventricle by electrode catheters. A review and report of nine cases. Ann Surg 168:1048, 1968

100. Meyer JA, Miller K: Malplacement of pacemaker catheters in the coronary sinus. J Thorac Cardiovasc Surg 57:511, 1969

101. Mickley H, Andersen C, Nielsen LH: Runaway pacemaker: A still existing complication and therapeutic guidelines. Clin Cardiol 12:412, 1989

102. Mindt W, Schaldach M: Electrochemical as-

pects of pacing electrodes. p. 297. In Schaldach M, Furman S (eds): Advances in Pacemaker Technology. Springer-Verlag, New York, 1975

103. Mond HG, Stuckey JG, Sloman G: The diagnosis of right ventricular perforation by an endocardial pacemaker electrode. PACE 1:62, 1978

104. Moss AJ, Rivers RJ Jr: Atrial pacing from the coronary vein: Ten-year experience in 50 patients with implanted pervenous pacemakers. Circulation 57:103, 1978

105. Mullen DC, Porter JM, Thompson HK, Silver D: Cardiac tamponade from ventricular perforation by a transvenous pacemaker. JAMA 203:164, 1968

106. Mymin D, Cuddy TE, Sinha SN, Winer DA: Inhibition of demand pacemakers by skeletal muscle potentials. JAMA 223:527, 1973

107. Nasrallah A, Hall RJ, Garcia E, et al: Runaway pacemaker in seven patients: A persisting problem. J Thorac Cardiovasc Surg 69:365, 1975

108. Nicolosi GL, Charmet PA, Zanuttini D: Large right atrial thrombosis. Rare complication during permanent transvenous endocardial pacing. Br Heart J 43:199, 1980

109. Odabashian HC, Brown DF: "Runaway" in a modern generation pacemaker. PACE 2:152, 1979

110. Ohm OJ, Bruland H, Pedersen OM, and Waerness E: Interference effect of myopotentials and function of unipolar demand pacemakers. Br Heart J 36:77, 1974

111. Parsonnet V: A stretch fabric pouch for implanted pacemakers. Arch Surg 105:654, 1972

112. Parsonnet V: Cardiac pacing and pacemakers. VII. Power sources for implantable pacemakers. Am Heart J 94:517(pt 1), 658(pt 2), 1977

113. Paull DL, Fellows CL, Guyton SW, Anderson RP: Early experience with the automatic implantable cardioverter defibrillator in sudden death survivors. Am J Surg 157:516, 1989

114. Peters RW, Scheinman MM, Raskin S, Thomas AN: Unusual complications of epicardial pacemakers: Recurrent pericarditis, cardiac tamponade and pericardial constriction. Am J Cardiol 45:1088, 1980

115. Petterson SR, Small JB, Reeves G, Kocot SL: Tricuspid valve perforation by endocardial pacing electrode. Chest 63:125, 1973

116. Phillips R, Frey M, Martin RO: Long-term performance of polyurethane pacing leads: Mechanisms of design-related failures. PACE 9:1166, 1986

117. Piller LW, Kennelly BM: Myopotential inhibition of demand pacemakers. Chest 66:418, 1974

118. Pirzada FA, Moschitto LJ, Diorio D: Clinical experience with steroid-eluting unipolar electrodes. PACE 11:1739, 1988

119. Platia EV, Griffith LSC, Watkins L Jr, et al: Treatment of malignant ventricular arrhythmias with endocardial resection and implantation of the automatic cardioverter-defibrillator. N Engl J Med 314:213, 1986

120. Preston TA: Anodal stimulation as a cause of pacemaker-induced ventricular fibrillation. Am Heart J 86:366, 1973

121. Preston TA, Fletcher RD, Lucchesi BR, Judge RD: Changes in myocardial threshold: Physiologic and pharmacologic factors in patients with implanted pacemakers. Am Heart J 74:235, 1967

122. Radovsky AS, Van Vleet JF, Stokes KB, Taker WA Jr: Paired comparisons of steroid-eluting and nonsteroid endocardial pacemaker leads in dogs: Electrical performance and morphologic alterations. PACE 11:1085, 1988

123. Robboy S, Hawthorne JW, Leinbach RC, et al: Autopsy findings with permanent pervenous pacemakers. Circulation 39:495, 1969

124. Rose ME, Ludwig G, Protos A: Transvenous pacemaker implantation by way of an anomalous left superior vena cava. J Thorac Cardiovasc Surg 62:965, 1971

125. Rotem CE, Greig MB, Walters MB: Air embolism to the pulmonary artery during insertion of a transvenous endocardial pacemaker. J Thorac Cardiovasc Surg 53:562, 1967

126. Roy OZ: The current status of cardiac pacing. CRC Crit Rev Bioeng 2:259, 1975

127. Rubenfire M, Anbe DT, Drake EH, Ormond RS: Clinical evaluation of myocardial perforation as a complication of permanent transvenous pacemakers. Chest 63:185, 1973

128. Rubenfire M, Evangelista J, Wajszezuk WJ: Implication of a persistent left superior vena cava in transvenous pacemaker therapy and cardiac hemodynamic monitoring. Chest 65:145, 1973

129. Ruiter JH, Degener JE, Van Mechelen R, Bos R: Late pululent pacemaker pocket in-

fection caused by staphylococcus epidermidis: Serious complications of in situ management. PACE 8:903, 1985

130. Schaldach M: New pacemaker electrodes. Trans Am Soc Artif Int Organs 29:29, 1971

131. Schatz JW, Wiener L, Brest AN: Pacemaker "nonsense." Am Heart J 90:677, 1975

132. Schwartz IS, Pervez N: Bacterial endocarditis associated with a permanent transvenous cardiac pacemaker. JAMA 218:736, 1971

133. Schwartzel EL, Crastnopol P, Hamby RI: Catheter extrusion with infection complicating permanent endocardial pacing. Dis Chest 54:28, 1968

134. Sedaghart A: Permanent transvenous pacemaker infection with septicemia. NY State J Med 74:868, 1974

135. Seeger W, Scherer K: Asymptomatic pulmonary embolism following pacemaker implantation. PACE 9:196, 1986

136. Serwer GA, Mericle JM, Armstrong BE: Epicardial ventricular pacing electrode longevity in children. Am J Cardiol 61:104, 1988

137. Shepard RB, Russo AG, Breland VC: Radiofrequency electro-coagulator hemostasis and chronically elevated pacing thresholds in cardiopulmonary bypass patients. In Meere C (ed): Proceedings of the Sixth World Symposium on Cardiac Pacing. Montreal. Laplante and Langevin, Montreal, 1979

138. Sheridan DJ, Reid DS, Williams DO, Gold RG: Mechanical failure causing current leakage with unipolar pacemakers: Significance and detection. Eur J Cardiol 8:1, 1978

139. Siddons H, Nowak K: Surgical complications of implanting pacemakers. Br J Surg 62:929, 1975

140. Singer I, Hutchins GM, Mirowski M, et al: Pathological findings related to the lead system and repeated defibrillations in patients with the automatic implantable cardioverter-defibrillator. J Am Coll Cardiol 10:382, 1987

141. Snell RC, Luchsinger PC, Shugol GG: The relationship between the timing of atrial systole and the useful work in the left ventricle in man. Am Heart J 72:653, 1966

142. Spitzberg JW, Milstoc M, Wertheim AR: An unusual site of ventricular pacing occurring during the use of a transvenous catheter pacemaker. Am Heart J 77:529, 1969

143. Stewart S, Cohen J, Murphy G: Sutureless

epicardial pacemaker lead: A satisfactory preliminary experience. Chest 67:564, 1975

144. Stokes KB: Preliminary studies on a new steroid eluting epicardial electrode. PACE 11:1797, 1988

145. Stokes KB, Church T: Ten-year experience with implanted polyurethane lead insulation. PACE 9:1160, 1986

146. Stokes K, Cobian K, Lathrop T: Polyurethane insulators, a design approach to small pacing leads. In Meere C (ed): Proceedings of the Sixth World Symposium on Cardiac Pacing, Montreal. Laplante and Langevin, Montreal, 1979

147. Stoney WS, Addlestone RB, Alford WC Jr, et al: The incidence of venous thrombosis following long-term transvenous pacing. Ann Thorac Surg 22:166, 1976

148. Swerdlow CD, Winkle RA, Mason JW: Determinants of survival in patients with ventricular tachyarrhythmias. N Engl J Med 308:1436, 1983

149. Szuman J, Lorkiewicz Z: Superior vena caval stenosis: A rare complication in permanent transvenous cardiac pacing. J Cardiovasc Surg 26:79, 1985

150. Taube MA, Elsberry DD, Exworthy KW: Physiological effects of DC fibrillation on pacemaker function. In Meere C (ed): Proceedings of the Sixth World Symposium on Cardiac Pacing. Montreal. Laplante and Langevin, Montreal, 1979

151. Tegtmeyer CJ: Roentgenographic assessment of causes of cardiac pacemaker failure and complications. CRC Crit Rev Diagn Imag 3:1, 1977

152. Tegtmeyer CJ, Deigman JM: The cardiac pacemaker: A different twist. AJR 228:1017, 1976

153. Tegtmeyer CJ, Hunter JG Jr, Keates TE: Bronchocutaneous fistula as late complication of permanent epicardial pacing. AJR 121:614, 1974

154. Thadani U, Pratt AE: Profunda femoral arteriovenous fistula after percutaneous atrial and venous catheterization. Br Heart J 33:803, 1971

155. Upton JE: New pacing lead conductors. In Meere C (ed): Proceedings of the Sixth World Symposium on Cardiac Pacing. Montreal. Laplante and Langevin, Montreal, 1979

156. Vecht RJ, Fontaine CJ, Bradfield JWB: Fatal

outcome arising from the use of a sutureless "corkscrew" epicardial pacing electrode inserted into apex of left ventricle. Br Heart J 38:1359, 1976

157. Venselaar JL, Van Kerkoerle HL, Vet AJ: Radiation damage to pacemakers from radiotherapy. PACE 10:538, 1987

158. Walker WJ: Serum potassium levels and myocardial threshold of excitability. JAMA 228:1638, 1974

159. Watnick M, Hooshmand I, Spindola-France H: Migration of epicardial pacemaker leads. Clin Radiol 26:483, 1975

160. Weirick WI, Gott VL, Lillihei W: The treatment of complete heart block by the combined use of a myocardial electrode and an artificial pacemaker. Surg Forum 8:360, 1957

161. Weiss D, Lorber A: Pacemaker twiddler's syndrome. Int J Cardiol 15:357, 1987

162. Wheelis RF, Cobb LA: Pathologic findings in perforation of the myocardium by a permanent endocardial electrode. JAMA 210:1278, 1969

163. Williams WG, Hesslein PS, Kormos R: Exit block in children with pacemakers. Clin Prog Electrophys Pacing 4:478, 1986

164. Williams WG, Izukawa T, Olley PM, et al: Permanent cardiac pacing in infants and children. PACE 1:439, 1978

165. Wilson GJ, MacGregor DC, Bobyn JD, et al: Tissue response to porous-surfaced electrodes: Basis for a new atrial lead design. In Meere C (ed): Proceedings of the Sixth World Symposium on Cardiac Pacing, Montreal. Laplante and Langevin, Montreal, 1979

166. Yarnoz MD, Attai LA, Furman S: Infection of pacemaker electrode and removal with cardiopulmonary bypass. J Thorac Cardiovasc Surg 68:43, 1974

167. Yongson GG, McKenzie FN, Nichol PM: Superior vena cava syndrome: Case report. A complication of permanent transvenous endocardial cardiac pacing requiring surgical correction. Am Heart J 99:503, 1980

168. Zafiracopoulos P: Breast cancer at site of implantation of pacemaker generator. Lancet 1:1114, 1974

169. Zeft HJ, Harley A, Whalen RE, McIntosh HD: Pulmonary air embolism during insertion of a permanent transvenous cardiac pacemaker. Circulation 36:456, 1967

170. Zoll PM: Resuscitation of the heart in ventricular standstill by external electrical stimulation. N Engl J Med 247:768, 1952

39

Role of Endomyocardial Biopsy in Diagnosis and Treatment of Heart Disease

Margaret E. Billingham

Biopsies of the kidney, liver, and bone marrow are routinely performed in clinical medicine. Endomyocardial biopsy has also now become a routine diagnostic procedure in many medical centers around the world.[36,42,45,46,59,61,83,87,90] This chapter reviews the role of endomyocardial biopsy in the diagnosis and treatment of heart disease.

Published techniques for obtaining myocardial biopsies have include transthoracic needle biopsy of the left ventricle using Menghini or Vim-Silverman needles, catheter needle biopsy of the interventricular septum, and open thoracotomy.[6,66,67,82,86,90] The morbidity and mortality associated with these methods have precluded their widespread acceptance. In 1962, a technique for obtaining transvenous endomyocardial biopsies with a catheter bioptome was first described by Konno and Sakakibara.[46,75,76] After some initial resistance, the potential of the endomyocardial biopsy was realized, and several groups began to describe their experiences using this intravenous method of myocardial

biopsy. Reports of several modifications of the original bioptome also emerged. Among them were the Caves-Shultz-Stanford bioptome,[26,28–30] the modified Olympus bioptome,[2] the King's endomyocardial bioptome, and, more recently,[68–70,72] the Cordis M bioptome. The experience with these individual bioptomes and descriptions of the various techniques have been reported by the different groups.

The predominant experience of endomyocardial biopsies in North America has involved the use of a new instrument and a new technique for obtaining the biopsies. In 1972, at Stanford University Medical School in California, Philip Caves developed a new transvenous catheter biopsy forceps,[28,30] shorter and more flexible than the original Konno catheter. More important, he designed a new technique for serial percutaneous transvenous biopsy of the right ventricle in humans via the right internal jugular vein. This method, which has been reported previously,[28,30] has the advantage of a percutaneous method of insertion through a catheter sheath following local anesthesia only, eliminating any need for venous cutdown, ligation, and sutures. This approach can be performed safely on an outpatient basis and is readily accepted by patients; in one case, 32 serial biopsies were performed on a patient.

For the first time, the endomyocardial biopsy has made possible the earliest morphologic detection of cardiac disease in the living patient, allowed the evolution of the disease to be followed, and documented its reversal morphologically following a course of treatment.

ENDOMYOCARDIAL BIOPSY SAFETY

At Stanford, since 1973, more than 10,000 endomyocardial biopsies have been performed with no deaths and with less morbidity than that accompanying liver and renal biopsies.[51] The most serious complication is cardiac perforation, which at Stanford has occurred five times in 10,000 biopsies; however, all five patients made uneventful recoveries without major surgery. Other complications include right pneumothorax, transient paralysis of the right recurrent laryngeal nerve, Horner's syndrome, and refractory atrial arrhythmias.[53] Most groups have also reported a safe record using endomyocardial bioptomes.[36,60,61,81,83] Some groups,[43] in the light of their own experience, have cautioned that ventricular biopsies are potentially dangerous and may cause complications when performed during the final stages of disease. Peter and colleagues[63] described postpericardiotomy syndrome, and Brooksby et al.[24] described cardiac perforations. When considering endomyocardial biopsy, the potential benefit to the patient should therefore be weighed against possible complications.

TISSUE HANDLING AND PRESERVATION

To obtain reliable results with the endomyocardial biopsy, the tissue should be handled very carefully so as to minimize artifacts. The myocardial fragment should be picked up with a needle point; even fine forceps can cause artifactual damage to the tissue. Although biopsies may be divided by a single stroke of a sharp blade, this also causes crush artifacts and should be avoided. Because the biopsy specimen is so small (usually not more than 2 to 3 mm, depending on the type of bioptome used), contraction artifact is one of the biggest nuisances. Contraction can be avoided in two ways:

1. The tissue fragment can be placed immediately in glutaraldehyde or formalin at room temperature rather than in an ice-cold solution (which seems to accentuate contraction).
2. The tissue fragment can be left on a piece of gauze dampened with normal saline for 10 minutes before fixing. This will ensure relaxation of the myocardium to the point of I-band formation, but it may also cause early mitochondrial change.

In any case, contraction of the myocardial fragment should not be interpreted as a feature of ischemia in endomyocardial biopsies, as it is also seen in endomyocardial biopsies of normal, young, disease-free hearts from patients who have become organ donors[1] (Fig. 39–1).

For light microscopic examination, the endomyocardial biopsy tissue should be fixed in 10-percent phosphate buffered formalin and processed in the usual way. All endomyocardial biopsies should be stained with hematoxylin and eosin (H&E) and with Masson's trichrome stain. Masson's trichrome better reveals fibrous tissue, myocyte morphology, and early myocytolysis and ischemia. Appropriate special stains should be used for indi-

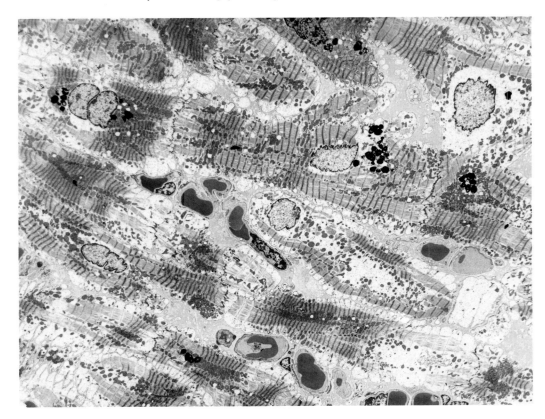

Fig. 39–1. Electron micrograph of a normal human heart (adolescent accident victim) obtained by endomyocardial biopsy. Note numerous myofibrillar contraction bands without evidence of ischemia. (× 1,600.)

vidually suspected diseases—for example, Perl's iron stain for hemochromatosis and Congo red or thioflavine T for amyloidosis. Methyl green pyronin stain is useful in certain circumstances, such as acute rejection.

For electron microscopy the endomyocardial biopsies should be fixed in buffered 2.5-percent glutaraldehyde and 2-percent paraformaldehyde solution and embedded in Epon or Marglas for thin sectioning. Whether to use uranyl acetate en bloc staining is a matter of personal preference, but it should not be used when it is necessary to show intracellular glycogen. Thick sections (0.5 to 1.0 μm thick) stained with toluidine blue provide excellent diagnostic information; at least 5 to

10 such blocks should be screened carefully for every diagnostic endomyocardial biopsy. In the case of biopsies for anthracycline toxicity grading, it is mandatory to screen not less than 10 blocks.

Endomyocardial biopsies can also be "snap frozen" in liquid nitrogen or isopentane (2-methylbutane) and dry ice for histochemical and immunofluorescent studies. It is convenient to freeze these minute biopsies by placing them in a plastic Beem capsule (the type used for plastic embedding for electron microscopy) filled with an embedding medium for frozen tissue specimens, closing the lid firmly, and plunging the whole capsule into the freezing mixture. Once labeled, the tissue can be stored indefinitely at −70°C. Frozen tissue is also required for immunohistochemical studies and in situ hybridization for the detection of cytomegalovirus or other viruses.

Whenever myocarditis is suspected clinically, or there is a history from the patient of a recent flulike syndrome, another fragment of the biopsy can be placed in a vial of Earle's or other suitable medium for viral culture, although success with this technique has been limited.

ENDOMYOCARDIAL BIOPSY TISSUE INTERPRETATION

The extent to which an accurate diagnosis can be made on the basis of endomyocardial biopsy is variable. Pieces from at least three different biopsy sites should be examined to ensure as representative a study as possible. In many cases, light microscopic evaluation is sufficient for diagnosis; in others, ultrastructural examination is necessary. Ultrastructural interpretation relies heavily on the pathologist's experience and the availability of control human endomyocardial biopsies for comparison. In most medical centers, control biopsies can be obtained during open heart surgery on certain congenital heart anomalies, but it is preferable to have controls obtained from the healthy hearts of young accident victims who have become organ donors. In many patients a definite diagnosis cannot be made from the endomyocardial biopsy, but it is often useful to the clinician if a statement can be made to rule out a suspected disease such as myocarditis, or to substantiate a suspected clinical diagnosis by a statement that the diagnosis is "consistent with but not necessarily diagnostic of . . ." the disease in question— for example, congestive cardiomyopathy. Following treatment for a particular disease entity such as myocarditis or acute cardiac rejection, a repeat endomyocardial biopsy will help by establishing ongoing active disease or reversal to normal after treatment. In our experience, clinicians often seek confirmation of an already clinically suspected cardiac condition as there are well-known clinical lookalikes; for example, cardiomyopathy and sarcoidosis. It is clear that even a negative biopsy diagnosis is useful to clinicians, in the same way as for liver and bone marrow biopsies.

In the Stanford series of 3,000 nontransplant cardiac biopsies, a firm conclusion, either by confirmation or exclusion of a clinical diagnosis, was achieved in 65 percent of cases; in 13 percent, a new and previously unsuspected diagnosis was made.[8] These figures are similar to those published in a report by Olsen[61] in a series of 81 patients biopsied where a confirmation or exclusion of a clinical diagnosis was made in 70 percent of cases.

It is appropriate here to include some observations on the pitfalls of biopsy interpretation. Myocyte contraction bands should not be used as evidence of ischemia in endomyocardial biopsies; the myocyte fragments obtained in this way often show severe contraction artifact, and studies of biopsies in normal "control" hearts frequently displayed contraction[1] (see Fig. 39–1). It is also necessary to caution against the diagnosis of interstitial edema in endomyocardial biopsies, as myocyte separation can easily occur during handling of the biopsies; this does not necessarily denote edema. In contrast, the diagnosis of intracellular edema can be made on the basis of enhanced perinuclear clear zones and myofibrillar separation. If the endocardium is not seen on light microscopic examination, the paraffin blocks can be turned in order to find the endocardial surface, as theoretically every biopsy should contain endocardium. Some pathologists are surprised to see adipose tissue in endomyocardial biopsies. If a biopsy is taken from the apex of the right ventricle rather than from the interventricular septum, the thinness of the myocardium at this point (as thin as 3 mm) will allow inclusion of subvisceral pericardial adipose tissue. If the pericardium is inadvertently biopsied, the characteristic appearance of pericardial mesothelial cells ("string of beads" appearance) can be recognized. It should be noted that pockets of subendocardial adipose tissue can also occur. Fibrosis is another area of difficulty in endomyocardial biopsies, as there are normally focal increases in subendocardial fibrosis or intertrabecular septal thickenings, which should not be interpreted as an abnormal increase in fibrous tissue. It is not unusual, at our institution, to biopsy a previous biopsy site, which can clearly lead to misinterpretation. This sometimes occurs because a particular configuration of ventricular trabeculae guides the bioptome to the same locus. Caution should be exercised in making a diagnosis of myocarditis on the basis of a few lymphocytes, and occasional macrophages can be seen in biopsies from normal hearts. Occasionally, foreign body granulomata related to talc or cloth fiber may be seen near old biopsy sites.

INDICATIONS FOR ENDOMYOCARDIAL BIOPSY

The indications for endomyocardial biopsy in humans[16,53] are tabulated in Table 39–1. Each will be considered separately. The indications for left versus right ventricular biopsy depend on the suspected cardiac abnormality[23,24,40,53,72]; for example, lesions producing pressure or volume overloading of the left ventricle are best evaluated by left ventricular biopsy. Radiation changes may be less obvious in the left endomyocardium because of thicker ventricular free walls. Carcinoid changes are more likely to be found on the right side. For diffuse disease processes such as hemochromatosis neither side has an advantage over the other. In our experience, there tends to be more fibrosis and a thicker endocardium in biopsies from the left ventricle. The Caves-Stanford technique of biop-

Table 39–1.   Indications for Endomyocardial Biopsy in Humans

1. Diagnosis, grading, and follow-up of rejection in cardiac allograft recipients
2. Diagnosis and grading of anthracycline-induced cardiotoxicity
3. Diagnosis and follow-up of acute myocarditis
4. Diagnosis or confirmation of idiopathic cardiomyopathies
5. Diagnosis and follow-up of specific heart muscle disease
6. Diagnostic aid in idiopathic chest pain and/or arrhythmias
7. Differentiation of restrictive versus constrictive heart disease

sying the right ventricular septum is easier, quicker, and safer than biopsy of the left side; emboli are less likely. Other groups feel strongly that there is less danger of ventricular perforation in a left ventricular biopsy where the heart wall is thicker.

The technique of endomyocardial biopsy has obvious potential as a research tool. The use of serial biopsies to follow the progress of certain disease states and their response to different therapeutic approaches can now be studied for the first time. Reliable ultrastructural, biochemical, and elemental analyses are now being performed on the diseased living myocardium.[50,65,66,92] Such studies were not previously possible on cadaver hearts.

Human Cardiac Allograft Recipients

In 1971, a serial transvenous biopsy of an orthotopically transplanted canine heart was performed to define the morphologic changes in acute cardiac rejection.[4] More than 7,000 endomyocardial biopsies have now been performed on more than 500 human cardiac transplant recipients at Stanford. On the basis of this experience, the histopathologic features of acute cardiac rejection in humans have also

Table 39–2. Histopathology of Endomyocardial Biopsies in Acute Human Cardiac Rejection

---

Mild rejection (reversible)
    Endocardial and interstitial edema
    Scanty perivascular and endocardial infiltrate of pyroninophilic lymphocytes

Moderate rejection (reversible)
    More pronounced perivascular, endocardial, and interstitial infiltrate of pyroninophilic lymphocytes and eosinophils
    Early focal myocytolysis

Severe rejection (difficult to reverse)
    Vascular and myocyte necrosis with interstitial hemorrhage
    Interstitial infiltrate of polymorphonuclear leukocytes and pyroninophilic lymphocytes

Resolving rejection
    Active fibrosis
    Residual small, nonpyroninophilic lymphocytes, plasma cells, and hemosiderin

---

been defined and graded[8,25,27] (Table 39.2) (see also Ch. 43).

Mild or early acute rejection is characterized by endocardial and/or interstitial edema with a scanty interstitial and endocardial, but predominantly perivascular, infiltrate of pyroninophilic lymphocytes with prominent nucleoli (immunoblasts). This lymphocytic infiltrate has been shown to be predominantly of the T-cell type.[17,91] Early acute rejection is also heralded by a significant increase in pyroninophilia of both endocardial cells and endothelial cells of small vessels seen in the biopsies. This sign is not present in donor biopsies at the time of transplantation, but it develops with rejection and may linger for a few days following reversal of rejection with immunosuppressive therapy or in rejection-free, long-term survivors.

In *moderate* acute rejection, the perivascular and interstitial inflammatory cell infiltrate is similar to that in the mild acute rejection but is significantly increased in amount (Fig. 39–2). The interstitial cellular infiltrate is frequently in clumps and may extend to the endocardium. In cyclosporine-treated recip-

ients, eosinophils are also seen in the infiltrate. Early focal degenerative myocytolysis can be seen adjacent to the clumps of inflammatory cells. The early degenerative myocyte change is easily recognized when the biopsy is stained with Masson's trichrome by the shrunken, more basophilic cells with pyknotic nuclei, as compared to the more eosinophilic staining of normal myocardial myocytes.

Severe acute rejection can readily be recognized on endomyocardial biopsy by changes similar to those of moderate acute rejection described above, but with a cellular infiltrate consisting of large pyroninophilic lymphocytes, polymorphonuclear leukocytes, and interstitial hemorrhage due to vascular damage, sometimes with microthrombi. Frank myocyte necrosis may be evident in areas of maximum cellular infiltrate.

Following treatment for acute rejection, reversal of most of the changes described above can be seen as early as 72 hours after the initiation of treatment. A biopsy of *resolving* acute rejection typically has many spindle-shaped fibroblasts, an area of scar, residual lymphocytes (which are smaller and nonpyroninophilic), plasma cells, and hemosiderin deposits. Recently, other grading systems for endomyocardial biopsy interpretation of acute rejection have been described.[41,57] The newer systems favor numeric rather than descriptive terms and are easier to computerize in data banks.

The changes of acute rejection described above relate to cardiac recipients treated with conventional immunosuppressive therapy, that is, antithymocyte globulin, steroids, and azathioprine. Since January 1981, cardiac allograft recipients at Stanford University Medical Center have been treated with the immunosuppresive drug cyclosporin-A, a selective inhibitor of certain subsets of T cells. These patients also develop acute rejection, but the morphologic changes are slightly different from those seen with conventional treatment.[9]

Endomyocardial biopsies from cyclosporin-A-treated cardiac recipients usually show a

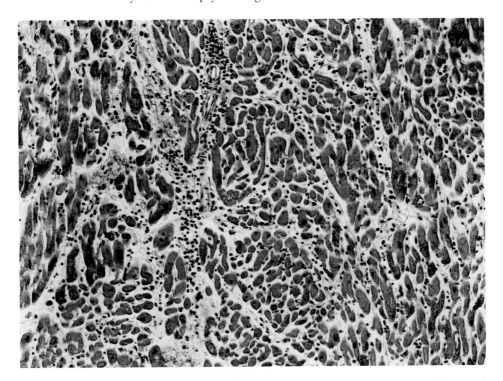

Fig. 39–2. Endomyocardial biopsy showing a perivascular and interstitial lymphocytic infiltrate in human acute cardiac allograft rejection. (H&E, × 120.)

widely scattered sparse infiltration of small mononuclear cells that do not portend acute rejection. Early morphologic change of acute rejection in these patients is also manifested by an increase in perivascular and interstitial mononuclear cells that are plump and pyroninophilic. Moderate acute rejection seems to be accompanied with more eosinophils that are seen with conventionally treated recipients, but is otherwise much the same. Severe acute rejection includes a neutrophilic infiltrate, more hemorrhage, and myocyte necrosis.[9]

Acute rejection is much less in cyclosporine-treated patients. It also develops more slowly, over a week instead of 2 days, and once established, takes much longer to resolve.[9] Even after augmented immunosuppression, myocyte damage and the infiltrate may be ongoing for 2 to 3 weeks before clearing. In addition, many of the recipients

treated with cyclosporine show a fine, perimyocytic fibrosis that is quite characteristic, whether they develop acute rejection episodes or not. This fine fibrosis is dose related and is not seen so much now that the cyclosporine levels are reduced with triple therapy. Acute rejection occurring in patients treated with OKT3 is not different from that described with other immunosuppressive treatments.

The pitfalls of endomyocardial biopsy grading for acute rejection include previous biopsy sites, which often contain fibrin and granulation tissue as well as myocyte disarray at the base of the lesion. Biopsies during the first 2 weeks post-transplantation often have evidence of ischemia and/or catecholamine (pressor) effect. Endocardial infiltrates (the "Quilty" phenomenon) do not require treatment if there is no other evidence of acute rejection.

Immunofluorescence is unreliable in the

assessment of acute rejection by endomyocardial biopsy. Although sarcolemmal immunoglobulin G (IgG), C'3, and fibrinogen can be detected in severe end-stage rejection, this is neither predictive of acute rejection nor of its severity; this may be due to the high dose of immunosuppressive agents in the early postoperative phase.

Transvenous endomyocardial biopsy has contributed significantly to the clinical management of human cardiac recipients. It provides an objective histologic index of host immune response to the cardiac allograft and allows an "on-line" assessment of the response of immunosuppressive therapy during acute rejection episodes. In this way, immunosuppressive therapy can be tailored to individual patients by direct histologic examination of the graft. Pulmonary infection is often associated with a decrease in externally measured QRS voltages in the standard electrocardiographic leads, but a voltage change is also a clinical sign of acute rejection; atrial arrythmias, though often associated with acute graft rejection episodes, do not inevitably indicate this process. In both these instances, morphologic assessment provides an independent, clear-cut evaluation of graft status so that an unnecessary and dangerous augmentation of immunosuppressive agents can be prevented. One of the most useful aspects of endomyocardial biopsies clearly lies in the management of cardiac transplant recipients and accounts, in a real sense, for the success of the cardiac transplant program at Stanford, where more than 500 patients have received cardiac transplants and where there is an 82 percent 1-year survival and a 65 percent 5-year survival. This group includes the longest living cardiac recipient survivor who is now 20 years post-transplantation.

Anthracycline-induced Cardiotoxicity

Anthracycline antibiotics such as Adriamycin and Daunomycin have a marked antineoplastic effect in adult and childhood solid tumors and in hematologic malignancies.[18] The toxic side effects produced by these drugs are clinically manageable and reversible—with the exception of severe cardiotoxicity, which can lead to congestive cardiomyopathy, heart failure, and death.[49] By use of endomyocardial biopsy, the histopathologic changes of anthracycline cardiotoxicity have been described *as they develop*[8,9,13,15] (see also Ch. 32). In this way a morphologic grading system has been developed that allows an accurate prediction of the development of cardiotoxicity, thus allowing patients to have the maximum amount of antitumor effect from the anthracyclines without the risk of death from heart failure. The grading system is tabulated in Table 39–3. The morphologic changes due to anthracyclines are both focal and disseminated. Early change in a biopsy may show

Table 39–3.   Morphologic Grading System for Cardiotoxicity

Grade*	Morphology
0	Normal myocardial ultrastructural morphology
1	Isolated myocytes affected by distended sarcotubular system and/or early myofibrillar loss; damage to <5 percent of all cells in 10 plastic blocks
1.5	Changes similar to those in grade 1 but with damage to 6 to 15 percent of all cells in 10 plastic blocks
2.0	Clusters of myocytes affected by myofibrillar loss and/or vacuolization, with damage to 16 to 25 percent of all cells in 10 plastic blocks
2.5	Many myocytes, ≤26 to 35 percent of all cells in 10 plastic blocks, affected by vacuolization and/or myofibrillar loss
3.0	Severe and diffuse myocyte damage (>35 percent of all cells in 10 plastic blocks) affected by vacuolization and/or myofibrillar loss

* At grade 2.5, only one more dose of anthracycline should be given without further evaluation. At grade 3.0, no more anthracycline should be given.

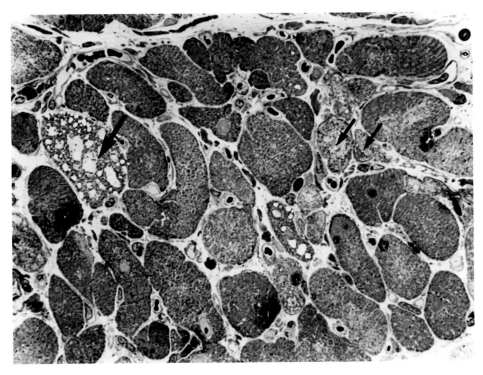

Fig. 39–3. Endomyocardial biopsy from an Adriamycin-treated patient showing myocytes with myofibrillar loss (small arrows) and with sarcotubular swelling. (Epon, toluidine blue, × 480.)

only isolated affected myocytes. It is interesting to note that the earliest changes tend to occur in the subendocardium and are therefore readily picked up by an endomyocardial biopsy.

In humans, two main types of lesions in myocytes are caused by anthracyclines.[18,22] In the first, myofibrillar loss occurs. It may be partial, but is more usually total, with only Z-band remnants remaining. In these myocytes, the nucleus may appear normal and the mitochondria tend to be fewer and smaller but with normal compact cristae. These cells can be recognized with practice on light microscopy, where they appear shrunken with a homogeneous pale cytoplasm; they are readily recognized in 1 μm-thick plastic sections stained with toluidine blue (Fig. 39–3) or, of course, by ultrastructural examination (Fig. 39–4). (See also Fig. 32–8.)

In the second type of anthracycline myocyte injury, well described in animal models,[38] the sarcoplasmic reticulum and T-tubule system dilate and may coalesce into large, membrane-bound vacuoles in the cytoplasm, but the mitochondria and nucleus may remain unaffected (see Fig. 39–4). These two types of degeneration may occur in the same cell or in separate cells. There does not appear to be a relationship between the two types of cell damage and the severity or course of the cardiotoxicity. Both types should be sought in the biopsy screening, as both are used in the grading system. In very severe grade 3 cardiotoxicity actual myocyte necrosis may occur; at this point, the nucleus becomes pyknotic, myelin figures denoting membrane destruction occur, and mitochondria exhibit degenerative changes. Interstitial fibrosis does occur with anthracycline-induced cardiotoxicity, but is not included as a factor in the grading system because it is a relatively nonspecific finding that can have other causes, such as radiation effect. Inflammatory infil-

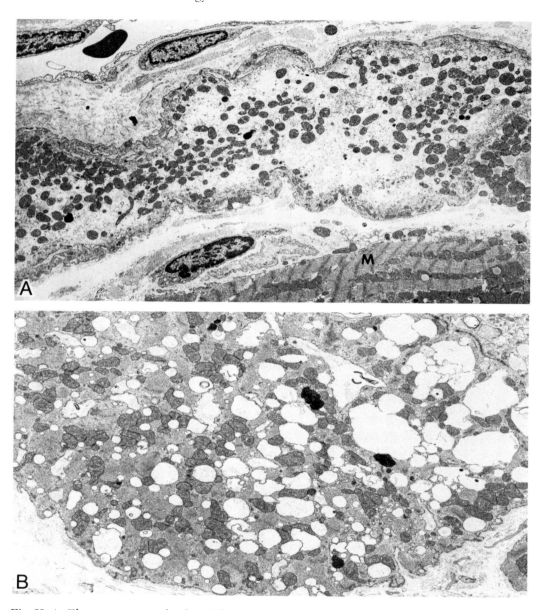

Fig. 39–4. Electron micrographs, from Adriamycin-treated patients. (**A**) Myofibrillar loss compared with normal myocyte (**M**). (**B**) Myocyte showing sarcotubular distension (note intact mitochondria.) (Figs. A and B, uranyl acetate and osmium, × 4,382.)

trates are not seen in anthracycline cardio-toxicity, even in grade 3 cardiotoxicity, and small vessels and nerves also appear to be unaffected in the therapeutic dose range.

The endomyocardial biopsy has also pro-vided a means of evaluating cardiotoxicity of Adriamycin analogues being developed and tested in clinical trials.[5,37] For example, the anthracycline analogues Adria-DNA, Dau-norubicin, Rubidazone, 4′ epirubicin, and mitoxantrone have caused changes similar to those seen in patients treated with Adriamycin alone, although the changes occurred at very different dose levels. In this respect, and with regard to testing the mitigating effects of different dose delivery systems and pharmacologic antagonists, the endomyocardial biopsy is a remarkable research tool.

Although the histopathologic ultrastructural changes of anthracycline administration are very characteristic and can be easily recognized and graded, they are not necessarily specific; similar degenerative changes in myocytes can be seen in end-stage primary cardiomyopathies. Recent morphometric studies show that myocyte nuclear sizes in anthracycline cardiotoxicity do not attain the size or bizarre shapes as those in cardiomyopathy. The changes caused by anthracyclines are seen long before biventricular dilation occurs, and the anthracycline-treated patients have normal cardiac evaluations before the onset of treatment.

Using this grading system, certain risk factors for anthracycline-treated patients have become obvious. Radiation to the mediastinum, either before or following anthracycline treatment, potentiates the risk of cardiotoxicity.[7,9,12] Furthermore, anthracycline will evoke a recall phenomenon of acute radiation effect in the myocardium, even if the radiation was given up to 14 years previously. Patients older than 70 years are at high risk for anthracycline-related cardiotoxicity. Those with a history of hypertension tend to be more prone to cardiotoxicity.

Clinicopathologic correlations made for biopsied patients have been described in detail in several publications.[5,8,15,20,21,33,54] Results indicate endomyocardial biopsy is helpful in scoring the degree of myocardial damage due to anthracycline administration and also show that even low cumulative doses of anthracycline can cause minor degrees of damage, detectable before any clinical, hemodynamic, or electrophysiologic signs are apparent.[11] The biopsy results demonstrate unequivocally that considerable biologic variation exists between individuals with regard to the degree of anthracycline toxicity—hence, the desirability of morphologic assessment.

In summary, endomyocardial biopsy provides an accurate and useful guide to the administration of anthracyclines in both adult patients and children and is a useful tool for arriving at a rational dose optimization. It is also useful in monitoring the results of clinical trials of anthracycline analogues, pharmacologic antagonists, and different dose delivery schedules.[88]

Diagnosis of Myocarditis

Endomyocardial biopsy is useful in cases of clinically suspected myocarditis following a history of a recent viral illness. Because focal infiltrates frequently are seen in viral myocarditis, a negative biopsy does not rule out the diagnosis, but a positive biopsy with an unequivocal lymphocytic interstitial or perivascular infiltrate will provide very suggestive evidence of myocarditis (Fig. 39–5). A biopsy fragment can be tested by in situ hybridization or cultured for virus, providing even more sensitive diagnostic tests.[47] In biopsies of acute myocarditis, immunofluorescence techniques of frozen biopsy specimens often are positive of IgG and C′3. Electron microscopy is neither necessary nor useful in myocarditis, as viral particles are seldom seen. In a few cases in our experience, treatment of myocarditis with steroids has produced dramatic clinical and hemodynamic cardiac improvement as well as an improved or negative follow-up endomyocardial biopsy.[56] Treatment with steroids for myocarditis is controversial and for this reason a 28-center randomized myocarditis trial was designed.

There are many pitfalls to the diagnosis of acute myocarditis by endomyocardial biopsy (Table 39–4), so the "Dallas criteria" have been outlined to guide diagnosis by biopsy and *specifically* for the purpose of the randomized myocarditis trial.[3] Table 39–5 out-

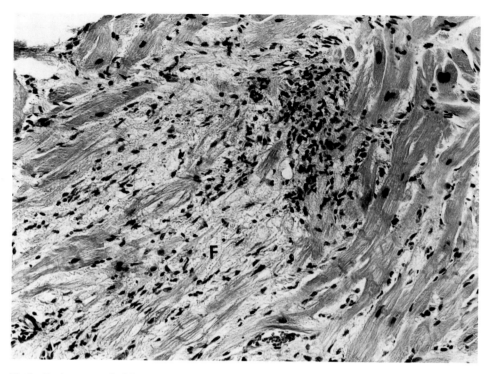

Fig. 39–5. Endomyocardial biopsy from a patient with suspected myocarditis. Note the lymphocytic infiltrate and recently formed fibrous tissue (F). (H&E, × 192.)

Table 39–4.   Histopathologic Pitfalls
in the Endomyocardial Biopsy Diagnosis
of Acute Myocarditis

1. Sampling error; insufficient number of biopsy fragments
2. Endothelial cell nuclei masquerading as lymphocytes
3. Focal ischemia, "catecholamine effect," drug reaction (toxic myocarditis)
4. "Tip of the iceberg" effect with an underlying unseen granuloma
5. Drug-induced myocarditis (toxic or hypersensitivity)
6. Lymphomatous infiltrate
7. Secondary myocarditis, Chaga's disease, etc.

lines the grading of acute myocarditis as used in the Dallas criteria.

Idiopathic Cardiomyopathies

Endomyocardial biopsies in cases of dilated/congestive cardiomyopathies show nonspecific features of increased endocardial and interstitial fibrosis and a mixture of hypertrophied and attenuated myocytes with large, bizarre, hyperchromatic nuclei on light microscopy (Fig. 39–6). Ultrastructural changes are characteristic, with myocardial cells show-

Table 39–5.   Endomyocardial Biopsy Diagnosis of Acute Myocarditis ("Dallas" Grading Criteria)

First Biopsy	*Second or Subsequent Biopsies*
No evidence of myocarditis	Ongoing myocarditis
Borderline myocarditis (requires rebiopsy)	Healing myocarditis (resolving)
Acute myocarditis	Healed myocarditis (may look like cardiomyopathy)

ing partial or complete myofibrillar loss, frequently with an increased number of small, compact mitochondria. In addition, there is dilation of the sarcotubular system, often starting adjacent to the intercalated disc. Mitochondrial morphology may also be pleomorphic, and the nuclear degenerative changes of chromatin clumping, margination, and crenation of the nuclear membrane are frequently seen. Cytosegresomes, vacuoles, and sarcolemmal blebs may be present. Myelin figures are frequent and indicate membrane degeneration. These changes are based on our own experience but are similar to those described by other groups.[31,32,48,62,78,79] At least three groups have described semiquantitative methods for the morphologic scoring of endomyocardial biopsies in an attempt to grade the severity and prognosis of congestive cardiomyopathy.[4,19,48,49,80]

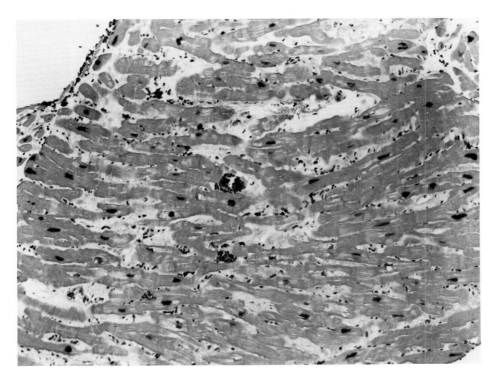

Fig. 39–6. Endomyocardial biopsy from a patient with end-stage congestive cardiomyopathy. Note the interstitial fibrosis, marked myocyte hypertrophy and bizarre hyperchromatic nuclei. (H&E, × 120.)

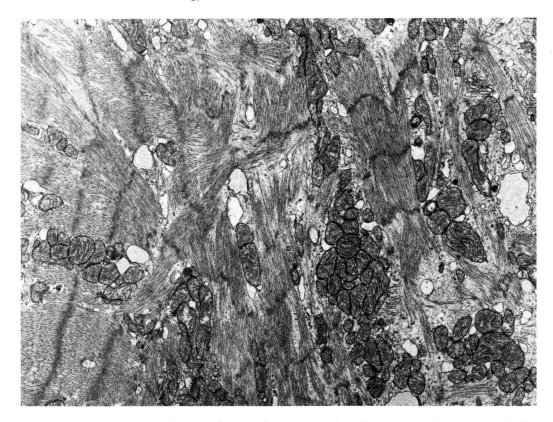

Fig. 39–7. Electron micrograph from a biopsy of a patient with cardiomyopathy showing myofibrillar disarray. (Uranyl acetate and osmium, × 14,959.)

There have been reports of the diagnosis of hypertrophic cardiomyopathy made by endomyocardial biopsy. Although myocyte and myofibrillar disarray is not infrequently seen on endomyocardial biopsies (Fig. 39–7), it is unlikely that this is pathognomonic of hypertrophic cardiomyopathy as myocardial disarray in this cardiomyopathy occurs in the middle third of the interventricular septum when seen at autopsy or on a surgical specimen.[85] Furthermore, in the left ventricle the septal bulge is usually covered by thick endocardial fibrous tissue that would be difficult for a bioptome to penetrate. A biopsy of the right ventricle is more likely to reach the middle of the interventricular septum because the endocardium is not necessarily thickened in the right ventricle.

Other cardiomyopathies, such as "postpartum" and alcoholic cardiomyopathy, have morphologic changes similar to those of congestive dilated cardiomyopathy. Recently, some changes have been described in familial cardiomyopathy that appear to be characteristic but may not be specific.[89] We have made the diagnosis of endocardial fibroelastosis by endomyocardial biopsy in a child with idiopathic congestive heart failure. The diagnosis was later confirmed at autopsy. It is readily made by biopsy.[83]

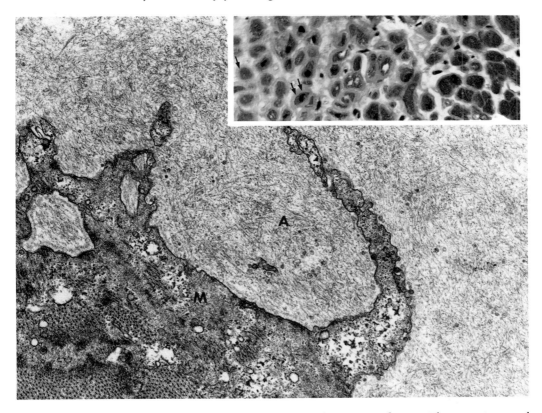

Fig. 39–8. Endomyocardial biopsy from patient presenting with restrictive disease. Electron micrograph shows degenerating myocyte (M) and amyloid fibrils (A). (× 29,946.) (Inset) Light microscopy showing amyloid (arrows) surrounding myocytes. (Masson's trichrome, × 130.)

Specific Heart Muscle Disease

Endomyocardial biopsy has yielded many useful diagnoses in specific heart muscle diseases (the category of secondary cardiomyopathies using Roberts and Ferrans' classification.)[73] Amyloidosis[34,77] (Fig. 39–8) and hemochromatosis[73] (Fig. 39–9) have been the most frequent diagnoses, although we have had several cases of previously unsuspected sarcoidosis (Fig. 39–10), glycogen storage disease, and hypothyroid heart disease. Opportunistic organisms seen on biopsies in immunosuppressed patients have included toxoplasma, cytomegalic viral inclusions, cryptococcus, blastomycosis, and coccidioidomycosis. We have observed metastatic neoplastic disease in biopsies and acute and chronic radiation effect. Acute cardiac allograft rejection and drug cardiotoxicities have already been mentioned. Eosinophilic myocarditis (hypersensitivity myocarditis) and drug-related toxic myocarditis have been seen on biopsies. Catecholamine effect (focal myocyte necrosis) may be observed in cocaine users.[39] The endomyocardial biopsy has been used to describe cardiac changes in myotonic dystrophy,[58] methysergide-induced heart disease,[52] mitral valve prolapse,[55] and giant cell myocarditis.

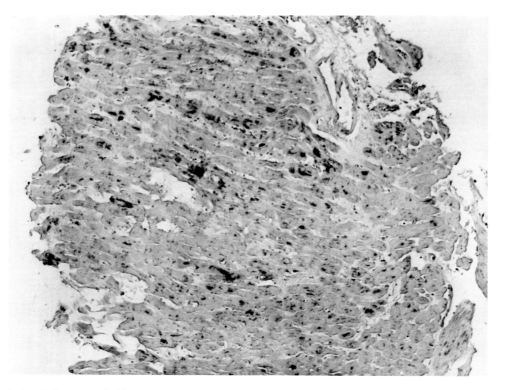

Fig. 39–9. Endomyocardial biopsy showing hemosiderin deposits (dark areas) in a patient with hemo-chromotosis. (Perl's iron, × 120.)

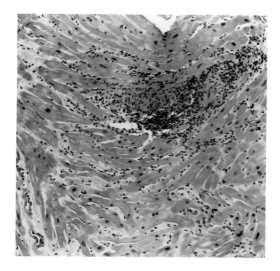

Fig. 39–10. Endomyocardial biopsy showing a noncaseating granuloma with giant cells in an un-suspected case of sarcoidosis. (H&E, × 120.)

Diagnostic Aid in Idiopathic Chest Pain

Occasionally the endomyocardial biopsy will throw light on idiopathic chest pain in a patient with angina-like chest pain but with normal angiograms or treadmill tests. The biopsy may show ischemic change (Fig. 39–11) or unsuspected myocarditis, which would account for the pain. In this group of patients, widening of the subendothelial lamina has been demonstrated in small intramyocardial vessels;[16] it may also be the cause of chest pain[44,71] (Fig. 39–12). Severe mitochondrial degenerative changes or ultrastructural myocyte changes will suggest an organic basis for the chest pain and thus avoid the unfortunate diagnosis of hysteria sometimes applied to these patients.

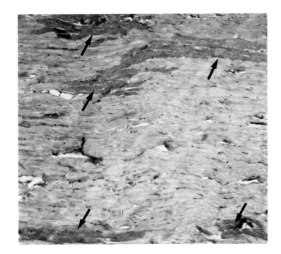

Fig. 39–11. Endomyocardial biopsy showing focal myocyte ischemia (arrows), highlighted. (Masson's trichrome, × 120.)

Differentiation of Restrictive versus Constrictive Heart Disease

Physical examination and cardiac catheterization data may not provide a definite differential diagnosis between restrictive and constrictive myocardial disease. Confirmation by endomyocardial biopsy, which is easier, quicker, and safer than open chest pericardial biopsy to demonstrate cardiac amyloidosis,[34,77] will assist by providing optimum diagnostic and therapeutic care for these patients. Occasionally, endomyocardial fibrosis (e.g., from previous radiation) may cause diastolic failure and present as restrictive disease; this can also be diagnosed by endomyocardial biopsy.

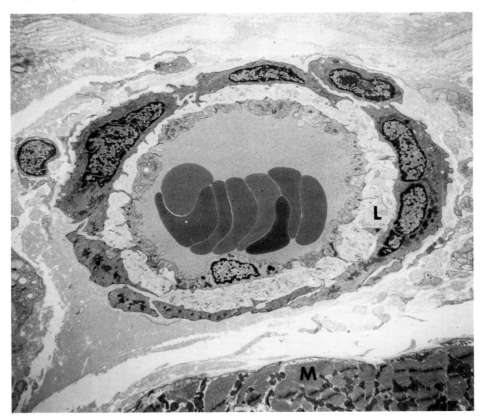

Fig. 39–12. Electron micrograph of intramyocardial vessel (22 μm diameter), showing a thickened subendothelial lamina (L) and an adjacent myocyte (M). (Uranyl acetate and osmium, × 2,900.)

SUMMARY

There is real potential for endomyocardial biopsy in the diagnosis and treatment of cardiovascular disease. The indications for endomyocardial biopsy in Table 39–1 are realistic and have been effectively applied in 10,000 biopsies at Stanford. The biopsy information has yielded useful information (as defined earlier) in more than 70 percent of cases. In cardiac rejection and cardiotoxicity due to anthracycline drugs, biopsies have yielded useful information in 100 percent of cases for both groups and have played a major part in improving the management and survival of those patients.

The safety record for endomyocardial biopsies at Stanford has been better than for liver or renal biopsies, with no mortality and a morbidity below 0.3 percent. Most other groups have also had a safe record. The safety of the technique depends, of course, on the skill and experience of the cardiologist performing the biopsy, although the technique can readily be taught to others. The question of whether the biopsies are representative of the heart as a whole requires comment. Obviously, in a focal condition a negative biopsy may not be representative. At least three pieces of myocardium from different sites on the septum should be sampled in order to reduce the likelihood of this error.[84] Most of the indications for endomyocardial biopsy are for diffuse myocardial diseases, some of which have a predilection for the endomyocardium—for example, acute rejection and anthracycline cardiotoxicity.

The future usefulness of endomyocardial biopsy in both clinical and research applications depends on the ability of pathologists, biochemists, and perhaps immunologists to develop accurate quantitative analyses of the small myocardial specimens and thereby advance the present analytic capacities of the technique. These advances will help clinicians in the diagnosis of myocardial disease and in the development of criteria for their prognosis and treatment.

With the exception of tissue taken during cardiac surgery, pathologists have had to rely in the past on postmortem tissue for studies of the morphology and biochemistry of the human heart. There were two obvious drawbacks: postmortem artifact, particularly for ultrastructural morphology; and the inability to follow the course of cardiac disease in vivo. Both problems have been significantly ameliorated with the advent of the transvenous endomyocardial biopsy. As a result, ultrastructural, biochemical, and elemental analyses are now being performed on diseased myocardium in vivo;[50,65,66,92] such studies were not previously possible on cadaver hearts. Above and beyond the clinical benefits of diagnosis of certain myocardial diseases, the more widespread use of the endomyocardial biopsy technique promises to reveal much about the fundamental mechanisms of heart disease in humans.

REFERENCES

1. Adomian GD, Laks MM, Billingham ME: The incidence and significance of contraction bands in endomyocardial biopsies from normal human hearts. Am Heart J 95:348, 1978
2. Ali N: Transvenous endomyocardial biopsy using the gastrointestinal biopsy (Olympus GFB) catheter. Am Heart J 87:294, 1974
3. Aretz HT, Billingham ME, Edwards WD, et al: Myocarditis: A histopathologic definition and classification. Am J Cardiovasc Pathol 1:47, 1986
4. Baandrup U, Olsen EGJ: Critical analysis of endomyocardial biopsies from patients suspect of having cardiomyopathy. I: Morphological and morphometric aspects. Br Heart J 45:475, 1981
5. Benjamin R, Billingham M, Mason J: Cardiotoxicity of Adriamycin-DNA and Rubidazone: evaluation by ECG and endomyocardial biopsy. Cancer Treat Rep 62:935, 1978
6. Berçu B, Heinz J, Choudhry AS, et al: Myo-

cardial biopsy—a new technique utilizing the ventricular septum. Am J Cardiol 14:675, 1964

7. Billingham ME: Endomyocardial changes in anthracycline-treated patients with and without irradiation. Front Rad Ther Oncol 13:67, 1979

8. Billingham ME: Some recent advances in cardiac pathology. Hum Pathol 10:367, 1979

9. Billingham ME: Diagnosis of cardiac rejection by endomyocardial biopsy. Heart Trans 1:25, 1982

10. Billingham ME: The post-surgical heart. Am J Cardiovasc Pathol 1(3):319, 1988

11. Billingham ME, Bristow MR: Evaluation of anthracycline cardiotoxicity: predictive ability and functional correlation of endomyocardial biopsy. Cancer Treat Symposia 3:71, 1984

12. Billingham ME, Bristow M, Glatstein E, et al: Adriamycin cardiotoxicity: endomyocardial biopsy evidence of enhancement by radiation. Am J Surg Pathol 1:17, 1977

13. Billingham M, Bristow M, Mason M, Friedman M: Endomyocardial biopsy findings in Adriamycin-treated patients. Am Soc Oncol Proc 17:281, 1976

14. Billingham ME, Caves PK, Dong E Jr, Shumway NE: Diagnosis of canine orthotopic cardiac allograft rejection by transvenous endomyocardial biopsy. Transplant Proc 10:741, 1973

15. Billingham ME, Mason JW, Bristow MR, Daniels JR: Anthracycline cardiomyopathy monitored by morphologic changes. Can Treat Rep 62:865, 1978

16. Billingham M, Schwartz B, Rider A, Harrison D: An ultrastructural study of age-related changes in intramyocardial arterioles. Proceedings of the 66th Scientific Sessions of IAP, Toronto, Canada, March 1977. Lab Invest 36:331, 1977

17. Billingham M, Warnke R, Weissman I: The cellular infiltrate in cardiac allograft rejection in mice. Transplantation 23:171, 1977

18. Blum RH, Carter SK: Adriamycin: A new anticancer drug with significant clinical activity. Ann Intern Med 80:249, 1974

19. Breithardt G, Kuhn H, Knieriem H-J: Prognostic significance of endomyocardial biopsy in patients with congestive cardiomyopathy. p. 258. In Kaltenbach M, Loogen F, Olsen EGJ, (eds): Cardiomyopathy and Myocardial Biopsy. Springer-Verlag, New York, 1976

20. Bristow MR, Billingham ME, Mason JW, Daniels JR: The clinical spectrum of anthracycline antibiotic cardiotoxicity. Cancer Treat Rep 62:875, 1978

21. Bristow MR, Mason J, Billingham ME, Daniels JR: Dauxorubicin cardiomyopathy: Evaluation by phonocardiography, endomyocardial biopsy and cardiac catheterization. Ann Intern Med 8:168, 1978

22. Bristow MR, Thompson PD, Martin PR, et al: Early anthracycline cardiotoxicity. Am J Med 65:823, 1978

23. Brooksby IAB, Jenkins BS, Coltart DJ, Webb-Peploe MM: Left ventricular endomyocardial biopsy. Lancet 2:1222, 1974

24. Brooksby I, Jenkins S, Coltart J, Webb-Peploe M, Davies M: Myocardial biopsy: Description of technique, comparison of right and left ventricular biopsy. Br Heart J 37:555, 1975 (abst)

25. Caves PK, Billingham ME, Stinson EB, Shumway NE: Serial transvenous biopsy of the transplanted human heart—improved management of acute rejection episodes. Lancet 1:821, 1974

26. Caves PE, Schulz WP, Dong E Jr, et al: A new instrument for transvenous cardiac biopsy. Am J Cardiol 33:264, 1974

27. Caves PK, Stinson EB, Billingham ME, et al: Diagnosis of human cardiac allograft rejection by serial cardiac biopsy. J Thorac Cardiovasc Surg 66:461, 1973

28. Caves PK, Stinson EB, Billingham ME, Shumway NE: Percutaneous transvenous endomyocardial biopsy in human heart recipients (experience with a new technique). Ann Thorac Surg 16:325, 1973

29. Caves PK, Stinson EB, Billingham ME, Shumway NE: Transvenous intracardiac biopsy using a new catheter forceps. Heart Lung 4:69, 1975

30. Caves PK, Stinson EB, Graham AF, et al: Percutaneous transvenous endomyocardial biopsy. JAMA 225, 1973

31. Ferrans VJ, Massumi RA, Shugoll GI, et al: Ultrastructural studies of myocardial biopsies in 45 patients with obstructive or congestive cardiomyopathies. p. 231. In Brink AJ, Bajuisz E (eds): Recent Advances in Studies of Cardiac Structure and Metabolism. University Park Press, Baltimore, 1973

32. Ferrans VJ, Morrow AG, Roberts WC: Myocardial ultrastructure in idiopathic hypertro-

phic subaortic stenosis. Circulation 45:769, 1972

33. Friedman M, Bozdech M, Billingham ME, Rider A: Doxorubicin cardiotoxicity: serial endomyocardial biopsies and systolic time intervals. JAMA 240:1603, 1978

34. Galichia JP, Gobel FL, Alexander CS: Cardiac amyloidosis in hereditary neuropathic amyloidosis diagnosed by endomyocardial biopsy. Hum Pathol 9:429, 1978

35. Harmjanz D, Reale E, Luciano L, Ostertag P: Die Endomyokardbiopsie als Hifsmittel in der Diagnostik von Myokarderkrankungen. 77 Tagung der deutschen Gesselschaft fur Innere medizin, 22 April. Cited by Sekiguchi M: J Molec Cell Cardiol 6:111, 1974

36. Harmanjz D: Problems of myocardial biopsy. Postgrad Med J 51:291, 1975

37. Henderson I, Billingham M, Israel A, et al: Comparative cardiotoxicity studies with adriamycin and AD_{32} in rabbits. Am Assoc Canc Res Proc 19:158, 1978

38. Jaenke RS: An anthracycline antibiotic-induced cardiomyopathy in rabbits. Lab Invest 30:292, 1974

39. Karch SB, Billingham ME: The pathology and etiology of cocaine-induced heart disease. Arch Pathol Lab Med 112:225, 1988

40. Kawai C, Kitaura Y: New endomyocardial biopsy catheter for the left ventricle. Am J Cardiol 40:63, 1977

41. Kemnitz J, Cohnert T, Schafers H-J, et al: A classification of cardiac allograft rejection. Am J Surg Pathol 7:503, 1987

42. Kin G, Combes S, Miray D, Grosgogeat Y: La biopsie endomyocardique. Technique, résultats et indications. Nouv Presse Med 2(64):3117, 1973

43. Kober G, Kunkel B, Becker H-J, et al: Technical aspects, experiences and complication of right-left ventricular endomyocardial biopsy. p. 40. In Kaltenbach M, Loogen F, Olsen EGJ (eds): Cardiomyopathy and Myocardial Biopsy. Springer-Verlag, New York, 1978

44. Koch F, Billingham M, Rider A, et al: Pathophysiology of "angina" with normal coronary angiograms. Proceedings of AHA 49th Scientific Sessions, Miami Beach, FL, Nov, 1976

45. Konno S, Sakakibara S: Endomyocardial biopsy. Dis Chest 44:345, 1963

46. Konno S, Sekiguchi M, Sakakibara S: Catheter biopsy of the heart. Radiol Clin North Am, 9:491, 1971

47. Kuhn H, Breithardt G, Knierem H-H, et al: Die Bedentung der endomyokardialen Katheterbiopsie fur die diagnostik und die Beurteilung der prognose derk kongestiven kardiomyopathie. Dtsch Med Wschr 100:717, 1975

48. Kunkel B, Lapp H, Kober G, Kaltenbach M: Correlations between clinical and morphologic findings and natural history in congestive cardiomyopathy. p. 271. In Kaltenbach M, Loogen F, Olsen EGJ (eds): Cardiomyopathy and Myocardial Biopsy. Springer-Verlag, New York, 1978

49. Lefrak EA, Pittra J, Rosenheim S, Gottlieb JA: A clinicopathologic analysis of Adriamycin cardiotoxicity. Cancer 32:302, 1973

50. Lucena GE, Schettel M, Azar M, et al: Serum enzyme activity following cardiac catheterization and endomyocardial biopsy. J Lab Clin Med 84:6, 1974

51. Mason JW: Techniques for right and left endomyocardial biopsy. Am J Cardiol 41:887, 1978

52. Mason JW, Billingham ME, Friedman JP: Methysergide-induced heart disease: a case of multivalvular and myocardial fibrosis. Circulation 56:889, 1977

53. Mason JW, Billingham ME, Rider AK, Harrison DC: Myocardial biopsy. p. 606. In Willerson JT, Sanders CA (eds): Clinical Cardiology, Grune & Stratton, Orlando, FL, 1977

54. Mason JW, Bristow MR, Billingham ME, Daniels JR: Invasive and non-invasive methods of assessing Adriamycin cardiotoxicity in man: Superiority of histopathologic assessment using endomyocardial biopsy. Cancer Treat Rep 62:857, 1978

55. Mason JW, Koch FH, Billingham ME, Winkle RA: Cardiac biopsy evidence for a cardiomyopathy associated with symptomatic mitral valve prolapse. Am J Cardiol 42:557, 1978

56. Mason JW, Ricci DR, Billingham ME: Effective therapy for acute inflammatory myocarditis. Am J Cardiol 43:408, 1979

57. McAllister HA, Schree MJ, Radovanceivc B, Frazier H: A system for grading cardiac allograft rejection. Texas Heart Inst J 13:1, 1986

58. Motta J, Guilleminault C, Billingham M, et al: Cardiac abnormalities in myotonic dystro-

phy: electrophysiologic and histopathologic studies. Am J Med 67:467, 1979

59. Muller SA, Muller P, Richter G: Herzbiopsie mit Kaheter-Bioptom. Z Gesamte Inn Med 36:107, 1971

60. Olsen EGJ: Diagnostic value of the endomyocardial bioptome. Lancet 1:658, 1974

61. Olsen EGJ: Myocardial biopsies. p. 349. In Hamen J (ed): Recent Advances in Cardiology. Churchill Livingstone, Edinburgh, 1977

62. Olsen EGJ: Postmortem findings and histologic, histochemical and electron microscopic findings of myocardial biopsies. p. 52. In Kaltenbach M, Loogen F, Olsen EGJ (eds): Cardiomyopathy and Myocardial Biopsy. Springer-Verlag, New York, 1978

63. Peter RH, Whalen RE, Orgain ES, McIntosh HD: Postpericardiotomy syndrome as a complication of percutaneous left ventricular puncture. Am J Cardiol 17:86, 1966

64. Peters JJ, Wells G, Oakley CM, et al: Enzymatic analysis of endomyocardial biopsy specimens from patients with cardiomyopathies. Br Heart J 39:1333, 1977

65. Peters TJ, Brooksby IAB, Webb-Peploe MM, et al: Enzymatic analysis of cardiac biopsy material from patients with valvular heart disease. Lancet 1:269, 1976

66. Price KC, Weiss JM, Hata JM, et al: Experimental needle biopsy of the myocardium of dogs with particular reference to histological study by electron microscopy. J Exp Med 101:687, 1955

67. Rattensperger J, Driscol J, Sutton G, Weinberg M Jr: Myocardial biopsy. Arch Surg 89:1021, 1964

68. Richardson PJ: Catheter technique for endomyocardial biopsy. J Cardiovasc Technol 16(2):31, 1974

69. Richardson PJ: King's endomyocardial bioptome. Lancet 1:660, 1974

70. Richardson PJ: Technique of endomyocardial biopsy—including a description of a new form of endomyocardial bioptome. Postgrad Med J 51:282, 1975

71. Richardson PJ, Livesley B, Oram S, et al: Angina pectoris with normal coronary arteries. Transvenous myocardial biopsy in diagnosis. Lancet 2:667, 1974

72. Richardson PJ, Olsen EGJ, Jewitt DE, Oram S: Percutaneous technique of left ventricular biopsy and comparison between right and left ventricular myocardial samples. Br Heart J 37:556, 1975 (abst)

73. Roberts WC, Ferrans VJ: Pathologic anatomy of the cardiomyopathies. Hum Pathol 6:287, 1975

74. Rowan R, Masek M, Billingham ME: Ultrastructural morphometric analysis of endomyocardial biopsies. Am J Cardiovasc Pathol 2:137, 1988

75. Sakakibara S, Konno S: Endomyocardial biopsy. Jpn Heart J 3:537, 1962

76. Sakakibara S, Konno S: Intracardiac heart biopsy. JPN Circ J 30:1582

77. Schroeder SS, Billingham ME, Rider AK: Cardiac amyloidosis: Diagnosis by transvenous endomyocardial biopsy. Am J Med 59:269, 1975

78. Sekiguchi M: Electron microscopical observation of the myocardium in patients with idiopathic cardiomyopathy using endomyocardial biopsy. J Mol Cell Cardiol 6:111, 1974

79. Sekiguchi M, Konno S: Histopathological differentiation employing endomyocardial biopsy in the assessment of primary myocardial disease. Jpn Heart J 10:30, 1969

80. Sekiguchi M, Konno S: Diagnosis and classification of primary myocardial disease with the aid of endomyocardial biopsy. Jpn Circ J 35:737, 1971

81. Sekiguchi M, Konno S, Hasegawa F, Hirosawa K: Some characteristic electron microscopic pictures of diseased myocardium obtained by endomyocardial biopsy. Bull Heart Inst Jpn 14:30, 1972/73

82. Shirey EK, Hawk WA, Mukerji D, Effler DB: Percutaneous myocardial biopsy of the left ventricle. Experience in 198 patients. Circulation 46:112, 1972

83. Somers K, Hutt MSR, Patel AK, D'Arbela PG: Endomyocardial biopsy in diagnosis of cardiomyopathies. Br Heart J 33:822, 1971

84. Spiegelhalter DJ, Stoven PGI: An analysis of repeated biopsies following cardiac transplantation. Stats Med 2:33, 1983

85. Tazelaar H, Billingham ME: The surgical pathology of hypertrophic cardiomyopathy. Arch Pathol Lab 3:257, 1987

86. Timmin CG, Gordon S, Baron RH, Brough AJ: Percutaneous myocardial biopsy. Am Heart J 70:499, 1965

87. Torp A: Endomyocardial biopsy. Scand J Thorac Cardiovasc Surg 7:253, 1973

88. Torti F, Bristow M, Hawes A, et al: Reduced cardiotoxicity of Doxorubicin delivered on a weekly schedule: Assessment by endomyocardial biopsy. Ann Intern Med 99:745, 1983

89. Urie PM, Billingham ME: Ultrastructural features of familial cardiomyopathy. Am J Cardiol 62:325, 1988

90. Weinberg M, Egbert HF, Lynfield J: Diagnostic biopsy of the pericardium and myocardium. Arch Surg 76:825, 1958

91. Weintraub D, Masek M, Billingham ME: Lymphocyte subpopulations in cyclosporine-related human cardiac rejection. Heart Transpl 4(2):213, 1985

92. Yarom R, Maunder CA, Oakley CM: Electron microscopic microanalysis of localized element concentrations in human cardiomyopathies: a pilot study. Human Pathol 9:531, 1978

40

Pathology of Mechanical Heart Valve Prostheses and Vascular Grafts Made of Artificial Materials

Malcolm D. Silver
Gregory J. Wilson

The modern aggressive medical and surgical approaches used to investigate and treat congenital and acquired cardiovascular and acquired cardiovascular disease have seen an increasing number and variety of prostheses inserted into the cardiovascular system. Each is the end result of much imagination and thought and is manufactured, to exacting specifications, of materials thought most suitable. Often, such devices function eminently, but each is a foreign body that the human organism, after implantation, may treat in a manner not predicted from prior testing on the bench or in animals; flaws in design or an unfortunate choice of material for manufacture may become obvious. Alternatively, host–prosthesis interactions may be bizarre, with adverse effects. If these effects are severe, use of a prosthesis may be abandoned, or the prosthesis may have to be redesigned or manufactured of different materials. Such problems are responsible, in part, for the pathology associated with the use of prostheses.

Their recognition in the past, with an appropriate response by a manufacturer aided by technologic advances, has produced a continuing improvement in these devices with the objective and technologic challenge being to achieve maximal function and durability without adverse effects.

Historically, the use of human or animal tissue often provided the first means of correcting a cardiovascular lesion; consequently, and as technology advanced, suitable prostheses of manufactured materials and in a range of sizes became available and are preferred.

The earliest prostheses were tested by insertion in humans and, in some instances, unexpected problems caused disasters. Nowadays, if we consider heart valve prostheses (HVPs), governmental regulations demand extensive animal and laboratory testing, including accelerated bench tests, before a new HVP is licensed for insertion. Once completed, the tests define a valve that has promising characteristics and performance. Clinical trials are still required because such tests do not, for example, accurately mimic physiologic conditions or reflect the hundreds of physical positions a human may assume in any day; nor is the testing fluid blood. In vivo, problems associated with a HVP may not be those demonstrated by accelerated bench testing; alternatively, those revealed by testing may evolve at a faster rates in humans. Such testing has undoubtedly aided HVP development, but it is expensive.

Gersh and colleagues[76] call for guidelines that would clarify procedures used to evaluate HVP before market release and standardize initial clinical evaluation. They believe that this approach would facilitate introduction of new models and aid clinicians making comparisons among HVPs. Rahimtoola[177] and Grunkemeier and Rahimtoola[85] discuss lessons learned about determinants of the results of valvular surgery, whereas Grunkemeier and Starr[86] emphasize pitfalls in the statistical analysis of heart valve prostheses.

While pathologic changes associated with prosthetic devices may be due in part to inherent problems, a range of other lesions are found associated with them. They are produced during preoperative investigation, during insertion, or subsequently. Such lesions either are located in the immediate vicinity of an implant or are obvious in the adjacent tissues or distal organs. They may be acute or evolve as the prosthesis or patient ages and cause or contribute to a patient's death, cause morbidity, or produce no symptoms. Some are likely to occur in any patient, irrespective of the type of prosthesis inserted, whereas others are uniquely associated with a particular implant because of problems with its design or the materials used in its manufacture. Then, too, different patients deal with their prostheses differently.

Therefore, when examining a surgically excised implant or a patient bearing one at autopsy, a pathologist must be able to (1) identify the particular device inserted, (2) examine it properly, and (3) make careful clinical path-

ologic correlations. Then the significance of any lesion may be properly assessed. Only in this manner will the pathology of prostheses be fully revealed. With this knowledge, better and safer means of preoperative diagnosis, methods of insertion, and improvements in the implants themselves evolve.

Pathologists have had, and continue to have, an important role in the evolution of prostheses. Again considering HVP, pathologists will detect prosthetic valve problems or dysfunction or provide complementary evidence of problems defined by other diagnostic methods. The interest of individual pathologists has enabled in-depth analyses, while collaborative studies with colleagues in other scientific disciplines have advanced knowledge. Even without an individual interest the referral of a prosthesis with a defect, or of one that has functioned a long time, to an interested colleague or to the manufacturer may allow detailed examination, using a wide variety of techniques. Alternatively, it could permit biomechanical theories to be tested or defined and so help improve design.[154] Please keep this in mind when next examining a prosthetic device.

This chapter discusses complications associated with the insertion of mechanical heart valves and some vascular grafts. Further discussion of other prostheses, devices, and grafts used in the current treatment of cardiovascular diseases and of pathology associated with them is found in Chs. 38, 41, 42, 44, and 45.

MECHANICAL HEART VALVE PROSTHESES

Prosthetic heart valves currently in use are constructed of either human or animal tissue (tissue valves) or have all components manufactured of nonbiologic material (nontissue or mechanical valves). Thus, an individual valve may be said to belong to one of two families.

Tissue HVPs are usually like native semilunar ones and have three cusps that allow central flow through their lumens. Schoen describes them and the pathology associated with them in Chapter 41. Currently, they are of three types, porcine, pericardial, and homograft.[84]

Mechanical HVPs, discussed in this chapter, have flow characteristics that also allow their separation into three types: (1) those in which blood passing through the valve orifice hits a centrally placed occluder and must swirl around it (lateral flow prostheses); (2) those in which a tilting occluder permits a semicentral flow; and (3) those of hinged, bileaflet construction and a greater degree of central flow.[84]

Ideal Characteristics

The ideal characteristics of an aortic HVP, enumerated by Harken and colleagues in 1962,[94] early in the era of heart valve prosthesis insertion, may be applied to any HVP. They are that a prosthesis must

1. Be chemically inert and not damage blood elements
2. Offer no resistance to physiologic flow
3. Close properly and remain closed during the appropriate phase of the cardiac cycle
4. Have lasting physical and geometric features
5. Be capable of permanent fixation
6. Be technically practical to insert at a physiologic site
7. Not annoy the patient
8. Not propagate emboli

To these caveats should be added the proviso that an HVP should be inexpensive, in view of the frequency of valvular heart disease in third world countries and the state of their economies. Angell and colleagues[67] commented on the need for

1. Durability
2. Central flow characteristics without a transvalvular gradient

3. The absence of a host reaction deleterious to the prosthesis
4. Nonthrombogenicity, without a need for anticoagulants
5. A resistance to infection

Another consideration is that a patient have only one HVP inserted in a lifetime. The insertion of a HVP induces both morbidity and mortality. For example, in a single-valve replacement 2 to 5 percent of patients die during the operation or in the immediate postoperative period, usually, not from complications directly related to the inserted prosthesis, but from iatrogenic problems.[215] That mortality and associated morbidity are not reduced at subsequent operation.[48,134,234,251] Mortality associated with initial double- and triple-valve replacements is approximately double and triple the figures for single-valve replacement. Mitchell et al.[150] found that many *patient-related factors* were significant predictors of the probability of certain patient groups sustaining *valve-related complications*. They indicate that comparison of results of valve performance from different institutions may be misleading, unless patient populations are comparable.

Morphology

The variation in the design of HVPs aimed at achieving these objectives is truly amazing. Cohn,[51] Lefrak and Starr,[127] and Rose[203] provide brief histories of cardiac valve replacement. Illustrations of many models, some no longer in use, are found in the literature.[36,120,144,155,156,200,223,243] Some prostheses are illustrated in Figure 40–1.

In general, a mechanical HVP has a cufflike sewing ring of cloth that is used by the surgeon to attach the prosthesis to the valve annulus. The sewing ring presents both inflow and outflow surfaces to the blood and has an outer rim that forms the peripheral margin of the prosthesis and an inner ring that defines

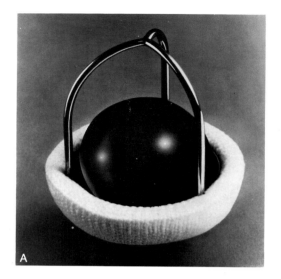

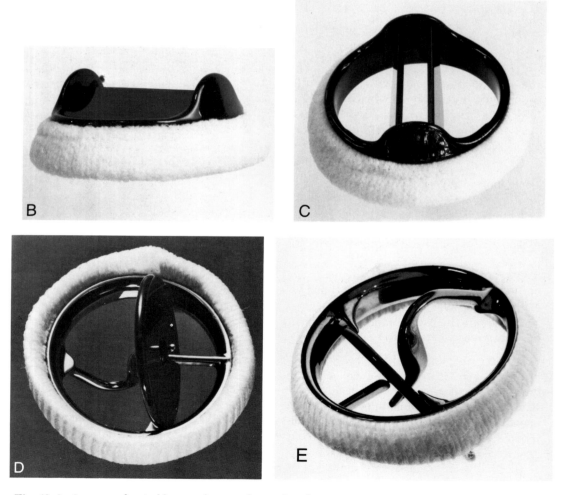

Fig. 40–1. Some mechanical heart valve prostheses that illustrate points in the text. (**A**) The De Bakey–Surgitool ball-valve prosthesis, showing most of its components covered with black pyrolytic carbon. (**B&C**) The Medtronic Hall prosthesis[101] and (**D&E**) the Omniscience prosthesis both have tilting disc occluders of a different design. (*Figure continues.*)

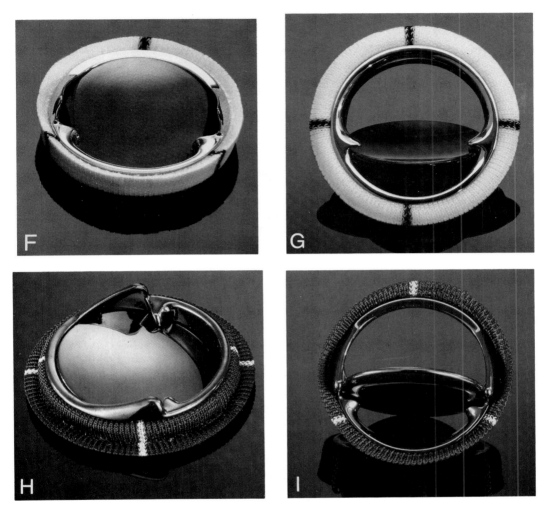

Fig. 40–1 (*Continued*). The Omnicarbon prosthesis also differs in design from the De Bakey–Surgitool ball-valve prosthesis. Note the curvilinear occluder of the Omniscience and Omnicarbon models and that all components of the Omnicarbon prostheses are covered by pyrolytic carbon. Compare these disc valves with the ball valve and note the reduction in cage size or its elimination in these prostheses. **(H&I)** The St. Jude Medical prosthesis has two small hinged leaflets that achieve occlusion. (Photographs courtesy of respective manufactures.)

the valve orifice. Prosthesis occlusion is achieved by an occluder or poppet, which may be a ball or a disc or have a hinged bi-leaflet construction (Fig. 40–1). An occluder may fill the lumen of an HVP or overlie it. In the former instance, occlusion may be at a ball occluder's equator or near its pole. Some disc occluders allow slight regurgitation

when they occlude a valve's orifice. The place of occlusion is called the seat.

Early HVP models had struts that projected from the inner ring on the outflow surface to form a cage that limited movement of the occluder contained within it (Fig. 40–2). In some early model prostheses, occluder movement warranted a second, smaller cage pro-

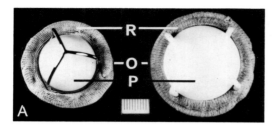 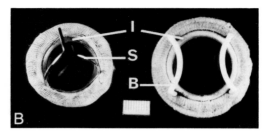

Fig. 40–2. Outflow surfaces of Starr-Edwards (1200) ball valve (*left*) and Beall (104) disc valve prostheses, illustrating the anatomy of HVPs in some older models. (**A**) Prostheses with occluders or poppets (P) in situ. (**B**) The occluders or poppets have been removed. Cloth sewing rings (R) have an outer rim (O) and an inner ring (I). The inner ring defines the valve orifice. Struts (S) form cage controlling poppet movement. Note different configuration of closed cages, especially struts forming horizontal bars (B) in disc prosthesis. Compare this structure with modern tilting disc prostheses illustrated in Fig. 40–1. Scale indicates 1 cm. (From Silver et al.,[223] with permission.)

jecting from the inflow surface of the inner ring. The cage of disc and bileaflet prostheses has been much reduced or eliminated completely. In them, one or more occluders pivot on an axis to permit opening and closing (Fig. 40–1).

Older model mechanical HVPs are composed of metal, cloth, and synthetic materials chosen for both their durability and their low thrombogenic activity. Prostheses introduced more recently are constructed such that the components that are exposed to blood are covered with black pyrolytic carbon. It is a very hard material, wears well, and has excellent thromboresistant properties.[26,27,98]

Identification

The need for a pathologist to identify a prosthesis has been stated. Several previous publications have provided methods of doing this, either by naked eye examination or radiologically.[27,49,144,145,155,200,223]

Most mechanical HVPs are identifiable by naked eye examination. Figures 40–3 and 40–4 provide keys for doing so. Some of these prostheses are no longer marketed (see Mehlman[144]), but a diminishing cohort of patients may bear them because they had one

inserted when the prostheses was "in fashion." Other prostheses listed may not be licensed for use in all countries.

Tissue prostheses, on the other hand, are hard to distinguish by the naked eye once they have been in situ some time and are best identified radiologically. Schoen (Ch. 41) indicates that this is also a good method for assessing the degree of calcification in such HVPs. Mehlman's 1988 article[144] is most useful for this, although, as Walley[245] points out the radiographic structure of the *low* profile Ionescu-Shiley valve, which has three thin metal semilunes in its base, was omitted from the illustrations in Mehlman's paper. A copy of Mehlman's article should be on hand in both surgical pathology and autopsy suites to aid HVP identification.

Examination

In examining an HVP in the heart at autopsy, radiographic studies of the body or of the prosthesis in situ may be indicated once the heart is excised. It is best to open the chamber or vessel proximal and distal to a HVP (not through the valve annulus). Then the prosthesis is viewed and its relationships to surrounding anatomic structures is assessed for evidence of tilting or disproportion; relation-

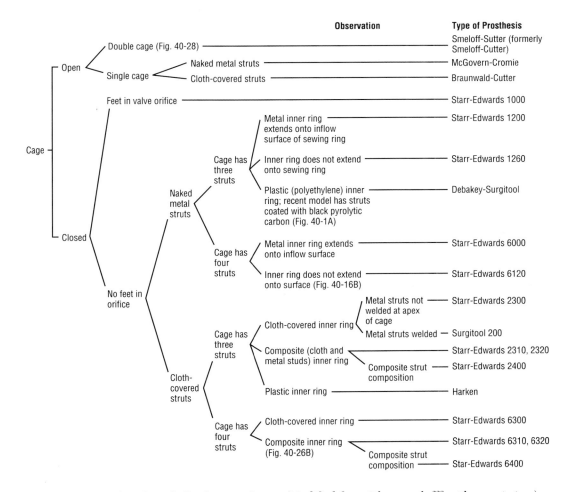

Fig. 40–3. Key for identifying ball valve prostheses. (Modified from Silver et al.,[223] with permission.)

ships to surgical wounds and sutures can be reviewed; vegetations attached to a HVP can be seen and sampled for microbiologic culture and histology; and both the function of valve components and the integrity of the prosthesis' attachment can be assessed. Subsequently, the annulus can be opened and the prosthesis removed by snipping sutures at its perimeter. Then the bed where the prosthesis lay and the annulus may be examined. Zeien and Klatt also discuss examination of a prosthesis at autopsy.[267]

Once in hand, whether in surgical pathology or the autopsy suite, the prosthesis must

be identified. This is important because some types of HVPs are prone to particular complications. Subsequent examination should be both detailed and thorough,[203,214,267] with a photographic record of abnormal findings. We recommend examining a prosthesis' surfaces with a dissecting microscope. Other sophisticated techniques may have to be used. Schoen[214] provides a useful chart for such analyses. Not all the techniques may be available to a pathologist, but colleagues interested in HVP or the manufacturer should be able to do them, or arrange for them to be done.

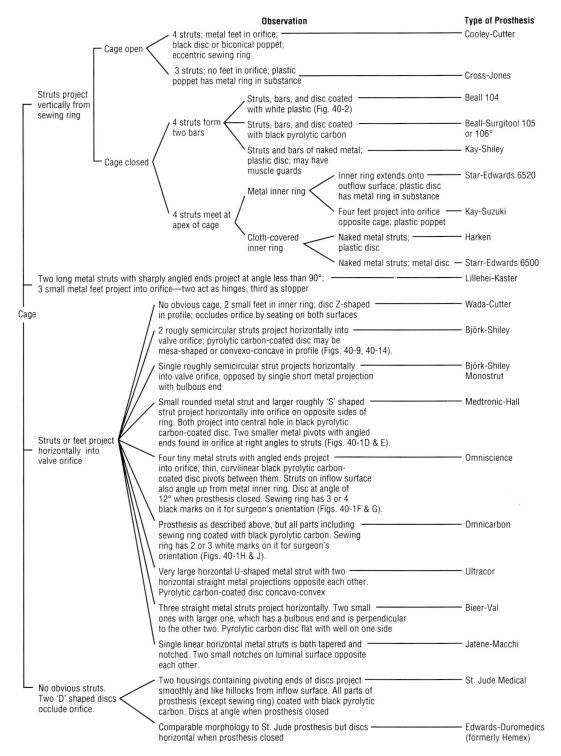

Fig. 40–4. Key for identifying disc valve prostheses. Beall model 106 has same appearance as 105 but struts are thicker. (Modified from Silver et al.,[223] with permission.)

Each mechanical HVP bears a serial number that identifies it. The number is usually found on the base of the metal stent, under the sewing ring.

Clinical Pathologic Correlations

To make good and useful clinical pathologic correlations, it is essential to understand the patient's history and the operative procedure that was done (see subsequent discussion). Discussions with clinical colleagues, either about a specific case or at regular rounds, will help prevent wrong conclusions being drawn from pathologic findings. Other authors stress this point.[203,220,267]

Insertion and Sequelae

The insertion of an HVP is now a common event. In the past, a patient received the prosthesis that a surgeon had invented, or thought was the best then available. Now, when selecting an HVP for a particular patient, choice is governed by many considerations. They include such things as the patient's cardiac anatomy, medical history, age, life-style, and access to medical care. In addition, perceived advantages and disadvantages of particular prostheses related to orifice size, flow characteristics through and across the valve, thrombogenesis, and infection control govern selection.[67,127,156,248] The objective is to obtain the best match between patient and prosthesis. Magilligan[138] provides key references for this topic.

Insertion of an HVP exposes a patient to a series of hazards associated with placing a foreign body in the bloodstream. For subsequent discussion, they are grouped as (1) those related to investigative procedures; (2) those arising from surgery and associated activities; and (3) those associated with the prosthesis itself, either because of its design or structure or because of an interaction between the HVP and body tissues.

Complications associated with HVPs can be classified into those that occur within a month of insertion (early complications) or those that occur after that (late complications). Either group may induce death, morbidity, or cause no clinical symptoms. Nowadays, these problems are infrequent, with a diminution in risk becoming apparent in the more than 30 years that HVPs have been used. The reduction in fatal and other complications is related both to increasing sophistication in diagnostic methods and to improvements in the preoperative, intraoperative, and postoperative management of patients. Also, improved valve design has eliminated some complications so that they now have only historic interest, while markedly reducing the likelihood of others occurring.

Pathology of Acute Complications

The successful replacement of a diseased heart valve with a prosthesis demands

1. A precise diagnosis
2. Appropriate medical and psychological preparation of the patient for the surgical procedure
3. Meticulous attention to anesthetic, perfusion and surgical techniques
4. Exacting postoperative care

A pathologist, examining at autopsy a patient who died in the early postoperative period or within a month of prosthesis insertion, will likely find morphologic changes to explain the patient's death in the majority of cases (85 to 95 percent). However, no satisfactory morphologic explanation may be forthcoming, despite an exacting examination. For example, Antunes et al.[8] reported intermittent aortic valve regurgitation in 4 of 160 Hall-Kaster prostheses following their insertion. The authors related valve dysfunction to the position of the prostheses and occluder in the open position and the latter's relation to the axis of blood flow. Each case was dealt with in the operating room. Sometimes, a single lesion

Table 40–1. Acute Complications Associated with Insertion of Heart Valve Prostheses (Lesions with Morphological Equivalents)

Due to error in preoperative diagnosis

Due to error in operative technique
    Related to anesthetic or extracorporeal perfusion
    Related to surgical technique and affecting prosthesis
        Dehiscence
        Disproportion
        Angulation
        Fixation
        Misplaced sutures
    Related to surgical technique and affecting pump (heart)
        Myocardial injury
            Caused by emboli
            Caused by iatrogenic damage of coronary arteries
            Due to direct traumatic damage
            Due to poor or absent perfusion during cardiopulmonary bypass
    Related to surgical technique and affecting other structures
        Annular and periannular injuries
        Vessels
        Conducting system

Due to problems inherent in heart valve prostheses
    Thrombus formation (with related thromboemboli)
    Infection
    Problems with prosthesis design/structure

Due to postoperative complications
    Related to surgery and affecting organs other than heart
    General
    Unique to open heart surgery

Unrelated to operative procedure

---

will have caused death, but more frequently a combination of events will have occurred. In such an examination one might ask whether the death was (1) due to an error in diagnosis or therapy preoperatively; (2) due to an operative complication related to anesthetic, perfusion, or surgical technique; (3) due to inherent problems with a prosthesis; (4) a result of postoperative complications; or (5) un-

related to the operative procedure (Table 40–1). In the last instance, an unrelated problem may have preceded surgery or developed subsequent to it.

To provide satisfactory answers to these questions, the pathologist must be aware of the techniques and procedures used by cardiologists, anesthetists, perfusionists, and surgeons before, during, or after cardiac surgery and of the pathophysiology that these may induce. An understanding of the patient's clinical behavior before death may indicate that the main problem resided in a particular organ, or it may give clues as to possible mechanisms of death. The pathologist must know that a complication may not be recognized clinically and cause death directly or, having been recognized and corrected during surgery, still cause death by the pathophysiology induced before it was corrected. Thus, very careful clinicopathologic correlations must be made before assigning a cause of death. As indicated earlier, this is best done by discussing each case with clinical colleagues so that a cause of death obvious to the clinician but possibly not to the pathologist is not missed and so that autopsy findings are not misinterpreted. Also, such discussions or presentations are of value in teaching all concerned and in providing a stimulus for research.

Pathologic studies of the causes of acute fatal complications following heart valve replacement are found in the literature.[52,63,107,113,116,163,189,190,193,202,203,214,267] A comparison between them is difficult because different methods of classifying the causes of death were used by the authors, operative techniques differed, different prostheses were inserted, and the studies were reported in different years. Also, in the interim between reports, new techniques were adopted in cardiovascular surgery that helped to minimize or eliminate some complications and to change mortality figures. Thus, in subsequent discussions no attempt will be made, except in general terms, to indicate the frequency of complications found at autopsy.

Complications Due to Errors in Preoperative Diagnoses

The frequency of this type of problem has diminished as the level of sophistication in diagnostic techniques has risen. Such problems are now extremely rare. Nevertheless, an overlooked or misdiagnosed lesion may assume a sinister, possibly lethal role once one that is recognized has been treated. The importance of a detailed and complete autopsy examination cannot be overemphasized.

Intraoperative Deaths/ Complications

Another method of reviewing causes of early deaths following HVP is to ask whether the death was related to (1) the anesthetic, (2) perfusion problems, (3) the operative procedure, (4) pump or heart failure, (5) the prosthesis, or (6) events not associated with the operative procedure.

Early deaths, especially those occurring in the first 2 weeks after HVP insertion, should be regarded as iatrogenic until proven otherwise. Problems directly attributable to the prosthesis are uncommon at this juncture, as are those resulting from unrelated diseases.[215]

Anesthetic/Perfusion Problems

Very often the lethal effects of complications of anesthetic or perfusion techniques produce no morphologic changes obvious to a pathologist. However, the pathologist's clinical colleagues, monitoring the patient in the operating room, are often aware of the cause of death. This re-emphasizes the need for careful clinicopathologic correlations.

Anesthetic Deaths. Operative deaths caused by anesthetic problems are rare. They are beyond the scope of this chapter; refer to Orkin and Cooperman.[168]

Deaths Related to Perfusion Techniques. Current perfusion techniques involve body cooling, the use of a heart-lung machine to provide dilute oxygenated blood to the body, and cold cardioplegic solutions.

"Priming the pump" for perfusion demands large quantities of blood. With this comes a risk of a mismatched blood transfusion, the development of isoimmunization that may cause hemolysis at subsequent surgical procedures, and a risk of transmitting bacterial or viral diseases to the patient. Again, any patient subjected to a blood transfusion faces these risks. Nevertheless, this led to the development of blood substitutes as a priming fluid for the pump, which was stimulated by a need to operate on patients whose religious beliefs prohibited blood transfusion. At most centers, a "bloodless" prime is now preferred to whole blood.

In general, both morbidity and mortality rise when perfusion exceeds 2 hours and increases markedly when pump time exceeds 3 to 4 hours.[249] Cardioplegic arrest up to 60 minutes is usually well tolerated but longer periods are likely to induce myocardial damage.[249]

With the exception of problems engendered by hypoperfusion of the myocardium (see later in this section), fatal complications associated with perfusion are uncommon. Most lethal or nonlethal complications result from hemorrhage or the formation of emboli.

Hemorrhage. Hemorrhage may occur at cannulation sites. It can be a result of the damage, depletion or activation of blood components during perfusion, or from insufficient neutralization of heparin with protamine sulfate at the end of a procedure. Such hemorrhage, unlike that associated with a leaking surgical wound that is focal, is usually diffuse and may be found in areas of surgical dissection, particularly if adhesions have been separated. Dobell and Jain[65] discuss catastrophic hemorrhage occurring at second sternotomy procedures and offer advice on management. Possibly, the normally negative pressure in the thoracic cavity encourages a continuation of venous bleeding in the chest. In the latter context it must be remembered that a pericardial drainage tube is not necessarily a guarantee against cardiac tamponade developing if the patient bleeds into the pericardium. However, a hemorrhage may affect tissues elsewhere in the body. In some series hemorrhage was a common cause of acute death following HVP replacement.[52,113,116,189,193]

Activation of plasma and cellular factors during perfusion with a resultant release of chemical substances may induce other pathology, for example, shock lung.[123] One notes that children who have deep hypothemia during open heart surgery may develop multifocal areas of subcutaneous fat necrosis.[77]

Emboli.   Emboli of the following types can occur during open heart surgery: air,[74] bone marrow[188] (Fig. 14–10), or fat derived from pericardial suction; calcium (Fig. 14–8), atheromatous material, talc, silicone particles, platelets or other debris derived from the perfusion apparatus; or other foreign material[237] (Fig. 14–9). Fat emboli, in particular, are commonly found in the brain (see also Ch. 28) and kidney if fat stains of frozen sections are prepared. They are rarely fatal. However, they and other cerebral emboli may cause morbidity and, if massive, death. Coronary artery emboli may also induce myocardial injury or death (see also Ch. 14).

Emboli arising from the perfusion apparatus have been much reduced by using efficient filters. Occasionally, they develop during cannulation procedures.

Deaths Related to Operative Techniques

Most preventable surgical complications capable of causing death produce morphologic changes that are usually obvious. They may be manifested clinically by hemorrhage, heart failure and/or low-output syndrome, or prosthesis dysfunction. These complications cause the patient's death in the operating room or subsequently, often with a low-output syndrome.

Such complications may occur with any HVP insertion. They can be related to (1) the manner in which a prosthesis is inserted and, in particular, to (a) its lie or disproportion, (b)

annular injury, or (c) problems with native valve remnants and long or misplaced sutures, or (d) prosthesis dehiscence; (2) myocardial injury; (3) vascular injury and hemorrhage; (4) damage to the conducting system and, uncommonly, to (5) general surgical complications; (6) reaction between prosthesis and host tissues; or to (7) inherent problems with an HVP.

Prosthesis Lie and Disproportion

Rarely, an HVP may not be positioned ideally, that is, it has an abnormal lie. This is likely if the annulus is heavily calcified or distorted by previous surgery. The resultant angulation may interfere with the HVP's function and cause a low-output syndrome postoperatively. It is important to study the prosthesis' position and the movements of its components at autopsy because resultant functional disturbances may be transient rather than permanent. Malfunction often encourages thrombus formation. A prosthesis may be angled on insertion or placed in a position proximal or distal to an ideal one. An acute dehiscence can also angle a prosthesis. I (M.D.S.) have seen one inserted upside down; it did not function.

A badly positioned and angled mitral prosthesis may cause left ventricular outflow tract obstruction. This complication is more likely if the prosthesis has a high profile. Rarely, such an angled prosthesis can interfere with the function of another in the aortic area. Furthermore, an angled aortic prosthesis can obstruct the coronary artery ostia. If a patient survives the acute insult caused by dysfunction, persistence of the problem can induce changes such as those described next under disproportion.

Disproportion.   Disproportion is caused by too large a prosthesis projecting into too small a distal chamber or vessel; poppet movement is usually interfered with and prosthesis dysfunction results. This may be manifested by a low-output syndrome or, if the prosthesis is in the aortic area, by severe hemolysis.[182]

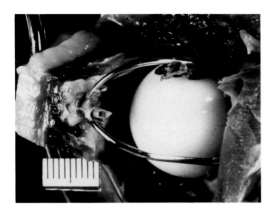

Fig. 40–5. Starr-Edwards prosthesis in tricuspid area with disproportion causing the incorporation of the apex of the cage and third strut into the right ventricular wall. This interfered with poppet movement and led to intractable right heart valve. The patient died 8 days after surgery. Note the thrombus extending along the strut. (Scale indicates 1 cm.)

Disproportion caused in this manner may induce:

1. Ulceration of the chamber or vessel wall by part of the prosthesis,[109,126,221] which may
   a. Perforate it
   b. Become incorporated into the wall of the chamber (Fig. 40–5) or vessel
   c. Cause a fatal arrhythmia
   Alternatively, the ulcer may provide a site of thrombus formation with subsequent thromboembolism.
2. Left ventricular outflow tract obstruction.[116,193]
3. Stretching and angulation of the elastic aorta about a prosthesis' cage so that it causes a relative stenosis of the ascending aorta that interferes with poppet movement.[163,175,189,195,218]

A prosthesis may be relatively large because of its configuration—for example, the relative length of the cage of a ball valve prosthesis (Fig. 40–5) or of the struts of a Lillehei Kaster prosthesis—compared to that of a low-profile disc-type prosthesis; it may also cause

disproportion. Nevertheless, disproportion occurs with disc valves.[188,189] Alternatively, disproportion may develop because of a peculiar configuration of the left ventricular septal wall—the so-called sigmoid septum or in hypertrophic cardiomyopathy.[81] Cardiac massage, too, can induce left ventricular laceration if a patient bears a stented prosthesis.[257]

At autopsy, disproportion can only be assessed by careful examination of the prosthesis in situ. The variation in frequency, from one published series to another, with which disproportion is recorded as a cause of early death following prosthesis insertion, mirrors the care expended in searching for the complication. The possibility of a mitral valve prosthesis causing left ventricular outflow tract obstruction should be assessed carefully at autopsy.

Nowadays, a surgeon will likely recognize severe disproportion in the operating room and replace the prosthesis. Alternatively, a cloth gusset may be inserted into the aortic wall to overcome disproportion in the aortic valve area[158,175] (Fig. 40–6). Such adaptive surgery will necessarily change morphologic findings at autopsy. Minor forms of disproportion may be seen as a late change in the form of endocardial thickening (Fig. 40–7; see Fig. 40–22) or as an indentation in the endocardium or aortic wall corresponding in location to parts of the prosthesis' cage.

The close proximity of aortic and mitral valve prostheses can allow components of one to impinge on the other with a similar result, despite whether disproportion exists. Interference is particularly likely with angulation or if a very large prosthesis is placed in the mitral area. When they were used, open-caged prostheses become fixed or tethered when the free end of their struts "engaged" the ventricular myocardium.[109,119]

Acute Annular Injury

Acute annular injury may occur to the aortic annulus, but more often occurs in the

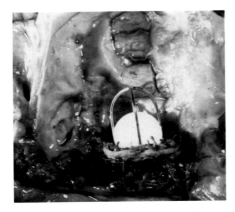

Fig. 40–6. Massive dehiscence of Starr-Edwards prosthesis in aorta associated with infectious endocarditis caused by *Staphylococcus aureus* with associated annular abscess. The patient died 3 weeks after prosthesis insertion. Note the cloth gusset in the ascending aorta used to increase its surface area.

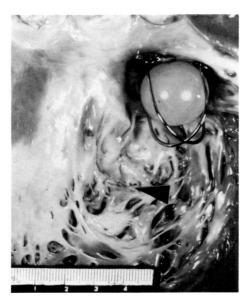

Fig. 40–7. Minor disproportion caused by the strut of the Starr-Edwards prosthesis impinging on and indenting endocardium on the septal wall of the left ventricle (lower marker), found at autopsy 10 years after prosthesis insertion. Note marked left ventricular endocardial thickening, thought to be caused by turbulence. (Scale indicates 4 cm.).

mitral annulus. Overall, it is uncommon.[31,137,190,204,236,260,265] It may occur as a result of too much tissue being removed when a valve is heavily calcified, or when annular tissues are unduly stretched over the ring of a large prosthesis. In all instances blood dissects through the weakened annular area, leading to a rupture with a massive intraoperative hemorrhage that is often fatal, if through the aortic annulus. However, a lesion in the mitral area may be repaired and the patient may survive. Alternatively, the hemorrhage can cause a false aneurysm that does not rupture or cause an epicardial hematoma subsequently rupturing in the early postoperative period.

Secondary complications arise if, during the emergency repair, coronary arteries are occluded by sutures. Comparable lesions occur when myocardial tears develop or are repaired (see below).

At autopsy the pathologist finds tissue disruption and hemorrhage in the area with or without formation of a large hematoma in the epicardial tissue and, possibly, signs of an attempted surgical repair (Fig. 40–8).

Problems Caused by Native Valve Remnants or Long or Misplaced Sutures

Sometimes, native valve remnants, which may be heavily calcified, stenose the lumen of a HVP or interfere with occluder movement by projecting into the cage of a ball valve or the lumen of a disc valve (Fig. 40–9).

Long sutures, suture knots, or remnants of native valves, especially chordae tendineae may reach the orifice of an HVP. There they can be jammed between the occluder and lumen margin of a disc valve and interfere with poppet movement either intermittently or permanently. Reports of such cases affecting a variety of disc valves located in mitral or aortic areas are found in the literature.[114,244,258] Folds of ventricular myocardium can produce the same effect. I (M.D.S.) have seen the free end of a generous suture

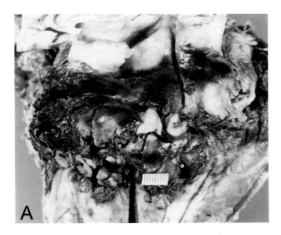

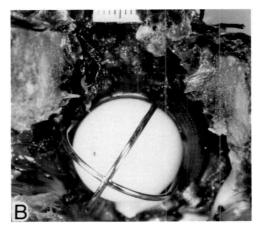

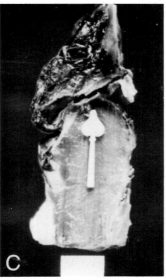

Fig. 40–8. Hematoma and numerous pledgetted sutures in the posterior atrioventricular groove marking a reparative attempt at (**A**) the site of acute annular injury with subsequent hemorrhagic dissection and fatal hemorrhage. (**B&C**) Section of posterior wall of left ventricle showing site of annular injury with acute hemorrhage dissecting through the area and into the epicardial fat (*upper part of photograph in Fig. B, arrow in Fig. C*). The prosthesis was removed to facilitate photography in Fig. C. A healed part of lesion of this type is illustrated in Fig. 40–23. (Scale indicates 1 cm.)

act as a nidus for thrombus formation and infection.

Sutures from an adjacent surgical wound or site or that encompass a generous amount of tissue sometimes impinge on adjacent structures and destroy or tether them; alternatively, they may stenose or occlude a vascular channel (see below). If part of a prosthesis becomes fixed by a suture in this manner, it may be affected and HVP dysfunction may result. Alternatively, a mass of several pledgetted sutures may stenose the orifice of a prosthesis.

Dehiscence

The acute dehiscence of a prosthesis from annular tissue, with the production of a large paravalvular leak leading to a patient's death in heart failure, is usually the result of sutures being inserted into annular tissue that provides an unsatisfactory anchor for them. Thus, the annulus may be the site of a pre-existing infection, myxomatous change, or heavy calcification. Surgeons are aware of these problems and take steps to overcome them, either by using pledgetted sutures or by inserting

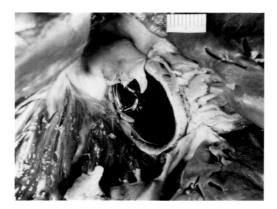

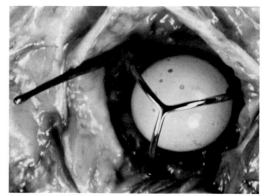

Fig. 40–9. Björk-Shiley prosthesis in mitral area showing remnant of anterior mitral valve leaflet, thickened by rheumatic disease, that caused acute prosthesis dysfunction by interfering with disc movement. The patient died 5 days after surgery. (Scale indicates 1 cm.)

Fig. 40–10. Small peripheral dehiscence (containing probe) associated with Starr-Edwards prosthesis in aortic areas. The patient died of bronchopneumonia 14 days after surgery.

more sutures into the area; as a result, major dehiscences due to these causes are infrequent.

Rarely, suture knots may slip and untie spontaneously or sutures are inserted with insufficient tension,[116] or a calcified nodule in the annulus interferes with their appropriate location. All these problems can cause a paravalvular leak.

An acute dehiscence may also be caused by an infection acquired at operation or immediately thereafter (Fig. 40–6).

Small dehiscences, 2 to 3 mm in diameter, that are due to tissue retraction during healing are a not uncommon finding if the patient dies of other causes in the first month following surgery (Fig. 40–10).

Dehiscences often increase hemolysis and may or may not be associated with an audible cardiac murmur. Small ones usually do not seriously affect cardiac function, but large ones do. In the latter instance a prominent regurgitant murmur is heard and a "dancing" or "rocking" HVP may be seen on fluoroscopy or echocardiography. Creation of the bypass channel allows thrombus formation and may foster endocarditis.

Myocardial Injury

Many patients undergoing heart valve replacement have heart failure that, at the time of operation, may or may not be controlled medically. In addition, a patient who is middle-aged or older may have had heart failure for many years and likely will have coronary atherosclerosis, often of severe degree. The latter may also affect cardiac function. A careful preoperative clinical assessment provides some measurements of cardiac function that help a clinician determine if valve replacement should be attempted and, if it is, its likely outcome. Furthermore, such assessments may dictate a need to modify surgical technique and, perhaps, for concomitant coronary artery bypass surgery or the use of ventricular assist devices. However, the predictive value of such assessments is still less than ideal. This not only indicates a need for further research in the area but also raises the question of earlier surgical intervention, perhaps before heart failure or coronary atherosclerosis is so advanced.

Clinically, the heart of a patient who sustains extensive myocardial injury during open heart surgery may not restart at the end of the procedure, be subject to repeated arrhythmias, or manifest a "low cardiac output syndrome." Often a combination of the two latter events occurs in patients to whom any of the following applies:

1. They cannot be weaned from the heart-lung machine
2. They must be replaced on the heart-lung machine
3. They can be weaned from cardiopulmonary bypass with difficulty, and they require large doses of vasopressor therapeutic agents or mechanical assistance to maintain an effective cardiac output

A low cardiac output syndrome is characterized by hypotension, cyanosis, and a low urinary output in the *presence* of a normal blood volume and in the *absence* of cardiac tamponade, a prosthetic valve problem, residual valvular lesions, or metabolic acidosis. It is the result of ineffective myocardial contraction and is usually associated with severe left ventricular damage. The syndrome mimics a shock-like state and causes hypoperfusion of distal organs. Thus, it may lead to:

1. Cerebral symptoms with findings at autopsy of eosinophilia of neurons, or frank necrosis of the brain or pituitary
2. An aggravation of myocardial ischemia with further subendocardial necrosis
3. Kidney failure with associated acute tubular necrosis
4. Ischemic bowel disease that in rare instances affects the small bowel or stomach
5. Liver malfunction with jaundice due to an apparent intrahepatic cholestasis
6. Pancreatitis and fat necrosis—sometimes severe
7. Adrenal cortical infarcts

The pathologist should search for all these changes in a patient who dies of a low-output syndrome.

Myocardial injury was once a very common finding in patients dying after open heart surgery.[52,61,100,153,183,203,215,227] Most commonly it was ischemic in origin and related to (1) embolic phenomena; (2) iatrogenic damage to either the coronary arteries or direct trauma to the myocardium itself; or (3) to poor or absent coronary artery or myocardial perfusion during cardiopulmonary bypass (which

was the most frequent cause). However, improved techniques of myocardial protection during cardiac surgery—in particular, use of cold cardioplegic solutions of various chemical compositions—have greatly reduced the incidence of myocardial injury, especially its most dreaded manifestations of "stone heart" and "circumferential hemorrhagic necrosis."

Caused by Emboli or Iatrogenic Damage to Coronary Arteries. Embolic episodes have been mentioned, and iatrogenic coronary artery damage will be discussed subsequently. They are both infrequent causes of major myocardial injury and death. However, the exact frequency with which emboli induce focal, nonfatal myocardial injury is uncertain.

Due to Direct Traumatic Damage. Very rarely the myocardium is ruptured during open heart surgery. This usually causes a massive hemorrhage, with death on the operating table, but it may lead to false aneurysm formation, with the aneurysm rupturing subsequently or persisting until the patient dies of some other condition.

Lesions comparable to those occurring in acute annular injury (discussed earlier) are seen on the posterior or lateral wall of the left ventricle following mitral valve replacement. They result from endocardial and myocardial tears. Some authors include acute annular injuries when discussing them.[58,120,193,203,236,260,265] In that circumstance, lesions are said to occur in the annular region at the midventricular wall related to the base of the papillary muscle or between those sites (types 1 and 2 of Treasure et al.[236] and type 3, defined by Miller et al.[149] [see discussion in Karlson et al.[120]]). Lesions at the midventricular wall are initiated by an excessive removal of papillary muscle tissue. The papillary muscle is pulled upward as it is being excised, and a volume of left ventricular wall is removed with it, thus weakening the wall and predisposing it to rupture. Ruptures between annulus and midventricular wall are usually associated with transverse endocardial tears caused by the tips of scissors during excision of the posterior mitral leaflet or chordae. However, a cardiotomy sucker, the prosthesis itself, or other mechanisms may be the culprit.[120,190a]

Due to Poor or Absent Perfusion During Cardiopulmonary Bypass. A patient may sustain a classical myocardial infarction with coagulation necrosis during the course of open heart surgery.[215] This is associated with a subsequent outpouring of polymorphonuclear leukocytes and heals by scarring. It is usually the result of myocardial ischemia, in the presence or absence of severe coronary atherosclerosis, but other causes—for example, an iatrogenic injury to a coronary vessel—must be excluded.

Another morphologic form of myocardial necrosis—contraction band change[13,153,183] [Baroldi (Ch. 17) prefers the term coagulative myocytolysis for this lesion.]—was an extremely common finding in the hearts of patients dying within the first 30 days of prosthesis insertion.[52,215] A pathologist could roughly correlate the extent of these lesions with a patient's postoperative course. They were particularly frequent and extensive when a patient had a low cardiac output syndrome or repeated bouts of cardiac arrythmia. Their frequency has diminished with the use of cold cardioplegia techniques for myocardial protection, but they are still found in the hearts of patients dying of pump failure after open heart surgery.[215]

Contraction band changes may affect fibers in any area of the myocardium but are particularly common in the subendocardium of the left ventricle. They may be focal, in which case sections of the left ventricular papillary muscles are a particularly useful site to demonstrate them, or affect extensive areas of the myocardium. In that case, they may indicate poor perfusion in a particular coronary bed.

Histologically, affected myocardial fibers are slightly more acidophilic than usual and have condensed cytoplasmic bands of various widths crossing them (see Figs. 17–5 through 17–7). The change is best seen by scanning hematoxylin and eosin-stained sections of the myocardium under reduced light when the anisotropism caused by the lesion is obvious, or by using Masson's trichrome or a phosphotungstic acid-hematoxylin stain. The lesions do not promote much, if any, polymorphonuclear leukocyte infiltrate but have mononuclear cells at their periphery. They may calcify very rapidly and heal by phagocytosis of the dead muscle fibers, leaving empty sarcolemmal sheaths (myocytolysis)[13,213] with subsequent condensation of the sheaths and fibrosis. Buja (Ch. 16) and Baroldi (Ch. 17) discuss these lesions in greater detail.

Contraction band myocardial damage is found associated with a distinct clinical syndrome called stone heart. Also, it is a common finding in circumferential hemorrhagic necrosis, which presents a distinct morphologic form of myocardial damage on gross examination. A gradation of damage, perhaps related to the duration or severity of anoxia or to subsequent events following the period of anoxia, seems likely in these conditions. Fortunately, in recent years both stone heart and circumferential hemorrhagic necrosis have become very uncommon.

Stone Heart. A "stone" or "muscle-bound" heart caused the patient's death in the operating room.[56] The condition was so named because the cardiac muscle developed a tetanic contraction during or at the end of the operative procedure and the affected heart did not respond to any of the various therapeutic regimens used in attempts to overcome it. The condition was likely in a patient who had severe aortic stenosis and marked left ventricular hypertrophy without severe coronary disease and developed if the period of coronary perfusion or anoxic cardiac arrest was prolonged.

At autopsy the left ventricular chamber of the stone heart was reduced to a slit by the hypertrophied contracted muscle (Fig. 40–11). In some patients the subaortic septal wall appeared to bulge into the cavity but did not cause functional subaortic stenosis. Also, the

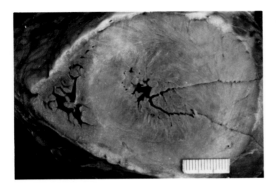

Fig. 40–11. Stone heart following replacement of calcified stenosed, congenitally bicuspid aortic valve. Note hypertrophied left ventricle clamped down onto the lumen in this view of the cut surface of both ventricles approximately two-thirds of the distance toward the apex. (Scale indicates 15 mm.)

deeper layers of the myocardium often appeared pale. Histologically, muscle fibers were hypertrophied and showed diffuse interstitial fibrosis,[56,254] and foci of contraction band necrosis were common.[14,130] Lie and Sun[130] examined the ultrastructural findings in two cases biopsied at surgery. They found widespread myofibrillar degeneration, interstitial hemorrhages, and prominent lymphedema, suggesting to them that a continuum existed between stone heart and circumferential hemorrhagic necrosis.

Stone hearts have been observed in adults, under both normothermic and hypothermic conditions,[261] and in neonates who have had congenital heart lesions corrected under hypothermic conditions (unpublished observations). Why this phenomenon should be observed clinically under hypothermic conditions when contraction band change can be prevented at low temperatures in experimental models is not known. However, it suggests that what is happening clinically is more complex than is modeled experimentally. This complication has become rarer with the widespread use of cold cardioplegic solutions in cardiac surgery. Again, see Chapter 16 and 17 for further discussion.

Circumferential Hemorrhagic Necrosis. This complication was another myocardial cause of early death; it is now rare. The majority of patients with this condition had a low cardiac output and died within the first 24 hours of surgery. The complication was found most often in those who had a stenosed aortic valve replaced or an aortic valve replacement combined with that of a second valve.[157]

Grossly and in transverse sections of the heart, the full-blown lesion presented a red, beefy, swollen zone of hemorrhagic muscle circling the left ventricular lumen (Fig. 40–12A). Its width was fairly uniform, and the change confined to the subendocardial third or two-thirds of the wall. The change extended from apex to base in the left ventricle and did not affect the right ventricle. Usually, the patient did not have severe coronary artery disease.

Gotlieb and colleagues[82] described developing and end stages of the lesion. Histologically (Fig. 40–12B), there was a variable combination of contraction band change and coagulation necrosis of muscle fibers in the affected area, with marked edema and interstitial hemorrhage. An exudate of polymorphonuclear leukocytes could be present, but was never marked when the patient survived less than 24 hours. The walls of small vessels might be necrotic, and fibrin or platelet thrombi might occlude their lumens. Healing was by scarring. In this condition ischemic injury is associated with reflow (see Chs. 16 and 17 for additional discussion).

Vascular Injuries

A vessel can be accidentally torn or perforated during insertion of cannulae, or a cannula itself can perforate a vessel[20,25,71,99,137,141,203,238,259] (see also Ch. 36).

A dissecting aneurysm may result if a perfusion cannula enters the media, either during insertion or through an atherosclerotic plaque while being passed along the vessel. In such cases the vessel shows no medial

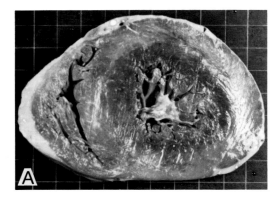

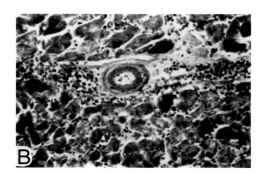

Fig. 40–12. (**A**) Circumferential hemorrhage necrosis shown in a heart slice from a man whose calcified, stenosed, congenitally bicuspid aortic valve was replaced by a Starr-Edwards prosthesis. A 35-minute period of anoxic cardiac arrest was used during the operation. Note the red, beefy muscle in the subendocardial part of the left ventricle. The lines on the background are each 1 cm apart. (**B**) Histology of the subendocardial muscle from this case showing hemorrhage, contraction bands, and fibrin deposit in small blood vessel. (H&E, × 16.)

changes that would predispose it to a dissection. Alternatively, an intimal tear at the site of a vascular wound or clamp site may permit blood to enter the media, with a resultant hemorrhagic dissection (Fig. 40–13). These dissections are likely in an area of poststenotic dilation in the ascending aorta or may occur in a hypertensive patient. In that case, the ascending aorta may show an increased amount of mucopolysaccharide material with or without muscle and elastic tissue changes in the media.

The ostia of coronary arteries may be damaged acutely during surgery, but the effects are not usually manifest until months or years later (see later discussion).

Fatal hemorrhages occur within the first postoperative month if a surgical wound in a vessel or a false aneurysm resulting from a hemorrhage subsequently ruptures. Alternatively, and rarely, a vascular wound may be the site of an infection or an infection may spread to it from an adjacent site (e.g., ascending aortic wound infected from endocarditis on an aortic prosthesis) and subsequently rupture (see also Ch. 36). Pressure necrosis caused by a clamp injury may also cause vessel rupture.

Sutures may impinge on a vessel and distort or stenose its lumen or act as a nidus for thrombus, which then is a source of distal emboli or occludes the vessel. Rarely, the circumflex coronary artery is occluded by a suture during mitral valve replacement.[60,240] In its course this vessel passes close to the mitral valve annulus, and, if the annulus is heavily calcified, a surgeon's need to extend sutures to achieve satisfactory attachment of a prosthesis may cause the vessel to be in-

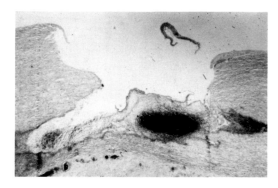

Fig. 40–13. Acute injury with localized dissection caused by an aortic clamp. (H&E × 6.) A healed lesion of this type is illustrated in Fig. 40–20.

corporated in a ligature. The result of the arterial occlusion depends, to some extent, on the anatomy of the artery.[15] In particular, if its left marginal branch arises early in the course of the artery, the occlusion may have little effect. However, if the occlusive ligature is placed on the vessel before it gives origin to the marginal branch, an acute myocardial infarction that affects the posteroseptal left ventricular wall near the base of the left ventricle usually results (Fig. 40–14). Roberts and colleagues[188] described an anomalous circumflex coronary artery arising from the right coronary artery that was compressed between two rigid frame-caged ball valve prostheses in mitral and aortic areas with resultant occlusion and necrosis of the lateral wall of the left ventricle.

Conducting System Injury

Hemorrhage in the atrioventricular node is a common finding after open heart surgery. It may not cause an arrythmia. The main cause of complete heart block is injury caused by sutures[62,73,75,107,160,203] (see also Ch. 37).

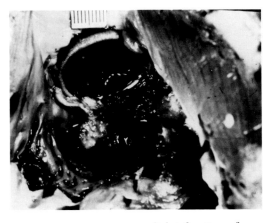

Fig. 40–14. Acute myocardial infarction of posterior left ventricular wall near the base of the heart resulting from an iatrogenic occlusion of the circumflex coronary artery during insection of a Beall disc valve prosthesis. (Scale indicates 1 cm.) A healed lesion of this type is illustrated in Fig. 40–24.

General Surgical Complications

Some general surgical complications affect organs other than the heart and are sometimes fatal. Some affect any patient following a surgical procedure and are uncommon; others, which are more frequent, may be directly related to the open heart surgery. In general, most are the result of either embolic phenomena, anoxia, or a combination of these processes.[1,37,70,92,100,102,105,115] Again, it should be remembered that some clinical conditions that kill patients do not necessarily produce morphologic equivalents—for example, metabolic acidosis or electrolyte imbalance.

Reath and colleagues[180] reviewed general surgical complications that developed among 3,200 patients who had cardiac surgery with cardiopulmonary bypass, only three had an HVP inserted. Overall, the incidence of complications was 0.8 percent. Gastrointestinal hemorrhage was the most frequent. Those complications seen were related to (1) an aggravation of a pre-existing disease, (2) hypoperfusion and/or the use of vasopressors, (3) iatrogenic factors, or (4) stress. Often, a combination of factors triggered a complication.

Postoperative Jaundice. The body of a patient dead of acute postoperative complications following heart valve replacement may be jaundiced. In these cases, both the clinician in life and the pathologist at autopsy must exclude such etiologic factors as (1) anesthesia, including halothane sensitivity; (2) increased pigment load following massive blood transfusion; (3) infection and septicemia; and (4) hemolysis; (5) the effects of drugs; (6) congestive heart failure; (7) extravasated blood; (8) underlying liver or gallbladder disease; (9) viral hepatitis, and (10) hepatic anoxia.

Hepatic anoxia is the likely cause of a mild jaundice that develops 1 to 12 days after operation and is characterized by bilirubinemia (mainly conjugated bilirubin) and bilirubinuria with a simultaneous elevation in serum alkaline phosphatase or glutamic oxaloacetic transaminase levels. The mechanism seems to involve an excretion defect producing intrahepatic cholestasis. A possible aggravating factor is the extra load of blood pigments associated with blood transfusions or extravasated blood that the liver must handle following open heart surgery. The condition usually resolves without inducing liver damage, but if the patient dies and death is usually caused by factors other than liver failure, the biliribin level in the blood usually exceeds 30 mg/100 ml before death. The histologic features are those of centrilobular congestion with, added to it, variable liver cell necrosis, polymorphonuclear leukocyte infiltrates, and erthrophagocytosis. A striking feature is bile, forming plugs in canaliculi and ductules.[163,171,207,230]

Postperfusion Lung. Following heart valve replacement, very few patients develop progressive pulmonary insufficiency or adult respiratory distress syndrome. However, this is likely if the period of extracorporeal circulation was prolonged.[19,110] The exact mechanism is obscure, but the lodgment of microaggregates of platelets and leukocytes in the pulmonary microcirculation with probable release of biologically active substances and obstructive effects on the microcirculation seem important factors. Secondary effects due to alteration in surfactant levels may complicate matters. The pulmonary lesions observed following extracorporeal circulation are similar to those found in adult respiratory distress syndrome caused by many other mechanisms[53,174,179,208] and, if prolonged before death, fibrosis of the lung may develop.[174,266] Pratt indicated the difficulty in determining those of the observed changes due to the original insult and those due to subsequent vigorous respiratory therapy.[174]

Postpericardotomy Syndrome. This is discussed in Chapter 22.

Complications Resulting from an Interaction Between Prosthesis and Host

Thrombus Formation. Thrombus formation is an inherent risk associated with placing a foreign body, such as an HVP, in the bloodstream. Very rarely, acute thrombus formation stenoses a prosthesis and contributes to a patient's death, especially if the patient suffers from a low cardiac output. Smaller thrombi may give rise to thromboemboli. The frequency of these complications as a cause of death seems to be diminishing with new model prostheses.

Sometimes, thrombus forms in the left atrium postoperatively and gives rise to emboli.[191] This may occur when protracted mitral valve stenosis is relieved and the dilated left atrium, which has had its wall replaced by fibrous tissue, is unable to function adequately. Alternatively, obstruction of left atrial emptying induced by other mechanisms or valve incompetence (Fig. 40–15) may aggravate thrombus formation.

Infection. A risk of infection at any operative wound is associated with the insertion of an HVP but, in practice, infection occurs rarely. Infections in an anterior chest wound may cause its dehiscence or lead to osteomyelitis or osteochrondritis of the sternum. The infection or its effects are usually obvious at autopsy.

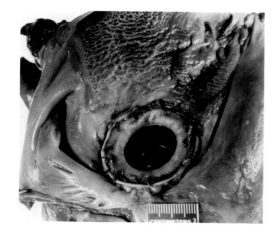

Fig. 40–15. Mural thrombus formed acutely in the left atrium following insertion 1 week earlier of a mitral Starr-Edwards prosthesis made incompetent by heavily calcified valve remnant interfering with poppet movement.

Infective endocarditis may develop soon after an HVP is inserted, either from such sources of if microorganisms are introduced at surgery. More often, infective endocarditis is a late complication of HVP insertion (see later discussion).

Infections on vascular wounds were mentioned earlier.

Inherent Problems with HVPs

Heart valve prostheses are manufactured to such demanding standards that acute complications, caused by abnormalities of a prosthesis itself and due to manufacture, are exquisitely rare. Nevertheless, prostheses may be damaged during sterilization or by manipulation during insertion and either not function normally or fail catastrophically if components are fractured or so strained that fracture is an inevitable consequence.[22,147]

Table 40–2. Late Complications Associated with Insertion of Heart Valve Prostheses (Lesions with Morphological Equivalents)

Complications common to all prostheses
    Related to prosthesis being located in bloodstream
        Thrombus formation/thromboemboli
        Infection
        Dehiscence
        Turbulence
        Hemolysis
    Caused during investigation or surgical treatment
        Foreign body emboli
        Vascular injury
        Disproportion
        Annular and myocardial injury
    Sudden death
Complications peculiar to particular prosthesis
    Related to anticoagulant therapy
    Related to prosthesis design and durability
Other complications

Late Complications

As a result of improved valve design and patient care, those bearing HVPs are living longer. Many will die of pathologic conditions that are not related to their prosthesis. Those who do develop late complications are likely to have problems directly related to the prosthesis itself because of host–prosthesis interactions or related to the design or structure of the HVP. Nevertheless, the pathologist may find the effects of pathology induced during investigation or surgery at autopsy. Again, late complications may cause no symptoms, morbidity, or the patient's death.

Many late complications encountered after a heart valve prosthesis has been in situ for more than a month are similar to early ones. Some late complications may be observed in any patient with an HVP, irrespective of its type, whereas others are associated with a particular prosthesis (see Table 40–2). As indicated above, the emphasis shifts, in the frequency of late compared with early complications, from iatrogenic lesions created during insertion to those that are (1) related

to a heart valve prosthesis being introduced in the bloodstream; (2) related to anticoagulant therapy; or (3) caused by poor prosthesis durability.

Late complications occur with all HVPs currently in use. Nevertheless, over the years since prostheses were first used clinically their frequency has been reduced considerably by improved prosthesis design and changes in the composition of their components. Indeed, some late complications have been eliminated completely and are mentioned only for historic interest. On the latter point, both clinician and pathologist must remember that when a surgical colleague is extolling the virtues of the most recently introduced valve prosthesis and is inserting it, many other patients, possibly thousands, bear an "old" model, prone to the complication(s) eliminated by the new one. Clinicians must carefully monitor the cohort of patients with the old prosthesis to detect the expected complications and determine the best time to replace the prosthesis. For patient monitoring, the value of a computerized patient registry cannot be overemphasized.[135]

Pathologists may encounter at autopsy an "old" prosthesis and its complications, long after its use has been discontinued and surgeons have come to regard both the prosthesis and its complications in a historic sense only. The reasons are that the rate of evolution of recognized changes in an old prosthesis may vary both with its site of insertion and from patient to patient.

Several studies deal with pathologic findings in patients dying of late complications.[63,106,117,163,188–190,194,195,202,203,214] The difficulties of comparison among these investigations, as far as determining the frequency of a particular complication at autopsy, are those described above in relation to acute complications. Also, findings at autopsy, because of their bias, may not be related to the frequency of complications in life. In attempts to determine the latter, clinicians have adapted actuarial methods. These are useful for both inter- and intragroup comparison providing a standard definition of an untoward event is accepted and used.[9] Unfortunately, to this point none has been adopted, except that of death. Also, actuarial comparisons of clinical events are based on clinical diagnosis not necessarily authenticated by pathologic ones. This is a further point of concern in interpreting results because of the recognized 8 to 10 percent variation between clinical diagnosis and pathologic finding at autopsy when "major" diagnoses are made and a 25 to 30 percent variation in "minor" diagnoses.[37,187] Again, in discussing late complication, only a broad indication of their frequency at autopsy is given. The inherent difficulties that exist in comparing the results of clinical studies have been mentioned previously.

Complications Common to All Prostheses

Complications Related to Prostheses Being Located in the Bloodstream (Prosthesis-Host Interactions)

Thrombus Formation/Thromboemboli. Thrombus deposition on the surfaces of the sewing ring of an HVP is both desirable and probably beneficial. With time, host tissue grows through and across it to cover the cloth. Histologic section reveals mature collagen associated with mononuclear cells and occasional giant cells. At the advancing edge recently deposited and/or organized thrombi are found. The gradual covering of HVP surfaces may be a factor in reducing thromboembolic episodes. However, deposition of thrombus or an associated pannus at other sites is undesirable and could be dangerous because of the location or the thrombus being a source of thromboemboli or a nidus or infection. Indeed, any thrombus found attached to an HVP at autopsy should be considered infected until proven otherwise.

Thrombi form on HVPs in areas where design allows relative stasis[264] or at component interfaces, especially where cloth and metal components meet.[59] They are a major problem associated with the use of mechanical HVPs and, although reduced in number in recent years as a result of improved valve design, they are the main cause of morbidity and mortality following valve replacement. Most modern prostheses engender thromboembolic rates of 1 to 4 percent per patient year.

The tendency to thrombosis associated with HVP increases if a patient has atrial fibrillation or if anticoagulant therapy is inadequate or in the "rebound" period following cessation of that therapy. A shortened platelet half-life, prosthetic valve dysfunction, and previous mitral valve operation all favour thromboembolic events. The risk of thrombosis is said to diminish slightly with the number of years a prosthesis has been in situ, for reasons given above, and then maintains a steady state. However, the point is controversial.

A thrombus may form soon after a prosthesis is inserted or at any time subsequently. Gradually, manufacturers altered prosthesis design to prevent stasis and moved to eliminate metal surfaces either by covering them with cloth (on the assumption that the cloth would become coated by tissue that was not thrombogenic) or by coating all surfaces with pyrolytic carbon, a very hard thromboresistant material[26,27,98] (see Fig. 40–1). The use of porous metal surfaces on HVPs is another step in this direction.[24] Modifications made to mechanical valves have reduced the frequency of thrombi and their clinical effects in patients bearing second- or third-generation prostheses, but it is still necessary for most bearing this type of HVP to receive anticoagulation therapy.

At autopsy, thrombi attached to older-style mechanical HVPs were usually small and found where the struts of the cage met the inner ring or at the junction of the cloth sewing ring and the metal inner ring (Fig. 40–16A & B). Rarely, they formed at the apex of the cage of ball valve prostheses in the mitral position (Fig. 40–16C & D). A thrombus could also spread across a valve orifice to stenose or occlude it (Fig. 40–16E & F)—this was a particular problem of disc valves—or onto or along the struts of a cage (Figs. 40–5, 40–16A–C) whether cloth covered or not and produce prosthesis dysfunction by inhibiting occluder movement ("poppet sticking," Fig. 40–16E) or by preventing it completely (poppet "entrapment" or "freezing," Fig. 40–16B). In this the poppet was trapped at an angle of about 45 degrees in some old disc valves.[63,174] Thrombi could also prevent the proper seating of a cage, cause a poppet to stick to the seat temporarily or permanently (Fig. 40–16B).

Thrombi are found much less often with valves coated with pyrolytic carbon. They may form at interfaces or in relationship to the pivot point of disc of leaflets. There they hinder occluder movement or entrap it.[3,54,165]

Seemingly, and unless the process is interrupted by embolization, a thrombus associated with a prosthesis that reaches a critical size becomes self-perpetuating because its bulk produces areas of stasis and leads to further thrombus accumulation. Thus, thrombi are not static. Those surrounding a valve orifice in older-model ball valves become organized and gradually encroach on the lumen. This process is a frequent cause of inflow tract obstruction long after an HVP is inserted.

Thromboembolic complications of such thrombi attached to HVPs are much more likely than those induced locally by the bulk of a thrombus itself. Their frequency seems to diminish after a mechanical HVP has been in place 12 months.[68] This is attributed to a gradual coating of the cloth sewing ring by connective tissue. Nevertheless thromboembolic complications associated with HVPs may occur at any time after insertion. In general, thromboemboli arise more frequently from mitral than aortic HVPs (4 per 100 patient-years versus 2 per 100 patient-years).[68]

Early-model ball valve prostheses, where cage and struts were not cloth-covered, had the highest incidence of thromboembolic complications clinically.[29,228] Fewer emboli were produced with clot-covered ball valve prostheses and tilting disc valves, in decreasing order.[22,35,45,206] In life, most thromboemboli must be tiny and cause no symptoms or only transient ones following lodgement. Unfortunately, many lodge in the brain.[58,71] Of thromboembolic complications that do cause symptoms, 40 to 50 percent produce severe or fatal effects, with many episodes (80 percent) presenting with cerebral symtpoms.[68] Coronary artery emboli, producing myocardial infarctions, are uncommon.[18]

Complications caused by valve thrombosis or associated thromboemboli evolve slowly or rapidly. They are recognized by the symptoms and signs that they evince. Valve function may be affected or symptoms *referred* to distal organs. If HVP function is affected, opening or closing sounds may change or murmurs may develop.[2,29,173]

Thrombotic vegetations attached to prostheses are recognizable by echocardiography or angiography. They may be removed from mechanical HVPs by fibrinolytic therapy,[27,235] or debridement.[167,237] Adequate anticoagulation is essential following lysis or debridement. However, if a thrombus is organized and forms a tough pannus stenosing or occluding the lumen, it cannot be removed by such methods and the prosthesis may have to be replaced.

Anticoagulant-Associated   Hemorrhage. Coumarin anticoagulants are the usual ther-

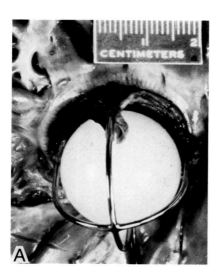

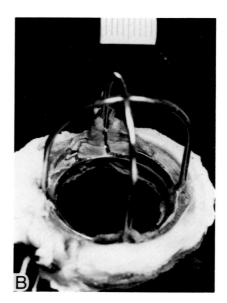

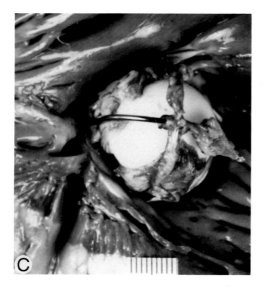

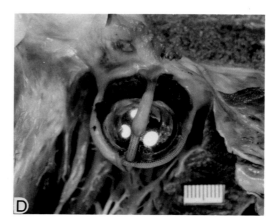

Fig. 40–16. Thrombi attached to an HVP and their effect on its function. (**A&B**) Deposits are visible at cloth-metal interfaces in older-model ball prostheses. As seen in Fig. B they extended onto the seat of the prosthesis, where they interfered with poppet seating and prosthesis occlusion. Figs. A and B show thrombi extending along the struts of the cage (see also Fig. 40–5) to (**C**) reach the cage apex. The accumulation seen in Figs. C and D represents thrombus on cloth-covered struts or the organized tissue that replaces it. Such accumulation may interfere with poppet movement (**D**) Thrombus at the apex of a cage caused the metal poppet to stick there permanently. Note that the sewing ring of this prothesis is completely covered by tissue. (Specimen in Fig. D courtesy of D. F. V. Brunsdon, M.D., Mississauga, Ontario.) (*Figure continues.*)

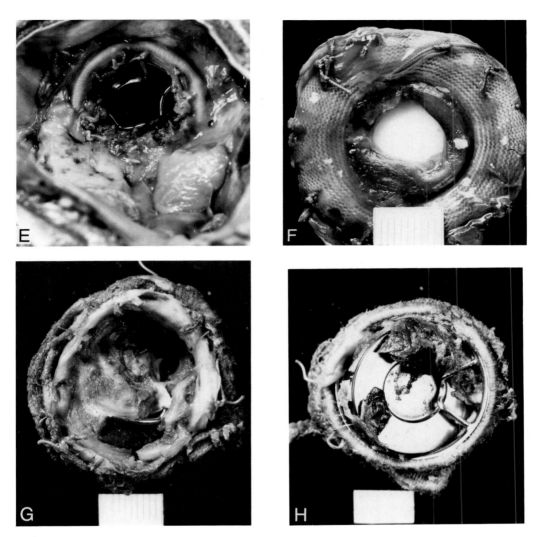

Fig. 40–16 (*Continued*). Thrombi may also stenose the valve lumen of (**E**) a disc prosthesis or (**F**) a ball valve prosthesis. Subsequent organization of the thrombus, seen in Fig. F, to form a pannus, is a common cause of late valve stenosis (see text). (Specimen in Fig. F courtesy of M. Provost, M.D., Sudbury, Ontario.) Thrombus build-up in an early model Björk-Shiley prothesis trapped the poppet at a 45° angle, rendering it immobile ("discentrapment"). Both (**G**) inflow and (**H**) outflow surfaces of the prothesis are illustrated.

apeutic means of maintaining long-term anticoagulation in patients with mechanical HVPs. The aim is to prolong the prothrombin time 2 to 2.5 times over control values. Some clinicians add antiplatelet drugs to the regimen.[46,125] Anticoagulation treatment promotes the risk of hemorrhage. Trauma and a markedly prolonged prothrombin time are the usual precursors of such an event. When a hemorrhage occurs, it is most likely to affect the central nervous system or either the genitourinary or gastrointestinal tract. Nonfatal hemorrhages have an instance of 0.5 to 6.3 per 100 patient-years, whereas the incidence of fatal bleeding is 0.1 to 0.2 per 100 patient-years. Most fatal episodes are the result of bleeding into the central nervous system.

Infective Endocarditis. Infective endocarditis is an infrequent but dreaded complication. Most centers report an incidence of 1 to 4 percent. No particular type of prosthesis is more prone to infection than another. However, those located in the aortic area seem more likely to be infected than those in mitral or tricuspid positions.

Thrombus-covered surfaces existing soon after an HVP is inserted, or a thrombus attached to a prosthesis subsequently, may act as a nidus for infection[250] (see also Ch. 23). Thus, infection of a prosthetic heart valve may be either an acute or a late complication (Fig. 40–17).

In acute infections, the infecting agent (usually a staphylococcus) is likely introduced during surgery, or an organism may have contaminated a prosthesis at insertion.[250] Late infective endocarditis developing months or years after a prosthesis is inserted may be caused by almost any microorganism. How-

ever, staphylococci and streptococci cause most cases, but yeasts or fungi may be the infective agent. Unfortunately, the risk of infection does not diminish with time. Schoen[214] cites a case that occurred after 22 years. The incidence is estimated at 0.2 to 0.5 percent per annum[95] affecting up to 3 percent of patients with prosthetic valves.[247]

Infected thrombotic vegetations on mechanical HVPs may stenose (Fig. 40–17A) or occlude the lumen or interfere with poppet function. Also, infection spreading from a prosthetic valve may cause an annular abscess[8] (Figs. 40–6, 40–17B), with subsequent valve dehiscence and paravalvular leak. The abscess may burrow into surrounding tissue and extend to the epicardium, aorta, or other heart chambers, causing sinuses or fistulae[69] (see also Ch. 23). Alternatively, it may destroy the conducting system.

Annular abscesses are more often a complication of an infection of an aortic prosthesis than one in the mitral area. Annular abscesses are difficult to treat either medically or surgically; but prosthetic valve endocarditis may be treated successfully and pathologists find

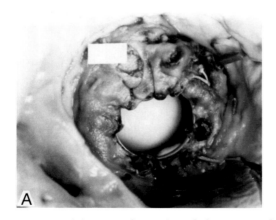 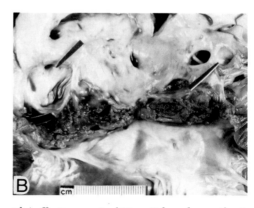

Fig. 40–17. (**A**) Acute infection (*Staphylococcus epidermidis*) affecting a mitral Starr-Edwards prosthesis. The infected vegetations cover the sewing ring and extend across the valve orifice to stenose it slightly. Spread of the infection to the annulus caused a small dehiscence (marker at upper right of photograph). (**B**) A healed aortitis with sinus formation. This followed a previous, successfully treated endocarditis (*Streptococcus viridans*) associated with an aortic Starr-Edwards prosthesis. The patient developed endocarditis (*Staph. aureus*) a second time with associated annular abscess and sinus formation (*lower marker defines ostium*). This occurred 2 years after the first attack and was fatal. The prosthesis was removed to reveal the annular abscess. (Scales indicate 1 cm.)

healed lesions at autopsy. Rarely, an aortic infection spreads to involve an aortotomy wound (Fig. 40–17B) (see also Ch. 36).

As already indicated, any thrombus attached to a heart valve prosthesis at autopsy or any thromboembolus removed surgically from a patient with a heart valve prosthesis should be regarded as infected until it is proved bland. Both microbiologic and histologic studies must be done. In the former, positive results are more likely if part of a vegetation is forwarded for culture, rather than a swab of its surface. Gram and Gomori methenamine-silver nitrate (GMS) stains are required histologically. A bacterial organism may not stain or may stain in an abberant fashion with Gram's but may be obvious in the GMS stain. The exact reason for this is not certain, but the results may indicate that the organisms are dead or, possibly, affected by previous antibiotic therapy.

The signs and symptoms of prosthetic valve endocarditis are a result of (1) microorganisms proliferating in the bloodstream, (2) local or distal complications of the disease, and (3) a loss of HVP function. A new cardiac murmur or manifestations of neurologic complications are the most frequent symptoms.[95,104,129,247] Indeed, fever is such a common presenting symptom that it should always raise the suspicion of infective endocarditis.[95] Blood cultures are usually positive if a patient has symptoms[94,104,247]; the bacteremia associated with prosthetic valve endocarditis is continuous. Several separate cultures should be collected because bacteremia may occur in a patient with an HVP, without the valve being infected. The recovery of microorganisms from a blood culture should raise the possibility of an infection, but the finding must be related to the patient's history and the likelihood of culture contamination. Isolation of similar microorganisms from two or more separate blood cultures makes contamination less likely.

Echocardiography may define vegetations, but interference by echoes arising from the prosthesis may make interpretation difficult.[39,66,95,247] The technique does help define complications of the infection, such as valve dehiscence or annular abscess.[39,66,95,247] Cinefluoroscopy may reveal valve instability resulting from dehiscence. Cardiac catheterization may be dangerous.

Treatment involves using the appropriate antibiotic(s) in cidal doses. Medical treatment cures some cases, but combined medical and surgical treatment is often required. Controversy surrounds aspects of surgical treatment. Indications for HVP replacement during active infective endocarditis include severe heart failure, persistent sepsis, recurrent emboli, or an unstable valve.[11,16] Relative indications include early disease and an associated periprosthetic leak.[11] The operative mortality is high.

Dehiscence. Many of the small dehiscences (less than 5 mm in diameter) found at the perimeter of a prosthesis at autopsy are caused by tissue retraction during healing (Fig. 40–10). They are not repaired surgically because they cause minor morbidity. Thus, they are are found as a late complication, sometimes associated with an endocardial "jet" lesion if the regurgitant stream through the dehiscence had been at high pressure. Theoretically, such jet lesions may act as a nidus for infection, but this occurs uncommonly.

If a large dehiscence is found as a late complication, it is likely to be of recent origin and an active infection of the prosthesis should be suspected. In such cases, appropriate microbiologic and histologic samples must be collected. The freedom of movement allowed a prosthesis by a major dehiscence explains its rocking movement seen by fluoroscopy. Such pivoting of an aortic valve prosthesis can affect the function of a native mitral valve.[232] If the dehiscence is large enough, it may permit a prosthesis to tilt across a valve orifice with resultant interference with poppet function.

Turbulence. Insertion of any HVP causes some degree of stenosis at its orifice.[34,176] The amount varies with prosthesis design and is reflected in the pressure gradient measurable across the orifice. Semicentral or central flow prostheses cause less turbulence than ones with lateral flow characteristics. Over the years, the turbulence induces fibromuscular thickening in the aortic intima or in the endocardium of a heart chamber distal to the prosthesis (Fig. 40–7). Usually, the thickening is of minor degree, but it may be aggravated in the presence of a concomitant paravalvular leak. Minor thickening causes no functional problems, but a markedly thickened endocardium may interfere with the nutrition of the subendocardial muscle layer. Roberts and Morrow[196] postulated that this is a factor aggravating heart failure. Also, coronary ostial stenosis has been thought due to aortic intimal thickening resulting from turbulence.[23,193]

Hemolysis. All prostheses cause intravascular hemolysis because of turbulence, the degree being affected by their design and structure. For example, covering the surfaces of an HVP with cloth aggravated hemolysis[29,226] while the least aggravation is caused by tilting-disc prostheses and those coated with pyrolytic carbon.[178,206,243] Also, hemolysis is aggravated if an associated paravalvular leak exists. Trauma and fragmentation of red cells during their passage through an HVP causes the hemolysis.

Disruption of the red blood cell (RBC) membrane occurs when its limited capacity to withstand strain is exceeded. This occurs, experimentally, at sheer stresses in excess of 3,000 dynes/cm.[4,162] Such stresses are commonly exceeded in the turbulent flow across an HVP orifice. Forces generated by the occluder striking its seat seem of importance too, because valves with absent poppets mounted in the aorta cause little hemolysis. Intravascular coagulation has no role in the hemolysis, as it does in microangiopathic hemolytic anemia, and the fibrinogen turnover rate is not increased in prosthetic valve hemolysis. The Coombs test may be positive occasionally, but is negative in most patients; this makes an immunologic component to RBC destruction, as suggested by Hjelm et al.[103] and Pirofsky et al,[172] an unlikely mechanism.

The RBC membrane has a remarkable capacity to reseal, with relatively little loss of free hemoglobin; it is through this mechanism that the helmet, triangle, and other bizarrely shaped RBCs that are seen on the blood smear are produced. These bizarrely shaped cells, although nonspecific, aid diagnosis. The damage to the RBCs diminishes their survival time in the circulation. Also, lactic dehydrogenase is released, and its level in the serum provides a rough guide to the severity of hemolysis.

The RBC fragments are trapped in their passage through the sinusoidal circulation of the spleen, and to a lesser extent in the liver, and are destroyed. Hemoglobin in them is processed in the normal manner by cells of the reticuloendothelial (RE) system with the release of iron, to be used over again in hemoglobin synthesis and with the eventual formation of bilirubin. The plasma protein transferrin (a β_1-globulin) carries iron from the surfaces of the cells of the RE system to developing RBCs. Transferring has *no* role in the handling of free hemoglobin.

Free hemoglobin is also released from RBC in mechanical hemolysis. There are two mechanisms for its clearance. First, haptoglobin—an α_2 globulin in the plasma—specifically binds free hemoglobin. The hemoglobin-haptoglobin complex is rapidly cleared by the RE system (mainly in the liver). Clearance occurs at a fixed rate of about 15 mg hemoglobin/100 ml plasma per hour and results in the degradation of both hemoglobin (which is desirable) and haptoglobin (which is not). Normal haptoglobin levels in serum range from 30 to 190 mg/100 ml. Decreased haptoglobin levels are reported in almost all conditions where hemolysis occurs.

When available haptoglobin is saturated with hemoglobin, unbound hemoglobin circulates. Second, unbound tetrameric hemoglobin in the blood freely dissociates into α,β dimers, the molecular weights of which are about 32,000, permitting glomerular filtration. Within limits, hemoglobin is reabsorbed by proximal renal tubular cells and, if plasma free hemoglobin is 30 mg/100 ml or less, no hemoglobin appears in the urine. Hemoglobin consists of three components: globin, porphyrin, and iron. The porphyrin and globin are rapidly catabolized in tubule cells with half-lives of less than 1 hour. The iron then finds its way into ferritin and hemosiderin, its two storage forms, in the tubule cells.

Ferritin is a complex molecule (molecular weight, 480,000) consisting of an iron core surrounded by 20 to 24 spherical polypeptide subunits. The apoferritin polypeptides are produced by the tubule cells. The ferritin iron is easily mobilized and, in fact, iron is transported out of tubule cells with a half-life of about 30 days. Because tubule cells are continually lost and may be demonstrated as siderocytes in the urine, patients with severe HVP hemolysis need iron replacement. Hemosiderin is an amorphous iron-containing granular substance formed by aggregation and polymerization of nonferritin iron with proteins. Hemosiderin granules are much larger than ferritin molecules and are easily seen by light microscopy when stained with Prussian blue (Fig. 40–18).

An appreciation of the pathophysiology by which iron is deposited in renal tubule cells provides a firm basis for understanding the methods used clinically to both diagnose and monitor hemolysis in a patient with an HVP.

Generally, patients compensate for hemolysis by increasing bone marrow function. A loss of compensation may herald a new complication of an HVP, for example, a paravalvular leak or degeneration of valve components.

Few patients with modern prostheses develop anemia. A minority (10 to 15 percent) of those bearing older prostheses do present with either a hemolytic or an iron-deficiency anemia. Treatment with supplementary iron by mouth may suffice, but blood transfusion or valve replacement may be indicated.

Renal hemosiderosis, with iron deposition in renal tubule cells but with no associated iron deposits in liver, spleen, or elsewhere, is the usual accompanying morphologic finding (see Fig. 40–18).[192,202] On the other hand, in the rare instance that an anemia develops and a patient requires repeated blood transfusions, iron deposits may be demonstrable in organs other than the kidney. An iron stain done on kidney tissue histologically should be routine in all patients coming to autopsy and bearing an HVP. Harrison and colleagues[96] drew attention to a higher frequency of cholelithiases in patients with HVPs.

Complications Caused During Investigation or Surgical Treatment

Lesions caused during preoperative investigation or surgical treatment may occur in any patient undergoing heart valve replacement. Alternatively, the lesion may be related to a particular surgical procedure used by an individual surgeon.

Foreign Body Emboli. We found foreign body emboli at autopsy in the hearts of 10 percent of patients dying with late complications but they were less frequent in other organs (unpublished observations). In the heart, such emboli may be attached to the endocardium between trabeculae carneae or be found in small intramyocardial blood vessels. Some are distinct emboli of calcium (Fig.

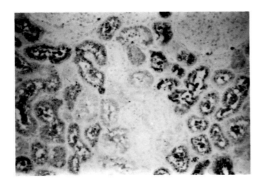

Fig. 40–18. Renal hemosiderosis in a patient with mitral and aortic Starr-Edwards prostheses in situ 5 years. A small paravalvular leak was associated with the aortic prosthesis. (Prussian blue stain, × 4.)

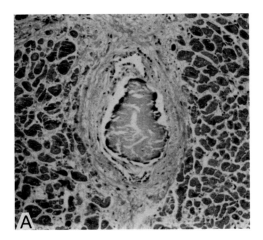 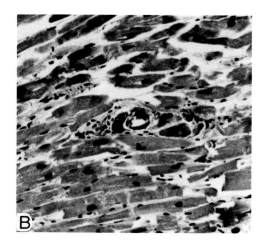

Fig. 40–19. (**A**) Calcium and (**B**) foreign body emboli following open heart surgery. Note the granuloma related to emboli in Fig. B. (H&E; Fig. A, × 16; Fig. B, × 25.)

40–19A) or of foreign material that may or may not be doubly refractile (see also Ch. 14). Many appear as granulomata related to and involving small intramyocardial coronary arteries but without an obvious associated foreign body (Fig. 40–19B).

The number of emboli and granulomata found may increase and become more widespread in distribution if a prosthesis wears during its lifetime, thus allowing component embolization.

Vascular Injury.   Vascular injuries usually cause acute complications, but some may heal

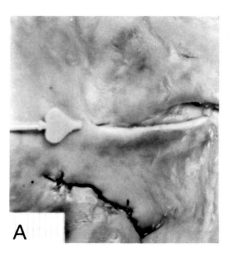 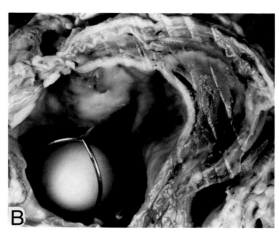

Fig. 40–20. (**A**) Healed surgical clamp wound in ascending aorta (defined by arrow and related to recent surgical wound), found 47 months after original aortic valve insertion. Patient died (of bronchopneumonia) 4 days after second valve insertion. (**B**) False aneurysm in ascending aorta found 6 years after insertion of aortic Starr-Edwards prosthesis. Note corrugated cloth (inserted at the time of surgery) at periphery of aneurysm. (Specimen in Fig. B courtesy of T. Dexter, M.D., St. John, New Brunswick.)

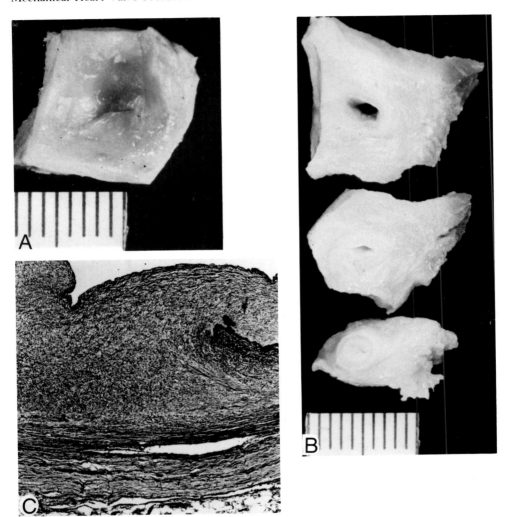

Fig. 40–21. (**A**) Ostium of left coronary artery and (**B**) sections of proximal part of right coronary artery in a patient with iatrogenic coronary ostial stenosis associated with coronary artery perfusion at surgery 6 months before the patient's sudden death. (Scales indicate 8 mm in Fig. A. 1 cm in Fig. B). (**C**) Site of coronary artery injury with medial rupture and proliferative repair process causing thickened intima. (Verhoeff elastic–Masson's trichrome stain, × 6).

and be found at autopsy months or years after operation. For example, a clamp injury can produce a healed transverse wound in the aorta (Fig. 40–20A); or diverticulae or false aneurysms may develop at the sites of surgical wounds (Fig. 40–20B).

Coronary ostial stenosis was a rare complication seen when coronary artery catheters were used for myocardial perfusion during bypass[23,148,159,181,193,223,263] (Fig. 40–21A & B). Presumably, the introduction of a catheter into the coronary ostium caused an intimal and/or medial injury that was followed by a flamboyant fibromuscular reparative response that encroached on the lumen, causing stenosis (Fig. 40–21C).

Both Roberts and Morrow[193] and Bjork et al.[23] question whether coronary ostial stenosis may also occur as part of the intimal thickening formed in the ascending aorta due to turbulence around an aortic ball valve prosthesis. Moreover, Yates et al.[263] reported one patient who had right coronary artery stenosis but who did not have an intraoperative perfusion of that vessel. This raises another possibility: that ostial injury could be induced during investigation.

The usual clinical history was that a patient who had normal coronary arteries before surgery, developed disabling angina or myocardial infarction within 6 months of prosthesis insertion. The lesion may be treated by aortocoronary bypass surgery.

The complication, as a cause of angina or sudden death, virtually disappeared with the introduction of newer methods of myocardial preservation not needing coronary artery perfusion. However, it recurred with use of intermittent intracoronary cardioplegia.[151] Minor forms may be found at autopsy. A careful gross and histologic examination of the ostia and proximal 1 to 3 mm of the major coronary arteries is needed to discern the change. Differentiation from atherosclerosis, which develops secondarily in the area of intimal proliferation, may be difficult.

Obvious late changes include stenosis, distortion, or occlusion of vessels produced by sutures impinging on them and healed localized dissections or other healed injuries at cannulation sites or elsewhere.

Disproportion. Major disproportion, where the struts of a prosthesis cage become incorporated into a chamber or vessel wall and interfere with poppet movement, is usually an acute complication. If a prosthesis has been in for many years and was disproportionate, the effects produced are likely to be minor, with the disproportion causing a slight intimal or endocardial thickening or indentation where it was in contact with aorta or heart chamber wall (Figs. 40–7, 40–22); such minor disproportion usually does not cause prosthesis dysfunction. Nevertheless, in rare instances, major disproportion may be en-

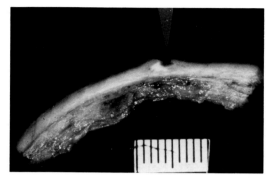

Fig. 40–22. Minor disproportion caused by strut of Starr-Edwards prosthesis producing ulceration of intima of ascending aorta 3½ years after insertion. (Scale indicates 1 cm.) (See also Fig. 40–8.)

countered long after a prosthesis with long struts is inserted. Possibly this is related to the gradual diminution in heart size that follows in the 18 months or so after a successful prosthetic valve insertion.[122,217]

Also, fatal arrythmias have been reported as a late complication of disproportion.[197] As indicated, the risk of disproportion is greater when ball valves are inserted than when low-profile disc or tilting disc valves are used.

Annular and Myocardial Injury. A patient may survive the disruption of tissue in the mitral annular region or left ventricular myocardium with subsequent dissection of blood through the disrupted tissue. If so, a false aneurysm passing a variable distance from the lumen of the left ventricle toward the pericardial fat will be found in the lateral or posterior part of the mitral annulus (Fig. 40–23) or left ventricle.

True aneurysms found in the left ventricle following heart surgery and caused by the operative procedure are infrequent. They are caused by removal of too much papillary muscle or by the occlusion of the circumflex coronary artery with a suture placed during a mitral valve insertion (Fig. 40–24) or develop at ventriculotomy sites.

Small foci of fibrosis, found mainly in the subendocardial half of the left ventricular

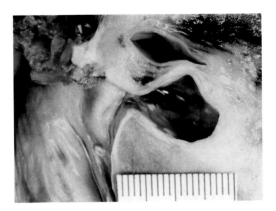

Fig. 40–23. False aneurysm on posterior aspect of mitral annulus, resulting from blood dissection following annular injury caused at valve replacement 4 years before death. (Scale indicates 2 cm.)

wall, were common in those patients who had their prostheses inserted before cold cardioplegia was introduced as a method of myocardial protection. In those without associated coronary artery disease, the fibrosis is

probably a residuum from small foci of myocardial necrosis related to cardiac ischemia at the time of prosthesis implantation. On the other hand, if the patient has associated coronary artery disease, one is less certain of the cause of the fibrosis. Overall, the frequency of this finding is diminishing as methods of myocardial preservation improve.

Many patients with HVPs eventually die of myocardial failure. In some, an abnormality of the prosthesis is a cause or a contributing factor, but in others no obvious prosthetic abnormality is detected. Some patients may have severe coronary artery disease that aggravates heart failure, but others do not show this condition. Rather, focal fibrosis of the myocardium, thought related to myocardial injury caused during surgery, is the only finding. Their deaths pose an intriguing question: Were they caused by the patient being operated on too late in the course of the valvular heart disease, or was the muscle injury and resultant heart failure iatrogenic in origin?

Sudden Death

Patients who have had an HVP in situ many years may die suddenly as a late complication and be subject to a medical examiner's or coroner's necropsy. This may reveal that the death is a result of coronary atherosclerosis and its complications, caused by other cardiovascular disease not related to the prosthesis, or was the result of other, obvious pathologic causes.

In other instances the cause is obvious and related to the prosthesis. For example, we have seen such sudden deaths caused by obstruction of poppet movement caused by entrapment by thrombi or disproportion (we note that relative stenosis[176] or transient obstruction may cause sudden death); chordal remnants obstructing a disc valve; thrombus occluding a valve orifice; component failure with poppet embolization; dehiscence inducing sudden and massive valvular incompetence with or without prosthesis embolization; emboli from thrombi or valve

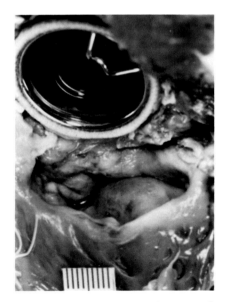

Fig. 40–24. Healed posterior left ventricular infarct with associated aneurysm caused by iatrogenic occlusion of circumflex coronary artery during mitral valve replacement 18 months before death. (Scale indicates 1 cm.)

components occluding coronary arteries and causing acute myocardial infarction; cerebral or other hemorrhages associated with anticoagulation therapy; and heart or vessel rupture and meningitis associated with infective endocarditis on an HVP. Manipulation of an HVP at autopsy may be required to reveal a transient but fatal problem.

Poppet "variance" is now of historic interest, except that a surgeon or pathologist may encounter one of the rapidly diminishing number of patients who had early-model ball or disc valve prostheses inserted.[85] Variance could produce complete prosthesis obstruction and sudden death when a swollen variant poppet impacted in an orifice.[143] Variance was caused when silicone rubber of a poppet absorbed lipids, mainly cholesterol, and cholesteryl ester, fatty acids, and triglycerides[47] and, as a result, become yellow, swollen, and soft. The swelling changed the poppet shape, while associated softening permitted pitting and splits to develop in its surface (Fig. 40–25), eroding it. Each of the latter changes could alter poppet shape, causing it to stick or impact in a valve orifice or, if the poppet diameter was reduced sufficiently, to escape

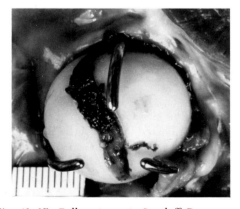

Fig. 40–25. Ball variance in Smeloff-Cutter prosthesis in mitral area for 7 years. Note split in poppet with thrombus filling it. *Streptococcus viridans* was cultured from this site, explaining the patient's symptoms of infective endocarditis; no other site of infection was found. (Scale indicates 1 cm.)

from the cage causing sudden valvular inefficiency. Fragments of a poppet that embolized readily,[92,185] and thrombi that developed in splits in the poppet surface could give origin to thromboemboli. We saw an infection confined to such a thrombus on a variant poppet. An alteration to the method of curing the silicone during manufacture eliminated variance.[108] However, such silastic poppets, in situ for many years, show tiny pits with associated shallow surface ulcerations. We have not yet seen these cause poppet dysfunction. Some patients who bear prostheses and die suddenly do not show a cause of death related to their prosthesis or other obvious pathologic causes.

Complications Peculiar to Particular Prostheses

An HVP must open and close 35 to 40 million times a year. Thus, its design and construction must allow for this great demand and be such to minimize the risk of the complications described above. One can only marvel at the excellence of prostheses currently in use. Nevertheless, flaws in design and/or manufacture that cause prostheses to wear or break apart,[79,126,161,164,186,199,217] thereby affecting functions, have occurred. Thus, durability is a prime factor in prosthesis design.

Some complications related to design faults have been described previously. Many are now of historic interest. When recognized, a prosthesis was withdrawn from use or it was modified. Unfortunately, some modifications themselves induced late problems.

Thus, coating the surfaces of prostheses with cloth to diminish thrombus formation was thought to be a successful innovation, but the cloth aggravated hemolysis and, as illustrated, provided a site where thrombus and/or organized tissue accumulated, interfering with poppet function (Fig. 46–16D). Also with time the cloth could wear and fragment, embolize, prolapse, or occlude adjacent coronary artery ostia.[6,140]

This innovation was associated with an-

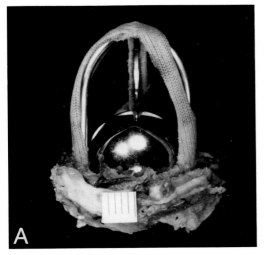 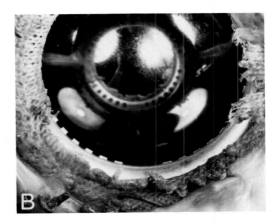

Fig. 40–26. **(A)** Cloth wear on struts of Starr-Edwards model 6300 prosthesis in situ 5½ years. (Scale indicates 5 mm.) **(B)** Wear of metal studs with subsequent cloth wear in composite seat of Starr-Edwards model 6310 prosthesis in situ 7 years.

other—the use of a hollow metal.("Stellite") poppet (Figs. 40–16D, 40–26). The function of the metal poppet was noisy and could disturb a patient who became morbidly concerned that the clicking noise produced by the poppet should continue. Also, with time, the metal poppet caused wear of the cloth lining the struts of a cage (Fig. 40–26A) and in the seat. This fragmented and freed the cloth covering to cause emboli, aggravate hemolysis, and induce prosthesis dysfunction.

A further development, to overcome cloth wear, was the introduction of composite metal/cloth struts and of metal studs in the seat so that a metal poppet would be in contact with metal rather than cloth during its function. However, metal studs also wore with time, eventually permitting the metal poppet to come into contact with cloth in the seat and to wear through it (Fig. 40–26B)

Open-ended cages in ball valve prostheses reduced turbulence but allowed the free end of the strut to engage trabeculae carneae.[109,119] with their impingement on the prosthesis lumen and interference with poppet function. The use of two open-ended cages, a design to allow the ball to occlude at

its equator rather than partway toward its pole, thereby increasing orifice size, doubled the risk of this latter complication. Changing a ball poppet to a disc or conical shape may permit it to stick or tilt and interfere with its function.[133,190]

Disc valves were designed to increase orifice size and reduce cage height, thereby reducing transprosthesis pressure gradients and both the risk of hemolysis and disproportion. However, as indicated, a disc may tilt or stick in a cage. In some early models discs were formed of Deludrin or Teflon, with the latter introduced to overcome poppet variance, then a problem, and because it was thromboresistant. Deludrin wore with time, as did Teflon. Teflon wear led to increased hemolysis, prosthesis dysfunction, and, in rare instances, allowed poppet escape[226] (Fig. 40–27D). Silicone poppets used in early disc valve prostheses also wore.[189]

Newer tilting disc valves were designed to achieve a more central blood flow, to reduce cage size, to provide large valve orifices, and to reduce both thrombosis and hemolysis. Most of these ideals were achieved, but areas of stasis existed.

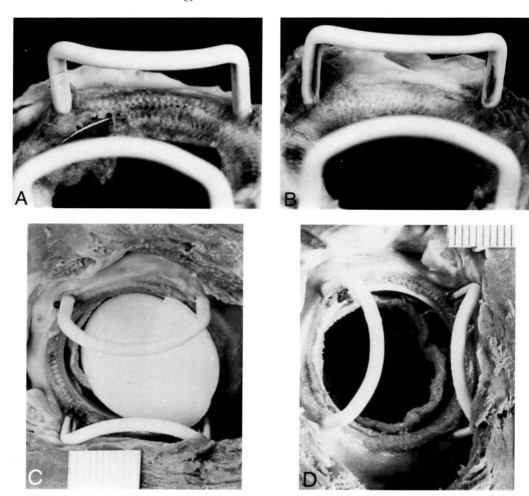

Fig. 40–27. Wear in model 104 Beall prosthesis. (**A&B**) Teflon wear on struts, showing more severe wear on the dependent struts seen in Fig. B. Prosthesis was in situ for 3½ years. (**C&D**) Wear of cloth seat, exposing underlying metal of the prosthesis stent seen in Fig. D. Torn cloth herniating into orifice (seen in both Figs. C and D), accentuating hemolysis and causing relative stenosis of orifice. Exposed metal accentuated wear of Teflon disc, permitting it to tilt into the orifice (Fig. C) or escape (Fig. D). Prosthesis seen in Fig. C had been in situ 6 years, that seen in Fig. D, 4 years. (Scales in Figs. C and D indicate 1 cm.) (Specimen in Fig. D courtesy of R. J. Sawchuck, M.D., Owen Sound, Ontario.)

Metal Fatigue and Component Brittleness

The frame of most mechanical HVPs, including struts or components that allow a disc to pivot, is made of metal or a metal alloy. Generally, metal withstands wear well and for long periods, but degrees of metal wear have been described in several HVPs (Fig. 40–28) with time.[222,224,226] We reported a corrugated pattern of wear seen on the strut of Lilllihei-Kaster HVPs. This caused no functional impairment and was thought to result from the formation of a layer of protein between moving disc occluder and metal with resultant "stick-slip" wear[224] (Fig. 40–29).

Where metal components are welded to the frame and/or can vibrate, metal fatigue may develop, with sudden and catastrophic results. For example, P. Blais M.D. (Bureau of Mechanical Devices, Ottawa, Ontario), in a

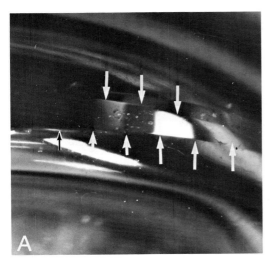
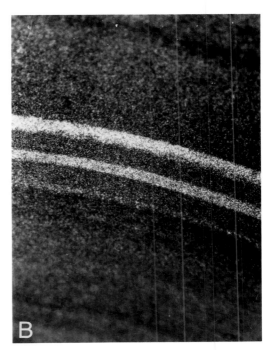

Fig. 40–28. (A) Bevelling of metal (highlight and between arrows) causing flattening of the rounded arm of the inflow strut of a Björk-Shiley prosthesis near its junction with the arch of the strut. Such wear is thought caused by contact with the pyrolytic carbon of the disc illustrated here (**B**) as circular white marks eroding the sloping surface of the disc. (From Silver,[222] with permission.)

personal communication, drew attention to metal fatigue occurring at the base of a strut of the cloth covered Starr Edwards model 2300 prosthesis. The struts of the prosthesis are not welded together at the apex of their cage. Presumably, their slight movement over many years caused metal fatigue, strut fracture, and sudden death.[64] Fractures of the struts of other ball valves have been reported.

The welding of the minor strut in some 60-degree and 70 degree opening Björk-Shiley prostheses led, over years, to metal fatigue and strut fracture at the site of the weld (Fig. 40–30). This caused poppet escape and sudden valve incompetence. If suspected in a fatal case, radiographs of the whole body should be taken before autopsy to locate the escaped disc. (It is recognized by the opaque metal ring it contains in its substance or minor strut [Fig. 40–30B].) Rockelein and colleagues[198] and Sachs et al.[205] discuss the

metallurgic aspects of such fractures. Two groups of this prosthesis were especially affected by the complication: the 23-mm aortic 60-degree convexo-concave valve (5-year actuarial incidence 2.2 percent) and the 29- to 31-mm mitral 70-degree convexo-concave valve (5-year actuarial incidence 8.3 percent).[132] The problem has been overcome in the newer, monostrut design of this valve.

Pyrolytic carbon may wear. This has been demonstrated on the disc of the Björk-Shiley prosthesis (Fig. 40–28B). Hertzian impact wear theory provides a rational basis for the wear. It is estimated that in vivo total dynamic loads of the order of 1 to 22 newtons (0.2 to 5 lb.f) act in the occluder.[154] Also, pyrolytic carbon is brittle under certain circumstances. In the past the Beall model 105 prosthesis was mishandled by surgeons, in some instances, stressing the struts and leading to their fracture at their junction with the cross

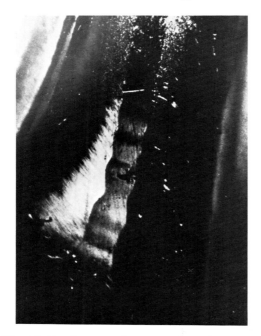

Fig. 40–29. Corrugated pattern of metal wear on luminal aspect of strut of Lillehei-Kuster prosthesis in situ for 5 years in the mitral area. This pattern of wear is thought to be caused by velocity controlled stick-slip abrasive wear resulting from an interaction between the edge of the moving pyrolytic carbon disc, the strut's titanium surface, and protein coating that surface. (From Silver et al.,[224] with permission.)

piece of the cage. This problem usually occurred within the year of insertion but was overcome by redesigning the HVP and putting a warning label on the container that housed the prosthesis. We[224a] described some Beall model valves in which the pyrolytic carbon at the base of the struts was cracked (Fig. 40–31). We assumed that one fatal case, in which a strut was fractured at that site, with disc escape, was a consequence. However, in that instance we were not certain whether the morphologic change was the result of brittleness of pyrolytic carbon or due to metal fatigue and rupture of the underlying strut promoting secondary changes in the carbon coating. Leaflet fracture of Edwards-Duromedics bileaflet HVPs has been reported.[124] The loss of a single disc of a bileaflet prosthesis[166] may represent a unique defect in a particular valve, an iatrogenic problem caused at insertion, or an example of a valve subject to an unusual stress.

That such problems related to wear and component fatigue are being observed is, in a way, a compliment to designers and manufacturers and an indication of component durability. Obviously, these HVPs are allowing patients to live long enough for these defects to become manifest. More of these complications should be expected. HVP modification, with a widening of tolerances, may be needed in the future.

We emphasize that this discussion is aimed at the pathologist who may encounter these complications, either in explanted valve prostheses seen in surgical pathology or in prostheses examined at autopsy. Obviously, the pathologist deals with a biased population and, in clinical practice, such complications may be relatively uncommon. For example, Isom and colleagues,[111] from their experience of more than 1,000 patients with Starr-Edwards cloth-covered steel ball prostheses, believed that the significance and frequency of hemolytic and cloth wear complications associated with this type of prosthesis have been overemphasized.

In general, the durability of materials used to make nontissue valves is known and predictable. In those materials prone to wear, it is inevitable and predictable but its rate may vary with prosthesis location and the host.

VASCULAR GRAFTS AND PATCHES

Vascular Grafts

Discussion in this section is limited to grafts manufactured of artificial materials. The pathology of vein grafts and conduits is presented in Chapter 42.

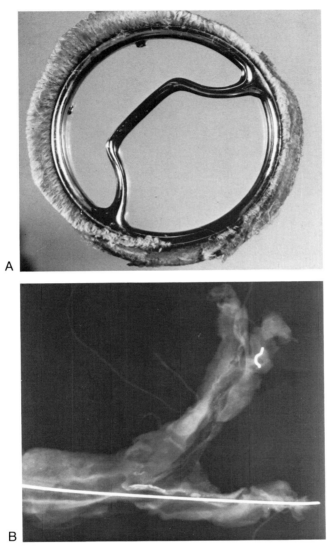

Fig. 40–30. (A&B) Case of 34-year-old woman who had both aortic and mitral valves replaced with Björk-Shiley prostheses and a tricuspid valvuloplasty done in 1983 to treat rheumatic valve disease. Ten days before she died (7 years later) she developed headaches, nausea, and vomiting and visited a hospital twice, being sent home on both occasions. She then, suddenly, developed left-sided chest pain and severe dyspnea and became hypotensive. Chest radiography revealed pulmonary edema, and echocardiograms demonstrated a possible mass in the left ventricle and erratic movement of the disc of the mitral prosthesis. Emergency surgery was done, successfully, to replace a suspected, fractured, prosthesis, but the patient died 5 days later with neurologic damage due to hypoxia related to her severe mitral insufficiency. Fig. A illustrates the stumps of the broken minor strut in the prosthesis, recovered at surgery. The disc occluder had escaped and was removed from the left ventricular cavity at operation. In Fig. B the minor strut is observed in the right iliac artery in a postmortem radiograph. It is the opaque U-shaped object in the upper part of the photograph. (Specimen courtesy of J. Butany, M.D. Toronto, Ontario, Canada.)

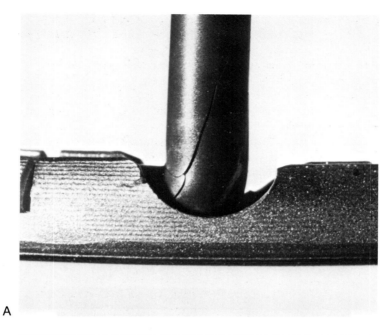

A

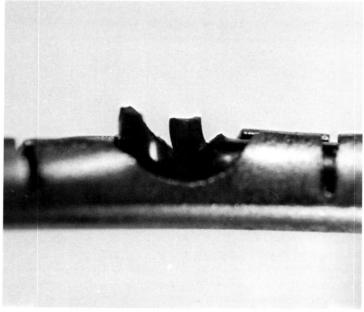

B

Fig. 40–31. (**A**) Fractured pyrolytic carbon coating at base of a strut of a Beall Model 105 prosthesis. (**B**) Fracture of both carbon and metal parts of another strut. The latter prosthesis had been in situ 10 years. (From Silver et al.,[224a] with permission.)

Historic and Technical Background

The replacement of segments of diseased or damaged arteries dates from 1894 when Gluck,[78] working in Germany, placed a vein graft in the carotid artery of a patient. A few years later, Carrel developed techniques for suturing large arteries and veins[44] and experimented with aortic segmental replacement.[43] Arterial allografts were introduced in the late 1940s, but degenerative tissue changes interfered with their function.[211] Arterial xenografts met the same fate, with a high incidence of graft aneurysms and rupture.[91,211] Rigid or semirigid materials were bound to fail. Satisfactory vascular prostheses had to await the development of synthetic polymers.

Optimal specifications for a material to be used for a graft were defined.[212] They included that the material should (1) not be physically modified by tissue fluids, (2) be technically inert, (3) not excite an inflammatory or foreign body response in the tissues, (4) be noncarcinogenic, (5) not cause hypersensitivity, (6) stand up to mechanical strains, (7) be sterilizable without alteration, and (8) be manufactured with reasonable ease and relative low cost. Guidoin and colleagues[88] modified one of these provisos by suggesting that the insertion of a graft should not cause undesirable reactions that were beyond the capacity of the recipient to handle and correct and added another that the durability of the implant should exceed the life expectancy of the recipient.

The modern era of prosthetic vascular reconstructive surgery dates from 1952, when Voorhees and colleagues introduced a porous polymer prosthesis.[241] After some false starts using materials such as nylon or Ivalon, which lost strength in the body leading to graft aneurysms or rupture.[83,167] Success was achieved with prostheses made of Telfon or Dacron.

Early designers of vascular prostheses found that graft porosity had greater impor-

tance in determining the tissue response of the host to the graft than the choice of material used in manufacture.[33,97,255] Wesolowski and colleagues[255] recommended that the biologic permeability of an "ideal" vascular graft should exceed 5,000 ml of water per minute per square centimeter of graft wall at a pressure head of 120 mm Hg. Most knitted grafts have porosities in the range of 1,200 to 1,900 ml/cm^2/min. Flexibility, durability, and tissue reactivity are also essential in the clinical setting. Flexibility was achieved by crimping the yarn, although both flexibility and elasticity disappear with incorporation of a graft into the tissues. Dacron proved closest to the ideal in achieving a balance between inertness in the tissues and provoking cellular growth and incorporation; Teflon did not stimulate adequate fibroblast invasion.[32,254] Table 40–3 presents current specifications of an ideal vascular prosthesis.

Manufacturing techniques used to construct the Dacron yarn from which grafts are made involve weaving the yarn in a simple over/under arrangement. The porosity of woven material is less than that of knitted fabrics because woven threads must be placed close together to reduce their tendency to slide and gather. Furthermore, woven fabric tends to

Table 40–3. Specifications for an Ideal Vascular Prosthesis

Absence of toxicity, allergenic or carcinogenic potential, or any other adverse chemical reactivity

Durability, implying complete resistance to biodegradation and resistance to aneurysm formation

A nonthrombogenic blood interface, implying no risk of thromboemboli

Resistance to infection

Maintenance of a uniform, patent lumen throughout the prosthesis and across anastomotic lines, implying an absence of significant intimal hyperplasia or atheromatous change

Desirable handling properties, including,
Conformability, for ease in performing the anastomosis
Pliability, for resistance to kinking

be inelastic. Braiding is a spiral weaving that produces a fabric with both a low porosity and a bulky yarn. Both woven and braided fabrics require heat sealing to prevent fraying of their cut edges. In contrast, knitting involves the looping of threads to form a continuous interconnecting chain (Fig. 40–32A) providing a fabric that is the most versatile with regard to porosity and elasticity. Indeed, only knitted fabrics provide porosities close to the ideal. A manufacturing variation in knitting allows loops of yarn to extend perpendicularly from the fabric, producing the velvety surface of velour (Fig. 40–32B). Velours have advantages in anchoring tissue and preventing undue hemorrhage through the interstices of the graft when a prosthesis is implanted. A velour has been used as both the inner and outer covering of a prosthesis with an intervening layer of highly porous knitted fabric.[209]

Dacron vascular prostheses have proved acceptable when used in the aortic and aortoiliac positions. However, grafts of the same fabric in the femoral-popliteal position have a dismal record in long-term patency, the reason being that grafts of knitted construction and less than 5 mm in diameter thrombose rapidly.[112] When a fabric graft is inserted, blood will clot in the interstices of the porous fabric and extend into the lumen. If blood flow is rapid enough to dilute the thrombin formed, the clot stops growing and platelet-fibrin deposition then occurs on the luminal surface. Accumulation of platelet-fibrin aggregate must itself be controlled by local hemodynamic factors[153]; in a graft of small caliber, continued accumulation and graft occlusion is favored. Platelet accumulation can be reduced in short-term vascular grafts in humans by administering aspirin and dipyridamole.[232] The authors also concluded from their studies that aspirin (325 mg tid) plus dipyridamole (75 mg tid) reduces platelet accumulation on long-term Dacron grafts. The development of synthetic vascular materials for the venous system and for arterial grafting in vessels smaller than 6 mm in internal diameter is an unsolved problem.

The quest for an ideal vascular prosthesis has stimulated a variety of imaginative approaches.[87] Many have not withstood the test of time; of these only expanded polytetrafluorethylene (PTFE) will be mentioned.[41,42,80,89,142] (Fig. 40–33) This carbon and fluorine polymer has electronegative and hydrophobic properties, good porosity, and

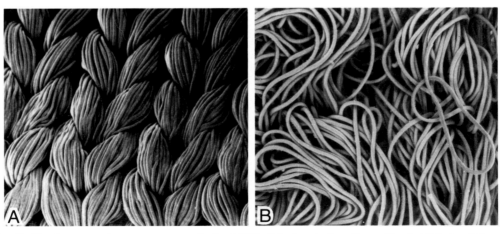

Fig. 40–32. Scanning electron micrographs (× 1000) of the luminal surfaces of both (**A**) knitted Dacron and (**B**) Dacron velour. (Photographs courtesy of Robert Guidoin, M.D., Laboratory of Experimental Surgery, Laval University, Quebec City.)

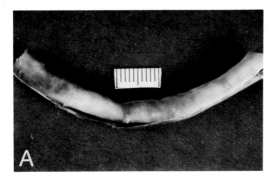

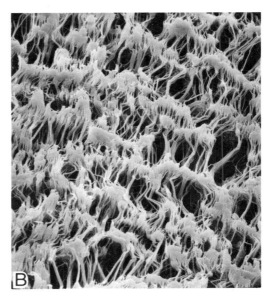

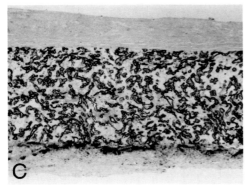

Fig. 40–33. (A) Gross and (B) scanning electron microscopic appearance (× 1,000) of PTFE (Goretex) graft at time of insertion. (C) Histology of graft in situ as aortocoronary bypass graft for 2 years showing pseudointima lining lumen and connective tissue sheath encasing adventitial aspect. (H&E, × 16.)

durability but a flexibility less than Dacron. Tissue ingrowth and neointimal development seem related to pore size, with best results with a size of 22. The aim of creating a perfect vascular substitute with live endothelium and permanently elastic walls remains elusive, if actively pursued.[87]

Healing in Vascular Prostheses

The tissue processes that occur when a vascular prosthesis is implanted must be understood if complications that may develop are to be appreciated. The experimental and human autopsy studies done by Wesolowski,[251,253] Sauvage,[210] and their colleagues have provided much knowledge in this area.

At implantation in humans the interstices of a cloth vascular prosthesis are rapidly filled by erythrocytes, leukocytes, and proteinaceous fluid. When blood comes in contact with the graft material it clots, and a platelet-fibrin aggregate eventually covers both luminal and outer surface of the prosthesis. Within weeks the fibrinous outer capsule and the interstices of the graft wall (usually referred to as tufts or bridges) are replaced by granulation tissue. Attempted organization of the luminal or inner capsule layer is associated with a histiocytic infiltration of its basal portions, through the graft interstices. Organization of the outer capsule and bridges between the inner and outer capsules is well developed at 1 month. However, organization of the luminal lining is very slow, and almost never heals completely. The delay is associated with the repeated deposition of fresh fibrin in the intercapsular bridges and basal portions of the inner capsule. The intercapsular bridges fracture, with resultant autolysis and hyalinization of the inner capsule. Coincident with fracture, new layers of fibrin are deposited on the luminal surface of the inner capsule. If bridge fracture and autolysis are extensive, portions of the inner capsule may detach and embolize. This explains how one can observe, in prostheses implanted for many years, areas of compact inner capsule adjacent to other areas where the intercapsular bridges have been replaced by granulation tissue and the inner capsule is composed entirely of fresh fibrin. Bridge fracture can also cause hemorrhage in the plane of the prosthesis itself, either in the basal layer of the inner capsule or between the prosthesis and the outer capsule.

Breakdown of intercapsular bridges at the outer capsule generally does not occur when the graft has firm contact with surrounding tissues. However, if a hematoma forms around the graft at insertion and its size exceeds the capacity of the local tissue to remove it, a pseudocyst or seroma[17] results with the graft floating in fluid. In such circumstances, bridge breakdown at the outer capsule may develop.

As long as healing of a vascular graft remains incomplete, and the bloodstream interface consists of layers of platelet-fibrin aggregate, the risk of distal embolization or graft stenosis with ultimate occlusion remains. Only when the entire graft is incorporated in a fibrous tissue matrix, and its luminal surface is covered by endothelium, can healing be considered complete.

The human ability to heal prostheses in the cardiovascular system seems limited when compared with that of animals such as the dog, pig, calf, and baboon.[210] Nevertheless, full healing and endothelialization of arterial prostheses are feasible. For example, Sauvage et al.[209] observed endothelialization in an axillary-femoral graft of knitted Dacron recovered after 20 months' implantation, with endothelium far removed from anastomotic lines and covering about one-third of the luminal surface.

There are three potential sources of endothelium in graft healing: (1) ingrowth across anastomotic sites from the host vessel, (2) differentiation of cells growing through the interstices of the graft wall, and (3) differentiation of pluripotent mononuclear cells deposited from the flowing blood. Although the first mechanism is undisputed, the role of the other two is controversial. There is evidence for a source of endothelium from the bloodstream in vascular grafts placed in experimental animals.[136] Also, the observation of endothelium distant from anastomotic sites in humans[209] is circumstantial evidence for such a source. What is clear is that, of all species studied, humans are least able to endothelialize prostheses across an anastomosis. Typically, endothelial cells extend 10 to 15 mm. This allows humans to heal fabric patches placed in the heart as well as the sewing rings of HVPs (see Fig. 40–16D) and to coat the cloth surface of the various metal rings, and such, used to reconstruct diseased heart valves (Fig. 40–34)—but not to heal long, synthetic vascular grafts.

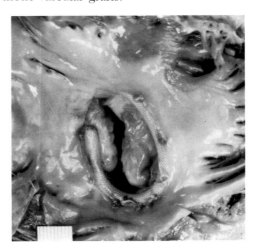

Fig. 40–34. Carpentier ring used in annuloplasty of tricuspid valve and in situ for 3 years. Note tissue coating its cloth surface. Some pathologists call this tissue ingrowth pannus. (Scale indicates 1 cm.)

Whether or not, in the future, humans may completely heal vascular grafts will depend on other sources of endothelium and improved graft design to encourage their development.

Another aspect of graft healing is smooth muscle cell proliferation, which occurs at anastomotic sites with the host artery. In large-caliber grafts, such tissue buildup at the anastomosis is a relatively minor problem, but

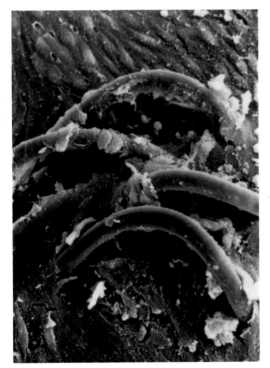

Fig. 40–35. Scanning electron micrograph ($\times$ 500) of the luminal surface of an aortoiliac graft obtained at autopsy. The specimen had been fixed in 10 percent buffered formaldehyde for several days before examination. Although fixation is not ideal, the image quality is good, allowing appreciation of the area of endothelialization on the upper side of the protruding loops of Dacron from this velour graft as contrasted with the fibrinous surface, indicative of incomplete healing, on the lower side. (Photograph courtesy of Robert Guidoin, M.D., Laboratory of Experimental Surgery, Laval University, Quebec City.)

at small caliber anastomoses (e.g., the femoral ends of an aortic-bifemoral graft), it can be important. The complications are graft stenosis and, ultimately, occlusion. The internal capsule (pseudointima) that forms in a vascular prosthesis may also develop lipid deposits and eventually demonstrate all the complications of atherosclerotic plaques in a native artery.

PTFE grafts heal in a similar manner. Histologically, pink serous fluid is found between the sectioned polymer fibers initially. Subsequently, a giant cell foreign body reaction of varying intensity extends into the graft mainly from the adventitial surface. This is associated with fibrosis. Luminal changes are those described above[1] (see Fig. 40–33C). Clowes et al.[50] found that rapid transmural capillary ingrowth provided a source of intimal endothelium and smooth muscle in the healing of PTFE vascular prostheses in baboons.

When vascular grafts are examined at autopsy, incomplete healing may be obvious with large exposed areas of graft intima. However, it is easy to mistake the smooth, glistening surface of compacted fibrin for an endothelialized intima. Before making statements regarding endothelialization it is best to examine the flow surface, either by light microscopy of conventional paraffin-embedded sections or, preferably, by scanning electron microscopy which allows detailed examination of large areas of the graft intima. An example is shown in Figure 40–35.

Complications of Vascular Grafts.

A variety of complications (Table 40–4) can occur with vascular grafts. As with HVPs, complications may occur early, or later.

Early Complications

The early failure of a prosthetic vascular graft is almost entirely from technical errors at implantation. Other complications arise from poor judgment in assessing operability, with

Table 40-4 Complications of Vascular Grafts

Mechanical failure at an anastomotic site, with
    Rupture and hemorrhage
    Rupture and false aneurysm formation within
    the graft, with
        Aneurysm formation involving the graft
        itself
        Rupture and hemorrhage
        Rupture and false aneurysm formation
Kinking with
    Graft stenosis
    Occlusion
Incomplete healing with
    Sloughing of the luminal surface
    Stenosis and occlusion
    Perigraft seroma
Infection with
    Septicemic shock
    Septic emboli
    Anastomotic separation and hemorrhage
Erosion into an adjacent viscus
Hemolysis

the patient succumbing to complications not directly related to the graft itself. Thus, when early graft failure occurs it is usually from separation at its sites of attachment and for the same reasons HVPs dehisce. Fatal hemorrhage may result or a hematoma may form at the site and produce a false aneurysm. Thrombosis is also a problem.

Late Complications

Mechanical Failure. Graft separation at an anastomotic site may also be a late complication, with a hemorrhage or a false aneurysm[88] the result. Wesolowski[252] described three causes of mechanical failure of tissues/materials at prosthesis-arterial anastomoses. They are

1. Fracture of sutures, which may lose strength after weeks to years in the body
2. Failure of the fabric of the graft due to yarn slippage or deterioration of the graft material (a particular problem in woven prostheses when the graft has been cut on the bias)

3. Tearing of the host arterial wall as the result of either (a) progression of the patient's disease—usually atherosclerosis, or (b) aseptic necrosis of the suture line resulting from devascularization of the host artery, the latter occurring if periadventitial tissues are stripped at the time of graft placement. Tearing of the host artery, due to progression of atherosclerosis or to aseptic necrosis, can be diagnosed at autopsy by an intact suture line attached to the edge of the prosthesis.

Deterioration of a prosthesis can cause mechanical failure at the anastomosis site or in the prosthesis itself with aneurysm formation or rupture involving the graft. The causes of such delayed deterioration include the following[252]:

1. Chemical, thermal, or mechanical damage to the polymeric materials forming the yarn during manufacture
2. Failure of fabric or damage to yarn fibers at manufacture (e.g., a dropped stitch) or insertion (e.g., injudicious application of hemostatic forceps to the graft)
3. Biodegradation of graft material in the patient's body

However, experience with Dacron now suggests that biodegradation is a minor problem. In fact, the intrinsic failure of vascular prostheses from any cause is unusual. However, in considering the quality control needed in graft fabrication, it is sobering to note that a single dropped stitch in an aortobilateral/common iliac artery prosthesis caused a fatal retroperitoneal hemorrhage.[262] In such cases of primary graft failure, the pathologist should make arrangements for the prosthesis to be analyzed by both optical stereoscopic microscopy and scanning electron microscopy to assess the cause, and the manufacturer should be notified.

Kinking. The fabric of a vascular graft may develop kinks where the graft is angulated in its anatomic course. If they are severe, the resulting stenosis can be a factor in causing graft occlusion. However, almost all large-caliber vascular grafts are corrugated to prevent kinking.

Incomplete Healing.   The problem of incomplete healing and complications that may arise from it are discussed above.

Thrombosis.   Thrombosis is observed in every type of graft. Late thrombosis is usually due to an extension of peripheral vascular disease with increased distal vascular resistance.[87]

Atherosclerosis.   Lipid accumulation in vascular grafts increases with their age, independent of the nature of the plastic fibers used or the manner of fabrication.[246] Walton et al.[246] found on immunopathologic analyses that the lipid in the atherosclerotic lesions in grafts derived from plasma LpB rather than platelets. Sometimes such atherosclerotic lesions contribute to graft failure.

Infection, Erosion and Hemolysis.   Infection is the most dreaded complication associated with prosthetic arterial grafts. The reported incidence varies from 0.25 to 6.0 percent and averages 1 to 2 percent, with mortality rates varying from 30 to 50 percent.[131] If an aortic anastomotic line is infected, the mortality rate is close to 100 percent.

Infection may be considered a complication of incomplete healing. In animal experiments, newly implanted prosthetic vascular grafts can be consistently infected by a transient bacteremia,[152] and a wide variety of prostheses are susceptible to bacteremic infection until they are completely lined by a fully developed neointima.[139] For example, Kaebnick et al.[118] isolated microorganisms from 19 of 21 grafts undergoing revision from associated anastomotic aneurysms and from 18 of 26 thrombosed grafts *Staphylococcus epidermidis* was the prevalent microorganism. No patient had signs of graft infection. They concluded that organisms of low virulence can colonize valvular grafts yet not provoke signs of graft infection.

Table 40–5.   Factors Contributing to Prosthetic Vascular Graft Infection

Reoperation
For graft occlusion
Unrelated to the graft
Chronic regional infection
Postoperative wound complication
Related to the graft (e.g., seroma)
Infection
Graft erosion of an adjacent viscus

Yet despite the absence of complete healing in vascular prostheses in humans, most do not become infected; some other contributing factor is present in most cases of infection (Table 40–5). A vascular graft may be infected at insertion, but infection usually develops months or years later after a subsequent surgical procedure, whether reoperation for graft occlusion or surgery unrelated to the graft. A postoperative wound complication, such as a perigraft seroma, predisposes to infection as does a chronic regional infection, most commonly in the groin. Paraprosthetic fistulas, which occur when a vascular graft erodes into an adjacent viscus, most commonly the ileum or duodenum but also the ureter, are associated with graft infections by gram-negative organisms. Prostheses in the groin are more likely to be infected by staphylococci. Most graft infections should be preventable by eliminating predisposing factors.

The infected graft can give rise to further complications, which include: (1) septicemic shock: (2) septic emboli, most often observed in the skin of the legs; and (3) anastomotic separation with hemorrhage.

In examining a patient coming to autopsy with an arterial prosthesis, the likelihood of a graft infection should always be suspected. A history of a fever of unknown cause should be thought to indicate graft infection until proven otherwise by gross and microscopic examination and submission of portions of the graft for microbiologic culture. Ancillary techniques, such as scanning electron microscopy,

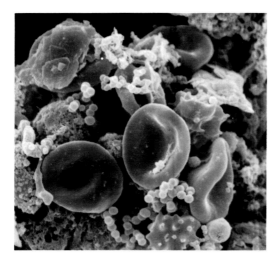

Fig. 40–36. Scanning electron micrograph (× 500) of the intima of an infected vascular graft showing the unhealed surface with red and white blood cells attached. Note, too, the grape-like clusters of cocci proven by culture to be *Staphylococcus aureus*. (Photograph courtesy of Robert Guidoin, M.D., Laboratory of Experimental Surgery, Laval University, Quebec City.)

can sometimes provide graphic demonstration of an infection (Fig. 40–36).

Erosion of adjacent tissues by vascular grafts is discussed in Chapter 8. Vascular grafts induce hemolysis infrequently. The mechanisms are comparable to those that occur in hemolysis associated with HVPs (see above).

Malignancy. A malignant fibrous histiocytomia has been reported associated with a Dacron vascular prosthesis.[169]

Cardiovascular Patches

Patches are used to repair atrial and ventricular septal defects or to provide a baffle where anomalous vascular drainage exists (e.g., transposition of the great vessels). They are made of autologous pericardial tissue or fabric.

If a patch has been in situ for several months when examined at autopsy, its location and size may be easily defined. However, if pres-

ent for many years, the patch will be totally encased in tissue and its location may not be obvious. On gross examination, the location, size, and diameter of a patch should be recorded and any dehiscences at its perimeter noted. Large thrombi attached to it should be cultured.

Patches are also prone to the complications listed in Table 40–4. Separation of a patch will lead to an intercardiac shunt. A fabric patch is also susceptible to infection until fully endothelialized. Furthermore, the exposed fabric may cause marked hemolysis.[219] Surprisingly, even though large-caliber vascular grafts present a great surface area to the bloodstream, significant associated hemolysis is rare. The reason for this difference is not apparent but presumably relates to blood flowing over cardiac patches in certain orientations and being exposed to particularly high shear stresses. If thrombi should form on a patch, they can embolize or form a nidus for infection. Fortunately, all these complications are uncommon.

REFERENCES

1. Abrams LD: Neurological complications of cardiac surgery and respiratory disorders. Proc R Soc Med 60:855, 1967
2. Acar J, Enriquez-Sarano J, Farah E, et al: Recurrent systemic embolic events with valve prostheses. Eur Heart J 5(suppl. D):33, 1984
3. Agozzino L, Bellitti R, Schettini S, Cotrufo M: Acute thrombosis of Sorin tilting disc mitral prostheses. Int J Cardiol 5:351, 1984
4. Akbarian M, Austen WG, Yurchak PM, Schannell JG: Thromboembolic complications of prosthetic cardiac valves. Circulation 37:826, 1968
5. Allwork SP, Norton R: Surface ultrastructure of silicone rubber aortic valve poppets after long-term implantation. Thorax 31:742, 1976
6. Angelini GD, Kulatilake ENP, Armistead SH: Right coronary artery occlusion by cloth from Starr-Edwards aortic valve prosthesis. Thorac Cardiovasc Surg 32:379, 1984
7. Angell WW, Angell JD, Kosek JC: Clinical and experimental comparisons establishing the glutaraldehyde treated xenograft as the

standard for tissue heart valve replacement. p. 89. In Ionescu MI (ed): Tissue Heart Valves. Butterworth (Publishers), London, 1978

8. Antunes MJ, Colsen PR, Kinsley RH: Intermittent aortic regurgitation following aortic valve replacement with the Hall-Kaster prosthesis. J Thorac Cardiovasc Surg 84:751, 1982

9. Armitage P: The comparison of survival curves. J R Stat Assoc 122:12, 1959

10. Arnett EN, Roberts WC: Valve ring abscess in active infective endocarditis. Frequency, location and clues to clinical diagnosis from the study of 95 necropsy patients. Circulation 54:140, 1976

11. Aslip SG, Blackstone EH, Kirklin JW, et al: Indications for cardiac surgery in patients with active infective endocarditis. Am J Med 78(suppl. 6B):138, 1985

12. Baba N, McKissick TL: Mycotic false aneurysm of the aorta following aortic valvular prosthesis. Circulation 31:575, 1965

13. Baroldi G: Different types of myocardial necrosis in coronary heart disease: A pathophysiologic review of their functional significance. Am Heart J 89:742, 1975

14. Baroldi G, Milam JD, Wukasch DC, et al: Myocardial cell damage in "stone hearts." J Mol Cell Cardiol 6:395, 1974

15. Baroldi G, Scomazzoni G: Coronary circulation in the normal and pathologic heart. Office of the Surgeon General, Department of the Army, Washington, 1967

16. Baumgartner WA, Miller DC, Reitz BA, et al: Surgical treatment of prosthetic valve endocarditis. Ann Thorac Surg 35:87, 1983

17. Bellenot F, Chatenet T, Kantelip B, et al: Aseptic periprosthetic fluid collection: A late complication of Dacron arterial bypass. Ann Vasc Surg 2:220, 1988

18. Benchimol A, Sandoval J: Coronary embolism in patients with mitral valve prosthesis. Chest 60:431, 1971

19. Bernard GR, Brigham KL: The adult respiratory distress syndrome. Ann Rev Med 36:195, 1985

20. Berroya RB, Mannix EP, Jr: Coronary artery dissection during aortic valve operation. Ann Thorac Surg 9:468, 1970

21. Björk VO: The improved Bjork-Shiley tilting disc valve prosthesis. Scand J Thorac Cardiovasc Surg 12:81, 1978

22. Björk VO, Henze A: Prosthetic heart valve replacement. Nine years experience with the Björk-Shiley tilting disc valve. p. 1. In Ionescu MI (ed): Tissue Heart Valves. Butterworth (Publishers), London, 1979

23. Björk VO, Henze A, Szamosi A: Coronary ostial stenosis. Scand J Thorac Cardiovasc Surg 10:1, 1976

24. Björk VO, Wilson GJ, Sternlieb JJ, Kaminsky DB: The porous metal-surfaced heart valve. J Thorac Cardiovasc Surg 95:1067, 1988

25. Black LL, McComb RJ, Silver MD: Vascular injury following heart valve replacement. Ann Thorac Surg 16:19, 1973

26. Bokros JC, Abins AJ, Shim HS, et al: Carbon in prosthetic devices. Petroleum derived carbon. p. 237. In Devaney ML, O'Grady TM (eds): ACS Symposium Series 21. American Chemical Society, Washington, 1975

27. Bokros JC, LaGrange LD, Schoen FJ: Control of structure of carbon for use in bioengineering. Chem Phys Carbon 9:103, 1973

28. Bonchek LI, Dobbs JL, Matar AF, et al: Roentgenographic identification of Starr-Edwards prostheses. Circulation 47:154, 1973

29. Bonchek LI, Starr A: Ball valve prosthesis: Current appraisal of late results. Am J Cardiol 35:843, 1975

30. Boskovic D, Elezovic I, Boskovic D, et al: Late thrombosis of the Björk-Shiley tilting disc valve prosthesis. J Thorac Cardiovasc Surg 91:1, 1986

31. Bowes VF, Datta BN, Silver MD, Minielly JA: Annular injuries following the insertion of heart valve prostheses. Thorax, 29:530, 1974

32. Boyd DP, Midell AI: Woven Teflon aortic grafts: An unsatisfactory prosthesis. Vasc Surg 5:148, 1971

33. Bradham RR: The importance of porosity in vascular prostheses. Am J Surg 100:557, 1960

34. Braunwald E Valvular heart disease. p. 1023. In Braunwald E (ed): Heart Disease: A Textbook of Cardiouscular Medicine. 3rd ed. WB Saunders, Philadelphia, 1988

35. Brawley RK, Donahoo JS, Gott VL: Current status of the Beall, Björk-Shiley, Braunwald-Cutter, Lillehei-Kaster and Smelloff-Cutter cardiac valve prostheses. Am J Cardiol, 35:855, 1975

36. Brewer LA, III (ed): Prosthetic Heart Valves. Charles C Thomas, Springfield, IL, 1969

37. Brierly JB: Brain damage complicating open heart surgery, a neuropathological study of 46 patients. Proc R Soc Med 60:858, 1967

38. Britton M: Clinical diagnostics: Experience from 383 autopsied cases. Acta Med Scand 196:211, 1974

39. Brottier E, Gin E, Brottier L, et al: Prosthetic valve endocarditis: Diagnosis and prognosis. Eur Heart J 5(suppl. C):123, 1984

40. Burkel WE: The challenge of small diameter vascular grafts. Med Prog Technol 14:165, 1988–89

41. Campbell CD, Brooks DH, Webster MW, et al: Expanded microporous polytetrafluoroethylene as a vascular substitute: A two year follow-up. Surgery 85:177, 1979

42. Campbell CD, Goldfarb D, Roe R: A small arterial substitute: Expanded microporous polytetrafluoroethylene: Patency versus porosity. Ann Surg 182:138, 1975

43. Carrel A: Graft of the vena cava on the abdominal aorta. Ann Surg 52:462, 1910

44. Carrel A, Guthrie CC: Results of biterminal transplantations of veins. Am J Med Sci 132:415, 1906

45. Cévese PG, Gallucci V, Morea M, et al: Heart valve replacement with the Hancock bioprosthesis: Analysis of long-term results. Circulation, 56(suppl. II):II-III.

46. Chesbro JH, Fuster V, Elveback LR, et al: Trial of combined warfarin plus dipyridamole or aspirin therapy in prosthetic valve replacement. Danger of aspirin compared with dipyridamole. Am J Cardiol 51:1537, 1983

47. Chin HP, Harrison EC, Blankenhorn DH, Moacanin J: Lipids in silicone rubber valve prostheses after human implantation. Circulation 43–44 (suppl. 1):I-51, 1971

48. Christakis GT, Weisel RD, Fermes SE, et al: Can the results of contemporary aortic valve replacement be improved? J Thorac Cardiovasc Surg 92:37, 1986

49. Chun PKC, Nelson WP: Common cardiac prosthetic valves. JAMA 238:401, 1977

50. Clowes AW, Kirkman TR, Reidy MA: Mechanisms of arterial graft healing. Rapid transmural capillary ingrowth provides a source of intimal endothelium and smooth muscle in porous PTFE prostheses. Am J Pathol 123:220, 1986

51. Cohn LH: Surgical treatment of valvular heart disease. Am J Surg 135:444, 1978

52. Colapinto ND, Silver MD: Prosthetic heart valve replacement. Causes of early postoperative death. J Thorac Cardiovasc Surg 61:938, 1971

53. Collins JA: The acute respiratory distress syndrome. Adv Surg 11:171, 1977

54. Commerford PJ, Lloyd EA, De Nobrega JA: Thrombosis of St. Jude Medical cardiac valve in the mitral position. Chest 3:326, 1981

55. Cooley DA, Bloodwell RD, Beall AC, Jr, Hallman GL: Cardiac valve replacement without blood transfusion. Am J Surg 112:743, 1966

56. Cooley DA, Reul GJ, Wukasch DC: Ischemic contracture of the heart: "Stone heart." Am J Cardiol 29:575, 1972

57. Copans H, Lakier JB, Kinsley RH, et al: Thrombosed Björk-Shiley mitral prostheses. Circulation 61:169, 1980

58. Craver JM, Jones EL, Guyton RA, et al: Avoidance of transverse midventricular disruption following mitral valve replacement. Ann Thorac Surg 40:163, 1985

59. Dale J: Arterial thromboembolic complications in patients with Starr-Edwards aortic ball valve prostheses. Am Heart J 91:653, 1976

60. Danielson GK, Cooper E, Tweeddale DN: Circumflex coronary artery injury during mitral valve replacement. Ann Thorac Surg 4:53, 1969

61. Datta BN, Gujral JS, Aikat BK: Histologic lesions in the myocardium following cardiac surgery. Indian J Pathol Bacteriol 13:136, 1970

62. Davies MJ: Pathology of Conducting Tissue of the Heart. Butterworth (Publishers), London, 1971

63. Davies MJ, Pomerance A: Surgical traumatic and iatrogenic heart disease. p. 441. In Pomeronce A, Davies MJ (eds): The Pathology of the Heart. Blackwell Scientific Publications, UK, 1975

64. Dilello F, Flemma RJ, Mullen DC, et al: Strut fracture of the Starr-Edwards cloth-covered metallic ball prosthesis. J Thorac Cardiovasc Surg 95:1020, 1988

65. Dobell ARC, Jain AK: Catastrophic hemorrhage during redo sternotomy. Ann Thorac Surg 37:273, 1984

66. Donaldson RM, Westgate C, Bennett JG, et al: The role of echocardiography in suspected

bacterial endocarditis. Eur Heart J 5(suppl. C):53, 1984

67. Editorial: Which heart valve prosthesis? Lancet 2:756, 1985

68. Edmonds LH: Thromboembolic complications of current cardiac valvular prostheses. Ann Thorac Surg 34:96, 1982

69. Edwards JE, Burchell HB: The pathological anatomy of deficiencies between the aortic root and heart including aortic sinus aneurysm. Thorax 12:125, 1957

70. Ehrenhaft JL, Claman MA: Cerebral complications of open-heart surgery. J Thorac Cardiovasc Surg 41:503, 1961

71. Eliot RS, Levy MJ, Lillehei CW, Edwards JE: False aneurysm of the ascending aorta following needle puncture and cross-clamping. J Thorac Cardiovasc Surg 47:248, 1964

72. Friedli B, Aerichide N, Grondin P, Campeau L: Thromboembolic complications of heart valve prostheses. Am Heart J 81:702, 1971

73. Fukuda T, Hawley RL, Edwards JE: Lesions of conducting tissue complicating aortic valve replacement. Chest 69:605, 1976

74. Gallagher EG, Pearson DT: Ultrasonic identification of sources of gaseous microemboli during open heart surgery. Thorax 28:295, 1973

75. Gannon PG, Sellers RD, Kanjuh, VI, Edwards JE, Lillehei C: Complete heart block following replacement of the aortic valve. Circulation, 33 (suppl. 1):152, 1966

76. Gersh BJ, Fisher LD, Schaff HV, et al: Issues concerning the clinical evaluation of new prosthetic valves. J Thorac Cardiovasc Surg 91:460, 1986

77. Gill B, Page-Goetz S: Deep hypothermic arrest in children undergoing heart surgery. Heart Lung 15:28, 1986

78. Gluck T: Die Moderne Chirugie des circulation apparates. Berl Klin 70:1, 1898

79. Gold H, Hertz L: Death caused by fracture of Beall mitral prosthesis. Am J Cardiol 34:371, 1974

80. Goldfarb D, Houk JA, Moore JL, Sr, Gain DL: Graphite-expanded polytetrafluoroethylene: An improved small artery prosthesis. Trans Am Soc Artif Intern Organs 23:268, 1977

81. Goor D, Lillehei CW, Edwards JE: The sigmoid septum. Variation in the contour of the left ventricular outlet. AJR 107:366, 1969

82. Gotlieb A, Masse S, Allard J, et al: Concentric hemorrhagic necrosis of the myocardium. Hum Pathol 8:27, 1977

83. Greech O, Jr, Deterling RA, Jr, Sterling E, et al: Vascular prostheses. Report of the Committee for the Study of Vascular Prostheses of the Society of Vascular Surgery, 41:62, 1957

84. Grunkemeier GL, Rahimtoola SH: Artificial heart valves. Ann Rev Med 41:251, 1990

85. Grunkemeier GL, Starr A: Late ball variance with the model 1000 Starr-Edwards aortic valve prosthesis. J Thorac Cardiovasc Surg 91:918, 1986

86. Grunkemeier GL, Starr A: Pitfalls in statistical analysis of heart valve prostheses. Ann Thorac Surg 48:514, 1989

87. Guidoin R, Couture J, Assayed F, Gosselin C: New frontiers of vascular grafting. Int Surg 73:241, 1988

88. Guidoin R, Downs AR, Barral X, et al: Anastomotic false aneurysms with aortic Dacron graft after twenty-five years. Ann Vasc Surg 1:369, 1986

89. Haimov H, Giron F, Jacobson JH: The expanded polytetrafluoroethylene graft. Arch Surg 114:673, 1979

90. Hall KV, Kaster RL, Wøien A: An improved pivotal disc-type prosthetic heart valve. J Oslo City Hosp 29:3, 1979

91. Halpert B, De Bakey ME, Gordon GL, Jr, Henly WS: The fate of vascular homografts and prostheses of the human aorta. Surg Gynecol Obstet 111:659, 1960

92. Hameed K, Ashfaq S, Waugh DOW: Ball fracture and extrusion in Starr-Edwards aortic valve prosthesis with dissemination of ball material. Arch Pathol (Chicago) 86:520, 1968

93. Hardy JD (Ed): Rhoads Textbook of Surgery. 5th Ed. JB Lippincott, Toronto, 1977

94. Harken DE, Taylor WJ, Lefemine AA, et al: Aortic valve replacement with a caged ball valve. Am J Cardiol 9:292, 1962

95. Harris RL, Wilson WR, Williams TW, Jr: Infections associated with prosthetic heart valves. p. 89. In Sugarman B, Young EJ (eds): Infections associated with Prosthetic Devices. CRC Press, Boca Raton, FL, 1984

96. Harrison EC, Roschke EJ, Meyers HI, et al: Cholelithiasis: A frequent complication of artificial heart valve replacement. Am Heart J 95:483, 1978

97. Harrison JH, Davalos PA: Influence of porosity on synthetic grafts. Arch Surg 82:9, 1961

98. Haubold A: Carbon in prosthetics. Ann NY Acad Sci 283:383, 1977

99. Heilbrunn A, Zimmerman JM: Coronary artery dissection. A complication of cannulation. J Thorac Cardiovasc Surg 49:767, 1965

100. Henson DE, Najafi H, Callaghan R, et al: Myocardial lesions following open heart surgery. Arch Pathol 88:423, 1969

101. Hill JD, Aguilar MJ, Baranco A, et al: Neuropathological manifestations of cardiac surgery. Ann Thorac Surg 7:409, 1969

102. Hill JD, Mittal AK, Kerth WJ, Gerbode F: Syndrome of acute hemorrhagic intestinal infection and renal insufficiency following aortic valve replacement for aortic insufficiency. J Thorac Cardiovasc Surg 61:430, 1971

103. Hjelm M, Hogman CF, Finnson M, Malers E: transient auto-antibody formation in a case of open heart surgery with no sign of increased red-cell destruction. Vox Sang 9:505, 1964

104. Horstcotte D, Korfer R, Loogen F, et al: Prosthetic valve endocarditis: Clinical findings and management. Eur Heart J 5(suppl. C):117, 1984

105. Horton EH, Murthy SK, Seal RME: Hemorrhagic necrosis of the small intestine and acute pancreatitis following open heart surgery. Thorax 23:438, 1968

106. Hudson REB: Pathology of the human aortic valve homograft. Br Heart J 28:291, 1966

107. Hudson REB: Cardiac Pathology, Vols. 1, 2, and 3. Edward Arnold Ltd., London, 1965, 1970

108. Hylen JC, Hodam RP, Kloster FE: Changes in the durability of silicone rubber in ball-valve prostheses. Ann Thorac Surg 13:324, 1972

109. Ibarra-Pérez C, Rodriquez-Trujillo F, Pérez-Redondo H: Engagement of ventricular myocardium by struts of mitral prosthesis. Fatal complication of use of open-cage cardiac valves. J Thorac Cardiovasc Surg 61:403, 1971

110. Ingram RH, Jr, Braunwald E: Pulmonary edema: Cardiogenic and noncardiogenic. p. 544. In Braunwald E (ed): Heart Disease. A Textbook of Cardiovascular Medicine. 3rd Ed. WB Saunders, Philadelphia, 1988

111. Isom OW, Spencer FC, Glassman E, et al: Long-term results in 1375 patients undergoing valve replacement with the Starr-Edwards cloth-covered steel ball prosthesis. Ann Surg 186:310, 1977

112. Jacobson JH, Suarez E, Katsumura T: Influence of prosthesis diameter in small arterial replacement. Circulation 28:742, 1963

113. Jaen R, Grossman-Siegert V, Ortega MA, et al: Complications in open-heart surgery. J Cardiovasc Surg 11:129, 1970

114. Järvinen A, Virtanen K, Peltola K, et al: Postoperative disc entrapment following cardiac valve replacement—a report of ten cases. Thorac Cardiovasc Surg 32:152, 1984

115. Javid H, Tufo HM, Najafi H, et al: Neurological abnormalities following open-heart surgery. J Thorac Cardiovasc Surg 58:502, 1969

116. Joassin A, Edwards JE: Cause of death within 30 days of mitral valvular replacement: Analysis of 93 cases. Cardiovasc Clin 1(2):170, 1973

117. Joassin A, Edwards JE: Late causes of death after mitral valve replacement: Analysis of 36 cases. J Thorac Cardiovasc surg 65:255, 1973

118. Kaebnick HW, Bandyk DF, Bergamini TW, Towne JB: The microbiology of explanted vascular prostheses. Surgery 102:756, 1987

119. Kalke B, Korns ME, Goott B, et al: Engagement of ventricular myocardium by open-cage atrioventricular valvular prostheses. J Thorac Cardiovasc Surg 58:92, 1969

120. Karlson KJ, Ashraf MM, Berger RL: Rupture of left ventricle following mitral valve replacement. Ann Thorac Surg 46:590, 1988

121. Katske G, Golding LR, Tubbs RR, Loop FD: Posterior mid-ventricular rupture after mitral valve replacement. Ann Thorac Surg 27:130, 1979

122. Kennedy JW, Doces J, Stewart DR: Left ventricular function before and following aortic valve replacement. Circulation 56:944, 1977

123. Kirklin JK, Westaby S, Blackstone EH, et al: Complement and damaging effects of cardiopulmonary bypass. J Thorac Cardiovasc Surg 86:845, 1983

124. Klepetko W, Moritz A, Mlczoch J, et al: Leaflet fracture in Edwards-Duromedics bileaflet valves. J Thorac Cardiovasc Surg 97:90, 1989

125. Kontos GJ, Jr, Schaff HV: Thrombotic occlusion of a prosthetic heart valve: Diagnosis and

management. Mayo Clin Proc 60:118, 1985

126. Larmi TKI, Kärkölä P: Shrinkage and degradation of the Delrin occluder in the tilting-disc valve prosthesis. J Thorac Cardiovasc Surg 68:66, 1974

127. Lefrak EA, Starr A: Cardiac Valve Prostheses. Appleton-Century-Crofts, East Norwalk, CT

128. Leonard EF: The role of flow in thrombogenesis. Bull NY Acad Med 48:273, 1972

129. Leport C, Vilde JL, Bricaire F, et al: Late prosthetic valve endocarditis. Bacteriological findings and managements. Eur Heart J 5(suppl. C):117, 1984

130. Lie JT, Sun SC: Ultrastructure of ischemic contracture of the left ventricle ("Stone Heart"). Mayo Clin Proc 51:785, 1976

131. Liekweg WG, Jr, Greenfield LJ: Vascular prosthetic infections: Collected experience and results of treatment. Surgery 81:335, 1979

132. Lindblom D, Rodriguez L, Björk VO: Mechanical failure of the Björk-Shiley valve. J Thorac Cardiovasc Surg 87:95, 1989

133. Low HBC, Lefemine AA: Acute mitral insufficiency due to jamming of disc-valve prosthesis. Ann Thorac Surg 4:71, 1967

134. Lytle BW, Cosgrove DM, Taylor PC, et al: Reoperations for valve surgery: Perioperative mortality and determinants of risk for 1000 patients, 1958–1984. Ann Thorac Surg 42:632, 1986

135. MacGregor DC, Covvey HD, Wilson GJ, et al: Computer-assisted reporting system for the follow-up of patients with prosthetic heart valves. Am J Cardiol 42:444, 1978

136. Mackenzie JR, Hackett M, Topuzlus C, et al: Origin of arterial prosthesis lining from circulating blood cells. Arch Surg 97:879, 1968

137. MacVaugh H, III, Joyner CR, Johnson J: Unusual complications during mitral valve replacement in the presence of calcification of the annulus. Ann Thorac Surg 11:336, 1971

138. Magilligan DJ: Present problems in selection of cardiac valves. Ann Thorac Surg 42:346, 1986

139. Malone JM, Moore WS, Campagna G, Bean B: Bacteremic infectability of vascular grafts: The influence of pseudointimal integrity and duration of graft function. Surgery, 78:211, 1975

140. Maroñas JM, Sich M, Sánchez P, et al: Fatal coronary obstruction due to cloth wear of a cloth covered Starr-Edwards aortic valve prosthesis. Chest 82:645, 1982

141. Matar AF, Ross DN: traumatic arterial dissection in open-heart surgery. Thorax 22:82, 1967

142. Matsumoto H, Hasegawa T, Fuse K, et al: A new vascular prosthesis for a small caliber artery. Surgery 74:519, 1973

143. McHenry MM, Smeloff EA, Fong WY, et al: Critical obstruction of prosthetic heart valves due to lipid absorption by silastic. J Thorac Cardiovasc Surg 59:413, 1970

144. Mehlman DJ: A pictorial and radiographic guide for identification of prosthetic heart valve devices. Prog Cardiovasc Dis 30:441, 1988

145. Mehlman DJ, Resnekov L: A guide to the radiographic identification of prosthetic heart valves. Circulation 57:613, 1978

146. Messmer BJ, Okies JE, Hallman GL, Cooley DA: Early and late thromboembolic complications after mitral valve replacement. A comparative study of various prostheses. J Cardiovasc Surg 13:281, 1972

147. Messmer BJ, Rothlin M, Senning A: Early disc dislodgement. An unusual complication after insertion of a Björk-Shiley mitral valve prosthesis. J Thorac Cardiovasc Surg 65:386, 1973

148. Midell AI, DeBoer A, Bermudez G: Postperfusion coronary ostial stenosis. Incidence and significance. J Thorac Cardiovasc Surg 72:80, 1976

149. Miller DW, Jr, Johnson DD, Ivey TD: Does preservation of the posterior chordae tendineae enhance survival during mitral valve replacement? Ann Thorac Surg 28:22, 1979

150. Mitchell RS, Miller DC, Stinson EB, et al: Significant patient-related determinants of prosthetic valve performance. J Thorac Cardiovasc Surg 91:807, 1986

151. Molina JE: Coronary stenosis following aortic valve replacement (Correspondence). Ann Thorac Surg 31:473, 1983

152. Moore WS, Rosson CT, Hall AD, Thomas AN: transient bacteremia: A cause of infection in prosthetic vascular grafts. Am J Surg 117:342, 1969

153. Morales AR, Fine G, Taber RE: Cardiac sur-

gery and myocardial necrosis. Arch Pathol 83:71, 1967

154. More RB, Silver MD: Pyrolytic carbon prosthetic heart valve occluder wear: *In vivo* vs *In vitro* results from the Björk-Shiley prostheses. J Appl Biomater 1:267, 1990

155. Morse D, Steiner RM: The Pacemaker and Valve Identification Guide. Medical Examination Publishing, New York, 1978

156. Morse D, Steiner RM: Cardiac valve identification atlas and guide. p. 257. In Morse D, Steiner RM, Fernandez J (eds): Guide to Prosthetic Cardiac Valves, Springer-Verlag, New York, 1985

157. Najafi H, Henson D, Dye WS, et al: Left ventricular hemorrhagic necrosis, Ann Thorac Surg 7:555, 1969

158. Najafi H, Ostermiller WE, Jr, Javid H, et al: Narrow aortic root complicating aortic valve replacement. Arch Surg 99:690, 1969

159. Nakhjavan FK, Maranhao V, Goldberg H: Iatrogenic stenosis of the proximal portion of the coronary arteries. Am Heart J 83:318, 1972

160. Natali J: Vascular prosthesis: Past, present and future. Int Surg 73:206, 1988

161. Nathan MJ: Strut fracture. Ann Thorac Surg 16:610, 1973

162. Nevaril CG, Lynch EC, Alfrey CP, Jr, Hellums JD: Erythrocyte damage and destruction induced by shearing stress. J Lab Clin Med 71:784, 1968

163. Niles NR, Sandilands JR: Pathology of heart valve replacement surgery: Autopsies of 62 patients with Starr-Edwards prostheses. Dis Chest 56:373, 1969

164. Norenberg DD, Evans RW, Gundersen AE, Abellera RN: Fracture and embolization of a Björk-Shiley disc. J Thorac Cardiovasc Surg 74:925, 1977

165. Nunez L, Inglesias A, Sotillo J: Entrapment of leaflet of St Jude Medical cardiac valve prosthesis by miniscule thrombus: Report of two cases. Ann Thorac Surg 29:567, 1980

166. Odell JA, Durandt J, Sharma DM, Vythilingum S: Spontaneous embolization of a St. Jude prosthetic mitral valve leaflet. Ann Thorac Surg 39:569, 1985

167. O'Hara I, Nakand S: Rupture of arterial plastic prosthesis. Arch Surg 77:55, 1958

168. Orkin FH, cooperman LM (eds): Complications in Anesthesiology. JB Lippincott, Philadelphia, 1983

169. Paterson HS: Malignant fibrous histiocytoma associated with a Dacron vascular prosthesis. Ann Thorac Surg 47:772, 1989

170. Pavie A, Bors V, Baud F, et al: Surgery of prosthetic valve thrombosis. Eur Heart J 5(suppl. D):39, 1984

171. Phillips MJ, Poucell S, Patterson J, Valencia P: The Liver. An atlas and text of ultrastructural pathology. Raven Press, New York, 1987

172. Pirofsky B, Sutherland DW, Starr A, Griswold HD: Hemolytic anemia complicating aortic-valve surgery. An autoimmune syndrome. New Eng J Med 272:235, 1965

173. Prabhus S, Friday KJ, Reynolds D, et al: Thrombosis of aortic St. Jude valve. Ann Thorac Surg 41:332, 1986

174. Pratt PC: Pathology of adult respiratory distress syndrome. Monogr Pathol 19:43, 1978

175. Quattlebaum FW, Kalke B, Edwards JE, Lillehei CW: Obstruction of the aorta by prosthetic aortic valve. J Thorac Cardiovasc Surg 55:231, 1968

176. Rahimtoola SH: The problem of valve prosthesis-patient mismatch. Circulation 58:20, 1978

177. Rahimtoola SH: Lessons learned about the determinants of the results of valve surgery. Circulation 78:1503, 1988

178. Rao KMS, Learoyd PA, Rao RS, et al: Chronic hemolysis after Lillehei-Kaster valve replacement. Thorax 35:290, 1980

179. Ratcliff NB, Young WJ, Jr, Hackel DB, et al: Pulmonary injury secondary to extracorporeal circulation. An ultrastructural study. J Thorac Cardiovasc Surg 65:425, 1973

180. Reath DB, Maull KI, Wolfgang TC: General surgical complications following cardiac surgery. Am Surg 49:11, 1983

181. Reed GE, Spencer FC, Boyd AD, et al: Late complications of intraoperative coronary artery perfusion. Circulation 47-48(suppl. III):III-80, 1973

182. Reed WA, Dunn M: fatal hemolysis following ball valve replacement of the aortic valve. J Thorac Cardiovasc Surg 48:436, 1964

183. Reichenbach DD, Benditt EP: Myofibrillar degeneration. Arch Pathol 85:189, 1968

184. Richardson JV, Kouchoukos NT, Wright JO, III, Karp RB: Combined aortic valve replace-

ment and myocardial revascularization: Results in 220 patients. Circulation 59:75, 1979

185. Ridolfi RL, Hutchins GM: Detection of ball variance in prosthetic heart valves by liver biopsy. Johns Hopkins Med J 134:131, 1974

186. Roberts AK, Lambert CJ, Mitchell BF: Embolization of disc occluder of a Wada-Cutter mitral prosthesis with survival. Ann Thorac Surg 21:361, 1976

187. Roberts WC: The autopsy: Its decline and a suggestion for its revival. N Engl J Med 299:332, 1978

188. Roberts WC, Bulkley BH, Morrow AG: Pathologic anatomy of cardiac valve replacement: A study of 224 necropsy patients. Progr Cardiovasc Dis 15:539, 1973

189. Roberts WC, Fishbein MC, Golden A: Cardiac pathology after valve replacement by disc prosthesis. Am J Cardiol 35:740, 1975

190. Roberts WC, Hammer WJ: Cardiac pathology after valve replacement with a tilting disc prosthesis (Björk-Shiley type). Am J Cardiol 37:1024, 1976

190a. Roberts WC, Isner JM, Virmani R: Left ventricular incision midway between the mitral annulus and the stumps of the papillary muscles during mitral valve excision with or without rupture or aneurysmal formation: Analysis of 10 necropsy patients. Am Heart J 104:1278, 1982

191. Roberts WC, Morrow AG: Mechanisms of acute left atrial thrombus after mitral valve replacement. Pathologic findings indicating obstruction to left atrial emptying. Am J Cardiol 18:497, 1966

192. Roberts WC, Morrow AG: Renal hemosiderosis in patients with prosthetic aortic valves. Circulation, 33:390, 1966

193. Roberts WC, Morrow AG: Cause of early postoperative death following pathologic correlations in 64 patients studied at necropsy. J Thorac Cardiovasc Surg 54:422, 1967

194. Roberts WC, Morrow AG: Late postoperative pathological findings after cardiac valve replacement. Circulation 35, 36(suppl. I):I-48, 1967

195. Roberts WC, Morrow AG: Topics in clinical medicine. Anatomic studies of hearts containing caged-ball prosthetic valves. Johns Hopkins Med J 121:271, 1967

196. Roberts WC, Morrow AG: Secondary left ventricular endocardial fibroelastosis follow-

ing mitral valve replacement. Cause of cardiac failure in the late postoperative period. Circulation, 37, 38(suppl. II):II-101, 1968

197. Robicsek F, Sanger PW, Daugherty HK, et al: Fatal arrhythmias caused by the pressure of the ball-valve prosthesis upon the left ventricular myocardium. Dis Chest 52:813, 1967

198. Röckelein G, Breme J, von der Emde J: Lethal blockage of a Björk-Shiley artificial heart valve caused by strut fracture—the metallurgical aspect. Thorac Cardiovasc Surg 37:47, 1989

199. Roe BB, Fishman NH, Hutchinson JC, Goodenough SH: Occluder disruption of Wada-Cutter valve prosthesis. Ann Thorac Surg 20:256, 1975

200. Roschke EJ: An engineer's view of prosthetic heart valve performance. Biomater Med Devices Artif Organs 1:249, 1973

201. Rose AG: Renal hemosiderosis in patients with prosthetic heart valves S Afr Med J 48:721, 1974

202. Rose AG: Pathology of aortic valve replacement. S Afr Med J 52:55, 1977

203. Rose AG: Pathology of Heart Valve Replacement. MTP Press Ltd. Lancaster, England, 1987

204. Rose AG, Losman JG: Subvalvular left ventricular false aneurysm complicating mitral valve replacement. Arch Pathol Lab Med 102:285, 1978

205. Sachs SH, Harrison M, Bischler PJE, et al: Metallurgical analysis of failed Björk-Shiley cardiac valve prostheses. Thorax 41:142, 1986

206. Salomon NW, Stinson FB, Greipp RB, Shumway NE: Mitral valve replacement: Longterm evaluation of prosthesis-related mortality and morbidity. Circulation 56(suppl. II):II-94, 1977

207. Sanderson RG, Ellison JH, Benson JA, Starr A: Jaundice following open-heart surgery. Ann Surg 165, 217, 1967

208. Sandritter W, Mittermayer C, Riede UN, et al: Shock lung syndrome. (A general review). Pathol Res Pract 162:7, 1978

209. Sauvage LR, Berger K, Beilin LB, et al: Presence of endothelium in an axillary-femoral graft of knitted dacron with an external velour surface. Ann Surg 182:749, 1975

210. Sauvage LR, Berger K, Wood SJ, et al: Interspecies healing of porous arterial prosthe-

ses: Observations, 1960–1974. Arch Surg 109:698, 1974

211. Sauvage LR, Wesolowski SA: The healing and fate of arterial grafts. Surgery 38:1090, 1955

212. Scales JT: Tissue reactions to synthetic materials. Proc Soc Med 46:647, 1953

213. Schlesinger MJ, Reiner L: Focal myocytolysis of the Heart Am J Pathol 31:443, 1955

214. Schoen FJ: Pathology of cardiac valve replacement. p. 209. In Morse D, Steiner RM, Fernandez J (eds): Guide to Prosthetic Cardiac Valves. Springer-Verlag, New York, 1985

215. Schoen FJ, Titus JL, Lawrie FM: Autopsy-determined causes of death after cardiac valve replacement. JAMA 249:899, 1983

216. Schwarz F, Flameng W, Schaper J, et al: Myocardial structure and function in patients with aortic valve diseases and their relation to postoperative results. Am J Cardiol 41:661, 1978

217. Scott SM, Sethi GK, Paulson DM, Takaro T: Insidious strut fractures in a DeBakey-Surgitool aortic valve prosthesis. Ann Thorac Surg 25:382, 1978

218. Seningen RP, Bulkley BH, Roberts WC: Prosthetic aortic stenosis. A method to prevent its occurrence by measurement of aortic size from preoperative aortogram. Circulation 49:921, 1974

219. Sigler AT, Forman EN, Zinkham WH, Neill CA: Severe intravascular hemolysis following surgical repair of endocardial cushion defects. Am J Med 35:467, 1963

220. Silver MA, Winters GL: Evaluation of operatively excised prosthetic mechanical valves. p. 331. In Waller BF (ed): Pathology of the Heart and Great Vessels. Churchill Livingstone, New York, 1988

221. Silver MD: Erosion of the left ventricular wall caused by a ball-valve prosthesis. Can Med Assoc J 99:1143, 1968

222. Silver MD: Wear in Björk-Shiley heart valve prostheses recovered at necropsy or operation. J Thorac Cardiovasc Surg 79:693, 1980

223. Silver MD, Datta BN, Bowes VF: A key to identify heart valve prostheses. Arch Pathol 99:132, 1975

224. Silver MD, Koppenhoeffer H, Heggtveit HA, et al: Metal wear in Lillehei-Kaster heart valve prostheses. Artif Organs 9:270, 1985

224a. Silver MD, Torok PR, Slinger RP, et al:

225. Silver MD, Wigle ED, Trimble AS, Bigelow WG: Iatrogenic coronary ostial stenosis. Arch Pathol 88:73, 1969

226. Silver MD, Wilson GJ: The pathology of wear in the Beall model 104 heart valve prosthesis. Circulation 56:617, 1977

227. Singh HM, Horton EH: Myocardial damage and valve replacements. Thorax 26:89, 1971

228. Starr A, Grunkemeier GL, Lambert LE, et al: Aortic valve replacement. A ten year follow-up of non-cloth-covered vs. cloth-covered caged-ball prostheses. Circulation 56(suppl. II):II-133, 1977

229. Starr A, Herr RH, Wood JA: Mitral replacement: Review of six years' experience. J Thorac Cardiovasc 333, 1967

230. Strasberg SM, Silver MD: Postoperative hepatogenic jaundice. Surg Gynecol Obstet 132:81, 1971

231. Stratton JR, Ritchie JL: Reduction of indium-111 platelet deposition on Dacron vascular grafts in humans by asprin plus dipyridamole. Circulation 73:325, 1986

232. Sutherland RD, Guynes WA, Nichol CT, et al: Excessive strut wear allowing ball-poppet embolization in a De Bakey-Surgitool aortic valve prosthesis. J Cardiovasc Surg 23:179, 1982

233. Sutton GC, Wright JEC: Major detachment of aortic prosthetic valves. Br Heart J 32:337, 1970

234. Teoh KH, Christakis GT, Weisel RD, et al: The determinants of mortality and morbidity after multiple-valve operations. Ann Thorac Surg 43:353, 1987

235. Thornburn CW, Morgan JJ, Shanahan MX, et al: Long-term results of tricuspid valve replacement and the problem of prosthetic valve thrombosis. Am J Cardiol 51:1128, 1983

236. Treasure RL, Rainer WG, Strevey TE, Sadler TR: Intraoperative left ventricular rupture associated with mitral valve replacement. Chest 66:511, 1974

237. Tubbs RR, Picha GC, Levin HS, et al: Cotton emboli (cellulose II polymorph. "Rayon") of the coronary arteries. Hum Pathol 11:76, 1980

238. Van der Woude R, Iticovicci H: Retroperitoneal hemorrhage as a complication of femoral artery cannulation for extracorporeal

Late strut fracture of the Beall model 105 disc valve prosthesis. J Thorac Cardiovasc Surg 96:448, 1988 circulation. J Thorac Cardiovasc Surg 44:540, 1962

239. Venugopal P, Kaul U, Iyer KS, et al: Fate of thrombectomized Björk-Shiley valves. A long-term circumfluoroscopic, echocardiographic and hemodynamic evaluation. J Thorac Cardiovasc Surg 91:168, 1986

240. Virmani R, Chun PKC, Parker J, et al: Suture obliteration of the circumflex coronary artery in three patients undergoing mitral valve operation. J Thorac Cardiovasc Surg 84:773, 1982

241. Voorhees AB, Jr, Jaretzki A, Blakemore AH: The use of tubes constructed from Vinyon "N" cloth in bridging arterial defects. Ann Surg 135:332, 1952

242. Vroman L, Leonard EF (eds): The Behaviour of Blood and Its Components at Interfaces. Ann NY Acad Sciences Vol. 283, 1977

243. Wallace RB: Prosthetic valves: Available types. p. 18. In Brest AN: Heart Substitutes: Mechanical and Transplants. Charles C. Thomas, Springfield, IL, 1966

244. Waller BF, Jones M, Roberts WC: Postoperative aortic regurgitation from incomplete seating of tilting disc occluders due to overhanging knots or sutures. Chest 78:565, 1980

245. Walley VM: The Low-profile Ionescu-Shiley valve (Letter to Editor). J Thorac Cardiovasc Surg 96:969, 1988

246. Walton KW, Slaney G, Ashton F: Atherosclerosis in vascular grafts for peripheral vascular disease, Part 2. Synthetic arterial prostheses. Atherosclerosis 61:155, 1986

247. Watanakunakorn C: Prosthetic valve infective endocarditis. Prog Cardiovasc Dis 23:181, 1979

248. Weiland AP: A review of cardiac valve prostheses and their selection. Heart Lung 12:498, 1983

249. Weiland AP, Walker WE: Physiologic principles and clinical sequelae of cardiopulmonary bypass. Heart Lung 15:34, 1986

250. Weinstein L: Infective endocarditis. p. 1093. In Braunweld E (ed): Heart Disease: A Text in Cardiovascular Medicine. 3rd Ed. WB Saunders, Philadelphia, 1988

251. Wesolowski SA: Performance of materials as prosthetic blood vessels. Bull NY Acad Med 48:331, 1972

252. Wesolowski SA: A plea for early recognition of late vascular prosthetic failure. Surgery 84:575, 1978

253. Wesolowski SA: Foundation of modern vascular grafts. p. 27. In Sawyer PN, Kaplit MJ (eds): Vascular Grafts. Appleton-Century-Crofts. East Norwalk, CT, 1978

254. Wesolowski SA, Dennis C: Fundamental Vascular Grafting. McGraw-Hill, New York, 1963

295. Wesolowski SA, Fries CC, Karlson KE, et al: Porosity: Primary determinant of ultimate fate of synthetic vascular grafts. Surgery 50:91, 1961

256. Wideman FE, Blackstone EH, Kirklin JW, et al: Hospital mortality of re-replacement of the aortic valve. Incremental risk factors. J Thorac Cardiovasc Surg 82:692, 1981

257. Wild LM, Lajos TZ, Lee AB, Jr, Wright J: Left ventricular laceration due to stented prosthesis. Chest 77:216, 1980

258. Williams DB, Plutt JJ, Orszulak TA: Extrinsic obstruction of the Björk-Shiley valve in the mitral position. Ann Thorac Surg 32:58, 1981

259. Windsor HM, Shanahan MX: Unusual aneurysms of the root of the aorta. J Thorac Cardiovasc Surg 53:830, 1967

260. Wolpowitz A, Barnard MS, Sanchez HE, Barnard CN: Intraoperative posterior left ventricular wall rupture associated with mitral valve replacement. Ann Thorac Surg 25:551, 1978

261. Wukasch DC, Reul GJ, Milam JD, et al: The "stone heart" syndrome. Surgery 72:1071, 1972

262. Yashar JJ, Richman MH, Dyckman J, et al: Failure of Dacron prostheses caused by structural defect. Surgery 84:659, 1978

263. Yates JD, Kirsch MM, Sodeman TM, et al: Coronary ostial stenosis. A complication of aortic valve replacement. Circulation 49:530, 1974

264. Yoganathan AP, Corcoran WH, Harrison EC, Carl JR: The Bjork-Shiley aortic prosthesis: Flow characteristics, thrombus formation and tissue. Circulation 58:70, 1978

265. Zacharias A, Groves LK, Cheanvechai CT, et al: Rupture of the posterior wall of the left ventricle after mitral valve replacement. J Thorac Cardiovasc Surg 69:259, 1975

266. Zapol WM, Trelstad RL, Coffey JW, et al: Pulmonary fibrosis in severe acute respiratory failure. Am Rev Respir Dis 119:547, 1979

267. Zeien LB, Klatt EC: Cardiac valve prostheses at autopsy. Arch Pathol Lab Med 114:933, 1990

41

Pathology of Bioprostheses and Other Tissue Heart Valve Replacements

Frederick J. Schoen

Diseased cardiac valves are commonly replaced by either mechanical prostheses (composed completely of nonphysiologic materials: metals, plastics, or synthetic carbons) or tissue-derived prostheses (composed, at least in part, of animal or human tissues).[20,137,173,175,231] This chapter summarizes pathologic considerations pertinent to cardiac valve substitutes made from animal and human tissues; those relative to mechanical valve prostheses are discussed in Chapter 40.

Topics discussed in this chapter are the various tissue valves presently and previously available; their clinical results, modes of failure, and other pathologic characteristics, especially mineralization (the major pathologic process contributing to failure of the widely used bioprosthetic valves); and an approach to the evaluation of removed tissue valves. Because problems with "obsolete" prostheses may prompt reoperation or cause death in the present era, thereby yielding a surgical pathology or autopsy specimen for study, pathologists (like clinicians) must be mindful of problems encountered not only with presently implanted prostheses, but also with valves previously used. Moreover, an appreciation by pathologists of both the clinical con-text in which tissue valves are used and an understanding of the pathology of prominent modes of failure can facilitate the demonstration and communication of clinically relevant pathologic findings. It is hoped that this base of knowledge will allow pathologists to contribute to better patient management as well as the development and effective application of improved substitute valves.

TISSUE VALVES: GENERAL CONSIDERATIONS

Valvular or nonvalvular tissue used to fashion replacement valves is generally obtained fresh and implanted either untreated or treated with an antibiotic to ensure sterility, or sterilized and preserved by chemical cross-linking and/or other treatments. Terminology used to describe tissue valves and their components is summarized in Table 41–1. Tissue heart valve substitutes have included heterografts/xenografts (usually, aldehyde cross-linked porcine aortic valve or bovine pericardial tissue), homografts/allografts (aortic valves harvested from human cadavers, variably

Table 41–1.   Tissue Heart Valve Terminology

Term	Meaning
Related to tissue/source/treatment/support	
Tissue (tissue-derived) valve	Any valve in which the primary functional components are derived from animal or human tissues, valvular or otherwise (see below)
Biologic valve	Tissue-derived valve in which most of the cells are viable at the time of, and remain viable following, implantation (e.g., pulmonic valve autograft, some homografts) (see below)
Bioprosthesis	Valve composed of tissue, usually but not necessarily chemically treated, mounted on a prosthetic stent (e.g., porcine aortic valve or bovine pericardial bioprostheses, autologous fascia lata valve)
Heterograft/xenograft	Valve or tissue transplanted from an individual of one species to that of another (e.g., porcine aortic valve or bovine pericardium implanted into a patient)
Homograft/allograft	Valve or tissue implanted in individual of the same species (e.g., a valve from a human cadaver implanted into a patient)
Autograft	Valve or tissue moved from one site to another in the same individual (e.g., a patient's own pericardium or fascia lata fashioned into valve cusps and mounted on a stent, or the pulmonic valve transplanted to the aortic root)
Related to valve structure	
Cusps	Flexible, moving tissue components
Stent/struts	Support structures of a tissue valve
Sewing ring	Cloth that surrounds the base of a valve, through which sutures are placed to anchor it in the annulus
Coaptation (alignment) sutures	Sutures necessary to maintain coaptation of cusps, placed at or near the commissures of tissue valves composed of nonvalvular tissue

treated, or glycerol-treated dura mater), or autografts (the patient's own pulmonic valve transplanted to the aortic valve site, or valves fabricated from fascia lata or pericardium). Heart valve replacements derived from human or animal tissues have been used clinically for several decades since the first homograft aortic valve replacements were done in the early 1960s.[50,231]

Contemporary tissue valves, like mechanical prostheses, function passively, responding to pressure and flow changes within the heart. Although homografts and pulmonary autografts are usually sewn freehand into the surgically prepared aortic valve annulus, most tissue valves are mounted on a metal or plastic stent for support. Stent-mounted valves can be used as replacements in any valve site; therefore, an aortic valve bioprosthesis can be used as a mitral valve substitute. In general, the morphologic features before and after insertion, and indeed, the clinical success and specific modes of failure of cardiac valvular tissue grafts depend primarily on the type and source of the tissue, the preservation and handling before insertion, and the method of tissue attachment and support.

The advantages of tissue valves include central flow and low thrombogenicity. Although chronic anticoagulation is critical for minimizing thromboembolic complications in patients with mechanical valve prostheses, this therapy is not necessary in most tissue valve recipients. Thus, tissue valves provide an attractive alternative to mechanical prosthetic valves for many patients in whom anticoagulation is either contraindicated or undesirable. However, the anatomic and functional resemblance of tissue valve substitutes to natural valves is deceptive. In general, tissue valves require some means of both chemical pretreatment and structural support, which to some extent distorts natural anatomic features and compromises valvular hemodynamic function. In addition, unlike natural valves, most tissue valves are composed of nonliving cells and altered surrounding extracellular matrix, and are thus incapable of physiologic processes that could repair progressive degenerative changes during function. In fact, limitations to durability are the major impediment to the long-term success of commercially available, glutaraldehyde-pretreated porcine aortic valve-derived bioprostheses and most other tissue valve substitutes.[20,62,65,98,133,137,173,174,181,231] In contrast, pulmonary autografts and some homografts likely retain some viability of the valvular connective tissue cells and have minimal loss of extracellular matrix,[145,162] features that could enhance long-term performance.

STRUCTURE AND FUNCTION OF BIOPROSTHETIC HEART VALVES

Structural Components

The most widely used tissue valves are *bioprostheses*, fabricated from chemically treated animal tissues (porcine aortic valve or bovine pericardium) mounted on a plastic or metallic frame (the stent). However, a valve fashioned from tissue not cross-linked (e.g., autologous pericardium or fascia lata) is also, by strict definition, a bioprosthesis. Thus, bioprostheses are hybrid structures, partly biologic (cuspal tissue) and partly synthetic (the stent supports and fabric [usually Dacron] sewing ring). The stents on which bioprosthetic tissue are mounted vary in structural design, flexibility, and composition among manufacturers and models. The portions of the stent that extend distally from its base and support the cuspal commissures are called *struts*. The techniques by which tissues are attached to the stents also vary among designs. Because of anatomic considerations, sewing ring configuration differs slightly among valves available from different manufacturers and among valves intended for implantation into atrioventricular versus semilunar sites. For virtually all tissue heart valves except all autografts and "fresh" homografts, some form of preservation has been used, so that most tissue valves have a stable "shelf-life" of several years. In contemporary practice, this includes chemical preservation (xenograft bioprostheses) and cryopreservation (allografts). Chemical preservation not only permits the surgeon to have valves of various sizes available at all times, but also minimizes the potential problem of immunologic rejection.

Glutaraldehyde (1,5 pentanedialdehyde; $CHO[CH2]_3CHO$), used since antiquity for tanning leather, and more recently as a fixative for electron microscopy, is the usual chemical preservative for bioprosthetic tissue. This dialdehyde forms complex, degradation-resistant, Schiff base-derived and pyridinium salt cross-links between protein molecules, especially collagen.[6,37,38,85,229] In contrast, methylene-based protein cross-links induced by formaldehyde are unstable, and previously used formaldehyde-pretreated bioprostheses frequently developed premature material failure.[31,160,197]

Porcine aortic valve bioprostheses, each fabricated from a glutaraldehyde-preserved pig aortic valve mounted on a flexible stent, continue to be the most commonly used tissue-derived valve. The aortic wall immediately adjacent to the valve cusps and the intervening natural cuspal attachments are incorporated into the valve. Approximately 500,000 porcine valves have been implanted

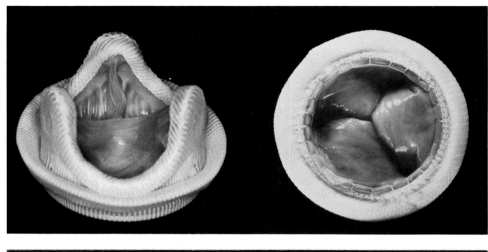

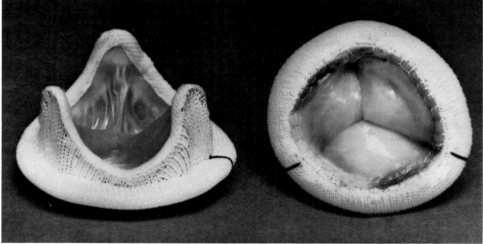

Fig. 41–1. Porcine aortic valve bioprostheses. (**A**) Hancock valve. (Courtesy of Medtronic Blood Systems, Minneapolis.) (**B**) Carpentier-Edwards valve. (Courtesy of Baxter Healthcare, Santa Ana, CA.)

worldwide since general use began in 1971, largely as two commercially available products: the Hancock valve (presently manufactured by Medtronic Blood Systems, Anaheim, CA) and the Carpentier-Edwards valve (presently manufactured by Baxter Cardiovascular, Santa Ana, CA) (Fig. 41–1). They differ primarily in the concentration of glutaraldehyde used to cross-link the pig valve (0.2 percent for the Hancock valve and 0.6 percent for the Carpentier-Edwards valve) and in stent composition (polypropylene in the Hancock, poly-

acetal [Delrin] in the Hancock II [under clinical investigation],[148,230] and Elgiloy metal alloy in the Carpentier-Edwards valve). Overall durability, failure rates, and nature of complications are similar for both types of prostheses.[141] Other porcine valves have been previously available or are under investigation.[49,53,97,148,149,227]

In contrast to the human anatomy, the right coronary cusp of the porcine aortic valve is partially supported by an extension of muscle from the interventricular septum. Consequently, both the Hancock and Carpentier-Edwards valves have a muscular shelf, noted as dark, firm tissue, within the right coronary cusp. It variably narrows the inlet orifice (Fig. 41–2). The muscle shelf can cause delayed and incomplete opening of the right coronary cusp, and the incorporated myocytes can become the site of late calcific deposits. The effect of the muscle shelf is minimized by careful and ingenious mounting of the valve on the stent and exclusion during fabrication of unsuitable valves. The Carpentier-Edwards design further minimizes the amount of septal muscle incorporated in the prosthesis through an asymmetric orifice that is contoured to the shape of the porcine valve (see Fig. 41–1,

bottom right). A "modified orifice" Hancock prosthesis for small sizes has a cusp without a muscular ridge from another valve substituted for the right coronary cusp as a means of widening the valve inlet area.[53] As in humans, the leaflets of the normal porcine aortic valve are generally unequal in size; the noncoronary cusp is usually the smallest.[191]

Glutaraldehyde-preserved bovine pericardial bioprostheses, used first in 1977, were developed with the rationale that a precisely "tailored" valve could optimize hemodynamics, especially in prostheses of small size. In a pericardial valve, each cusp is individually selected from the parietal pericardial sac of a cow. The most frequently implanted model,

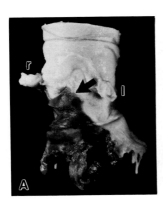
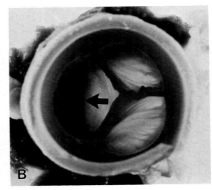
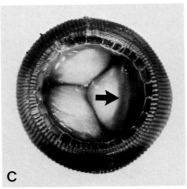

Fig. 41–2. Right coronary cusp muscle shelf in porcine valve. (**A**) Side view of partially dissected aortic root demonstrating right (r) and left (l) coronary arteries and extension of muscle into right coronary cusp (arrow). (**B**) Same as Fig. A, but from distal aspect with transillumination, demonstrating extension of muscle shelf into right coronary cusp (arrow). (**C**) Completed valve, transilluminated, showing cardiac muscle in right coronary cusp (arrow).

the Ionescu-Shiley bovine pericardial valve, is constructed of glutaraldehyde-treated bovine pericardium mounted on a Dacron-covered titanium frame[88] (Fig. 41–3). Other types have also been used.[96,150,188] Like porcine valve bioprostheses, pericardial valves have favorable hemodynamics and low rates of thromboembolism. However, recent recognition of problems associated with intrinsic deterioration has dampened clinical enthusiasm for bovine pericardial valves.[68,142,156,177,221,225] Nevertheless, without the inherent anatomic constraints of porcine valves, novel design configurations are feasible. Although porcine and most other tissue valves are trileaflet, regardless of the valve position in which they are implanted, unicuspid and bicuspid pericardial valves can be fabricated and are under investigation[19,69] (Fig. 41–4).

Structure-Function Correlations

The normal aortic valve allows unidirectional passage of blood without obstruction or regurgitation, trauma to molecular or formed blood elements, thromboembolism, or excessive stress concentrations in the cuspal tissue or supports. Aortic valve cusps open against the aortic wall during systole and close rapidly and completely under minimal reverse pressure, rendering the closed valve fully competent throughout diastole. Although the pressure differential across the closed valve induces a large load on the cusps, the fibrous network within the cusps effectively transfers the resultant stresses to the annulus.[205] The functional movements of the natural aortic valve cusps and supporting structures are complex.[199,205,206,207] The movement of bioprosthetic valve cusps is altered by and depends on details of fixation conditions (chemistry of solution, pressure relationships) and the method of mounting the valve on the stent.[28,29,152,198]

Optimal aortic valve function is achieved by means of a highly specialized inhomogeneous structure, which includes three well-defined tissue layers:[30,41,59,61,172] (1) the *ventricularis*, facing the inflow surface, predominantly collagenous with radially aligned elastic fibers; (2) the centrally located *spongiosa*, composed of loosely arranged collagen and abundant proteoglycans; and (3) the *fibrosa*, facing the outflow surface, composed predominantly of circumferentially aligned, macroscopically crimped, densely packed collagen fibers, largely arranged parallel to the cuspal free edge (see below). The cross-sectional structure of a porcine aortic valve

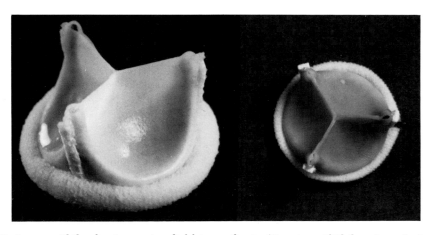

Fig. 41–3. Ionescu-Shiley bovine pericardial bioprosthesis. (Courtesy of Shiley, Inc., Irvine, CA.)

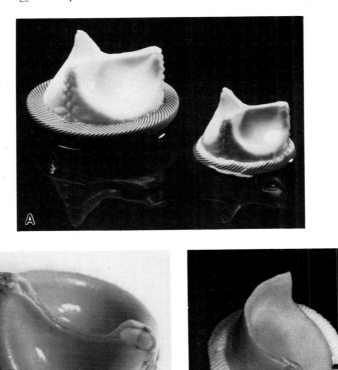

Fig. 41–4. Pericardial valve designs under investigation, demonstrating a valve with three cusps and the potential for novel configurations with either two cusps or a single cusp. (**A**) Mitroflow pericardial bioprosthesis. (Courtesy of Symbion Medical, Richmond, British Columbia, Canada.) (**B**) Brownlee bicuspid pericardial bioprosthesis. (Courtesy of Richard Brownlee, M.D., Victoria, British Columbia, Canada.) (**C**) Gabbay-Meadox unicusp pericardial bioprosthesis. (Courtesy of Meadox Biomedical, Oakland, NJ.)

bioprosthetic cusp is illustrated in Figure 41–5. The fibrosa is the primary strength component. In contrast, the spongiosa has only negligible structural strength, but appears to minimize mechanical interaction (i.e., lubricate relative movement) between the two fibrous layers and dissipate energy by acting as a shock absorber during closure. Fibrosa and spongiosa layers are most prominent; each is sparsely cellular, with approximately equal cell density.[184] The ventricularis is thin; nevertheless, its elastin enables the cusps to have minimal surface area when the valve is open but still stretch to form a large coaptation area when back pressure is applied. The predominant cells in porcine aortic valve are fibroblasts, but myofibroblasts and smooth muscle cells are present. Porcine valve cusps, like those of the normal human aortic valve, are nearly avascular.

Aortic valve cusps have highly *anisotropic* material properties in the plane of the tissue

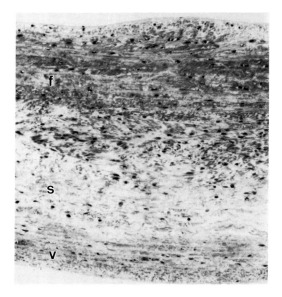

Fig. 41–5. Structure of porcine bioprosthetic aortic valve cusp. The structure is layered, with fibrosa (f), spongiosa (s), and ventricularis (v). The inflow surface is at the bottom and the outflow surface is at the top. (H&E, × 200.)

(i.e., properties are not the same in all directions), reflecting the nonrandom orientation of architectural elements (Fig. 41–6).[29,198] The predominant alignment of collagen in the fibrosa is parallel to the cuspal free margin. There are several structural specializations of collagen orientation and fibrosa architecture. The collagen fibers are *crimped* along their length. *Corrugations* in the fibrosa produce a grossly visible surface rippling. The ridges of the corrugations are approximately parallel to the collagen fiber bundles in the fibrosa (i.e., perpendicular to those of the crimp ridges). Collagen crimp and corrugations enable cusps to be extremely soft and pliable when unloaded (i.e., when these structures are contracted) but virtually inextensible when pressure is applied (i.e., when crimp and corrugations are extended), thereby allowing cusps to have different shape and dimension at different phases of the cardiac cycle. The fibrosa is reinforced by the presence of *cords* comprised of focal thickening of collagen fibers arranged in bundles oriented toward the commissures and points near the cuspal base.

During opening, as the cusp moves up and outward in the direction of the aortic wall, the ventricularis must stretch while the fibrosa undergoes compression. Stresses caused by this differential movement are largely dissipated in the spongiosa. During closure, the corrugations expand in the radial direction (i.e., perpendicular to the free margin) and promote cuspal coaptation. Tissue compliance in the radial direction (due to flattening of corrugations) is very much greater than that in the circumferential direction, (due to direct extension of the crimp). Through the stiffening induced by extended collagen crimp, flattened corrugations, and taut collagen cords, exaggerated sag of the cusp centers is prevented when the valve is shut, thereby preserving maximum coaptation. The resultant coaptation area of the natural aortic valve is substantial and can be as much as 50 percent of the loaded cusp surface area.

The structure of bovine pericardium used for bioprosthetic valve cusps differs from that of porcine valve. Pericardial tissue is a relatively homogeneous sheet of laminated collagen that is compact but not as tightly arranged as porcine valve fibrosa (Fig. 41–7). Parietal pericardium is composed of (1) a smooth serosal layer, originally covered by mesothelial cells; (2) fibrosa (accounting for almost the entire thickness), which contains collagen, elastic fibers, nerves, blood vessels, and lymphatics; and (3) rough epipericardial connective tissue, with loosely arranged collagen and elastic fibers.[3,91,93] Pericardial valves are fabricated with the smooth surface as the outflow aspect; thus, the inflow surface is relatively rough. Practically all pericardium for bioprostheses is derived from a bovine source. The thickness of pericardial valve cusps is greater than that in porcine bioprostheses (usually 0.3 to 0.5 versus 0.2 mm, respectively).

The complex array of connective tissue fibers in the fibrosa of a natural porcine valve

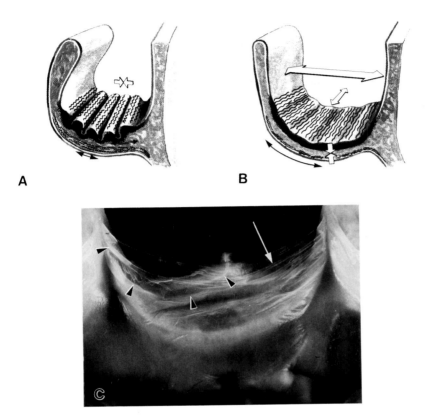

Fig. 41–6. Effect of structure on the biomechanical characteristics of the aortic valve. Force distribution on a cusp during phases of the cardiac cycle: (**A**) opening and (**B**) closing. (**B**) demonstrates the straightening of collagen crimp and flattening of corrugations that occur during valve closure. (**C**) Close-up photograph of a cusp in an opened porcine aortic valve bioprosthesis, demonstrating collagen cords (arrow) on half of the cusp, and lower margin of coaptation surface (arrowheads) on the other half. (Figs. A and B courtesy of Medtronic Blood Systems, Minneapolis, MN.)

ensures that excessive stress is not concentrated at the commissures, provided that normal coaptation is maintained. However, cuspal stresses at the valve commissures would increase sharply with decreasing coaptation area, or with decreasing anisotropy of the cusp material (tending toward *isotropic*, i.e., same properties in all directions). The collagen fibrils in parietal pericardium form relatively short, multidirectional and overlapping bundles, parallel to the surfaces but otherwise randomly oriented in the plane of the tissue. Therefore, pericardium has practically isotro-

pic mechanical properties.[28,214] Detailed studies of porcine and pericardial valve collagen have been done using polarized light microscopy, permitted by the intrinsic birefringence of collagen. This allows assessment of collagen configuration, degree of crimping, and bundle orientation.[86] Collagen is the most abundant protein in both tissues, but collagen chemistry in aortic valve and pericardium is different. Although porcine valve contains type I and type III collagens, bovine pericardial collagen is almost entirely type I.[125,186]

Thus, bioprostheses fabricated from bovine

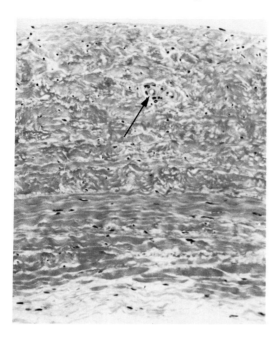

Fig. 41–7. Structure of bovine pericardial bioprosthetic tissue. There is fibrosa throughout, with occasional blood vessels (arrow). The inflow surface is at the bottom and the outflow surface is at the top. (H&E, × 200.)

pericardium and porcine valve differ in several important respects. First, as discussed above, pericardial tissue differs from aortic valve cusps in both architecture and mechanical properties; pericardium has approxi-

mately isotropic structure and mechanical properties in the plane of the tissue, and the cross section of pericardium is not as clearly differentiated into distinct layers that have different mechanical properties. Moreover, in contrast with aortic valve cusps whose natural attachments to the supporting aortic wall are preserved in a porcine bioprosthesis, pericardial bioprosthetic valve cusps are composed of individually obtained pieces of tissue that must be artifically and nonanatomically attached to stent supports. Consequently, stress in pericardial valves is directed toward the natural focal point, the commissure, leading to high stress concentrations in tissue at that site. These are not encountered in a natural valve. Sutures placed in the tissue near the free edge at the stent post during valve fabrication to maintain cuspal alignment, commissural apposition, and coaptation can exacerbate stress concentrations that occur during cusp flexure. It is, therefore, not surprising that cuspal tearing initiated near the top of the stent post is a common mode of pericardial valve failure.[23,68,173,174,177,203,225]

In addition, the edges of pericardial cusps used in bioprosthetic valves are cut, rather than being natural edges as in a porcine valve; during function, collagen bundles at these edges tend to splay, allowing host cells and fluid to enter and react with cuspal tissue. Key structural differences between porcine aortic valve and pericardial bioprostheses are summarized in Table 41–2.

Table 41–2.   Structural Differences between Bioprosthetic Valves Fabricated from Porcine Aortic Valve and Bovine Pericardium

	Porcine Valve	*Pericardium*
Cuspal cross section	Layered	Near homogeneous
Fibrosa connective tissue	Highly oriented in tissue plane	Random in tissue plane
Cuspal properties	Anisotropic	Isotropic
Free cuspal edges	Natural	Fabricated by cutting
Stent attachments	Natural	Artificial

PREIMPLANTATION CHANGES INDUCED BY TISSUE TREATMENT AND FABRICATION OF BIOPROSTHETIC VALVES

Aldehyde pretreatment of bioprosthetic tissue is intended to enhance material stability and decrease antigenicity, while maintaining both thromboresistance and the antimicrobial sterility characteristic of the native tissue. Chemical reactions of glutaraldehyde with tissue result in cross-linking of proteins, especially collagen, the most abundant structural protein of porcine aortic valves and bovine pericardium.[6,37,38,85,229] Because the antibacterial and antifungal (especially against spores) action of low concentrations of glutaraldehyde is poor, the sterility of some types of glutaraldehyde-treated bioprostheses is enhanced by either storage in dilute formaldehyde solution after processing, or transient treatment with alcoholic glutaraldehyde solutions. Inadequately sterilized valves contaminated with *Myobacterium chelonei* were encountered approximately a decade ago;[36,108,164] but no valve processed since then has been contaminated.[158]

Histologic alterations observed following manipulation and glutaraldehyde treatment of bioprosthetic valves include near-complete or complete loss of surface endothelium or mesothelium (aortic valve or pericardial bioprostheses, respectively), autolytic disruption of porcine or bovine connective tissue cells, collagen bundle loosening, and loss of ground substance (largely acid mucopolysaccharides)[34,59,61,62,157] (Table 41–3). In standard porcine valves, the quality of structural preservation of valve fibroblasts is especially poor, as judged by usual standards of electron microscopic fixation with glutaraldehyde, with loss of integrity of cytoplasmic membranes and disruption of organelles.[59,61,62] Moreover, the endothelial cell layer is virtually completely lost on the inflow surface and partially on the outflow surface; the denuded valve surfaces are composed of subendothelial connective tissue components, including basement membrane-like material, collagen fibrils, and a few elastic fibrils.[34,92,157] Small textile fibers occasionally noted adherent to, and entangled in, the superficial collagen bundles of bioprosthetic valve cusps are probably derived from materials used to pack valves; they can persist following implantation.[62] Anticalcification treatments, including pretreatment with surfactants (e.g., T6 and PV2), devised to mitigate calcific deposits developing in bioprostheses, do not detectably alter the morphology of unimplanted bioprostheses.[62] Clinical trials of valves prepared according to these processes are currently in progress.[97,148]

The functional/mechanical characteristics of the natural aortic valve and other tissues used in bioprostheses are altered by glutaraldehyde cross-linking procedures.[28–30,41,110,198,207,214] The specific alterations in collagen morphology and mechanical properties depend on the techniques of fixation. During glutaraldehyde-induced cross-linking, the aortic valve is usually preloaded by a hydrostatic back pressure, which locks the valve structure into a geometric configuration characteristic of that of a closed valve (diastole),[28,41,198] and both corrugations and crimp waveform are fully straightened. When crimp and corrugations are preloaded in an

Table 41–3. Preimplantation Structural Changes in Bioprosthetic Tissue

Cross-linking of proteins

Loss of endothelium (porcine valve) or mesothelium (pericardium)

Fragmentation of cuspal cell membranes

Loosening of collagen bundles

Loss of ground substance

Loss of compliance with resultant stiffening

Adherent textile fibers from packing

elongated state, stresses must be absorbed by the collagen fibers, which themselves have little compliance. Moreover, following fixation under back pressure, the leaflet surface area is near maximal even when the load is removed. Porcine valve or bovine pericardial cusps fixed under load are relatively stiff and inflexible and have poor hemodynamic function and potentiated tissue fatigue at points of sharp bending. The cusps of valves previously fixed under back pressure do not open smoothly. Instead of dispersing stress over a large area, such cusps open by bending in a series of kinks. During each subsequent cycle the cusps hinge, thereby inducing substantial mechanical stresses repetitively, exactly at the same site. Moreover, buckling of the fully stretched fibrosa probably contributes to mechanical failure.[218] This led to the concept of "low-pressure" fixation in which the hydrostatic back pressure during fixation is sharply reduced, to better preserve leaflet microstructure and anatomy.[198] Although altered (straightened) corrugations and crimp, and reduced radial and circumferential compliance, occur despite minimal hydrostatic back pressure during fixation as low as 2 to 4 mmHg,[28,198] some data suggest that the mechanical properties of cusps are improved when fixation occurs without any back pressure at all (i.e., 0 mmHg), thereby retaining full crimp and corrugation geometry.[28] Valves with this treatment are under investigation.[227] The effects of glutaraldehyde interaction with elastic and ground substance have not been described in detail.

POSTIMPLANTATION CHANGES IN BIOPROSTHETIC TISSUE

Following implantation, pathologic changes occur to a variable degree in all types of bioprostheses[34,59,61,62,78,177,180] (Table 41–4). The alterations largely reflect that (1) the cusp/

Table 41–4. Pathologic Changes in Bioprosthetic Tissue Following Implantation

Deposition of platelets and fibrin

Superficial or deep mononuclear inflammatory cells

Endothelialization

Pannus overgrowth

Fluid insudation

Superficial collagen fragmentation

Generalized architectural homogenization and loss of staining

Delamination

Mechanical fatigue damage

Abrasion

Calcification

Cuspal sagging

Intracuspal hematomas

Infiltration of lipid and amyloid

Involvement with systemic disease (e.g., Whipple's disease, carcinoid heart disease)

Colonization by infectious organisms

Cuspal destruction by infection

blood interface is not a natural biologic surface; (2) collagen is the most important structural element; (3) bioprostheses have no synthetic or renewal mechanism to replace collagen gradually degraded by proteolysis or mechanical damage (such as that provided by fibroblasts present in native valves); and (4) bioprostheses tend to undergo time-dependent superimposed pathologic processes, particularly calcification.

The most characteristic histologic changes that occur following implantation are illustrated in Figure 41–8. Within a few days of implantation, bioprostheses become covered with a layer of fibrin, platelets, leukocytes, and a few erythrocytes. Inflammatory cells usually consist mainly of monocytes/macrophages and multinucleated giant cells; neutrophils, lymphocytes, and plasma cells are scarce. Leukocytes remain confined to the surfaces in most bioprostheses, but deep mononuclear inflammation in the absence of infection is occasionally noted, especially at the cut edges of pericardial valves. The presence of superficial or deep neutrophils in association with implanted bioprostheses is unusual and suggests infection. Clusters of lymphocytes, macrophages, and a few plasma cells are sometimes found in the connective tissue of host origin at the junction between valve tissue and sewing ring, particularly associated with the muscle shelf of the right coronary cusp of porcine valves. Foreign body giant cells may be associated with suture materials traversing the base of a valve.

The basal regions of the cusps may become covered with a variably thick fibrous sheath of host origin (pannus), which, when excessive, can lead to valve failure (discussed below). Endothelialization of porcine valves is slow, focal, and confined to the basal attachments of the cusps, despite prolonged postoperative intervals.[92] Like vascular grafts and other prosthetic materials elsewhere in the cardiovascular system, endothelialization is probably limited to a distance less than approximately 1 cm from a tissue source, as deposition of endothelial cells from blood does not occur to any appreciable degree.[175] Endothelialization of pericardial valves has not been demonstrated. Aggregates of platelets also may form on the nonendothelialized regions of the valves, in direct contact with exposed collagen fibrils, which form part of the surfaces.[34,61,196] Focal superficial microthrombi are frequently noted along the cusps and at junctions of the cuspal bases with the frame, especially in pericardial valves.[51,177] Moreover, proteins and other constituents of plasma penetrate into the substance of the bioprostheses, probably in part because of the absence of a functional endothelial cell barrier. Nevertheless, although endothelialization of a bioprosthetic valve might decrease the propensity toward thrombosis, infection, or calcific or noncalcific degeneration, no evidence exists that endothelialization of a bio-

prosthesis would be necessarily beneficial. Moreover, demonstration of the presence of an endothelial cell layer would not ensure its proper function, because perturbed but morphologically normal endothelial cells can have abnormal function, including thrombogenicity ("endothelial dysfunction").[138] Erythrocytes are commonly noted deep in cuspal connective tissue of removed porcine valve bioprostheses; large accumulations of blood may yield grossly visible hematomas, which could stiffen cusps or possibly provide sites for mineralization.[89,202]

Valve function in vivo also induces generalized architectural homogenization with connective tissue disruption, mineralization, and, in some cases, lipid accumulation (sometimes with cholesterol crystals) and/or amyloid deposition.[34,62,77–79,177] These changes are accentuated near cuspal tears and other defects. With all types of bioprostheses, intrinsic cuspal architecture is often disrupted with the large collagen bundles appearing separated, distorted, indistinct, and hyalinized. After several months of function, there is loss of definition of virtually all components of a valve that appear basophilic on routine hematoxylin and eosin (H&E) histologic staining before implantation. The valve structure becomes homogeneously eosinophilic without staining of connective tissue nuclei. Except for mineralization and collagen degeneration, which frequently make major contributions to valve failure (and are described in detail below), the extent to which the nonspecific pathologic processes described above contribute to late failure modes has not been determined.

Some processes are largely specific to, or are accentuated in, pericardial valves. With pericardial valves, deep fluid insudation with resultant stiffening may contribute to stenosis, and the inflow surface of pericardial valve cusps often appears rough and granular following long-term implantation, due to fragmentation of superficial collagen bundles.[177] Attached macrophages and deep inflammatory infiltration with focal destruction of the

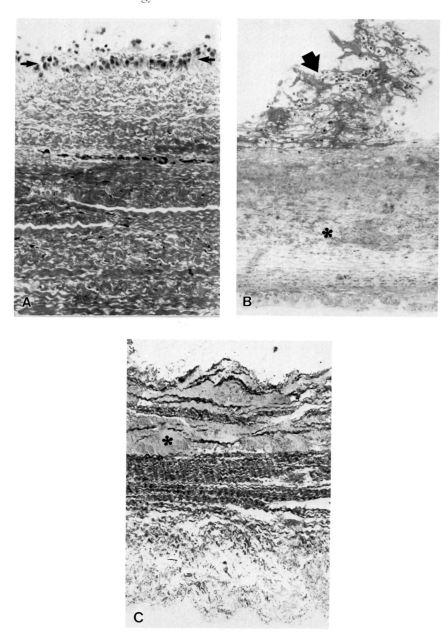

Fig. 41–8. Typical changes in porcine valve and bovine pericardial bioprostheses following implantation. (A) Macrophages lining surface of valve (between arrows) (pericardial). (B) Mural thrombotic deposit (arrow) and structural homogenization (asterisk), with loss of basophilic staining characteristics of the cuspal connective tissue (porcine). (C) Deep cuspal pooling of plasma-derived fluid (asterisk), with separation of large collagen bundles (pericardial). (*Figure continues.*)

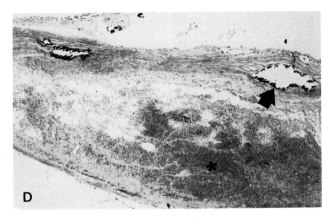

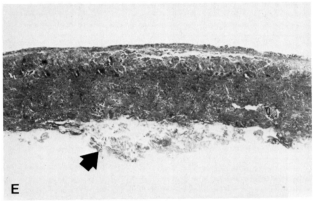

Fig. 41–8 (*Continued*). (**D**) Calcification (arrow) and cuspal hematoma (asterisk) (porcine). (**E**) Loose, splayed collagen bundles on inflow pericardial surface (arrow), correlating with gross appearance of roughened inflow surface of valve after long-term function. (All H&E, except Fig. C [Masson's trichrome]; Figs. A & B: × 200; Fig. C: × 150; Figs. D & E: × 60.)

cuspal architecture of pericardial bioprosthetic tissue by mononuclear cells, predominantly macrophages, is frequently noted, especially at cuspal edges. Clinical and experimental studies of pericardial valves also demonstrate cuspal stretching ("sagging"), in which dynamic creep of this viscoelastic material allows progressive stretching of the tissue, leading to permanent cusp deformation and occasionally valvular incompetence.[109,177,189,215] The cause of pericardial stretching is unknown, although data suggest that the mechanical properties of pericardial tissue are heterogeneous among sites within a pericardial sac, that one site has particularly

increased deformability, and that details of elastic tissue morphology may predict a propensity toward stretching.[214]

Immunologic rejection has been an obstacle to the use of some natural materials and reconstituted tissue macromolecules in nonvalvular bioprostheses.[14,140] However, although cross-linking reduces but does not eliminate the antigenicity of bioprosthetic material, no immunologic basis for bioprosthetic valve failure has been demonstrated. The significance of observations that experimental animals can be sensitized to both fresh and cross-linked heart valve tissues,[14] and that antibodies to valve components are detected in some children following valve dysfunction,[159] is unknown, as second valve replacements fail no sooner than the first.[122] Moreover, lymphocytes or plasma cells noted in failed valves are not specific evidence of an immunologic cause of failure.

Glutaraldehyde toxicity could compromise the outcome of bioprosthetic valve replacement. Because aldehydes are extremely reactive compounds that can produce significant toxic effects, it has been suggested that reactions to cross-linked collagenous proteins are due to both a slow leaching of unreactive glutaraldehyde and, in part, to the reactivity of free aldehyde groups persisting in the cross-linked polymeric network.[75] Low concentrations of glutaraldehyde are toxic to endothelial cells.[226] Thus, endothelialization after implantation could conceivably be inhibited by local toxicity. Formaldehyde is more toxic than glutaraldehyde, because it forms less stable cross-links and can leach more readily from implants. The concentrations of glutaraldehyde in bioprosthetic tissue and potential toxicity may vary, depending on the period of rinsing of a glutaraldehyde-fixed valve before surgical implantation.

Systemic diseases may affect bioprostheses. Whipple's disease involving the cusps of a porcine bioprosthesis has been reported,[154] and plaque characteristic of carcinoid heart disease has been noted on the right atrial surface of a bioprosthetic tricuspid valve, implanted 8 months previously for carcinoid valve dysfunction.[179] The plaque on the prosthesis was not hemodynamically significant, but extended survival with continued plaque deposition on valve cusps could eventually lead to prosthetic valvular dysfunction.

Tissue mechanical properties are likely further altered during function in vivo, due to pure mechanical effects[187] or biologic interactions, or to both. Explanted pericardial valve is thicker and less extensible than unimplanted tissue, but specific chemical and mechanical effects of interactions of blood with bioprosthetic tissue remain largely unknown.

CLINICAL PERFORMANCE OF BIOPROSTHETIC VALVES

Most patients with severe valvular heart disease who undergo valve replacement with either mechanical or tissue valves experience enhanced survival and functional improvement for extended periods. The hemodynamic performance of bioprostheses and other tissue valves is comparable or superior to that of mechanical prostheses, except in small-size bioprostheses.[104] Moreover, with contemporary bioprosthetic heart valves hemolysis is generally not present or is slight and well compensated for, but it may become accentuated or in some cases decompensated with the onset of paravalvular leaks or bioprosthetic valve dysfunction.[107,155]

The overall probability of porcine bioprosthetic valve failure from all causes in adults (defined as death or reoperation owing to periprosthetic leak, thromboembolic complications, infective endocarditis, structural deterioration, or other valve-related causes),[55] predicted at various institutions by actuarial statistics, is approximately 35 to 50 percent at 10 years and 50 to 75 percent at 15 years.[45,46,65,74,84,98,123,133] Large comparative studies suggest the incidence of failure of mechanical and bioprosthetic valve replacements is approximately the same at 10 years postoperatively.[45,46,84] However, both the *nature* and *consequences* of major modes of failure differ markedly between mechanical prosthetic and bioprosthetic valves. Structural deterioration leading to stenosis or regurgitation, or both, is the predominant late valve-related complication with porcine bioprostheses, and calcification is contributory in most cases. Most studies demonstrate that lower rates of thromboembolic complications with bioprostheses (relative to mechanical prostheses) are balanced by more frequent reoperations for intrinsic structural deterioration. However, mechanical valve problems (largely thromboembolic) are often catastrophic and occur in the early postoperative years, whereas bioprosthetic structural dysfunction generally occurs 5 years or later postoperatively and generally induces slow patient deterioration. Thus, when studies consider the overall outcome for a patient 5 to 10 years postoperatively, such that problems that can be managed successfully by reoperation are still considered a "successful" treatment, bioprosthetic valves emerge, statistically, in a more favorable light.[42]

The reported clinical experience with bovine pericardial prostheses remains limited. Thus the long-term fate of these valves remains largely undetermined. Nevertheless, despite favorable clinical results reported in some series,[88,188] calcific and noncalcific degenerative failures occur frequently.[23,67,68,73,142,156,177,203,221,225]

Table 41–5. Modes of Bioprosthesis Failure

Thrombosis/thromboembolism
Endocarditis
Paravalvular leak
Structural deterioration
    Cuspal tearing and defects, noncalcific
        Fatigue
        Abrasion
        Commissural suture-related damage
    Calcification, leading to
        Stiffening
        Tearing
        Emboli
Fibrous tissue overgrowth
Suture perforation/entrapment
Prosthetic disproportion or malposition
Other obstruction (intrinsic and progressive)
Hemolysis

CAUSES AND PATHOLOGIC CHARACTERISTICS OF BIOPROSTHETIC HEART VALVE FAILURE

The most frequent indications for reoperation or causes of death in patients with mechanical or bioprosthetic valve prostheses are thromboembolic complications, infective endocarditis, paravalvular leak, tissue overgrowth, and degenerative dysfunction.[42,45,46,73,74,84,123,134,173–175,180] Table 41–5 lists the major modes of failure of contemporary bioprostheses. The cause of dysfunction in 112 consecutive porcine bioprostheses surgically removed at our hospital from July 1980 through December 1985 are summarized in Figure 41–9, and compared with those of 45 mechanical valves removed during the same period. In agreement with results from other studies, the overwhelming cause of bioprosthetic valve failure was sterile structural degeneration (74 percent of bioprosthetic valve failures). Bioprosthetic valve re-

moval was required for endocarditis in 11 patients (9 percent) and for thrombosis in 4 (4 percent). In contrast, thrombosis was a major cause of mechanical valve dysfunction (18 percent of failures), but infrequent with bioprostheses. Sterile paravalvular leak and prosthetic infective endocarditis were equally frequent with mechanical and bioprosthetic valves, each accounting for 12 percent of removed valves. Clinicopathologic features of these and other failure modes are described below.

Thromboembolic Complications

Contemporary substitute heart valves generally have thromboembolic rates of 1 to 4 percent per patient year.[54] Thromboembolic complications (fatal and nonfatal thromboembolism and local thrombosis as well as anticoagulation-related hemorrhage) occur less frequently in patients with porcine bioprostheses who are not receiving anticoagulation then they do in patients who have received contemporary mechanical valve prostheses and are anticoagulated.[54] How-

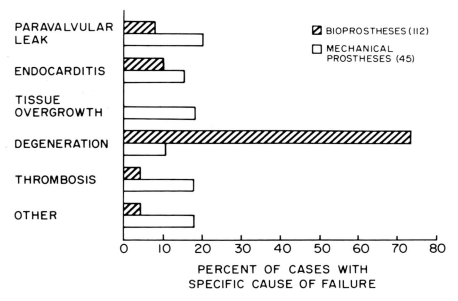

Fig. 41–9. Causes of failure of surgically removed mechanical prosthetic and bioprosthetic heart valves, 1980–1985. Failure modes of mechanical valves are diverse; in contrast, bioprosthetic valves fail most frequently by degenerative processes. (From Schoen,[174] with permission.)

ever, patients with bioprostheses in atrial fibrillation are at increased risk of thromboembolic complications, because patients with atrial fibrillation, irrespective of its cause, have a substantially increased risk of cerebrovascular emboli.[72,228] Such patients generally receive anticoagulants, as thromboemboli in patients with arrhythmias presumably arise from nonvalvular atrial sites.

Early postoperative thrombosis occurs rarely in patients with mitral bioprostheses, usually in the presence of low cardiac output. In these cases, thrombotic deposits initially involve the host tissue/interface at the sewing ring, the sewing ring itself, or the left atrial wall. Early thrombogenicity of the fabric sewing cuff is alleviated by tissue ingrowth occurring over the first several months following implantation; this provides the rationale for transient postoperative anticoagulation used in some patients. In contrast, late thrombosis can occur at the bioprosthetic cusps, with large thrombotic deposits present in one or more of the prosthetic sinuses of Valsalva (Fig. 41–10).[180,201] In most cases, there is no

demonstrable underlying cuspal pathology. Bioprosthetic valves sewn freehand into conduits have small spaces between the valve struts and the conduit wall that can provoke thrombus formation in proximity to the orifices of reimplanted coronary arteries or aortocoronary grafts.[47]

The lack of adjacent vascularized tissue retards the histologic organization of thrombi on bioprosthetic or mechanical valves. Therefore, microscopic evaluation often underestimates their age. For similar reasons, such thrombi maintain their friability and embolic potential for extended periods. Moreover, clinical fibrinolytic treatment of prosthetic valve thrombi might be effective in some cases, despite temporal delay from onset of thrombus-induced dysfunction.

Platelet deposition dominates initial blood/surface interaction when valves or other devices with nonphysiologic (artificial) surfaces are exposed to blood at high-fluid shear stresses, and there is a strong relationship of prosthetic valve thromboembolism to altered platelet function.[5,175] Although gross meas-

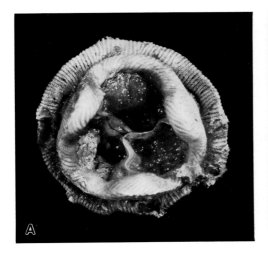
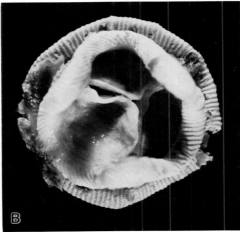

Fig. 41–10. Bioprosthetic valve thrombosis, shown with porcine bioprostheses. (**A**) Thrombosis involving outflow surfaces of all three cusps. (**B**) Thrombosis involving the outflow portion of one cusp only. (Fig. A from Schoen,[180] with permission.)

ures (e.g., platelet survival studies) are generally not clinically abnormal in patients with bioprosthetic valves, platelet deposition has been observed by scanning electron microscopy and radiolabeled platelet deposition has been directly observed on bioprosthetic valve surfaces and on immediately adjacent damaged vascular walls.[51,61,157,196] Experimental work suggests that there is no difference in platelet adherence to porcine aortic valve or bovine pericardium.[124]

Endocarditis

Infective endocarditis is a serious complication of valve replacement in general. It occurs in up to 4 to 6 percent of patients with prostheses.[32,48,95] Rates of infection do not differ consistently among bioprostheses and mechanical valves. Because synthetic biomaterials used in mechanical prostheses generally cannot support bacterial or fungal growth, mechanical prosthetic valve infection is almost always localized to the prosthesis/tissue interface at the sewing ring.[4,13,173,175] The resultant tissue destruction around the prosthesis causes a *ring abscess*.

The pathologic features of bioprosthetic valve endocarditis are demonstrated in Figure 41–11. Bioprosthetic valve endocarditis is often localized to tissue adjacent to the prosthesis sewing ring and complicated by ring abscess, analogous to endocarditis on mechanical valves. However, infections on bioprosthetic valves may involve and indeed are occasionally limited to the cuspal tissue; such infections can be complicated by valve obstruction caused by bulky vegetations or secondary cuspal tearing or perforation with valve incompetence.[25,57,60,176,232] Histologic examination of the cusps of infected bioprosthetic valves often demonstrates deep clumps of bacterial or fungal organisms with few inflammatory cells. Four stages of bioprosthetic valve cuspal infection have been described.[60] Stage I is characterized by localization of organisms only on thrombotic deposits adherent to the cuspal surfaces; stage II, by extension of organisms to immediately subjacent cuspal collagen; stage III, by penetration of organisms into central areas of cuspal tissue (i.e., the spongiosa of porcine bioprostheses and the middle third of the fibrosa in pericardial bioprostheses); and stage IV, by frank perforation of the cusp (Fig. 41–12).

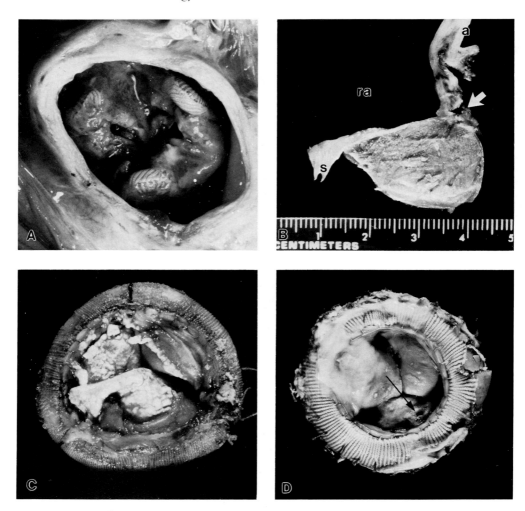

Fig. 41–11. Bioprosthetic valve endocarditis. (**A**) Aortic aspect of porcine valve showing vegetation with extensive superimposed thrombus, associated with streptococcal endocarditis. (**B**) Same case, sectioned through medial aortic wall with proximal atrioventricular conduction system demonstrating ring abscess. Patient died of sudden-onset complete heart block. Legend: a, aorta; ra, right atrium; s, septal leaflet of the tricuspid valve; arrow, area of necrosis, which involves the bundle of His. (**C**) Extensive cuspal vegetations on valve from another patient. (**D**) Cuspal perforation by organism-induced necrosis (arrow) in an additional patient. (*Figure continues.*)

Cuspal perforations due to endocarditis on bioprosthetic valves resemble those on natural valves. Cusp-limited infection can be sterilized by antibiotic therapy in early cases[163]; in contrast, mechanical prosthetic or bioprosthetic valve endocarditis with ring ab-scess is less frequently cured without surgery. Interestingly, recurrent infection following valve replacement for active endocarditis is greater when a bioprosthesis rather than a mechanical valve is used.[200]

Bioprosthetic valve endocarditis is caused

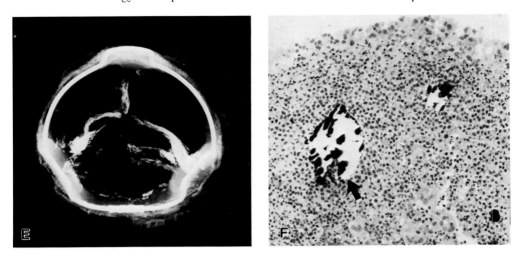

Fig. 41–11 (*Continued*). (**E**) Typical radiographic appearance in a bioprosthesis of dystrophic mineralization within extensive cuspal vegetations (extrinsic calcification). The pattern of mineralization is diffuse, primarily on the free edges of valve cusps. (**F**) Histologic demonstration of calcification in vegetation on bioprosthesis (arrow). (H&E, × 200.) (Figs. A & D from Schoen,[176] with permission; Fig. B from Schoen,[172a] with permission; Fig. C from Schoen and Hobson,[180] with permission.)

by a microbiologic spectrum similar to that of other prosthetic valve endocarditis, including *Staphylococcus aureus* and *epidermidis*, fungi, gram-negative bacteria, and other organisms unusual for natural valve endocarditis.[173,174] *Legionella pneumophila* and the organism causing Q fever have been recognized as bioprosthetic valve pathogens.[56,212]

Calcification can occur in platelets, degenerating bacteria, and inflammatory cells

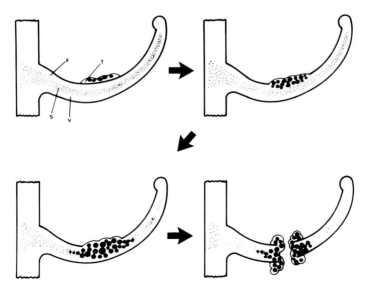

Fig. 41–12. Progression of bioprosthetic valve endocarditis involving cusps: Stage I, upper left; stage II, upper right; stage III, lower left; and stage IV, lower right. (From Ferrans et al.,[60] with permission.)

within endocarditic cuspal vegetations (*extrinsic calcification*).[58,176] Specimen radiography often demonstrates a characteristic morphology of calcification in infected bioprosthetic valves with diffuse mineral deposits along the free edge of the cusps (see Fig. 41–11E).

Paravalvular Leaks

Considerations for paravalvular leaks are nearly identical for bioprostheses and mechanical valves. Paravalvular defects may be clinically inconsequential, aggravate hemolysis, or cause heart failure through regurgitation. An early paravalvular leak usually results from suture knot failure, inadequate suture placement, or separation of sutures from a pathologic annulus in endocarditis with ring abscess, myxomatous valvular degeneration (i.e., floppy mitral valve), or calcified valvular annulus (i.e., calcific aortic stenosis or mitral annular calcification).[52] Late paravalvular leaks are generally small and are caused, during healing, by anomalous tissue retraction from the sewing ring and between sutures. It has been suggested that paraval-

vular leak associated with a glutaraldehyde-pretreated bioprosthetic valve could be caused by necrosis of tissues adjacent to the sewing ring resulting from the toxic effects of residual glutaraldehyde.[62] Small paravalvular defects may be overlooked by the surgeon or by pathologic examination at autopsy unless the perimeter of a prosthesis is carefully examined with a probe.

Tissue Overgrowth

Following implantation of a bioprosthesis, host fibrous tissue grows from tissues adjacent to the annulus over the sewing ring to partially cover the prosthesis. It is composed of fibrous connective tissue, with collagen and elastic fibers, and is generally lined partly or completely by endothelium; organization of microthrombi might contribute to its formation. The fibrous sheath thickens and stiffens the cusps, causes commissural fusion or compromises the area of the orifice (Fig. 41–13). In some instances, encasement can more than double cuspal thickness. Ensheathing tissue is usually easily distinguished from cuspal matrix because the new collagen is less eosino-

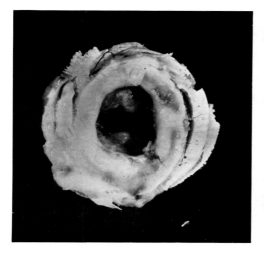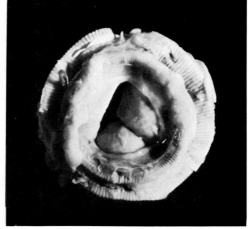

Fig. 41–13. (**A, B**) Tissue overgrowth causing stenosis of porcine bioprostheses. In both valves shown, tissue overgrowing the sewing ring compromises a significant portion of the original valve lumen.

philic than cuspal collagen and cells stain normally, in contrast to the poor or nonexistent staining of cuspal cells following prolonged implantation. Calcification,[58] and in experimental models, metaplastic cartilage,[9] can occur in the fibrous tissue. Tissue overgrowth is a particular problem in right-sided valves, particularly valved right ventricular-pulmonary artery conduits in children. In them, fibrosis can not only cause stenosis but also retraction of cusps with wide-open valve regurgitation.[139] Similar fibrous sheathing can occur with dura mater, fascia lata, and homograft valves (see below).

Disproportion, Misplacement, Hemodynamic Obstruction, and Miscellaneous Effects

There are many potential causes of bioprosthetic valve obstruction. They may be present at implantation or develop progressively during function (Table 41–6). In a particular case, valve stenosis can be multifactorial and assessment of the relative importance of contributory factors difficult.[24] Although the central flow pattern of bioprosthetic valves generally promotes good hemodynamic function, bioprosthetic valves, like mechanical valves, partially obstruct forward flow and have a small amount of regurgitant flow. The intrinsic stiffness of bioprosthetic valve cusps renders the extent of valve opening dependent on cardiac output.[71] The presence of a right coronary cuspal muscle shelf and uneven opening of cusps are additional inherent factors. Obstruction is potentiated in small bioprostheses, in which the base and struts occupy a greater fraction of the orifice area than in ones of larger size. As large a prosthesis as possible is often implanted into a fixed-sized annulus because of its perceived tendency to be less obstructive than a smaller-sized prosthesis. However, the stents of such an oversized valve could interfere with ventricular

Table 41–6. Causes of Obstruction in Bioprosthetic Valves

Present at implantation
  Strut bulk relative to orifice area (obstructive at small sizes)
  Intrinsic cuspal stiffness due to glutaraldehyde fixation under pressure
  Cardiac output dependence of cuspal opening
  Right coronary cuspal muscle shelf
  Disproportion
  Malposition
  Suture looping
  Strut from mitral prosthesis causing left ventricular outflow tract obstruction
Progressive during function
  Tissue overgrowth occluding orifice
  Cuspal stiffening
    Fluid insudation
    Thrombus
    Calcification
  Stent creep

contraction, irritate the ventricular wall to cause arrhythmias, or even perforate the myocardium or aorta.[102] Angulation can result from insertion of the valve away from the usual axis. This possibility is potentiated when the annulus is distorted by scarring, infection, or calcification. Cuspal motion can be restricted by sutures looped around bioprosthetic valve stents. This is seen particularly in pericardial bioprostheses, where the commissural cuspal attachments are not protected by bulky struts (Fig. 41–14A).[103,173] Exuberant fibrous tissue overgrowth may obstruct the inflow orifice of any valve, preventing full mechanical valve occluder excursion or causing stenosis of a bioprosthesis (see above). Specific details of valve orientation may alleviate or potentiate extrinsic interactions. Obstruction to a coronary ostium can result from the malpositioning of a stent of an aortic bioprosthesis. The left ventricular outflow tract can be obstructed by a stent of an improperly oriented mitral bioprosthesis.[99]

Progressive inward deflection of the stent posts (*stent creep*) of porcine aortic valve bioprostheses is commonly observed to variable degree, but is infrequently a cause of valve

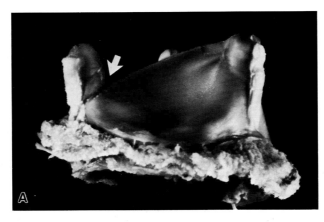

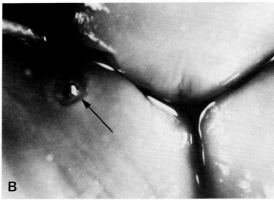

Fig. 41–14. Suture interactions with bioprosthetic valves. **(A)** Suture around stent post (arrow) of mitral bovine pericardial bioprosthetic valve, causing stenosis. **(B)** Perforation of porcine valve cusp (arrow) by long suture. (From Schoen,[173] with permission.)

dysfunction (Fig. 41–15). Reported cases include instances of reoperation required for secondary valvar thrombosis due to strut compression in the aortic root,[168] and severe hemolytic anemia[121]; both cases were probably due to extrinsic stent post compression. In another case, permanent centripetal stent post deformation resulted in relative mitral stenosis after mitral valve replacement.[21] Recent studies of the relative frequency and hemodynamic significance of stent creep have concluded that: (1) clinically important progressive geometric reduction of the outflow orifice is infrequent; (2) stent creep is not specifically related to the constructional materials or design of the stent post; (3) stent defor-

mation increases slowly with functional duration; (4) the major causes of stent post bending are compression of the left ventricular wall, aortic outflow tract, and/or tissue overgrowth (i.e., extrinsic factors); and (5) the degree of inward bending of stent posts noted clinically does not usually affect hemodynamic valvular dysfunction with geometric change of up to a 15-degree inward bending angle of the struts.[1,2,185]

Fracture of the wire stents of the Carpentier-Edwards bioprosthetic valve has been noted in several instances, but its clinical significance is uncertain. Several cases of porcine valve dysfunction caused by cusps in a fixed-opened position have been reported.[170,209]

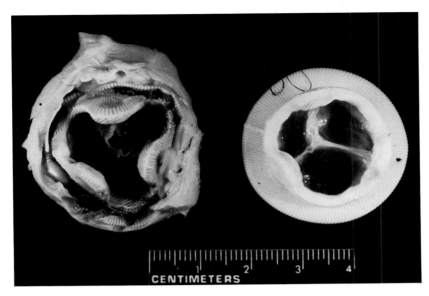

Fig. 41–15. Stent creep of aortic bioprosthesis implanted 36 months (left); an unimplanted prosthesis of the same size is shown for comparison (right). The reduction in outflow orifice of the removed valve is apparent. (From Schoen et al.,[185] with permission.)

Cuspal performations can be caused by long suture ends, especially those stiffened by fibrous tissue encapsulation. Uncommon in clinical Hancock valves, except experimentally in the mitral position,[103] suture perforations have been reported in clinical aortic Carpentier-Edwards valves, where the cusps have less peripheral protection by the stent.[143]

Structural Deterioration

Prosthetic valve dysfunction caused by degradation of materials frequently prompts reoperation or causes death in patients who have had a valve replaced by mechanical bioprosthetic devices.[173–175] The durability of mechanical prosthetic valves and bioprostheses varies widely and for specific types of each.

An intrinsic structural deterioration (often termed *primary tissue failure*) is the most frequent cause of dysfunction of cardiac valve bioprostheses derived from either porcine aortic valve or bovine pericardium.[42,45,46,68,73,74,84,123,134,142,156,173–175,177,180,221,225] Bioprosthetic valve deterioration is usually the result of cuspal mineralization, but noncalcific mechanical dysfunction (due to tears, fenestrations, abrasions, etc.) also occurs. A diagnosis of primary tissue failure presupposes the absence of antecedent infective endocarditis. Porcine aortic bioprosthetic valve deterioration, with cuspal tears or calcification or both, is strongly time dependent and accounts for an accelerated valve failure rate following 4 to 5 years of function (Fig. 41–16). Structural dysfunction occurs in approximately 50 percent of porcine valves by 15 years postoperatively. The most frequent clinicopathologic mode of failure in porcine valves is regurgitation through tears secondary to calcification. This causes approximately three-fourths of degenerative failures (Fig. 41–17). Pure stenosis due to calcific cuspal stiffening (Fig. 41–18) and cuspal tears or perforations unrelated to either calcification or endocarditis (Fig. 41–19) occur less frequently (approximately 10 to 15 percent each). The mech-

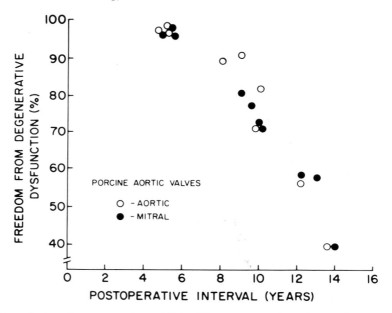

Fig. 41–16. Compilation of representative published data on actuarial incidence of porcine valve intrinsic structural deterioration (primary tissue failure). Data adapted from references 45, 46, 65, 74, 98, 123, 133, and 173.

anisms of very late valve failure (after more than 15 years) appear similar to those in the 5 to 10 year interval. Figure 41–20 illustrates a valve functioning for over 16 years that was removed surgically because of tearing superimposed on mild mineralization. The clinical presentation of bioprosthetic valve failure is heterogeneous; most patients develop cardiac dysfunction insidiously, permitting elective reoperation, but 5 to 10 per-

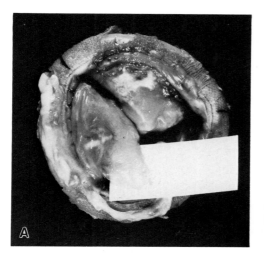

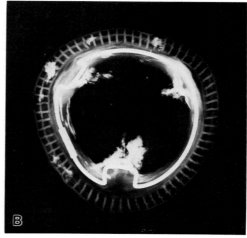

Fig. 41–17. Porcine valve, primary tissue failure due to calcification with secondary cuspal tear leading to severe regurgitation. (**A**) Gross specimen. (**B**) Specimen radiograph. Dense calcific deposits are apparent at commissures. (From Schoen and Hobson,[180] with permission.)

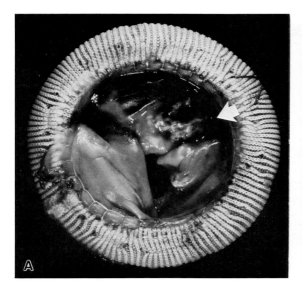
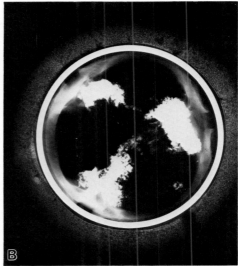

Fig. 41–18. Calcific stenosis of porcine bioprosthesis. (**A**) Gross specimen showing stiff cusps. Incidentally, there is a cuspal hematoma (arrow), which is probably of no functional significance in this case. (**B**) Specimen radiograph demonstrating the extensive mineralization that characterizes most valves with calcific stenosis. (From Schoen and Hobson,[180] with permission.)

cent of them deteriorate rapidly and require urgent surgery.[22] Calcific valve failure is more frequent in young recipients, and studies suggest that increased risk continues to age 35.[98,123]

A unified model for clinical porcine bioprosthetic heart failure has been proposed (Fig. 41–21).[183] Calcification, mediated by a complex interplay of host and implant factors, can cause failures directly through stenosis or

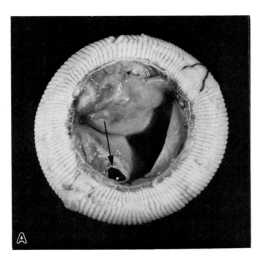
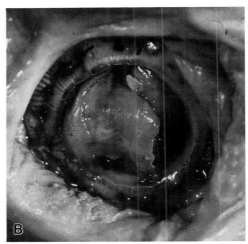

Fig. 41–19. Noncalcific cuspal defects causing regurgitation of porcine aortic valves implanted at the mitral site. (**A**) Perforation (arrow). (**B**) Tear. (From Schoen et al.,[176] with permission.)

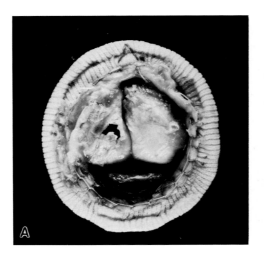
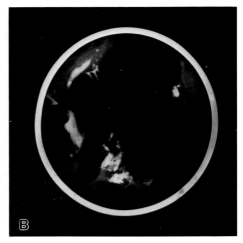

Fig. 41–20. Porcine bioprosthetic valve failure with calcification and cuspal tear 16 years after implantation. (**A**) Gross specimen. (**B**) Specimen radiograph.

can induce sites of stress concentration vulnerable to superimposed tearing. The pathophysiology and specific determinants of bioprosthetic valve calcification are discussed below. Alternatively, collagen degradation, induced primarily by mechanical factors, may cause failure without any contribution from calcification. Degradative failure of clinical bioprostheses relates to an interplay of these mechanisms, with one usually dominant.

Pericardial bioprostheses also fail by calcific and noncalcific deterioration.[23,68,142,156,177,203,221,225] The actuarial rate of structural dysfunction has not yet been established, due to an insufficient number of valves reaching the most susceptible postoperative interval. However, bovine pericardial bioprostheses could have an even greater propensity for late primary tissue failure than porcine valves.[73] Calcification makes an important contribution to failure through stiffening or secondary tearing (Fig. 41–22). The morphology of calcific deposits in pericardial valves is remarkably similar to that found in failed porcine valves.[177,225] Moreover, noncalcific structural changes are likely to be more important in pericardial than in porcine bioprostheses and to comprise a major source of failures. Figure

41–23 illustrates the most frequent type of noncalcific pericardial valve structural defect, a large tear at the attachment margin of the cusp to the stent.[23,68,142,203,225] The mechanisms contributing to these tears are discussed below.

Both mechanical and biologic factors are important in most cases of structural valve dysfunction.[173,174] Biologic factors are uniformly degradative, because reparative events cannot occur in bioprosthetic valves. Studies of durability in vitro clearly highlight some specific modes of failure and design flaws,[70] but such tests disregard and potentially fail to reveal important mechanisms of materials degeneration dependent on an interaction with host biologic processes.[173,174] This suggests that in vitro accelerated testing occasionally predicts, but most often overestimates, the fatigue life of a bioprosthetic valve.

Calcification

Mineral deposits located within the boundaries of a cusp are called *intrinsic*. In contrast, *extrinsic* mineralization is associated with elements or tissue not initially implanted (e.g.,

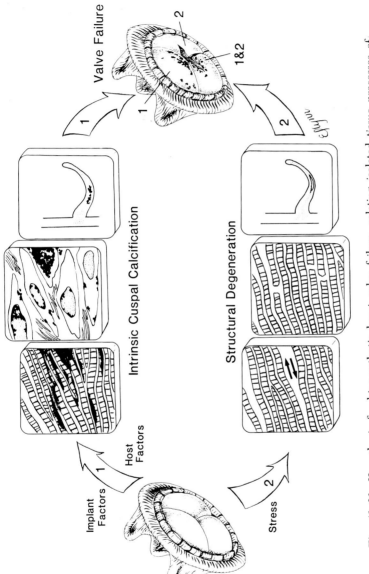

Fig. 41–21. Hypothesis for bioprosthetic heart valve failure, relating isolated tissue processes of mineralization (pathway 1) and collagen degeneration (pathway 2) to gross clinical failures. Such failures have calcification with cuspal stiffening (1), cuspal defects without calcific deposits (2), or cuspal tears associated with mineralization (1 & 2). These processes can occur independently or may be synergistic. (From Schoen and Levy,[183] with permission.)

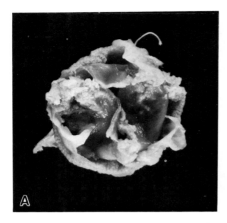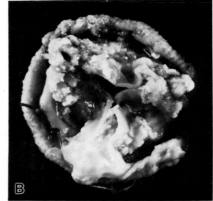

Fig. 41–22. Pericardial valve failure with calcification. **(A)** Calcification with tearing of clinical mitral bovine pericardial bioprosthesis (Ionescu-Shiley standard valve). **(B)** Calcific stenosis of clinical mitral bovine pericardial bioprosthesis (Ionescu-Shiley standard valve). (Fig. A from Schoen, et al.,[177] with permission; Fig. B from Schoen,[173] with permission.)

ulcerated calcific deposits) or calcification within thrombus, vegetations, or tissue overgrowth.[178] Intrinsic calcific deposits are generally only noted in valves implanted in patients 3 to 4 years or longer; in contrast, extrinsic mineral deposits can develop in thrombi or infected vegetations in several days.[178] The multiple specific sites in which calcific deposits can occur in bioprosthetic valves are listed in Table 41–7. Dysfunction due to structural deterioration of bioprosthetic heart valves is almost always caused by intrinsic mineralization (i.e., extrinsic mineralization per se unusually causes dysfunction). Degenerative cuspal calcific deposits

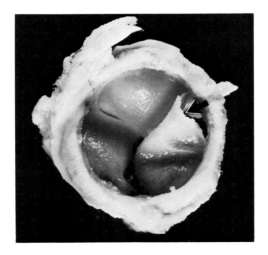

Fig. 41–23. Clinical mitral bovine pericardial bioprosthesis with extensive tear of one cusp (arrow), involving cuspal free edge. (From Schoen,[173] with permission.)

Table 41–7. Sites of Calcification in Bioprosthetic Valves

Intrinsic to the cusps
    Porcine aortic valve
        Fibrosa
        Spongiosa
        Ventricularis
        Muscle shelf
    Bovine pericardium
        Fibrosa
        Blood vessels
    Cells
    Collagen
    Ground substance
    Insudated fluid and cells

Extrinsic to the cusps
    Thrombi
    Vegetations
        Platelets
        Inflammatory cells
        Bacteria
    Tissue overgrowth

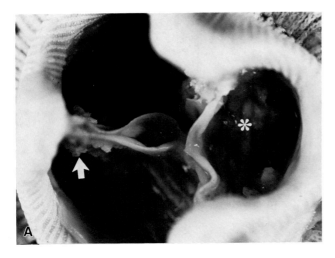

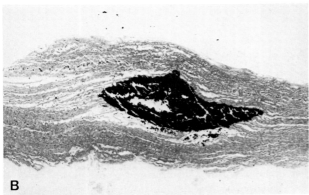

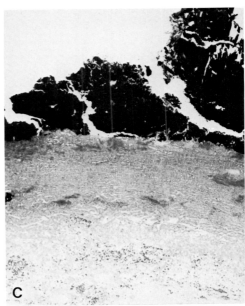

Fig. 41–24. Morphology of calcification in bioprosthetic valves. (**A**) Close-range photograph of calcified porcine bioprosthesis, demonstrating ulcerated commissural calcific nodules (arrow) and deep intrinsic cuspal calcific deposits (asterisk). Photomicrographs of (**B**) intrinsic and (**C**) extrinsic mineralization in bovine pericardial bioprostheses. (Figs. B & C: von Kossa stain [calcium phosphates black]; Fig. B: × 60; Fig. C: × 150.)

are grossly visible as nodular gray/white masses that often ulcerate through cuspal tissue. Generally, they predominate at cuspal commissures and near basal attachments (Fig. 41–24), the sites of most intense mechanical deformation during function. Light microscopic examination demonstrates the most extensive mineral in the spongiosa layer of porcine valves. Ultrastructurally, calcific deposits are related to cuspal connective tissue cells and collagen.[58,217] The mineral phase in bioprosthetic valves is a carbonate-substituted

apatite, similar to, but less crystalline than, the hydroxyapatite phase in bone and dental enamel.[211] The chemical composition and structural characteristics of bioprosthetic heart valve deposits are very similar to dystrophic calcific deposits that occur in atherosclerosis, natural aortic valves, and mechanical blood pumps.[178,210]

The extent of calcification of removed bioprosthetic valves varies widely among patients after long-term implantation (Fig. 41–25).[182] Calcification rarely causes dysfunction of

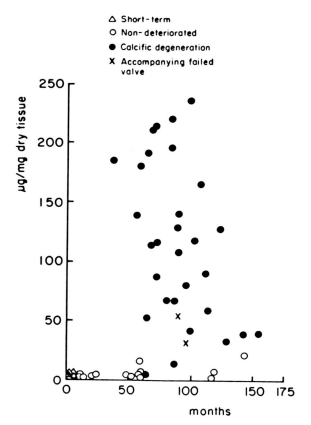

Fig. 41–25. Calcium concentration measured by atomic absorption spectroscopy, plotted against duration of function of removed porcine valves. (From Schoen et al.,[182] with permission.)

valves implanted less than 4 years in adults, but most failed valves removed following at least 4 years are mineralized. Nevertheless, some bioprostheses with tears have minimal or no radiographically demonstrable calcific deposits after implantation for 10 years or longer. Moreover, some nonfailed valves examined after long periods of entirely adequate function (e.g., valves removed at cardiac transplantation for progressive ventricular dysfunction or at autopsy following late noncardiac death) show little or no mineral. This emphasizes that there is considerable patient-to-patient and valve-to-valve variability in mineralization, the basis for which is poorly understood. The calcium content of 32 porcine bioprostheses functioning for 36 to 156

months (mean 87) and removed because of calcific failure was measured by atomic absorption spectroscopy as 113 ± 68 μm/mg (mean ± standard deviation). In contrast, nondeteriorated valves (functioning for 8 to 145 months [mean 57]) had 5 ± 6 μm/mg calcium. Stenotic, calcific valves tend to have more mineralization than calcified, torn, and hence regurgitant valves. There is a strong spatial relationship of porcine valve tears with underlying calcific deposits.[194] Although cuspal tearing and stiffening are the most frequent consequences of bioprosthetic valve calcification, calcific deposits in bioprosthetic valves can also dislodge and result in embolic damage.[100]

Percutaneous transluminal balloon dilation

of stenotic valves by catheter, now widely done for natural mitral and aortic valves,[153] has been used to dilate stenotic right-sided, conduit-mounted, and left-sided porcine bioprosthetic valves.[33,120,219] In catheter balloon valvuloplasty of native calcific aortic stenosis, the mechanism of dilation is usually fracture of calcific nodules.[94] In calcified, stenotic porcine bioprostheses, balloon inflation induces commissural splitting, leaflet cracks and fractures, and leaflet tearing. Balloon-induced breakage of friable commissural calcific deposits in calcified, stenotic bioprostheses could lead to calcific emboli and dislodge thrombotic deposits when present.[132] Large cuspal tears occurring during balloon treatment of stenotic valves could precipitate rapid deterioration. In this respect, dilation of right-sided valves in children would likely be more efficacious and safer, as stenosis is more frequently the problem with such valves, and the consequences of tearing and embolization are less.

Cuspal Tears and Perforations

Tears and other defects in bioprosthetic valves have many causes (Table 41–8). Factors contributing to cuspal defects and tears can be (1) inherent in valve fabrication, design, and

Table 41–8.   Factors Potentially Contributing to Cuspal Defects or Tears in Bioprosthetic Valves

Related to factors in manufacture and design
    Manufacturing defects
    Tissue fatigue
    Abrasion
    Stress concentrations at commissures
    Stress concentrations at sutures
    Delamination
Related to interactions with the recipient
    Infection
    Calcification
    Suture perforation
    Inflammation
Artifactual
    Valve trauma during removal

otherwise uncomplicated functional interactions; (2) caused by factors related to patient/prosthesis interactions, such as calcification, infection, or sutures; or (3) artifactual. Noncalcific tissue defects in porcine aortic valve bioprostheses usually reflect direct mechanical destruction of collagen architecture during function. They are revealed by scanning and transmission electron microscopy as fraying of the tips and disruption of collagen fibers,[90,157,196] can occur almost any time postoperatively, and appear to be more frequent in valves implanted in the mitral than the aortic site. Certainly, mechanical and possibly chemical processes degrade the connective tissue framework during function of bioprosthetic valves. Mechanical disruption of collagen fibrils occurs as a consequence of cyclical cuspal bending during function.[218] Particularly deleterious are compressive stresses along the outflow surface of the cusps during opening, which in the porcine valve have been previously fixed in the closed position.[28,198] Accelerated breakdown occurs at sites where there are stress concentrations, particularly at cuspal attachment sites. The effect on degradation of collagen by proteolytic enzymes is unknown. Both calcification and infection can also precipitate cuspal defects (see above). Moreover, a tear may be inadvertently induced or extended during surgical removal.

Classification schema for cuspal defects in bioprosthetic valves have been presented.[67,90] The scheme described in Figure 41–26 was developed primarily from observations on failed porcine valves but is equally applicable for pericardial valves.[90] In this classification, type I tears involve the free edge of a cusp; type II lesions are linear perforations that extend along the base of a cusp, forming an arc parallel to the annular margin; type III lesions are large, round or oval defects that occupy the central body of the cusp, often in association with severe cuspal destruction; and type IV lesions are small pinholes, often multiple, that appear in the central regions of the cusps. Any type of defect can be associated with calcific deposits. Moreover, each of the

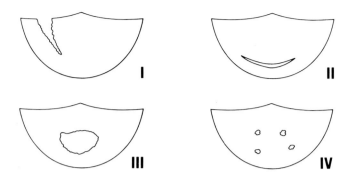

Fig. 41–26. Types of cuspal tears and perforations that occur in cardiac valve bioprostheses. See the text for details. (From Ishihara et al.,[90] with permission.)

four types of cuspal defects can be reproduced by in vitro durability testing.

Type I lesions are particularly frequent near the stent post in standard pericardial bioprostheses. They occur because the free edges of pericardial valves are composed of sharply transected, multidirectional bundles of collagen without reinforcement, the commissural attachments are contrived, and stresses at the commissures are high. Because the cuspal free edges of porcine aortic valves are reinforced by collagenous cords, which run from one commissure to the another and commissural stresses are thereby low, noncalcific type I lesions are infrequent in porcine valves. Breakage and degeneration of collagen fibrils are severe along the edges of type I lesions, but it can be extremely difficult to distinguish cuspal pathology that occurred before, from that which occurred after, tearing. Type II lesions are thought to be related to "hinging" in which the cusps do not open evenly, but tend to open by bending excessively at one localized site near the cuspal base with damage and separation of collagen bundles and formation of a linear defect along the cusp base. Type III lesions usually result from infection and have extensive destruction and necrosis of cuspal tissue at their edges, but also can be produced by the confluence of several type IV lesions. Type IV lesions usually occur in the vicinity of calcific deposits

and presumably result from mechanical stress concentrations at the edges of such deposits.

Tears in pericardial valves along the attachment points of cusps could be related to the continuous trauma of the tissue against bare Dacron cloth ("abrasion") or to tissue fatigue along these repetitive flexure sites (Fig. 41–27). Although the specific cause of such a tear often cannot be determined by gross or microscopic examination of a removed valve specimen, abrasion is suggested by systematic tapering of the tissue cross section with an attrition of collagen bundles. Cuspal perforations and tears are also frequently associated with a commissural suture ("alignment stitch"), a feature unique to the Ionescu-Shiley design, which holds cusps in apposition near the free edge and adjacent to the stent post (Fig. 41–28). Loss of commissural apposition may increase leaflet excursions and potentiate fatigue or abrasion damage. Because pericardial valves depend on an artificial attachment at the commissures, cusp tears at this site may be difficult to avoid in any tricusped pericardial valve design. Other pericardial, dura mater, and fascia lata bioprosthesis designs (see below) also fail with tears causing severe regurgitation.[23,203] A general comparison of the pathologic features observed with porcine valve and bovine pericardial bioprostheses is summarized in Table 41–9.

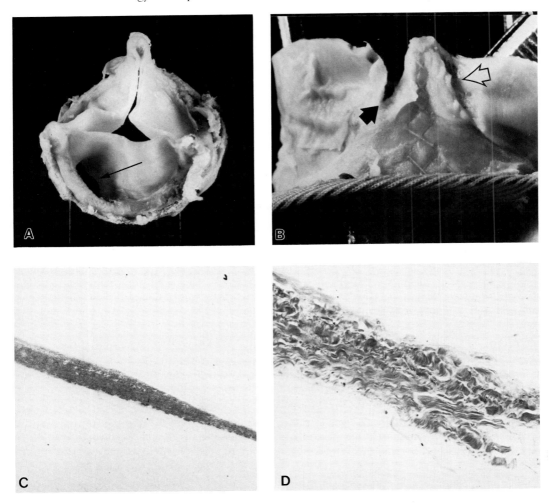

Fig. 41–27.   Fatigue and abrasion causing tearing of pericardial valves. **(A)** Basal cuspal tear in Ionescu-Shiley pericardial bioprosthesis (arrow) not involving free edge. **(B)** Tear at free edge (closed arrow) and abrasion causing thinning and incipient tear of pericardial bioprosthesis at commissural attachment (open arrow) (Gross photograph). **(C)** and **(D)** Photomicrographs of valve shown in Fig. B through area indicated by open arrow, indicating thinning and loss of pericardial tissue. (Figs. C & D: H&E; Fig. C: × 15; Fig. D: × 60.)

BIOPROSTHETIC VALVE CALCIFICATION: BASIC CONSIDERATIONS

The pathophysiology and prevention of bioprosthetic tissue calcification have been investigated using experimental models, including orthotopic and conduit-mounted valves in the circulatory system, particularly in calves and sheep, and heterotopic implantation, including subcutaneous locations, largely in rodents.[64,66,112–118,184,186,216] In these models, using immature and rapidly growing animals, bioprosthetic tissue calcifies progressively, with a morphology similar to

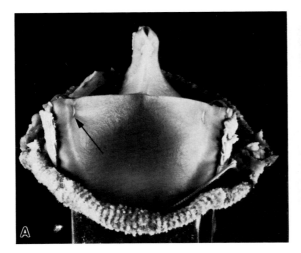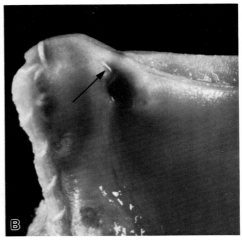

Fig. 41–28. Perforation/tearing of Ionescu-Shiley standard pericardial bioprosthetic valve cusps in area of commissural alignment stitch. (**A**) Original configuration of valve; alignment stitch indicated by arrow. (**B**) Close-up photograph of valve following long-term function demonstrating early hole at alignment suture (arrow). (*Figure continues.*)

that observed in clinical specimens, but with markedly accelerated kinetics. Studies using subcutaneous implantation of bioprosthetic tissue in weanling rats have allowed detailed investigation of mechanisms and preventive strategies. Both the morphology and extent of calcification in subcutaneous implants are analogous to those observed in clinical and experimental circulatory studies, despite the absence of dynamic mechanical activity and blood contact characteristic of the circulatory environment. Calcification of porcine valve and bovine pericardial tissue are identical in this model, both morphologically and kinetically.[181,184,186] Initial calcific deposits are almost exclusively localized to transplanted connective tissue cells and their fragments, particularly at membranes, the nucleus, and intracellular organelles such as mitochondria (Fig. 41–29). In pericardial tissue, early calcific deposits also involve endothelial cells of intrapericardial blood vessels. With increasing duration of implantation, cell-associated deposits progressively increase in size and number, obliterating cells and dissecting among collagen bundles. Direct collagen involvement is subsequently noted. Calcific de-

posits in experimental porcine valves, as in clinical valves, are greater in the spongiosa than in the fibrosa.[184] Proliferation of nucleation sites and crystal growth in both porcine valve and bovine pericardium result in a progressive confluence of diffusely distributed microcrystals into macroscopic nodules. Analogous to those responsible for clinical valve failures, gross calcific nodules focally obliterate implant architecture and ulcerate through the cuspal surface.

Pathobiology

Mineralization of bioprosthetic valves has mechanical, host, and implant determinants.[173,178,181,183,184] Mechanical deformation during function accelerates their calcification. Calcification of functioning clinical and experimental bioprosthetic valves begins and is enhanced in areas of leaflet flexion where deformations are maximal, especially at cuspal commissures and bases.[166,167,204] Some, but not all, data suggest that the degree of calcification in clinical porcine valves varies according to pressure differential across the

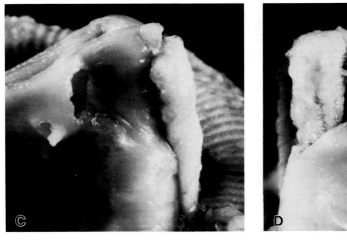
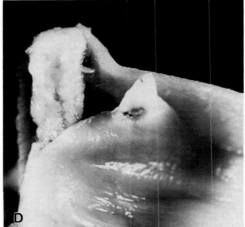
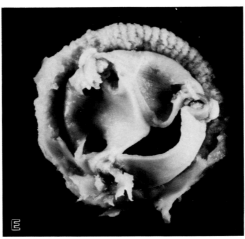

Fig. 41–28 *(Continued).* **(C)** Close-up of cuspal defect near commissure, at alignment suture site, following long-term function. **(D)** Close-up of tear initiated near but not through alignment suture hole, possibly following loss of commissural apposition. **(E)** Valve with numerous alignment suture-related tears. (Figs. A, C–E from Schoen,[177] with permission; Fig. B from Schoen et al.,[173] with permission.)

valve during the closed phase of the cardiac cycle (i.e., mitral > aortic > tricuspid).[15,39,44,182,222]

The effects of mechanical deformation on calcification are complex. In the subcutaneous model, mineralization occurs despite an absence of cyclical bending, but enhanced mineral deposition is noted in areas of tissue folds,[113] suggesting that static (as well as dynamic) mechanical deformation potentiates mineralization. The mechanisms by which

stress enhances calcification are unknown, but contributory factors could include stress-generated crystal nucleation sites, structural disruption of the collagen architecture creating internal spaces that facilitate crystal growth, piezoelectric crystal augmentation, or increased fluid insudation deep into bioprosthetic valve cusps due to a pumping action. Cuspal stiffening by calcific deposits induces new and substantial sites of stress concentration between the deposits and the surround-

Table 41–9.   Comparison of Pathologic Features: Porcine Aortic Valve vs. Bovine Pericardial Bioprostheses

	Porcine Aortic Valve	*Bovine Pericardial*
Cuspal calcification	+	+
Cuspal tears	+	+
Tissue fatigue	+	+
Cuspal abrasion	0	+
Alignment suture-related holes/tears	0	+
Cuspal stretching/sagging	0	+
Tissue overgrowth	+	+
Endocarditis involving cusps	+	+
Endocarditis with ring abscess	+	+
Adherent macrophages	+	+
Deep inflammation	Minimal	+
Deep fluid insudation	Minimal	+
Inflow surface collagen fragmentation	0	+
Focal thrombi	Minimal	+
Endothelialization	Minimal	0
Suture entrapment	0	+
Suture perforation	+	Minimal

ing tissue, potentiating leaflet rupture.[166,167]

The rate of clinical and experimental bioprosthetic tissue calcification is dependent on host metabolic factors. Calcification in particular, and valve failure in general, is markedly accelerated in children, adolescents, and young adults, with either left- of right-sided intracardiac or conduit-mounted bioprostheses.[98,105,123,135,169] Fewer than 60 percent of valves implanted in the right heart or pulmonary circulation in this population remain intact 3 to 5 years postoperatively, and the failure rate is almost total for left-sided valves.[105,135] Some data suggest that the increased risk may continue to approximately age 35.[98,123] Calcification is dramatically accelerated in younger experimental animals, simulating clinically accelerated calcification in young patients.[115] Other host factors that can cause hypercalcemia, such as renal failure[63] or calcium carbonate therapy,[136] likely promote mineralization. Whether anticoagulation retards bioprosthetic valve and

other pathologic calcification remains a controversial and unsettled issue.[115,195]

Neither nonspecific inflammation nor specific immunologic responses appear to mediate bioprosthetic tissue calcification. Inflammation induces neither mineral deposition nor resorption.[115] Morphologic examination of both circulatory and subcutaneous porcine valve implants reveals a classic foreign body response primarily composed of nonlymphocytic mononuclear cells, virtually always external to the implant. Inflammatory cell penetration into bioprosthetic tissue tends to be more pronounced in pericardial valves[177,189] and host cell reaction to mineral deposits are minimal and inconsistent. In experiments in which enclosure of valve cusps and chambers prevents host cell contact with tissue but allows free diffusion of extracellular fluid, neither the extent nor morphology of mineralization is altered.[115] Moreover, valve tissue implanted in congenitally athymic ("nude") mice, in whom T-cell function is

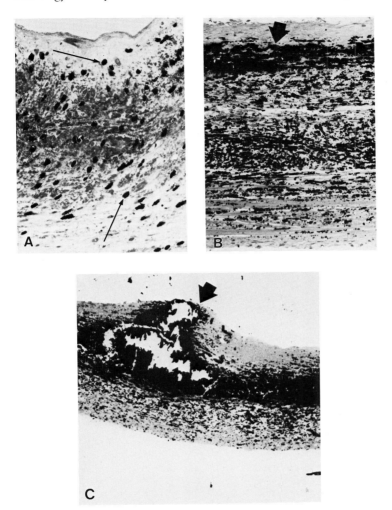

Fig. 41–29. Experimental bioprosthetic valve calcification (subcutaneous implantation in rats). Figs. A–C: Light photomicrographs. (**A**) 3-day porcine valve implant with focal well-localized deposits (arrows). (**B**) 21-day implant demonstrating early nodule formation (arrow) in pericardium. (**C**) 84-day implant demonstrating ulceration of nodule through cuspal surface (arrow) of porcine aortic valve. (*Figure continues.*)

grossly diminished, calcifies to the same extent as implants in immunologically competent hosts.[114] Second bioprosthetic valve replacements in patients fail by calcification no sooner than initial replacements.[122]

A calcifiable substrate is a prerequisite for tissue mineralization; its nature can be altered by tissue preparation details. Pretreatment of tissue with an aldehyde cross-linking agent is needed for calcification in the subcutaneous experimental environment.[81,115] Short-term delays in processing, typical of those that occur in the fabrication of commercially available valves (i.e., to 34 hours) do not appreciably potentiate mineralization.[126]

The striking similarities between physiologic and pathologic calcification are particularly germane to bioprosthetic tissue

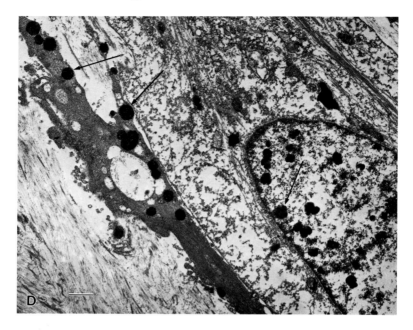

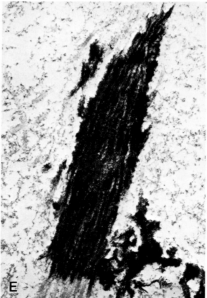

Fig. 41–29 (*Continued*). Figs. D and E: Ultrastructural features of calcification. (**D**) Focal deposits at cell surface, nucleus, and cytoplasm (arrows). (**E**) Collagen calcification. (Figs. A–C: von Kossa [calcium phosphates black]; Fig. A: × 200; Fig. B: × 150; Fig. C: × 60; Figs. D & E: Bar—1 μm.) (Figs. A, C–E from Schoen et al.,[184] with permission.)

mineralization.[178] The deposits in usual pathologic (i.e., dystrophic) calcification are almost always poorly crystalline calcium phosphate related to hydroxyapatite, which forms in physiologic (i.e., skeletal and dental) mineralization. A second feature common to virtually all forms of calcification is crystal formation associated with cell membranes, usually in the form of extracellular vesicles, often called *matrix vesicles*. A potential role in valve mineralization for the enzyme alkaline phosphatase, likely important in skeletal mineralization, is under investigation.[127] Thus, intrinsic and extrinsic biomaterial-associated mineralization, other dystrophic calcifications, and physiologic mineralization may occur via a common mechanism.[178]

Dystrophic calcification in general, and mineralization of bioprosthetic valves in particular, likely occurs in situations where the normally low calcium content of cells cannot be maintained relative to the extracellular environment.[178,186] The intracellular free calcium concentration of intact living animal cells is approximately 10^{-7} M, whereas extracellular calcium is approximately 10^{-3} M (i.e., a 10,000-fold gradient across the plasma membrane). Low cellular calcium is usually maintained by an intact cellular envelope and by energy-requiring metabolic pumps that extrude Ca^{++}, as well as intracellular buffering mechanisms. Nevertheless, calcium and phosphorus levels are relatively high in membrane-bound organelles, such as mitochondria, and phosphorous is prevalent both within the organelles and plasma membranes themselves, largely in phospholipids, and within the nucleus in nucleic acids.

Hypothesized mechanisms and determinants of bioprosthetic valve mineralization are detailed in Figure 41–30. In cells modified by aldehyde cross-linking or mechanical injury, cell membranes are disrupted, permeability is increased, and the mechanisms for calcium extrusion are no longer fully functional. Moreover, high-energy phosphates required to fuel these mechanisms are largely unavailable. Thus, calcium accumulation occurs un-impeded, but extrusion is prevented, resulting in a dramatic increase in intracellular calcium concentration, eventuating in crystal nucleation and growth. The mechanism of calcification suggested in Figure 41–30 indicates that modification of influential host or implant factors or interruption of the critical events summarized could reduce bioprosthetic valve mineralization.

Prevention

Several approaches are under investigation to reduce calcific bioprosthetic valve failure by modifying host, implant, or mechanical determinants of the mineralization process. Design changes, which include modifications in the cuspal number, configuration, and attachment to the stents, as well as alteration of pretreatment procedures, might enhance overall durability through lower mechanical stresses, as well as reduce calcification.[19,28,69,97,198,227] A complementary strategy employs exogenous mineralization inhibitors. Diphosphonate compounds, used to treat metabolic bone disease, are potent inhibitors of physiologic and pathologic calcification. They function through a retardation of calcium phosphate crystal growth.[165] In rats with subcutaneously implanted bioprosthetic tissue, either systemic therapy with such drugs (e.g., ethanehydroxydiphosphonate [EHDP])[116,118] or EHDP administered in the vicinity of the valve tissue from controlled-release drug delivery polymers loaded with the drug[80,117] inhibit leaflet calcification. Local administration of a physiologic inhibitor also mitigates mineralization.[216] Cuspal modification through incubation in solutions of the trivalent ion of aluminum (Al^{+++}),[224] an element associated with osteomalacia in renal dialysis patients, or preloading with anticalcification agents (e.g., EHDP or aminopropanehydroxydiphosphonate [APDP]),[113,223] inhibit bioprosthetic valve calcification. Pretreatment of bioprosthetic valve cusps with

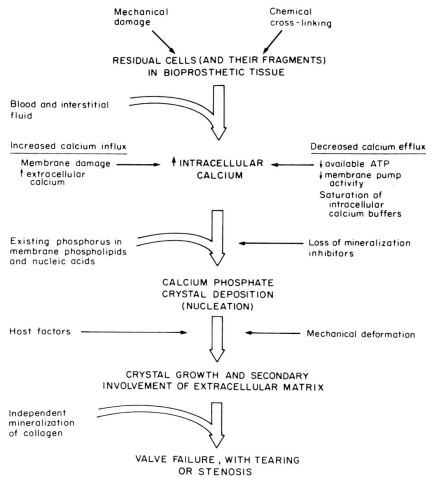

Fig. 41–30. Hypothetic model for the calcification of bioprosthetic tissue. This model considers host factors, implant factors, and mechanical damage, and relates initial sites of mineral nucleation to increased intracellular calcium in residual cells and cell fragments in bioprosthetic tissue. The ultimate result of calcification is valve failure with tear or stenosis. (From Schoen,[175] with permission.)

detergent compounds inhibits their calcification in some models.[10,35,112] Nevertheless, studies using various surfactants have shown inconsistent efficacy, possibly due to reaccumulation of blood-borne components, which negates the advantage of phospholipid extraction (i.e., removal of nucleation sites from the substrate), or charge modification, thought to be the major modes of calcification inhibition by detergents, such as sodium dodecyl sulfate (SDS). Moreover, the extent to which cuspal structural integrity could be compromised by detergent exposure has not been carefully studied.

VALVULAR HOMOGRAFTS (ALLOGRAFTS)

Cadaver-derived, unstented, antibiotic-sterilized aortic and pulmonary valvular homografts have been used as aortic valve replacements and in right ventricular or aortic outflow tract reconstructions (Fig. 41–31).[131,213,231] When implanted in semilunar sites, such valvular homografts do not require a stent. Homografts are not treated with aldehyde fixatives but are sterilized, usually with antibiotics; previous methods of sterilization and preservation proved less satisfactory.[82,220] Analogous to natural aortic valves, valvular homografts have central, unimpeded blood flow; thromboembolic complications are rare, despite the lack of anticoagulation therapy in virtually all recipients.[17,128,146] The disadvantages of homograft valves are the relatively difficult technique of insertion, progressive degeneration, and the logistic difficulties in having them available as needed.

Major factors in the fate of a homograft are the source of the graft and its treatment before insertion.[16,82,111,161,213,220,231] Some allograft valves retrieved aseptically and implanted within several weeks are likely to be partially viable. In contrast, valves sterilized either chemically or by irradiation in preparation for storage following nonsterile procurement are clearly nonviable. Implantation following chemical sterilization in formaldehyde, chlorhexadine, β-propiolactone, or ethylene oxide,

or long-term storage at −70° C or freeze-drying yield valves that frequently developed leaflet calcification and rupture, making reoperation necessary.[16,82,111,161,220] Antibiotic sterilized homograft valves are often considered "fresh," but their viability is inconsistent. Cryopreserved valves may have enhanced viability relative to antibiotic-sterilized "fresh valves."[146]

Although homograft valves are virtually free of most usual failure modes of valve substitutes, aortic homografts frequently undergo slowly progressive deterioration due to wear and tear, and occasionally calcification. The frequency of valve failure is reported as 38 to 50 percent at 10 years and 57 to 75 percent at 15 years.[17,128,146] The rate of failure of allografts implanted on the right side of the heart is less.[171] Calcification is a late degenerative feature of homografts, but it usually involves the aortic wall more prominently than the valve itself,[26,171] and frequently it appears to begin in elastic tissue. Figure 41–32 illustrates a right-sided "fresh" homograft aortic valve and conduit that was removed for extrinsic compression; valve function was otherwise normal. The valve had severely altered morphology, whereas the aortic wall segment was markedly calcified.

The role of viability of various allograft components at the time of implantation is now undergoing a critical assessment. It has been concluded that with "fresh," antibiotic-treated homografts, donor fibroblasts, whether or not viable at implantation, usually die within months.[145] Tissue reaction is variable among grafts prepared by different means. The pathology of human aortic valve homografts includes morphologic degenerative cuspal changes with cuspal architectural homogenization, thickening of the bases of the cusps, calcification, and cuspal rupture.[8,50,87,106,193] Although continued function of "fresh" grafts (with nonviable cells) following implantation could be enhanced by colonization of their cusps by host fibrous connective tissue, the cusps of valves prepared by techniques currently used are not detectably invaded to any extent by host elements

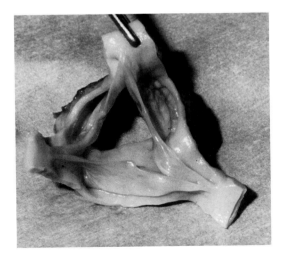

Fig. 41–31. Unimplanted homograft aortic valve replacement. (Courtesy of Cryolife, Inc., Marietta, GA.)

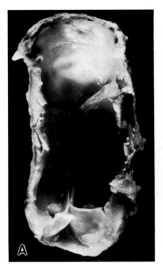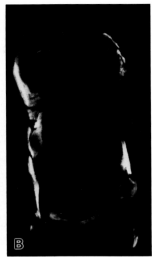

Fig. 41–32. Aortic root homograft used as a right-sided valved conduit in a patient with congenital heart disease, demonstrating diffuse dilation and mineralization of aortic wall portion. The valve was intact. (**A**) Gross specimen (valve at bottom). (**B**) Specimen radiograph, same orientation as in Fig. A.   (*Figure continues.*)

(see Fig. 41–32).[11,130,147] Evolving antibiotic treatments may be superior.[11] Valvular ground substance might play an important role in restructuring, and this ground substance may be modified by antibiotics used in graft preparation. Assessment of fibroblast viability is multifaceted and can be useful,[27] but it does not guarantee overall integrity of the aortic valve homograft because it does not assess the status of the ground substance. Moreover, endothelium is virtually completely lost during homograft valve preparation; it is unknown whether maintenance of this cell layer would improve performance.

The resurgence of interest in the use of valvular homografts is largely due to the introduction of a technique of freezing valves with dimethylsulfoxide cryoprotectant to liquid nitrogen temperatures. This yields valves that can be thawed and used following storage of more than a year.[7,130,145,146] The preservation technique does not produce demonstrable deleterious morphologic or functional changes in cusp tissue. It also appears superior to simple storage in fluid and is of potential for the development of valve banks.[12,83] Recent results suggest this technique yields

valves comparable or superior to those prepared by other modes of treatment and procurement yielding "fresh" valves and that some donor cells remain viable.[101,145]

Despite the antigenicity of allograft tissue, host reactions and pathologic changes in cardiac valvular homografts are not generally considered to be those of tissue rejection as classically seen in solid organ grafts.[18] Histocompatibility considerations are largely ignored in transplanting heart valve allografts, and it is not clear whether improved tissue matching would yield superior results.

Stent-mounted aortic allografts are occasionally used for mitral valve replacement, but detachment of the allograft tissue from the supporting stent post is a potential mode of failure.[43]

OTHER TISSUE VALVES

Fascia lata valves were used mounted on a cloth-covered metal stent. Early experimental data suggested that fascia lata had limited durability due to progressive fibrous thick-

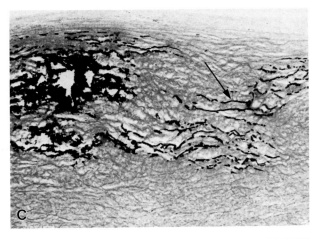

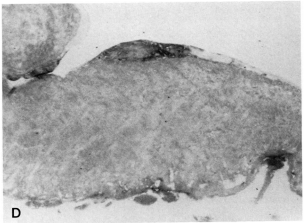

Fig. 41–32 (*Continued*). (**C**) Photomicrograph demonstrating nodular calcification in aortic wall portion largely involving elastic tissue (arrow). (**D**) Photomicrograph of valve portion demonstrating bland structure without inflammatory infiltrate or calcification. (Fig. C: von Kossa [calcium phosphates black], × 250; Fig. D: H&E, × 150.) (Specimen courtesy of R. A. Jonas, M.D., Boston, MA.) (From Schoen,[175] with permission.)

ening of the cusps, collagen degeneration, and commissural fusion.[76] Clinical studies revealed extremely high failure rates.[144] Removed valves showed calcification and a thick connective tissue covering that caused leaflet shrinkage, retraction, and loss of mobility (Fig. 41–33).[129,192]

In response to the discouraging results obtained with fascia lata prostheses, and as a potentially less expensive alternative to commercially prepared bioprostheses, the dura mater valve was developed. This valve was made of homologous dura obtained fresh from

victims of traumatic death. The dura was prepared in glycerol, a compound previously used to preserve erythrocytes and spermatozoa during frozen storage.[147] The tissue was mounted on a Dacron-covered rigid steel stent. Normal human dura mater is composed of two distinct layers; an outer (endosteal) layer and an inner (meningeal) layer.[62] The outer layer contains large bundles of loosely oriented collagenous fibers and constitutes about two-thirds of the total thickness of the dura. The inner layer is thinner and has smaller, irregularly oriented bundles of col-

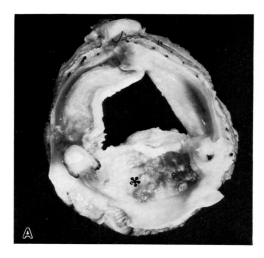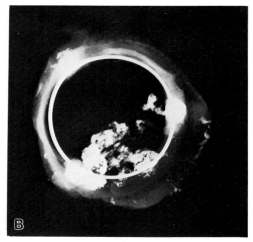

Fig. 41–33. Autologous fascia lata valve removed after 13 years. This valve has one stiff, heavily calcified cusp (asterisk in Fig. A). (**A**) Gross specimen. (**B**) Radiograph. (Specimen courtesy of M. I. Ionescu, M.D., Leeds, England.) (From Schoen,[175] with permission.)

lagen. In some areas, the two layers are closely apposed; in others they are separated by spaces of variable width, many with blood vessels. In both layers the collagen is wavy, elastic fibers are few and small, proteoglycan content is low, and fibroblasts are scarce. Despite a low rate of thromboembolism without anticoagulation, these valves had high failure rates, which were due particularly to calcification, cuspal tears, and endocarditis.[151]

PATHOLOGIC ANALYSIS OF BIOPROSTHESES AND OTHER TISSUE VALVES

General considerations for the analysis of retrieved mechanical and bioprosthetic valves are described in Chapter 40 and elsewhere.[173–175] This section emphasizes several issues particularly relevant to bioprostheses and other tissue valves.

Informed valve analysis considers the data presented in Tables 41–3 through 41–9. Complete evaluation of clinical and experimental bioprostheses and homografts includes careful and close-range gross examination, photography, radiography, and light microscopy of representative histologic sections. During gross inspection of bioprostheses and other tissue valves, special attention should be paid to cuspal flexibility, areas of thickening or thinning, vegetations, thrombi, tissue overgrowth, tears, or calcification. Some abnormalities are diagnosed by examination of the bioprosthesis in situ, and thus can be assessed by the pathologist only at necropsy; these include paravalvular leak, left ventricular outflow tract or coronary ostial obstruction, disproportion, abnormal angulation, and some types of suture interaction. Photographic documentation should include close-up views from both proximal and distal aspects, as well as pertinent lateral views. Close-range photography using a bellows and/or transillumination may be helpful in some cases. A representative gross and histologic valve evaluation data-recording form to be used for detailed clinicopathologic studies or experimental studies of new valve configurations and design modifications of existing valves is illustrated in Figure 41–34 for porcine aortic valve or other bioprostheses. This can be modified for novel structural features and anticipated complications of particular designs.

Specific pathologic features to be assessed in the evaluation of tissue valves are outlined

BIOPROSTHESIS PATHOLOGIC EVALUATION

SURGEON SPECIMEN #_____   CARDIAC PATHOLOGY LABORATORY #_____

SPECIES_____   VALVE REPLACED (CIRCLE ONE)   T   M   A

DATE RECEIVED_____

DATES OF ANALYSIS: GROSS _____   PHOTOS _____   MICROSCOPIC _____

GROSS DESCRIPTION

CALCIFICATION (RADIOGRAPHIC) 0 1+ 2+ 3+ 4+   DATE _____

  LOCATION

THROMBUS

VEGETATIONS

CUSPAL REDUNDANCY (STRETCHING)

TEARS/FENESTRATIONS

TISSUE OVERGROWTH

PARAVALVULAR LEAK

MYOCARDIAL LESIONS

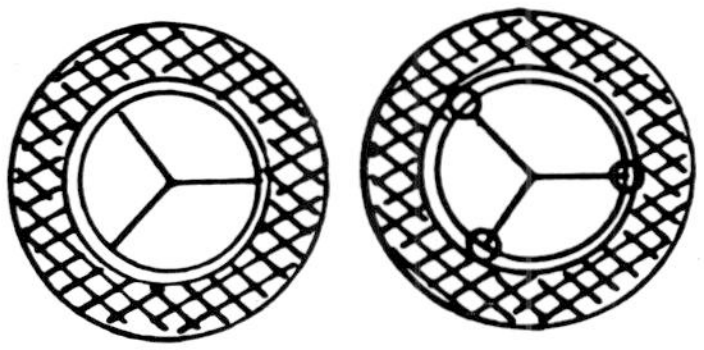

FEATURES OF SYSTEMIC NECROPSY (IF APPLICABLE)

OTHER FINDINGS

MICROSCOPIC DESCRIPTION (H&E____; GRAM____; VON KOSSA____; OTHER____)

(DEFINE SITE OF SECTIONS)

SECTION A

SECTION B

SECTION C

ETC.

(PROXIMAL EDGES LABELED WITH INDIA INK)

COMMENTS (INCLUDES OVERALL SUMMARY,

  ADDITIONAL HISTOLOGIC SECTIONS,   PATHOLOGIST - DATE
                                         CARDIAC PATHOLOGY LABORATORY
  UNUSUAL FEATURES)   BRIGHAM AND WOMEN'S HOSPITAL

Fig. 41–34. Data recording form for pathologic analysis of explanted clinical and experimental cardiac valve bioprostheses. (Modified from Schoen,[175] with permission.)

in Table 41–10. Findings may be graded semiquantitatively (0, not present; 1+, mild through 4+, most severe) for comparative studies. The use of preselected standards is encouraged for semiquantitative grading of pathologic features that are essentially subjective. The detailed extent and location of vegetations, thrombi, tissue overgrowth, fenestrations, tears, cuspal hematomas, and calcific nodules are important pathologic features. Tears are an important finding, and should be described according to size and location, but the pathologist must consider that tears might be inadvertently introduced by a surgeon during valve removal. The mor-

phology of tears may be characterized using one of the schemes previously published and discussed above.[67,90] Other features such as tissue overgrowth and altered strut relationships, including central migration, are noted.

Specimen radiography (we use the Faxitron, Hewlett-Packard, McMinnville, OR, 1.0 minute × 35 Kv) allows identification of valve type (Fig. 41–35), as well as semiquantitation of the degree of calcification (usually, 0, not present; 1+, mild through 4+, most severe) (Fig. 41–36). Correlation of semiquantitative radiographic grading of calcification with chemically determined valve mineral is good.[182] The gross localization of

Table 41–10. Pathologic Analysis of Bioprosthetic Valves

Gross Examination	Histology	Radiography
Thrombi	Vegetations/organisms	Valve type identification
Vegetations	Thrombi	Calcification
Paravalvular leak	Host cell interactions	Degree
Tissue overgrowth	Endothelialization	Morphology
Cuspal stiffness	Pannus overgrowth	Location
Cuspal hematomas	Degeneration	Ring or stent fracture
Calcification	Calcification	
Cuspal fenestrations and tears	Degree	
Cuspal abrasions	Morphology	
Cuspal stretching	Location	
Strut relationships		
Extrinsic interference or damage		

calcification can be specifically described (e.g., cuspal bodies, commissures, basal attachment sites, and/or free cuspal edges).[40] Radiography allows correlation of sites of tearing with those of calcific deposits, as well as suggesting the diagnosis of endocarditis by the pattern of characteristic mineralization (recall Fig. 41–11E).

Specimens for histologic analysis are obtained from the cuspal centers and commissures and mounted in cross section, either in glycolmethacrylate medium (JB-4, Polysciences, Inc., Warrington, PA) or conventionally in paraffin. Plastic embedding enhances morphologic detail, particularly when calcification is present. Plastic or paraffin sections are stained routinely with hematoxylin and eosin for overall morphology and selected duplicate sections are stained by von Kossa's method (for calcium phosphate), as well as other special stains such as Masson's trichrome (for collagen), Verhoeff van Gieson

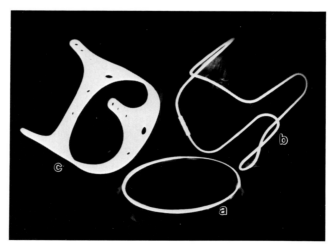

Fig. 41–35. Radiographs of Hancock (a), Carpentier-Edwards (b), and Ionescu-Shiley (c) bioprosthetic valves, demonstrating identification by stent configuration. (From Schoen,[175] with permission.)

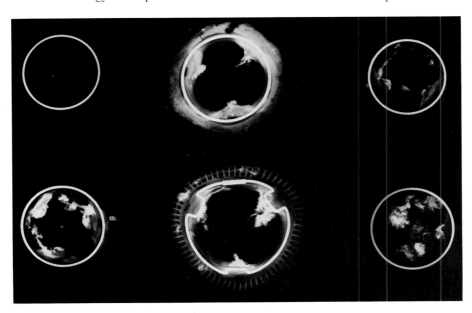

Fig. 41–36. Composite radiograph of calcified porcine aortic valve bioprostheses, demonstrating the various levels of mineralization, 1 + through 4 +, and providing radiographic standards for examination. Uncalcified (0), 1 +, and 2 + (top). 3 +, 3 + and 4 + (bottom). (From Schoen et al.,[182] with permission.)

(for elastin), and stains for microorganisms. Histologic analysis is directed toward determination of general morphology of tissue-prosthesis interactions as well as degree and specific morphology of calcific deposits.

Additional studies can be useful to address specific questions of an investigative nature. Examination under polarized light may assist definition of collagen morphology.[86] Polarized light microscopy can be performed on intact, wet-valve cusps, without embedding and sectioning. Surface scanning electron microscopy with the use of energy-dispersive radiographic analysis,[184] if available, or transmission electron microscopy,[58,217] may be done, if desired and permitted by specimen fixation conditions. Scanning electron microscopy (SEM) is useful to demonstrate overall surface morphology,[61,157,196] but SEM cannot absolutely identify endothelium. Demonstration of endothelial cells requires specific staining methods such as immunohistochemical staining with factor VIII antigen/von Willebrand Factor [vWF] or *Ulex europaeus* lectin.[175] Im-

munohistochemical techniques also provide definitive identification of macrophages, lymphocytes, and other cells, and extracellular components. Transmission electron microscopy can demonstrate overall ultrastructural morphology[34,59,61] as well as indicate sites of calcific deposits.[58,115,184,186,217] Chemical determination of the concentration of calcium and phosphorus[115,180,182,184,186] or determination of mineral crystal structure and composition[210,211] may also be done. Biochemical analysis of collagen or ground substance may be useful for some studies.[186] For studies of homograft valve cellular viability and origin, cell culture, cytogenetics, DNA fingerprinting, and other techniques may be important.[27,83,145,146]

REFERENCES

1. Akiyama K, Sawatani O, Imamura E, et al: Stent creep of porcine bioprosthesis in the mitral position. Ann Thorac Surg 46:73, 1988
2. Akiyama K, Sawatani O, Imamura E, et al:

In vitro analysis of performance of porcine xenografts with inward bending of stent posts: real-time measurement of valve orifice area using an area meter. Ann Thorac Surg 46:331, 1988

3. Allen DJ, Didio LJ, Zacharias A, et al: Microscopic study of normal parietal pericardium and unimplanted Puig-Zerbini pericardial valvular heterografts. J Thorac Cardiovasc Surg 87:744, 1984

4. Anderson DJ, Bulkley BH, Hutchins GM: A clinicopathological study of prosthetic valve endocarditis in 22 patients: morphologic basis for diagnosis and therapy. Am Heart J 94:324, 1977

5. Anderson JM, Kottke-Marchant K: Platelet interactions with biomaterials and artificial devices. CRC Crit Rev Biocompat 1:111, 1985

6. Angell WW, Angell JD: Porcine valves. Prog Cardiovasc Dis 23:141, 1980

7. Angell WW, Angell JD, Oury JH, et al: Long-term follow-up of viable frozen aortic homograft. A viable homograft valve bank. J Thorac Cardiovasc Surg 93:815, 1987

8. Aparicio SR, Donnelly RJ, Dexter F, Watson DA: Light and electron microscopy studies on homograft and heterograft heart valves. J Pathol 115:147, 1975

9. Arbustini E, Jones M, Ferrans VJ: Formation of cartilage in bioprosthetic cardiac valves implanted in sheep: a morphologic study. Am J Cardiol 52:632, 1983

10. Arbustini EI, Jones M, Moses RD, et al: Modification by the Hancock T6 process of calcification of bioprosthetic cardiac valves implanted in sheep. Am J Cardiol 53:1388, 1984

11. Armiger LC, Gavin JB, Barratt-Boyes BG: Histologic assessment of orthotopic aortic valve leaflet allografts. Its role in selecting graft pretreatment. Pathology 15:67, 1983

12. Armiger LC, Thomson RW, Strickett MG, Barratt-Boyes BG: Morphology of heart valves preserved by liquid nitrogen freezing. Thorax 40:778, 1985

13. Arnett EN, Roberts WC: Prosthetic valve endocarditis. Clinicopathological analysis of 22 necropsy patients with active infective endocarditis involving natural left-sided cardiac valves. Am J Cardiol 38:281, 1976

14. Bajpai PK: Immunological aspects of treated natural tissue prostheses. p. 5. In Williams DF (ed): Biocompatibility of Tissue Analogs. Vol. 1. CRC Press, Boca Raton, FL, 1985

15. Barbour DJ, McIntosh CL, Roberts WC: Extensive calcification of a bioprosthesis in the tricuspid valve position and minimal calcification of a simultaneously implanted bioprosthesis in the mitral valve position. Am J Cardiol 59:179, 1987

16. Barratt-Boyes BG: Cardiac surgery in the Antipodes. J Thorac Cardiovasc Surg 73:804, 1979

17. Barratt-Boyes BG, Roche AHG, Subramanyan R, et al: Long-term follow-up of patients with the antibiotic sterilized aortic homograft valve inserted free-hand into the aortic position. Circulation 75:768, 1987

18. Baue AE, Donawick WJ, Blakemore WS: The immunologic response to heterotopic allovital aortic valve transplants in presensitized and nonsensitized recipients. J Thorac Cardiovasc Surg 56:775, 1968

19. Bodnar E, Bowden NL, Drury PJ, et al: Bicuspid mitral bioprosthesis. Thorax 36:45, 1981

20. Bodnar E, Yacoub M: Biologic and Bioprosthetic Valves. Yorke Medical Books, New York, 1986

21. Borkon AM, McIntosh CL, Jones M, et al: Inward stent-post bending of a porcine bioprosthesis in the mitral position. Cause of bioprosthetic dysfunction. J Thorac Cardiovasc Surg 83:105, 1982

22. Bortolotti U, Guerra F, Magni A, et al: Emergency reoperation for primary tissue failure of porcine bioprostheses. Am J Cardiol 60:920, 1987

23. Bortolotti U, Milano A, Thiene G, et al: Early mechanical failures of the Hancock pericardial xenograft. J Thorac Cardiovasc Surg 94:200, 1987

24. Bortolotti U, Milano A, Valfre C, Thiene G: Multifactorial stenosis of a porcine aortic valve. Am Heart J 106:166, 1983

25. Bortolotti U, Thiene G, Milano A, et al: Pathological study of infective endocarditis on Hancock porcine bioprostheses. J Thorac Cardiovasc Surg 81:934, 1981

26. Brock L: Long-term degenerative changes in aortic segment homografts, with particular reference to calcification. Thorax 23:249, 1968

27. Brockbank KGM, Bank HL: Measurement of postcryopreservation viability. J Cardiac Surg 2(suppl):145, 1987

28. Broom N, Christie GW: The structure/function relationship of fresh and glutaraldehyde-

fixed aortic valve leaflets. p. 476. In Cohn LH, Gallucci V (eds): Cardiac Bioprostheses. Yorke Medical Books, New York, 1982

29. Broom ND, Marra D: Effect of glutaraldehyde fixation and valve constraint conditions on porcine aortic valve leaflet coaptation. Thorax 37:620, 1982

30. Broom ND, Thompson FJ: Influence of fixation conditions on the performance of glutaraldehyde-treated porcine aortic valves. Towards a more scientific basis. Thorax 34:166, 1979

31. Buch WS, Kosek J, Angell WW: Deterioration of formalin treated aortic valve heterografts. J Thorac Cardiovasc Surg 60:673, 1970

32. Calderwood SB, Swinski LA, Waternaux CM, et al: Risk factors for the development of prosthetic valve endocarditis. Circulation 72:31, 1985

33. Calvo OL, Sobrino N, Gamallo C, et al: Balloon percutaneous valvuloplasty for stenotic bioprosthetic valves in the mitral position. Am J Cardiol 60:736, 1987

34. Camilleri JP, Porin B, Carpentier A: Structural changes of glutaraldehyde-treated porcine bioprosthetic valves. Arch Pathol Lab Med 106:490, 1982

35. Carpentier A, Nashef A, Carpentier S, et al: Techniques for prevention of calcification of valvular bioprostheses. Circulation 70(suppl I):I165, 1984

36. Centers for Disease Control: Isolation of mycobacteria species from porcine heart valve prostheses. MMWR 26:42, 1977

37. Cheung DT, Nimni ME: Mechanism of crosslinking of proteins by glutaraldehyde: II. Reaction with monomeric and polymeric collagen. Connect Tissue Res 10:201, 1982

38. Cheung DT, Perelman N, Ko EC, Nimni ME: Mechanism of crosslinking of proteins by glutaraldehyde: III. Reactions with collagen in tissues. Connect Tissue Res 13:109, 1985

39. Cipriano PR, Billingham ME, Miller DC: Calcification of aortic versus mitral porcine bioprosthetic heart valves: A radiographic study comparing amounts of calcific deposits in valves explanted from the same patient. Am J Cardiol 54:1030, 1984

40. Cipriano PR, Billingham ME, Oyer PE, et al: Calcification of porcine prosthetic heart valves: A radiographic and light microscopic study. Circulation 66:1100, 1982

41. Clark RE, Finke EH: Scanning and light microscopy of human aortic leaflets in stressed and relaxed states. J Thorac Cardiovasc Surg 67:792, 1974

42. Cobanoglu A, Jamieson WRE, Miller DC, et al: A tri-institutional comparison of tissue and mechanical valves using a patient-oriented definition of "treatment failure." Ann Thorac Surg 43:245, 1987

43. Christie GW, Gavin JB, Barratt-Boyes BG: Graft detachment: A cause of incompetence in stent-mounted aortic valve allografts. J Thorac Cardiovasc Surg 90:901, 1985

44. Cohen SR, Silver MA, McIntosh CL, Roberts WC: Comparison of late (62 to 140 months) degenerative changes in simultaneously implanted and explanted porcine (Hancock) bioprostheses in the tricuspid and mitral valve positions in six patients. Am J Cardiol 53:1599, 1984

45. Cohn LH, Allred EN, Cohn LA, et al: Early and late risk of mitral valve replacement. A 12-year concomitant comparison of the porcine bioprosthetic and prosthetic disc mitral valves. J Thorac Cardiovasc Surg 90:872, 1985

46. Cohn LH, Allred EN, DiSesa VJ, et al: Early and late risk of aortic valve replacement. A 12-year concomitant comparison of the porcine bioprosthetic and tilting disc prosthetic aortic valves. J Thorac Cardiovasc Surg 88:695, 1984

47. Collins T, Schoen FJ, Mudge GH, Collins JJ: Thrombosis associated with a porcine bioprosthesis and ascending aortic graft in a patient with the Marfan syndrome. J Thorac Cardiovasc Surg 85:794, 1983

48. Cowgill LD, Addonizio VP, Hopeman AR, Harken A: A practical approach to prosthetic valve endocarditis. Ann Thorac Surg 43:450, 1987

49. David TE, Ropchan GC, Butany JW: Aortic valve replacement with stentless porcine bioprostheses. J Cardiac Surg 3:501, 1988

50. Davies H, Missen GAK, Blandford G, et al: Homograft replacement of the aortic valve. A clinical and pathologic study. Am J Cardiol 22:195, 1968

51. Dewanjee M, Solis E, Mackey ST, et al: Quantification of regional platelet and calcium deposition on pericardial tissue valve prostheses in calves and effect of hydroxyethylene diphosphonate. J Thorac Cardiovasc Surg 92:337, 1986

52. Dhasmana JP, Blackstone EH, Kirklin JW, Kouchoukos NT: Factors associated with periprosthetic leakage following primary mitral valve replacement: With special consideration of the suture technique. Ann Thorac Surg 35:170, 1983

53. DiSesa VJ, Allred EN, Kowalker W, et al: Performance of a fabricated trileaflet porcine bioprosthesis. Midterm follow-up of the Hancock modified-orifice valve. J Thorac Cardiovasc Surg 94:220, 1987

54. Edmunds LH: Thrombotic and bleeding complications of prosthetic heart valves. Ann Thorac Surg 44:430, 1987

55. Edmunds LH, Clark RE, Cohn LH, et al: Guidelines for reporting morbidity and mortality after cardiac valvular operations. J Thorac Cardiovasc Surg 96:351, 1988

56. Fernandez-Guerrero ML, Muelas JM, Aguado JM, et al: Q fever endocarditis on porcine bioprosthetic valves. Clinicopathologic features and microbiologic findings in three patients treated with doxycycline, cotrimoxazole, and valve replacement. Ann Intern Med 108:209, 1988

57. Ferrans VJ, Boyce SW, Billingham ME, et al: Infection of glutaraldehyde-preserved porcine valve heterografts. Am J Cardiol 43:1123, 1979

58. Ferrans VJ, Boyce SW, Billingham ME, et al: Calcific deposits in porcine bioprostheses: Structure and pathogenesis. Am J Cardiol 46:721, 1980

59. Ferrans VJ, Hilbert SL, Tomita Y, et al: Morphology of collagen in bioprosthetic heart valves. p. 145. In Nimni ME (ed): Collagen. Vol. 3, Biotechnology. CRC Press, Boca Raton, FL, 1988

60. Ferrans VJ, Ishihara T, Jones M, et al: Pathogenesis and stages of bioprosthetic infection. p. 346. In Cohn LH, Gallucci V (eds): Cardiac Bioprostheses. Yorke Medical Books, New York, 1982

61. Ferrans VJ, Spray TL, Billingham ME, Roberts WC: Structural changes in glutaraldehyde-treated porcine heterografts used as substitute cardiac valves. Transmission and scanning electron microscopic observations in 12 patients. Am J Cardiol 41:1159, 1978

62. Ferrans VJ, Tomita Y, Hilbert SL, et al: Pathology of bioprosthetic cardiac valves. Human Pathol 18:586, 1987

63. Fishbein MC, Gissen SA, Collins JJ, et al: Pathologic findings after cardiac valve replacement with glutaraldehyde-fixed porcine valves. Am J Cardiol 40:331, 1977

64. Fishbein MC, Levy RJ, Ferrans VJ, et al: Calcification of cardiac valve bioprotheses: Biochemical, histologic and ultrastructural observations in a subcutaneous implantation model system. J Thorac Cardiovasc Surg 83:602, 1982

65. Foster AH, Greenberg GJ, Underhill DJ, et al: Intrinsic failure of Hancock mitral bioprostheses: 10- to 15-year experience. Ann Thorac Surg 44:568, 1987

66. Gabbay S, Bortolotti U, Factor S, et al: Calcification of implanted xenograft pericardium: Influence of site and function. J Thorac Cardiovasc Surg 87:782, 1984

67. Gabbay S, Bortolotti U, Strom J, et al: Fatigue-induced failure of the Ionescu-Shiley pericardial xenograft in the mitral position. In-vivo and in-vitro correlation and a proposed classification. J Thorac Cardiovasc Surg 87:836, 1984

68. Gabbay S, Bortolotti U, Wasserman F, et al: Long-term follow-up of the Ionescu-Shiley mitral pericardial xenograft. J Thorac Cardiovasc Surg 88:758, 1984

69. Gabbay S, Frater RW: The unileaflet heart valve bioprosthesis: New concept. p. 411. In Cohn LH, Gallucci V (eds): Cardiac Bioprostheses. Yorke Medical Books, New York, 1982

70. Gabbay S, Kadam P, Factor S, et al: Do heart valve bioprostheses degenerate for metabolic or mechanical reasons? J Thorac Cardiovasc Surg 95:208, 1988

71. Gabbay S, McQueen DM, Yellin EL, Frater RWM: In vitro hydrodynamic comparison of mitral valve bioprostheses. Circulation 60(suppl 2):17, 1978

72. Gajewski J, Singer RB: Mortality in an insured population with atrial fibrillation. JAMA 245:1540, 1981

73. Gallo I, Nistal F, Arbe E, Artinano E: Comparative study of primary tissue failure between porcine (Hancock and Carpentier-Edwards) and bovine pericardial (Ionescu-Shiley) bioprostheses in the aortic position at five- to nine-year follow-up. Am J Cardiol 61:812, 1988

74. Gallucci V, Mazzucco A, Bortolotti U, et al:

The standard Hancock porcine bioprosthesis: Overall experience at the University of Padova. J Cardiac Surg 3(suppl):337, 1988

75. Gendler E, Gendler S, Nimni ME: Toxic reactions evoked by glutaraldehyde-fixed pericardium and cardiac valve tissue bioprosthesis. J Biomed Mater Res 18:727, 1984

76. Gilbert JW, Mansour K, Sanders S, Gravanis MB: Experimental reconstruction of the tricuspid valve with autologous fascia lata. Arch Surg 97:149, 1968

77. Goffin YA, Bartik MA, Hilbert SL: Porcine aortic vs. bovine pericardial valves. A morphologic study of the Xenomedica and Mitroflow bioprostheses. Z Kardiol 75(suppl 2):213, 1986

78. Goffin YA, Deuvaert F, Wellens F, et al: Normally and abnormally functioning left-sided porcine bioprosthetic valves after long-term implantation in patients: distinct spectra of histologic and histochemical changes. J Am Coll Cardiol 4:324, 1984

79. Goffin YA, Gruys E, Sorenson GD, Wellens F: Amyloid deposits in bioprosthetic cardiac valves after long-term implantation in man. A new localization of amyloidosis. Am J Pathol 114:431, 1984

80. Golomb G, Langer R, Schoen FJ, et al: Controlled-release of diphosphonate to inhibit bioprosthetic heart valve calcification: Dose-response and mechanistic studies. J Control Release 4:181, 1986

81. Golomb G, Schoen FJ, Smith MS, et al: The role of glutaraldehyde-induced crosslinks in calcification of bovine pericardium used in cardiac valve bioprostheses. Am J Pathol 127:122, 1987

82. Gonzalez-Lavin L, Al-Janabi N, Ross DN: Long-term results after aortic valve replacement with preserved aortic homografts. Ann Thorac Surg 13:594, 1972

83. Gonzalez-Lavin L, McGrath LB, Amini S, Graf D: Homograft valve preparation and predicting viability at implantation. J Cardiac Surg 3(suppl):309, 1988

84. Hammond GL, Geha AS, Kopf GS, Hashim SW: Biological versus mechanical valves. Analysis of 1,116 valves inserted in 1,012 adult patients with a 4,818 patient-year and a 5,327 valve-year follow-up. J Thorac Cardiovasc Surg 93:182, 1987

85. Hayat MA (ed): Fixation for Electron Microscopy. Academic Press, San Diego, p. 64, 1981

86. Hilbert SL, Ferrans VJ, Swanson WM: Optical methods for the nondestructive evaluation of collagen morphology in bioprosthetic heart valves. J Biomed Mater Res 20:1411, 1986

87. Hudson REB: Pathology of the human aortic valve homograft. Br Heart J 28:291, 1966

88. Ionescu MI, Smith DR, Hasan SS, et al: Clinical durability of the pericardial xenograft valve: Ten years' experience with mitral replacement. Ann Thorac Surg 34:268, 1982

89. Ishihara T, Ferrans VJ, Barnhart GR, et al: Intracuspal hematomas in implanted porcine valvular bioprostheses. J Thorac Cardiovasc Surg 83:399, 1982

90. Ishihara T, Ferrans VJ, Boyce SW, et al: Structure and classification of cuspal tears and perforations in porcine bioprosthetic cardiac valves implanted in patients. Am J Cardiol 48:665, 1981

91. Ishihara T, Ferrans VJ, Jones M, et al: Histologic and ultrastructural features of normal human parietal pericardium. Am J Cardiol 46:744, 1980

92. Ishihara T, Ferrans VJ, Jones M, et al: Occurrence and significance of endothelial cells in implanted porcine bioprosthetic valves. Am J Cardiol 48:443, 1981

93. Ishihara T, Ferrans VJ, Jones M, et al: Structure of bovine parietal pericardium and of unimplanted Ionescu-Shiley pericardial valvular bioprostheses. J Thorac Cardiovasc Surg 81:747, 1981

94. Isner JM, Samuels DA, Slovenkai GA, et al: Mechanism of aortic balloon valvuloplasty: Fracture of valvular calcific deposits. Ann Intern Med 108:377, 1988

95. Ivert TSA, Dismukes WE, Cobbs CG, et al: Prosthetic valve endocarditis. Circulation 69:223, 1984

96. Jamieson WRE, Gerein AN, Ling H, et al: The Mitral Medical pericardial bioprosthesis: New generation bovine pericardial prosthesis. J Cardiac Surg 3(suppl):413, 1988

97. Jamieson WRE, Munro AI, Miyagishima RT, et al: The Carpentier-Edwards supra-annular porcine bioprosthesis: New generation low pressure glutaraldehyde fixed prosthesis. J Cardiac Surg 3(suppl):507, 1988

98. Jamieson WRE, Rosado LJ, Munro AI, et al:

Carpentier-Edwards standard porcine bio-prosthesis: Primary tissue failure (structural valve deterioration) by age groups. Ann Thorac Surg 46:155, 1988

99. Jett GK, Jett MD, Bosco P, et al: Left ventricular outflow tract obstruction following mitral valve replacement. Effect of strut height and orientation. Ann Thorac Surg 42:299, 1986

100. Johnson D, Gonzalez-Lavin L: Myocardial infarction secondary to calcific embolization: An unusual complication of bioprosthetic valve degeneration. Ann Thorac Surg 42:102, 1986

101. Jonas RA, Ziemer G, Britton L, Armiger LC: Cryopreserved and fresh antibiotic-sterilized valved aortic homograft conduits in a long-term sheep model. Hemodynamic, angiographic, and histologic comparisons. J Thorac Cardiovasc Surg 96:746, 1988

102. Jones M, Eidbo EE, Rodriguez ER, et al: Ventricular aneurysms and other lesions produced by the struts of bioprosthetic valves implanted in sheep. J Thorac Cardiovasc Surg 95:729, 1988

103. Jones M, Rodriguez ER, Eidbo EE, Ferrans VJ: Cuspal perforations caused by long suture ends in implanted bioprosthetic valves. J Thorac Cardiovasc Surg 90:557, 1985

104. Khuri SF, Folland ED, Sethi G, et al: Six month postoperative hemodynamics of the Hancock heterograft and the Bjork-Shiley prosthesis: Results of a Veterans Administration Cooperative Prospective Randomized Trial. J Am Coll Cardiol 12:8, 1988

105. Kopf GS, Geha AS, Hellenbrand WE, Kleinman CS: Fate of left-sided cardiac bioprosthesis valves in children. Arch Surg 121:488, 1986

106. Kosek JC, Iben AB, Shumway NE, Angell WW: Morphology of fresh heart valve homografts. Surgery 66:269, 1969

107. Lader E, Kronzon I, Trehan N, et al: Severe hemolytic anemia in patients with a porcine aortic valve prosthesis. J Am Coll Cardiol 1:1174, 1983

108. Laskowski LF, Marr JJ, Spernoga JF, et al: Fastidious mycobacteria grown from porcine prosthetic-heart-valve cultures. New Engl J Med 297:101, 1977

109. Lawford PV, Black MM, Drury PJ, et al: The in vivo durability of bioprosthetic heart valves-modes of failure observed in explanted valves. Engin Med 16:95, 1987

110. Lee JM, Boughner DR, Courtman DW: The glutaraldehyde-stabilized porcine aortic valve xenograft. II. Effect of fixation with or without pressure on the tensile viscoelastic properties of the leaflet material. J Biomed Mater Res 18:79, 1984

111. Lefrak EA, Starr A: Cardiac Valve Prostheses. Appleton-Century-Crofts, East Norwalk, CT, 1979

112. Lentz DJ, Pollock EM, Olsen DB, Andrews EJ: Prevention of intrinsic calcification in porcine and bovine xenograft materials. Trans Am Soc Artif Intern Organs 28:494, 1982

113. Levy RJ, Hawley MA, Schoen FJ, et al: Inhibition by diphosphonate compounds of calcification of porcine bioprosthetic heart valve cusps implanted subcutaneously in rats. Circulation 71:349, 1985

114. Levy RJ, Schoen FJ, Howard SL: Mechanism of calcification of porcine bioprosthetic aortic valve cusps: Role of T-lymphocytes. Am J Cardiol 52:629, 1983

115. Levy RJ, Schoen FJ, Levy JT, et al: Biologic determinants of dystrophic calcification and osteocalcin deposition in glutaraldehyde-preserved porcine aortic valve leaflets implanted subcutaneously in rats. Am J Pathol 113:143, 1983

116. Levy RJ, Schoen FJ, Lund SA, Smith MS: Prevention of leaflet calcification of bioprosthetic heart valves with diphosphonate injection therapy. Experimental studies of optimal dosages and therapeutic durations. J Thorac Cardiovasc Surg 94:551, 1987

117. Levy RJ, Wolfrum J, Schoen FJ, et al: Inhibition of calcification of bioprosthetic heart valves by local controlled-released diphosphonate. Science 227:190, 1985

118. Levy RJ, Zenker JA, Bernhard WF: Porcine bioprosthetic valve calcification in bovine left ventricle-aorta shunts: Studies of the deposition of vitamin K-dependent proteins. Ann Thorac Surg 36:187, 1983

119. Lian JB, Levy RJ, Bernhard W, et al: LVAD mineralization of gammacarboxyglutamic acid containing proteins in normal and pathologically mineralized tissue. Trans Am Soc Artif Intern Organs 27:683, 1981

120. Lloyd TR, Marvin WJ, Mahoney LT, Lauer RM: Balloon dilation valvuloplasty of bio-

prosthetic valves in extracardiac conduits. Am Heart J 114:268, 1987

121. Magilligan DJ, Fisher E, Alam M: Hemolytic anemia with porcine xenograft aortic and mitral valves. J Thorac Cardiovasc Surg 79:628, 1980

122. Magilligan DJ, Lewis JW, Heinzerling RH, Smith D: Fate of a second porcine bioprosthetic valve. J Thorac Cardiovasc Surg 85:362, 1983

123. Magilligan DJ, Lewis JW, Tilley B, Peterson E: The porcine bioprosthetic valve. Twelve years later. J Thorac Cardiovasc Surg 89:499, 1985

124. Magilligan DJ, Oyama C, Klein S, et al: Platelet adherence to bioprosthetic cardiac valves. Am J Cardiol 53:945, 1984

125. Mannschott P, Herbage D, Weiss M, et al: Collagen heterogeneity in pig heart valves. Biochem Biophys Acta 434:177, 1976

126. Maranto A, Schoen FJ: Effect of delay between tissue harvest and glutaraldehyde pretreatment on mineralization of bovine pericardium used in bioprosthetic heart valves. J Biomed Mater Res 72:819, 1988

127. Maranto AR, Schoen FJ: Alkaline phosphatase activity of glutaraldehyde-treated bovine pericardium used in bioprosthetic cardiac valves. Circ Res 63:844, 1988

128. Matsuki O, Robles A, Gibbs S, et al: Longterm performance of 555 aortic homografts in the aortic position. Ann Thorac Surg 46:187, 1988

129. McEnany MT, Ross DN, Yates AK: Valve failure in seventy-two frame-supported autologous fascia lata mitral valves: Two year follow-up. J Thorac Cardiovasc Surg 63:199, 1972

130. McGiffin DC, O'Brien MF, Stafford EG, et al: Long-term results of the viable cryopreserved allograft aortic valve: Continuing evidence for superior valve durability. J Cardiac Surg 3(suppl):289, 1988

131. McGrath LB, Gonzalez-Lavin L, Graf D: Pulmonary homograft implantation for ventricular outflow tract reconstruction: Early phase results. Ann Thorac Surg 45:273, 1988

132. McKay CR, Waller BF, Hong R, et al: Problems encountered with catheter balloon valvuloplasty of bioprosthetic aortic valves. Am Heart J 115:463, 1988

133. Milano AD, Bortolotti U, Mazzucco A, et al: Performance of the Hancock porcine bioprosthesis following aortic valve replacement: Considerations based on a 15-year experience. Ann Thorac Surg 46:216, 1988

134. Milano A, Bortolotti U, Talenti E, et al: Calcific degeneration as the main cause of porcine bioprosthetic valve failure. Am J Cardiol 53:1066, 1984

135. Miller DC, Stinson EB, Oyer PE, et al: The durability of porcine xenograft valves and conduits in children. Circulation 66(suppl I):I, 1982

136. Moront MG, Katz KM: Early degeneration of a porcine aortic valve bioprosthesis in the mitral valve position in an elderly woman and its association with long-term calcium carbonate therapy. Am J Cardiol 59:1006, 1987

137. Morse D, Steiner RM, Fernandez J: Guide to Prosthetic Cardiac Valves. Springer-Verlag, New York, 1985

138. Munro JM, Cotran RS: The pathogenesis of atherosclerosis: Atherogenesis and inflammation. Lab Invest 58:249, 1988

139. Murphy SK, Rogler WC, Fleming WH, McManus BM: Retraction of bioprosthetic heart valve cusps: A cause of wide-open regurgitation in right-sided heart valves. Hum Pathol 19:140, 1988

140. Nimni ME: The cross-linking and structure modification of the collagen matrix in the design of cardiovascular prostheses. J Cardiac Surg 3:523, 1988

141. Nistal N, Artinano E, Gallo I: Primary tissue valve degeneration in glutaraldehyde-preserved porcine bioprostheses: Hancock I versus Carpentier-Edwards at 4- to 7-years' follow-up. Ann Thorac Surg 42:568, 1986

142. Nistal F, Garcia-Martinez V, Fernandez D, et al: Degenerative pathologic findings after long-term implantation of bovine pericardial bioprosthetic heart valves. J Thorac Cardiovasc Surg 96:642, 1988

143. Nunez L, Iglesias A, Aguado MG, et al: Early leaflet perforation as a cause of bioprosthetic dysfunction. Scand J Thorac Cardiovasc Surg 16:17, 1982

144. Obituary for fascia lata heart valves. Editorial. Br Med J 1:115, 1976

145. O'Brien MF, Johnston N, Stafford G, et al: A study of the cells in the explanted viable cryopreserved allograft valve. J Cardiac Surg 3(suppl):279, 1988

146. O'Brien MF, Stafford EG, Gardner MAH, et al: Comparison of aortic valve replacement with viable cryopreserved and fresh allograft valves, with a note on chromosomal studies. J Thorac Cardiovasc Surg 94:812, 1987

147. Osinowo O, Monro JL, Ross JK: The use of glycerol-preserved homologous dura mater grafts in cardiac surgery. The Southampton experience. Ann Thorac Surg 39:367, 1985

148. Oury JH, Angell WW, Koziol JA: Comparison of Hancock I and Hancock II bioprostheses. J Cardiac Surg 3(suppl):375, 1988

149. Pavie A, Bors V, Piazza C, et al: Mid-term results of the Liotta-Bioimplant low profile bioprosthesis. J Cardiac Surg 3(suppl):353, 1988

150. Pelletier LC, Leclerc Y, Bonan R, et al: Aortic valve replacement with the Carpentier-Edwards pericardial bioprosthesis: Clinical and hemodynamic results. J Cardiac Surg 3(suppl):405, 1988

151. Permanyer-Miralda G, Soler-Soler J, Casan-Cava JM, Tornos-Mas MP: Medium term fate of dura mater valvular bioprostheses. Eur Heart J 1:195, 1980

152. Pohlner PG, Thomson FJ, Hjelms E, Barratt-Boyes BG: Experimental evaluation of aortic homograft valves mounted on flexible support frames and comparison with glutaraldehyde-treated porcine valves. J Thorac Cardiovasc Surg 77:287, 1979

153. Rahimtoola SH: Catheter balloon valvuloplasty of aortic and mitral stenosis in adults: 1987. Circulation 75:895, 1987

154. Ratliff NB, McMahon JT, Naab TJ, Cosgrove DM: Whipple's disease in the porcine leaflets of a Carpentier-Edwards prosthetic mitral valve. New Engl J Med 311:902, 1984

155. Reddy SB, Pater JL, Pym J, Armstrong PW: Hemolytic anemia following insertion of Ionescu-Shiley mitral valve bioprostheses. Can Med Assoc J 131:1469, 1984

156. Reul GJ, Cooley DA, Duncan JM, et al: Valve failure with the Ionescu-Shiley bovine pericardial bioprosthesis: Analysis of 2680 patients. J Vasc Surg 2:192, 1985

157. Riddle JM, Magilligan DJ, Stein PD: Surface morphology of degenerated porcine bioprosthetic valves four to seven years following implantation. J Thorac Cardiovasc Surg 81:279, 1981

158. Robicsek F, Hoffman PC, Masters TN, et al: Rapidly growing nontuberculous mycobacteria: A new enemy of the cardiac surgeon. Ann Thorac Surg 46:703, 1988

159. Rocchini AP, Weesner KM, Heidelberger K, et al: Porcine xenograft valve failure in children: An immunologic response. Circulation 64(suppl II):II, 1981

160. Rose AG: Pathology of the formalin-treated heterograft porcine aortic valve in the mitral position. Thorax 27:401, 1972

161. Rose AG: Pathology of Heart Valve Replacement. MTP Press Limited, Lancaster, England, 1987

162. Ross D: Pulmonary valve autotransplantation (The Ross operation). J Cardiac Surg 3(suppl):313, 1988

163. Rossiter SJ, Stinson EB, Oyer PE, et al: Prosthetic valve endocarditis. Comparison of heterograft tissue valves and mechanical valves. J Thorac Cardiovasc Surg 76:795, 1978

164. Rumisek JD, Albus RA, Clarke JS: Late *Mycobacterium chelonei* bioprosthetic valve endocarditis: Activation of implanted contaminant? Ann Thorac Surg 39:277, 1985

165. Russell RGG, Smith R: Diphosphonates: Experimental and clinical aspects. J Bone Joint Surg 55:66, 1973

166. Sabbah HN, Hamid MS, Stein PD: Estimation of mechanical stresses on closed cusps of porcine bioprosthetic valves: Effects of stiffening, focal calcium and focal thinning. Am J Cardiol 55:1091, 1985

167. Sabbah HN, Hamid MS, Stein PD: Mechanical stresses on closed cusps of porcine bioprosthetic valves: Correlation with sites of calcification. Ann Thorac Surg 42:93, 1986

168. Salomon NW, Copeland JG, Goldman S, Larson DF: Unusual complications of the Hancock porcine heterograft: Strut compression in the aortic root. J Thorac Cardiovasc Surg 77:294, 1979

169. Sanders SP, Levy RJ, Freed MD, et al: Use of Hancock porcine xenografts in children and adolescents. Am J Cardiol 46:429, 1980

170. Sarabu MR, Parker FB: Unusual complication of porcine heterograft. Ann Thorac Surg 35:553, 1983

171. Saravalli OA, Somerville J, Jefferson KE: Calcification of aortic homografts used for reconstruction of the right ventricular outflow tract. J Thorac Cardiovasc Surg 80:909, 1980

172. Sauren AAHJ, Kuijpers W, van Steenhoven

AA, Veldpaus FE: Aortic valve histology and its relation with mechanics—preliminary report. J Biomech 13:97, 1980

172a. Schoen FJ: Pathology of cardiac valve replacement. p. 209. In Morse D, Steiner RM, Fernandez J (eds): Guide to Prosthetic Cardiac Valves. Springer-Verlag, New York, 1985

173. Schoen FJ: Cardiac valve prostheses: Pathological and bioengineering considerations. J Cardiac Surg 2:65, 1987

174. Schoen FJ: Surgical pathology of removed natural and prosthetic heart valves. Hum Pathol 18:558, 1987

175. Schoen FJ: Interventional and Surgical Cardiovascular Pathology: Clinical Correlations and Basic Principles. WB Saunders, Philadelphia, 1989

176. Schoen FJ, Collins JJ, Cohn LH: Long-term failure rate and morphologic correlations in porcine bioprosthetic heart valves. Am J Cardiol 51:957, 1983

177. Schoen FJ, Fernandez J, Gonzalez-Lavin L, Cernaianu A: Causes of failure and pathologic findings in surgically removed Ionescu-Shiley standard bovine pericardial heart valve bioprostheses: Emphasis on progressive structural deterioration. Circulation 76:618, 1987

178. Schoen FJ, Harasaki H, Kim KM, et al: Biomaterials-associated calcification: Pathology, mechanisms and strategies for prevention. J Biomed Mater Res Appl Biomater 22(A1):11, 1988

179. Schoen FJ, Hausner RJ, Howell JF, et al: Porcine heterograft valve replacement in carcinoid heart disease. J Thorac Cardiovasc Surg 81:100, 1981

180. Schoen FJ, Hobson CE: Anatomic analysis of removed prosthetic heart valves: Causes of failure of 33 mechanical valves and 58 bioprostheses, 1980 to 1983. Hum Pathol 16:549, 1985

181. Schoen FJ, Kujovich JL, Levy RJ, St. John Sutton M: Bioprosthetic valve failure. Cardiovasc Clin 18:289, 1988

182. Schoen FJ, Kujovich JL, Webb CL, Levy RJ: Chemically determined mineral content of explanted porcine aortic valve bioprostheses: Correlation with radiographic assessment of calcification and clinical data. Circulation 76:1061, 1987

183. Schoen FJ, Levy RJ: Bioprosthetic heart

valve failure: Pathology and pathogenesis. Cardiol Clin 2:717, 1984

184. Schoen FJ, Levy RJ, Nelson AC, et al: Onset and progression of experimental bioprosthetic heart valve calcification. Lab Invest 52:523, 1985

185. Schoen FJ, Schulman LJ, Cohn LH: Quantitative anatomic analysis of "stent creep" of explanted Hancock standard porcine bioprostheses used for cardiac valve replacement. Am J Cardiol 56:110, 1985

186. Schoen FJ, Tsao JW, Levy RJ: Calcification of bovine pericardium used in cardiac valve bioprostheses: Implications for the mechanisms of bioprosthetic tissue mineralization. Am J Pathol 123:134, 1986

187. Schuster PR, Wagner JW: A preliminary durability study of two types of low-profile pericardial bioprosthetic valves through the use of accelerated fatigue testing and flow characterization. J Biomed Mater Res 23:207, 1989

188. Scully H, Goldman B, Fulop J, et al: Five-year follow-up of Hancock pericardial valves: Management of premature failure. J Cardiac Surg 3(suppl):397, 1988

189. Shemin RJ, Schoen FJ, Hein R, et al: Hemodynamic and pathologic evaluation of a unileaflet pericardial bioprosthetic valve. J Thorac Cardiovasc Surg 95:912, 1988

190. Silver MA, Oranburg PR, Roberts WC: Severe mitral regurgitation immediately after mitral valve replacement with a parietal pericardial bovine bioprosthesis. Am J Cardiol 52:218, 1983

191. Silver MA, Roberts WC: Detailed anatomy of the normally functioning aortic valve in hearts of normal and increased weight. Am J Cardiol 55:454, 1985

192. Silver MD, Hudson REB, Trimble AS: Morphologic observations on heart valve prostheses made of fascia lata. J Thorac Cardiovasc Surg 70:360, 1975

193. Smith JC: The pathology of human aortic valve homografts. Thorax 22:114, 1967

194. Stein PD, Kemp SR, Riddle JM, et al: Relation of calcification to torn leaflets of spontaneously degenerated porcine bioprosthetic valves. Ann Thorac Surg 40:175, 1985

195. Stein PD, Riddle JM, Kemp SR, et al: Effect of warfarin on calcification of spontaneously

degenerated porcine bioprosthetic valves. J Thorac Cardiovasc Surg 90:119, 1985

196. Stein PD, Wang CH, Riddle JM, Magilligan DJ: Leukocytes, platelets, and surface microstructure of spontaneously degenerated porcine bioprosthetic valves. J Cardiac Surg 3:253, 1988

197. Stephens BJ, O'Brien MF: Pathology of xenografts in aortic valve replacement. Pathology 4:167, 1972

198. Stress-free Fixation. Technical monograph, Medtronic, Inc., Minneapolis, 1987

199. Swanson WM, Clark RE: Dimensions and geometric relationships of the human aortic valve as a function of pressure. Circ Res 35:871, 1974

200. Sweeney MS, Reul GJ, Cooley DA, et al: Comparison of bioprosthetic and mechanical valve replacement for active endocarditis. J Thorac Cardiovasc Surg 90:676, 1985

201. Thiene G, Bortolotti U, Panizzon G, et al: Pathological substrates of thrombus formation after heart valve replacement with the Hancock bioprosthesis. J Thorac Cardiovasc Surg 80:414, 1980

202. Thiene G, Bortolotti U, Talenti E, et al: Dissecting cuspal hematomas. A rare form of porcine bioprosthetic valve dysfunction. Arch Pathol Lab Med 111:964, 1987

203. Thiene G, Bortolotti U, Valente M, et al: Mode of failure of the Hancock pericardial valve xenograft. Am J Cardiol 63:129, 1989

204. Thubrikar MJ, Deck JD, Aouad J, Nolan SP: Role of mechanical stress in calcification of aortic bioprosthetic valves. J Thorac Cardiovasc Surg 86:115, 1983

205. Thubrikar MJ, Nolan SP, Aouad J, Deck JD: Stress sharing between the sinus and leaflets of canine aortic valve. Ann Thorac Surg 42:434, 1986

206. Thubrikar M, Nolan SP, Bosher LP, Deck JD: The cyclic changes and structure of the base of the aortic valve. Am Heart J 99:217, 1980

207. Thubrikar M, Piepgrass WC, Bosher LP, Nolan SP: The elastic modulus of canine aortic valve leaflets in vivo and in vitro. Circ Res 47:792, 1980

208. Thubrikar M, Piepgrass WC, Shaner TW, Nolan SP: The design of the normal aortic valve. Am J Physiol 241:H795, 1981

209. Tolis GA, Michalis A, Pouliou A, et al: Un-usual complication of a Carpentier-Edwards porcine valve. Texas Heart Inst J 13:337, 1986

210. Tomazic BB, Brown WE, Queral LA, Sadovnik M: Physicochemical characterization of cardiovascular calcified deposits. I. Isolation, purification and instrumental analysis. Atherosclerosis 69:5, 1988

211. Tomazic BB, Brown WE, Queral LA, Schoen FJ: Cardiovascular calcified deposits: Characterization of properties and mechanism of formation. Presented at the 8th Symposium on Atherosclerosis, Rome, October 9–13, 1988

212. Tompkins LS, Roessler BJ, Redd SC, et al: *Legionella* prosthetic-valve endocarditis. New Engl J Med 318:530, 1988

213. Transplantation techniques and use of cryopreserved allograft cardiac valves: A symposium. J Cardiac Surg 2(suppl), 1987

214. Trowbridge EA, Lawford PV, Crofts CE, Roberts KM: Pericardial heterografts: Why do these valves fail? J Thorac Cardiovasc Surg 95:577, 1988

215. Trowbridge EA, Roberts KM, Crofts CE, Lawford PV: Pericardial heterografts. Toward quality control of the mechanical properties of glutaraldehyde-fixed leaflets. J Thorac Cardiovasc Surg 92:21, 1986

216. Tsao JW, Schoen FJ, Shankar R, et al: Retardation of calcification of bovine pericardium used in bioprosthetic heart valves by phosphocitrate and a synthetic analogue. Biomaterials 9:393, 1988

217. Valente M, Bortolotti U, Thiene G: Ultrastructural substrates of dystrophic calcification in porcine bioprosthetic valve failure. Am J Pathol 119:12, 1985

218. Vesely I, Boughner D, Song T: Tissue buckling as a mechanism of bioprosthetic valve failure. Ann Thorac Surg 46:302, 1988

219. Waldman JD, Schoen FJ, George L, et al: Balloon dilatation of porcine bioprosthetic valves in the pulmonary position. Circulation 76:109, 1987

220. Wallace RB, Londe SP, Titus JL: Aortic valve replacement with preserved aortic valve homografts. J Thorac Cardiovasc Surg 67:44, 1974

221. Walley VM, Keon WJ: Patterns of failure in Ionescu-Shiley bovine pericardial bioprosthetic valves. J Thorac Cardiovasc Surg 93:925, 1987

222. Warnes CA, Scott ML, Silver GM, et al: Comparison of late degenerative changes in porcine bioprostheses in the mitral and aortic valve position in the same patient. Am J Cardiol 51:965, 1983

223. Webb CL, Benedict JJ, Schoen FJ, et al: Inhibition of bioprosthetic heart valve calcification with aminodiphosphonate covalently bound to residual aldehyde groups. Ann Thorac Surg 46:309, 1988

224. Webb CL, Schoen FJ, Levy RJ: Al^{+++} preincubation inhibits calcification of bioprosthetic heart valve tissue in the rat subdermal model. Trans Am Soc Artif Intern Organs 34:855, 1988

225. Wheatley DJ, Fisher J, Reece IJ, et al: Primary tissue failure in pericardial heart valves. J Thorac Cardiovasc Surg 94:367, 1987

226. Wiebe D, Megerman J, L'Italien GJ, Abbott WM: Glutaraldehyde release from vascular prostheses of biologic origin. Surgery 104:26, 1988

227. Williams MA: The Intact bioprosthesis—early results. J Cardiac Surg 3(suppl):347, 1988

228. Wolf PA, Dawber TR, Thomas E, et al: Epidemiologic assessment of chronic atrial fibrillation and risk of stroke: The Framingham Study. Neurology 28:973, 1978

229. Woodroof EA: The chemistry and biology of aldehyde treated tissue heart valve xenografts. p. 347. In Ionescu MI (ed): Tissue Heart Valves. Butterworth, London, 1979

230. Wright JTM, Eberhardt CE, Gibbs ML, et al: Hancock II—An improved bioprosthesis. p. 425. In Cohn LH, Gallucci V (eds): Cardiac Bioprostheses. Yorke Medical Books, New York, 1982

231. Yankah AC, Hetzer R, Miller DC, et al: Cardiac Valve Allografts 1962–1987. Current Concepts on the Use of Aortic and Pulmonary Allografts for Heart Valve Substitutes, Springer-Verlag, New York, 1988

232. Zussa C, Galloni MR, Zattera G, et al: Endocarditis in patients with bioprostheses. Pathology and clinical correlations. Int J Cardiol 6:719, 1984

42

Aortocoronary Bypass Grafts and Extracardiac Conduits

Renu Virmani
James B. Atkinson
Mervyn B. Forman

In the United States nearly 5 million people are afflicted with ischemic heart disease and nearly 1.5 million of them suffer an acute myocardial infarction each year.[4] Approximately 200,000 Americans under the age of 65 die annually with "premature" coronary atherosclerosis.[4] The mortality from coronary heart disease reached its peak in the late 1960s in most industrialized countries. There has since been a significant downward trend.[102] The decline may be due to a reduced incidence of disease, effective preventive programs, or a change in fatality rates from improved medical and surgical management. Ischemic heart disease has varied presentations, ranging from transient chest discomfort/pain (angina pectoris), unstable or variant angina, acute myocardial infarction, cardiac arrhythmias, and congestive heart failure to the most dramatic, sudden cardiac death.

Interest in the surgical relief of angina dates back more than 50 years. First attempts to relieve pain by dorsal sympathectomy were not successful.[148] In 1935, Beck revascularized the heart by implanting a portion of the pectoral muscle into the pericardium,[16] and O'Shaughnessy implanted omentum into the pericardium.[120] These procedures were followed by others such as scarifying the pericardium by introducing phenol or talcum powder. Perhaps the most bizarre was ligation of the distal internal mammary artery, with the hope of stimulating increased flow into its pericardial branch.[148] In 1946, Vineberg implanted an open end of the internal mammary artery into the myocardium.[172] However, this procedure did not attract attention until two decades later when contrast visualization of the implanted artery showed anastomoses between it and branches of the coronary arteries.[162]

The use of saphenous veins as aortocoronary artery bypass grafts was developed by De-Bakey in the 1960s, refined in the 1970s, and helped dramatically change the management of patients with ischemic heart disease.[60,102] However, the role of these grafts remains controversial, despite numerous clinical trials. There is little doubt that such surgery prolongs life in patients with left main coronary artery disease, three-vessel disease, and left ventricular dysfunction. Data on patients with less severe coronary artery disease are controversial.

RANDOMIZED TRIALS IN CORONARY BYPASS SURGERY

The goals of both medical and surgical treatment in ischemic heart disease are constant: improvement in the quality of life by reducing attacks of angina, improvement in left ventricular function, elimination of resistent ventricular tachyarrhythmias, reduction in the incidence of myocardial infarction, and an increased and productive life span.[126] The last decade has seen major advances in both the medical and surgical treatment of coronary heart disease, with the introduction of calcium channel blockers, thrombolytic therapy, decreased perioperative mortality, wide-spread use of internal mammary artery grafts, and percutaneous transluminal coronary angioplasty.[39] As a result, an increasing number of patients are being treated simultaneously or sequentially with both coronary artery bypass grafts and nonsurgical procedures. This means that randomized trials are confounded by crossover from medical to surgical therapy, with this occurring, on average, in about 5 percent of cases a year. Therefore, comparisons between surgical and medical management are applicable to the early years of a study, but the advantages of surgery over medical therapy decline with longer follow-up.[82] Comparisons are also difficult today because of the changing profiles of patients undergoing coronary artery bypass surgery. In one study, those receiving isolated coronary artery bypass surgery in 1975 were compared with identically selected groups from 1985.[115] There was a significant worsening of preoperative conditions with increased age, increased congestive heart failure, greater severity of coronary artery disease, and a higher incidence of emergency operations. In 1985, more patients had associated medical diseases such as diabetes, chronic lung disease, hypertension, renal dysfunction, peripheral and cerebrovascular disease.[115]

The Veterans Administration Coronary Bypass Cooperative Study (1972 to 1974),[45,114,146,160,170] the European Coronary Surgery Study (ECSS) (1973 to 1976),[54] and the Coronary Artery Surgery Study (CASS) (1974 to 1979)[30,31,80] were randomized trials aimed to determine whether assignment to medical or surgical therapy offers a significant advantage for long-term survival. Despite obvious differences in study populations, the time of the investigation, the number of grafts anastomosed, differences in medical and surgical mortality, and differences in medical management, certain conclusions can be drawn[83]:

1. Bypass surgery improves survival in patients with significant left main coronary artery disease.
2. Bypass surgery improves survival in patients with three-vessel disease and reduced ventricular function.[121]
3. Bypass surgery prolongs and improves the quality of life in patients with "left main equivalent" disease (proximal left anterior descending and proximal left circumflex).
4. Bypass surgery does not protect patients from the risk of subsequent myocardial infarction.
5. Graft patency deteriorates with time.
6. Accelerated changes of atherosclerosis develop in bypassed vessels.

OPERATIVE MORTALITY

Overall, the operative mortality associated with treating coronary ischemic heart disease with coronary bypass surgery has been declining, despite an increase of 15 years in the median age of patients being operated on today.[95] In the CASS study, mortality for patients operated on between 1975 and 1978 was 2.3 percent, with mortality increasing with left ventricular dysfunction and age: 0 percent in patients younger than 30 years, 7.0 percent among patients older than 70 years. Elderly patients have an increased mortality that does not correlate with the severity of coronary artery disease, anginal pattern, or diminished left ventricular function. The major causes of increased mortality are pulmonary and/or renal failure, sepsis, and neurologic complications.[1] For elective surgery the operative mortality is 1.7 percent, for urgent surgery 3.5 percent, and for emergency surgery 10.8 percent.[81] Urgent surgical revascularization in acute evolving myocardial infarction has been shown to be safe and an effective procedure with reduced early (2.9 percent) and late death (compared to medical 20 percent), but it does not improve left ventricular function.[87]

The risk of death is greater at reoperation for coronary artery disease than at initial operation.[33,100] At the Cleveland Clinic Foundation, during the years 1982 through 1984, the risk of death for primary cases was 1 percent and for perioperative infarction 0.6 percent compared to 3.4 percent and 8 percent, respectively for reoperative cases. Left main vessel stenosis, decreased left ventricular function, and incomplete revascularization were predictors of increased in-hospital mortality.[100] The in-hospital mortality is even greater for coronary artery bypass grafting done the third time or more (12.0 percent).[23]

NATURAL HISTORY OF SAPHENOUS VEIN BYPASS GRAFTS

At the introduction of coronary artery bypass grafting, the long-term patency of grafted veins was not known. Subsequently, we learned that in the first 5 years following surgery, graft patency rates appeared to be high, and atherosclerosis within grafts was a minor problem.[36] Attrition rates between 7 and 12 percent occur less than 1 month after surgery, an additional 10 percent failure rate occurs between 1 month and 1 year. Beyond the first year and up to 6 years, the attrition rate is approximately 2.5 percent a year.[19,20,63] Similar rates have been reported by other groups of investigators.[66,90,147] Currently, patency rates of approximately 65 and 75 percent can be expected at 5 and 7 years, respectively, and 50 to 60 percent at 10 years.[35] At an 11-year follow-up at the Montreal Heart Institute, only 60 percent of grafts were patent and, of these, 46 percent showed relatively severe atherosclerosis.[19,20]

Duke University investigators, in analyzing their data, argue that surgical techniques have advanced more rapidly than medical and,

therefore, results of surgical treatment have become progressively better.[125] However, the recent recognition that internal mammary artery (IMA) grafts have a patency rate of 90 percent at 10 years, which is far higher than that of vein grafts (25 to 50 percent), will change surgical results when compared to those of medical therapy. Also, IMA grafts were initially used for a single anastomosis; with better surgical techniques, they are now used to bypass several coronary arteries.[140]

Coronary artery bypass surgery has been reported superior to medical therapy for unstable angina and to control ischemic pain, but it does not appear to improve survival.[127] Coronary angioplasty compared favorably with bypass surgery in terms of in-hospital mortality (0 versus 11 percent), late mortality (2.8 versus 7.7 percent), freedom from angina (62 versus 69 percent), and subsequent employment (44 versus 27 percent) at 18-months-follow-up.[91] This study demonstrated that there is an increasing role for angioplasty in treating medically refractory patients and that angioplasty offers a good alternative to bypass surgery.[91] However, randomized trials are needed to answer this question: is percutaneous transluminal coronary angioplasty used as an initial therapeutic strategy reasonable for patients with multivessel disease or is bypass surgery better? Currently, two trials sponsored by the National Institutes of Health to answer the question are underway: The Emory Angioplasty Surgery Trial (EAST) and Bypass Angioplasty Revascularization Investigation (BARI Trial).

EXAMINATION OF BYPASS GRAFTS

When removing the heart at autopsy, care must be taken to avoid injury to saphenous vein bypass grafts or an IMA graft. A longer segment of the ascending aorta than usual is left in continuity with the heart to enable examination of vein grafts from their aortic or-

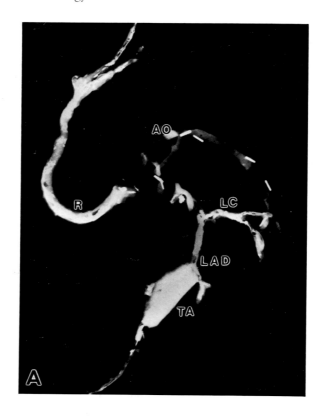

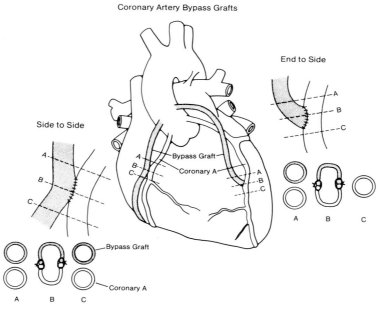

Coronary Artery Bypass Grafts

ifice to their distal anastomosis. Twists, as well as excessive tautness in their course between aorta and distal anastomosis, are noted.[134] As with native coronary arteries, saphenous vein grafts are best visualized by postmortem radiographs. Inject all vein grafts simultaneously with a barium-gelatin mixture[65,70] and radiograph them before injecting the coronary arteries. This enables a more detailed study of the native coronary arteries distal to the grafts as well as at the coronary/graft anastomosis.[174] Measurements of lumen diameters may be made from the radiographs. Where an IMA is anastomosed to the left coronary system, the internal mammary artery is injected at the point where it was severed during removal of the heart. The native coronary arteries are injected, fixed, and radiographed to evaluate the extent of disease in them. The grafts and native arteries may then be removed from the heart, radiographed again (Fig. 42–1A), and cut at 5-mm intervals to determine the extent of luminal narrowing, the presence or absence of thrombi, and/or the extent of atherosclerosis in vein or IMA grafts and coronary arteries. If it is not possible to inject the vessels, fix the heart in 10 percent buffered formaldehyde overnight before dissecting the grafts and native vessels.

When no lesions are identifiable grossly, randomly section the entire length of a graft for histologic study. Anastomotic sites are sectioned in different ways depending on whether the connection is end-to-end or end-to-side (Fig. 42–1B).[28]

PATHOLOGY OF SAPHENOUS VEIN GRAFTS
Causes of Early Graft Closure (Within 3 Days)

Early graft closure can result from mechanical problems, including faulty surgical technique, inadequate size of the coronary vessels, and poor run-off.[35] A fine deposit of platelets, fibrin, erythrocytes, and polymorphonuclear leukocytes is consistently seen in the intima of vein grafts from patients who die shortly after operation (Fig. 42–2). Also, various blood elements may be seen within the intima of some grafts, suggesting insudation of blood elements secondary to increased permeability of the endothelium, probably from high arterial pressure within the lumen.[166] In an animal model of saphenous vein grafts,[24] it was shown that the endothelium sloughs and platelet microthrombi form and that these findings may be related to vessel wall injury caused by high flow or "jet" lesions. Noera et al.[117] compared two surgical techniques for preserving vein grafts. Half the veins were removed by conventional surgical techniques and the other half by atraumatic procedures; tonic vasodilators, distension of the vein with autologous blood at 150 mmHg, and storage at room temperature were also employed. Veins prepared by atraumatic techniques were better preserved when examined by light and electron microscopy.[117] In humans, thrombus deposition is probably a response to endothelial injury, an unavoidable conse-

Fig. 42–1. (A) Radiograph of epicardial coronary arteries and saphenous vein bypass graft (course marked by radiopaque clips) to left circumflex (LC) removed at autopsy. Note calcification in native coronary arteries and absence of calcification in the vein graft. Also, a portion of the left anterior descending coronary artery was surrounded by myocardium (bridging or tunneled coronary artery [TA]). Ao, aorta; LAD, left anterior descending; R, right. (B) Diagram illustrating coronary bypass grafts that have end-to-side and side-to-side anatomosis in two separate grafts (shaded areas) to left anterior descending and right coronary arteries, respectively. The figure illustrates the method used for sectioning anastomotic sites with end-to-side or side-to-side anastomoses to demonstrate if any of the three mechanisms for obstruction at the anastomotic site are present (i.e., compression or loss of arterial lumen, which may occur if the majority of the arterial wall has been used for anastomosis; thrombosis at the anastomosis site; or dissection of the native coronary artery at the site of anastomosis) and if the coronary artery has severe narrowing at the site of anastomosis because of severe atherosclerotic change. (Modified from Bulkley and Hutchins,[28] with permission.)

quence of manipulation and preparation of the graft.[26] The incidence of a fine layer of fibrin/thrombus on the intima of saphenous vein grafts has been reported in as many as 73 percent of patients who die within 24 hours of surgery.[28]

Whereas occlusive luminal thrombi rarely form within 24 hours of graft implantation, they are a major cause (33 percent) of occlusion within 30 days of operation.[62] The incidence of thrombus reached 75 percent in patients who died more than 1 month after operation.[62] Patients treated with dipyridamole and aspirin or warfarin have a higher graft patency rate.[38,104] Also, the level of plasma anticardiolipin antibody (ACA) has been correlated with the incidence of early (1 to 2 weeks) and late (12 month) graft closure, as judged by angiography. The ACA level was higher in patients who had had a myocardial infarction in the past than in those with a history of angina only. This observation supports the concept that one mechanism of ACA production is an immune response to myocardial injury and that ACA may play a part in progression of coronary vessel disease.[113]

Another cause of early graft closure is compression; that is, a loss of circumference of a coronary artery that occurs when part of the intrinsic coronary wall is everted or compressed by suturing during construction of the graft/artery anastomosis.[62] Griffith and associates calculated the percent reduction in luminal area for coronary arteries with an internal diameter of 2 mm or 1 mm.[62] In a 2-mm artery, suture "bites" that are 0.5 mm or 1.0 mm from the edge of the arteriotomy reduce the cross-sectional area of the coronary lumen by 29 and 54 percent, respectively. In a 1-mm artery, on the other hand, the same sutures reduce the area by 52 and 89 percent, respectively. This obviously occurs only where the wall is everted.

Another important factor in early graft closure is severe atherosclerosis in the distal segment of the bypassed coronary artery. Plaque reduces the internal circumference of the arterial wall available for anasto-

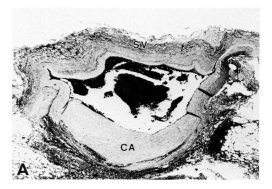
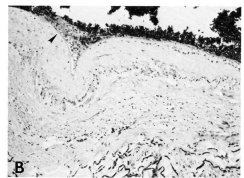
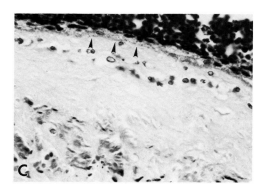

Fig. 42–2. A 60-year-old man underwent saphenous vein bypass surgery for unstable angina and died 6 hours after surgery with postoperative difficulty in maintaining systemic pressures. At autopsy the heart weighed 540 g. The bypass grafts were intact, but all vein grafts proximal and at site of anastomosis showed a thin layer of platelet deposition on the endothelial surface. (A) Anastomotic site of vein graft (SV) to left obtuse marginal coronary artery (CA). (B) Platelet-fibrin deposit close to the anastomotic site in the vein graft (arrowhead). (C) Vein graft with a fine layer of platelet deposition (arrowheads). (Movat's pentachrome; Fig. A: × 15; Fig. B: × 160; Fig. C: × 600; reduced 44 percent.) (From Virmani,[173] with permission.)

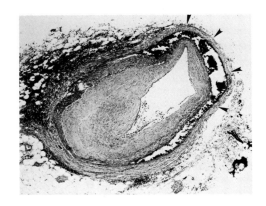

Fig. 42–3. Histologic section of coronary artery taken distal to the anastomic site. Note dissection (arrowheads) involving 50 percent of the circumference of the artery. The media is dissected; however, the dissection extended less than 1 cm. (Movat's pentachrome, × 40.) (From Virmani,[173] with permission.)

mosis; if plaque is present distal to the anastomosis, it will decrease coronary artery lumen, reduce flow, and thereby predispose to thrombosis.[62] Also, if atherosclerotic plaque is present at the site of an anastomosis, it may detach from the coronary wall when the anastomosis is being created and cause dissection in the vein graft, as well as distal to the anastomosis (Fig. 42–3). The length of dissection, however, is usually short. Spray and Roberts[155] reported a 17 percent incidence of this complication, whereas Griffith and co-workers[62] reported an 8 percent incidence. Although the frequency of dissection is low, it is another cause of lumen compression.

Changes in Long-Term Grafts

Between 1 Month and 1 Year of Surgery

Grafts that are in place for up to 1 year uniformly demonstrate intimal proliferation, characterized by a highly cellular connective tissue composed of proliferating cells in a loose matrix of acid mucopolysaccharide and collagen (Fig. 42–4). Electron microscopy has shown that the cellular component is a smooth muscle cell, with myofibrils, dense bodies, and basement membranes.[166] However, Kern and co-workers[81] considered the cell with rough endoplasmic reticulum a fibroblast. The pathogenesis of fibrointimal proliferation is speculative; it may represent a reparative response to ischemia or to hemodynamic stresses (such as systemic hypertension), resulting in endothelial damage with platelet

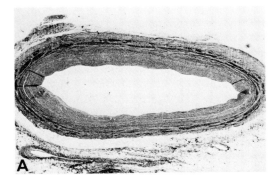

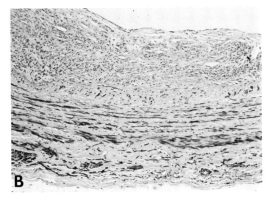

Fig. 42–4. **(A)** Section of a saphenous vein graft in place for 8 months. There is uniform concentric circumferential intimal proliferation. **(B)** Higher magnification. Note elastic fibers in adventitia (black) but not in the media; the intima shows smooth muscle cells (dark gray) and collagen in a background of acid mucopolysaccharide. (Movat's pentachrome; Fig. A: × 15; Fig. B: × 100.) (From Virmani,[173] with permission.)

aggregation, smooth muscle proliferation, and intimal thickening.[27] Brody and colleagues,[25] employing a canine model of vein to vein and artery-vein-artery anastomosis, concluded that the initial necrosis and inflammatory changes in the media are ischemic in origin and that the disruption of vasa vasorum may be responsible for the resultant intimal thickening. Inasmuch as the degree of fibrointimal proliferation may vary along the length of a vein graft or even among different grafts in the same patient,[25,103,107] ischemia alone cannot entirely account for these changes. Tsukada et al.,[165] using HHF35 antibody (which exhibits specificity to smooth muscle cells), demonstrated that fibrointimal thickening in vein grafts was inevitably smooth muscle cell in origin. Flow rate may modify the extent of the fibrointimal proliferation, inasmuch as increased flow may produce recurrent endothelial damage, resulting in fibrin-platelet deposition, thrombosis, and repair.[156] However, we and others[8,153] have not observed mural thrombus (fibrin, erythrocytes, iron) in vein grafts manifesting fibrointimal proliferation.

The fibrointimal proliferation observed in grafts from humans and experimental animals shows progression and fibrosis at varying rates and varies in intensity at different locations along a graft. During the early phase of graft implantation, fibrointimal proliferation is uneven and patchy in distribution; with time it becomes circumferential and diffuse.[12] Its presence may be beneficial, because it induces a moderate reduction of a graft's internal diameter and reduces it to the approximate size of the recipient artery, thereby promoting a greater velocity of flow.[12]

More Than 1 Year After Surgery

We[8] have recently reported our findings in 117 saphenous vein grafts that had been in place 12 to 168 months before death (mean 62.7 ± 37.5 months). They came from 56 patients (50 men, 6 women) of mean age 59.6 ± 9.1 years. Death was sudden in 21, caused by acute myocardial infarction in 11, and congestive heart failure in 5. Six patients died during or shortly after reoperation for coronary artery bypass. Other causes of death included malignant neoplasms in 4 patients, pulmonary embolism in 2, rupture of an aortic aneurysm in 1, sepsis in 2, cerebrovascular accident in 1, and poisoning in 1.

All patients had one or more risk factors for accelerated coronary atherosclerosis (Table 42–1). Thirty-two (57 percent) had systemic hypertension, 15 (27 percent) diabetes mellitus, 17 patients (30 percent) a documented history of hyperlipidemia, and 19 (34 percent) had a family history of premature coronary heart disease. The majority had an-

Table 42–1. Cardiovascular History in 56 Patients with Saphenous Vein Aortocoronary Bypass Grafts, at Necropsy

Risk Factors for Accelerated Coronary Artery Disease[a]	No. of Patients
Systemic hypertension	32
Diabetes mellitus	15
Hyperlipidemia	
Hypercholesterolemia	13
Hypercholesterolemia and hypertriglyceridemia	4
Smoking	33
Family history of premature coronary heart disease	19
Cardiovascular history	
Angina pectoris	44
Acute myocardial infarction	37
Congestive heart failure	21

[a] Risk factors had been clearly documented in these patients subsequent to placement of aortocoronary bypass grafts. Systemic hypertension was defined as blood pressure greater than 140/90 mmHg; diabetes mellitus was assessed by determining whether patients were being treated at the time of death or had a serum glucose level greater than 130 mg/dl. Hypercholesterolemia was defined as a serum cholesterol level greater than 240 mg/dl, and hypertriglyceridemia was a serum triglyceride level greater than 200 mg/dl. (From Atkinson et al.,[8] with permission.)

Table 42–2.   Morphology of 117 Saphenous Vein Grafts Implanted Longer Than 12 Months in 56 Patients, at Necropsy

Morphology of Graft Implants	No. of Grafts
Atherosclerosis	25
Recent Thrombus	10
Aneurysm	1
Fibrointimal proliferation	66
Fibrosis with total occlusion	26

Distribution of Vein Grafts	No. of Patients
Fibrointimal proliferation	25
Atherosclerosis	9
Fibrosis	6
Fibrointimal proliferation + atherosclerosis	3
Fibrointimal proliferation + fibrosis	10
Atherosclerosis + fibrosis	2
Atherosclerosis + fibrointimal proliferation + fibrosis	1

No. of Grafts with Various Degrees of Cross-sectional Area Luminal Narrowing				
	0–25%	*26–50%*	*51–75%*	*>75%*
Atherosclerosis	0	4(16%)	5(20%)	16(64%)
Fibrointimal proliferation	17(26%)	29(44%)	14(21%)	6(9%)
Total	17(18%)	33(36%)	19(21%)	22(24%)

(From Atkinson et al.,[8] with permission.)

gina pectoris (44 patients), and 37 had suffered an acute myocardial infarction as documented by electrocardiographic and/or enzyme changes. Twenty-one patients (38 percent) were symptomatic from their congestive heart failure.

Morphologic Findings

Three characteristic types of morphologic changes were found (Table 42–2). Atherosclerosis, as defined by the World Health Organization,[178] was present in 25 vein grafts (Fig. 42–5). Ten atherosclerotic grafts were occluded by a recent thrombus, and the others had varying degrees of luminal narrowing secondary to atherosclerosis. One atherosclerotic vein graft had an aneurysmal dilation. Sixty-six vein grafts had various degrees of fibrointimal proliferation in the absence of atherosclerotic change, with prominent internal elastic laminae, smooth muscle cell proliferation, collagen, and acid mucopolysaccharide

ground substance (Fig. 42–6). Twenty-six saphenous vein grafts were totally occluded with fibrous tissue (Fig. 42–7). Atherosclerotic vein grafts had been in place longer than those with fibrointimal proliferation (Table 42–2).

Fibrointimal proliferation occurred exclusively in 25 patients, atherosclerotic change alone in 9, and fibrosis alone in 6. Most patients had one type of lesion in their grafts, although 16 had more than one morphologic lesion (see Table 42–2). Some degree of fibrointimal proliferation was found in all the atherosclerotic grafts, but significant fibrointimal proliferation (greater than 25 percent cross-sectional area narrowing) was never noted in atherosclerotic grafts.

The degree of cross-sectional area luminal narrowing of saphenous vein grafts determined at autopsy is shown in Table 42–2. Nearly one-fourth of grafts with atherosclerosis and fibrointimal proliferation had significant narrowing at necropsy (greater than 75 percent cross-sectional area luminal narrowing). Total occlusion was secondary to fi-

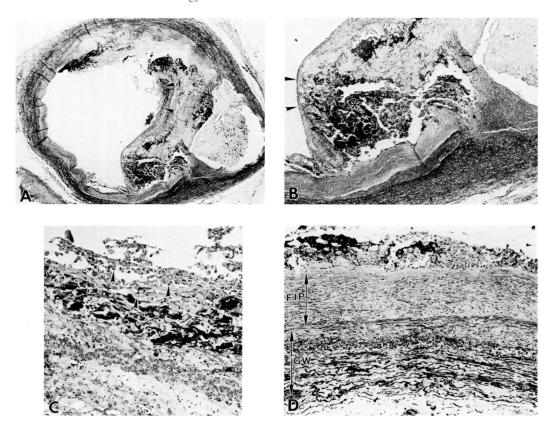

Fig. 42–5. Atherosclerotic saphenous vein graft from a 62-year-old man. It had been in situ 56 months. His risk factors included diabetes mellitus and systemic hypertension. (**A**) Photomicrograph showing eccentric atherosclerotic plaque with a fibrous cap (arrowheads) and hemorrhage within a plaque (asterisk). (**B**) Higher magnification of hemorrhage (asterisk) into a plaque, which is covered by a thin layer of fibrous cap (arrowheads). (**C**) Extensive foam cell deposition (arrowheads) in the subintimal region with fibrin interspersed (black areas). (**D**) Saphenous vein graft wall (GW) and superimposed fibrointimal proliferation (FIP) with foam cells in the superficial layers of the intima interspersed with fibrin deposits (black areas). (Movat's pentachrome; Fig. A: × 15; Fig. B: × 40; Fig. C: × 160; Fig. D: × 100; reduced 45 percent.) (From Virmani et al.,[173] with permission.)

brointimal proliferation in 2 vein grafts and to atherosclerosis in 8.

There was no statistical difference when comparing mean heart weight with the type of morphologic change (Table 42–3). The mean number of four major coronary arteries (left main, left anterior descending, left circumflex, and right) with greater than 75 percent cross-sectional area luminal narrowing is

shown in Table 42–3 and was similar among the three groups. Histologic evidence of acute and/or healed myocardial infarction was found at necropsy in 12 of the 15 patients with atherosclerotic vein grafts, 33 of 39 patients with fibrointimal proliferation in their grafts, and 18 of 19 patients with fibrotic vein grafts. Ten patients had no evidence of infarction, either healed or acute.

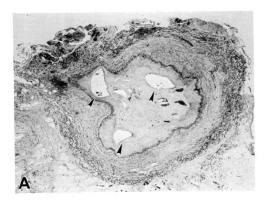

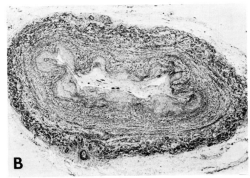

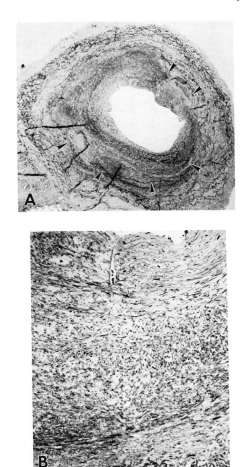

Fig. 42–6. Fibrointimal proliferation in a saphenous vein graft in place 12 months. The patient had a history of systemic hypertension and was a smoker. (**A**) Note extensive fibrointimal tissue within the vein wall (arrowheads). (**B**) Higher magnification showing smooth muscle cells (dark gray) in a background of acid mucopolysaccharide. There was almost total absence of collagen. (Movat's pentachrome; Fig. A: × 25; Fig. B: × 160.) (From Virmani et al.,[173] with permission.)

Fig. 42–7. (**A**) Fibrotic saphenous vein grafts. Note total occlusion of the lumen by fibrous tissue with interspersed multiluminal channels (arrowheads), representing recanalized thrombus. (**B**) Collapsed fibrotic vein graft with the lumen occupied by fibrous tissue. The compression of the vein graft could be secondary to fibrous tissue retraction. Only a few multiluminal channels are seen. (Movat's pentachrome, × 25.) (From Virmani et al.,[173] with permission.)

Correlation of Graft Morphology with Cardiovascular Risk Factors

Cardiovascular risk factors were correlated with the specific type of vein graft morphology (atherosclerosis or fibrointimal proliferation)

(Table 42–4). Systemic hypertension was present in 76 percent of patients with saphenous vein grafts showing fibrointimal proliferation, as compared with 24 percent of atherosclerotic grafts. Forty percent of atherosclerotic vein grafts occurred in patients with diabetes mellitus, as compared with 18 percent of grafts with fibrointimal proliferation. Sixty-eight percent of atherosclerotic vein grafts were found in patients with hypercholesterolemia in contrast to only 15 percent with fibrointimal

Table 42–3.   Morphologic Features in Hearts from 56 Patients with Saphenous Vein Graft Implants

	Athero-sclerotic Grafts (15 pts)[a]	Fibrointimal Proliferation Grafts (39 pts)[a]	Fibrotic Grafts (19 pts)[a]	Total
Duration of vein graft[b]	75.9 ± 42.7	57.4 ± 33.4	56.4 ± 41.2	62.7 ± 37.5
Heart weight (g)	520 ± 96	609 ± 168	640 ± 172	598 ± 150
Graft implantation[c]				
Right coronary artery	10	25	9	44
Left anterior descending[d]	7	28	9	44
Left circumflex[e]	8	13	8	29
Mean number of coronary arteries > 75% narrowed	2.7 ± 1.0	2.4 ± 1.1	2.8 ± 0.9	2.6 ± 1.1
Myocardial infarction (MI)				
Acute MI	1(7%)	0	1(5%)	2(4%)
Healed MI	4(27%)	24(62%)	11(58%)	39(70%)
Acute and healed MI	7(47%)	9(23%)	6(32%)	22(41%)

[a] Patients with more than one type of lesion in vein grafts were counted twice, according to the type of morphologic change.
[b] $P < 0.05$ for atherosclerotic versus fibrointimal proliferation grafts.
[c] Includes posterior descending branch in hearts with dominant right coronary artery.
[d] Includes left diagonal branches.
[e] Includes left obtuse marginal branch.
(From Atkinson et al.,[8] with permission.)

Table 42–4.   Correlation of Saphenous Vein Graft Morphology with Cardiovascular Risk Factors in 56 Patients

Risk Factors	Atherosclerosis (Total Grafts 25) No.(%) of Grafts	Fibrointimal Proliferation (Total Grafts 66) No.(%) of Grafts
Systemic hypertension	6(24)	50(76)
Diabetes mellitus	10(40)	12(18)
Hypercholesterolemia	17(68)	10(15)
Smoking	15(60)	40(61)
Family history of premature coronary heart disease	9(36)	17(26)
History of		
Acute myocardial infarction	17(68)	44(67)
Angina pectoris	23(92)	48(73)
Congestive heart failure	9(36)	23(35)

(From Atkinson et al.,[8] with permission.)

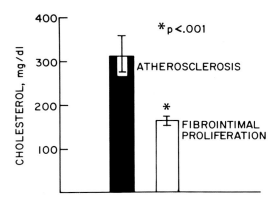

Fig. 42–8. Total serum cholesterol levels in patients with atherosclerotic grafts, as compared with those in patients with fibrointimal proliferation. Values were obtained from 44 patients, representing a total of 74 grafts (25 with atherosclerosis and 49 with fibrointimal proliferation). (From Atkinson et al.,[8] with permission.)

proliferation. The differences between atherosclerotic grafts and those with fibrointimal proliferation for the two risk factors (systemic hypertension, hypercholesterolemia) were statistically significant (Table 42–4). The majority of grafts (17 of 22) from hypertensive patients that did not demonstrate fibrointimal proliferation were fibrotic. No statistically significant differences were noted between these two morphologic groups with regard to history of smoking, family history of premature coronary heart disease, acute myocardial infarction, or congestive heart failure.

In 8 of our 56 patients, accurate documentation of cardiovascular risk factors and/or values for total serum cholesterol, serum glucose, and blood pressure was not available. We therefore excluded these patients from statistical analysis. Grafts with less than 25 percent cross-sectional area luminal narrowing by fibrointimal proliferation in four patients were also excluded, because mild degrees of fibrointimal proliferation (phlebosclerosis) can be seen in saphenous veins at the time of implantation. Of the re-

maining 74 grafts in 44 patients, statistically significant differences were seen in the atherosclerotic and fibrointimal proliferation groups with regard to elevated cholesterol and systemic hypertension, but no statistically significant differences were noted for diabetes mellitus. The mean total serum cholesterol levels obtained after surgery were significantly higher in patients with atherosclerotic grafts, compared with those with fibrointimal proliferation ($P < 0.001$) (Fig. 42–8). Although the mean serum glucose level was also higher in patients with atherosclerotic grafts (163 ± 38 mg/dl) than in patients with fibrointimal proliferation (127 ± 10 mg/dl), the differences were not statistically significant. Patients with fibrointimal proliferation had higher systolic and diastolic blood pressures than did patients with atherosclerotic grafts, but these differences reached statistical significance only for systolic blood pressure ($P < 0.05$) (Fig. 42–9). The number of separate measurements made (subsequent to coronary artery bypass graft placement) for cholesterol, glucose, and blood pressure were 5.4 ± 0.7, 5.0 ± 0.7, and 4.1 ± 0.6 per patient, respectively.

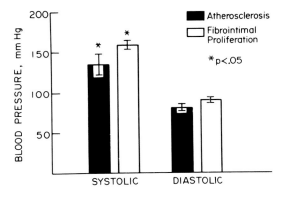

Fig. 42–9. Graph showing systolic and diastolic blood pressures in patients with atherosclerotic vein grafts, compared with those with fibrointimal proliferation. Values were obtained from 44 patients, representing a total of 74 grafts (25 with atherosclerosis and 49 with fibrointimal proliferation). (From Atkinson et al.,[8] with permission.)

Role of Risk Factors in the Development of Atherosclerosis Versus Diffuse Intimal Change

The role of hyperlipidemia in inducing atherosclerosis in grafts is now well accepted (Table 42–5). In hypercholesterolemic animals, there is a greater propensity for atherosclerosis to develop in vein grafts,[58,84,138,141,145] than in the native coronary arteries or grafted internal mammary arteries.[138] In vitro, canine venous grafts incorporate lipids at accelerated rates compared with normal arteries and veins.[88] However, the role of hyperlipidemia in the pathogenesis of atherosclerosis in human grafts is less clear, although some studies have confirmed the animal data. Lie and associates found atherosclerosis in 78 percent of grafts implanted longer than 12 months in hyperlipidemic patients, compared with 11.5 percent in patients with normal lipids.[93] This was confirmed by Barboriak and colleagues[13];

however, in other morphologic[15,116,153] and angiographic[64] studies, no correlation between hyperlipidemia and atherosclerosis was present, suggesting that other etiologic factors may also be involved. Campeau and associates[35] recently reported progression of new lesions in saphenous vein grafts after 1 year of implantation in patients who had high levels of very low-density and low-density lipoproteins and low levels of high-density lipoproteins. Total plasma cholesterol and triglyceride levels were also higher in patients with new lesions. All lesions that appeared after 1 year were designated "atherosclerotic" based on patterns of irregularity observed by angiography.[34]

Our study, which was based on histologic confirmation of atherosclerosis, demonstrated that "atherosclerosis" is not the predominant change in vein grafts that have been in place for more than 1 year; in fact, fibrointimal proliferation is encountered more frequently.

Table 42–5.   Reports of Morphologic Changes in Long-term Saphenous Vein Bypass Grafts

Author	Year	No. of Patients	Duration of SVBG	DIT	Athero-sclerosis	Thrombus
Barboriak[12]	1976	11[a]	23.7 ± 3.1 months	11	1	4
Lie[93]	1977	23	13–75 months	14	9[b]	0
Bulkley[26]	1977	9	1–54 months	8	4	6
Batayias[15]	1977	12	6 to > 36 months	12	3	2
Walts[176]	1982	5	5–8 years		5	5
Bourassa[19]	1983	19	> 24 months		8	
Smith[153]	1983	24	7–116 months	21	11	3
Atkinson[8]	1985	56	62.7 ± 37.5 months	39	15[c]	9
Neitzel[116]	1986	42	72–144 months		71%	

[a] Eight patients had hyperlipidemia, one had systemic hypertension.

[b] Only 11.5% of grafts of normolipemic patients manifested histologic changes of atherosclerosis compared with 78.6% of those from hyperlipemic patients.

[c] Elevated cholesterol was present in 67% compared with 16% in patients with DIT.

Abbreviations: DIT, diffuse intimal thickening; SVBG, saphenous vein bypass graft; Thrombus, recent thrombus.

(From Virmani et al.,[173] with permission.)

However, the natural progression of fibrointimal proliferation may be affected by the presence of risk factors, with hypercholesterolemia producing atherosclerotic change and systemic hypertension leading to greater luminal narrowing by unrelenting proliferation of fibrointimal tissue.

Although there are inherent problems in a retrospective study of a selected patient population such as ours, this was the first study, to our knowledge, to show a relationship between the presence of systemic hypertension and the development of significant (greater than 25 percent cross-sectional area luminal narrowing) fibrointimal proliferation. Hypertension may lead to hemodynamic and/or ischemic endothelial damage with resultant repair and intimal hyperplasia. Although a relationship between hyperlipidemia and development of atherosclerosis in vein grafts has been demonstrated by others, this study is among the few in which atherosclerosis in vein grafts has been confirmed morphologically. Inasmuch as morphologic lesions vary from graft to graft in the same patient, it is likely that other risk factors may also be important etiologically. Technical, hemodynamic, or pre-existing changes in vein grafts may all contribute to the development of either fibrointimal proliferation or atherosclerosis. Because known cardiac risk factors play a contributory role in the development of different morphologic lesions, continued reduction in risk factors in patients who have undergone bypass surgery may help prolong the patency of these grafts.

Atherosclerotic Plaque in Saphenous Vein Grafts

Early atherosclerotic lesions in saphenous vein grafts are rich in foam cells, which are located within the intima and the media. The lesions tend to be focal. As a plaque progresses, it becomes rich in lipid and contains numerous cholesterol clefts with and without giant cell reaction, foam cells, and blood elements. The pultaceous debris is overlaid by a thin fibrous cap that is delicate and easily disrupts. The plaque is generally soft and friable rather than densely fibrotic and calcified as in native coronary arteries. Even when graft plaques are small, it is not uncommon to see hemorrhage and mild calcific areas within them.

Plaque rupture, with disruption of the fibrous cap and superimposed occlusive thrombus occurs in patients with grafts who present with acute events such as unstable angina or acute myocardial infarction. The thrombosis is said to result from plaque disruption and endothelial injury, which lead to release of thrombogenic substances. As with native coronary arteries, the cause of rupture of saphenous vein graft plaques is unknown. It is not unusual to see destruction of the media with extension of atherosclerotic plaque into the adventitia, where it focally elicits an inflammatory response. The recognition of sudden thrombotic occlusion of vein grafts allows nonsurgical intervention such as use of thrombolytic therapy and emergency transluminal balloon angioplasty.[10,176]

Correlation of Saphenous Vein Bypass Graft Angiograms with Histologic Changes at Necropsy

Previous studies of saphenous vein bypass grafts have either been angiographic or morphologic, and few have correlated angiograms with histology. Nine necropsy patients who had received 21 saphenous vein implants 12 to 120 (mean 67 ± 42) months before death were studied (Table 42–6).[7] All had severe coronary artery disease. Three types of histologic changes were found: atherosclerosis in 9 grafts, fibrointimal proliferation in 8, and total occlusion with fibrosis in 4 (Table 42–7). All patients had premortem angiograms 0 to 3 (mean 0.8 ± 0.1) months before death.

Table 42–6.   Clinical Findings in Nine Patients with Long-term Saphenous Vein Bypass Grafts

No.	Age (yrs)	Sex	DM	TC	SH	FH	CS	AP	AMI	CHF	Duration SVBG (mo)	Interval between Angiography and Death (days)
1	65	M	0	0	+	0	+	+	0	0	12	30
2	69	M	0	+	+	0	+	+	+	0	39	2
3	58	M	0	0	+	+	+	+	0	+	45	30
4	64	M	0	0	+	+	0	+	0	0	120	2
5	62	F	+	0	+	+	0	+	+	+	14	90
6	64	M	0	0	0	+	0	+	+	0	64	5
7	67	M	0	0	+	0	+	+	+	0	105	4
8	49	M	+	+	+	0	0	+	+	0	96	60
9	52	M	0	0	0	0	+	+	+	+	111	3

Abbreviations: AMI, acute myocardial infarction; AP, angina pectoris; CHF, congestive heart failure; CS, cigarette smoking; DM, diabetes mellitus; F, female; FH, family history of coronary disease; M, male; SH, systemic hypertension; SVBG, saphenous vein bypass graft; TC, total serum cholesterol > 250 mg/dl.
(From Atkinson et al.,[7] with permission.)

Premortem Angiography

Two patterns were found at angiography. Five saphenous vein (SV) grafts demonstrated a generalized irregularity with or without localized stenotic lesions and were interpreted as having atheromatous change (Fig. 42–10). Eight grafts had smooth walls with areas of tubular narrowing of a variable length, believed to represent fibrointimal hyperplasia (Fig. 42–11). Eight grafts were totally occluded at their origin.

Morphologic Evaluation

Three characteristic lesions were found: fibrointimal proliferation in 8, total fibrotic occlusion in 4, and atherosclerosis in 9. Planimetry confirmed the extent of luminal narrowing estimated by visual inspection in

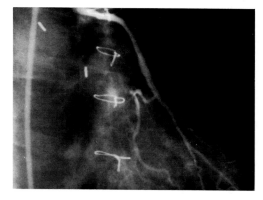

Fig. 42–10. Cineangiogram in the left anterior oblique projection showing generalized irregularity of an obtuse marginal graft, believed to represent atherosclerotic change in the graft, confirmed at autopsy. Selective angiography was performed 4 days before death. (From Atkinson et al.,[8] with permission.)

all cases. Three grafts were narrowed in diameter (greater than 50 percent) by atherosclerosis, whereas 5 were totally occluded

Table 42–7. Correlation of Angiographic Findings and Morphologic Changes in Long-term Saphenous Vein Bypass Grafts

No.	Angiographic Narrowing of SVBG (% Diameter)	Anatomic Narrowing of SVBG (% XSA)[a]	No. CAs >75% Narrowing in XSA	AMI	HMI	Postmortem Angiography
1	OM: 100 R: 100 LAD:NORMAL	100(F) 100(F) 72(FIP)[b]	4	+	0	+
2	LD:NORMAL LAD: 50 OM:NORMAL R: 100	25(FP) 19(FP)[c] 25(FP) 100(F)	3	0	0	+
3	LAD: 50 R:NORMAL	53(FIP)[c] 54(FIP)[b]	4	0	0	+
4	R: 100 LAD: 95 OM:NORMAL	100(A) 39(FP)[c] 25(A)	3	0	0	+
5	LAD:100 PD: 50	100(A) 38(A)[c]	4	0	0	+
6	R: 50 LAD:100	75(A) 100(F)	4	0	+	+
7	R: 50 LAD: 90 OM:NORMAL	100(A) 100(A) 50(A)	3	+	0	+
8	LAD:NORMAL	63(FIP)[b]	4	+	+	0
9	OM: 75	80(A)	4	+	+	0

[a] Values for anatomic narrowing at necropsy were obtained by computer-linked planimetry.
[b] Underestimation by premortem angiography.
[c] Overestimation by premortem angiography.
Abbreviations: AMI, acute myocardial infarction; A, atherosclerosis; CAs, coronary arteries; F, fibrosis; FIP, fibrointimal proliferation; HMI, healed myocardial infarction; LAD, left anterior descending coronary artery; LC, left circumflex coronary artery; LD, left diagonal branch of left anterior descending coronary artery; OM, obtuse marginal coronary artery; PD, posterior descending branch of right coronary artery; R, right coronary artery; SVBG, saphenous vein bypass graft; XSA, cross-sectional area.
(From Atkinson et al.,[7] with permission.)

with hemorrhage into plaques and superimposed thrombosis.

Correlation of Premortem Angiograms and Necropsy Findings. In seven grafts, premortem angiograms incorrectly assessed the extent of luminal narrowing—three underestimations (Fig. 42–11) and four over-estimations (Fig. 42–12). Six incorrectly assessed grafts had fibrointimal proliferation, and one had atherosclerosis with 26 to 50 percent cross-sectional narrowing at necropsy. Postmortem angiograms in seven hearts confirmed the correlations between the premortem angiographic and postmortem histologic findings.

Causes of Underestimation and Overestimation of Degrees of Luminal Narrowing by Angiography Versus Histology

Compared with histology, angiography underestimates the degree of coronary narrowing by 5 to 33 percent.[75] Possible causes for this discrepancy have been listed as nonperfusion of coronary arteries at necropsy, diffuse atherosclerosis, eccentric slitlike lumens and postmortem shrinkage, and fixation artifacts. Atherosclerosis in vein grafts is usually diffuse and could result in underestimation, but only one of the seven vein grafts that were incorrectly assessed in this study had atherosclerosis. Postmortem shrinkage artifacts have also been incriminated and may result in reduction of tissue size of up to 20 percent. Smooth muscle and elastic fibers in grafts with fibrointimal proliferation may accentuate these changes. Shrinkage artifacts were minimized by performing postmortem angiography in 7 of 8 of our patients. Angiography also has its limitations, because it permits only a two-dimensional view of a three-dimensional structure.

In 6 of 8 grafts with fibrointimal proliferation in our study,[7] angiograms tended to overestimate or underestimate luminal narrowing. Smooth muscle, a prominent component of the intima of saphenous veins that develop fibrointimal proliferation, may undergo transient spasm or dilation, resulting in incorrect assessment of the grafts at angiography. Focal spasm in saphenous vein grafts has been reported in two patients[171,175]; both had recurrent Prinzmetal's angina following coronary bypass surgery. The increased number of smooth muscle cells present in the intima of many grafts may have a hyperreactive response to either endogenous vasoconstrictors or dilators.[52,77,139]

Our results[7] indicate that selective angiography of saphenous vein grafts is a precise and reliable means of assessing graft patency in the majority of patients. However, grafts narrowed by fibrointimal proliferation are

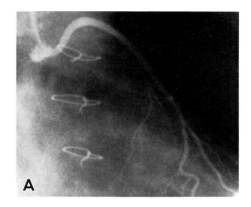

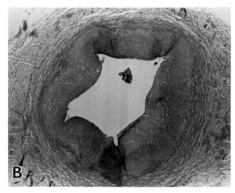

Fig. 42–11. Patient 1 (see Tables 42–6 and 42–7) underwent catheterization 3 weeks before death. **(A)** Angiogram of the anterior descending coronary graft in the left anterior oblique projection, showing tubular narrowing with no focal stenotic lesions; the graft was estimated to have less than 25 percent diameter reduction. **(B)** At autopsy, there was up to 75 percent cross-sectional area narrowing by fibrointimal proliferation. The angiogram underestimated the extent of narrowing in this graft. (Movat's pentachrome, × 30.) (From Atkinson et al.,[8] with permission.)

prone to erroneous assessment by angiography, perhaps due to spasm or dilation. Spasm had not been recognized in any of our patients clinically, and other factors may certainly be responsible for the angiographic findings.

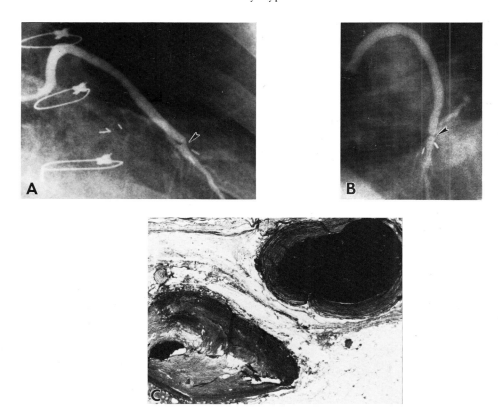

Fig. 42–12. Patient 2 (see Tables 42–6 and 42–7) underwent angiography 2 days before death. The **(A)** right and **(B)** left anterior oblique projections revealed generalized tubular narrowing of the anterior descending graft with focal stenotic lesions of up to 50 percent diameter reduction (arrowheads). **(C)** Histologic section at autopsy through the site of maximal narrowing of the vein graft showed less than 25 percent cross-sectional area reduction by fibrointimal proliferation, but a 90 percent cross-sectional luminal narrowing of the native left anterior descending coronary artery occurred just proximal to the anastomotic site. The angiogram therefore overestimated the extent of narrowing in the vein graft. (Fig. C: Movat's pentachrome, × 18, reduced 28 percent.) (From Atkinson et al.,[8] with permission.)

Atherosclerotic Aneurysm of Saphenous Vein Grafts

Saphenous vein aneurysms have been described at 4 to 6 months after grafting and are related to venous valves,[133] whereas late graft aneurysms, reported 5 to 12 years after grafting, are associated with atherosclerosis.[92,123,161] The frequency of such atherosclerotic aneurysms in vein grafts is unknown. Angiographically, vein grafts appear tortuous with relative luminal narrowing and multiple areas of focal dilation. The graft lumen appears as large as that of a native vein; however, the flow of contrast material is slow, and there are often surrounding round soft tissue densities and focal constriction. All affected vein grafts show severe atherosclerosis and grossly contain multiple aneurysms.[161] All aneurysms are composed of complicated atherosclerotic plaque and poorly organizing thrombi that almost completely fill the lumen. The wall of the aneurysm is atheromatous with medial atrophy, and loss of elastic tissue.[161] Rarely, there may even be a false aneurysm.[161]

INTERNAL MAMMARY ARTERY VERSUS SAPHENOUS VEIN AS A BYPASS GRAFT

The use of the internal mammary artery (IMA) as a graft to improve myocardial perfusion has had a checkered history. The Vineberg operation—implantation of the left IMA into a tunnel of left ventricular muscle—demonstrated that the implanted artery could remain patent over a long time.[154] At the Cleveland Clinic from 1960 to 1965, the Vineberg procedure was increasingly used, because Sones confirmed patency by angiography.[51] In 1968, Spencer and associates demonstrated in animals that the IMA could be directly anastomosed to the left anterior descending coronary artery, and that year the first IMA anastomosis was performed in a human being.[154] However, its routine use was inhibited because of concerns about the adequacy of flow rates. Finally, in 1984, reports from Montreal of 10-year angiographic studies comparing vein graft patency with mammary artery patency showed that 30 percent of vein grafts became occluded and that another 30 percent developed atherosclerosis, whereas 95 percent of IMA grafts remained patent.[64] This led to an increased use of IMA anastomoses, including sequential anastomoses and bilateral mammary anastomoses.[154] Also, it has been shown that the IMA can enlarge, probably in response to increased peripheral resistance to blood flow as atherosclerosis further occludes native vessels.[154]

In a recent report, Loop and co-workers[97] compared retrospectively 2,306 mammary artery anastomoses with 3,625 saphenous vein grafts to the left anterior descending coronary artery over 10 years, representing the largest data currently available. The 10-year actuarial survival rate among the group receiving the IMA graft as compared to the group receiving vein grafts was 93.4 percent versus 88 percent ($P = 0.05$) for one vessel disease; 90 percent versus 79.5 percent ($P < 0.0001$) for two vessel disease; and 82.6 percent versus 71 percent ($P < 0.0001$) for those with three-vessel disease. The frequency of myocardial infarction was also decreased, but not the frequency of recurrent angina or arrhythmias. This study shows that most patients undergoing bypass surgery who have severe stenosis of the anterior descending artery should receive an IMA graft to that artery, along with vein grafts to other vessels as indicated. Loop and co-workers[97] used free (aorta to coronary) IMA grafts with only 0.6 percent hospital mortality. At 18 months postoperatively (mean 9.4 months) graft patency was 91 percent: 92 percent of those restudied at 60 months were open. There were no irregularities or late stenosis to indicate presence of atherosclerosis. Therefore, longevity of free IMA grafts appears comparable to in situ IMA grafts.[97] The overwhelming superiority of IMA grafts versus saphenous vein grafts has encouraged more extensive use of bilateral and sequential IMA grafts (Fig. 42–13).

Bilateral IMA grafting is technically more difficult and is associated with a slightly increased perioperative morbidity (stroke, wound complications, respiratory complications, and bleeding).[98] However, comparison of early experience (1971 to 1982) with late (1982 to 1984) showed a decrease in complication rates from 7.2 percent to 2.7 percent. This did not correlate with gender, diabetes, number of grafts, or preoperative left ventricular function but was associated with increasing age and previous surgery.[98] Using sequential, bilateral, and free IMA grafts, a total of 4:1 grafts per patient has been achieved,[99] with early excellent graft patency rates for left IMA to left ascending coronary artery (LAD), left IMA to circumflex mar-

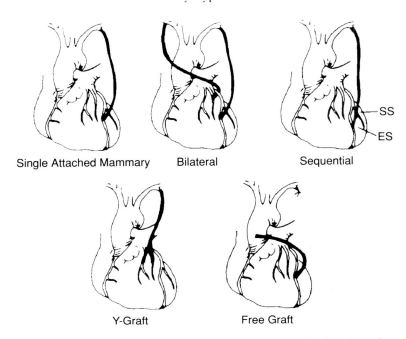

Single Attached Mammary   Bilateral   Sequential

SS
ES

Y-Graft   Free Graft

Fig. 42–13. Different types of IMA grafts. A single attached IMA graft (either the right or left) remains attached proximally to the subclavian artery and is connected to the coronary arteries. Bilateral IMA grafts (right and left) are joined end-to-side to coronary arteries. Sequential IMA grafts consist of an attached or free IMA with one or more side-to-side (SS) anastomoses and one end-to-side (ES) anastomosis. The IMA graft has two terminal branches of either the attached or free IMA sutured to two coronary arteries. A free IMA graft is placed by transecting the right or left IMA near its origin from the subclavian artery, and the proximal artery is then anastomosed to the aorta and the distal end to the coronary artery. (From Tector et al.,[162a] with permission.)

ginal, right IMA to right coronary, right IMA to LAD, sequential IMA to LAD, sequential IMA to circumflex marginal system, free IMA, free sequential IMA. Only right IMA to circumflex marginal artery graft patency was suboptimal. Therefore, expanded use of more complicated types of mammary grafts is justified.[128] During a 15-year follow-up of patients with IMA grafts and those with saphenous vein grafts, those with IMA grafts had a better cumulative survival, less recurrence of angina, fewer myocardial infarcts, fewer reoperations, and better cumulative event-free survival. Patients with double IMA grafts had the best survival rates and lowest recurrence of angina and rate of late myocardial infarcts with no need for reoperation.[32]

Histologic Studies of Long-Term Internal Mammary Artery Grafts

Histologic studies of IMA grafts have reported an extremely low incidence of atherosclerosis in the graft.[78,109,152] We studied 18 patients, 16 male and 2 female, with a mean age of 56 ± 9 years (range 43 to 70).[150] All had 1 or greater risk factor for accelerated coronary atherosclerosis. Hypercholesterolemia was present in 15 patients, diabetes mellitus in two, and systemic hypertension in 7. A positive family history of premature coronary disease was found in 10, and 13 were smokers.

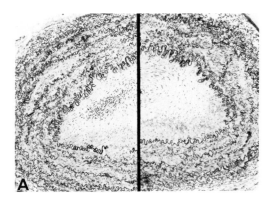

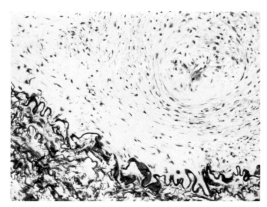

Fig. 42–15. Excised IMA graft in place 33 months in a 53-year-old man. The lumen is totally occluded by concentric layers of smooth muscle, collagen, and ground substance typical of fibrointimal proliferation. (Movat's pentachrome, × 250.)

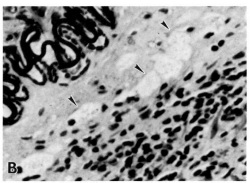

Fig. 42–14. The cineangiogram from a 53-year-old man, whose grafts had been in place 36 months, showed subtotal occlusion of a left IMA graft. Two days later the patient underwent coronary artery bypass surgery, and the IMA graft was excised. (**A**) Histologic section shows subtotal occlusion by fibrointimal proliferation (right, left). (**B**) Occasional foam cells (arrowheads) and inflammatory cells are present in the intima. (Movat's pentachrome; Fig. A: × 100; Fig. B: × 300.)

The 18 IMA grafts had been in place 12 to 118 months (mean 56 ± 9) before either excision (12) or autopsy (6). Three characteristic morphologic changes were found. Atherosclerosis was present in only 1 of the 18 grafts; plaques showed only occasional foam cells (Fig. 42–14); 8 grafts had fibrointimal proliferation without atherosclerotic change (with or without occlusion) (Fig. 42–15), with prominent internal elastic laminae and a thickened intima due to smooth muscle proliferation, collagen accumulation, and acid mucopoly-

saccharide ground substance; and 8 were occluded by fibrosis representing organized thrombus (Fig. 42–16). One internal mammary graft was histologically normal. Acute thrombus formation was not found in any graft. The various degrees of cross-sectional luminal area narrowing of IMA grafts are shown in Tables 42–8 to 42–10.

Findings in Associated Saphenous Vein Grafts

A total of 15 saphenous vein grafts were available from 11 of the 18 study patients. Ten grafts had atherosclerosis and, of these, three had acute thrombotic occlusion, four had fibrointimal proliferation, and one had fibrosis (see Tables 42–8 to 42–10). Atherosclerosis was significantly more frequent in saphenous vein grafts than in internal mammary artery grafts (10 of 14 versus 1 of 18; $P < 0.01$). In 11 cases both an IMA graft sample and at least one saphenous vein graft sample were available from the same patient. The results from these 11 patients again demonstrated the low incidence of atherosclerosis in IMA grafts (0 of 11), whereas 9 of 15 saphenous vein grafts had atherosclerosis (Table 42–10). Fibrointimal proliferation was more frequent in inter-

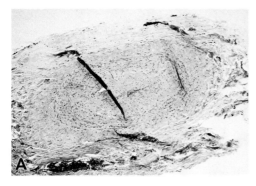

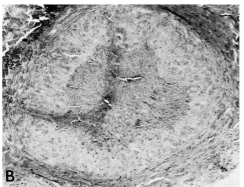

nal mammary artery than in saphenous vein grafts (8 of 18, 44 percent, versus 4 of 15, 27 percent; *P* was not significant). Figure 42–17 shows an example of minimal fibrointimal proliferation in an IMA graft taken from a patient with severe atherosclerosis in a saphenous vein graft.

Correlation of Premortem Angiograms and Necropsy Findings in IMA and Saphenous Vein Bypass Grafts

Premortem angiography of both IMA and saphenous vein grafts showed a good positive relation with the morphologic estimates of area narrowing (d = 0.90 and d = 0.71, respectively). In only one IMA graft did angiography overestimate the stenosis found morphologically (30 percent narrowing caused by fibrointimal proliferation was interpreted to be 60 percent diameter reduction by angiography).

Fig. 42–16. Cineangiogram from a 44-year-old man, showed total occlusion of a left IMA graft that had been placed 87 months earlier. (**A**) The excised IMA graft was totally occluded by fibrosis. (**B**) The excised radial artery graft was totally occluded by fibrous tissue with focal necrosis and occasional inflammatory cells present in the wall (Both H&E, × 60.)

Correlation of IMA and Saphenous Vein Bypass Graft Morphology and Atherosclerosis Risk Factors

The average serum cholesterol in all 18 patients was 241 ± 8.8 mg/dl. In 5 of the 11 patients with atherosclerotic saphenous vein

Table 42–8. Morphologic Narrowing (%) of Internal Mammary Artery and Saphenous Vein Grafts Implanted Greater Than 12 Months in 18 Patients

	0–25%	26–50%	51–75%	76–99%	100%	Total
Internal mammary artery grafts (n = 18[a])						
Fibrointimal proliferation	2	4	1	0	1	8
Atherosclerosis	0	0	0	1	0	1
Fibrosis	0	0	0	1	7	8
Saphenous vein grafts (n = 15)						
Fibrointimal proliferation	2	0	0	2	0	4
Atherosclerosis	0	0	3	0	7	10[b]
Fibrosis	0	0	0	0	1	1

[a] One internal mammary graft manifested no pathologic changes
[b] *P* = 0.01, Fisher's exact test; 3 of the 10 patients had fresh thrombus
(From Shelton et al.,[150] with permission.)

Table 42–9.   Correlation of Angiographic Findings and Morphologic Changes in Long-term Internal Mammary Artery and Saphenous Vein Bypass Grafts in Each Patient[a]

| No. Patients | Internal Mammary Artery Grafts | | | | Saphenous Vein Bypass Grafts | | |
	Duration of Bypass Graft (mo)	Angiographic Narrowing (% Diameter)	Anatomic Narrowing (% XSA)	Graft Lesion	Angiographic Narrowing (% Diameter)	Anatomic Narrowing (% XSA)	Graft Lesion
1	37	100	100	F			
2	27	100	100	F			
3	21	50	50	FIP			
4	24	60	35	FIP	100	99	FIP
5	33	100	100	F	>90	99	FIP
6	53	>90	100	F	50	50	A
7	54	100	100	F			
8	36	>90	99	FOCAL A	<25	<25	N
9	87	100	100	F	100	99	F
10	70	75	95	F	70	50	A
					100	100	A
11	64	<25	25	FIP	<25	25	FIP
					100	100	A
12	118	<25	<25	FIP	70	100	A,T
					90	100	A,T
13	95	<25	<25	N	100	100	A,T
14	80	<25	30	FIP	100	100	A,F
15	102	100	100	F			
16	24	25	40	FIP	100	100	F
17	12	25	25	FIP	40	50	A
18	72	100	100	FIP			

[a] Values for anatomic narrowing were obtained by computer-linked planimetry; angiographic narrowing measurements have been normalized to anatomic cross-sectional stenosis.

Abbreviations: A, atherosclerosis; F, fibrosis representing organized thrombus; FIP, fibrointimal proliferation; N, normal; T, acute thrombus; XSA, cross-sectional area.

(From Shelton et al.,[150] with permission.)

Table 42–10.   Morphologic Narrowing (%) of Internal Mammary Artery and Saphenous Vein Grafts in the Same Patient (n = 11)

	0 to 25%	26 to 50%	51 to 75%	>75%	Total
Internal mammary artery grafts[a]					
Fibrointimal proliferation	2	3	0	0	5
Atherosclerosis	0	0	0	0	0
Fibrosis	0	0	0	5	5
Saphenous vein grafts					
Fibrointimal proliferation	2	0	0	2	4
Atherosclerosis	0	0	3	6	9
Fibrosis	0	0	0	2	2

[a] One internal mammary graft manifested no pathologic changes.

(From Shelton et al.,[150] with permission.)

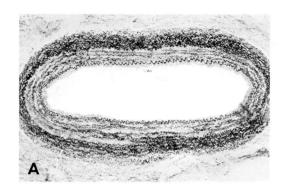

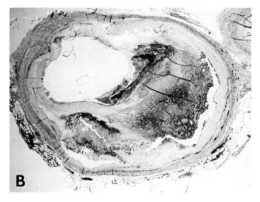

Fig. 42–17. Cineangiograms from a 52-year-old man who had bypass grafts for 118 months demonstrated a less than 25 percent stenosis of the IMA graft on angiography and a greater than 75 percent stenosis of the saphenous vein graft to the right coronary artery. The patient died of an acute myocardial infarction 4 days after cardiac catheterization. **(A)** Histologic section of the IMA graft at the anastomotic site demonstrates minimal fibrointimal hyperplasia. **(B)** There is greater than 75 percent reduction in cross-sectional area of the saphenous vein graft by atherosclerosis. (Both Movat's pentachrome, × 60.)

grafts, cholesterol levels were higher (253 ± 22 mg/dl, n = 5) than in the 6 patients with nonatherosclerotic saphenous vein grafts (219 ± 10 mg/dl, n = 6, P not significant).

There was no apparent correlation of hypertension with the presence of fibrointimal proliferation in the IMA or saphenous vein grafts studied, and none of the other risk factors for accelerated atherosclerosis correlated with specific morphology in these grafts.

Three types of morphologic changes (fibrointimal proliferation, atherosclerosis, fibrosis representing organized thrombus) were observed in the IMA grafts in our 18 patients. A high incidence (44 percent) of fibrointimal proliferation was found in these 18 IMA grafts, and there was a very low rate (5 percent) of atherosclerosis. Conversely, there was a significantly higher rate (71 percent) of atherosclerosis in saphenous vein grafts. Acute thrombi were observed only in saphenous vein grafts (three cases). Our study revealed a good correlation between the amount of narrowing estimated by angiographic and histologic measurements. Angiography overestimated the degree of IMA graft narrowing recorded on histologic study in only 1 of the 18 cases. These results were comparable with those observed (5 to 33 percent) in saphenous vein grafts and native coronary arteries.[5,7,75]

Pathogenesis of Morphologic Changes in Saphenous Vein and IMA Grafts

Hypercholesterolemia has been associated by others[99] with increased atherosclerosis in saphenous vein grafts. Our study confirmed that total serum cholesterol in patients with atherosclerotic saphenous vein grafts tended to be higher than that in patients with nonatherosclerotic saphenous vein grafts, but the difference did not reach statistical significance, possibly because of the small sample. The low incidence rate (5 percent) of atherosclerosis in IMA grafts was observed despite the group having a high average serum cholesterol (241 mg/dl). Although hypertension was associated in a previous study[8] with increased fibrointimal proliferation in saphenous vein grafts, this pathologic change in IMA grafts did not correlate with hypertension in our study. The explanation for the differences in incidence of fibrointimal proliferation and atherosclerosis in these two types of grafts cannot be attributed solely to known risk factors for accelerated coronary artery disease, because the two phenomena were observed at the same time in the same patients.

Possible Factors Involved in the Varied Morphologic Responses of Saphenous Vein and Internal Mammary Artery Grafts

Several possible factors may contribute to qualitative histologic difference noted between saphenous vein and IMA grafts. The intact vasa vasorum and lymphatics present in the internal mammary artery pedicle graft may be a major advantage over "free" radial artery, "free" internal mammary, or saphenous vein grafts. Free grafts of the radial artery have very poor angiographic patency rates compared with those of IMA grafts.[154] Free grafts of the internal mammary artery have been used as well, but, to date, there has been no long-term follow-up. Because there have been no long-term anatomic studies of either free IMA grafts or free radial artery grafts, we cannot yet conclude that live pedicle grafts age in a qualitatively different way than do free artery grafts. One patient in our study had both a free radial and a pedicle internal mammary artery graft. The wall of the radial artery showed necrosis with polymorphonuclear leukocyte infiltrate, whereas that of the mammary graft was free of necrosis or inflammatory infiltrate (Fig. 42–16).

Another potentially important difference between the IMA graft and the saphenous vein graft is that the saphenous vein must undergo adaptive changes ("arterialization") when placed in the high left-sided pressure aortocoronary circulation,[173] whereas the internal mammary artery is already accustomed to such high pressures. The size of an IMA also more closely approximates that of the coronary vessels. This may result in a less turbulent flow than in the larger saphenous vein

conduits. The IMA graft may also have the ability to enlarge substantially over a number of years[14] and maintain vasoregulatory properties.[46] Finally, the IMA itself seems to have a lower incidence of inherent atherosclerosis than do other arteries in the same patients.[78,152] This has been attributed to the vessel's abundant collateral blood supply to its runoff bed, which protects the intima.[78]

The Incidence or Rate of Acceleration of Atherosclerosis in the IMA May Change When the Artery Is Used As a Graft

The attachment of the distal mammary artery to the diseased coronary artery system may well expose the IMA to a higher pressure and initiate a time when the mammary artery begins to be more comparable with other medium-sized arteries. It is possible that our observation of minimal atherosclerosis formation in IMA grafts over the time of our study (12 to 118 months) is consistent with the natural history of the development of atherosclerosis in other arteries, because one generally expects only fatty streaks to occur in the first decade of life and the progression to significant disease to take 30 to 40 years.[72]

SYNTHETIC CONDUITS FOR AORTOCORONARY BYPASS GRAFTING

Conduits of choice for aortocoronary bypass grafting are the IMA and long saphenous vein. If they are unavailable, however, the next choices are short saphenous veins, upper limb veins (usually cephalic), preserved human umbilical veins, the radial artery, and splenic or gastroepiploic vessels, all of which have been used in humans with only limited success.

Synthetic grafts, particularly expanded

polytetrafluoroethylene (PTFE, or Gore-tex) grafts, have been successfully used in substituting or bypassing small arteries. The use of synthetic grafts in the coronary position has been reported in only a small number of patients; long-term studies are lacking.

The short-term patency rates of PTFE grafts for aortocoronary bypass are reported to be 61 percent at 3 months in one series[142] and 64 percent at 12 months by others.[37] PTFE grafts that have failed have shown bridging of neointima across side-to-side anastomoses, with total obstruction of the lumen of the graft by neointima and thrombus.[37] The pathogenesis of these changes is presumably obstruction at the distal anastomosis by neointima, resulting in reduced runoff and subsequent thrombosis.[37]

The use of Dacron grafts for aortocoronary bypass is even more limited, with only one reported case,[144] as Dacron grafts have been historically less efficient for bypassing small-caliber arteries than PTFE grafts.

The mortality and complication rates of PTFE grafts in the coronary position are considered unacceptably high when compared to saphenous vein or IMA grafts.[37,111,142] Although they may remain patent from 18 months to more than 2 years,[74,142] it is recommended that they be used for aortocoronary bypass only as a last resort. With increasing use of the IMA graft, it seems unlikely that use of synthetic conduits in the coronary position will become widespread in the near future.

EXTRACARDIAC CONDUITS

A major advance in the treatment of congenital heart disease occurred with the development of extracardiac conduits. In 1965, Rastelli et al.[130] reported the first placement of a valveless (pericardial) conduit from the right ventricle to main pulmonary artery to correct pulmonary atresia. A year later, Ross and Somerville described use of a valved aortic homograft to repair a case of tetralogy of Fallot with pulmonary atresia.[137] Subsequently, this technique was extended to repair truncus arteriosus[86] and complex transposition of the great vessels.[129] The major indications for the use of extracardiac conduits are (1) truncus arteriosus, (2) tetralogy of Fallot with pulmonary valvular stenosis, (3) transposition of the great arteries with pulmonary valvular stenosis, (4) pulmonary atresia, (5) tricuspid atresia, and (6) severe left ventricular outflow disease (fibrous tunnel obstruction of the left ventricular outflow tract, severe hypoplasia of the aortic annulus, tubular hypoplasia of the ascending aorta) not easily amenable to valvotomy or annular augmentation.[49,57,89,101,106,131,132,159]

The patient of Ross and Somerville had an antibiotic-sterilized aortic homograft inserted.[137] Subsequently, an alternative technique of x-ray sterilization of aortic homografts was adopted by many. It was soon discovered, however, that irradiated aortic homografts became severely calcified and stenotic,[11,112] so their use was abandoned. Fresh antibiotic-sterilized homografts, which are not as susceptible to calcification during the first 5 to 10 years after implantation,[143] have continued to be used despite limited availability.[25,105,149] In 1971, glutaraldehyde-treated porcine-valved Dacron conduits became available.[21] Although the Dacron heterograft is stiff and more difficult to suture than the aortic homograft,[49] its availability in a variety of sizes led to its widespread use. Despite the popularity of tissue valves (which allow freedom from anticoagulation) in children, calcification and a lack of durability limit their use.[136] Because of early valve failures, nonvalved conduits are used in certain clinical situations, especially in the absence of increased pulmonary vascular resistance. However, conduits also fail due to compression and formation of an obstructive fibrous "peel" within the Dacron tube, and this is reflected in the pathology of explanted conduits or those encountered at necropsy.

Complications of Extracardiac Conduits

Silver and Wilson[151] have listed the major complications of vascular grafts as (1) mechanical failure with rupture, hemorrhage, or aneurysm formation, (2) kinking with graft stenosis or occlusion, (3) incomplete healing with detachment of the luminal surface thrombus leading to stenosis, (4) infection, (5) erosion into an adjacent viscus, and (6) hemolysis. Several long-term postoperative studies have demonstrated that conduit stenosis may be a significant complication. The potential mechanisms of conduit stenosis are listed in Table 42–11. It can occur at the proximal anastomosis, the valve, within the conduit itself, at the distal anastomosis, or in the pulmonary artery (or aorta). Obstruction at the proximal anastomosis may be caused by abnormal angulation of the conduit.[22] Although an oversized conduit may alleviate the problem of a patient outgrowing a prosthesis, larger conduits carry a greater risk of anastomotic angulation.[22] Bailey et al.[11] found compression of conduits between the sternum and heart in 5 of 7 patients who required reoperation for obstruction. Placing the conduit lateral to the sternum eliminates this type of obstruction and prevents anastomotic angulation. All patients with small conduits placed early in life will eventually require reoperation. Its timing is determined by the development of graft obstruction and growth of the patient.[22]

Table 42–11. Mechanisms of Conduit Stenosis

Intraoperative and early postoperative
    Conduit too small for patient
    Extrinsic compression by sternum
    Obstruction at proximal and/or distal anastomosis
    Thrombosis
Late postoperative
    Patient outgrows conduit
    Valvular stenosis
    Fibrous peel (neointima)
    Thrombosis

(Adapted from Edwards et al.,[50] with permission.)

Unfortunately, bioprosthetic valves, which diminish the need for continuous anticoagulation and improve hemodynamics, undergo degeneration.[9] Calcification is the leading cause of bioprosthetic valve failure,[168] and calcification is accelerated in valves implanted in children.[119] Bioprosthetic valves in extracardiac conduits may develop stenosis, insufficiency, or both. Valvular stenosis may be due to degenerative changes in the valve cusps, which can lead to thrombosis of valvular commissures or calcification of commissures or cusps. Valvular incompetence may be due to flail valve resulting from degeneration and calcification leading to tears, thrombosis of valvular pockets causing cusp retraction and fusion to the conduit wall, or valve destruction by endocarditis.[50] Mechanical valves are avoided in conduits used to reconstruct the right ventricular outflow tract because of neointimal proliferative stenosis and subsequent valve malfunction.[108]

Several studies have identified the frequency of conduit failure. Bisset et al.[18] found a 30 percent incidence of xenograft conduit failure over a short follow-up period, whereas Geha et al.[61] reported a 12 percent failure rate for extracardiac conduits. Dunn[48] found better durability of porcine valves in pulmonary conduits when compared to those in the aortic or mitral position, although younger children had a higher incidence of calcification and valve dysfunction. Catheterization studies have demonstrated significant conduit obstruction even in patients who are asymptomatic. Heck et al.[68] observed a 57 percent incidence of conduit obstruction following the Rastelli procedure in 13 patients who underwent catheterization at 1 year, despite an absence of symptoms in 88 percent of these patients. Stewart et al.[158] studied 15 asymptomatic patients 6 to 9 years after placement of Hancock right ventricle-to-pulmonary conduits. A significant gradient was observed in 2 patients at 1 year and in 7 at 6 years. In a large series of 201 patients who had received synthetic right heart conduits (predominantly porcine-valved Dacron conduits), actuarial freedom from conduit replacement was 81 percent at 5 years, 61 percent at 7 years, and 0 percent at 10 years for valved conduits; patients with nonvalved conduits were reoperation-free at 4 years.[76] McGoon et al.[105] from the Mayo Clinic reported follow-up of 333 patients who had received Hancock conduits, 130 patients received frozen irradiated conduits, and 5 had nonvalved conduits. Ninety patients who underwent serial catheterization to determine the transconduit gradient change from the completion of conduit insertion to the most recent cardiac catheterization showed an increase of 32 mmHg for homograft aortic conduit and 0 for Hancock conduit. However, the average postoperative interval was 4 to 5 years for the former and 1.7 years for the latter. Reoperation was required in 16 percent of patients and most commonly because of progressive conduit stenosis. Need for reoperation was greater for homograft than for Hancock conduits.[105]

Fresh antibiotic-sterilized homografts may develop fewer complications than composite conduits. In short-term follow-up, Kirklin et al.[85] found that actuarial freedom from reoperation for obstruction in 147 patients receiving cryopreserved or fresh allograft valved conduits was 94 percent at 3.5 years. In longer studies, others have reported that at 15 years, 70 percent of patients with aortic homografts may be free from obstruction requiring conduit replacement at 15 years.[56,79] Pericardial valved conduits, first described in a large series of patients in 1971,[69] may function as well as fresh allograft valved conduits. Among 21 patients who received a pericardial conduit, 87 percent of survivors were free from reoperation at 16 years.[73]

The complications seen in valved conduits used for reconstruction of the left ventricular outflow tract (apical left ventricular to aortic valved conduits) differ from conduits placed from the right ventricle to the pulmonary artery. Four well-recognized complications of apicoaortic conduits are (1) endocarditis,[118,157] (2) pseudoaneurysm formation of the left ventricular apex-graft anastomosis,[135,165] (3) thromboembolism,[157] and (4) deterioration of the bioprosthetic porcine valve.[61,135,156] Although most reported cases of endocarditis of the prosthetic valve have been due to bacteria,[118,157] we have observed candidal myocarditis in a patient who had undergone placement of a ventriculoaortic conduit for subaortic stenosis.[6] Late development of peripheral emboli was reported by Stansel[157]; however, Rocchini et al.[135] observed no such events in their series of 24 patients with apicoaortic conduits. Obstruction also occurs in ventriculoaortic conduits and is usually found at the egress of the left ventricle, at the valve level, or at the aortic-conduit junction.[135] Proximal conduit obstruction may be due to malorientation of the apical stent with respect to the long axis of the left ventricle.[135] In contrast to calcification and stenosis in porcine valves used for valve replacement, Rocchini et al.[135] observed that the major cause of valve dysfunction in patients with left ventricular apicoaortic conduits was insufficiency. In a series of 24 patients, these investigators found some degree of conduit obstruction in 11 of 15 patients at 1 to 5 years (mean 1.2), while 3 developed porcine valve insufficiency.

In addition to conduit obstruction and valvular degeneration, occasional reports of unusual complications have been published. They include fatal myocardial ischemia due to coronary artery compression by a metallic stent of the conduit valves, and complete obstruction by an organizing thrombus between the outer portion of the conduit and the adherent pericardial tissue, resulting, presumably, from a deceleration injury in an automobile accident 5 months before death.[44,167]

Pathology of Extracardiac Conduits

The pathology of extracardiac conduits can be considered in terms of whether they are valved or nonvalved and heterograft (Dacron) or aortic homografts (Table 42–12). Bioprosthetic valves in conduits undergo changes sim-

Table 42–12.   Pathologic Features
of Extracardiac Conduits

Aortic homografts
    Calcification
    Intimal peel (neointima)
    Endocarditis
    Thrombosis
Valved synthetic conduits
    Bioprosthetic valve
        Stenosis secondary to
            Calcification
            2° thrombosis at commissures or
                valve stenosis
            Fusion of cusps
        Insufficiency secondary to
            Degeneration, with cusp tears
            Thrombotic adhesions
            Endocarditis
            Fusion of cusps
    Conduit
        Fibrous peel (neointima)
        Thrombosis
        Pannus formation at anastomoses
Nonvalved synthetic conduits
    Fibrous peel (neointima)
    Thrombosis

ilar to those described for intracardiac bioprosthetic valves(see Ch. 41).[9] The pathologic changes seen in bioprosthetic valves can be classified as early and late. Short-term changes (less than 2 months) consist of plasma protein insudation, fibrin deposition, collections of platelets and/or erythrocytes, and deposition of macrophages and giant cells.[156] Late changes consist of collagen disruption, erosion of valve surfaces, platelet aggregation, and lipid accumulation. The cuspal surfaces may be partially covered with endothelium or fibrous tissue. Calcification may underlie valvular stenosis and usually begins at the commissures, progressing until the commissures are fixed in a semiclosed position[2] (Fig. 42–18). Osseous metaplasia may be seen as well. Thrombosis causing commissural fusion and fixation of the cusps leads to valvular stenosis. Cuspal tears occur secondary to calcification and degeneration of the cusps, and valvular incompetence may coexist with stenosis.[2,18,50] Four patterns of cusp degeneration are (1) tears involving the free edges of

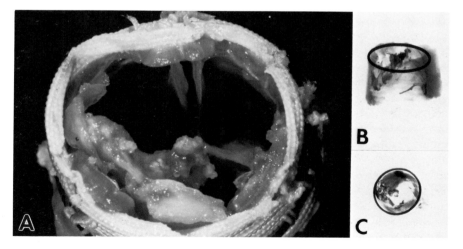

Fig. 42–18. (**A**) Calcified commissural fusion of one of the three commissures of a porcine valve from a conduit. This change caused valvular insufficiency. (**B, C**) Radiographs of the same with anteroposterior and superior views. Note calcific deposits involving one of the commissures with mild extension into one of the leaflets.

the cusp (50 percent), (2) linear perforations extending along the basal region of the cusp parallel to the sewing ring (rare), (3) large oval perforations in the central portion of the cusp (30 percent), and (4) small, often multiple perforations.[71] Edwards et al.[50] noted that the three interdependent mechanisms of valvular stenosis are (1) degenerative changes on porcine cusps and adjacent porcine aorta, (2) thrombosis of valvular commissures and pockets, and (3) destruction of the valve by endocarditis.

All conduits develop a luminal fibrous "peel," or neointima. The thickness may vary, resulting in major obstruction in some conduits or little or no obstruction in others. Nonobstructive neointima forms a thin, opalescent lining, whereas obstructive linings may consist of firm, thick fibrous tissue that may be focally calcified.[17,50] This neointima usually contains fenestrations that communicate from the lumen of the conduit to the interface between conduit and neointima. This interface may contain a layer of thrombus. The neointima may be adherent to the conduit but can easily be stripped away; in some cases, it may be almost totally separate from the conduit (Fig. 42–19). Occasionally, massive thrombus separates the fibrous peel, causing severe obstruction.[2] Conduit peels are similar microscopically, regardless of thickness or apparent age[2,50] and consist of (1) a luminal region comprised of dense collagen with only a few fibroblasts and occasional capillaries and (2) a conduit portion comprised of active granulation tissue with proliferating fibroblasts, neovascularization, focal collections of lymphocytes, neutrophils and/or plasma cells, and early collagen deposition (see Fig. 42–19). The thrombotic material between the peel and conduit wall varies in amount and ranges in age and content from a fresh platelet-fibrin thrombus to organizing thrombotic debris.[2] Varying amounts of fibrous tissue are found along the outer surface of the conduit, and within this external fibrous tissue layer occasional foreign body giant cells and thrombi may be seen (Fig. 42–20).

Conduit obstruction may be caused by a thick neointima that is either diffuse (see Fig. 42–19 and 42–20) or localized (pannus formation),[40] thrombotic separation of neointima from the conduit, or by formation of a flap-valve following dislodgement of neointima from the conduit.[50] In a series of 37 explanted porcine-valved extracardiac conduits from the Mayo Clinic,[50] calcific stenosis of the porcine valve accounted for conduit obstruction in 17 cases (46 percent), conduit stenosis was secondary to a thick fibrous neointima alone in 11 cases (30 percent), and both calcific valvular stenosis, and a thick neointima produced obstruction in six (16 percent) conduits. Two patients had outgrown their conduits (one also had extrinsic sternal compression), and one patient had obstruction only at the distal anastomosis.[50]

Pathogenesis of Conduit Obstruction

The etiology of accelerated calcification and degeneration of bioprosthetic valves implanted in children is unknown. Some factors that have been implicated include mechanical fatigue due to rapid heart rate, greater turbulence due to higher gradients in small valves, accelerated calcium turnover in children, and immunologic reactions.[9,169]

The pathogenesis of fibrous peel (neointima) formation is also unknown. Within the first day after implantation, a platelet-fibrin lining forms in extracardiac conduits, and a neointima develops as this lining becomes organized by migrating and proliferating fibroblasts.[2] The source of cells comprising the growing neointima is presumed to be from the proximal and distal anastomoses. Fibrous tissues may also grow throughout the interstices of the Dacron fabric.[18] It has been shown that endothelial and smooth muscle cells can be derived from transmural capillary ingrowth through porous polytetrafluoroeth-

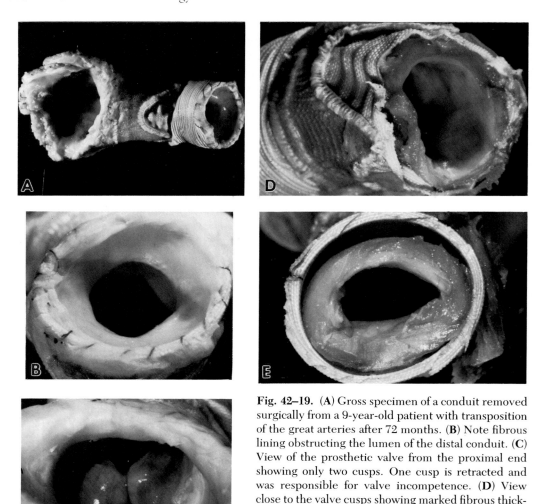

Fig. 42–19. (A) Gross specimen of a conduit removed surgically from a 9-year-old patient with transposition of the great arteries after 72 months. (B) Note fibrous lining obstructing the lumen of the distal conduit. (C) View of the prosthetic valve from the proximal end showing only two cusps. One cusp is retracted and was responsible for valve incompetence. (D) View close to the valve cusps showing marked fibrous thickening which incorporated the valve cusps (not visible). (E) Distal to the valve, the fibrous neointima retracted away from the conduit.

ylene grafts.[42,43] This mechanism may not account for the contribution of fibroblasts.[43] Growth and progressive thickening of the neointima is thought to occur from the surface that is in contact with the conduit and not from the portion in contact with the luminal flow of blood.[2,9] Agarwal et al.[3] suggested that, with each heartbeat, the corrugated conduit moves in an accordionlike fashion that loosens

neointima from the conduit and promotes the formation of fenestrations. The tight weave of the synthetic conduit precludes firm anchoring between the conduit and neointima, enabling blood to dissect through the interface with subsequent thrombosis and organization. Thus, the neointima undergoes progressive thickening at the surface in contact with the conduit. The type of connection for

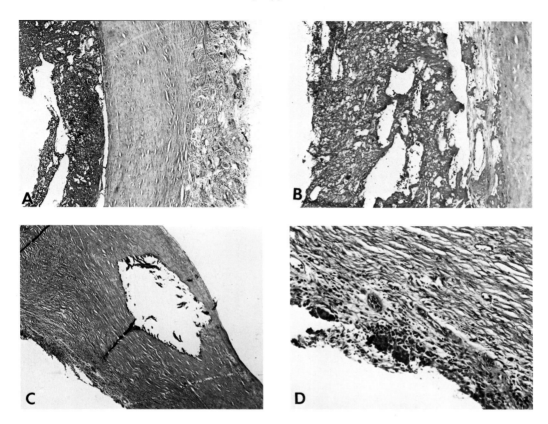

Fig. 42–20. Photomicrographs of (**A,B**) the fibrous covering of a conduit and (**C,D**) the neointima. Figs. A and B show fibrous lining outside the conduit with intervening fibrin clot that attached to the conduit. As seen in Fig. C, the neointima is fibrous. The portion near the lumen (upper right hand corner) is calcified focally. Fig. D is a close-up of the surface in contact with the conduit showing macrophages, chronic inflammatory cells, giant cells, and neovascularization. (H&E; Fig. A: × 40; Fig. B: × 100; Fig. C: × 40; Fig. D: × 198.)

which conduits are used (i.e., right atrium to pulmonary artery, right atrium to right ventricular infundibulum) may also influence the formation of a fibrous peel[59]; Geha et al.[61] did not find conduit or valve obstruction in patients who had undergone a modified Fontan correction, but they did observe obstruction in conduits subjected to higher pressures.

Attempts have been made to alter some factors that contribute to complications in conduits. For example, high-porosity knitted Dacron conduits may retard detachment of the fibrous peel more effectively than low-porosity woven Dacron,[41,67,76] although blood loss

through high-porosity grafts can be considerable in the immediate postoperative period, precluding their use in the repair of congenital heart defects.[110,124] Some investigators have administered acenocoumarol, which inhibits synthesis of γ-carboxyglutamic acid to slow calcification.[124] Experimental studies in which a calcification-retarding agent was evaluated in porcine-valved conduits failed to demonstrate prevention of calcification; furthermore, fibrous peel formation remained a significant problem.[163]

Despite the overwhelming success of extracardiac conduits in the treatment of serious congenital cardiac defects, the ideal conduit has yet to be developed. Valveless conduits would eliminate valvular complications, but the problem of obstructing neointima would remain, and valveless conduits are indicated only in the absence of pulmonary hypertension, hypoplastic pulmonary arteries, significant right ventricular dysfunction, or unrepaired tricuspid regurgitation.[47,55] Modifications in the Dacron weave to promote formation of fibrous anchors between the neointima and conduit wall may minimize neointimal proliferation.[3,50] Fresh aortic homografts appear promising, although their availability is limited. Experimental studies also suggest that pulmonary homografts may have use in right ventricular outflow tract reconstruction,[53,122] and the pulmonary homograft may be less prone to calcification.[94]

REFERENCES

1. Acinapura AJ, Rose DM, Cunningham JN, et al: Coronary artery bypass in septuagenarians. Analysis of mortality and morbidity. Circulation 78(suppl I):I-179, 1988

2. Agarwal KC, Edwards WD, Feldt RH, et al: Clinicopathological correlates of obstructed right-sided porcine-valved extracardiac conduits. J Thorac Cardiovasc Surg 81:591, 1981

3. Agarwal KC, Edwards WD, Feldt RH, et al: Pathogenesis of nonobstructive fibrous peels in right-sided porcine-valved extracardiac conduits. J Thorac Cardiovasc Surg 83:584, 1982

4. American Heart Association: 1987 Heart Facts. American Heart Association National Center, Dallas, 1987

5. Arnett EN, Isner JM, Redwood DR, et al: Coronary artery narrowing in coronary heart disease: Comparison of cineangiographic and necropsy findings. Ann Intern Med 91:350, 1979

6. Atkinson JB, Connor DH, Robinowitz M, et al: Cardiac fungal infections. Review of autopsy findings in 60 patients. Hum Pathol 15:935, 1984

7. Atkinson JB, Forman MB, Perry JM, et al: Correlation of saphenous vein bypass graft angiograms with histologic changes at necropsy. Am J Cardiol 55:952, 1985

8. Atkinson JB, Forman MB, Vaughn WK, et al: Morphologic changes in long-term saphenous vein bypass grafts. Chest 88:341, 1985

9. Atkinson JB, Virmani R: Complications of bioprosthetic heart valves. Primary Cardiol 12:46, 1986

10. Baber RS, Edwards WD, Holmes DR, et al: Balloon angioplasty of aortocoronary saphenous vein bypass grafts: A histologic study of six grafts from five patients, with emphasis on restenosis and embolic complications. J Am Coll Cardiol 12:1501, 1988

11. Bailey WW, Kirklin JW, Bargeron LM, et al: Late results with synthetic valved external conduits from venous ventricle to pulmonary arteries. Circulation 56(suppl II):II-73, 1976

12. Barboriak JJ, Batayias GE, Pintar K, et al: Pathological changes in surgically removed aortocoronary vein grafts. Ann Thorac Surg 21:524, 1976

13. Barboriak JJ, Pintar K, Korns ME: Atherosclerosis in aortocoronary vein grafts. Lancet 2:621, 1974

14. Bashour TT, Nanna ES, Mason DT: Myocardial revascularization with internal mammary artery bypass: An emerging treatment of choice. Am Heart J 111:143, 1986

15. Batayias GE, Barboriak JJ, Korns ME, et al: The spectrum of pathologic changes in aortocoronary saphenous vein grafts. Circulation 56(suppl II):II-18, 1977

16. Beck CS: The development of a new blood supply to the heart by operation. Ann Surg 102:801, 1935

17. Berger K, Sauvage LR, Rao AM, et al: Healing of arterial prosthesis in man. Its incompleteness. Ann Surg 175:118, 1972

18. Bisset GS, Schwartz DC, Benzing G, et al: Late results of reconstruction of the right ventricular outflow tract with porcine xenografts in children. Ann Thorac Surg 31:437, 1981

19. Bourassa MG, Campeau L, Lesperance J, et al: Changes in grafts and in coronary arteries after saphenous vein aortocoronary bypass surgery. p. 293. In Hammermeister KE (ed): Coronary Bypass Surgery. The Late Results. Praeger Publishers, New York, 1983

20. Bourassa MG, Fisher LD, Campeau L, et al: Long-term fate of bypass grafts. The coronary

artery surgery study (CASS) and Montreal Heart Institute experience. Circulation 72(suppl V):V-71, 1985

21. Bowman FO, Hancock WD, Malm JR: A valve containing Dacron prosthesis. Arch Surg 107:724, 1973

22. Boyce SW, Turley K, Yee ES, et al: The fate of the 12 mm porcine valved conduit from the right ventricle to the pulmonary artery. J Thorac Cardiovasc Surg 95:201, 1988

23. Brenowitz JB, Johnson WD, Kayser KL, et al: Coronary artery bypass grafting for the third time or more. Results of 150 consecutive cases. Circulation 78(suppl I):I-166, 1988

24. Brody WR, Angell WW, Kosek JC: Histologic fate of the venous coronary artery bypass in dogs. Am J Pathol 66:111, 1972

25. Brody WR, Kosek JC, Angell WW: Changes in vein grafts following aorto-coronary bypass induced by pressure and ischemia. J Thorac Cardiovasc Surg 68:847, 1972

26. Bulkley BH: Pathology of coronary artery bypass graft surgery. Am Heart J 98:539, 1979

27. Bulkley BH, Hutchins GM: Accelerated "atherosclerosis": A morphologic study of 97 saphenous vein coronary artery bypass grafts. Circulation 55:163, 1977

28. Bulkley BH, Hutchins GM: Pathology of coronary artery bypass graft surgery. Arch Pathol Lab Med 102:273, 1978

29. Bull SC, Macartney FJ, Horvath P, et al: Evaluation of long term results of homograft and heterograft valves in extracardiac conduits. J Thorac Cardiovasc Surg 94:12, 1987

30. CASS Principal Investigators: Coronary Artery Surgery Study (CASS): A randomized trial of coronary artery bypass surgery: Survival data. Circulation 68:939, 1983

31. CASS Principal Investigators: Comparison of coronary bypass surgery and medical therapy in patients 65 years of age or older. A nonrandomized study from the Coronary Artery Surgery Study (CASS) Registry. N Engl J Med 313:217, 1985

32. Cameron A, Kemp HG, Green GE: Bypass surgery with the internal mammary artery graft: 15 year follow-up. Circulation 74(suppl III):III-30, 1986

33. Cameron A, Kemp HG, Green GE: Reoperation for coronary artery disease 10 years of clinical follow-up. Circulation 78(suppl I):I-158, 1988

34. Campeau L, Enjalbert M, Lesperance J, et al: Atherosclerosis and late closure of aortocoronary saphenous vein grafts: sequential angiographic studies at 2 weeks, 1 year, 5 to 7 years and 10 to 12 years after surgery. Circulation 68(suppl II):II-1, 1983

35. Campeau L, Enjalbert M, Lesperance J, et al: The relation of risk factors to the development of atherosclerosis in saphenous vein bypass grafts and the progression of disease in the native circulation. A study 10 years after aortocoronary bypass surgery. N Engl J Med 311:1329, 1984

36. Campeau L, Lesperance J, Corbara J, et al: Aortocoronary saphenous vein bypass graft changes 5 to 7 years after surgery. Circulation 58(suppl I):I-170, 1978

37. Chard RB, Johnson DC, Nunn GR, et al: Aorta-coronary bypass grafting with polytetrafluoroethylene conduits. J Thorac Cardiovasc Surg 94:132, 1987

38. Chesebro JH, Fuster V, Elveback LR, et al: Effect of dipyridamole and aspirin on late vein-graft patency after coronary bypass operations. N Engl J Med 310:209, 1984

39. Christian CB, Mack JW, Wetstein L: Current status of coronary artery bypass grafting for coronary artery atherosclerosis. Surg Clin North Am 65(3):509, 1985

40. Chun PKC, Rocchini AP, Gibbs HR, et al: Pannus formation in a Hancock-valved conduit resulting in proximal intraconduit obstruction: Late complication of Rastelli procedure for complete transposition of the great vessels with ventricular septal defect and pulmonic stenosis. Am Heart J 101:855, 1981

41. Ciaravella JM, McGoon DC, Danielson GK, et al: Experience with the extracardiac conduit. J Thorac Cardiovasc Surg 78:920, 1979

42. Clowes AW, Gown AM, Hanson SR, et al: Mechanisms of arterial graft failure. 1. Role of cellular proliferation in early healing of PTFE prostheses. Am J Pathol 118:43, 1985

43. Clowes AW, Kirkman TR, Reidy MA: Mechanisms of arterial graft healing. Rapid transmural capillary ingrowth provides a source of intimal endothelium and smooth muscle in porous PTFE prostheses. Am J Pathol 123:220, 1986

44. Daskalopoulos DA, Edwards WD, Driscoll DJ, et al: Coronary artery compression with fatal myocardial ischemia. A rare complica-

tion of valved extracardiac conduits in children with congenital heart disease. J Thorac Cardiovasc Surg 85:546, 1983

45. Detre KM, Peduzzi P, Takaro T: Eleven-year survival in the Veterans Administration randomized trial of coronary bypass surgery for stable angina. N Engl J Med 311:1333, 1984

46. Dincer B, Barner HB: The "occluded" internal mammary artery graft: Restoration of patency after apparent occlusion associated with progression of coronary disease. J Thorac Cardiovasc Surg 85:318, 1983

47. Downing TP, Danielson GK, Schaff HV, et al: Replacement of obstructed right ventricular-pulmonary arterial valved conduits with nonvalved conduits in children. Circulation 72(suppl II):II-84, 1985

48. Dunn JM: Porcine valve durability in children. Ann Thorac Surg 32:357, 1981

49. Ebert PA: Conduits—indications, problems, and future use. Adv Cardiol 26:138, 1979

50. Edwards WD, Agarwal KC, Feldt RH, et al: Surgical pathology of obstructed, right-sided, porcine-valved extracardiac conduits. Arch Pathol Lab Med 107:400, 1983

51. Effler DB, Groves LK, Sones FM Jr, et al: Increased myocardial perfusion by internal mammary artery implant: Vineberg's operation. Am Surg 158:526, 1963

52. Ellis EF, Oelz O, Roberts LJ II, et al: Coronary arterial smooth muscle contraction by a substance released from platelets: Evidence that it is thromboxane A$_2$. Science 193:1135, 1976

53. Euguchi S, Asano K: Homograft of pulmonary artery or ascending aorta with valve as a right ventricular outflow. J Thorac Cardiovasc Surg 56:413, 1968

54. European Coronary Surgery Study Group: Long-term results of a prospective randomized study of coronary artery bypass surgery in stable angina pectoris. Lancet 2:1173, 1982

55. Fiore AC, Peigh PS, Robison RJ, et al: Valved and nonvalved right ventricular-pulmonary arterial extracardiac conduits. J Thorac Cardiovasc Surg 86:490, 1983

56. Fontan FM, Choussat A, Deville C, et al: Aortic valve homografts in the surgical treatment of complex cardiac malformations. J Thorac Cardiovasc Surg 87:649, 1984

57. Fontan F, Mounico F, Baudet E, et al: "Correction" de l'atresie tricuspidienne. Rapport

de deux cas "corriges" par l'autilisation d'une technique chirurgicale nouvelle. Ann Chir Thorac Cardiovasc 10:39, 1971

58. Friedman M: Spontaneous atherosclerosis and experimental thromboatherosclerosis. Arch Pathol 76:571, 1963

59. Gale AW, Danielson GK, McGoon DC, et al: Modified Fontan operation for univentricular heart and complicated congenital lesions. J Thorac Cardiovasc Surg 78:831, 1979

60. Garrett HE, Dennis EW, DeBakey M: Aortocoronary bypass with saphenous vein graft: Seven year follow-up. JAMA 223:792, 1973

61. Geha AS, Laks H, Stansel HC Jr, et al: Late failure of porcine valve heterografts in children. J Thorac Cardiovasc Surg 78:351, 1979

62. Griffith LSC, Bulkely BH, Hutchins GM, et al: Occlusive changes at the coronary artery bypass graft anastomosis. Morphologic study of 95 grafts. J Thorac Cardiovasc Surg 73:668, 1977

63. Grondin CM, Campeau L, Lesperance J, et al: Atherosclerotic changes in coronary vein grafts six years after operation: Angiographic aspect in 110 patients. J Thorac Cardiovasc Surg 77:24, 1979

64. Grondin CM, Campeau L, Lesperance J, et al: Comparison of late changes in internal mammary artery and saphenous vein grafts in two consecutive series of patients ten years after operation. Circulation 70(suppl I):I-208, 1984

65. Hales MR, Carrington CB: A pigment gelatin mass for vascular injection. Yale J Biol Med 43:257, 1971

66. Hamby RI, Aintablian A, Handler M, et al: Aortocoronary saphenous vein bypass grafts. Long-term patency, morphology and blood flow in patients with patent grafts early after surgery. Circulation 60:901, 1979

67. Haverich A, Oelert H, Maatz W, et al: Histopathological evaluation of woven and knitted Dacron grafts for right ventricular conduits: a comparative experimental study. Ann Thorac Surg 37:404, 1984

68. Heck HA Jr, Schieken RM, Lauer RM, et al: Conduit repair for complex congenital heart disease: late follow-up. J Thorac Cardiovasc Surg 75:806, 1978

69. Horiuchi T, Abe T, Okada Y, et al: Reconstruction of the main pulmonary artery with a valve-bearing tube graft made of autologous

pericardium. J Thorac Cardiovasc Surg 62:793, 1971

70. Hutchins GM, Bulkley BH, Ridolfi RL, et al: Correlation of coronary arteriograms and left ventriculograms with post mortem studies. Circulation 56:32, 1977

71. Ishihara T, Ferrans VJ, Boyce SW, et al: Structure and classification of cuspal tears and perforations in porcine bioprosthetic cardiac valves implanted in patients. p. 362. In Cohn LH, Gallucci V (eds): Cardiac Bioprosthesis. Yorke Medical Books, New York, 1982

72. Ishii T, Newman WP, Guzman MA, et al: Coronary and aortic atherosclerosis in young men from Tokyo and New Orleans. Lab Invest 54:561, 1986

73. Ishizawa E, Suzuki Y, Haneda K: Surgical management of pulmonary atresia and ventricular spetal defect. Nippon Kyobu Geka Gakkai Zasshi, 34:1292, 1986 (abst)

74. Islam MN, Zikria EA, Sullivan ME, et al: Aortocoronary Gore-Tex graft: 18-month patency. Ann Thorac Surg 31:569, 1981

75. Isner JM, Kishel J, Kent KM, et al: Accuracy of angiographic determination of left main coronary arterial narrowing. Angiographic-histologic correlative analysis in 28 patients. Circulation 63:1056, 1981

76. Jonas RA, Freed MD, Mayer JE, et al: Long term follow up of patients with synthetic right heart conduits. Circulation 72(suppl II):II-77, 1985

77. Kalsner S, Richard R: Coronary arteries of cardiac patients are hyperreactive and contain stores of amines: A mechanism for coronary spasm. Science 223:1435, 1981

78. Kay HR, Korns ME, Flemma RJ, et al: Atherosclerosis of the internal mammary artery. Ann Thorac Surg 21:504, 1976

79. Kay PH, Ross DN: Fifteen years' experience with the aortic homograft: The conduit of choice for right ventricular outflow tract reconstruction. Ann Thorac Surg 40:360, 1985

80. Kennedy JW, Kaiser GC, Fisher LD, et al: Clinical and angiographic predictors of operative mortality from the collaborative study in coronary artery surgery (CASS). Circulation 63:793, 1981

81. Kern WH, Dermer GB, Lindesmith GG: The intimal proliferation in aortic-coronary saphenous vein grafts. Light and electron microscopic studies. Am Heart J 84:771, 1972

82. Killip T: Twenty years of coronary bypass surgery. New Engl J Med 319:366, 1988

83. Killip T, Ryan TJ: Randomized trials in coronary bypass surgery. Circulation 71:418, 1985

84. King P, Royle JP: Autogenous vein grafting in atheromatous rabbits. Cardiovasc Res 6:627, 1972

85. Kirklin JW, Blackstone EH, Maehara T, et al: Intermediated-term fate of cryopreserved allograft and xenograft valved conduits. Ann Thorac Surg 44:598, 1987

86. Kiser JC, Ongley PA, Kirklin JW, et al: Surgical treatment of dextrocardia with inversion of ventricles and double-outlet right ventricle. J Thorac Cardiovasc Surg 55:6, 1968

87. Koshal A, Beaulands DS, Davies RA, et al: Urgent surgical reperfusion in acute evolving myocardial infarction. A randomized controlled study. Circulation 78(suppl I):I-171, 1988

88. Larson RM, Hagen PO, Fuchs JCA: Lipid biosynthesis in arteries, veins and venous grafts. Circulation 50(suppl III):III-139, 1974

89. Lawrie GM, Morris GC, Howell JF, et al: Results of coronary bypass more than 5 years after operation in 434 patients. Clinical, treadmill exercise and angiographic correlations. Am J Cardiol 40:665, 1977

90. Layton CA, McDonald A, McDonald L, et al: The syndrome of absent pulmonary valve. Total correction with aortic valvular homografts. J Thorac Cardiovasc Surg 63:800, 1972

91. Leeman DE, McCabe CH, Faxon DP, et al: Use of percutaneous transluminal coronary angioplasty and bypass surgery despite improved medical therapy for unstable angina pectoris. Am J Cardiol 61:33G, 1988

92. Liang BT, Antman EM, Taus R, et al: Atherosclerotic aneurysms of aortocoronary vein grafts. Am J Cardiol 61:185, 1988

93. Lie JT, Lawrie GM, Morris GC: Aortocoronary bypass saphenous vein graft atherosclerosis. Anatomic study of 99 vein grafts from normal and hyperlipoproteinemic patients up to 75 months postoperatively. Am J Cardiol 40:906, 1977

94. Livi U, Abdulla AK, Parker R, et al: Viability and morphology of aortic and pulmonary homografts. J Thorac Cardiovasc Surg 93:755, 1987

95. Loop FD: CASS continued. Circulation 72(suppl II):II-1, 1985

96. Loop FD, Lytle BW, Cosgrove DM, et al: Influence of the internal mammary artery graft on ten year survival and other cardiac events. N Engl J Med 314:1, 1986

97. Loop FD, Lytle BW, Cosgrove DM, et al: Free (aorto-coronary) internal mammary artery graft. J Thorac Cardiovasc Surg 92:827, 1986

98. Lytle BW, Cosgrove DM, Loop FD, et al: Perioperative risk of bilateral internal mammary artery grafting: Analysis of 500 cases from 1971 to 1984. Circulation 74(suppl III):III-37, 1986

99. Lytle BW, Loop FD, Cosgrove DM, et al: Long-term (5–12 years) serial studies of internal mammary artery and saphenous vein coronary bypass grafts. J Thorac Cardiovasc Surg 89:248, 1985

100. Lytle BW, Loop FD, Cosgrove DM, et al: Fifteen hundred coronary reoperations. Results and determinants of early and late survival. J Thorac Cardiovasc Surg 93:847, 1987

101. Marchand P: The use of a cusp bearing homograft patch to the outflow tract and pulmonary artery in Fallot's tetralogy and pulmonary valvular stenosis. Thorax 22:497, 1967

102. Marmot MG: Interpretation of trends in coronary heart disease mortality. Acta Med Scand (suppl) 701:58, 1985

103. Marti MC, Bouchardy B, Cox JN: Aortocoronary bypass with autogenous saphenous vein grafts: Histopathologic aspects. Virchows Arch [A] 352:255, 1971

104. McEnany MT, DeSanctis RW, Harthorne JW: Effect of antithrombolytic therapy on aortocoronary vein graft patency rates. Circulation 54(suppl II):II-124, 1976

105. McGoon DC, Danielson GK, Puga FJ, et al: Late results after extracardiac conduit repair for congenital cardiac defects. Am J Cardiol 49:1741, 1982

106. McGoon DC, Rastelli GC, Ongley PA: An operation for the correction of truncus arteriosus. JAMA 205:69, 1968

107. McNamara JJ, Darling RC, Linton RR: Segmental stenosis of saphenous vein autografts. N Engl J Med 277:290, 1967

108. Meldrum-Hanna W, Cartmill T, Johnson D,

et al: Late results of right ventricular outflow tract reconstruction with Bjork-Shiley valved conduits. Br Heart J 55:371, 1986

109. Mestres CA, Reves A, Igual A, et al: Atherosclerosis of internal mammary artery. Histopathologic analysis and implications on its results in coronary artery bypass graft surgery. Thorac Cardiovasc Surg 34(6):356, 1986

110. Miller DC, Stinson EB, Oyer PE, et al: The durability of porcine xenograft valves and conduits in children. Circulation 66(suppl I):I-172, 1982

111. Molina JE, Carr M, Yarnoz MD: Coronary bypass with Gore-Tex graft. J Thorac Cardiovasc Surg 75:769, 1978

112. Moodie DS, Mair DD, Fulton RE, et al: Aortic homograft obstruction. J Thorac Cardiovasc Surg 72:553, 1976

113. Morton KE, Gavaghan TP, Krilis SA, et al: Coronary artery bypass graft failure—an autoimmune phenomenon? Lancet 2:1353, 1986

114. Murphy ML, Hultgren HN, Detre K, et al: Treatment of chronic stable angina: A preliminary report of survival data of the randomized Veterans Administration cooperative study. N Engl J Med 297:621, 1977

115. Naunheim KS, Fiore AC, Wadley JA, et al: The changing profile of the patients undergoing coronary artery bypass surgery. J Am Coll Cardiol 11:494, 1988

116. Neitzel GF, Barboriak JJ, Pintar K, et al: Atherosclerosis in aortocornary bypass grafts. Morphologic study and risk factor analysis 6 to 12 years after surgery. Arteriosclerosis 6:594, 1986

117. Noera G, Massini C, Ferrini L, et al: Microscopic analysis for aortocoronary bypass. G Ital Cardiol 16:1037, 1986

118. Norman JC, Nihill MR, Cooley DA: Valved apico-aortic composite conduits for left ventricular outflow tract obstruction. A 4 year experience with 27 patients. Am J Cardiol 45:1265, 1980

119. Odell JA: Calcification of porcine bioprosthesis in children. p 231. In Cohn LH, Gallucci V (eds): Cardiac Bioprostheses. Yorke Medical Books, New York, 1982

120. O'Shaughnessy L: Surgical treatment of cardiac ischemia. Lancet 1:185, 1937

121. Passamani E, Davis KB, Gillispie MJ, et al:

A randomized trial of coronary artery bypass surgery. Survival of patients with a low ejection fraction. N Engl J Med 312:1665, 1985

122. Pierce WS, Thompson WM, Kazama S, et al: Replacement of the pulmonary outflow tract and valve with a formalin-treated porcine heterograft. J Thorac Cardiovasc Surg 61:924, 1971

123. Pintar K, Barboriak JJ, Johnson WD: Atherosclerotic aneurysm in aortocoronary vein graft. Arch Pathol Lab Med 102:287, 1978

124. Prenger KB, Hess J, Cromme-Dijkhuis AH, et al: Porcine-valved Dacron conduits in Fontan procedures. Ann Thorac Surg 46:526, 1988

125. Pryor DB, Harrel FE Jr, Rankin JS, et al: The changing survival benefit of coronary vascularization over time. Circulation 76(suppl V):V-13, 1987

126. Rahimtoola SH: Coronary bypass surgery—a perspective. p. 1. In Rahimtoola SH, Brest AN (eds): Coronary Bypass Surgery. FA Davis, Philadelphia, 1977

127. Rahimtoola SH: Coronary bypass surgery for unstable angina. Circulation 68:842, 1984

128. Rankin JS, Newman GE, Bashore TM, et al: Clinical and angiographic assessment of complex mammary artery bypass grafting. J Thorac Cardiovasc Surg 92:832, 1986

129. Rastelli GC: A new approach to "anatomic" repair of transposition of the great arteries. Mayo Clin Proc 44:1, 1969

130. Rastelli GC, Onlgey PA, Davis GD, et al: Surgical repair for pulmonary valve atresia with coronary-pulmonary artery fistula. Report of case. Mayo Clin Proc 40:521, 1965

131. Rastelli GC, Wallace RB, Ongley PA: Complete repair of transposition of the great arteries with pulmonary stenosis. A review and report of a case corrected by using a new surgical technique. Circulation, 39:83, 1969

132. Reder RF, Dimich I, Steinfeld L, et al: Left ventricle to aorta valved conduit for relief of diffuse left ventricular outflow tract obstruction. Am J Cardiol, 39:1068, 1977

133. Riahi M, Vasu CM, Tomatis LA, et al: aneurysm of saphenous vein bypass graft to coronary artery. J Thorac Cardiovasc Surg 70:358, 1975

134. Roberts WC, Lachman AS, Virmani R: Twisting of an aortic-coronary bypass conduit. A

complication of coronary surgery. J Thorac Cardiovasc Surg 75:722, 1978

135. Rocchini AP, Brown J, Crowley DC, et al: Clinical and hemodynamic follow-up of left ventricular to aortic conduits in patients with aortic stenosis. J Am Coll Cardiol 1:1135, 1983

136. Rose AG: Valve-containing conduits. p. 154. In Rose AG (ed): Pathology of Heart Valve Replacement. MTP Press, Lancaster, England, 1987

137. Ross DN, Somerville J: Correction of pulmonary atresia with a homograft aortic valve. Lancet 2:1446, 1966

138. Rossiter SJ, Brody WR, Kosek JC, et al: Internal mammary artery versus autogenous vein for coronary artery bypass graft. Circulation 50:1236, 1974

139. Roy L, Knapp HR, Robertson RM, et al: Endogenous prostacyclin (PGI_2) biosynthesis is stimulated by cardiac catherization and angiography in man. Circulation 68(suppl III):III-104, 1983 (abst)

140. Russo P, Orszulak TA, Schaff HV, et al: Use of internal mammary artery grafts for multiple coronary artery bypasses. Circulation 74(suppl III):III-48, 1986

141. Sako Y: Susceptibility of autologous vein grafts to atheromatous degeneration. Surg Forum 12:247, 1961

142. Sapsford RN, Oakely GD, Talbot S: Early and late patency of expanded polytetrafluoroethylene vascular grafts in aorta-coronary bypass. J Thorac Cardiovasc Surg 81:860, 1981

143. Saravalli OA, Somerville J, Jefferson KE: Calcification of aortic homografts used for reconstruction of the right ventricular outflow tract. J Thorac Cardiovasc Surg 80:909, 1980

144. Sauvage LR, Schloemer R, Wood SJ, et al: Successful interposition of synthetic graft between aorta and right coronary artery: Angiographic follow-up to 16 months. J Thorac Cardiovasc Surg 72:418, 1976

145. Scott HW Jr, Morgan CV, Bolasny BL, et al: Experimental atherosclerosis in autogenous venous grafts. Arch Surg 101:677, 1970

146. Scott SM, Luchi RJ, Deupree RH, et al: Veterans Administration Cooperative Study for the treatment of patients with unstable angina: Results in patients with abnormal left ventricular function. Circulation 78(suppl I):I-113, 1988

147. Seides SF, Borer JS, Kent KM, et al: Long-term anatomic fate of coronary artery bypass grafts and functional status of patients five years after operation. N Engl J Med 298:1213, 1978

148. Selzer A: Fifty years of progress in cardiology: A personal perspective. Circulation 77(5):955, 1988

149. Shabbo FP, Wain WH, Ross DN: Right ventricular outflow tract reconstruction with aortic homograft conduit: Analysis of the long term results. Thorac Cardiovasc Surg 28:21, 1980

150. Shelton ME, Forman MB, Virmani R, et al: A comparison of morphologic and angiographic findings in long-term internal mammary artery and saphenous vein bypass grafts. J Am Coll Cardiol 11:297, 1988

151. Silver MD, Wilson GJ: Pathology of cardiovascular prostheses including coronary artery bypass and other vascular grafts. p. 1225. In Silver MD (ed): Cardiovascular Pathology. Churchill Livingstone, New York, 1983

152. Simms FH: A comparison of coronary and internal mammary arteries and implications of the results in the etiology of arteriosclerosis. Am Heart J 105:560, 1983

153. Smith SH, Geer JC: Morphology of saphenous vein-coronary artery bypass grafts seven to 116 months after surgery. Arch Pathol Lab Med 107:13, 1983

154. Spencer FC: The internal mammary artery: The ideal coronary bypass graft? N Engl J Med 314:50, 1986

155. Spray TL, Roberts WC: Status of the grafts and the native coronary arteries proximal and distal to coronary anastomotic sites of aortocoronary bypass grafts. Circulation 55:741, 1977

156. Spray TL, Roberts WC: Structural changes in porcine xenografts used as substitute cardiac valves: Gross and histologic observations in 51 glutaraldehyde-preserved Hancock valves in 41 patients. Am J Cardiol 40:319, 1977

157. Stansel HC Jr, Tabry II, Hellenbrand WE, et al: Apical-aortic shunts in children. Am J Surg 135:547, 1978

158. Stewart S, Manning J, Alexson C, et al: The Hancock external valved conduit: A dichotomy between late clinical results and late cardiac catheterization findings. J Thorac Cardiovasc Surg 86:562, 1983

159. Sweeney MS, Walker WE, Cooley DA, et al: Apicoaortic conduits for complex left ventricular outflow obstruction: 10-year experience. Ann Thorac Surg 42:609, 1986

160. Takaro T, Hultgren HN, Lipton MJ, et al: The VA cooperative randomized study of surgery for coronary arterial occlusive disease. II. Subgroup with significant left main lesions. Circulation 54(suppl III):107, 1976

161. Talierico CP, Smith HC, Pluth JR, et al: Coronary artery venous bypass graft aneurysm with symptomatic coronary artery emboli. J Am Coll Cardiol 7:435, 1986

162. Taylor WJ, Gorlin R: Objective criteria for internal mammary artery implantation. Ann Thorac Surg 4:143, 1967

162a. Tector AJ, et al: Expanding the use of the internal mammary artery to improve patency in coronary artery bypass grafting. J Thorac Cardiovasc Surg 91:9, 1986

163. Thiene G, Laborde F, Valente M, et al: Experimental evaluation of porcine-valved conduits processed with a calcium-retarding agent (T6). J Thorac Cardiovasc Surg 91:215, 1986

164. Tsukada T, Tejima T, Amano J, et al: Immunocytochemical investigation of atherosclerotic changes observed in aortocoronary bypass grafts using monoclonal antibodies. Exp Mol Pathol 43(2):193, 1988

165. Ugori C, Cooley D, Norman J: Post-traumatic apical left ventricular aneurysm in a patient with left ventricular apical-abdominal aortic conduit: Case presentation. Cardiovasc Dis Bull Tex Heart Inst 6:439, 1979

166. Unni KK, Kottke BA, Titus JL, et al: Pathologic changes in aortocoronary saphenous vein grafts. Am J Cardiol 34:526, 1974

167. Ursell PC, Griffiths SP, Bowman FO Jr: Traumatic rupture of extracardiac valved conduit: Unusual late complication producing outflow tract obstruction. Ann Thorac Surg 46:351, 1988

168. Valente M, Bortolotti U, Arbustini E, et al: Glutaraldehyde-preserved porcine bioprostheses. Factors affecting performance as determined by pathologic studies. Chest 83:607, 1983

169. Vergesslich KA, Gersony WM, Steeg CN, et al: Postoperative assessment of porcine-

valved right ventricular-pulmonary artery conduits. Am J Cardiol 53:202, 1984

170. The Veterans Administration Coronary Artery Bypass Surgery Cooperative Study Group: Eleven-year survival in the Veterans Administration randomized trial of coronary artery bypass surgery for stable angina. N Engl J Med 311:1333, 1984

171. Victor MF, Kimbiris D, Iskandrian AS, et al: Spasm of a saphenous vein bypass graft. A possible mechanism for occlusion of the venous graft. Chest 80:413, 1981

172. Vineberg AM: Development of anastomoses between coronary vessels and transplanted internal mammary artery. Can Med Assoc J 55:117, 1946

173. Virmani R, Atkinson JB, Forman MB: Aortocoronary saphenous vein bypass grafts. p. 41. In Waller BF (ed): Contemporary Issues in Cardiovascular Pathology. FA Davis, Philadelphia, 1987

174. Virmani R, Ursell PC, Fenoglio JJ: Examination of the heart. Hum Pathol 18:432, 1987

175. Walinsky P: Angiographic documentation of spontaneous spasm of saphenous vein coronary artery bypass graft. Am Heart J 103:290, 1982

176. Walts AE, Fishbein MC, Sustaita H, et al: Ruptured atheromatous plaques in saphenous vein coronary artery bypass: A mechanism of acute, thrombotic, late graft occlusion. Circulation 65:197, 1982

177. World Health Organization: Classification of atherosclerotic lesions report of a study group. Technical Report Series. Publication 143, World Health Organization, Geneva, pp. 3–20, 1958

43

Pathology of Cardiac Transplantation

Alan G. Rose
C. J. Uys

This chapter emphasizes autopsy findings in patients who received heart transplants and presents aspects of findings in endomyocardial biopsies from their new hearts. The latter topic is also discussed in Chapter 39.

The first recorded cardiac transplant was that of Carrel and Guthrie,[20] who in 1905 transplanted a heart to the neck of a dog, where it beat spontaneously for 1 hour. Using a similar model, Mann et al.[73] in 1933 performed a series of transplants with the intact hearts of puppies. Three times out of four, the transplanted heart resumed beating promptly. The average survival time of these hearts was 4 days, although one heart survived 8 days. Mann et al. provided a brief description of the pathologic changes observed in the transplanted heart, which we recognize today as those of acute rejection. In 1964 James D. Hardy[49] of Jackson, Mississippi, in the absence of a suitable human donor transplanted the heart of a chimpanzee to a dying patient. The xenograft maintained function for approximately 1 hour.

The first human heart transplant was performed by Christiaan N. Barnards' team at Groote Schuur Hospital, Cape Town, South Africa, on December 3, 1967.[8] The recipient in this historic operation was 57-year-old Louis Washkansky; the donor heart (Fig. 43–1) was from an 18-year-old female motor vehicle accident victim. Washkansky survived for 18 days with the orthotopic transplant before dying of a combination of acute rejection and sepsis.[103]

Since that event, the operation has been performed at many centers throughout the world. In this procedure the donor atria are anastomosed to the upper atrial remnants of the recipient, which bear respectively the venae cavae and pulmonary veins; and the donor pulmonary artery and aorta are anastomosed to those of the recipient.

In 1975 Barnard and Losman[10,66] successfully applied in humans the technique of heterotopic transplantation, which, until then, had usually been employed in experimental cardiac transplantation. In the human heterotopic transplant, the recipient's heart is left in position and the donor heart is placed to the right of it. The donor superior and inferior venae cavae are ligated, the pulmonary artery is anastomosed to the recipient's by means of a tube graft, an end-to-side anastomosis is performed between donor and recipient aortae, and the donor left and right atria are anastomosed to the respective atria of the recipient (Fig. 43–2). Normal hemodynamics are re-

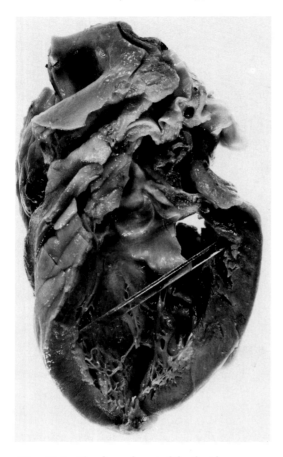

Fig. 43–1. The donor heart of the first human cardiac transplant, performed on Louis Washkansky by C. N. Barnard.

and total cardiac function will be assumed by the graft. Losman[66] reviewed the Cape Town experience with heterotopic cardiac transplantation.

Heterotopic transplantation is seldom applied currently, due to the potential danger of thromboembolism derived from stasis thrombi in the recipient's heart and infection of prosthetic heart valves if present in the latter. The development of cardiopulmonary transplantation as a treatment for pulmonary hypertension has also removed a prime indication for heterotopic cardiac transplantation. If the donor heart is too small for the recipient, heterotopic transplantation may be indicated.

EXPERIMENTAL HEART TRANSPLANTATION

Before the first human cardiac transplant in 1967, experimental cardiac transplantation, in a variety of animals, had been successfully and widely performed for almost 15 years. The knowledge gained from these procedures allowed the technique for both heterotopic and orthotopic transplantation to be standardized. The experiments gave insight into the clinical and histologic manifestations of rejection and enabled the effect of immunosuppressive agents on survival and the morphology of rejection to be studied and assessed.

Following the initial experiments of Carrel and Guthrie[20] and Mann et al.,[73] Downie[36] in 1953 established the technique of cardiac transplantation in the dog by placing a heterotopic graft in the neck and anastomosing the aorta to the carotid artery and the pulmonary artery to the jugular vein. These hearts pulsated regularly for an average of 129 hours.

In 1961, Lower, Stofer, and Shumway[71] described the technique for a successful orthotopic transplant in the dog. This was probably the first meaningful step toward human transplantation. One of their dogs survived 8 days.

stored and the recipient heart is left intact. The recipient's right ventricle will cope with pulmonary hypertension until the improved left heart function brings the pulmonary resistance back to normal. The recipient's left ventricle provides assistance during graft recovery from surgical anoxia and injury, as well as during episodes of rejection; this may be life-saving if the graft is totally rejected. In such an event the rejected organ may be resected without the use of extracorporeal circulation, avoiding further damage to the recipient's heart. Alternatively, should the recipient's heart cease to function and become a source of complication, it may be resected

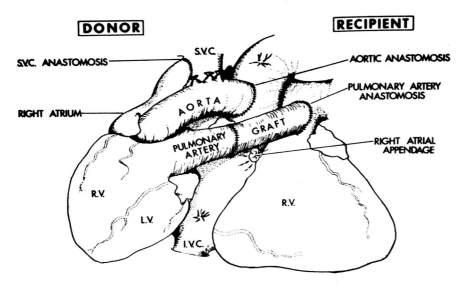

Fig. 43–2. Diagram illustrating the anastomoses in a heterotopic cardiac transplant.

Thereafter, Blumenstock et al.[17] performed orthotopic cardiac transplants on 50 unrelated mongrel dogs and demonstrated that methotrexate increased survival time and diminished rejection response in the heart, thereby acting as an immunosuppressive agent. Their longest survivor was 42 days. Lower and associates[68,69] followed their pioneering work by publishing, in 1965, their observations on untreated and treated dogs with orthotopic transplants, the treated group surviving up to 250 days.[68,69] In 1968, Lower et al.[70] drew attention to the proliferative and obliterative intimal changes of chronic rejection in the epicardial coronary arteries of long-surviving canine transplants.

Full descriptions of the pathology of experimental cardiac transplants[68-73] have been given for dogs,[16,17,23,27,36,53–56,62,83,96,114] rats,[1,60,61,72,98,105,113] rabbits,[5,60,61] and baboons.[34]

Changes occurring in the kidney and other transplants are discussed in Chapter 12.

Experimental cardiac transplantation allows the observation of either the changes of cardiac rejection unaltered by immunosuppressive therapy or the efficacy of different immunosuppressant regimens. The absence of immunosuppression severely limits the survival of a graft.

HUMAN HEART TRANSPLANTATION

The first description of the findings in a transplanted human heart was by Thomson.[103] In 1968, he presented the findings of Barnard's patient who survived the operation 18 days (see Fig. 43–1). This was followed, in the same year, by a report from Lower et al.[70] on a patient who had survived 7 days. In 1969, Thomson[104] described the donor heart of a patient who had survived 19½ months. This was the first description in a human donor heart of the obliterative vascular changes that characterize chronic rejection. Thereafter, detailed reports on cardiac findings and complications in series of orthotopic transplants followed. Bieber et al. presented their findings in 12 autopsies[13]; Levinsky et al.[64] in one; Milam et al.[76] in 13 autopsies[76]; Ellis et al. in three[38]; Kosek et al.[53] in 20 autopsies; and

Caves et al.[25] in biopsies from 16 patients. There have been fewer reports of autopsied patients with heterotopic cardiac allograft.[107]

In the majority of patients, the indication for transplantation was ischemic heart disease; cardiomyopathy and advanced rheumatic heart disease were indications only in occasional patients.[13,64,76,86,103,104,105,108] With a few exceptions, the donors were young people who were anticipated to have normal hearts and vessels free of degenerative disease.[76,86,108] This is not always the case. We examined several donor hearts that either were not transplanted because of poor tissue match or were recovered following the death of the recipient less than a few days posttransplantation and in which scanty, focal or solitary, severe coronary atherosclerosis was present. Such lesions in the donor heart, if encountered months or years after transplantation, could easily be misconstrued as representing accelerated atherosclerosis of chronic rejection. The occurrence of such coronary stenoses in young persons (younger than 25 years) is a reflection of the high incidence of atherosclerosis in the South African population.

Unfortunately, this problem is not confined to young South Africans. At some centers,

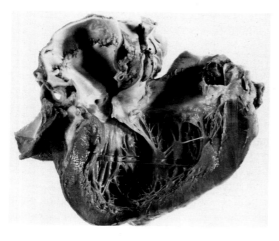

Fig. 43–3. Orthotopic transplant in which there is no evidence of rejection. The patient survived 61 days and died of a pulmonary infection.

because of the risk of atherosclerotic coronary artery lesions, coronary angiography is done before organ collection. The editor has seen an acute myocardial infarction 1 week after transplantation resulting from an occlusive thrombus developing in an area of a severe stenosis affecting a coronary artery of a donor heart obtained from a 19-year-old man.

The use of current immunosuppressive regimes as applied in the human situation and the longer survival associated with them do not totally eliminate the acute rejection response.[13,53,56,76] Rather, they allow development of a chronic rejection reaction, characterized by vascular occlusion, which, ultimately, is the prime cause of graft failure.

Acute Rejection

Macroscopic Appearance

Macroscopically, few donor hearts are remarkable (Fig. 43–3). The pericardium has been excised at operation, and the donor heart is usually attached by fibrous adhesions to the sternum and adjacent lungs. In heterotopic transplants in our series, the bulk of the two conjoined hearts is surprisingly well accommodated in the thoracic cavity. With time, sutures at the anastomotic sites become barely visible and are buried in endothelialized fibrous tissue (Fig. 43–4).

Occasionally, an anastomosis is the site of mural thrombus formation. Mild or moderate acute rejection may produce no naked-eye alterations in a donor heart. Those with severe acute rejection are flabby, their ventricular walls are thickened, the cavities dilated, and the myocardium of both ventricles has a mottled appearance with ill-defined, pale areas alternating with congested hemorrhagic areas. Subendocardial hemorrhages are noted in both ventricles and, occasionally, the cavity of the left ventricular apex is occupied by mural thrombus (Fig. 43–5).

In our cases, and in those of others,[38] changes of acute rejection are seen from 5 days

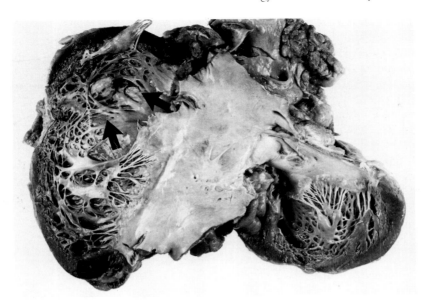

Fig. 43–4. Heterotopic transplant that survived 220 days before rejection supervened. The recipient heart shows an extensive, anteroseptal, healed, subendocardial myocardial infarction (arrows). Sutures at anastomotic sites are no longer visible.

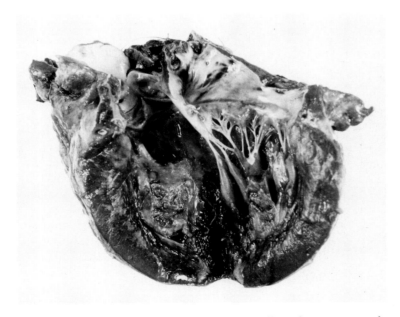

Fig. 43–5. Donor heart of heterotopic transplant removed surgically 81 days post-transplantation because of acute rejection. The left ventricle is thickened, the myocardium appears mottled and hemorrhagic, and the cavity is occupied by mural thrombus. This graft helped the recipient survive an episode of fulminating myocarditis.

post-transplantation onward, occurring later in conjunction with chronic changes. In most cases acute rejection does not occur during the first 2 postoperative weeks. Early chronic rejection may be manifest by 30 days postoperatively. However, this is an arbitrary period, because early intimal vascular thickening, regarded as a manifestation of chronic rejection, was seen after 20 days in one case. Bieber et al. reported a patient in whom this was observed after 9 days.[13]

Microscopic Appearance

The histologic changes of acute rejection are most obvious in the ventricular myocardium and affect both sides equally. In the atria of orthotopic transplants, operative changes overshadow those of rejection.

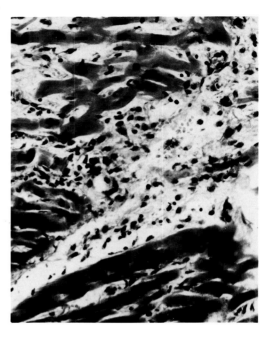

Fig. 43–7. Severe acute rejection. Edema and a moderate infiltrate of small lymphocytes are present in the interstitium. There is occasional loss of myofibers. (H&E, × 300.)

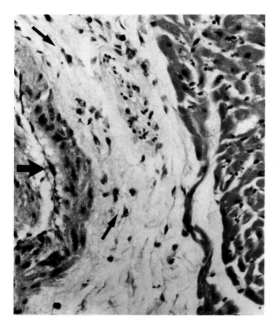

Fig. 43–6. Changes associated with early rejection. There is edema of interstitial connective tissue and swelling of endothelial cells lining a vessel (large arrow). In the perivascular connective tissue Anitschow myocytes are prominent and enlarged (small arrows). (H&E, × 255.)

The earliest histologic manifestation of acute rejection consists of diffuse interstitial edema of the myocardium, which is most obtrusive around intramural vessels (Fig. 43–6).

Interstitial edema is less obvious in patients receiving cyclosporine based immunosuppressive therapy. Others have attributed increased heart weight in patients receiving cyclosporine to edema.[102] Cyclosporine-associated hypertension may also contribute to increased heart weight.

Focal lymphocytic infiltration of varying intensity in the interstitium is the hallmark of acute rejection (Fig. 43–7). In nonimmunosuppressed animals, this infiltrate is intense and occurs within the first week post-transplantation. In humans who are immunosuppressed it is usually of mild to moderate intensity. The infiltrate is also prominent in the edematous subendocardial connective tissue

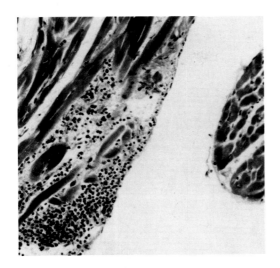

Fig. 43–8. Subendocardial lymphoid infiltrate of mild early acute rejection. (H&E, × 150.)

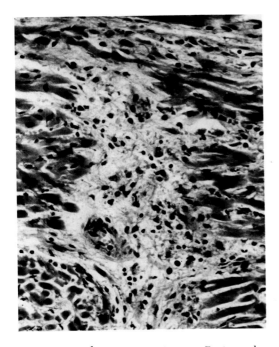

Fig. 43–9. Moderate acute rejection. Perivascular lymphoid infiltrate in which some cells are acquiring the cytoplasm of transformed lymphocytes. Interstitial edema, fibrin exudation, and early myofiber damage are noted. (H&E, × 300.)

and around small blood vessels (Figs. 43–8 and 43–9). Initially, the cellular infiltrate consists of small lymphocytes with little cytoplasm, occasional polymorphonuclear leukocytes, and a few eosinophils. With time, the nuclei of lymphocytes enlarge and acquire nucleoli, and their cytoplasm becomes more abundant and pyroninophilic (see Fig. 43–9); that is, the cells acquire the characteristics of immunoblasts. At the same time, Anitschow myocytes of the interstitium enlarge, acquire more cytoplasm, and appear unusually prominent. The central chromatin bar is a hallmark of these cells (see Fig. 43–6).

Concurrently, myofibers are affected in a patchy manner. Initially they show cytoplasmic swelling followed by vacuolization due to an increase of cytoplasmic lipid (Fig. 43–10). If rejection is mild, no more than this may be seen. If there is an increased intensity of rejection, focal areas of myocytolysis (Fig. 43–11) become evident. Groups of adjacent myofibers may show coagulative necrosis (Fig. 43–12). Muscle cells affected by myocytolysis show a loss of cytoplasm that is replaced by a clear space. The cells disintegrate and disappear, leaving focal areas of stroma devoid of myofibers but containing histiocytes with

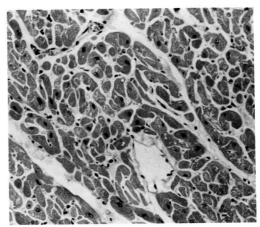

Fig. 43–10. Mild rejection showing vacuolization of myofibers and interstitial edema. (H&E, × 240.)

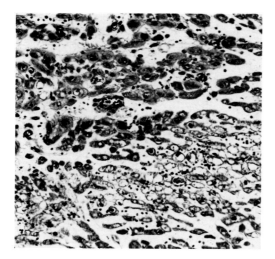

Fig. 43–11. Patchy myocytolysis in acute rejection. Affected fibers show a loss of cytoplasm with only the outlines of cells remaining. Edema and cellular infiltration are also present. (H&E, × 150.)

ingested lipofuscin released by necrotic cells and a variable lymphoid infiltrate. Next, there is collapse of the stromal network with the formation of small, fibrous scars (see Fig. 43–19; see also Ch. 17). In cases with the most severe rejection, areas of microinfarction are present throughout the myocardium (Figs. 43–12 and 43–13) accompanied by interstitial hemorrhage.

The earliest vascular changes consist of swelling of endothelial cells lining capillaries, arterioles, and small arteries with detachment of these cells. They become separated from the underlying media by edema fluid containing scattered mononuclear cells (Fig. 43–6 and Figs. 43–14 through 43–16). Similar cells may infiltrate the media and adventitia to a variable extent (Fig. 43–15). Platelet and fibrin plugs have been described in the lumina of small vessels thus affected,[19] although this was an inconspicuous feature in our cases. There is evidence that rejection may activate the coagulation mechanism.[63] Rejection is also associated with reduced myocardial fibrinolytic activity.[67] In severe acute rejection, observed in animals but seldom in human material, capillaries are disrupted with

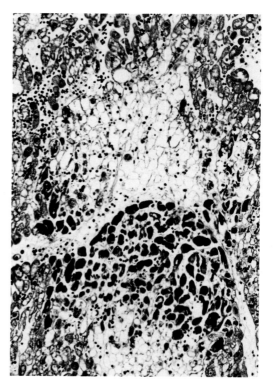

Fig. 43–12. Advanced myocytolysis in acute rejection. Myofibers show a range of appearances varying from early loss of cytoplasm to complete disintegration of cells. Other groups of myofibers show coagulative necrosis (darkly stained cells, lower half). Lymphocytic cellular infiltrate accompanies these changes. Myocyte necrosis is secondary to vascular changes. (H&E, × 150.)

accompanying patchy hemorrhage into the interstitial tissue[23,55] (see Fig. 43–13). More frequently, in severe rejection, the smaller radicals of coronary arteries show fibrinoid necrosis of the media with an exudation of eosinophilic proteinaceous material into the vessel wall (Figs. 43–15 and 43–17). Only in an isolated instance have we observed superadded thrombosis in vessels thus affected. Vessels of this size are usually not included in endomyocardial biopsies. On the whole, venules and veins are spared those changes, and only rarely have we observed venules partially occluded by thrombus (Fig. 43–18).

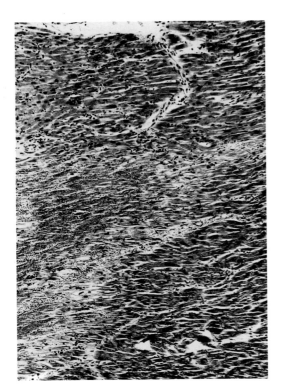

Fig. 43–13. Small infarct of myocardium and interstitial hemorrhage in severe acute rejection. (H&E, × 100.)

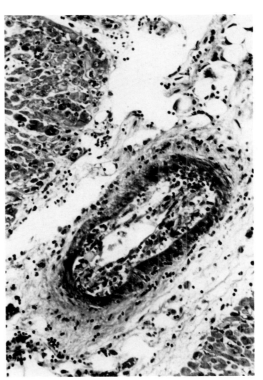

Fig. 43–15. Fibrinoid necrosis of media of a small artery in severe acute rejection. Separation of intimal cells and infiltration of the subintima, media, and adventitia by mononuclear cells. (H&E, × 150.)

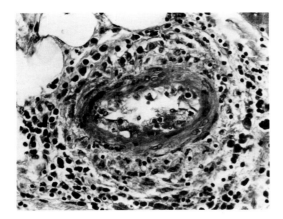

Fig. 43–14. Small arteriole in acute rejection showing swelling of endothelial cells and their separation from the media by edema fluid and mononuclear cells. An intense perivascular lymphoid and plasma cell infiltrate is present. (H&E, × 350.)

Role of Endomyocardial Biopsy in Diagnosis of Cardiac Rejection

Initially (pre-cyclosporine era), the clinical recognition of rejection in a transplanted human heart was based on the appearance of heart failure, a pericardial friction rub, electrocardiographic changes, malaise, a rise in serum lactate dehydrogenase, and the development of a third or fourth heart sound.[78,86] In patients with heterotopic transplants, heart failure due to rejection may be masked by residual function of the recipient's own heart.

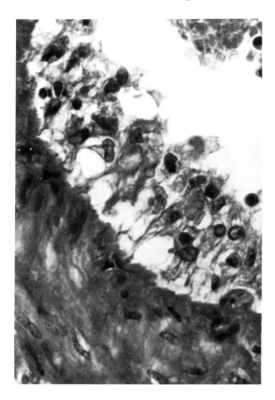

Fig. 43–16. Detachment of intimal lining cells of a coronary artery in acute rejection. Mononuclear inflammatory cells are also present. (H&E, × 600.)

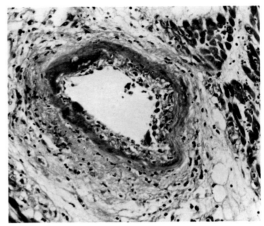

Fig. 43–17. Fibrinoid necrosis of small artery in severe acute rejection. A proteinaceous eosinophilic exudate infiltrates the damaged vessel wall. (H&E, × 200.)

biopsy samples a relatively circumscribed zone of endocardium of the apex and interventricular septum, serial biopsies have a good chance of sampling a previous biopsy site.[34,80,87,90,92,102] A localized lymphocytic response with or without some myocyte necrosis may be evoked around such sites (Fig. 43–

Electrocardiographic changes are not reliable for the early detection of rejection.[78]

The introduction of serial transvenous endomyocardial biopsy of the donor heart by the Stanford group[16,24,67] enabled early detection of cardiac rejection and improved management of rejection episodes.

Although rejection changes may be patchy, there is little chance of missing them if three to five samples are taken per biopsy procedure.[34,87,92,102] In our institution two samples are submitted fresh for frozen section for rapid recognition of severe acute rejection and so that lymphocytic subsets may be determined, if necessary. The other three samples are submitted in glutaraldehyde so that the option of performing electron microscopy is available.

Because right ventricular endomyocardial

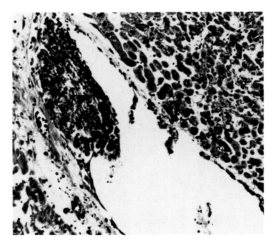

Fig. 43–18. Venule in acute rejection showing detached intimal lining cells and a small mural thrombus. (H&E, × 150.)

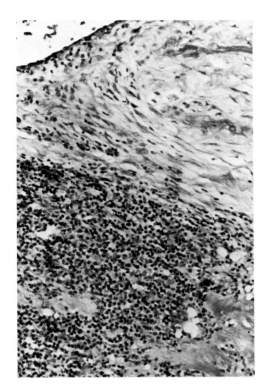

Fig. 43–19. Seven-day-old biopsy site in a baboon heart showing organizing fibrin and a prominent lymphocytic infiltrate (no transplant performed). (H&E, × 150.)

19). Sampling of a biopsy site may lead the unwary to diagnose acute rejection.

At present, donor heart biopsy continues to be the gold standard for the early recognition of acute rejection, despite various attempts to find other means of recognizing cardiac rejection, including radionuclide imaging, intramyocardial electrocardiogram (ECG) recordings, magnetic resonance imaging, antimyosin imaging, measurement of urinary polyamines, and assessment of peripheral blood lymphocytic activation and the levels of soluble interleukin-2 receptors and prolactin.[3,21,22,37,39,43,52,79,95,109,110,112] Indeed, the use of cyclosporine immunosuppression has led to an even greater reliance on biopsy, because the usual clinical signs of

acute rejection described above are less readily observable and only occur in association with severe acute rejection.

It is fortunate that donor heart biopsy is seldom required in the first 10 days after transplantation, because myocardial alterations due to brain death[81,91] (focal necrosis with a mononuclear cellular infiltration) or inadequate myocyte preservation (distal heart procurement) may pose problems for histologic interpretation.

Donor heart infection, for example, due to toxoplasmosis,[93] coccidiodomycosis, cytomegalic inclusion disease, Chagas' disease, or sarcocystis infection, is very rarely encountered. Rupture of pseudocysts of toxoplasmosis evokes a mononuclear inflammatory cellular response that may be confused with acute rejection. The infection has been transmitted by the donor heart in some instances.

In clinical practice the severity of acute rejection must be graded.[14,32,45,74,87,99] No matter what grading system is used, it is essential that there be good communication between the cardiac surgeon and pathologist to prevent misunderstanding and to avoid over- or under-immunosuppression.

In the Cape Town semiquantitative grading system for acute rejection,[32,87] the following five histologic criteria are assessed: (1) interstitial edema; (2) lymphocytic infiltration; (3) pyroninophilia of lymphocytic cytoplasm (Unna Pappenheim stain); (4) myocyte damage; and (5) evidence of vasculitis. Each feature is given a score of 0 to 3 as follows: 0, absent or normal; 1, 0.5 minimal change; mild change; 2, moderate change; and 3, severe change. Thus, each biopsy is given a total score based on the five criteria. Theoretically, the maximum is 15, but in practice one seldom has scores above 7. Interpretation is as follows: 0.5–2.0 denotes mild acute rejection; 2.5–4.0, moderate rejection; and a score greater than 4 indicates severe acute rejection.

The standard immunosuppressive regimen presently used is that based on cyclosporine. Whereas earlier steroid-based immunosuppressive regimens led to effective dissolution

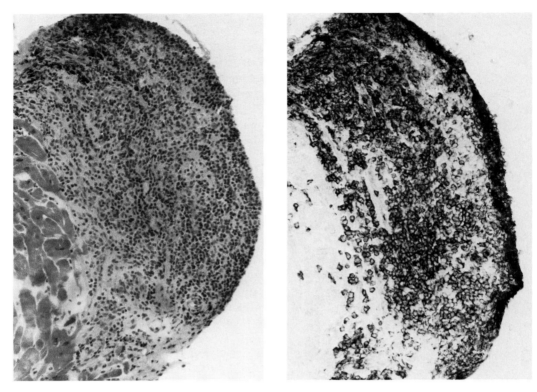

Fig. 43–20. (A) Endocardial lymphocytic aggregation in cyclosporine-treated patient. (B) The cells mark as cytotoxic-suppressor T lymphocytes. (Figs. A & B: Immunoperoxidase, × 150.)

of myocardial lymphocytic infiltrates, cyclosporine achieves its immunosuppressor effect by interfering with the generation of inducer-helper T lymphocytes. Therefore, lymphocyte exudates disappear more slowly. Focal collections of lymphocytes, particularly within the endocardium may be encountered (Fig. 43–20). These isolated groups of lymphocytes appear to be nonactivated and non-pyroninophilic. Their exact significance remains to be determined. The Stanford group calls these collections the "Quilty" effect (see Ch. 39).

Lymphocytic infiltrates that involve the myocardial interstitium, fan out between myocytes, and have lymphocytes closely applied to the surface of the myocytes indicate rejection.[63] Acute rejection is encountered less frequently in patients treated with cy-

closporine; however, once it develops in these patients, severe acute rejection is more difficult to ablate and takes longer to resolve, despite increased immunosuppression.

Myocyte necrosis[14,48] has been rarely observed in our biopsy material, but is a valuable indicator of significant (moderate or severe) acute rejection when present. A recent report[115] compares the reliability for rejection prediction when myocyte necrosis is present or absent. Ratliff et al[85] noted a unique form of reversible myocyte injury (which is similar to apoptosis) associated with acute rejection.

Refractory rejection is diagnosed if repeated biopsies show no reduction in severity of acute rejection despite augmented immunosuppression. Methotrexate has been used in such cases.[31]

Resolving acute rejection[28] can only be diagnosed if serial biopsies are performed after the initial biopsy diagnosis of acute rejection has been made. Features of note include a diminution of the interstitial lymphocytic infiltration, minimal pyroninophilia of the residual lymphocytes, and the presence of iron- and lipofuscin-containing histiocytes. Myocyte loss leads to fibrosis, caused by stromal collapse.

Fine, interstitial, perimyocyte fibrosis, which has been reported from some centers has hardly ever been encountered in our biopsy material. Possible causes include an idiosyncratic effect of cyclosporine (unlikely, as it does not affect the recipient heart in heterotopic transplants), poor donor heart preservation during distal heart procurement, and chronic rejection.

The presence of abundant fibrous tissue in a biopsy sample raises the possibility of chronic rejection[106] (see below), but other sources of fibrous tissue in biopsies may be encountered, for example, tricuspid valvular tissue,[88] sampling of a healed biopsy site, or fibrosed epicardial tissue, if the bioptome penetrates the right ventricular wall. Coronary artery—right ventricular fistulae have also complicated endomyocardial biopsy.[43,65]

Chronic Rejection

Macroscopic Appearance

In chronic rejection, the heart is usually enlarged and the myocardium appears fibrosed. The most striking change occurs in the epicardial branches of coronary arteries. The vessels appear prominent, their thickened walls show yellow lipid deposits, and their lumina are significantly reduced. Indeed, these appearances closely mimic those of diffuse atherosclerosis.[15,104,106] The altered lumen of a coronary artery may be further compromised by a recent, superadded thrombus. The vascular changes may lead to infarction of part of or all the graft. The anastomoses appear well healed. Myocardial scarring is usually most evident in the right ventricle.

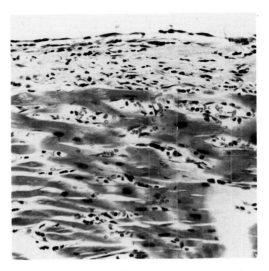

Fig. 43–21. Fibrous thickening of the endocardium (top of picture) in chronic rejection (593 days) accompanied by an infiltrate of lymphoid and plasma cells. (H&E, × 300.)

Microscopic Appearance

Histologically, with the onset of chronicity, many of the changes of acute rejection persist. The interstitial and subendocardial cellular infiltrates are still evident and may even be more obtrusive (Figs. 43–21 and 43–22). The cells, however, consist largely of activated lymphocytes with RNA-rich cytoplasm. Plasma cells are seen. At sites of myocytolysis, the collapsed stroma gives rise to small scars that are scattered throughout the myocardium and may also contain lymphoid infiltrates (see Fig. 43–22).

Vascular changes are prominent in chronic rejection (see Chs. 13 and 39). The main epicardial and medium-sized branches of the coronary arteries show progressive proliferation of intimal cells. This results in a markedly thickened intima composed of collagen and concentric layers of spindle-shaped cells in the early stages (Fig. 43–23). This process narrows the lumen, even to the point of almost complete occlusion (Figs. 43–24 to 43–26). Progressively there is increased collagen and deposition of lipids in the thickened intimal

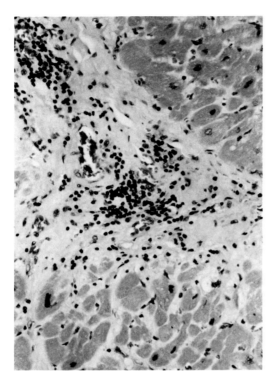

Fig. 43–22. Small myocardial scar of chronic rejection (593 days) infiltrated by activated lymphocytes and plasma cells. These scars may be induced by ischemia or follow myocytolysis with stromal collapse. (H&E, × 300.)

layer. The lipid occurs in smooth muscle cells and macrophages initially (see Fig. 43–27), but is released from them later and deposited in the intima in a free form. The internal elastic lamina may be intact or fragmented; the media shows complete or partial replacement of smooth muscle and elastica by connective tissue.

Cellular infiltration of arteries thus altered varies. In some vessels a lymphoid infiltrate in all layers of the vessel wall may be striking (Fig. 43–26), whereas in others there may be marked fibrous thickening of the intima with almost no cellular infiltrate (Fig. 43–23). Lipid deposition also varies in degree from being barely perceptible to being an obstrusive feature. The fully established vascular lesion, in

which lipid deposition is prominent, closely resembles advanced atherosclerosis (Figs. 43–26 through 43–28). At this stage the occlusive vascular lesions are responsible for ischemia, which contributes to the myocardial fibrosis and scarring observed.

The consensus is that the proliferative vascular changes are the result of previous, possibly repeated, immunologic damage followed by reparative myointimal proliferation.[5,13,53,76,98,115] The smooth muscle cells may be derived from the media[60] or from transformed intimal fibroblasts.[53] Thomson[104] and others[5,60,61] attributed lipid deposition in the thickened intima to sustained immune-related damage and coexistent hypercholesterolemia. However, Bieber et al.[13] state that

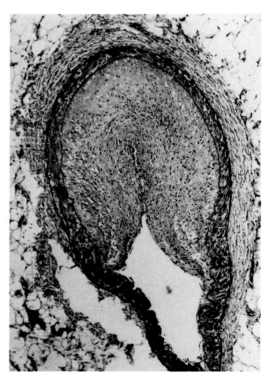

Fig. 43–23. Small coronary artery showing fibrous intimal thickening in chronic rejection, with narrowing of lumen. The spindle cells in the intima are myofibroblasts. No cellular infiltrate accompanies the myointimal proliferation. (H&E, × 60.)

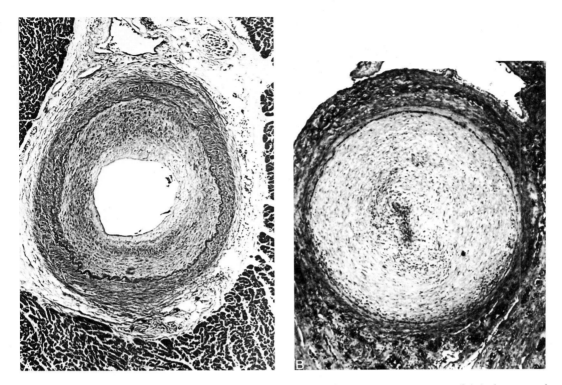

Fig. 43–24. Chronic rejection led to (**A**) partial narrowing of a penetrating artery and (**B**) almost total occlusion of an epicardial coronary artery. (Figs. A & B: H&E, × 60.)

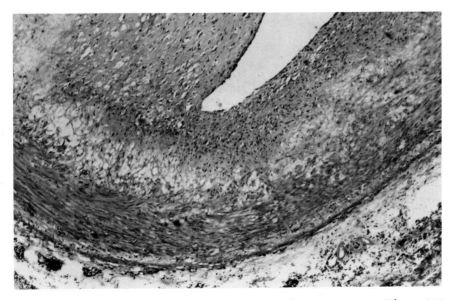

Fig. 43–25. Changes of advanced chronic rejection in epicardial coronary artery. Fibrous intimal thickening encroaching on the lumen is a notable feature. Prominent lipid deposits are present in the intima. The atrophied media shows fibrous replacement. (H&E, × 60.)

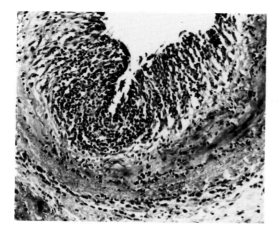

Fig. 43–26. A striking lymphoid cell infiltrate accompanies the myointimal proliferation of chronic rejection. The infiltrate also involves media and adventitia. (H&E, × 150.)

lipid deposition may occur in the absence of hypercholesterolemia. Steroid therapy may be an additional causative factor.[84]

Attempts to prevent vascular changes in chronic rejection have met limited success.[85] Accelerated atherosclerosis of chronic rejection differs from usual atherosclerosis in several ways. First, it develops rapidly and is much more diffuse in the affected coronary arteries. This makes its angiographic recognition more difficult because focal stenoses are not a usual feature. Then, calcification is rarely observed in the atherosclerosis of chronic rejection.[115] Also, the penetrating branches of epicardial coronary arteries, which are unaffected by ordinary atherosclerosis, develop more intimal thickening in chronic rejection, but lipid deposits are usually absent in these

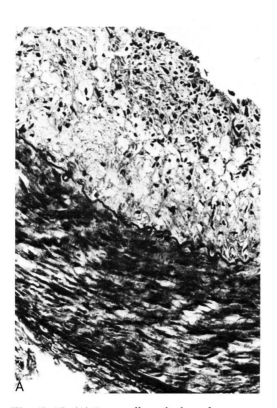

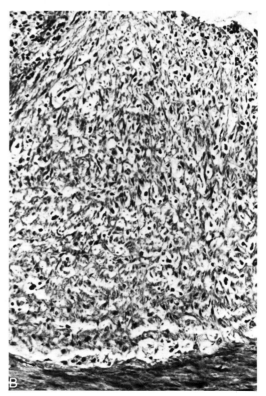

Fig. 43–27. (A) Foam cells in thickened coronary arterial intima in chronic rejection. **(B)** More advanced lesions in another coronary artery. (Both elastic van Gieson; Fig. A: × 150; Fig. B: × 60.)

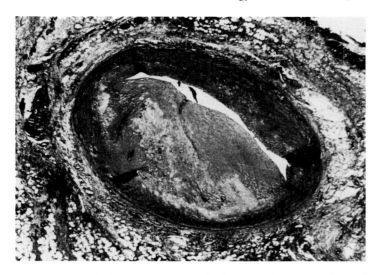

Fig. 43–28. Changes of advanced chronic rejection, which resemble severe atherosclerosis, in an epicardial coronary artery. They severely compromise the vascular lumen and occurred within 81 days in this heart from a donor aged 25 years. (H&E, × 14.)

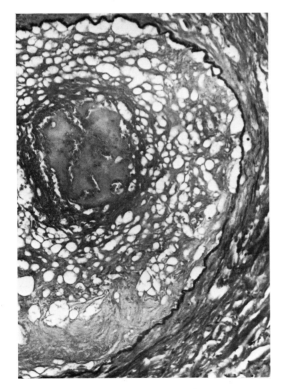

Fig. 43–29. A thrombus occludes the lumen of a coronary artery that is greatly narrowed as a result of chronic rejection. (Elastic van Gieson, × 60.)

vessels. Finally, occasional coronary arteries in accelerated atherosclerosis of chronic rejection show evidence of a previous, healed, necrotizing vasculitis as indicated by fibrous replacement of segments of the media and internal elastic lamina. Thrombosis (Fig. 43–29) may affect the narrowed arteries.

The degree of vascular occlusion and myocardial fibrosis (Fig. 43–30) in chronic rejection appears to bear no relationship to the severity or frequency of previous acute rejection episodes, or to the duration a graft has been in situ. In our patients these occlusive lesions took from 1.1 to 12.5 years to evolve. Not all arteries in the donor heart show accelerated atherosclerosis, which is surprising given the suspected immunologic etiology, in which humoral rejection is believed to be an important factor.

As in all conditions in which immune complexes are formed, a close relationship exists between the immunologically stimulated cascade of the complement enzymes and the clotting system.[63] In this type of immune response, the inflammatory process and the release of chemical mediators are followed by platelet aggregation and clotting, and the ef-

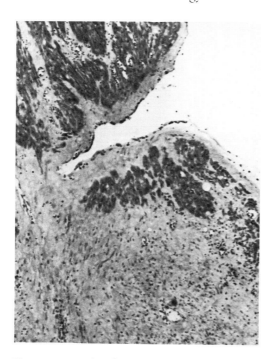

Fig. 43–30. Subendocardial myocyte survival in fibrosed right ventricle of chronic rejection. (H&E, × 20.)

fects of this are made worse by reduced fibrinolytic activity in the graft.[67] This justifies current attempts to use anticoagulant therapy and antiplatelet agents as an adjunct to immunosuppressive therapy. The Stanford group (results quoted by Rappaport, Converse, and Billingham[84]) tried to lower the incidence of graft coronary atherosclerosis by the prophylactic use of antithrombotic agents combined with weight reduction in their transplant patients. Differences were observed, in coronary angiograms done annually, between patients who were not receiving the regimen and those given prophylactic therapy. Their experience suggests that immune injury to the intima of coronary arteries may lead to fibrin and platelet microthrombi, followed by proliferative repair.

Other cardiac structures show little change. Epicardial fibrosis is evident in all cases, prob-

ably the end result of the operative trauma. The aorta and pulmonary arteries are little altered. No cellular infiltrate occurs in these vessels, but in long-term survivors a loss of smooth muscle fibers is observed in the media. The valves generally appear normal, except in isolated cases where the mitral leaflets, at the line of contact, show a focal lymphoid infiltrate and incipient platelet thrombus formation.

Endomyocardial biopsy is less useful in diagnosing chronic rejection compared with acute rejection, and chronic rejection is usually only diagnosed at autopsy. Chronic rejection may be diagnosed during life if a biopsy shows either severe myocyte injury that is out of proportion to the intensity of the inflammatory cell infiltrate[57] or if there are apparently normal (surviving subendocardial) myocytes in the presence of a very poorly functional graft.[87]

Immunofluorescence

Few immunofluorescent studies on transplanted hearts are reported in the literature, and in these the demonstration of immunoglobulins is inconsistent and disappointing, even in the face of severe rejection morphologically. Bieber et al.,[13] on the basis of immunofluorescence, concluded that in early rejection the role of antibodies was uncertain.[13] At this stage, immunoglobulin G (IgG) was demonstrable only within the cytoplasm of invading mononuclear cells, but when acute rejection was well developed IgG and βIC were found in the perivascular connective tissue of arterioles and arteries, within the media of larger coronary arteries, and focally within myocardial fibers. Intimal deposition of immunoglobulin was rarely seen. Deposition of IgG in vascular media was nearly always associated with severe degeneration or necrosis of these structures. In patients dying from severe chronic rejection injury, deposition of IgG and βIC was usually quantitatively less than that seen in severe acute rejection, or was absent entirely. In all their cases bar one, circulating antibodies could not be detected in the patient's serum. The one case with circulating antibodies cytotoxic to donor lymphocytes showed muscle necrosis of the media of the coronary arteries.

Sinclair et al.[99] examined vessels in heterotopic rat allografts. In some vessels showing fibrinoid necrosis complement (C3), IgG, and α globulin deposition could be demonstrated. Others showed cellular infiltration but did not reveal immune deposits. Weil et al.[113] transplanted mouse hearts heterotopically into rats; while an immediate rejection response was observed, there was no consistent deposition of IgG or C3 and only later was the deposition of these immunoglobulins more prominent.

In our series of 6 cases in which the immunoglobulins IgG, IgM, IgA, and C3 were looked for by fluorescence, none was demonstrated in the donor hearts of 5 cases at autopsy. Histologically, 1 showed severe rejection, 2 mild rejection, and 2 no rejection. In the one surgically removed heart that showed severe rejection, moderate amounts of complement (C3) and fibrinogen were demonstrated within the walls of the affected vessels.

The number of T lymphocytes[37,95] within grafts increases when acute rejection develops. The ratio of helper to suppressor T lymphocytes does not correlate with rejection. Few B lymphocytes are encountered in endomyocardial biopsies. Macrophages are evident in resolving acute rejection.

Ultrastructural Changes

Detailed descriptions of the ultrastructural changes observed in dogs have been given by Kosek et al. in acute and chronic rejection, in both immunosuppressed and nonimmunosuppressed animals.[53–55] In human transplants there are a few descriptions of ultrastructure by Levinsky et al.,[64] Kosek et al.,[53] and Uys et al.[107,108]

Experimental studies are valuable in that they give a picture of the early changes in nonimmunosuppressed animals, and these, of course, are not available from human studies. In vessels the changes consist of enlargement of endothelial cells resulting in a severe reduction in lumen size. The cells show hypertrophy of Golgi apparatus, an increase of ribosomes and granular endoplasmic reticulum, large numbers of pinocytic vesicles, and occasional dense bodies.[53] Later, this is followed by intraluminal rupture of endothelial cells with loss of organelles from the cells. Microthrombi of fibrin, platelets, red blood cells, and mononuclear cells become attached to the exposed internal elastic lamina. Medial smooth muscle cells show enlargement with hypertrophy of Golgi apparatus, prominence of granular endoplasmic reticulum, increased numbers of mitochondria and blebs, cytoplasmic lipid droplets, cytosegresomes, myelin figures, and frequent dense bodies. Smooth endoplasmic reticulum is dilated and forms vacuoles. Scattered myocytes show complete disintegration.[54]

The myocytes show dilation of the transverse tubular system and the cisternae of smooth endoplasmic reticulum. Lipid droplets are common. Nuclei show little change initially, but later there is margination of chromatin and excessive convolution. Mitochondria are generally normal, but in advanced lesions there is swelling, myelin figure formation, and focal mineralization progressing to complete opacification of organelles by deposits of iron and/or calcium salts. Dissolution of plasma membranes, fragmentation of myocytes, and phagocytosis by infiltrating monocytes are readily demonstrable in severe lesions.[55] Ratliff et al.[85] observed reversible myocyte injury in acute rejection. It was characterized by radially arranged myofilaments.

The presence of contraction bands in autopsy material is a reliable indication of myofiber damage before death. Their presence in a biopsy does not have the same significance because the biopsy procedure may induce this change, however, the presence of large num-

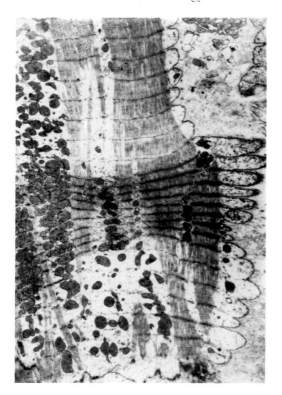

Fig. 43–31. Contraction bands are shown in a myofiber in this electron micrograph. Blebs that occur deep to the plasma membrane are accentuated by the contraction bands. Loss of myofilaments is also present. (Uranyl acetate and lead citrate, × 3,500.)

bers of contraction bands, especially away from the edge of the biopsy, may indicate some myocyte damage.

In our biopsy material myofilaments showed striking alterations. Contraction bands (probably artifactual) were noted in some myofibers (Fig. 43–31), but loss of myofilaments to varying degrees was most constantly present (Fig. 43–32). In these fibers the Z-bands lay free within the cytoplasm of the cell and had no attached myofilaments (Figs 43–31 through 33). Levinsky et al.[64] also comment on this manifestation. In addition, the Z-band may have a smudgy, ill defined appearance. With severe involvement, complete disintegration of myofibers occurred

with disruption of the intercalated discs (Fig. 43–33). Generally, mitochondria were slightly swollen and sometimes contained small, spherical electron-dense granules (Fig. 43–34), whereas in autopsy material these granules were present in almost every case. The transverse tubular system was often dilated. The fibers contained abundant glycogen, and cytoplastic lipid vacuoles were prominent. The number of lipofuscin granules were not significantly altered (see Figs. 43–32 and 34). The myofiber changes described above were not regarded as being specific for rejection as any cause of acute cellular damage may evoke them. For example, they may be caused by toxemia due to septicemia, which indeed was present in many of our cases. Again, anoxia,

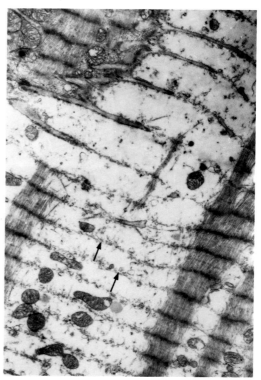

Fig. 43–32. A cell from which there is a general loss of myofilaments. The Z-bands (arrows) have a smudged appearance and appear to lie free in the cytoplasm. (Uranyl acetate and lead citrate, × 6,000.)

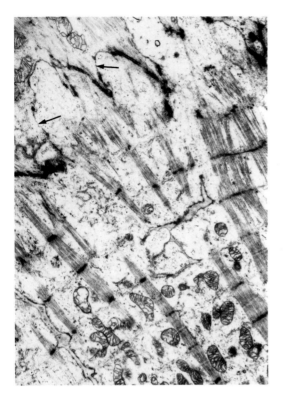

Fig. 43–33. This fiber shows loss of myofilaments, dilation of the transverse tubular system, and disruption of the intercalated disc (arrows). (Acute rejection, × 6,000.)

on an ischemic or central basis will induce the same changes,[54] and, in rejection, this may well be the mediating factor. The intramitochondrial dense bodies observed in some cases may also be the result of nonspecific cellular damage, as they have been described in early cardiac ischemia.[35]

The vascular changes were similar to those outlined in animal models. Small capillaries and arterioles sometimes showed necrosis of endothelial lining cells. More often there was swelling of endothelial cells due to acquisition of cytoplasm and their nuclei appeared excessively crenated. These enlarged endothelial cells significantly reduced capillary lumen size (Figs. 43–35 and 43–36). However, no platelet-fibrin aggregates were demonstrated in the capillary lumina. As in light microscopy

the interstitial infiltrate consisted of lymphocytes, activated lymphocytes, histocytes, and occasional plasma cells (Fig. 43–37).

Hyperacute Rejection

Knowledge of hyperacute rejection is mainly derived from experimental transplantation using noninbred models, particularly the dog.[23,59] This accelerated form of rejection is especially seen in a xenograft (formerly known as heterograft)–that is, a graft between members of different species. A donor heart from a different species has occasionally been used in humans as a desperate attempt to save the life of a patient when no human donor was available.[11,49] However, despite massive immunosuppressive therapy, rejection will cause xenograft destruction within 4 days.[11] The procedure is of use only when there is evidence that the patient's own heart function will recover or the possibility exists of obtaining a replacement human donor heart. Widespread platelet aggregations throughout the vasculature by 1 minute is the initial morphologic event in hyperacute cardiac allograft rejection.[42] At this early stage little endothelial damage is obvious, suggesting that platelet aggregation is triggered by an immunologic mechanism. Widespread endothelial cell damage rapidly follows. The mechanism for this damage is unknown; it may be mediated by lysosomal enzymes released from degranulating platelets,[103] or from the direct action of complement fixed to cell-bound antibody. Capillary destruction leads to extensive fresh interstitial hemorrhage. Other features noted include intravascular fibrin deposition, capillary rupture, interstitial edema, neutrophil margination and emigration, and ischemic myocardial damage.

We had the opportunity to examine two cardiac xenografts transplanted into human patients. The first was that of a chacma baboon (*Papio ursinus*).[11] This graft functioned 6 hours before fibrillating. By light microscopy there was no evidence of a classical hyperacute

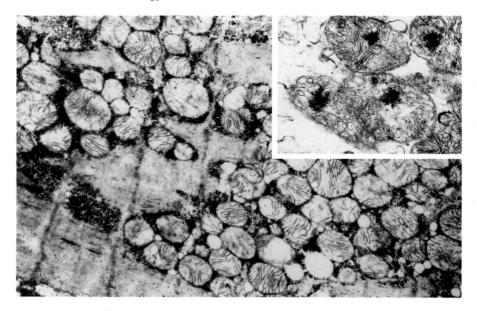

Fig. 43–34. Swollen mitochondria and prominent intracytoplasmic glycogen. ($\times$ 6,000.) **(Inset)** Electron-dense intramitochondrial granules. (Uranyl acetate and lead citrate, $\times$ 12,000.)

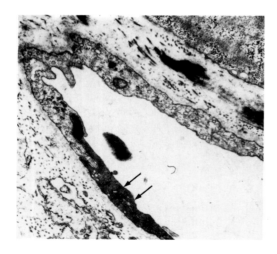

Fig. 43–35. Capillary lined partly by necrotic endothelium (arrows) and partly by viable endothelium. (Acute rejection, $\times$ 10,000.)

rejection. Ultrastructurally, capillaries showed loss of endothelial cells and their lumens contained cell debris and occasional basophils. The other xenograft was the heart of a chimpanzee (*Pan troglodytes*) that functioned for 3 days. This graft showed intracapillary platelet aggregates, endothelial cell damage, and interstitial edema and hemorrhage. Foci of myofiber degeneration were seen in relationship to groups of lymphocytes and immunoblasts.

Recent work from our laboratories provides new pathologic data regarding hyperacute rejection in a number of experimental animals.[89] Immunosuppression, which greatly delayed the onset of hyperacute rejection, led, ultimately, to a mixed picture of both acute and hyperacute rejection in concordant xenografts. Immunosuppression was less effective in prolonging concordant xenograft survival and had no effect on discordant xenograft survival.

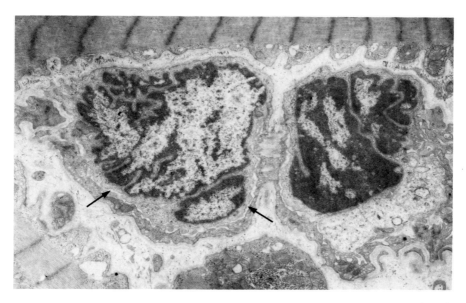

Fig. 43–36. Capillary lined by swollen endothelial cell that has an excessively crenated nucleus. The lumen (arrows) is virtually obliterated by the swollen cell. (Acute rejection, × 7,000.)

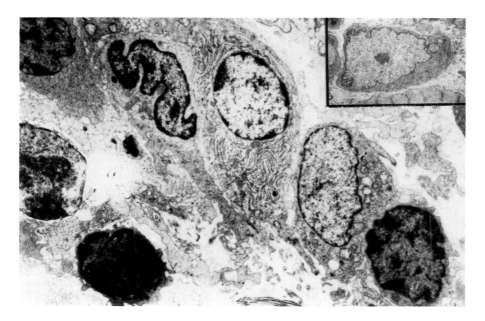

Fig. 43–37. The cellular infiltrate of the perivascular interstitial tissues includes lymphocytes, plasma cells, and histiocytes. (Acute rejection, × 2,500.) **(Inset)** Transformed lymphocyte may be a prominent component of the infiltrate in acute rejection. (Uranyl acetate and lead citrate, × 3,500.)

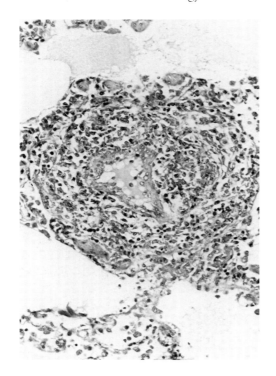

Fig. 43–38. Mild acute pulmonary rejection with perivascular lymphocytic infiltration. (H&E, × 150.)

HEART-LUNG TRANSPLANTATION

Non-neoplastic end-stage primary pulmonary disease or pulmonary hypertension may be treated by cardiopulmonary transplantation rather than by heterotopic cardiac transplantation. The presence of acute rejection in the transplanted heart and lungs is not always synchronous; pulmonary rejection may occur without cardiac rejection[75] and vice versa. There appears to be a reduced incidence of cardiac rejection if a combined heart-lung transplant has been performed.[96]

Glanville et al.[44] report a low incidence of acute rejection in their heart-lung transplantation patients. However, freedom from acute rejection did not correlate with freedom from obliterative broncholitis or coronary arterial

narrowing. They suggest that endomyocardial biopsy should only be performed for specific indications in long-term management. Transbronchial or open-lung biopsies have been performed in order to diagnose pulmonary rejection, but it is sometimes difficult to distinguish infections (e.g., viral or protozoal) from acute rejection, and the small biopsy may not be representative. Tuberculosis is a problem in Third World populations, and immunosuppression may activate latent infection in the transplanted lungs. We have encountered several cases of infection by cytomegalovirus (CMV) and *Pneumocystis carinii* as well as disseminated subacute tuberculosis in two patients.

Mild acute pulmonary rejection (Fig. 43–38) is characterized by scanty perivascular col-

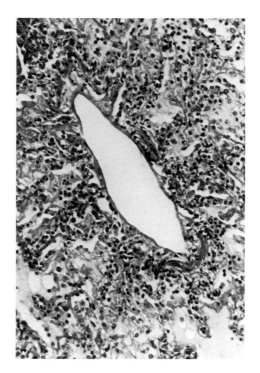

Fig. 43–39. Moderate acute rejection of the lung shows lymphocytic infiltration spreading away from the central blood vessel. (H&E, × 150.)

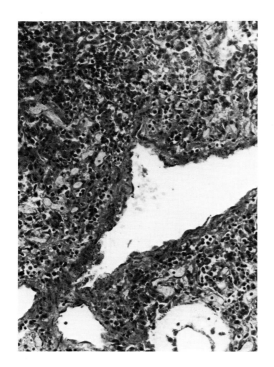

Fig. 43–40. Massive lymphocytic infiltration of the lung in severe chronic rejection. (H&E, × 150.)

lections of lymphocytes. In moderate rejection (Fig. 43–39) the lymphocytes spread to infiltrate many alveolar walls. Severe acute rejection (Fig. 43–40) is characterized by an extensive lymphocytic infiltration of the alveolar walls, accummulation of cells and fibrin within alveoli, as well as evidence of a septal venulitis. Bronchioles show mucosal infiltration by lymphocytes, and broncholitis obliterans is an important feature of chronic pulmonary rejection. Pulmonary arterial changes are usually minimal.

Bronchoalveolar lavage is used to monitor rejection in lung transplants. Rejection produces increased numbers of lymphocytes and macrophages and polymorphonuclear cells in the lavage. Quantitative and qualitative differences separate patients who are well from those with rejection or various types of infection.

GENERAL AUTOPSY FINDINGS

The general autopsy findings in patients bearing heart transplants fall into the groups discussed below.

Pathologic Features of Congestive Cardiac Failure

Pathologic features of cardiac failure will be more evident the shorter the duration of the postoperative period, and also if cardiac failure has again supervened and includes brown induration of the lungs (interstitial fibrosis with iron-laden histiocytes), passive congestion (nutmeg) liver, a congested spleen, and peripheral edema.

Advanced Development of Original Pathology in Heterotopic Transplant

If a heterotopic cardiac transplant has been performed, the recipient heart will show advanced development of the original pathology, far beyond that usually compatible with life. Ischemic heart disease progresses to total occlusion of all three major epicardial coronary arteries with massive replacement fibrosis of the left ventricle. Cardiac function may have ceased months or years before, and the cardiac chambers may contain abundant stasis thrombi. Similarly, dilated cardiomyopathy may advance to massive dilation with abundant stasis thrombi. Recipient hearts with valvular prostheses may show thrombotic obstruction with host tissue overgrowth.

Increased Incidence of Neoplasia in Immunosuppressed Patients

There is an increased incidence of neoplasia, for example, Kaposi's sarcoma (Fig. 43–41), non-Hodgkin's lymphoma (especially of the

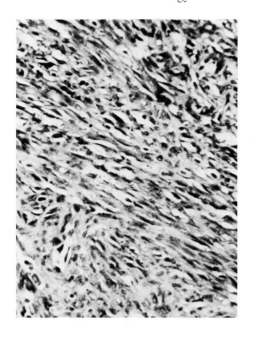

Fig. 43–41. Kaposi's sarcoma in a lymph node biopsy from a heart transplant patient. (H&E, × 150.)

central nervous system),[82] and malignancies of the skin, including squamous and basal cell carcinomas and malignant melanoma, in immunosuppressed patients.[34,58] The reasons for this have not been clearly established. Impaired immune surveillance of mutating cells is a possible cause. Immunosuppression may also reactivate a latent Epstein-Barr virus infection. This virus selectively infects B lymphocytes, and it is a known cause of Burkitt's lymphoma and nasopharyngeal carcinoma. Cyclosporine therapy may lead to reactivation of infection or predispose to a primary Epstein-Barr virus infection by inhibiting the cytotoxic response of T cells to Epstein-Barr virus-infected cells. The Stanford group[34,58] has claimed that patients with cardiomyopathy who undergo transplantation have an increased risk for developing a lymphoma. With increasing survival after heart transplantation there is a greater risk of developing a malignant tumor.[58] Patients who undergo a second

heart transplantation seem to have an even higher incidence of tumors.

The non-Hodgkin's lymphomas that develop in transplant patients are the most common type of malignant tumor encountered in these patients, who tend to be young. Histologically the tumors are large-cell lymphomas of the B-cell type. Clonal analysis, using immunoglobulin-gene arrangement techniques, reveals a uniform clonal rearrangement of immunoglobulin-gene DNA as observed in malignant B-cell lymphomas.[29,30]

Because immunosuppression interferes with rejection of transplanted malignant tumor cells, any patient with extracranial malignant disease cannot be an organ donor. The risk of developing a malignant tumor in the individual transplant patient is relatively low, but the risk appears to increase with time.

Cyclosporine-Induced Infection (Morbidity and Mortality)

Although infection is less of a problem with cyclosporine-azathioprine versus steroid-azathioprine therapy, it still is an important cause of morbidity and mortality in cardiac transplant patients. In some reports it accounts for more than 50 percent of postoperative deaths.[47] Pulmonary infections,[46,86] especially bacterial infections (*Klebsiella*, *Pseudomonas*), as well as infections caused by fungi (Fig. 43–42) (aspergillus and *Nocardia* species), protozoa (Fig. 43–43) (*Toxoplasma gondii* and *Pneumyocytis carinii*), and viruses (cytomegalovirus), have been encountered.[87] *Herpesvirus hominis* infection of the upper gastrointestinal tract was a common concomitant of earlier, steroid-based, regimens. Instances of fatal herpes encephalitis have also occurred. Unusual organisms,[111] for example, the rare fungus *Petriellidium boydii*, which ordinarily is responsible for localized soft tissue mycetomas, may lead to disseminated infection in immunosuppressed persons.

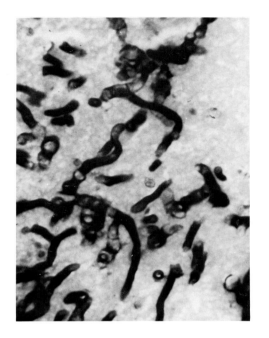

Fig. 43–42. Fungal elements within brain abscess. (Methenamine silver, × 600.)

In developing countries, where pulmonary tuberculosis is common, reactivation of dormant disease may occur. We encountered two heart-lung patients who developed reactivated tuberculous infection in donor lungs with subsequent subacute hematogenous dissemination. Repeated transbronchial biopsies during life were negative, and in both cases the diagnosis of tuberculosis was first made at autopsy.

We have also observed lobar consolidation with a zone of infarction in the lung of a patient with disseminated CMV infection. Although CMV infection usually produces a diffuse pneumonitis (Fig. 43–44) and may coexist with *Pneumocytis carinii* infection, other cases of lobar consolidation have been reported.[98] Muller et al.[77] recommend the use of early aggressive lung biopsy in cardiac transplant patients.

Skin and other tissues may become infected with mycobacteria other than *Mycobacterium tuberculosis*, as well as viruses, for example, *Herpes zoster*, varicella, and vaccinia.

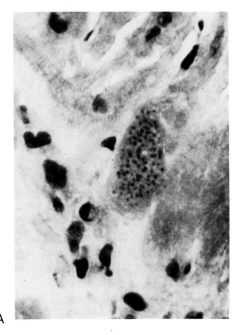
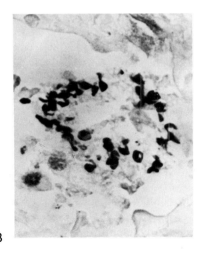

A   B

Fig. 43–43. **(A)** Toxoplasmosis of donor myocardium. (H&E, × 600.) **(B)** *Pneumocystis carinii* infection of the lung. (Methenamine silver, × 600.)

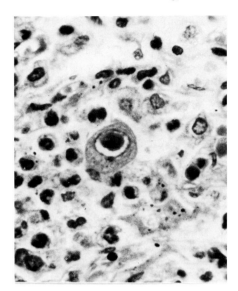

Fig. 43–44. Pneumonitis due to infection with CMV. A typical enlarged pneumocyte containing a prominent intranuclear inclusion is present at the center. (H&E, × 600.)

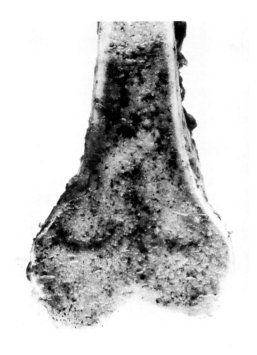

Fig. 43–45. Fat necrosis of the lower femoral bone marrow. (One-half of normal size.)

Morphologic Changes in Drug Therapy

Drug therapy may produce morphologic changes; cyclosporine[18,51] may induce hirsutism, gingival hyperplasia, and, in the kidney, one may observe interstitial nephritis, tubular atrophy, diffuse interstitial fibrosis, and an arteriolopathy, as well as fibrin thrombi within glomerular loops. Mild systemic hypertension is a frequent concomitant condition. Renal transplant patients receiving cyclosporine have heavier hearts than those receiving other immunosuppressive agents.[101]

Corticosteroid therapy may produce Cushing syndrome, a proximal large muscle myopathy, osteoporosis, bone infarcts,[19] fat necrosis in pancreas and bone marrow (Fig. 43–45), posterior subcapsular cataracts of the lens, adrenal gland cortical atrophy, and peptic ulceration.

HEART TRANSPLANTATION IN NEWBORNS AND CHILDREN

Heart transplantation is performed on newborns and children, but the overall experience is small. Bailey and colleagues detail short-term results (1 to 29 months follow-up) in a group of 14 neonates and young children (transplanted on days 79, 86 and 101, respectively) who received heart transplants because of hypoplastic aortic tract complex.[7] Three patients died in the perioperative period, one each of a perforated peptic ulcer, necrotizing pneumonitis, or graft failure not caused by rejection. The remainder were well, normotensive, and had no evidence of renal dysfunction. Rejection had been monitored mainly by noninvasive techniques, none of which alone was entirely reliable for diagnosing rejection. However, in combination and with clinical intuition the tests could be used to support a diagnosis of graft rejection with reasonable confidence. The importance of the transplanted patient being *well* is emphasized with deviation from wellness during the first 6 months of transplantion being highly suspicious of rejection, providing infection and/or drug toxicity could be excluded. Bailey et al. found, as they did in experimental studies, that rejection and infection seemed greatly reduced when transplantation is done early in life (0 to 30 days), but that "immunological privilege" did not extend much beyond 1 month of age. They indicate that cardiac transplantation is effective therapy for selected neonates and young infants with incurable congenital heart disease. However, heart procurement was a problem in dealing with this age group. One notes that the use of hearts from anencephalics is controversial.

Starnes et al.[100] present the Stanford experience in 17 children aged 5 months to 14 years. Transplantation was done most often for cardiomyopathy (13 cases), with congenital heart disease and endocardial fibroelastosis, less frequent indications. The children had been followed 2 months to 7 years with an average of 2.6 years. Of four hospital deaths, two were caused by infection, one by rejection, and one resulted from graft failure. The authors found that rejection occurred as often in these children as it did among adults with heart transplants. They note that the diagnosis of rejection in infants is a controversial matter. Although they monitor a child with serial echocardiograms and adjunctive noninvasive tests and do not biopsy as often as in adults, they advocate use of heart biopsies in diagnosing rejection in this age group. The authors noted an increased morbidity caused by current immunosuppressive therapy in children. They record problems with mildly depressed kidney function, growth retardation in two of five followed more than a year and a tumor in one patient. Graft function was normal with

arterial anastomoses growing without evidence of gradients. Their opinion is that heart transplantation is an effective therapeutic modality in children with end-stage heart disease. Graft atherosclerosis had occurred less frequently in children than in adults, but Starnes and colleagues warn that their observation may reflect an inadequately long follow-up rather than a true difference.

FINAL COMMENT

Cardiac transplantation is firmly established as an acceptable form of treatment for end-stage cardiac disease.[9] Cyclosporine-based immunosuppression has contributed to improved patient survival; thus, a 1-year survival rate of 22 percent for patients receiving transplants in 1968 has an equivalent, in 1989, of a 90 percent survival at 1 year and a 5-year survival of 75 percent. Endomyocardial biopsy maintains its pre-eminence in the diagnosis of acute rejection[41] and the procedure can also be applied in children.[12]

Rejection does not appear to be significantly influenced by a close histocompatibility of the graft, as mismatches have been followed by long survival and vice versa. Recent work suggests that impending acute rejection may be detected by examining the levels of major histocompatibility complex antigens on cardiac biopsies. Chronic rejection has emerged as the major long-term factor limiting successful graft function in patients who do not die from infection. Although retransplantation is feasible[33] and has been performed on many patients, the shortage of donor hearts raises ethical problems as to who should receive the few available donor organs. This problem could be overcome if xenografts could be used in human patients.

Infection, the other hazard to survival, is often pulmonary in location. Although most bacterial infections respond to treatment, disseminated fungal and viral infections are more difficult to control and may prove fatal. *Pneu-*

mocystis carinii pneumonitis responds well to appropriate therapy.

Cardiopulmonary transplantation and use of the artificial heart as a bridge to transplantation has removed several indications for heterotopic cardiac transplantation. The ideal indication for the latter is reversible myocardial disease (e.g., severe viral myocarditis as encountered in one of our patients), but such cases are very rare. Recently, there has been renewed interest in heterotopic cardiac transplantation. This procedure may make possible use of a smaller donor heart. Retransplantation has also sometimes been performed in the heterotopic position—the recipient then has two donor hearts.

REFERENCES

1. Abbott CP, De Witt CW, Creech O: The transplanted rat heart: Histologic and electrocardiographic changes. Transplantation 3:432, 1965

2. Adominian GE, Laks MM, Billingham ME: The incidence and significance of contraction bands in endomyocardial biopsies from normal human hearts. Am Heart J 93:348, 1978

3. Aherne T, Yee ES, Tscholakoff D, et al: Diagnosis of acute and chronic cardiac rejection by magnetic resonance imaging: a non-invasive in-vivo study. J Cardiovasc Surg 29:587, 1988

4. Ahmed-Ansari A, Tadros TS, Knopf WD, et al: Major histocompatibility complex class I and class II expression by myocytes in cardiac biopsies posttransplantation. Transplantation 45:972, 1988

5. Alonso DR, Storek PK, Minick CR: Studies in the pathogenesis of atheroarteriosclerosis induced rabbit cardiac allografts by the synergy of graft rejection and hypercholesterolaemia. Am J Pathol 87:415, 1977

6. Baldwin JC, Oyer PE, Stinson EB, et al: Comparison of cardiac rejection in heart and heart-lung transplantation. J Heart Transplant 6:352, 1987

7. Bailey LL, Assaad AN, Trimm AF, et al: Orthotopic transplantation during early infancy as therapy for incurable congenital heart disease. Ann Surg 208:279, 1988

8. Barnard CN: A human cardiac transplant. S Afr Med J 49:1271, 1967

9. Barnard CN: The present status of heart transplantation. S Afr Med J 49:213, 1975

10. Barnard CN, Losman JG: Left ventricular bypass. S Afr Med J 49:303, 1975

11. Barnard CN, Wolpowitz A, Losman JG: Heterotopic cardiac transplantation with a xenograft for assistance of the left heart in cardiogenic shock after cardiopulmonary bypass. S Afr Med J 52:1035, 1977

12. Bhargava H, Donner RM, Sanchez G, et al: Endomyocardial biopsy after heart transplantation in children. J Heart Transplant 6:298, 1987

13. Bieber CP, Stinson EB, Shumway NE, et al: Cardiac transplantation in man. VII. Cardiac allograft pathology. Circulation 41:753, 1970

14. Billingham ME: Diagnosis of cardiac rejection by endomyocardial biopsy. J Heart Transplant 1:25, 1982

15. Billingham ME: Cardiac transplant atherosclerosis. Transplant Proc 14:19, 1987

16. Billingham ME, Caves PK, Dong E, Shumway NE: The diagnosis of canine orthotopic allograft rejection by transvenous endomyocardial biopsy. Transplant Proc 5:741, 1973

17. Blumenstock DA, Hechtman HB, Collins JA, et al: Prolonged survival of orthotopic homotransplants of the heart in animals treated with methotrexate. J Thorac Cardiovasc Surg 46:616, 1963

18. Borel JF: Cyclosporin-A—Present experimental status. Transplant Proc 13:344, 1981

19. Burton DS, Machizuki RM, Holpern AA: Total hip arthroplasty in cardiac transplant patient. Clin Orthop 130:186, 1978

20. Carrel A, Guthrie CC: The transplantation of veins and organs. Am J Med 11:1101, 1905

21. Carrier M, Russell DH, Davis TP, et al: Urinary polyamines as markers of cardiac allograft rejection. A clinical evaluation. J Thorac Cardiovasc Surg 96:806, 1988

22. Carrier M, Russell DH, Wild JC, et al: Prolactin as a marker of rejection in human heart transplantation. J Heart Transplant 6:290, 1987

23. Caves PK, Dong E, Morris RE, Shumway NE: Hyperacute rejection of orthotopic car-

diac allografts in dogs following solubilized antigen pretreatment. Transplantation 16:2785, 1976

24. Caves PK, Stinson EB, Billingham ME, et al: Diagnosis of human cardiac allograft rejection by serial cardiac biopsy. J Thorac Cardiovasc Surg 66:461, 1973

25. Caves PK, Stinson EB, Billingham ME, Shumway NE: Serial transvenous biopsy of the transplanted human heart: Improved management of acute rejection episodes. Lancet 1:821, 1974

26. Caves PK, Stinson EB, Graham AF, et al: Percutaneous transvenous endomyocardial biopsy. JAMA 225:288, 1973

27. Chiba C, Wolf PL, Gudbjarneson S, et al: Studies in the transplanted heart. J Exp Med 115:853, 1962

28. Chomette G, Auriol M, Delcourt A, et al: Human cardiac transplants. Diagnosis of rejection by endomyocardial biopsy. Causes of death (about 30 autopsies). Virchows Arch [A] 407:295, 1985

29. Cleary ML, Sklar J: Lymphoproliferative disorders in cardiac transplant recipients are multiclonal lymphomas. Lancet 2:489, 1984

30. Cleary ML, Warnke R, Sklar J: Monoclonality of lymphoproliferative lesions in cardiac transplant recipients. N Engl J Med 310:477, 1984

31. Constanzo-Nordin MR, Grusk BB, Silver MA, et al: Reversal of recalcitrant cardiac allograft rejection with methotrexate. Circulation 78(suppl III):47, 1988

32. Cooper DKC, Fraser RC, Rose AG, et al: Technique, complications and clinical value of endomyocardial biopsy in patients with heterotopic heart transplants. Thorax 37:727, 1982

33. Copeland JG, Griepp RB, Bieber CP, et al: Successful retransplantation of the human heart. J Thorac Cardiovasc Surg 73:242, 1977

34. Copeland JG, Stinson JL, Bieber CP, et al: Human heart transplantation. Curr Probl Cardiol 4:1, 1979

35. Csapò Z, Dusek J, Rona G: Early alteration in the cardiac muscle cells in isoproterenol-induced necrosis. Arch Pathol 93:356, 1972

36. Downie HG: Homotransplantation of the dog heart. Arch Surg 66:624, 1953

37. Duquesnoy RJ, Zeevi A, Fung JJ, et al: Sequential infiltration of class I and class II spe-

cific alloreactive T cells in human cardiac allografts. Transplant Proc 19:2560, 1987

38. Ellis B, Madge G, Kolkatkar M, Still W: Clinical and pathological findings in human cardiac rejection. Arch Pathol 92:58, 1971

39. Fieguth HG, Haverich A, Schafers HJ, et al: Cytoimmunologic monitoring in early and late acute cardiac rejection. J Heart Transplant 7:95, 1988

40. Fitchett DH, Forbes C, Guerraty AJ: Repeated endomyocardial biopsy causing coronary arterial-right ventricular fistula after cardiac transplantation. Am J Cardiol 62:829, 1988

41. Foerster A, Simonsen S, Froysaker T: Heart transplantation in Norway. Morphological monitoring of cardiac allograft rejection. A 3-year follow-up. APMIS 96:14, 1988

42. Forbes RDC, Kuramochi T, Guttmann RD, et al: A controlled sequential morphologic study of hyperacute cardiac allograft rejection in the rat. Lab Invest 33:280, 1975

43. Frist W, Yasuda T, Segall G, et al: Non-invasive detection of human cardiac transplant rejection with indium-III antimyosin (Fab) imaging. Circulation 76:V-81, 1987

44. Glanville AR, Imoto E, Baldwin JC, et al: The role of right ventricular endomyocardial biopsy in the long-term management of heart-lung transplant recipients. J Heart Transplant 6:357, 1987

45. Gokel M, Reichart B, Struck E: Human cardiac transplantation—evaluation of morphological changes in serial endomyocardial biopsies. Pathol Res Pract 178:354, 1985

46. Griepp RB, Stinson EB, Bieber CP, et al: Control of graft arteriosclerosis in human heart transplant recipients. Surgery 81:262, 1977

47. Griepp RB, Stinson EG, Bieber CP, et al: Human heart transplantation: Current status. Ann Thorac Surg 22:171, 1976

48. Griffith BP, Hardesty RL, Bahnson HT, et al: Cardiac transplants with cyclosporin-A and low-dose prednisone: histologic graduation of rejection. Transplant Proc 15:1241, 1983

49. Hardy JD, Chavez CM, Kurrus FD, et al: Heart transplantation in man: developmental studies and a report of a case. JAMA 188:1132, 1964

50. Herskowitz A, Soule LM, Mellits ED, et al: Histologic predictors of acute cardiac rejec-

tion in human endomyocardial biopsies: a multivariate analysis. J Am Coll Cardiol 9:802, 1987

51. Keown PA, Essery GL, Stiller CR, et al: Mechanisms of immunosuppression by Cyclosporin. Transplant Proc 13:386, 1981

52. Klanke D, Hammer C, Dirschedyl P, et al: Sensitivity and specificity of cyto-immunological monitoring in correlation with endomyocardial biopsies in heart transplant patients. Transplant Proc 19:3781, 1987

53. Kosek JC, Bieber C, Lower RR: Heart graft arteriosclerosis. Transplant Proc 3:512, 1971

54. Kosek JC, Chartrand C, Hurley EJ, Lower RR: Arteries in canine cardiac homografts. Ultrastructure during acute rejection. Lab Invest 21:328, 1969

55. Kosek JC, Hurley EJ, Lower RR: Histopathology of orthotopic canine cardiac homografts. Lab Invest 19:97, 1968

56. Kosek JC, Hurley EJ, Sewell DH, Lower RR: Histopathology of orthotopic canine cardiac homografts and its clinical correlation. Transplant Proc 1:311, 1969

57. Kottke-Marchant K, Ratliff NB: Diagnosis of humoral (chronic) cardiac transplant rejection by endomyocardial biopsy. XVII International 8th World Congress of Academic and Environmental Pathology, Dublin, Ireland, September 4–9, 1988 (abst)

58. Krikorian JG, Anderson JL, Bieber CP, et al: Malignant neoplasms following cardiac transplantation. JAMA 240:639, 1978

59. Kuwahara O, Kondo Y, Juramochi I, et al: Organ specificity in hyperacute rejection of canine heart and kidney allografts. Ann Surg 180:72, 1977

60. Laden AMK: Experimental atherosclerosis in rat and rabbit cardiac allografts. Arch Pathol 93:240, 1973

61. Laden AMK, Sinclair RA, Ruskiewicz M: Vascular changes in experimental cardiac allografts. Transplant Proc 5:737, 1973

62. Leandri-Cesari J, Crepin Y, Cachera JP: Transplantation cardiaque chez le chien un cas de survie à ans. Nouv Presse Med 41:2785, 1976

63. Lessof M: Immunological reactions in heart disease. Br Heart J 40:211, 1978

64. Levinsky L, Kessler E, Lurie M, et al: Ultrastructural and histopathologic observa-tions of human cardiac transplant with features of rejection. Am J Clin Pathol 53:811, 1970

65. Locke TJ, Furniss SS, McGregor CG: Coronary artery-right ventricular fistula after endomyocardial biopsy. Br Heart J 60:81, 1988

66. Losman JG: Review of the Cape Town experience with heterotopic cardiac transplantation. Cardiovasc Dis Bull Tex Heart Inst 4:243, 1977

67. Losman JG, Rose AG, Barnard CN: Myocardial fibrinolytic activity in allogenic cardiac rejection. Transplantation 23:414, 1977

68. Lower RR, Dong E, Shumway NE: Long-term survival of cardiac homografts. Surgery 58:110, 1965

69. Lower RR, Dong E, Shumway NE: Suppression of rejection process in the cardiac homograft. Ann Thorac Surg 1:645, 1965

70. Lower RR, Kontos HA, Kosek JC, et al: Experiences in heart transplantation. Am J Cardiol 22:766, 1953

71. Lower RR, Stofer RC, Shumway NE: Homovital transplantation of the heart. J Thorac Cardiovasc Surg 41:196, 1961

72. MacSween RNM, Ono K, Thomasan CM: Immunological and histological studies of ectopic heart transplants in the rat. J Pathol 105:49, 1971

73. Mann FC, Priestley JT, Markowitz J, Yater WM: Transplantation of the intact mammalian heart. Arch Surg 26:219, 1933

74. McAllister HA, Schnee MJ, Radovancevic B, Frazier H: A system for grading cardiac allograft rejection. Tex Heart Inst J 13:1, 1986

75. McGregor CG, Baldwin JC, Jamieson SW, et al: Isolated pulmonary rejection after combined heart-lung transplantation. J Thorac Cardiovasc Surg 90:623, 1985

76. Milam JD, Shipkey FH, Lind CJ, et al: Morphological findings in human cardiac allografts. Circulation 41:519, 1970

77. Miller R, Burton NA, Karwande SV, et al: Early, aggressive open lung biopsy in heart transplant recipients. J Heart Transplant 6:96, 1987

78. Nora JJ, Cooley DA, Fernbach DJ, et al: Rejection of the transplanted human heart. Indexes of recognition and problems in prevention. N Engl J Med 280:1079, 1969

79. Novitzky D, Boniaszczuk J, Cooper DKC, et

al: Prediction of acute cardiac rejection using radionuclide techniques. S Afr Med J 65:5, 1984

80. Novitzky D, Rose AG, Cooper DKC, Reichart BA: Histopathologic changes at the site of endomyocardial biopsy: potential for confusion with acute rejection. Heart Transplant 5:79, 1986

81. Novitzky D, Wicomb WN, Cooper DKC, et al: Electrocardiographic and endocrine changes occurring during experimental brain death in the Chacma baboon. Heart Transplant 4:63, 1984

82. Penn I: Tumour incidence in human allograft recipients. Transplant Proc 11:1047, 1979

83. Penn OC, McDicken I, Leicher F, Bos E: Histopathology of rejection in DLA-identical canine orthotopic cardiac allografts. Transplantation 22:313, 1976

84. Rapaport FT, Converse JM, Billingham ME: Recent advances in clinical and experimental transplantation. JAMA 237:2835, 1977

85. Ratliff NB, Myles J, McMahan J, et al: Myocyte injury in acute cardiac transplant rejection and in lymphocytic myocarditis is similar and reversible. Transplant Proc 19:2568, 1987

86. Rider AK, Copeland JG, Hunt SA, et al: The status of cardiac transplantation. Circulation 52:531, 1975

87. Rose AG: Endomyocardial biopsy diagnosis of cardiac rejection. Heart Failure 2:64, 1986

88. Rose AG: Biopsy of tricuspid valve. Society for Cardiovascular Pathology. Core Notes 3:2, 1988

89. Rose AG, Cooper DKC, Human PA, et al: Histopathology of hyperacute rejection of the heart: Experimental and clinical observations in allografts and xenografts. Heart Transplant. In press

90. Rose AG, Novitzky D, Cooper DKC: Endomyocardial biopsy site morphology. An experimental study in baboons. Arch Pathol Lab Med 110:622, 1986

91. Rose AG, Novitzky D, Factor SM: Catecholamine-associated smooth muscle contraction bands in the media of coronary arteries of brain dead baboons. Am J Cardiovasc Pathol 2:63, 1988

92. Rose AG, Uys CJ, Losman JG, Barnard CN: Evaluation of endomyocardial biopsy in the diagnosis of cardiac rejection: A study using bioptome samples of formalin-fixed tissue. Transplantation 26:10, 1978

93. Rose AG, Uys CJ, Losman JG, Barnard CN: Morphological changes in 49 Chacma baboon cardiac allografts. S Afr Med J 56:880, 1979

94. Rose AG, Uys CJ, Novitzky D, et al: Toxoplasmosis of donor and recipient hearts after heterotopic cardiac transplantation. Arch Pathol Lab Med 107:368, 1983

95. Rose ML, Gracie JA, Fraser A, et al: Use of monoclonal antibodies to quantitate T lymphocyte subpopulations in human cardiac allografts. Transplant 38:230, 1984

96. Rowlands DT, Vanderbeek RB, Seigler HF, Ebert PA: Rejection of canine cardiac allografts. Am J Pathol 53:617, 1968

97. Schulman LL: Cytomegalovirus pneumonitis and lobar consolidation. Chest 91:558, 1987

98. Sinclair RA, Andres GA, Hsu KC: Immunofluorescent studies of the arterial lesion in rat cardiac allografts. Arch Pathol 94:331, 1972

99. Spiegelhalter DJ, Stovin PG: An analysis of repeated biopsies following cardiac transplantation. Statistics Med 2:23, 1983

100. Starnes VA, Bernstein D, Oyer PE, et al: Heart transplantation in children. J Heart Transplant 8:1, 1989

101. Stovin PG, English TA: Effects of cyclosporine on the transplanted human heart. J Heart Transplant 6:180, 1987

102. Thomas FJ, Lower RR: Heart transplantation—1978. Surg Clin N Am 58:335, 1978

103. Thomson JG: Heart transplantation in man—necropsy findings. Br Med J 2:511, 1968

104. Thomson JG: Production of severe atheroma in a transplanted human heart. Lancet 2:1088, 1969

105. Tilney NL, Bell PRF, MacSween RNM: Morphological changes in indefinitely surviving enhanced ectopic cardiac allografts. J Pathol 119:29, 1976

106. Uys CJ, Rose AG: Pathologic findings in long-term cardiac transplants. Arch Pathol Lab Med 108:112, 1984

107. Uys CJ, Rose AG, Barnard CN: The autopsy findings in a case of heterotopic cardiac transplantation with left ventricular bypass for ischaemic heart failure. S Afr Med J 49:2029, 1975

108. Uys CJ, Rose AG, Barnard CN: The pathology of human cardiac transplantation. An assessment after 11 years' experience at Groote Schuur Hospital, Cape Town. S Afr Med J 56:887, 1979

109. Valantine HA, Fowler MB, Hunt SA, et al: Changes in Doppler echocardiographic indexes of left ventricular function as potential markers of acute cardiac rejection. Circulation 76:V-86, 1987

110. Wahlers T, Haverich A, Busselberg C, et al: Electrocardiographic parameters in allograft rejection after orthotopic cardiac transplantation. Transplant Proc 190:3784, 1987

111. Walker DH, Adamec T, Krigman M: Disseminated petriellidosis. Arch Pathol Lab Med 102:158, 1978

112. Warnecke H, Schuler S, Goetze HJ, et al: Non-invasive monitoring of cardiac allograft rejection by intramyocardial electrocardiogram recordings. Circulation 74:III–72, 1986

113. Weil R, Nozawa M, Weber C, et al: Cardiac heterotransplantation: Morphological and immunohistological studies. Transplantation 19:1950, 1975

114. Wesolowski SA, Fennessey JF: Pattern of failure of the homografted canine heart. Circulation 8:750, 1953

115. Zerbe TR, Arena V: Diagnostic reliability of endomyocardial biopsy for assessment of cardiac allograft rejection. Hum Pathol 19:1307, 1988

44

Pathology of New Cardiovascular Interventional Procedures

Bruce F. Waller

The past 10 years have seen the development and continuing evolution of various devices and techniques used to treat patients with cardiac disease. Experimental and clinical results have stimulated interest in the pathologic changes produced by these procedures. As their use becomes widespread, many pathologists are asked to evaluate the tissue consequences. This chapter summarizes certain morphologic-histologic changes resulting from the experimental and/or clinical use of 11 new therapeutic interventions: (1) coronary artery and aortocoronary saphenous vein graft balloon angioplasty, (2) thrombolytic therapy for evolving acute myocardial infarction, (3) arterial stents, (4) atherectomy, (5) laser irradiation, (6) balloon pyroplasty, (7) ventricular endocardial resection and catheter oblation of sites causing chronic life-threatening ventricular arrhythmias, (8) automatic implantable cardioverter-defibrillators, (9) temporary left and right ventricular assist devices, (10) catheter balloon valvuloplasty of stenotic cardiac valves, and (11) the total artificial heart.

PERCUTANEOUS TRANSLUMINAL BALLOON ANGIOPLASTY

Several reports of percutaneous transluminal balloon angioplasty have demonstrated its clinical usefulness as a nonsurgical treatment of chronically and acutely obstructed coronary arteries and aortocoronary saphenous vein bypass grafts.

Atherosclerotic Coronary Arteries

Since its introduction in 1977,[85] coronary balloon angioplasty has gained wide acceptance as a nonsurgical therapy for acutely and chronically obstructed coronary arteries. Increased experience and advances in technology have increased primary success rate (90 to 95 percent) and lowered complication rate (4 to 5 percent).[10] Despite this, the precise mechanism(s) by which balloon angioplasty improves vessel patency remains unsettled. Morphologic and histologic observations in coronary arteries of patients undergoing percutaneous transluminal balloon angioplasty are limited,[9,26,39,66,128,168,201,231,243,246,249,250,253,257,258,260] but provide clues regarding the mechanism of action. These observations may be divided into (1) changes observed early (acute) (up to 30 days) after balloon angioplasty, and (2) changes observed late (chronic) (more than 30 days) after balloon angioplasty.

Early (Acute) Changes

Morphologic changes in coronary arteries dilated within 30 days of tissue examination have been reported by several investigators.[9,26,39,128,168,201,231,243,246,249,250,253,257,260]

Block and colleagues[26] initially reported atherosclerotic plaque "splitting" in two patients. In one patient, an extension of plaque "splitting" into the coronary media resulted in a dissecting hematoma. Waller and colleagues[246,250] subsequently reported morphologic and histologic observations in several patients who had undergone angioplasty procedures 4 hours to 30 days before tissue examination (Figs. 44–1 to 44–3). At each site, an intimal "crack," "tear," "fracture," or "break" was recognized, each having variable degrees of medial penetration. In some patients, medial involvement was localized (barely penetrating the internal elastic membrane); in others, it was extensive (dissection antegrade, retrograde, or both) (Figs. 44–1 and 44–3B). Adventitial disruption was not observed. Waller and colleagues[260] reported 9 additional autopsy subjects who had undergone transluminal balloon angioplasty procedures alone or in conjunction with a thrombolytic agent to treat an evolving acute myocardial infarction. Each showed intimal-medial tears but 4, with combined thrombolytic reperfusion and balloon angioplasty, had associated coronary wall and luminal hemorrhage. Colavita and colleagues[39] described coronary angioplasty findings at necropsy in

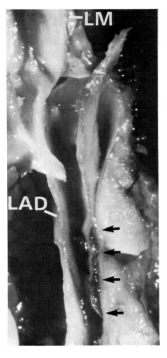

Fig. 44–1. Localized coronary artery dissection (arrows) at site of transluminal balloon angioplasty in the left descending coronary (LAD) artery. LM, left main coronary artery. (From Waller,[243] with permission.)

four patients undergoing dilation during acute myocardial infarction. Intimal hemorrhage and plaque disruption were found in all 4 cases but, in contrast to others, these investigators did not observe coronary artery medial dissection. Saffitz and colleagues[201] had a single patient in whom coronary artery rupture had developed during balloon angioplasty. Histologic observations at the site disclosed an eccentric, heavily calcified, plaque with rupture of the disease-free wall.

Mizuno and colleagues[168] serially sectioned the balloon angioplasty site in one autopsied subject and observed intimal and medial splitting that led to coronary artery dissection (Fig. 44–4). Soward and associates[231] noted plaque splitting, medial dissection, and "lifting" of the atherosclerotic plaque from the medial layer at the site of previous balloon angioplasty

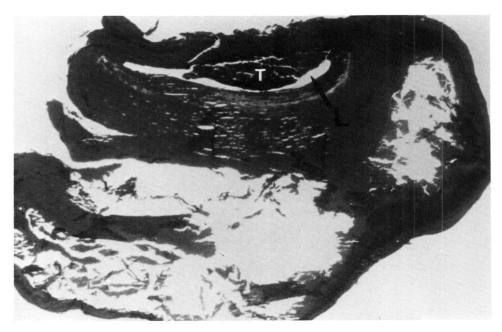

Fig. 44–2. Histologic section of an endarterectomy specimen from the area of an attempted transluminal balloon angioplasty showing severe plaque hemorrhage and thombus (T) in an already severely narrowed lumen (L). (van Gieson, × 28.) (From Waller,[243] with permission.)

(Fig. 44–5). La Delia and colleagues[128] reported histologic findings in the left anterior descending coronary artery of a patient receiving angioplasty and streptokinase for an evolving acute myocardial infarction. Atherosclerotic plaque "cleavage," subintimal leukocytic infiltrations, and medial and adventitial fractures with hemorrhage were observed (Fig. 44–6).

Late (Chronic) Changes

While little morphologic information is available concerning early changes in the coronary arteries of patients undergoing balloon angioplasty, even less is available about late changes.[9,66,243,253,257,258] To date, those observed in human coronary arteries may be divided into two categories: (1) no morphologic evidence of previous angioplasty injury (Figs. 44–7 to 44–9) and (2) intimal fibrous proliferation (Figs. 44–15 to 44–19).

No Morphologic Evidence of Previous Balloon Angioplasty Injury

Waller and colleagues[243,253,257] reported morphologic-histologic changes at the site of angioplasty in three patients in whom sudden death had occurred 80, 90, and 150 days (Figs. 44–7, 44–8, and 44–9, respectively) after clinically successful coronary angioplasty. In each of three men, the left anterior descending coronary artery had an increased angiographic luminal diameter and decreased transtenotic pressure gradient, and the patient achieved relief of angina pectoris and improved exercise tolerance. Of two clinically asymptomatic patients, one died suddenly at home (sudden coronary death), and the other was killed in an automobile accident while intoxicated with alcohol (noncardiac cause of death). The symptomatic patient died suddenly at work (sudden coronary death). At autopsy, the site of balloon angioplasty in the left anterior descending cor-

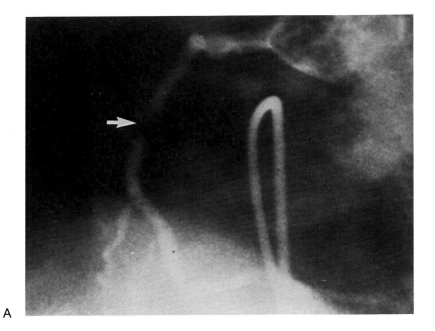

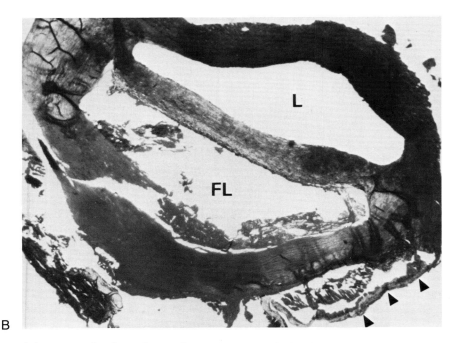

Fig. 44–3. (**A**) Angiographic frame from right coronary artery before balloon angioplasty. Arrow indicates site of dilation. (**B**) Histologic section of endarterectomy specimen at the site of angioplasty showing coronary dissection with an intimal flap separating true (L) and false lumen (FL). Extensive hemorrhage is present in the outer wall of the FL (arrowheads). (van Gieson, × 28.) (From Waller,[243] with permission.)

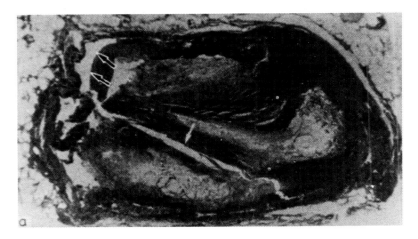

Fig. 44–4. Histologic appearance at the site of dilation of a left anterior descending artery showing intimal and medial splitting, which led to medial dissection (black arrows) and plaque fracture (white arrow). (From Mizuno et al.,[168] with permission.)

onary artery in each patient was narrowed 76 to 95 percent in cross-sectional area by fibrous atherosclerotic plaques. Each balloon angioplasty site was free of intraluminal thrombus and mural hemorrhage. Histologic assessment of atherosclerotic plaques in the areas of previous angioplasty compared with other areas of atherosclerotic plaque in the same artery or other arteries in the same patient disclosed no distinct morphologic differences. No distinctive acute morphologic lesions or healed modifications of the plaques were recognized in these patients.

In view of clinical evidence of successful angioplasty, the morphologic findings suggest recoil of overstretched concentric and eccentric lesions may have resulted in later restenosis. The absence of morphologic signs of healed angioplasty in the presence of severe atherosclerotic plaque should not be interpreted as indicating acceleration of underlying atherosclerotic plaque within a mere 80, 90, or 150 days.

Intimal Fibrous Proliferation

Essed and colleagues[66] were the first to report intimal fibrous hyperplasia at the site of coronary angioplasty, 5 months after dilation.

Cross sections of the left anterior descending coronary artery showed evidence of previous disruption of the media with extensive proximal and distal coronary dissection. A large intimal crack with partial flap formation created a false channel. After 5 months, the fibrocellular proliferation coated surrounding portions of atherosclerotic plaque in and at the area of previous plaque fracture producing a severely narrowed coronary artery (Fig. 44–10). Austin and colleagues[9] reported a late angioplasty site that appeared to have distinct intimal layers: an outer layer composed of hypocellular connective tissue with cholesterol clefts (atherosclerotic plaque), and an inner layer (luminal layer) composed of smooth muscle cells, fibroblasts, and a basophilic interstitial matrix (intimal fibrous proliferation). The outer atherosclerotic plaque layer contained gaps, which were presumed evidence of previous transluminal balloon angioplasty. These gaps were filled with the cellular proliferation from the inner layer. Waller and colleagues[258] presented histologic evidence of restenosis in a proximal left anterior descending coronary artery 4.5 months after a clinically successful angioplasty (Figs. 44–11 and 44–12). The sites of previous balloon angio-

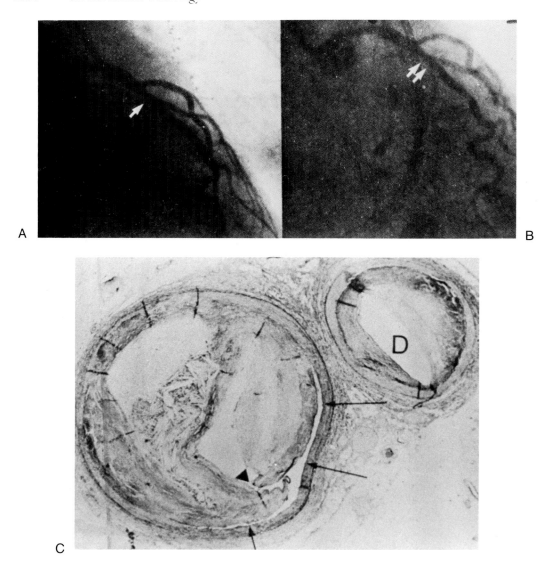

Fig. 44–5. Frames from coronary angiogram showing severe left anterior descending artery stenosis (arrows) before (**A**) and after (**B**) balloon angioplasty. (**C**) Histologic section of proximal left anterior descending artery and adjacent diagonal branch (D). Atherosclerotic plaque narrows the lumen (arrows). The plaque shows disruption and splitting (arrowhead) and is dissected and lifted from the media. (From Soward et al.,[231] with permission.)

plasty showed atherosclerotic plaque cracks or splits and localized medial dissection (disruption) similar to lesions observed in patients who died acutely after balloon angioplasty. The initial underlying atherosclerotic plaque

was still clearly identified, and the luminal channels created by the angioplasty were filled with fibrocellular tissue that also coated the denuded media and narrowed the coronary lumen 96 to 100 percent in cross-sec-

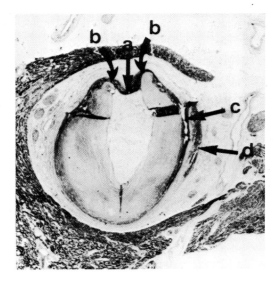

Fig. 44–6. Distal left anterior descending coronary artery angioplasty site, showing intimal fracture (a), plaque cleavage (b), medial fracture with hemorrhage (c), adventitial fracture with hemorrhage (d). (From La Delia,[128] with permission.)

tional area. Fibrocellular tissue proliferation involved 28 mm of the proximal left anterior descending artery and then abruptly disappeared, covering a distance corresponding to the lengths of the previously used angioplasty balloons.

Thus, at sites seen late after an angiographically successful balloon angioplasty, no distinctive lesion(s) may be seen or, more commonly, a concentric fibrocellular proliferation that is distinctly different from underlying atherosclerotic plaque is observed.

Mechanism(s) of Coronary Artery Balloon Angioplasty

Plaque Compression

In their original description of the procedure, Dotter and Judkins[61] (as well as Gruntzig,[84] 14 years later) attributed the mechanism of balloon angioplasty to redistribution and compression of intimal atherosclerotic plaque. Inflation of the angioplasty balloon within an arterial stenosis was thought to compress atherosclerotic plaque components against the arterial wall, thereby producing a larger vessel lumen. However, most atherosclerotic plaques in human coronary arteries are composed of dense fibrocollagenous tissue with varying amounts of calcific deposits and with far lower amounts of intracellular and extracellular lipid (i.e., hard plaques). Thus, it appears unlikely that plaque compression plays a major role in human coronary artery dilation associated with transluminal balloon angioplasty. In experimental animal models, vessel-induced injury plus high-cholesterol diets are used to create atherosclerotic lesions. Those so induced are composed almost entirely of lipid-laden foam cells without dense collagen and calcific deposits (i.e., soft plaques). Compression may play a role in balloon dilation of these experimental lesions.

Plaque Fracture

Data from angioplasty results in experimental models,[21,22,68] human autopsy coronary arteries,[17,25,35] and human vessels examined after successful or complicated angioplasty procedures.[61,168,231] suggest that a major mechanism of dilation by angioplasty is a result of atherosclerotic plaque breaking, cracking, splitting, or fracturing. Plaque fractures, breaks (also called dissection clefts), and cracks extending from the lumen into the plaque for variable lengths improve vessel patency by creating additional channels for coronary blood flow. Healing and repair at the angioplasty site eventually may remodel the acute pathologic lesion(s) to alter or modify their distinctive features, which were described previously. Healing at the angioplasty site may also increase (as has been noted angiographically[138]) or decrease luminal size (restenosis).

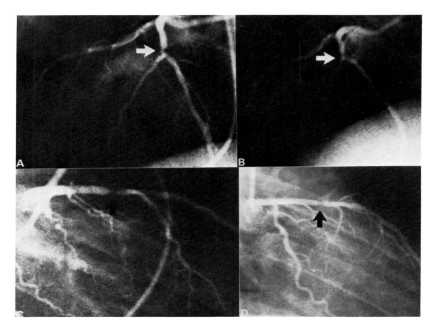

Fig. 44–7. Frames of coronary angiogram 80 days before death, showing (**A,C**) severe diameter reduction of the proximal left anterior descending coronary artery (arrows) with (**B,D**) an increased luminal diameter after balloon angioplasty. (*Figure continues.*)

Plaque Fracture, Intimal Flaps, and Localized Medial Dissection

Waller and colleagues[250] reported plaque fracture, intimal atherosclerotic flaps, and localized medial dissection as the major mechanism of balloon angioplasty in human coronary arteries from patients undergoing angioplasty during life (see Figs. 44–1, 44–3B, 44–4, 44–5C, 44–13). Initial and persistent luminal cross-sectional area expansion appears to require deep intimal fractures (occasionally creating intimal flaps) with localized tears or dissection of the underlying media. Failure to obtain localized and limited medial involvement in addition to the intimal cracks may cause an initially successful dilation but also an early return of a symptomatic patient with restenosis of the vessel.

Stretching of Plaque-Free Wall Segment

An additional mechanism of coronary artery dilation appears to be stretching of plaque-free wall segments of eccentric atherosclerotic lesions (Figs. 44–14 to 44–16). Inflation of angioplasty balloons across eccentric plaque lesions may distend or stretch the normal wall segment and produce little or no damage to the plaque. Stretching of the plaque-free wall segment may initially increase the coronary lumen (diameter and cross-sectional area), but several weeks later gradual relaxation of this overstretched segment (restitution of tone) decreases the lumen toward the predilation state. The decrease may provide another explanation for early restenosis after an initially angiographically successful dilation.[244,248] The high frequency of eccentric coronary lumen in severely diseased vessels[14,240,248] suggests that stretching of the plaque-free wall segment may be a more frequent mechanism of clinically successful coronary angioplasty than was previously thought. On examination of 200 atherosclerotic coronary artery sections, Vlodaver and Edwards[240] found an eccentric (i.e., eccentric polymorphous and eccentric slitlike) coronary lumen in 70 percent of cross sections and a concentric lumen in the re-

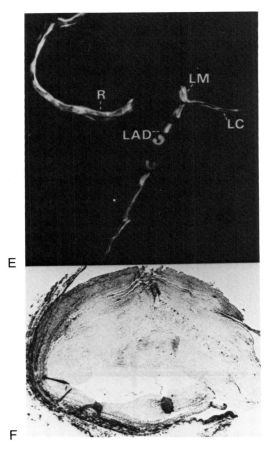

Fig. 44–7. (*Continued*). (**E**) Postmortem radiograph of excised coronary tree showing no calcific deposits. (**F**) Histologic section of the left anterior descending (LAD) coronary artery at the site of previous balloon angioplasty showing severe luminal narrowing by atherosclerotic plaque. (Movat's pentachrome, × 26.) LC, left circumflex; LM, left main; R, right coronary artery. (From Waller et al.,[253] with permission.)

maining 30 percent. Baroldi[14] examined 1,069 sites of severe (greater than 70 percent) diameter reduction in coronary arteries and found that 46 percent of lumens were concentric, 24 percent eccentric (lateral lumen position but still encircled by plaque), and 30 percent semilunar (a variable arc of disease-free wall). Saner and colleagues[203] studied 100 coronary artery segments narrowed 50 to 90 percent in cross-sectional area by atherosclerotic plaque. Of these, 17 to 23 percent (average, 20 percent) of the vessel circumference was free of disease. The percentage length of disease-free wall arc length did not differ significantly with increasing severity of coronary luminal obstruction, proximal or distal location of the lesion, or location of the lesion in various coronary arteries.[203] Waller[248] reported histologic observations in 500 coronary artery segments narrowed 76 to 95 percent in cross-sectional area by atherosclerotic plaque; 365 (73 percent) had an eccentric lumen and 185 (27 percent) were concentric. Of eccentric lesions, an arc of disease-free free wall accounted for 2.3 to 32 percent (mean 16.6 percent) of the circumference of the internal elastic membrane. Waller[248] also compared the thickness of the medial layer in diseased

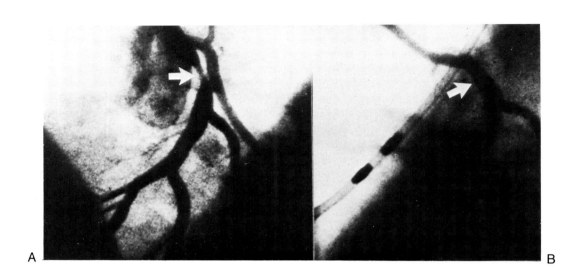

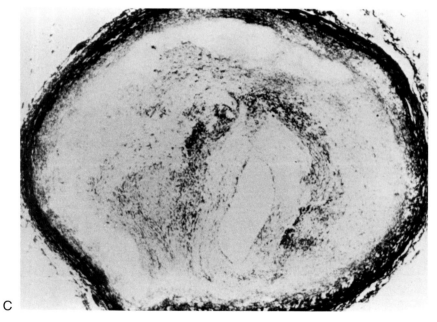

Fig. 44–8. **(A,B)** Frames of coronary angiogram 90 days before death, showing an increased diameter of the left anterior descending coronary artery after transluminal balloon angioplasty (arrows). **(C)** Histologic section of the artery at the site of angioplasty procedure, showing severe luminal narrowing by atherosclerotic plaque. (Movat's pentachrome, × 22.) (From Waller et al.,[253] with permission.)

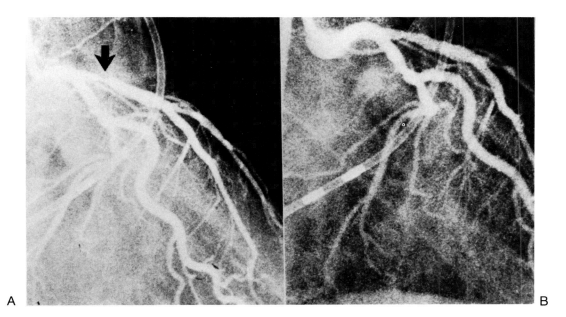

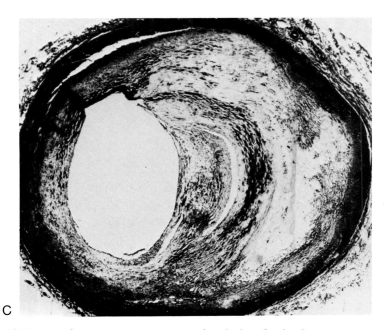

Fig. 44–9. (A,B) Frames of coronary angiogram 150 days before death, showing an increase in diameter of the left anterior descending coronary artery after transluminal balloon angioplasty (arrows). **(C)** Histologic section at the angioplasty site showing severe luminal narrowing by atherosclerotic plaque. (Movat's pentachrome, × 22.) (From Waller et al.,[253] with permission.)

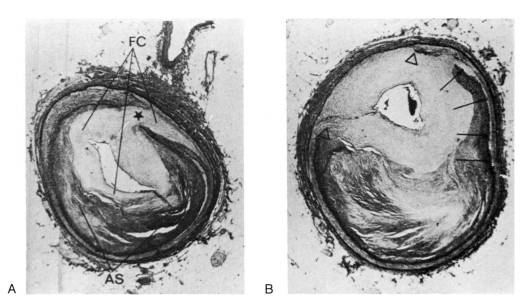

Fig. 44–10. Cross sections of left anterior descending artery. (**A**) Medial disruption (star) has caused a medial dissection. The false channel and lumen have filled with fibrocellular tissue (FC). AS, atherosclerotic plaque. (**B**) Distal arterial segment shows dehiscence of plaque from media (pointers) and localized medial interruption (open arrowheads). (From Essed et al.,[66] with permission.)

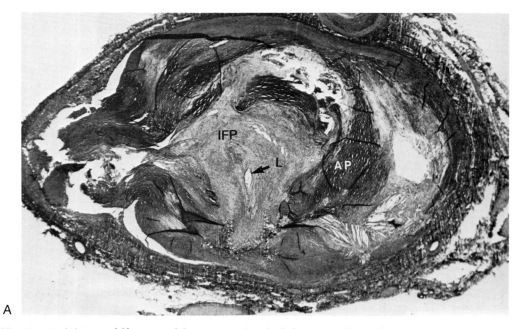

Fig. 44–11. (**A**) Intimal fibrous proliferation (IPF) in the left anterior descending coronary artery "coating" underlying atherosclerotic plaque (AP) 4½ months after balloon angioplasty. L, lumen. (*Figure continues.*)

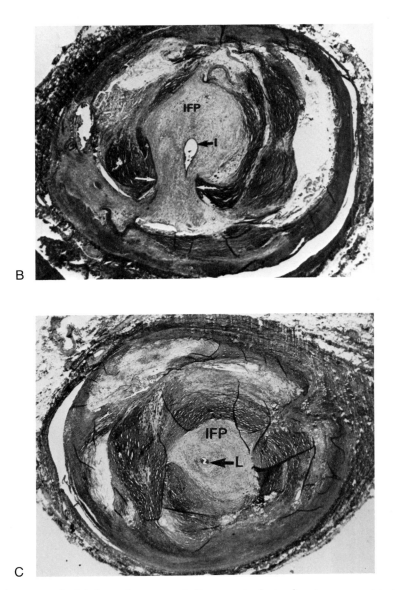

Fig. 44–11 (*Continued*). (**B**) Site of previous balloon angioplasty showing concentric intimal fibrous proliferation coating angioplasty "crack" (white arrows). (**C**) Concentric intimal fibrous proliferation severely narrowing the lumen. (Fig. A from Waller et al.,[258] with permission.)

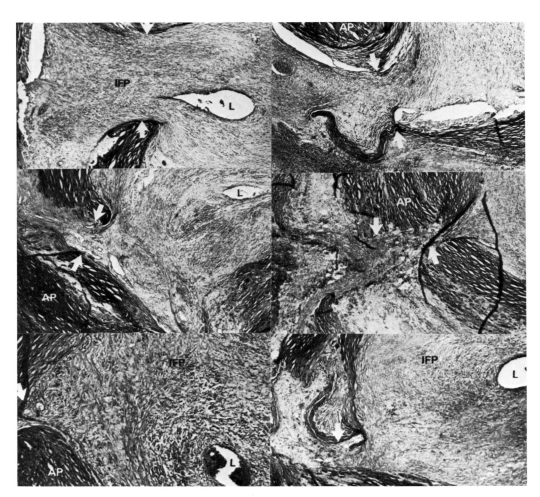

Fig. 44–12. Composite of zones of coronary restenosis lesions seen in Fig. 44–11. Intimal fibrous proliferation (IFP) coats undering atherosclerotic plaque (AP), projects into area of previous "cracks" (arrows) and severely narrows residual coronary lumen. (Trichrome-elastic, × 100.)

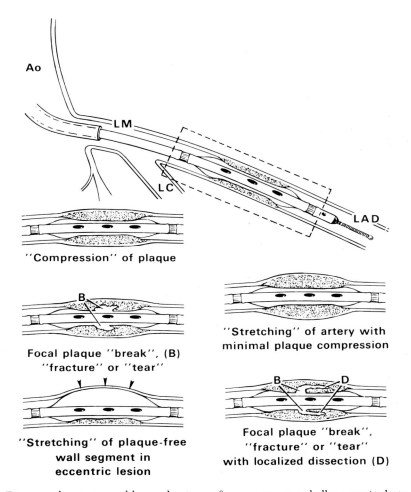

Ao

LM

LC

LAD

"Compression" of plaque

B

Focal plaque "break", (B)
"fracture" or "tear"

"Stretching" of plaque-free
wall segment in
eccentric lesion

"Stretching" of artery with
minimal plaque compression

B   D

Focal plaque "break",
"fracture" or "tear"
with localized dissection (D)

Fig. 44–13. Diagram showing possible mechanisms of coronary artery balloon angioplasty. Ao, aorta; LAD, left anterior descending coronary artery; LC, left circumflex coronary artery; LM, left main coronary artery. (From Waller,[244] with permission.)

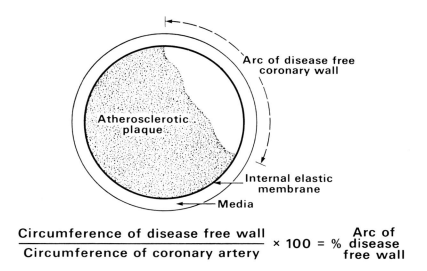

$$\frac{\text{Circumference of disease free wall}}{\text{Circumference of coronary artery}} \times 100 = \% \begin{array}{c}\text{Arc of}\\\text{disease}\\\text{free wall}\end{array}$$

Fig. 44–14. Diagram defining the disease-free segment of an eccentric coronary atherosclerotic lesion. (From Waller,[248] with permission.)

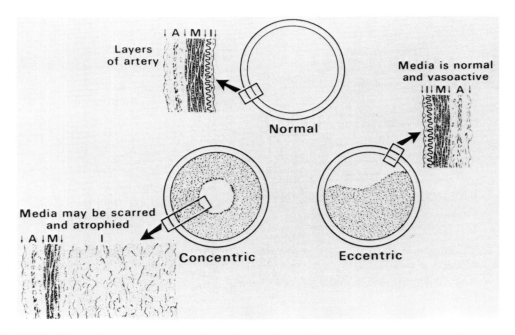

Fig. 44–15. Types of coronary artery atherosclerotic plaque lumen. Diagram compares the coronary media of the diseased segment and arc of disease-free wall. The disease-free wall has a media capable of reacting to various humoral or neurogenic stimuli (i.e., spasm). (From Waller,[248] with permission.)

and disease-free portions of the segments. The average thickness of the coronary artery media was thinner in diseased segments (mean 99.4 μm) compared with disease-free wall segments in the same vessel (mean 202.9 μm).

In addition to stretching, the normal or nearly normal arc of coronary wall with normal medial thickness is capable of reacting to various humoral or neurogenic stimuli (Figs. 44–15 and 44–16). The extent to which dynamic augmentation or contraction of the coronary wall (i.e., spasm) is possible appears to be a function of the amount and location of smooth muscle in the wall. The potential for spasm is unlikely along the diseased circumference

but is more likely along the disease-free segment of an eccentric lesion. Thus, balloon angioplasty of an eccentric plaque may be associated with coronary artery spasm of the disease-free segment. This may lead to an abrupt closure or severe luminal narrowing at the balloon angioplasty site.

Coronary angiographic recognition of an eccentric atherosclerotic plaque is limited at best. Figure 44–17 shows various luminal shapes that may be encountered with eccentric and concentric plaques. Simply observing a laterally displaced lumen on angiography does not define an eccentric plaque. Similarly, observing a centrally placed lumen angio-

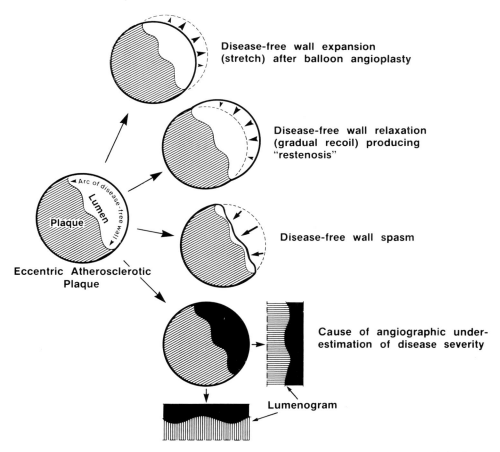

Fig. 44–16. Diagram showing the clinical relevance (angioplasty, spasm, angiography) of eccentric atherosclerotic plaques in patients with coronary artery disease. (From Waller,[248] with permission.)

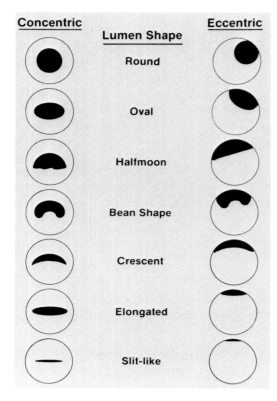

Fig. 44–17. Diagram showing various luminal configurations of eccentric and concentric coronary atherosclerotic plaques. Coronary angiography (lumenogram) cannot easily discern an anatomically eccentric plaque. (From Waller,[248] with permission.)

gioplasty balloon may stretch an entire coronary segment that is concentrically narrowed by fibrocollagenous plaque.

Morphologic Correlates of Coronary Angioplasty Patterns at the Site of Balloon Angioplasty

Since the introduction of percutaneous transluminal coronary angioplasty, there has been considerable interest in the angiographic recognition of successful dilation, complications of the technique, and various predictors of restenosis. Holmes and colleagues[99] addressed the classification of various coronary angiographic patterns produced by balloon angioplasty with an analysis of 100 consecutive patients (Table 44–1). Smooth-walled dilation was the most common (41 percent), followed by intimal flaps (splits) and dissection (22 percent), and intraluminal haziness (17 percent). Speculation on the anatomic basis of these patterns included alterations in endothelium and disruption of intimal and medial layers of the coronary vessel with or without associated intraluminal thrombus. Waller[247] recently completed an angiographic-histologic correlation of 76 coronary balloon angioplasty sites in 66 patients, all of whom died within 30 days of coronary angioplasty.

Morphologic Patterns

Of 76 coronary balloon angioplasty sites from the 66 patients, evidence of angioplasty injury was found at 67 (88 percent) (Table 44–2):

graphically does not define a concentric lesion. Thus, coronary angioplasty procedures may be performed on eccentric lesions interpreted as concentric and on concentric lesions interpreted to represent eccentric lesions. Advances in ultrasound-tipped vascular catheters will permit accurate recognition of eccentric and concentric lesions during life.

Stretching and Compression

A fifth mechanism for balloon angioplasty of coronary arteries is the combination of vessel stretching with minimal or mild plaque compression. In this situation, an oversized an-

Table 44–1. Angiographic Patterns Observed at the Site of Clinical Balloon Angioplasty[a]

Smooth-walled dilation
Intraluminal haziness
"Intimal" flaps or "splits"
Dissection
Extravasated contrast material

[a] See also Figures 44–18 to 44–22.

Table 44–2.   Angiographic-Morphologic Correlation at Sites of Percutaneous Transluminal Coronary Angioplasty in 66 Patients at 76 Sites

| Angiographic Appearance at PTCA Site | Sites | Anatomic Findings at PTCA Site Sites | | | | | No Injury | |
| | | Intimal Injury Only[a] | Intimal-Medial Tear | | Intimal-Medial-Adventitial Tear | | | |
			Localized Dissection	Extensive Dissection	Confined Rupture	Rupture	Eccentric Lesion	Concentric Lesion
Smooth-walled	10 (14)	2	0	0	0	0	7	1
Intraluminal haziness (ground-glass)	29 (38)	9 (31)	20[a] (69)	0	0	0	0	0
Intimal flap (Intimal Crack) (Intimal Dissection) (Localized Dissection)	33 (43)	0	29 (88)	4 (12)	0	0	0	0
Dissection (coronary dissection)	1 (1)	0	0	1	0	0	0	0
Spasm	1 (1)	0	0	0	0	0	1	0
Extravasated contrast material	2 (3)	0	0	0	1 (1.5)	1 (1.5)	0	0
Totals	76 (100)	11 (15)	49 (65)	5 (7)	1 (1)	1 (1)	8 (10)	1 (1)

[a] Includes one laminated thrombus.

shallow, superficial intimal cracks or splits (intimal injury), at 11 sites (16 percent); deeper intimal cracks or splits with localized medial dissection (intimal-medial injury), at 49 sites (73 percent); intimal cracks with extensive medial dissection, at 5 sites (7 percent); and adventitial perforation or rupture (intimal-medial-adventitial injury), at 2 sites (13 percent). Deep intimal-medial injury produced intimal flaps at 29 sites (43 percent). The remaining 9 balloon angioplasty sites (12 percent) had no morphologic evidence of dilation injury. Of these, 8 had eccentric lesions with an arc of disease-free wall, and 1 was a concentric atherosclerotic plaque.[247]

Angiographic Patterns

Of the 76 coronary balloon angioplasty sites from the 66 patients, the angiographic patterns were classified as follows (Table 44–1): smooth-walled dilation, at 10 sites (14 percent) (Fig. 44–18); intraluminal haziness, at 29 sites (38 percent) (Fig. 44–19); intimal flap, at 33 sites (43 percent) (Fig. 44–20); coronary dissection, at 1 site (1 percent) (Fig. 44–21); extravasated contrast material, at 2 sites (3 percent); and spasm at 1 site (1 percent). The two patients with extravasated contrast material had contrast material confined to the coronary wall in one (vessel staining) or leaked outside the vessel in the other (rupture into pericardial space) (Fig. 44–22).

Morphologic-Angiographic Correlations

Corresponding morphologic-angiographic patterns are summarized in Table 44–2. Of 10 balloon angioplasty sites with a smooth-walled appearance by coronary angiogram, 2 had shallow, superficial intimal cracks (intimal injury only) and 7 had eccentric lesions without morphologic evidence of injury (Fig. 44–18). Of 29 sites with angiographic intraluminal

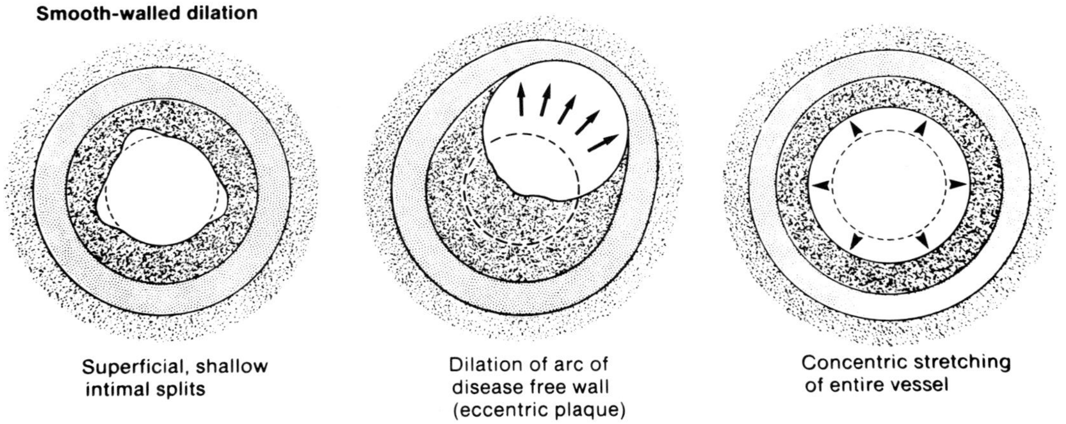

Smooth-walled dilation

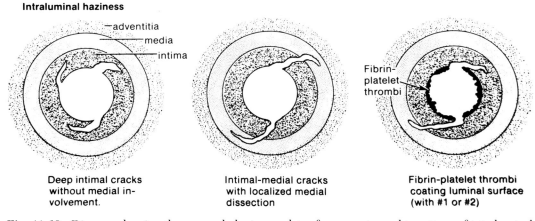

Superficial, shallow
intimal splits

Dilation of arc of
disease free wall
(eccentric plaque)

Concentric stretching
of entire vessel

Fig. 44–18. Diagram showing three morphologic correlates for an angiographic smooth-walled appearance of the site of balloon angioplasty. Shallow, superficial intimal injuries or no injury at all are the most common explanations for the smooth-walled appearance. (From Waller,[248] with permission.)

haziness or ground-glass appearance, 9 had intimal injuries only, 19 had intimal-medial injuries with localized medial dissection, and 1 had a similar intimal-medial tear, but the luminal surface are irregularly covered by fibrin-platelet thrombus (Fig. 44–19). Of 33 balloon angioplasty sites with an intimal flap or localized dissection, 29 had deep intimal-medial tears with medial dissection, and 4 had intimal-medial tears with extensive medial dissection (Fig. 44–20). In the single patient

with a coronary dissection, the balloon angioplasty site disclosed a deep intimal-medial tear with an extensive longitudinal medial dissection (Table 44–1, Fig. 44–21). The two patients with angiographic evidence of extravasated contrast material both had intimal-medial-adventitial involvement of the coronary artery. One site had localized adventitial involvement referred to as a coronary perforation or confined rupture. The other had adventitial separation (i.e., frank rupture)

Intraluminal haziness

adventitia
media
intima

Deep intimal cracks
without medial in-
volvement.

Intimal-medial cracks
with localized medial
dissection

Fibrin-
platelet
thrombi

Fibrin-platelet thrombi
coating luminal surface
(with #1 or #2)

Fig. 44–19. Diagram showing three morphologic correlates for an angiographic pattern of intraluminal haziness at the site of balloon angioplasty. Intimal-medial splits are the most common finding for this angiographic appearance. (From Waller,[247] with permission.)

Intimal flap

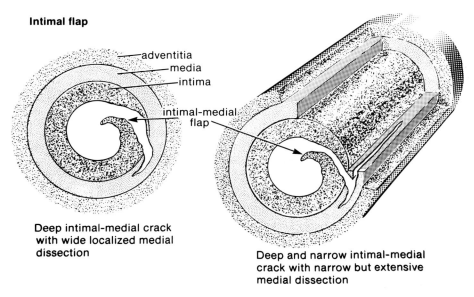

Deep intimal-medial crack
with wide localized medial
dissection

Deep and narrow intimal-medial
crack with narrow but extensive
medial dissection

Fig. 44–20. Diagram showing that the angiographic pattern of intimal splitting correlates morphologically with a deep intimal-medial tear with a localized medial dissection. Large intimal flaps may be associated with sudden closure of a vessel lumen at the angioplasty site. (From Waller,[247] with permission.)

Dissection

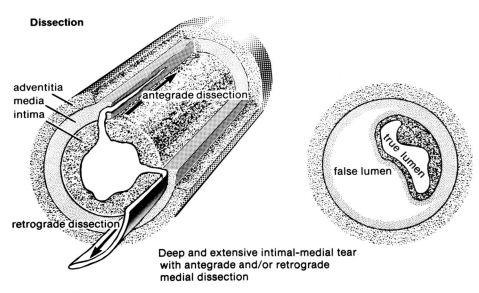

Deep and extensive intimal-medial tear
with antegrade and/or retrograde
medial dissection

Fig. 44–21. Diagram showing the morphologic correlate of angiographic coronary artery dissection. An intimal-medial tear with extensive medial dissection creates a false lumen that extends antegrade and/ or retrograde from the balloon angioplasty site. This anatomic finding appears to be a complication and/ or extension of the balloon angioplasty mechanism shown in Fig. 44–19. (From Waller,[247] with permission.)

(Fig. 44–22). Only one coronary angioplasty site had angiographic evidence of coronary spasm that correlated morphologically with an eccentric atherosclerotic plaque lesion (arc of disease-free wall) and no evidence of atherosclerotic plaque injury (see Fig. 44–18).

Results of the retrospective study indicated that intimal flaps and intraluminal haziness were the two most frequent angiographic patterns accounting for 43 percent and 38 percent of the sites, respectively. The most common anatomic correlate for both angiographic patterns was an intimal-medial split or crack with localized medial dissection (Figs. 44–13, 44–19, and 44–20). Of the 33 coronary balloon angioplasty sites with angiographic intimal flaps, all had varying degrees of intimal-medial tears, giving the appearance of intraluminal flaps. The deep cracks or breaks created by the balloon dilation produced luminal channels associated with a flap of intimal (plaque)-medial tissue. These flaps may be large at times and cause sudden or abrupt closure of the dilation site.[246]

Of the 29 balloon angioplasty sites with angiographic patterns of haziness, 19 (66 percent) had anatomic correlates of intimal-medial splits. However, the haziness pattern was also associated with purely intimal injuries (31 percent) and laminated fibrin-platelet thrombus coating an underlying intimal-medial injury (3 percent) (see Fig. 44–19). In the past,[25,35,99] angiographic haziness at an angioplasty site has been attributed to the dispersion of contrast media along multiple fissures or channels. The present study indicates that intimal irregularities (shallow, superficial splits) and/or irregular surfaces produced by adherent thrombus are also explanations for this angiographic pattern.

Intimal flaps created by deep intimal-medial cracks may be interpreted angiographically as either coronary dissections or intimal splits, or both. The angiographic term *coronary dissection* has generally been reserved for the situation in which clinical symptoms of ischemia are associated with this pattern or in which an extensive coronary intramural channel of contrast material is visible angiographically. By contrast, the terms *intimal dissection* or *intimal split* are used for the situations in which the split is localized to the angioplasty site and is not associated with clinical ischemia. From an anatomic point of view,

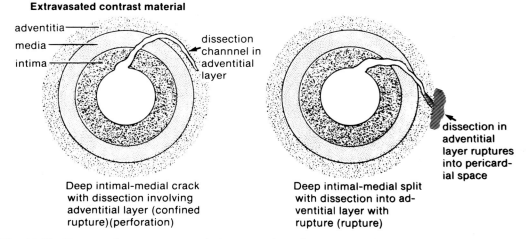

Extravasated contrast material

adventitia —
media —
intima —

dissection channnel in adventitial layer

Deep intimal-medial crack with dissection involving adventitial layer (confined rupture)(perforation)

dissection in adventitial layer ruptures into pericardial space

Deep intimal-medial split with dissection into adventitial layer with rupture (rupture)

Fig. 44–22. Diagram showing two morphologic correlates for extravasated contrast media at the site of balloon angioplasty. A dissection channel extends into the adventitial layer and remains confined to this zone (left) or the dissection channel perforates the adventitial layer and enters the pericardial space (right). (From Waller,[247] with permission.)

these localized intimal flaps are the result of a desirable intimal-medial split with localized medial dissection[15] (Figs. 44–13 and 44–20). Angiographic evidence of an intimal flap resulting from balloon angioplasty was initially considered an unfavorable outcome, but recent clinical studies suggest that their presence may indicate a substantial increase in coronary luminal cross-sectional area[272] and may be associated with a decreased frequency of restenosis.[135,152]

Angiographic coronary artery dissection is associated with an extensive intramural channel that is anatomically located in the vessel

media (Fig. 44–21). The intramural channel (false lumen) may extend antegrade or retrograde from the angioplasty site. An extensive pre-existing coronary artery dissection may be a relative contraindication to balloon angioplasty. I examined the right coronary artery of a 37-year-old woman who underwent balloon dilation of a focal, proximal, severe right coronary artery stenosis. Preceding the angioplasty, an extensive coronary artery dissection was created by the guiding catheter (Fig. 44–23). The intimal layer remained anchored to the vessel wall at the site of proximal stenosis. Subsequent successful balloon an-

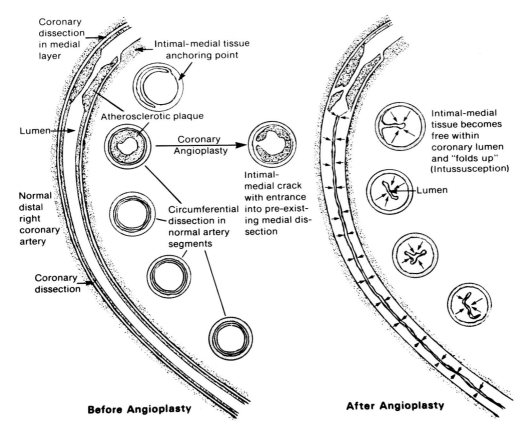

Fig. 44–23. Diagram showing the potential consequences of coronary angioplasty upon a pre-existing acute coronary artery dissection (left). Proximal atherosclerotic stenosis anchors the intimal layer to the vessel wall. Subsequent balloon angioplasty created an intimal-medial tear freeing the previously attached intimal layer (right). The intimal layer collapsed upon itself occluding the distal lumen. (From Waller,[247] with permission.)

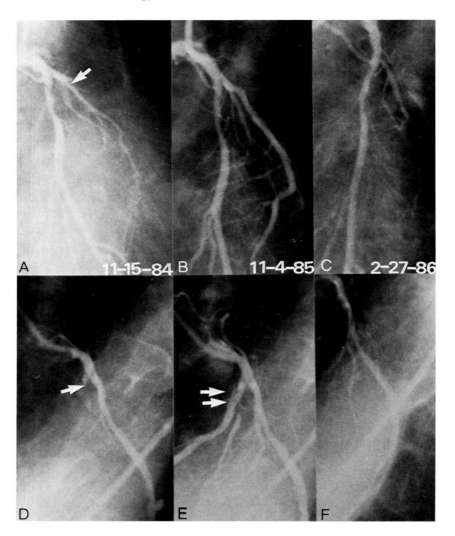

Fig. 44–24. Frames of coronary cineangiogram in (A–C) right anterior oblique and (D–F) left anterior oblique views obtained (**A,D**) about 1 year before percutaneous transluminal coronary angioplasty; (**B,E**) at the time of angioplasty; and (**C,F**) 6 days before death. The proximal left anterior descending artery is initially totally occluded (arrows in Figs. A and D), recanalized with balloon angioplasty (Figs. B and E), and is again totally occluded shortly before death (Figs. C and F). A plaque "crack" or "fracture" is visualized (arrows in Fig. E) after balloon dilation. In each of the three angiograms, the left main coronary artery has luminal irregularities. (From Waller et al.,[258] with permission.)

gioplasty of the proximal stenosis created the usual intimal-medial crack, but now the intimal layer became free within the coronary lumen and collapsed on itself, occluding the entire distal right coronary artery (intimal intussusception) (Fig. 44–23).

Formation of a coronary artery aneurysm after balloon angioplasty is an uncommon an-

giographic pattern reported by Hill and colleagues.[95] Aneurysmal dilation was not observed in patients studied by Holmes and associates,[99] nor was it found in the angiographic-morphologic study by Waller.[247] An anatomic explanation for the angiographic appearance of an aneurysm at an angioplasty site is probably related to overdilation of an arc

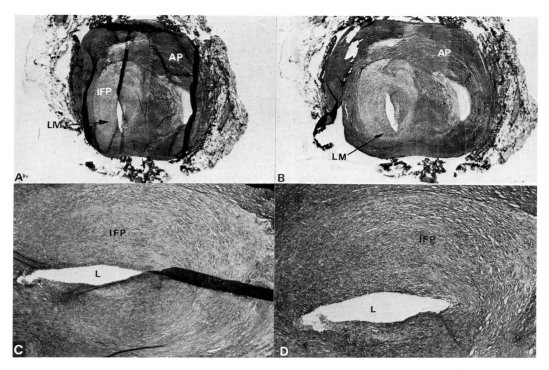

Fig. 44–25. (A–D) Two sections of left main coronary artery showing old atherosclerotic plaque (AP) with superimposed new intimal fibrous proliferation (IFP) severely narrowing the coronary lumen (L). The left main vessel (LM) was not subjected to angioplasty but developed accelerated narrowing as a complication of a previous balloon angioplasty of the proximal left anterior descending artery. (Figs. A&B, × 7; Figs. C&D, × 100.)

of disease-free wall in an eccentric plaque (Figs. 44–13 and 44–18) and less likely the result of perforation into the coronary adventitial layer (confined rupture, pseudoaneurysm) (Fig. 44–22). Thus, various coronary angiographic patterns following balloon angioplasty are associated with a spectrum of anatomic findings, but the most frequent morphologic finding is an intimal-medial split with localized medial dissection.

Effects of Balloon Angioplasty on Adjacent Nondilated Vessels

Angiographic reports have noted an accelerated development of coronary artery stenoses proximal to the site of a previous dilation.[15,83,228] In these, five patients received

proximal left anterior descending coronary balloon angioplasty and returned 6 to 14 months later with severe left main coronary artery lesions: morphologic evaluations were not available. Waller and colleagues[258] reported histologic observations in an accelerated stenosis occurring proximal to a previously dilated lesion (Figs. 44–24 and 44–25). The patient had balloon angioplasty of the proximal left anterior descending artery 4 months before returning with severe left main stenosis. At autopsy, two 5-mm-long segments of the left main coronary artery disclosed old atherosclerotic plaque narrowing the lumen 51 to 75 percent in cross-sectional area with superimposed (new) fibrocellular material, further narrowing it 76 to 100 percent. The fibrocellular tissue was identical to that observed in the proximal left anterior descending at the site of a previous balloon an-

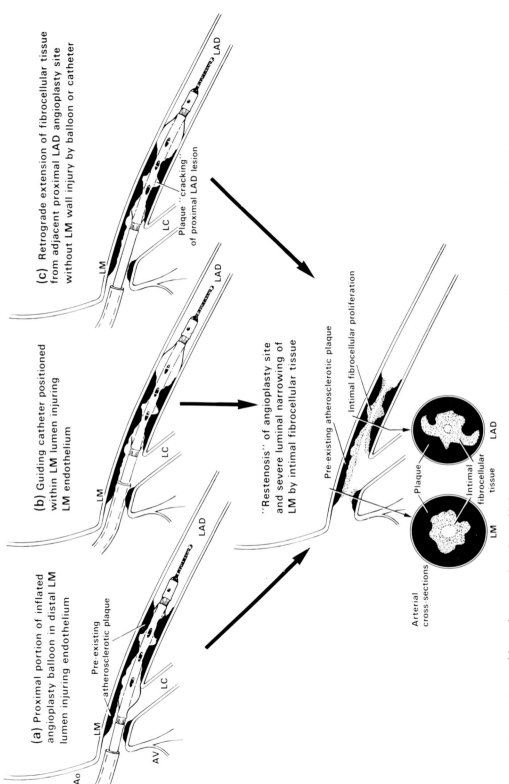

Fig. 44-26. Possible mechanisms of accelerated left main coronary narrowing occurring late after percutaneous transluminal balloon angioplasty of the proximal left anterior descending coronary artery (LAD). Ao, aorta; VA, aortic valve; LC, left circumflex; LM, left main coronary artery. (From Waller et al.,[258] with permission.)

(a) Proximal portion of inflated angioplasty balloon in distal LM lumen injuring endothelium

Pre-existing atherosclerotic plaque

(b) Guiding catheter positioned within LM lumen injuring LM endothelium

(c) Retrograde extension of fibrocellular tissue from adjacent proximal LAD angioplasty site without LM wall injury by balloon or catheter

Plaque "cracking" of proximal LAD lesion

"Restenosis" of angioplasty site and severe luminal narrowing of LM by intimal fibrocellular tissue

Pre-existing atherosclerotic plaque

Intimal fibrocellular proliferation

Arterial cross-sections

Plaque

Intimal fibrocellular tissue

LM   LAD

gioplasty (Fig. 44–26).

The acceleration of left main coronary narrowing by fibrocellular tissue proliferation may result from several mechanisms involving intimal injury or from retrograde extension of fibrocellular tissue from an adjacent site, without left main wall injury (Fig. 44–26). First, insertion of large-bore guiding catheters into the left main artery could certainly cause intimal injury. Then, positioning the proximal end of a dilating balloon in the distal left main artery while dilating a proximal anterior descending or left circumflex lesion may also

cause intimal damage. In addition, simple retrograde extension or "growth" of fibrocellular tissue into the adjacent left main artery from the proximally dilated left anterior descending is possible. Morphologic observations of left main endothelial injury in 9 of 11 patients with angioplasty of the left coronary system and the absence of injury in a single patient with dilation of only the right coronary artery suggest that the first and second mechanisms (Fig. 44–26) are more likely.

The incidence of progressive narrowing of the left main artery following percutaneous

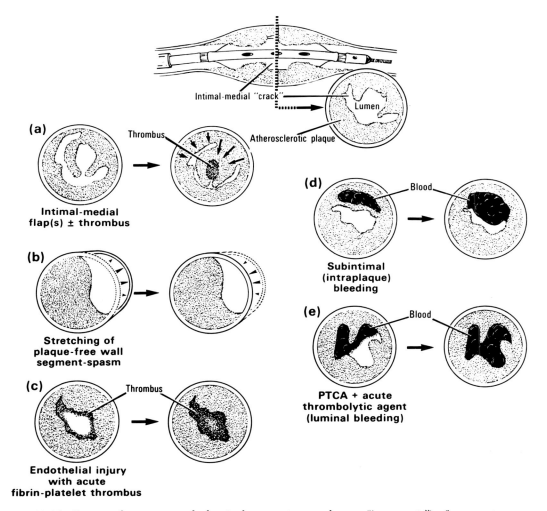

Fig. 44–27. Causes of acute or early luminal narrowing or closure ("restenosis") of a percutaneous transluminal coronary balloon angioplasty (PTCA) site. (From Waller,[249] with permission.)

transluminal coronary angioplasty of the left anterior descending and/or left circumflex arteries is unknown. Although detailed analysis of the left main artery in preangioplasty and follow-up angiograms has not been uniformly evaluated, the incidence of severe narrowing of the left main artery is probably low. Of more than 344 patients restudied angiographically within 1 year of previous coronary dilation in whom specific attention was given to the left main artery, only four (1 percent) were recognized with accelerated left main narrowing.[83,228]

Acute and Late Closure of the Angioplasty Site

Despite a highly successful technique, percutaneous balloon angioplasty has been plagued with two major problems at the an-

gioplasty site: (1) early (abrupt) closure (Fig. 44–27) and (2) late closure (restenosis) (Fig. 44–28). Various new interventional devices and techniques have been used to solve these problems (Figs. 44–29 and 44–30).

Acute (Abrupt) Closure of the Angioplasty Site

Despite improvement in equipment and technique, abrupt closure at the angioplasty site occurs in 2 to 6 percent of patients treated with balloon angioplasty.[12,29,45,223,227] Clinical explanations include coronary artery spasm (2 percent), localized thrombus (8 percent), and coronary dissection (34 percent).[6] Morphologic explanations are depicted in Figure 44–27. Acute vessel occlusion from a folded, curled-up, large intimal flap accounts for the majority of these cases (Fig. 44–27A). This

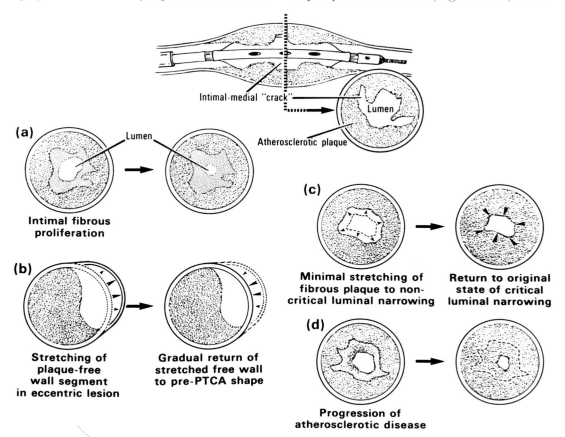

Fig. 44–28. Causes of late luminal narrowing or closure ("restenosis") of a percutaneous transluminal coronary balloon angioplasty (PTCA) site. (From Waller,[249] with permission.)

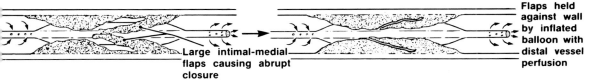

Fig. 44–29. Diagram showing the use of reperfusion balloons in the treatment of acute vessel closure following balloon angioplasty. (From Waller,[249] with permission.)

finding may correspond to the clinical category of dissection in that a large intimal flap is created by an extensive intimal-medial dissection plane. Acute closure may be produced by abrupt relaxation of an overstretched disease-free wall of an eccentric plaque (Fig. 44–27B). The coronary artery media of the disease-free wall contains smooth muscle and is capable of reacting to various humoral, neurogenic, or traumatic (balloon dilation)

stimuli. This morphologic mechanism may correspond to the clinical category of spasm. The potential for dynamic alteration of the coronary lumen (wall spasm) is more likely to occur with eccentric than with concentric atherosclerotic lesions.[248] Nonocclusive fibrin-platelet thrombus frequently layers the angioplasty site, but occlusive thrombus at the site is uncommon in patients dying within hours of coronary dilation[243,253,257] (Fig. 44–

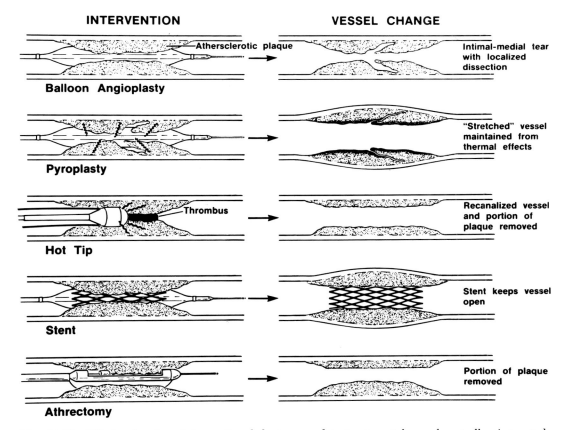

Fig. 44–30. Effects of various interventional devices used to treat acutely or chronically obstructed coronary arteries. (From Waller,[249] with permission.)

27C). Although thrombus may be associated with large, curled-up intimal flaps, the primary mechanism for abrupt closure is the intimal-medial flap. Subintimal hemorrhage from traumatic balloon injury of atherosclerotic plaque is a possible cause for abrupt closure. Subintimal plaque bleeding may acutely expand the plaque and severely narrow or occlude the angioplasty site (Fig. 44–27D). Intraplaque and intraluminal bleeding can acutely occlude an angioplasty site (Fig. 44–27E) but has been reported only in the setting of combined balloon angioplasty and thrombolytic therapy.[260]

Treatment of Abrupt Closure

Treatment of sites of abrupt closure has included repeated balloon angioplasty and prolonged (30 to 60 minutes) balloon inflation using perfusion catheters (bailout catheters, hemoperfusion catheters, autoperfusion catheters, shunt catheters[6,11,65,70,236,237] (Figs. 44–29 and 44–30). Perfusion catheters are placed across the occluded angioplasty site, so that arterial blood enters the catheter proximally and exits distally (Fig. 44–29).

Newer devices may have an important role in treating sites of abrupt closure (Fig. 44–29). Large intimal flaps may be sealed or welded against the adjacent vessel wall using thermal angioplasty balloons. Pyroplasty techniques (thermal welding) may employ laser or radiofrequency energy sources.[111,117,143,206–208,233,264] An advantage of pyroplasty techniques over perfusion catheters is the immediate repair of the intimal-medial flap without a need for coronary bypass grafting. Balloon-expandable intravascular stents (an intravascular mechanical support device) have also been used for abrupt closure of an angioplasty site[180–182,198,199,217,221] (Fig. 44–30D). Several types of these metal meshwork devices are being tested, and at least one has been used to treat abrupt closure of an angioplasty site.[221] The balloon-expandable stent also offers a rapid percutaneous technique to hold the intimal-medial flap permanently against the vessel wall without resorting to surgery and avoids the extra catheterization laboratory equipment needed for thermal angioplasty.

Thermal angioplasty including stents may be used at the site of abrupt closure where "spasm" is the culprit. Thermal injury to the segment of disease-free wall that is in spasm may permit long-term luminal distention. Hot-tipped lasers may be used to reopen an angioplasty site occluded by thrombus with or without intimal flaps.[50,75,204,205,209] (Fig. 44–30C). Atherectomy devices also can be used to remove either large intimal-medial flaps or thrombus, or both (Fig. 44–30E).

Late (Chronic) Closure (Restenosis)

Despite the widespread acceptance and use of percutaneous transluminal balloon angioplasty to treat severely narrowed coronary arteries in patients with symptomatic coronary heart disease, recurrence of stenoses (restenosis) at the angioplasty site within several months of the procedure has been a major problem (Fig. 44–28). The frequency of clinical restenosis ranges from 17 to 47 percent, depending on variations in the definition of restenosis (angiographic, clinical, anatomic, physiologic, statistical).[20,43,78,100,114,148,159,173,174,220,265] Multiple clinical-angiographic factors (number of vessels, site of angioplasty, pre- and postangioplasty diameter stenoses, transtenotic pressure gradients, lesion characteristics, i.e., diffuse, long, eccentric, calcified), technical factors (number of inflations, duration of inflation, pressure of inflation, balloon-vessel size ratio, intimal flap or dissection, incomplete revascularization), and pharmacologic factors (anticoagulants, vasodilators) have been analyzed to determine factors responsible for restenosis.[173] Despite the many parameters evaluated, studies diverge on their significance but concur on the significance of a few.[173]

The most widely accepted theory for the development of fibrocellular intimal proliferation (Figs. 44–10 to 44–12 and 44–28) involves responses of damaged vessel endothelium and media. A major participant appears to be the smooth muscle cells of the media and diseased intima (plaque).[4,66,78,258] The most common mechanism of balloon angioplasty, intimal-medial disruption likely initiates restenosis. The intimal fibrous proliferation may be stimulated by the release of thromboxane A_2, which leads to platelet deposition, release of platelet-derived growth factor (PDGF), and fibroblast and endothelial growth factors,[84] resulting in migration, proliferation, and alteration of smooth muscle cells from the media. The fibrocellular coating (Figs. 44–10 to 44–12) narrows the vessel lumen.

Other mechanisms of late luminal narrowing at the angioplasty site (restenosis) involve gradual elastic recoil of an overstretched disease-free wall of an eccentric lesion (Figs. 44–16 and 44–28B), return to predilation state of a stretched concentric lesion (Fig. 44–28C), and progression of atherosclerotic plaque (Fig. 44–28D). The latter appears unlikely in the short interval of 2 to 4 months following balloon angioplasty.

Treatment of Chronic Closure (Restenosis)

Treatment of restenosis has primarily involved repeated balloon angioplasty procedures two, three, and four times after the initial dilation.[11,163] Various pharmacologic approaches to prevent restenosis using antiplatelet agents (aspirin, dipyridamole) and calcium-channel blockers have so far proved unsuccessful in reducing the frequency of restenosis.[173] Newer clinical trials with other antiplatelet agents (prostacyclin analogues, ω-3-fatty acids), steroids, and PDGF blockers[36] are under way. Newer mechanical devices, too, may be used to delay or prevent intimal fibrous proliferation at the angioplasty site (Figs. 44–29 and 44–30). Balloon expandable intravascular stents (Fig. 44–30D) have been proposed as an alternate approach.[217,221] The mechanism of preventing restenosis with stents has not been established, but possible explanations include damage to smooth muscle cells of the vessel media or a purely mechanical effect of the stent, or both. Thermal angioplasty (Fig. 44–30B) may alter the vessel media to prevent, or at least delay, the smooth muscle response. Prolonged inflation time (30 to 60 minutes) with perfusion catheters is also being evaluated as a means of preventing restenosis (Fig. 44–29). Mechanical removal of the intimal fibrous hyperplasia by atherectomy devices is also being evaluated[224,225] (Fig. 44–30E). Simpson and colleagues[225] indicate that if all angiographically visible atheroma is removed, the rate of restenosis is as low as 14 percent.

Methodology for Clinical-Pathologic Correlations of the Balloon Angioplasty Site

To gain anatomic information from a coronary vessel receiving balloon angioplasty requires three special techniques: (1) precise location of the balloon angioplasty site, (2) cross-sectional analysis of the site, and (3) knowledge of vessel artifacts that can be confused with angioplasty-induced injury.

1. *Anatomic location:* Precise anatomic location can be determined by a review of the clinical coronary angiogram. The site is determined by locating the area of maximal diameter reduction on a pre-angioplasty coronary angiogram. The guide catheter diameter just proximal to its tip is measured (in millimeters) on a screen or black-and-white print. A magnification correction factor is determined by dividing the angiographic catheter diameter by the actual catheter diameter. The angiographic distance (in millimeters) from the origin of the artery to the site of balloon dilation is measured. To locate this area on the heart specimen, epicardial coronary arteries are dissected free of subepicardial fat and the

distance measured on the angiogram, divided by the magnification correction factor, is measured at autopsy. A 5-mm-long segment containing the angioplasty site is then removed for sectioning.

2. *Cross-sectional analysis of the coronary artery:* The coronary artery subjected to balloon angioplasty and the identified site of angioplasty are cut into 5-mm-long transverse sections. This permits proper assessment of the coronary lumen, evaluation of any intimal, medial, or adventitial changes, as well as an evaluation of any coronary dissection that might have been created. Opening the coronary vessel in a longitudinal fashion (parallel to the long axis of the vessel) will not provide the information required for proper assessment of the angioplasty procedure.

3. *Knowledge of vessel artifacts or nonangioplasty cracks:* Certain histologic artifacts can be created during section of coronary arteries. Isner and Fortin[107] reported morphologic observations in coronary arteries that had not been subjected to balloon angioplasty. In 34 of 70 patients examined (49 percent), plaque fractures and dissection clefts (or cracks) similar to those described in dilated arteries were observed. These findings emphasize a need for precise angiographic-morphologic correlations in the histologic evaluation of arteries subjected to balloon angioplasty. However, deeper intimal splits with adjacent localized medial dissection (many times associated with hemorrhage in the medial dissection) are rarely the result of sectioning artifacts.

Spontaneous plaque fissures are currently implicated as a connecting link between clinical subsets of patients with coronary heart disease.[249] In balloon angioplasty lesions in which the injury is confined to the intimal layer without medial disruption, distinguishing plaque fissures from superficial angioplasty splits is not always possible. Colavita and colleagues[39] provide certain characteristics that might help distinguish spontaneous plaque rupture from secondary plaque disruption caused by balloon angioplasty. These investigators indicate that when spontaneous plaque rupture occurs, the fibrous cap separating the arterial lumen from the underlying lipid plaque may be discontinuous, with the contents of the lipid plaque protruding through the fibrous cap and bulging into the lumen. By contrast, superficial plaque cracks associated with balloon angioplasty may be sharply demarcated, suggesting traumatic shearing or abrasion of the plaque. Finding plaque emboli is more likely in vessels with balloon angioplasty than in these with spontaneous plaque rupture.[39]

Angioplastic Treatment of Aortocoronary Saphenous Vein Bypass Grafts

Several reports have indicated that balloon angioplasty is useful in treating obstructed aortocoronary saphenous vein bypass grafts.[8,23,42,58,63,67,73,74,187,200,259] However, morphologic-histologic changes have received little attention.[67,73,200,259] To date, 10 saphenous vein grafts (9 patients) so treated have been studied histologically.[67,73,200,259] Waller and colleagues[259] were the first to define mechanisms, comparing dilation changes in grafts less or more than 1 year of age and discussing mechanisms of restenosis (Figs. 44–30 to 44–40).

Angioplasty of Saphenous Vein Graft Early After Bypass Surgery

Clinical Features

A 63-year-old man with angina pectoris had an unsuccessful balloon angioplasty of the left anterior descending coronary artery and an aortocoronary saphenous vein bypass graft inserted into the left anterior descending coronary artery. Seven weeks after surgery, the patient had recurrent angina; angiography disclosed a 95 percent symmetric diameter reduction of the bypass graft near its proximal (aortic) anastomosis (Fig. 44–31). The stenosed area was dilated by multiple balloon inflations, resulting in a marked increase in graft luminal diameter. Four weeks after successful graft angioplasty, the patient had recurrent angina. Repeat angiography disclosed severe graft narrowing (restenosis) at the previous dilation site. This time, however, the stenotic segment was not smooth and symmetric but appeared irregular and asymmetric (Fig. 44–31). The proximal portion of the graft was excised.

Morphologic Features

The excised specimen contained the proximal site of maximal balloon inflation and a short distal portion in which the catheter and guide wire had passed but in which balloon inflation had not occurred (Fig. 44–32). The excised graft was free of calcific deposits. The lumen was diffusely and severely (greater than 75 percent cross-sectional area) narrowed by cellular fibrocollagenous tissue without foam cells or cholesterol clefts (i.e., intimal fibrous hyperplasia or fibrous proliferation) (Fig. 44–

33). Areas of dilated and nondilated graft contained similar amounts of intimal thickening. Serial 10-μm sections of the angioplastic site did not disclose morphologic evidence (cracks, tears, and breaks) of previous balloon angioplasty (Figs. 44–32 to 44–34). Furthermore, histologic assessment did not reveal any significant or distinctive morphologic lesion(s) in the intimal, medial, or adventitial layers of dilated or nondilated portions.

Angioplasty of Saphenous Vein Graft Late After Bypass Surgery

Clinical Features

A 42-year-old man underwent aortocoronary bypass grafting for persistent pain following an acute myocardial infarction. Fifty-two months later, the patient had recurrent angina. Angiography disclosed a left circumflex saphenous vein bypass graft narrowed 95 percent in diameter in its mid-portion (body) (Fig. 44–35). Balloon angioplasty resulted in increased luminal diameter. Two months later (54 months after graft insertion), a second balloon angioplasty procedure was performed for the restenosis at the previous angioplasty site.

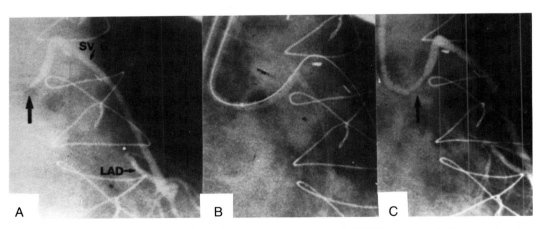

Fig. 44–31. Angiographic frames of a saphenous vein bypass graft (SVG) before and after transluminal balloon angioplasty (1 month before graft excision and 2 months after graft insertion). (**A**) Severe luminal narrowing of the bypass graft near the aortic anastomotic site (arrow). (**B**) Inflated angioplasty balloon located within the proximal SVG. (**C**) Marked increase in luminal diameter of graft following angioplasty (arrow). LAD, left anterior descending coronary artery. (From Waller et al.,[259] with permission.)

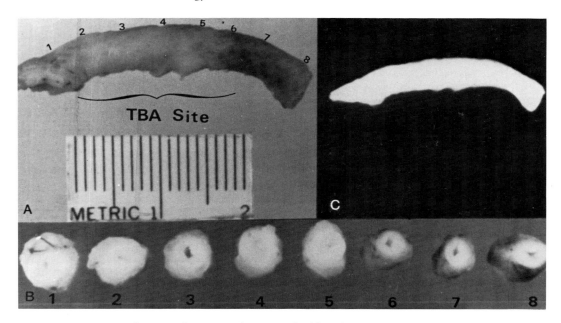

Fig. 44–32. Operatively excised portion of a 3-month-old saphenous vein graft. (**A**) Diameter of the proximal portion (aortic anastomotic end [1]) subjected to transluminal balloon angioplasty (TBA) is slightly wider than that of the distal nondilated segment. The numbers represent sites of transverse sections appearing in Fig. B and in Fig. 44–33. (**C**) Radiograph disclosed no calcific deposits. (From Waller et al.,[259] with permission.)

Multiple dilations again greatly improved graft luminal diameter (95 percent diameter reduction to 10 percent diameter reduction). During this angioplasty procedure, a localized dissection and crack (or fracture) was apparent at the angioplasty site (Fig. 44–35). Two months later (56 months after insertion and two previous balloon angioplasty procedures), the graft was again severely stenosed at the angioplasty site. Its mid-portion was excised.

Morphologic Features

The excised portion had foci of calcific deposits in the area of previous balloon angioplasty (Figs. 44–36 and 44–37). Its lumen was diffusely narrowed by variable degrees of intimal thickening. The maximal narrowing (in the area of angioplasty) consisted of foam cells, cholesterol clefts, fibrocollagenous tissue, foci of myofibroblasts, and calcific deposits characteristic of atherosclerotic plaque. Other areas of the graft were narrowed by predom-

inantly fibrocollagenous tissue. The site of angioplasty dissection (Figs. 44–37 and 44–38) showed partial separation of intima from media. This intimal flap had begun to reattach to the graft wall (healing of localized plaque tear).

Clinical-Morphologic Correlations in Saphenous Vein Graft Angioplasty

Each patient described above had one or more clinically successful percutaneous transluminal angioplasty dilations of a stenosed saphenous vein bypass graft early (2 months) or late (52 to 54 months) after graft insertion. *Angiographic similarities* between the early and late grafts included an increased luminal diameter associated with a decreased mean transtenotic gradient following angioplasty, and restenosis at the site of previous dilation 1 or 2 months later. *Angiographic differences* included the absence of cracks, breaks, or

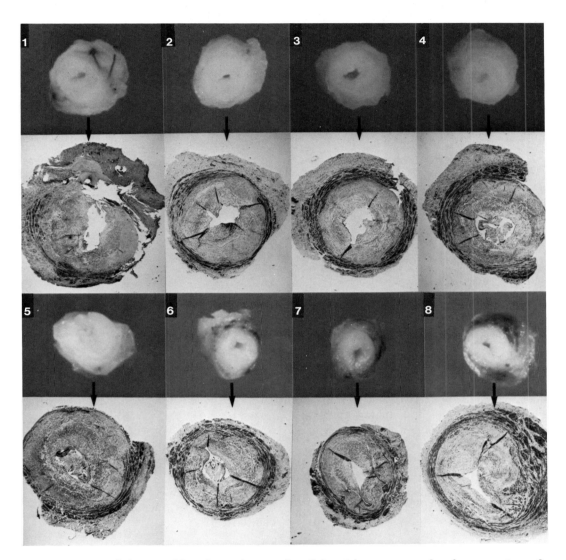

Fig. 44–33. Morphologic and histologic photographs of the eight segments of saphenous vein graft, corresponding to the sites labeled in Figure 43–32. Segments 1–6 are from the area of balloon inflation and dilation, and segments 7 and 8 are from nondilated portions of the graft (controls). Each segment had diffuse and severe cross-sectional area luminal narrowing by intimal thickening consisting of fibro-collagenous tissue. No segments contained atherosclerotic plaque or calcium deposits. No distinctive histologic changes were observed in the segments subjected to transluminal balloon angioplasty, compared with control segments. (Elastic van Gieson, × 6.) (From Waller et al.,[259] with permission.)

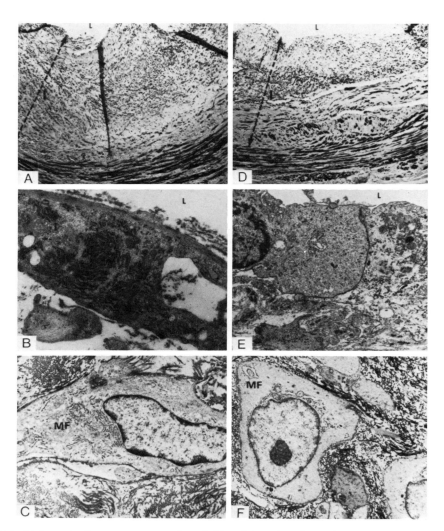

Fig. 44–34. Light and electron micrographs of dilated (**A–C**) and nondilated (**D–F**) portions of the saphenous vein graft (segments 2 and 8 from Figs. 44–32 and 44–33, respectively). Light micrographs of dilated (Fig. A) and nondilated (Fig. D) segments show that both segments have marked intimal thickening composed of smooth muscle cells and fibrocollagenous tissue. (Elastic × 40.) Electron micrographs at the luminal border of dilated (Fig. B) and nondilated (Fig. E) segments show a loss of endothelial cells, with micropinocytotic vesicles bordering the lumen (Fig. E). A short segment of basement membrane is visible at the lower right. (× 8,300.) Electron micrographs from deeper portions of the intimal thickening of the dilated (Fig. C), and nondilated (Fig. F) segments show similar types of myofibroblastic cells (MF) and dense bundles of collagen fibrils. (× 8,300.) (From Waller et al.,[259] with permission.)

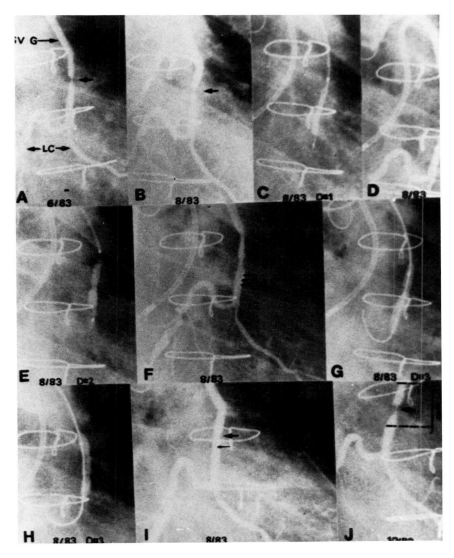

Fig. 44–35. Serial angiographic frames of a saphenous vein bypass graft (SVG) before and after two transluminal balloon angioplasty (TBA) procedures. (**A**) Severe luminal narrowing in the midportion of the SVG (arrow), 52 months after insertion. TBA (not shown) resulted in decreased luminal narrowing (from 95 percent to 20 percent). LC, left circumflex coronary artery. (**B**) Restenosis in graft, 2 months later at previous TBA site (arrow). (**C–I**) Second TBA, 54 months after insertion, showing serial dilations (D#1 to D#3) using progressively larger balloons, variable inflation pressures, and inflation durations. Figs. F and I show localized break, fracture, or dissection line at the site of TBA (small arrows). The second TBA resulted in decreased luminal narrowing (from 95 percent to 10 percent). (**J**) Restenosis of the graft 2 months later, (56 months after insertion) at the previous TBA sites. The boxed area indicates the operatively excised segment (Ex Sg) of the SVG. Month and year indicated in each frame. (From Waller et al.,[259] with permission.)

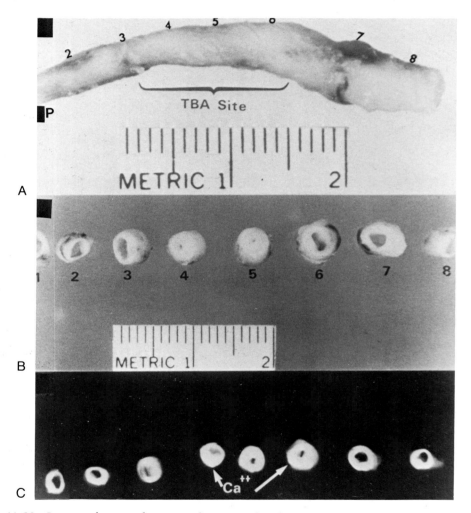

Fig. 44–36. Operatively excised portion of a 56-month-old saphenous vein graft. **(A)** Bracket indicates the site of two TBA procedures located in the mid-portion of the graft. P, proximal end. **(B)** Numbers represent sites of transverse sections (see also Fig. 44–38). **(C)** Radiograph of transverse section discloses foci of calcific deposits (Ca[++]). (From Waller et al.,[259] with permission.)

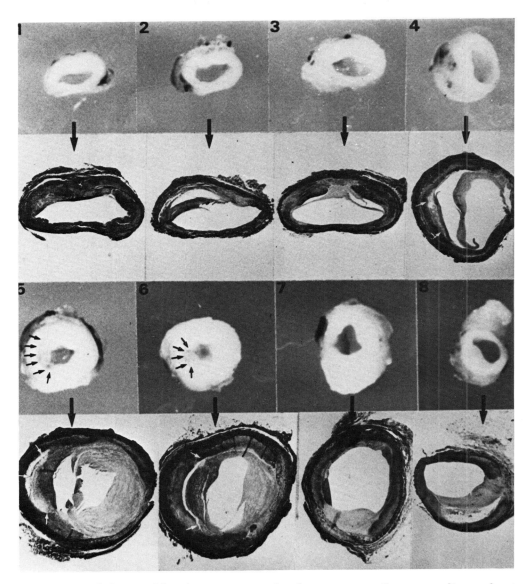

Fig. 44–37. Morphologic and histologic segments of saphenous vein graft corresponding to the sites labeled in Figure 44–36. Each segment shows diffuse but variable degrees of intimal thickening composed of atherosclerotic plaque. The segment with the most severe luminal narrowing (5) corresponds to the area of previous transluminal balloon angioplasty procedures (small arrows). (From Waller et al.,[259] with permission.)

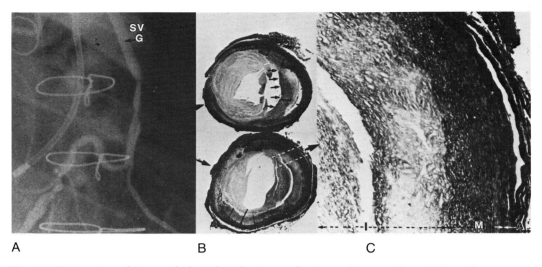

Fig. 44–38. Angiographic morphologic-histologic correlation at the site of angioplasty dissection, 2 months before graft excision. **(A)** Angiographic frame of saphenous vein bypass graft (SVG) after transluminal balloon angioplasty showing a line of dissection. **(B)** Corresponding morphologic segments (large arrows) of SVG in area of angiographic dissection showing severe luminal cross-sectional area narrowing with an intimal flap (small arrows) and a partially healed intimal fracture. **(C)** Higher magnification (× 80) of boxed area in Fig. B showing the intimal fracture site (I). The intimal thickening is composed of fibrocollagenous tissue, foam cells, and cholesterol clefts. M, media; A, adventitia. (Elastic stains.) (From Waller et al.,[259] with permission.)

splits following the second angioplasty in the early graft. An additional angiographic difference was the location of the stenosis. In the early graft, it was at the proximal end (aortic anastomosis), whereas in the late graft it was in the body of the graft (mid-portion). *Morphologic similarities* between grafts included diffuse intimal thickening by fibrocollagenous tissue with fibrotic medial and adventitial layers. *Morphologic differences* were distinctive: the early graft had a thickened intima without atherosclerotic plaque changes or calcific deposits and no morphologic evidence of previous dilations, whereas the late graft had thickened intima typical of atherosclerotic plaque with focal calcific deposits and morphologic evidence of balloon angioplasty injury.

Saber and colleagues[200] reported histologic changes in six grafts from five patients with graft ages ranging from 5 to 105 months (angioplasty to graft excision interval ranged from 6 hours to 24 months). Balloon angioplasty produced intimal fissures in three grafts initially obstructed by intimal fibromuscular pro-

liferation. Healing and restenosis resulted from filling of intimal lacerations with fibrocellular tissue and apparently also from restitution of muscular tone.[200] In two of three saphenous vein grafts narrowed by atherosclerotic plaque, balloon angioplasty caused extensive plaque rupture, and restenosis resulted from plaque debris and secondary luminal thrombosis. In the third graft, narrowed by atherosclerotic plaques, no distinctive lesions were found. Later restenosis in this graft was caused by progressive atherosclerosis. Evidence of embolization from atherosclerotic plaque was observed in 2 patients.

Therapeutic Implications for Saphenous Vein Angioplasty Derived from Morphologic Observations

The fate of an aortocoronary saphenous vein bypass graft appears to depend on several factors related to the interval from grafting to graft obstruction.[7,16,32,139,151,229,238,241,252,263] Graft occlusion developing within 1 month of insertion is almost invariably secondary to thrombosis related to technical factors, such as stenosis at aortic or coronary anastomotic sites, intraoperative vein trauma, or poor distal runoff secondary to severe atherosclerosis or reduced caliber of the distal native vessel.[33,193,245] These technical factors may limit the role of balloon angioplasty in successfully relieving saphenous vein graft obstruction occurring within 1 month of operation.

Functionally significant graft stenoses developing 1 month to 1 year after graft insertion are nearly always characterized by intimal thickening, histologically composed of cellular or acellular fibrocollagenous tissue. The venous medial and adventitial layers become fibrotic and the graft resembles a thick fibrous tube. Focally stenotic lesions produced appear amenable to dilation by balloon angioplasty, as illustrated in the first patient described above.[259] In view of the histologic composition of the intima, the dilating mechanism is probably not intimal compression or intimal fracture but, rather, graft stretching (Fig. 44–39). Depending on the degree of graft stretching, the dilating procedure may have limited therapeutic success (weeks or months), with graft restenosis representing gradual restitution of tone of an overstretched graft segment.

Saphenous vein graft stenoses occurring beyond 1 year and generally after 3 years following graft insertion usually consist of atherosclerotic plaque in addition to intimal fibrous thickening.[16,32,33,138,229] Atherosclerotic plaque in saphenous vein grafts appears histologically similar to that observed in native coronary arteries. They demonstrate foam cells, cholesterol clefts, blood product debris, fibrocollagenous tissue, and calcific deposits. This type of stenosis also appears amenable to dilation by balloon angioplasty, as illustrated in the second patient.[259] The mechanism of graft dilation in this setting appears to be similar to that proposed for coronary artery angioplasty, showing, for example, plaque splitting, cracking, or breaking with or without localized intimal-medial dissection (Fig. 44–40). Therapeutic limitations in dilating saphenous vein grafts narrowed by ath-

erosclerotic plaque should be similar to those observed in atherosclerotic coronary arteries subjected to TBA.

In addition to the age of a bypass graft, at least two other anatomic factors appear to influence the therapeutic success of balloon angioplasty in saphenous vein grafts: (1) length of stenosis, and (2) location of stenosis. Long stenotic segments (greater than 15 to 20 mm) are technically more difficult to dilate and are associated with a lower primary therapeutic success compared with short stenotic segments (up to 5 mm).[23] Graft stenoses may be located at the anastomotic sites (aorta or coronary grafts) or within the body of the graft (Fig. 44–40). Angiographic studies[23,63] suggest that dilation of graft stenoses at the coronary-graft anastomotic site have the best therapeutic results, followed by lesions in the graft body and at the aorta-graft anastomotic site. An anatomic factor supporting the relatively high success rate at dilating stenotic coronary-graft anastomotic sites is the presence of atherosclerotic plaque in the coronary portion of the anastomosis[258] (Fig. 44–40). Stenoses in the graft body or at aortic anastomotic site are less likely to have the potential angioplasty advantage of associated atherosclerotic plaque unless the graft is more than 3 years old. An additional adverse factor for successful dilation at the aortic anastomotic site is the presence of an aortic wall consisting of many layers of elastic fibers.[259]

In reporting thromboatheromatous emboli following balloon angioplasty of an aortocoronary bypass graft, Saber and colleagues[200] suggested that the plaques in vein grafts may be particularly vulnerable to disruption and to embolization of large fragments.

THROMBOLYSIS THERAPY FOR EVOLVING ACUTE MYOCARDIAL INFARCTION

Management of acute coronary thrombosis and evolving acute myocardial infarction (AMI) includes use of pharmacologic (strep-

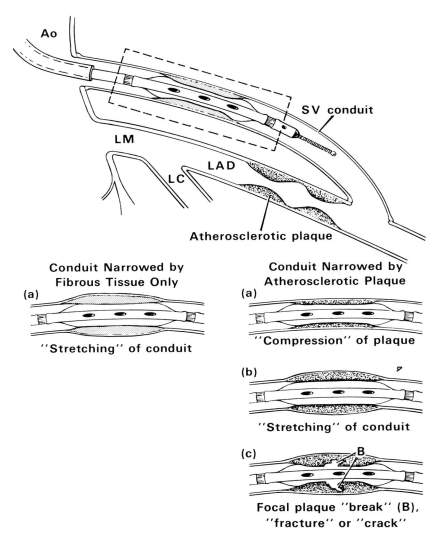

Fig. 44–39. Possible mechanisms of luminal balloon angiography in stenotic aortocoronary saphenous vein (SV) bypass grafts. Two types of lesions characterize SV stenoses, depending on the interval from graft insertion to early obstruction. Early (<1 year) grafts (a, left) contain intimal thickening composed primarily of fibrocollagenous tissue without calcium, and dilation is accomplished by conduit stretching. Late (>1 year) grafts (a,b,c right) contain intimal thickening composed of atherosclerotic plaque and calcium, and dilation is accomplished by "plaque compression" (unlikely), graft stretching, or plaque fracture or break (most likely). Ao, aorta; LAD, left anterior descending coronary artery; LC, left circumflex coronary artery; LM, left main coronary artery. (From Waller et al.,[259] with permission.)

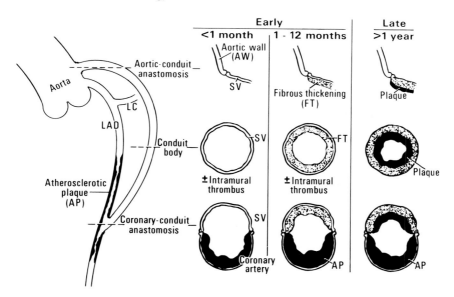

Fig. 44–40. Anatomic features of the saphenous vein (SV) bypass graft-native coronary artery unit with luminal changes developing with increasing graft age. Balloon angioplasty would be most successful in areas containing some element of atherosclerotic plaque (coronary-conduit anastomosis in the early and late grafts and the conduit body in the late grafts) and least successful in areas with primarily elastic tissue (aortic anastomotic sites). LAD, left anterior descending coronary artery; LC, left circumflex coronary artery. (From Waller,[246] with permission.)

tokinase, urokinase, tissue plasminogen activator), mechanical (balloon angioplasty, guide wire perforation), or combined therapies to re-establish coronary blood flow and limit infarct size.[245] Use of intracoronary thrombolytic therapy was first reported by Rentrop and colleagues[193] in 1979. The ability of this procedure to lyse an occlusive thrombus during the early hours of myocardial infarction has been confirmed by numerous subsequent studies[80,150,154,188,192] (Fig. 44–41). Streptokinase and urokinase were the first pharmacologic agents employed for this purpose. Intracoronary administration of streptokinase to patients with AMI results in recanalization of 60 to 94 percent of occluded arteries,[235] but streptokinase is not a perfect agent for this purpose. It is antigenic, has a relatively long half-life, has a low specificity for fibrin, and induces a generalized lytic state.[190] Interest has focused on the development of thrombolytic agents that would be

more specific and induce fewer systemic bleeding complications. Tissue plasminogen activator (now available in recombinant form), urokinase-type plasminogen activator (prourokinase), and acylated streptokinase-plasmogen complex are being evaluated to achieve therapeutic coronary thrombolysis with increased safety. Using percutaneous balloon angioplasty, Hartzler and associates[90,91] have taken a mechanical approach to acute coronary thrombolysis, avoiding the systemic lytic effects of currently available pharmacologic agents and treating the underlying severely stenosed coronary artery at the same procedure. Other strategies have combined both therapies, using pharmacologic therapy followed by balloon angioplasty[65,81,183,218] or balloon angioplasty followed by smaller doses of streptokinase.[90,91]

Despite widespread use of thrombolysis therapy, few autopsy observations regarding

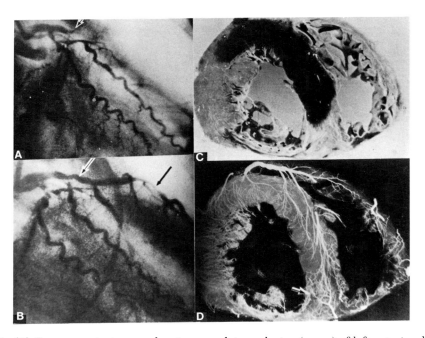

Fig. 44–41. (A) Coronary arteriogram showing complete occlusion (arrow) of left anterior descending artery prior to treatment with streptokinase. **(B)** Coronary arteriogram after streptokinase administration showing reopening of lumen of artery at site of previous occlusion (black and white arrow). Note point of marked distal narrowing (black arrow). **(C)** Upper surface of basal slice of ventricles showing severe hemorrhage (black) in anterior and septal regions of left ventricle. **(D)** Radiograph of slice in Fig. C, illustrating left anterior descending artery (LAD) (bottom) and bed supplied by this vessel. Note correspondence to hemorrhagic region in Fig. C. Arrows in Fig. D indicate margins of bed of LAD. (From Kao et al.,[116] with permission.)

myocardium or coronary arteries have been reported[19,77,88,98,108,116,154,155,165,210,235,239,269] (Figs. 44–42 to 44–55). With the exception of two cases,[153,165] all observations have been in patients receiving either streptokinase[19,88,98,108,116,154,155,210,239] or urokinase.[77,269] Some reports describe causes of death but do not provide autopsy data.[82,90,92,141,144,210,215,235] In 13 reports that include autopsy data, 99 patients received acute thrombolysis therapy (Table 44–3). Of these 66 patients (68 percent) received streptokinase alone, 31 (31 percent) received urokinase alone, and 2 (2 percent) received streptokinase plus balloon angioplasty.[153,165] Detailed information on the two patients who received combined pharmacologic and mechanical therapy was not provided. No reports have yet described autopsy findings in patients who had mechanical thrombolysis therapy alone, tissue-plasminogen activator thrombolysis therapy alone, or tissue plasminogen activator therapy combined with balloon angioplasty.

Clinical and morphologic information is incomplete for these 99 patients (see Table 44–3). In nine studies,[19,77,98,116,153,155,210,239,269] information was provided on the status of the myocardium. Of 93 patients, 43 (46 percent) had a hemorrhagic infarct. Explanations for the lack of hemorrhage in the remaining hearts were not provided. Eleven reports[19,77,88,98,108,116,153–155,210,239,269] included some information on the status of the treated coronary artery: 28 patients had residual thrombus and 46 had underlying atherosclerotic plaque of varying severity.

Fujiwara and colleagues[77] reported on 30

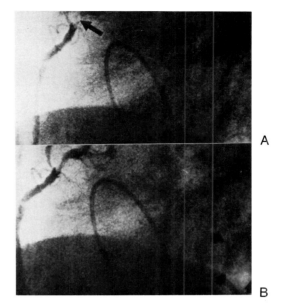

A

B

Fig. 44-42. Angiographic recognition of myocardial hemorrhage. (**A**) Initial right coronary arteriogram in the left anterior oblique projection showing subtotal occlusion at the proximal portion (arrow) and delayed distal flow. (**B**) Arteriogram after nitroglycerin infusion showing extravasation of the contrast medium at the inferoposterior wall of the left ventricle (see Fig. 44-43). (From Yasuno et al.,[269] with permission.)

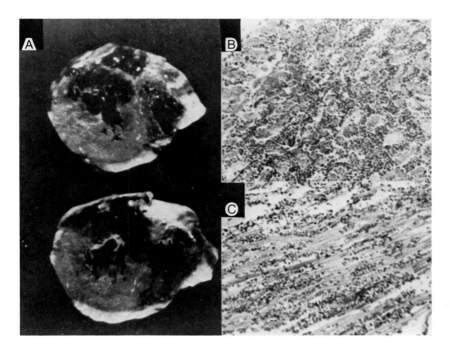

Fig. 44-43. Autopsy documentation of angiographically recognized hemorrhagic infarction during streptokinase thrombolysis therapy. (**A**) Transverse slices of the heart from the patient. Severe hemorrhagic transmural infarct is seen in the inferoposterior wall of the left ventricle. (**B,C**) Microscopic findings in the hemorrhagic infarct. Note coagulation necrosis of the myocytes and marked hemorrhage. (H&E, × 200.) (From Yasuno et al.,[269] with permission.)

Table 44–3. Clinical and Morphologic Findings in 99 Autopsy Cases from 13 Previous Reports with AMI Undergoing Acute Thrombolysis Therapy[a,b]

Observation	Schachenmayr & Haferkamp[210] (n = 6)	Berry[19] (n = 27)	Verstraete et al.[239] (n = 14)	Mathey et al.[153] (n = 3)	Meyer et al.[165] (n = 1)
1. Age, yr (mean)	43–67 (59)	—	—	71,	67
2. Sex	5M:1F	—	—	—	M
3. Location of AMI	—	—	8A, 2P, 1 UK	2A, 1P	—
4. Infarct vessel	1B, ILC, 3 LAD	—	—		
5. Interval of onset symptoms to reperfusion, hr	—	—			
6. Angiographically successful thrombolysis	—	—	—	0	
7. Interval of onset symptoms to death, days	0.08–5 (1.4)	—	—	2[d]	2
8. Thrombolysis method(s) (dose)	S (IV)	S (IV)	S (IV)	S	S
S/U	1–5 mil	2.5 mil	1.45 mil	[c]	160,000
S with FICA	0	0	0	0	+
9. Type of AMI					
Hemorrhagic	3	3 (11%)	3[g]	—	—
Anemic	2[h]	24 (89)	11	—	—
10. Histology of infarct coronary artery					
Residual thrombus Occlusive	4	11	9	1 / 1	[i] / —
Underlying atherosclerotic plaque	5	25	4	2	—

[a] Sixty-four streptokinase, 31 urokinase, 2 streptokinase with percutaneous transluminal coronary angioplasty (PTCA).

[b] One patient had an anterior and posterior infarct of similar age, one with and one without reperfusion.

[c] Delayed thrombolysis, detected on postmortem coronary angiogram.

[d] 1.5 Million U IV, followed by selective intracoronary infusion, 2,000–4,000 U/min.

[e] Of 27 hearts, 4 had myocardial rupture.

[f] Of 14 patients, 7 had myocardial rupture.

[g] Reperfusion in only 3 of 7 patients, including 1 of 2 with hemorrhagic infarct.

[h] Cardiac rupture.

[i] Angiographically recognized.

[j] Includes patients with slight, moderate, or marked bleeding (with moderate or marked called hemorrhagic infarct).

[k] Both died during administration of streptokinase with less than 1.3 million U infused. One patient with hemorrhagic infarct had cardiac rupture.

[l] Three of 5 patients with 3 hours of streptokinase infusion; 2 patients died 12 and 14 months, respectively, after streptokinase therapy.

[m] Simply described as "patient."

[n] Uncertain whether 5 findings represent angiographic or autopsy findings.

[o] Intraplaque hemorrhage in three, coronary artery dissection in 1. Abbreviations: A, anterior; AMI, acute myocardial infarction; C, combination; LC, left circumflex; LAD, left anterior descending; mil, million; P, posterior; UK, unknown; S, streptokinase; U, urokinase.

(From Waller,[245] with permission.)

Mathey et al.[154] (n = 6)	Isner et al. (n = 1)	Mattfeldt et al.[155] (n = 7)	Harrison et al.[88] (n = 1)	Hollander et al.[98] (n = 1)	Yasuno et al.[269] (n = 1)	Kao et al.[116] (n = 1)	Fujiwara et al.[77] (n = 30)
44–77 (67)	66	32–70 (56)	—	61	83	37	45–93 (68)
4M:2F	F	5M:2F	—	M	M	M	17M:13F
3P, 3A[b]	A	—	—	A	P	A	21A, 7P, 2L
2B, 1 LC, 3 LAD	LAD	3 LAD, 3B, 1 LC	—	LAD	R	LAD	
1.7–3.5 (2.9)		3.5–5.5	—	1	2.5	5	2–9 (4)
6	0[c]	3/7	—	c	c	c	
	1–9 (6)	0.35	0.25–21	—	0.54	0.62	1.24 Hr–12 Mo
S[e]	S	S	S	S	U	S	U
175,000–250,000	380,000	7[f]	—	100,000	240,000	380,000	240,000–1.2 mil
1	0	0	—	0	0	0	0
4	—	2[i]	—	j	k		25 (83%)[l]
2	—	5	—	0	0	0	5 (17%)[n]
0 (5)							
c (1)	c	1	c	0	—	0	—[h]
—	0	1	—		—		—
	c	6/6[o]	—	c	c	c	—

autopsies studied after selective intracoronary thrombolysis with urokinase. Three stages of infarcts were identified based on hours after the thrombolysis therapy. Hearts of patients in stage II (infarcts 9 hours to 11 days after thrombolysis therapy) had hemorrhagic infarction (15 of 18 hearts). These investigators concluded that myocardial hemorrhage increases gradually after thrombolysis, becoming moderately or markedly diffuse after 4 hours, and is apparently replaced by fibrous tissue after 3 to 4 weeks. The hemorrhagic infarct was caused by the combined effects of reperfusion and large doses of urokinase.

Analysis According to Type of Reperfusion Therapy

Waller and colleagues[260] reported autopsy observations in 19 cases in which various forms of acute reperfusion therapy have been given; 9 had received streptokinase (Figs. 44–44 and 44–45); 3, streptokinase plus percutaneous transluminal coronary angioplasty (PTCA) (Figs. 44–47 to 44–50); 1 patient, streptokinase plus guide wire perforation of clot; 1, recombinant tissue plasminogen activator (tPA) plus PTCA (Fig. 44–51); and 5, PTCA only (Fig. 44–46) (Table 44–3).[250] Patients who

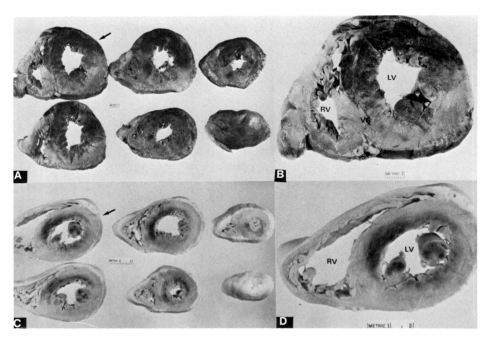

Fig. 44–44. Thrombolysis therapy with streptokinase alone. (**A,B**) Ventricular slices from hearts of two patients undergoing thrombolysis therapy with streptokinase infusion, showing extensive hemorrhagic infarct. (**C,D**) Ventricular slices indicated by arrows in Figs. A and B. LV, left ventricle; RV, right ventricle; VS, ventricular septum. (From Waller et al.,[245] with permission.)

received combined forms of reperfusion therapy (PTCA plus a lytic agent) had an acute PTCA initially, followed within minutes by intracoronary streptokinase or tPA. The interval from onset of symptoms to clinical or angiographic evidence of coronary reperfusion ranged from 2.5 to 4.5 hours. At autopsy, all 19 had transmural AMI. Observations separated the 19 patients into two distinct groups based on changes in the myocardium: 14 (74 percent) had hemorrhagic myocardial infarction (Figs. 44–44, 44–45, 44–47 to 44–51) and 5 (26 percent) had nonhemorrhagic (anemic) infarction (Fig. 44–46). Each of the 14 patients with a hemorrhagic infarct had been treated with pharmacologic (9 with streptokinase) or combined forms of reperfusion therapy (1 tPA plus PTCA, 1 streptokinase plus guide wire, three streptokinase plus PTCA). The 5 anemic infarcts were in hearts of patients who re-

ceived purely mechanical reperfusion therapy (PTCA).

Among patients who had received streptokinase therapy, hemorrhagic infarcts were grossly and histologically similar in nine who had received streptokinase only (Figs. 44–44 and 44–45), in three with combined streptokinase and balloon angioplasty (Figs. 44–47 to 44–50), and in the one who had received streptokinase and in whom guide wire perforation of coronary thrombus had been attempted. The hemorrhagic infarct in the patient who had received tPA was grossly and histologically comparable to those observed in patients who had received streptokinase therapy (Fig. 44–51).

Among the fourteen hearts with hemorrhagic infarction, no morphologic or histologic difference was apparent in the extent of hemorrhage with respect to the interval from onset

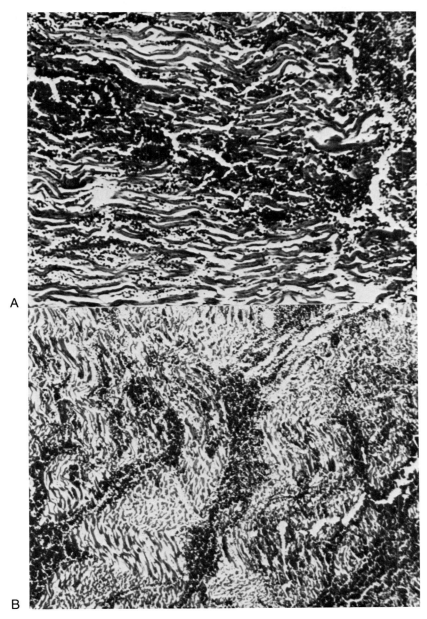

Fig. 44–45. (A,B) Histology sections from patients with streptokinase reperfusion showing extensive sheets of interstitial erythrocytes among necrotic myocardial fibers. (From Waller et al.,[260] with permission.)

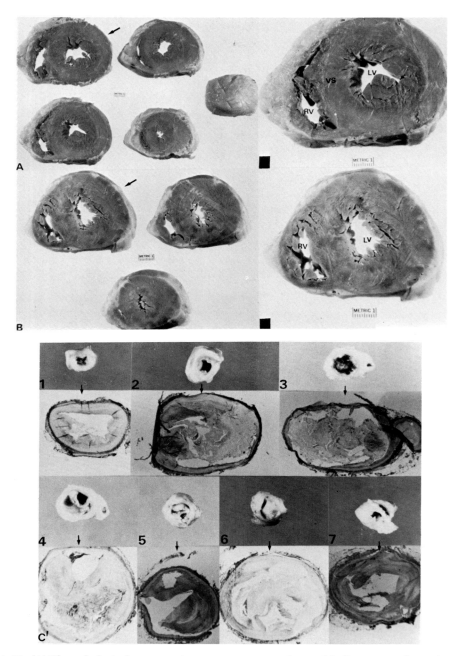

Fig. 44–46. (**A**) Thrombolysis therapy with percutaneous transluminal balloon angioplasty alone. (**A,B**) Ventricular slices from hearts of two patients receiving thrombolysis therapy with balloon angioplasty. Both hearts show a hemorrhagic infarct. Arrows indicate ventricular slice shown to the right. LV, left ventricle; RV, right ventricle (**C**) One through eight form a composite of cross sections of the left anterior descending coronary artery from the case seen in Fig. A. They show atherosclerotic plaque "cracks" and localized medial dissection (segment 5) from the balloon angioplasty. Segment 3 shows residual proximal thrombus. Histology sections correspond to macroscopic pictures. (From Waller et al.,[260] with permission.)

of symptoms to clinical reperfusion. Myocardial infarct hemorrhage in patients with reperfusion by 3.5 hours or less (range 2.5 to 3.5, mean 3.3) was qualitatively similar in extent and severity to myocardial hemorrhage in patients with reperfusion of 3.6 hours or longer (range 4.0 to 4.5, mean 4.2). One heart demonstrated only traces of myocardial hemorrhage suggesting either temporary or partial reperfusion, or both (Fig. 44–52). During systemic streptokinase administration, the patient had experienced a transient decrease in chest pain and ST-segment elevation, followed by a fatal, sudden ventricular fibrillation 72 hours later. At autopsy, the infarct-related right coronary artery was found to be occluded by severe atherosclerotic plaque and residual thrombus, explaining the myocardial observation of limited hemorrhagic necrosis from temporary and partial reperfusion.

Myocardial Histology

Histology sections from the central infarct zones showed coagulative necrosis involving myofibers and interstitial vessels (Figs. 44–45 and 44–49). In the 14 hearts with hemorrhagic infarction, the interstitial space was packed with extravasated erythrocytes. By contrast, histologic sections from the central infarct zones of three of five hearts with anemic infarcts disclosed scattered foci of erythrocytes confined to the zone of coagulative necrosis.

Clinical factors such as the use of intracoronary versus intravenous streptokinase infusion, of streptokinase versus tPA, or of purely lytic agents versus combined lytic agent plus PTCA did not alter the occurrence or appearance of hemorrhagic infarction. In view of the grossly anemic myocardial infarcts associated with PTCA only, the common denominator for patients with hemorrhagic myocardial infarction appears to be related to the lytic effects of the pharmacologic reperfusion agents, rather than a direct effect of the coronary reperfusion (Figs. 44–54 and 44–55).

Infarct Coronary Artery

In 19 autopsy subjects, the left anterior descending was the infarct artery in 13; the right vessel in four; the left main in one, and the left circumflex in one. In 16 hearts, residual thrombus was present at the site of previous occlusion and in 9 hearts, it was occlusive (Fig. 44–48). All reperfusion arteries had more than 50 percent cross-sectional area narrowing by pre-existing atherosclerotic plaque at the site of previous occlusion, and 10 had 76 to 100 percent cross-sectional area narrowing.

Intraplaque Hemorrhage and Plaque Rupture in the Infarct-Related Artery

The nine patients receiving acute angioplasty reperfusion therapy can be separated into two subgroups: those treated with angioplasty alone and those treated with angioplasty and thrombolytic agents. In the five treated by angioplasty alone, the site of angioplasty had plaque fractures and cracks without intimal or medial hemorrhage. In one patient, the fracture extended into the adventitia and caused coronary artery rupture. By contrast, four patients treated with angioplasty plus thrombolytic therapy had at the site of angioplasty, plaque fractures and cracks with hemorrhage involving the intimal, medial, and adventitial layers. In one, the hemorrhage was so extensive that it narrowed the coronary lumen at the angioplasty site (Figs. 44–47). In 10 patients receiving streptokinase therapy alone, intraplaque hemorrhage was absent. Thus, the use of combined angioplasty and thrombolytic agents in acute reperfusion therapy may produce localized bleeding at the angioplasty site, and the bleeding may cause additional luminal narrowing.

Hemorrhagic Infarct

Hemorrhagic infarct in association with surgical procedures requiring cardiopulmonary bypass has been recognized at autopsy for more than 20 years. Ten years ago, it was described with aortocoronary bypass surgery

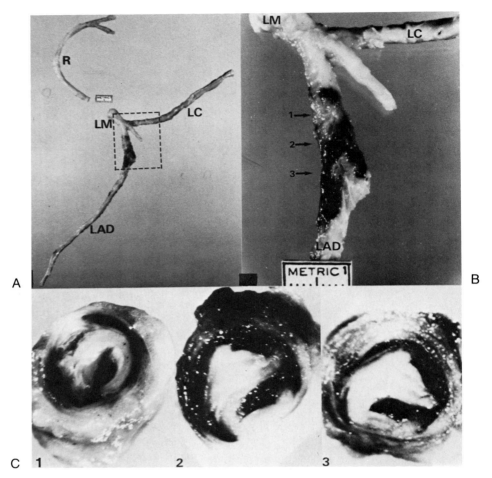

Fig. 44–47. Thrombolysis therapy with combined balloon angioplasty plus streptokinase. (**A,B**) Coronary arterial site of balloon angioplasty showing marked adventitial hemorrhage. Numbers in Fig. B correspond to (**C**) sites of cross sections. 1, prominent atherosclerotic plaque "crack" with surrounding hemorrhage; 2,3, marked bleeding into area of angioplasty severely narrows the coronary lumen. LAD, left anterior descending; LC, left circumflex; LM, left main; R, right coronary artery. (Figs. A through C from Waller et al.,[258] with permission.) (*Figure continues.*)

performed on patients with unrecognized preoperative evolving acute myocardial infarction or in patients with postoperative infarction.[102,140] More recently, management of acute coronary thrombosis and evolving acute myocardial infarction with various thrombolytic agents has been associated with hemorrhagic infarct.[19,34,77,98,116,154,155,210,239,260,269]

An infarction is defined as hemorrhagic if grossly visible blood is found within the myocardium at necropsy examination. Histologically, the hemorrhagic zones consist of extensive coagulative necrosis with interwoven sheets or pools of interstitial erythrocytes (Figs. 44–45 and 44–49). Focal areas of scattered interstitial erythrocytes present histologically within an area of myocardial necrosis do not produce grossly visible hemorrhagic infarct.[260]

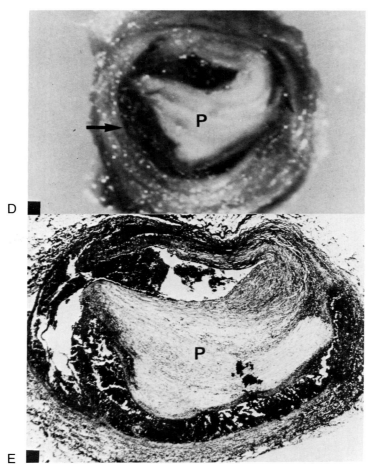

Fig. 44–47 (*Continued*). (**D**) Closeup of angioplasty site. Prominent plaque (P) crack with surrounding hemorrhage (arrow). (**E**) Histologic section of segment shows medial dissection and extensive adventitial blood. (Figs. D and E from Waller et al.,[245] with permission.)

Hemorrhagic infarct has been observed in about one-half of patients with acute reperfusion therapy for evolving myocardial infarction[14] (Table 44–3). In our study,[260] all patients receiving reperfusion with a thrombolytic agent (rTPA, streptokinase) with or without acute angioplasty had a hemorrhagic infarct (Figs. 44–54 and 44–55; Table 44–4).

As described previously, Fujiwara and co-workers[77] concluded that myocardial hemorrhage increases gradually after acute thrombolytic therapy, becoming moderately or markedly diffuse after 4 hours. They speculated that hemorrhagic infarct is a result of the combined effects of reperfusion and large doses of urokinase. Mathey et al.[154] described transmural, hemorrhagic myocardial infarction after intracoronary streptokinase in six patients who died 1 to 18 days after thrombolytic therapy. These investigators suggested that sudden reperfusion after three to four hours of coronary artery occlusion was a major determinant and that hemorrhage probably was not the consequence of streptokinase

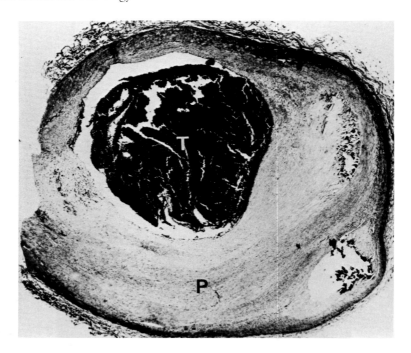

Fig. 44–48. Residual occluding thrombus in patient illustrated in Fig. 44–47. The artery is severely narrowed by atherosclerotic plaque (P) and thrombus (T). (From Waller,[245] with permission.)

use, as such. Colavita and colleagues[39] autopsied the hearts from four patients who had undergone balloon angioplasty and streptokinase reperfusion therapy 6 hours to 4 days before death. Two of the four hearts exhibited hemorrhagic infarct. In one of the remaining two hearts, the lack of hemorrhage in the area of infarction was explained by an occluded artery preventing the effects of reperfusion.[39]

Hemorrhagic Infarct Without Reperfusion

Hemorrhagic infarcts frequently coincide with reperfusion efforts during an evolving AMI or during aortocoronary bypass grafting; myocardial hemorrhage in acute myocardial infarction without intervening thrombolysis or revascularization therapy is unusual. Among 119 patients with fatal acute myocar-

dial infarction for whom the preceding interventions had not been performed, three (2 percent) had hemorrhagic infarcts.[245] In one patient, overwhelming sepsis with disseminated intravascular coagulation (DIC) developed, during repair of an abdominal aortic aneurysm. The coagulation abnormality may have provided a "natural" thrombolytic state similar to that induced therapeutically (Fig. 44–53). Reasons for the other two hemorrhagic infarcts were unknown. Mathey and associates[154] found a hemorrhagic infarct in none of 200 autopsied patients with fatal acute myocardial infarction without interventional therapy. Of 60 autopsied patients with acute myocardial infarction and without thrombolytic therapy studied by Fujiwara and colleagues, two (3 percent) had moderate diffuse hemorrhage (hemorrhagic infarct).[77]

To my knowledge, only two patients have been described in whom the clinical diagnosis of hemorrhagic infarct was made after acute thrombolytic therapy.[142,269] Little and Rogers[142] reported angiographic evidence of intramyocardial contrast pooling (representing interstitial extravasation of erythrocytes) after successful streptokinase therapy. The patient's condition subsequently deteriorated with infarct extension. Autopsy documentation of hemorrhagic infarct was not provided. Yasuno and colleagues[269] suggested stopping thrombolytic therapy if angiographic evidence of hemorrhagic infarct is observed (Figs. 44–42 and 44–43).

Significance of Hemorrhagic Myocardial Infarction

Debate continues as to whether hemorrhage within zones of necrosis delays[154] or accelerates[3] healing of infarcted myocardium or expands or accelerates myocardial necrosis.[129] Mathey and colleagues[154] described a patient with two infarcts of equal age in whom one infarct-related artery was reperfused and the other was not; at autopsy, the reperfused artery was associated with a hemorrhagic infarct and the nonreperfused artery with an anemic infarct. Distinct histologic differences were noted between the hemorrhagic and anemic infarcts in terms of removal of necrotic tissue and replacement by connective tissue. The hemorrhagic infarct showed no evidence of repair after 18 days, whereas the anemic infarct showed typical resorption and repair by granulation tissue. This difference indicated a marked delay in the usual healing process in the hemorrhagic infarct.[154]

Experimental and Clinical Differences

Experimental studies in rats, dogs, and pigs have been performed to define potential benefits and hazards of acute myocardial reperfusion. The results are divergent in areas of hemorrhagic infarct, infarct size reduction or expansion, wall-motion changes, and altered survival. Some investigators found hemor-

rhagic infarct confined to areas of necrosis, sparing the subepicardial zone (i.e., subendocardial infarction), and no evidence of infarct expansion.[3,34,37,71,113,122,124,189,197] Others[13,30,51,129] have suggested that myocardial hemorrhage is not strictly confined to the necrotic zone and that infarct expansion may occur with interstitial hemorrhage. Application of experimental reperfusion studies to humans has limitations with regard to the animal model used, the nature of coronary artery occlusion (coronary ligation versus occlusion by atherosclerotic plaque and thrombus), presence or absence of collateral circulation, and the rate of occlusion (slow versus fast). As a consequence, at least two major differences exist between hemorrhagic myocardial infarcts observed in humans and those observed in experimental animals. First, in patients the hemorrhagic infarction is transmural and not subendocardial, as described in animals. Second, extension of hemorrhage into areas of noninfarcted myocardium has been observed in autopsies and may not be confined to the central necrotic zone, as is described in most experimental models.[71,72,113,123]

Potential Effects on Functional Recovery

Significant improvement in left ventricular function after acute coronary reperfusion with streptokinase was not observed in several controlled trials of intracoronary or intravenous streptokinase therapy.[5,119,121,149,175] Only one study using intracoronary streptokinase in acute infarction showed improvement in serially assessed left ventricular ejection fraction. By contrast, comparing the use of intracoronary streptokinase and PTCA during evolving acute myocardial infarction, O'Neill and et al.[176] showed that left ventricular ejection fraction significantly improved during serial testing in the angioplasty-treated group but not in the streptokinase-treated group. These investigators also noted that residual luminal stenosis in the infarct-related artery was significantly greater angiographically after angioplasty than after streptokinase ther-

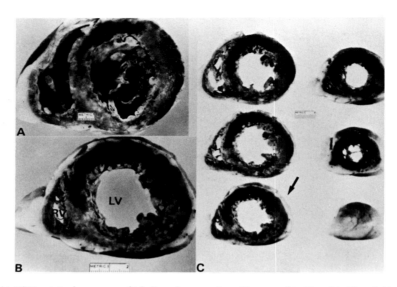

Fig. 44–49. (**A,B**) Ventricular myocardial slices from patient illustrated in Fig. 44–48 and 44–49. Markedly hemorrhagic infarct is present from base to apex. RV, right ventricle; LV, left ventricle. (**C**) Slice illustrated in Fig. B (arrow). (*Figure continues.*)

apy. O'Neill and co-workers suggested that acute angioplasty is significantly more effective than streptokinase infusion in alleviating the underlying coronary stenosis and that this may result in a more effective preservation of left ventricular function after acute reperfusion therapy. The striking difference between hemorrhagic infarcts present in our thrombolytic group compared with the anemic infarcts in our angioplasty group suggests that myocardial hemorrhage may be a factor determining a poor clinical improvement in left ventricular function in streptokinase-treated patients. However, additional factors, such as the time between onset of infarction and clinical reperfusion, the presence of collateral circulation, and the altered contractility of noninfarcted myocardium in the acute and follow-up state, may contribute.

Failure of Clot Lysis

Limited angiographic observations and few autopsy data are available in patients with streptokinase-resistant intracoronary thrombus. In 6 to 23 percent of patients with acute myocardial infarction, a totally occlusive intracoronary thrombus has been reported to persist despite administration of strepto-

kinase.[80,82,153,193] Autopsy studies have been limited to two patients.[108,153] Mathey and associates[108] described a 71-year-old patient in whom 2 hours of intracoronary steptokinase infusion had failed to reopen a totally occluded right coronary artery. At autopsy, the artery showed persistent occlusion caused by the superimposition of thrombus on severe atherosclerotic plaque. Isner and colleagues[153] studied a 66-year-old woman with a persistently occluded left anterior descending artery but severe narrowing by atherosclerotic plaque. These investigators interpreted this finding as evidence of "delayed" thrombolysis.

Distal Embolization of Atherosclerotic Plaque and/ or Thrombus During Balloon Angioplasty or Reperfusion Procedures

Balloon Angioplasty of Coronary Arteries

Embolic complications during or immediately following balloon angioplasty of stenosed coronary arteries have been mentioned

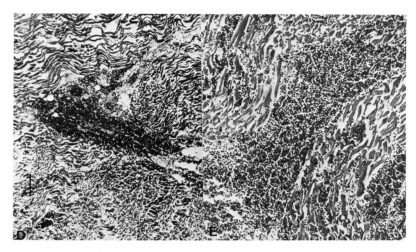

Fig. 44–49 (*Continued*). (**D,E**) Histologic sections showing severe interstitial hemorrhage with marked myocardial necrosis. (From Waller,[245] with permission.)

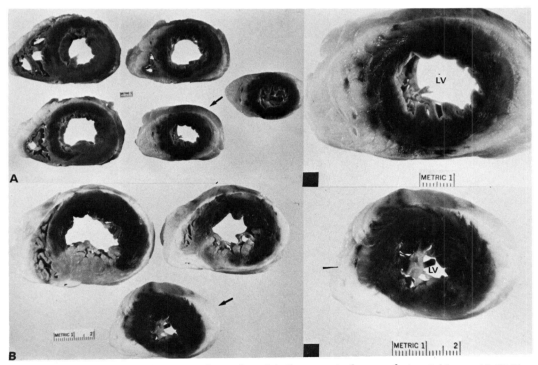

Fig. 44–50. Thrombolysis therapy with combined balloon angioplasty and streptokinase. (**A,B**) Two patients with combined therapy demonstrate severe hemorrhagic infarct. Compare these findings with those in Fig. 44–45 (streptokinase alone) and Fig. 44–47 (balloon angioplasty alone). Arrows indicate slices shown to the right. LV, left ventricle. (From Waller et al.,[260] with permission.)

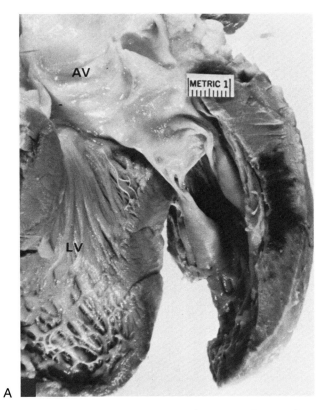
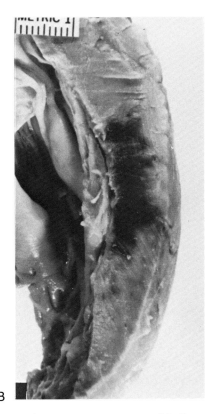

A   B

Fig. 44–51. (A,B) Thrombolysis therapy with recombinant tissue plasminogen activator and balloon angioplasty. Hemorrhagic infarct present in anterior left ventricular (LV) free wall. The patient died with artery rupture. AV, aortic valve. (From Waller et al.,[260] with permission.)

above. They are reported in experimental animals[24] and in 0.06 to 1.0 percent of patients.[44,57,87,97,120,135] Pathologic documentation has been provided in only two patients.[39,52]

Acute Reperfusion Therapy

Although angiographic evidence of distal coronary thromboembolism has been alluded to[91] or specifically excluded[81] during acute thrombolysis therapy, one report documented the final location of fragments of thrombus angiographically observed to stream distally. Menke and colleagues[164] studied at autopsy a 44-year-old patient who had histologic evidence of distal embolization after proximal left main artery thrombolysis therapy. Sections of the anterolateral papillary muscle disclosed several intramyo-

cardial coronary arteries occluded by thrombotic material identical in composition to that remaining in the left main artery (Fig. 44–56). In a study of 78 patients with AMI treated with coronary angioplasty (with and without previous streptokinase infusion), Hartzler and colleagues[91] rarely observed distal coronary embolization; when observed, it was without apparent clinical consequence. Gold and associates[81] performed coronary angioplasty in 28 patients with acute myocardial infarction immediately after intracoronary streptokinase infusion and reported no angiographic evidence of distal embolization of clot.

The consequences of distal migration of thrombus fragmented during pharmacologic or mechanical thrombolysis therapy for evolving myocardial infarction remain uncertain;

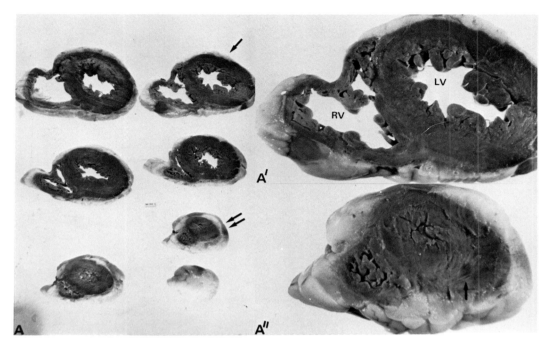

Fig. 44–52. Thrombolysis therapy with systemic streptokinase. In contrast with Fig. 44–45 and 44–59 which show hemorrhagic infarct with streptokinase therapy (solely or combined), the ventricular myocardium has only a hint of hemorrhage (double arrow) near the apex. Cross sections of the right coronary artery show total occlusion by atherosclerotic plaque and thrombus. The explanation for the absence of hemorrhagic infarct with streptokinase is unsuccessful reperfusion. (**A′**) Slice indicated by single arrow in Fig. A. (**A″**) Slice indicated by double arrow in Fig. A. LV, left ventricle; RV, right ventricle. (From Waller,[245] with permission.)

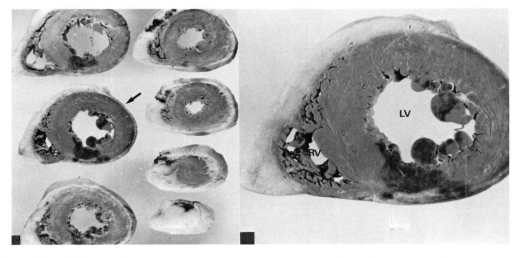

Fig. 44–53. (**A**) Hemorrhagic myocardial infarction in a patient without thrombolysis therapy in whom disseminated intravascular coagulation (DIC) developed from sepsis. The patient reperfused with the altered coagulation in the DIC process. (**B**) Closeup of slice indicated by arrow in Fig. A. LV, left ventricle; RV, right ventricle. (From Waller,[245] with permission.)

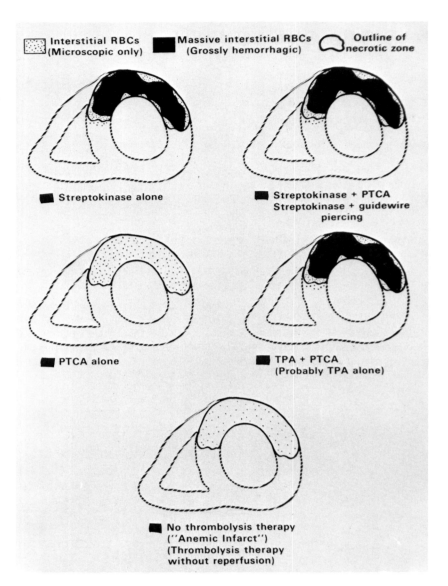

Fig. 44–54. Comparison of myocardial responses to various forms of thrombolysis therapy. Much of the hemorrhage is confined to the necrotic zone, but interstitial hemorrhage may be present in border zones, potentially compromising interstitial vascular channels. PTCA, percutaneous transluminal coronary angioplasty; TPA, tissue plasminogen activator. (From Waller et al.,[245] with permission.)

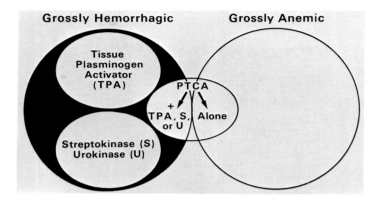

Fig. 44–55. Myocardial response in acute myocardial infarction (AMI) with various forms of acute thrombolysis therapy. PTCA, percutaneous transluminal coronary angioplasty. (From Waller,[245] with permission.)

they may be similar to those of primary coronary embolism.[195,251] In that situation, the smaller the embolus, the greater the chance that it will travel distally and lodge in a small coronary artery. Conversely, the larger the embolus, the greater the likelihood that it will impact proximally in a large coronary artery. An embolus so small that it occludes a single intramural coronary artery and is observed at autopsy by histologic examination alone is probably of limited clinical significance, whereas a larger embolus may occlude multiple intramural vessels and produce new or added myocardial dysfunction. In the setting of an evolving myocardial infarction, migration of a single small fragment of thrombus

Table 44–4.   Observations at Autopsy in 19 Patients with Acute Infarction Undergoing Reperfusion Therapies

Observation	Streptokinase Only (n = 9)	PTCA Only (n = 5)	S + PTCA (n = 3)	S + Guide Wire (n = 1)	tPA + PTCA (n = 1)
Type transmural infarct					
Anemic	0	5	0	0	0
Hemorrhagic	9[a]	0	3	+	+
Histology of AMI					
Contraction and necrosis	9	5	3	+	+
Coagulation necrosis	9	4	3	+	+
Interstitial necrosis	9	4	3	+	+
Interstitial extravasated RBC	4 + = 8	1	4 + = 3	4 +	4 +
(0–4 +)	1 + = 1	$\frac{1}{2}$ + = 1			
		1 + = 2			
		0 = 3			
Massive (grossly visible)	8	0	3	+	+
Focal (microscopic only)	1	3	0	0	0
Extravasated RBC limited to necrotic zone	6/10	3/3	3/3	0	+

[a] Minute trace of hemorrhage present grossly in one patient.
Abbreviations: AMI, acute myocardial infarction; PTCA, percutaneous transluminal coronary angioplasty; RBC, red blood cells; S, streptokinase; tPA, recombinant tissue plasminogen activator.

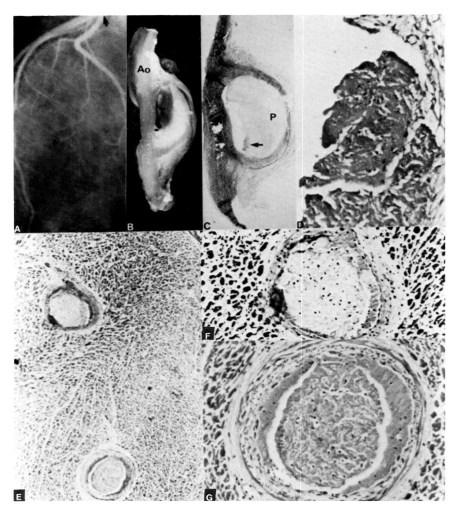

Fig. 44–56. Histologic evidence of distal coronary thromboembolism as a complication of acute proximal coronary artery thrombolysis therapy. **(A)** Angiographic view of left main coronary artery after initial streptokinase infusion and distal migration of thrombi fragments showing severe residual luminal diameter reduction (arrow). The left anterior descending and left circumflex arteries are normal. **(B)** Cross-sectional view of the severely narrowed left main artery. The lumen is narrowed by atherosclerotic plaque and residual thrombus (T). Ao, aorta. **(C)** Histologic cross section of segment shown in Fig. B, confirming the presence of underlying atherosclerotic plaque (P) and showing a residual amount of thrombus (arrow). **(D)** High-powered view of thrombus shown in Fig. C. **(E–G)** Photomicrographs of the anterolateral papillary muscle. **(E)** Low magnification (× 40) of intramural coronary arteries. **(F,G)** Higher magnification (× 400) showing that the luminal narrowing is the result of thromboemboli. The occluding thrombus is similar in composition to that remaining in the left main coronary artery **(D)**. (From Menke et al.,[164] with permission.)

into the distal infarct artery is likely to be clinically silent or clinically inseparable from the ongoing infarction and produce little additional myocardial damage. However, a single larger fragment impacting more proximally in the infarct artery could aggravate myocardial necrosis already in progress. Alternatively, larger thrombi that fragment and occlude many intramyocardial arteries may produce secondary thrombus of an epicardial coronary vessel feeding the obstructed arterioles or may compromise collateral flow from other major coronary arteries, or both. In either situation, extension of myocardial necrosis may occur.

Balloon Angioplasty of Aortocoronary Saphenous Vein Bypass Grafts

Coronary embolization as a complication of balloon angioplasty of saphenous vein grafts has been emphasized by several investigators and is discussed above.[8,187,200] Its frequency is higher than that in balloon angioplasty of native coronary arteries occurring in 2 (2.4 percent) of 82 patients reported by Reeder and colleagues[187] and in 2 (1.9 percent) of 103 cases reported by Saber and associates.[200] Pathologic documentation of coronary embolization after balloon angioplasty of saphenous vein bypass grafts has been reported by Saber and colleagues.[200] In one of their two cases, a large thromboatheromatous embolus obstructed the proximal left anterior descending artery and was removed at operation. In the second case, embolization of atheromatous and thrombotic debris resulted in obstruction of many intramural coronary artery branches and was thought to contribute to the patient's death.

Embolization of thrombotic or atheromatous material probably occurs more frequently after balloon angioplasty of coronary arteries than has been recognized but is clinically asymptomatic in most cases because of the small size and number of emboli. Balloon dilation of saphenous vein grafts, however, is probably more likely to produce symptomatic embolization because vein grafts are generally larger than the coronary arteries to which they are anastomosed and because atherosclerosis in grafts tends to involve dilated segments and to be more friable and less fibrocalcific than its counterpart in native coronary arteries. Saber and colleagues[200] concluded that percutaneous transluminal balloon angioplasty of aortocoronary saphenous vein bypass grafts more than 1 year old be performed with the realization that they are apt to be affected by friable atherosclerosis and that atheroembolization is a risk.

ARTERIAL STENTS

Intra-arterial stenting of dilated vessels has been used as a nonsurgical treatment for abrupt closure of balloon angioplasty sites.[31,60,62,131,146,147,179–182,198,199,212,217,221,234, 251,268] The principle was first described by Dotter in 1969.[60] Over the past few years, variants of the original technique using thermal-shaped memory alloy[62,234,251] expanding spring steel spirals,[147] expanding stainless steel stents,[31,146] and expanding woven stainless steel meshes[180–182,221] have been reported in animal experiments. Recently, intravascular stents have been implanted in humans to prevent occlusion and restenosis after balloon angioplasty.[179,180,221] The stenting device (endoprosthesis) is delivered to the arterial site by a balloon catheter. Upon balloon expansion, the meshwork expands against the arterial wall and becomes permanently embedded (Fig. 44–57). Histologic studies[60,147,180–182,212,221,234,251,268] in animals indicate that a neointimal layer covers the luminal aspect of the stent (Fig. 44–58). Stents appear to reduce luminal obstruction by displacing plaque, stretching vessel walls, and maintaining intimal-medial flaps against adjacent vessel wall. Serruys and colleagues[217] found an additional increase in cross-sectional area of a previously dilated ves-

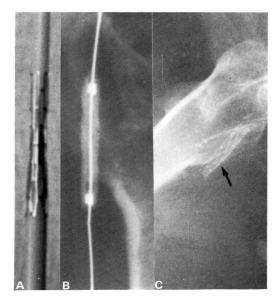
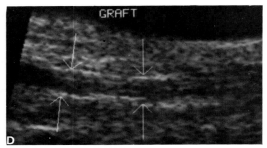

Fig. 44–57. Intravascular stents in an experimental model. (**A**) Housing and delivery catheter for stent. (**B**) Stent being "floated" into vessel via balloon catheter. (**C**) Radiograph showing stent in vessel (arrow). (**D**) Stents can also be recognized using ultrasound (arrows). (Courtesy of G. Becker, M.D., Indiana University.)

sel indicating the stenting device has a dilating function in addition to its stenting role. Long-term effects of stents, and their effects on altering the restenosis rate at balloon angio-plasty sites are under study. An initial report suggests a marked reduction in the rate of restenosis when stenting is used.[221]

Technical considerations for the histologic evaluation of stented vessels include cutting the stent. Cross-sectional or longitudinal section of the stent site with the wire meshwork in place requires diamond-cutting blades and special embedding materials. An alternate method involves removal of the stent mesh-work prior to sectioning. The latter technique may disrupt some of the intraluminal neointima and prevent accurate assessment of luminal patency.

ATHERECTOMY

Cutting instruments that can excise obstructing material in vessel lumen have recently been developed and used clinically (Fig. 44–59). Simpson and colleagues designed a catheter (Simpson Athero-Cath) that permits transluminal removal of occlusive arterial lesions, leaving a surgically smooth luminal surface. Simpson termed this procedure *atherectomy*. A transluminal atherectomy differs from a surgical endarterectomy in that only a portion of the atheroma is removed, whereas a surgical endarterectomy removes essentially all of a plaque. The Simpson atherotome consists of a circular blade rotating at a high speed. It is pressed against the diseased vessel wall by an inflated balloon.[96,224,225,270] The procedure can be repeated several times to remove atherosclerotic plaque, thrombus, or the hyperplastic intimal tissue responsible for a restenosis. Focal stenoses or short-segment total occlusions and ulcerative or calcified lesions can be treated. Intimal flaps creating abrupt closure of a balloon angioplasty site may also be excised. Specimens removed average 12 mm in length, 2 mm in width, and 0.25 mm in depth. Histology discloses atherosclerotic plaque, thrombus, internal elastic membrane, and portions of media.[270] Theoreti-

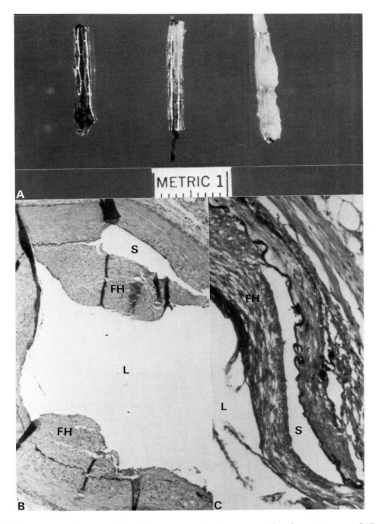

Fig. 44–58. (A) Three excised stents showing progressive fibrous with advancing age (left-to-right). (B,C) Histology of peripheral vessel following removal of stent wires (S) showing fibrous hyperplasia (FH) covering the luminal (L) surface of the stent. (H&E, × 200.) (From Waller,[249] with permission.)

cally, exposure of large segments of medial smooth muscle by atherectomy predisposes the site to a similar or higher frequency of intimal fibrous proliferation (restenosis) as seen with conventional balloon angioplasty. Actual removal of plaque, rather than simply cracking atheroma, increases the luminal cross-sectional area, which may then delay clinical expression of restenosis. Modifications of the Simpson Athero-Cath include the Kensey catheter, the Suth/Ritchie Rotablator, and the transluminal extraction catheter.

LASER IRRADIATION

Rapid advances are being achieved in the use of lasers (light amplification by stimulated emission of radiation) to treat coronary and peripheral atherosclerosis.[1,50,75,76,105,106,134,204,205,209] The capacity to conduct tremendous amounts of energy and focus it onto a relatively small area of tissue has made laser devices, combined with fiberoptic catheters, an intriguing means of ablating atherosclerotic plaque. Many types of lasers are being in-

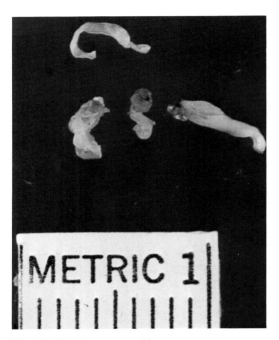

Fig. 44–59. Fragments of human coronary artery atherosclerotic plaque, including portions of vessel media removed by an atherectomy catheter.

vestigated, including neodymium-doped-yttrium aluminum garnet (Nd:YAG), argon, CO_2, and excimer (Fig. 44–60). Variation in biologic tissue response appears to depend on a number of factors, including physical characteristics of both the laser energy source and the target lesion. Laser irradiation appears to be a logical extension of therapies developed to treat coronary atherosclerosis: bypass grafting bypasses an obstruction, while lasers eliminate atherosclerotic plaque by converting plaque from a solid-phase matter to a water-soluble (or blood-soluble) gas. As pointed out by Isner and Clarke,[105] "Laser offers the promise of a percutaneous, definitive therapy for atherosclerosis." However, perforation of the coronary artery wall represents the principal risk, limiting routine clinical use.

Laser recanalization results in plaque removal by directed energy that is absorbed and converted into heat in the target tissue. The irradiated tissue evaporates, becomes carbonized (charred) or desiccated, or is thermally injured sufficiently to cause necrosis.[134]

The net result is a luminal expansion. The tissue that first absorbs the incident laser beam is explosively evaporated, resulting in a plaque crater.[134] Most early laser reaction probably represents thermal degradation rather than molecular photodissociation, since the gaseous byproducts of laser-irradiated plaque have been identified as hydrocarbon fragments.[134] Tissue that is not evaporated may persist as charred material. Hyalinized, fibrotic, and calcified plaques produce greater debris compared with lipid-laden (fatty) plaques.[134] Chronic changes in postirradiated lesions include replaced endothelium in the evacuated area and focal aneurysmal dilation at sites where medial injury has occurred.[134] In experimental models, the laser-induced crater is still evident several weeks later. In addition, full-thickness laser injury may either alter the adventitia or rupture an artery, or both.[134]

Laser light can be delivered as a continuous beam or as a pulse. Histology studies following use of a continuous-wave laser show that vascular tissue developed a cone-shaped crater surrounded by concentric zones of protein denaturation and tissue vacuolization.[75] The resulting charred, ragged endothelial surface is not desirable because it promotes thrombosis, and thermal diffusion leads to vessel perforation.[75] Laser research has now concentrated on ablating tissue by limiting thermal injury. Two methods have been used: (1) modified tip of the delivery system of continuous-wave lasers, and (2) pulsed lasers.

Hot-Tip Probes

Sanborn and colleagues[205] recanalized totally occluded peripheral arteries in human subjects using a hot-tip probe coupled to a continuous-wave argon laser. Abela and colleagues[1] used a hybrid hot-tip system to heat a metal cap and deliver laser energy through the center of the catheter. Histology of vessels subjected to hot-tip probes show thermally damaged plaque and media. Fouvier and associates[76] coupled an Nd:YAG laser to a sapphire tip, which diffuses the laser beam

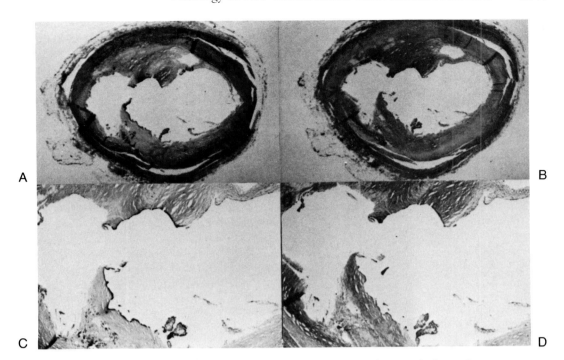

Fig. 44–60. (A–D) Light microscopic findings after excimer laser irradiation of atherosclerotic coronary artery plaque. There is a superficial zone of linear discoloration at the perimeter of the neolumen; otherwise, no remarkable alterations are observed. (Fig. A, Verhoeff's elastic tissue stain, × 10; Fig. B, Richardson's stain, × 10.) (From Isner et al.,[106] with permission.)

over a larger area than the bare wire. Advantages of hot-tip probes include rapid action, creation of a large orifice, and a tip shape that may reduce the frequency to vessel perforation. Disadvantages include limitations for use in small vessels and an associated increased frequency of spasm and thrombosis.[75] Radiofrequency energy is an alternate power source for thermal probes and has the advantage of being considerably cheaper.[143]

Pulsed Lasers

Pulsing the laser energy reduces thermal damage by limiting thermal diffusion.[75] Ultraviolet excimer laser light can be transmitted through a fiberoptic with enough pulsed energy to ablate an atheroma without a thermal effect. Tissue ablation occurs as a discrete, precise event. The mechanism appears to be disruption of molecular bonds; no thermal injury occurs because of a very rapid, highly localized heat effect.[75] Thus, while it is hypothesized that removal of atherosclerotic plaque by laser vaporization may be more effective than balloon angioplasty, the technique is still limited by inadequate delivery systems, a high frequency of vessel perforation and thrombosis, and the creation of small recanalized channels. Newer systems, employing fluorescence spectroscopy, will make use of tissue recognition before laser treatment begins. These "smart" lasers appear to reduce the frequency of vessel perforation.

BALLOON PYROPLASTY

Balloon pyroplasty, also known as thermal balloon angioplasty and biologic stenting (see Fig. 44–30), initially developed as laser-balloon angioplasty,[143,232] is another method of remolding or remodeling a stenosed atherosclerotic vessel to increase luminal area. Ther-

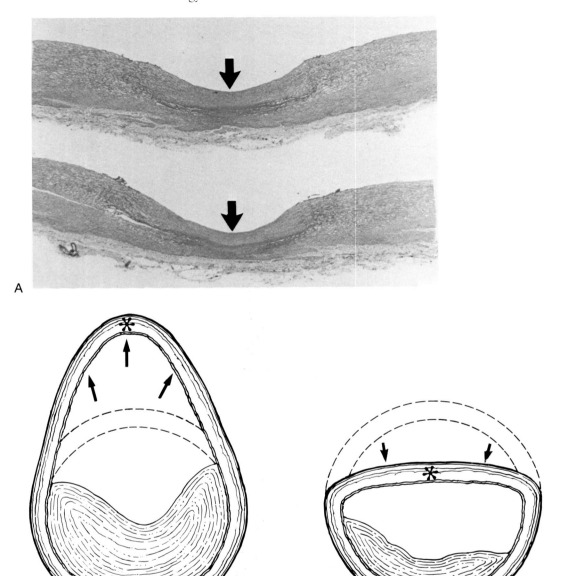

A

B

Fig. 44–61. (A) Thermoplasty of human aorta showing "molding" effects (arrows). Tissue within depressed areas is necrotic. **(B)** Diagram showing beneficial effects of thermal angioplasty (pyroplasty) on eccentric atherosclerotic plaques. (Left) Diagram of eccentric atherosclerotic vessel with segment of disease free wall (asterisks) "molded" to the size and shape of an inflated balloon by radiofrequency pyroplasty resulting in an increase in luminal area (arrows) above expected nondilated lumen (dashed lines). (Right) Eccentric plaque dilated without pyroplasty. Both vessels from which diagrams prepared were dilated when fresh, then fixed in formalin. The vessel treated by thermal angioplasty remained stretched, whereas the vessel dilated by angioplasty alone shrinks with formalin fixation. (From Lee et al.,[133] with permission.)

mal balloon angioplasty may use various energy sources (laser, radiofrequency, chemical, ultrasound) to produce a thermal injury on adjacent plaque. Laser balloon angioplasty features traditional balloon angioplasty followed by laser irradiation of the atherosclerotic plaque during final balloon dilation.[143,232] In one model, Nd:YAG laser energy fires through an ultrathin central fiber and is transmitted through the balloon to enter adjacent plaque as heat. Animal[143,226] and cadaver[110,133] studies have indicated that thermal balloon angioplasty decreases vessel elasticity at the dilation site and heat "molds" the arterial segment to the size and shape of the inflated angioplasty balloon (Fig. 44–61). This process essentially creates a biologic stent. In addition to the acute remolding, thermal effects to the underlying media may destroy smooth muscle cells involved in late restenosis.

Lee and colleagues[133] evaluated radiofrequency as an alternate energy source for balloon pyroplasty. Delivered in combination with angioplasty balloon inflation pressure, it effectively molded atherosclerotic plaque and vessels. Experimental studies on layers of human cadaver aorta showed tissue fusion (welding) of previously separated layers, indicating its clinical value in intraluminal intimal flaps (Fig. 44–62). Balloon pyroplasty has not been associated with subsequent aneurysm or rupture in the experimental model. Thermal angioplasty with lower-power homogeneous heating and simultaneous tissue compression may be better than thermal probes (hot-tipped probes), which apply an instaneous high heat to the luminal surface.

Thermal Probes (G-Lazing)

Conventional coronary balloon angioplasty may be followed by a laser thermal probe in an attempt to seal superficial intimal disruptions (see Fig. 44–30). The low-powered probe skims through the treated vessel, "glazing" the new lumen. Removal of tissue does

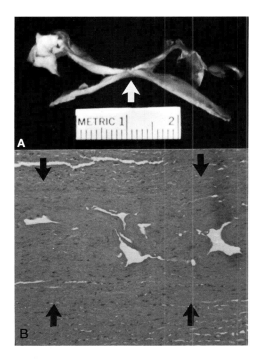

Fig. 44–62. Experimental studies on the effects of radiofrequency thermoplasty on layers of human cadaver aorta. **(A)** Tissue fusion (welding) (arrow) of previously separated layers. These results indicate a potential use to "weld" intraluminal flaps resulting from balloon angioplasty. **(B)** Histology section through fusion zone (arrows) showing melting of aortic layers.

not result, but a "finishing-touch" remodeling occurs.[172]

VENTRICULAR ENDOCARDIAL RESECTION AND CATHETER ABLATION FOR CHRONIC VENTRICULAR ARRHYTHMIAS

Even with the vast array of pharmacologic agents available for the treatment of recurrent ventricular arrhythmias, the clinical results have been disappointing.[261] Surgical treatment, with direct excision or ablation of a focus of ventricular tachycardia, has emerged as an alternative.[46,86,101,113,130,169,188,242] As a result, surgical pathologists now receive resected endocardial tissue for histologic evaluation (Fig. 44–63). Endocardial resection, described by Josephson and colleagues,[113] is a commonly used technique. However, it may fail to eliminate an arrhythmia, because ventricular arrhythmias arise from myocardial or subepicardial layers of the ventricular wall.[46] For this reason, endocardial electrical shocks, delivered through trans-

venous catheters, are used to improve results.[46,130,185]

Endocardial Resection

Morphologic-histologic features of excised left ventricular subendocardial regions have been described by Fenoglio and colleagues.[69] Bundles of apparently viable myocardial fibers embedded in dense fibrous tissue were identified throughout the endocardial resections from each of 23 patients. The cell bundles were separated by fibrous tissue but extended uninterrupted to the margins of the surgical resection. In 14 patients, Purkinje fibers were identified deep to the thickened endocardium, whereas the remaining bundles were composed of ventricular muscle. The Purkinje fibers appeared to have normal ultrastructure; ventricular cells exhibited both normal and abnormal ultrastructural changes. Abnormal muscle cells were characterized by loss of contractile elements, aggregates of dilated sarcoplasmic reticulum, and osmophilic dense bodies. Fenoglio and associates[69] suggested that the abnormal structure and arrangement of surviving cardiac fibers may be responsible for the abnormal electrophysiologic function that results in ventricular tachycardia.

Silver and colleagues[222] reported late autopsy findings in a 51-year-old man who had been treated with endomyocardial resection for recurrent ventricular tachycardia 19 months earlier. Ventricular tachycardia was successfully ablated, but the patient died of a postoperative wound infection. At autopsy, the resection site was covered with snow-white thickened endocardium that consisted of collagen and elastic fibers, similar to that seen in the acquired form of endocardial fibroelastosis.

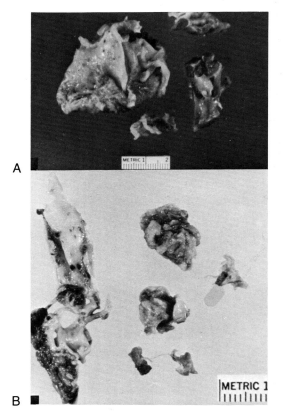

Fig. 44–63. (**A,B**) Operatively excised ventricular endocardium from two patients with chronic ventricular arrhythmia following myocardial infarction. The site of tachycardia was mapped at surgery before endocardial resection. (From Waller,[245] with permission.)

Catheter Ablation

Catheter ablation of ventricular arrhythmias resistant to medical therapy appears to be a promising technique. High-energy catheter-delivered electrical discharges are used to damage the previously mapped ventricular focus. Endocardial shocks produce local myocardial necrosis; the extent depends on the dose of energy delivered. Experimental models[222] have produced discrete transmural wedge-shaped zones of necrosis without perforation at necropsy. The extent of myocardial necrosis resulting from multiple endocardial shocks may contribute to congestive heart failure.

To date, several patients have undergone catheter ablation of ventricular tachycardia by endocardial shocks.[18,38,185,188] All had episodic, drug-resistant ventricular tachycardia, and in all cases, endocardial shocks prevented recurrence of the arrhythmia. We examined the explanted heart of a patient who had received catheter ablation before cardiac transplantation (Fig. 44–64). Despite several catheter shocks, the arrhythmia frequency was merely reduced, not eliminated.

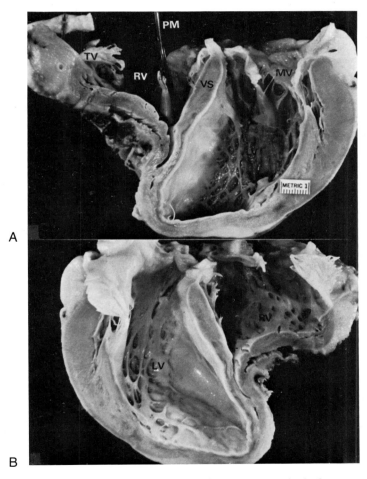

Fig. 44–64. (A,B) Explanted heart (transplant patient) from a patient who had previous catheter ablation therapy from recurrent ventricular tachycardia. The catheter shocks were delivered along the right and left ventricles (RV, LV). Note the healed myocardial infarction involving the ventricular septum (VS) with marked endocardial thickening (pearly white LV lining). MV, mitral valve; PM, pacemaker catheter; TV, tricuspid valve. (From Waller,[245] with permission.)

Chemical Ablation

Inoue and colleagues[103] established chemical ablative therapy experimentally. Intra-coronary injection of 25 percent phenol or 50 to 100 percent ethyl alcohol ablated aconitine-induced ventricular tachycardia in the dog.[103] Pathologic examination of the hearts and injected coronary arteries disclosed transmural myocardial necroses in 35 of 41 dogs that received phenol or alcohol. The myocardial necrosis apparently suppressed the tachycardia focus or prevented propagation or both. Fibrin or thrombus, or both, was present in six of the perfused coronary vessels. It was concluded that this approach could have value in selected cases, particularly in combination with drugs that (1) cause less necrosis, (2) are more specific for the arrhythmogenic site, or (3) that can be injected with greater accuracy into smaller coronary arteries supplying the arrhythmogenic area.[103]

I examined the heart of a patient who had undergone chemical ablation of a focus pro-ducing chronic refractory ventricular tachy-cardia. A marginal branch of the right coro-nary artery was injected with alcohol that stopped the ventricular arrhythmia. At au-topsy, two-thirds of the right coronary artery was occluded by thrombus, and the posterior walls of right and left ventricles in zones sup-plied by portions of the right coronary artery were necrotic.

AUTOMATIC IMPLANTABLE CARDIOVERTER-DEFIBRILLATOR

Patients who respond poorly to drug therapy and who are not candidates for surgery (en-docardial resection, cryoablation) may be treated with a combination of drug therapy and implantation of an automatic implantable cardioverter-defibrillator (AICD) (Figs. 44–65 to 44–68) (See Ch. 44 also.)

In the past, two devices were available for

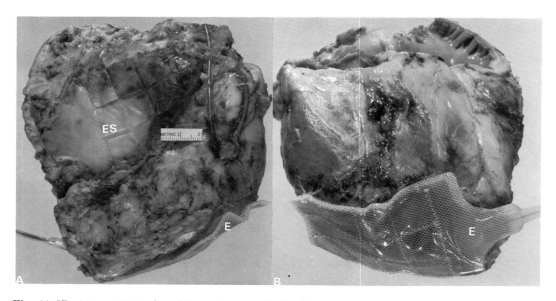

Fig. 44–65. Automatic implantable cardioverter-defibrillator (AICD) (CPI, Mirowski-Winkle). **(A)** Ex-ternal view of heart showing sites of two epicardial patch electrodes (E). One patch has been removed. ES, electrode site. A superior vena cava catheter is also seen on the epicardial surface. **(B)** Posterior-apical view of patch electrode.

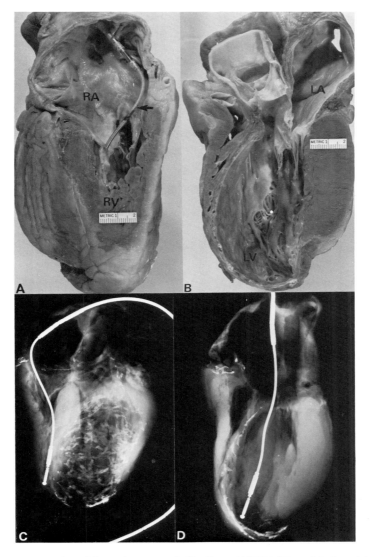

Fig. 44–66. Automatic implantable cardioverter-defibrillator (AICD) (Zipes Medtronic). (**A**) Right heart view showing AICD catheter (arrows) inserted in right ventricle (RV). (**B**) Left heart view showing large left ventricular (LV) aneurysm. (**C,D**) Postmortem radiographs showing AICD and calcific deposits in LV aneurysm. LA, left atrium; RA, right atrium.

clinical trials: the cardioverter-defibrillator (Cardiac Packemaker) and the cardioverter (Medtronic). The former device, conceived by Mirowski[166,167] and refined by Winkle[267] (Fig. 44–65), cardioverts and defibrillates but does not pace. The latter, devised by Zipes (Figs. 44–66 to 68), paces and cardioverts but cannot defibrillate. The first requires major surgery

to implant, the second a subcutaneous incision. Both units cost about $10,000 each. The Medtronic device has been suspended from use during patent debates. Recently, Ebstein and colleagues[64] reported the results of implantation of combined AICD and pacemaker systems.

The AICD includes a number of equipment

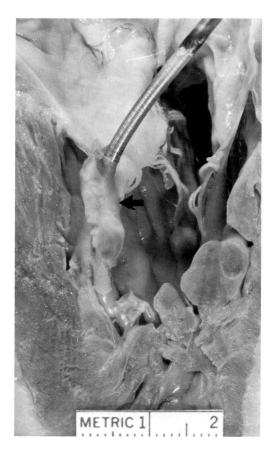

Fig. 44–67. Closeup of right ventricle shown in Fig. 44–66, showing increased fibrosis around AICD tip (arrow). Underlying right ventricle has no increased scar from repeated discharges.

options and surgical implantation techniques. The present unit consists of a pulse generator and electrodes. The transcardiac electrode system consists of a superior vena cava catheter and one or two epicardial apical patch electrodes (Fig. 44–65). With respect to the Zipes cardioverter, multiple shocks given by the cardioverter electrode positioned in the right ventricular apex were not associated with increased tissue damage at the myocardial-electrode interface (Fig. 44–66 to 44–68).

PERMANENT CARDIAC VENTRICULAR PACING

The historic and technical aspects of cardiac pacing are reviewed by Wilson[266] (see Ch. 44). Ongoing developments in generators, pacing leads and electrodes puts the pathologist in a key position to describe observations and complications associated with various systems. Morphologic changes of normally-functioning pacing leads and electrodes include encasement of a lead by a fibrocollagenous sheath as it passes from the superior vena cava to the right ventricle (Fig. 44–69), adherent thrombus, occasional adherence of tricuspid valve tissue to the pacing lead, and fibrosis at the electrode-endocardial insertion site (Fig. 44–70).

An endocardial pacing lead presents a foreign surface to the bloodstream. Some degree of thrombus formation is inevitable with conventional silicone rubber lead coatings and even with newer polyurethane coats.[266] The thrombi produce a sheath covering 30 to 80 percent of the length of the lead. The sheath is well formed within 12 hours and then undergoes organization over several months to form fibrous tissue. This fibrous sheath may extend from the site of electrode contact with the endocardium (usually at the right ventricular apex) across the chordae tendineae and tricuspid valve, to which it is fused, and into the right atrium. Such lead ensheathment with adhesions to the endocardium and tricuspid valve apparatus usually causes no valve dysfunction. If a lead is to be removed, avulsion of part of the tricuspid valve is a possible complication.[266]

Perforation of the ventricular walls (septum or free wall, or both) is an occasional complication of emergency placement of pacing catheters (Fig. 44–71). Delayed perforation can occur and results from gradual penetration of the electrode through the myocardium. A major predisposing factor in acute or late per-

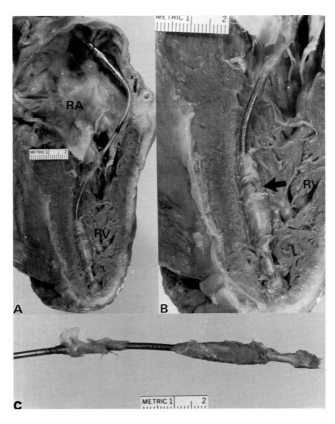

Fig. 44–68. Automatic implantable cardioverter-defibrillator (AICD) (Zipes Medtronic). (**A**) Right ventricular view showing AICD catheter inserting in right ventricle (RV). (**B**) Closeup of Fig. A, showing increased fibrosis around AICD catheter tip (arrows) that is unassociated with underlying myocardial fibrosis. (**C**) Autopsy excised AICD catheter.

foration is stiffness of the electrode lead. The stiffer the wire, the more likely the complication. Specific techniques with which to examine cardiac pacemakers at autopsy are presented by Wilson[266] (see Ch. 44).

TEMPORARY VENTRICULAR ASSIST DEVICES

Temporary left and right ventricular assist devices are currently used in patients who cannot be separated from cardiopulmonary

bypass or who have severe myocardial dysfunction. Relatively little morphologic information is available on their effects. Schoen and colleagues[213] reported pathologic findings in 21 patients receiving temporary left ventricular assist pump support (model X pump in 20 patients, model XI in one patient). The device was implanted after isolated valve replacement, coronary artery bypass grafting, or combined procedures. The duration of support was 1 to 190 hours (average, 61 hours). Myocardial biopsy specimens were obtained at implantation of the ventricular assist device. Correlation of findings in myocardial bi-

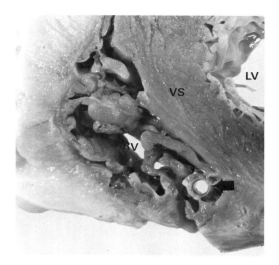

Fig. 44–69. Fibrous sheath in right ventricle (RV) encapsulates permanent pacemaker lead. LV, ventricular septum; VS, ventricular septum.

opsy specimens in 15 patients and autopsy findings in nonsurvivors suggested that myocardial dysfunction has a reversible component, apparently related to diminished compliance (probably edema), severe but reversible ischemic myocardial injury, or both.[213] No patient studied had thrombotic or biomaterial emboli or other pump-related complications. Schoen and associates[214] updated their findings in the evaluation of 41 patients, distributed among four centers, who had left (33 patients), right (5), or bilateral (3) temporary ventricular assist devices. Cardiac failure occurred in 39 postoperative patients, following aortocoronary bypass (23), valve replacement (4), both (9), or other surgical procedures (3). The cause of death in 35 cases was myocardial necrosis (14), hemorrhage (9), cerebrovascular accidents (3), infection (3), or other (6). The mean duration of support in all patients was 62 hours. In 16 patients (40 percent) who improved, cardiac assist duration was a mean of 127 hours (range, 44 to 264 hours), compared with a mean of 19 hours

(range, 1 to 120 hours) in 25 who did not. Of 17 patients in whom support exceeded 72 hours, 15 (88 percent) improved, 11 were weaned, and 6 survived in the long term. Tissue examination (in 33 patients) by biopsy at pump implantation or autopsy revealed coagulation or contraction band myocyte necrosis, with or without hemorrhage, in 26 cases; of these, 10 improved, and 6 were long-term survivors. Pump-related complications included one patient each with pulmonary embolism (most likely related to a cannulation site thrombus) and an aortic cannulation site infection. This study suggests that mechanical

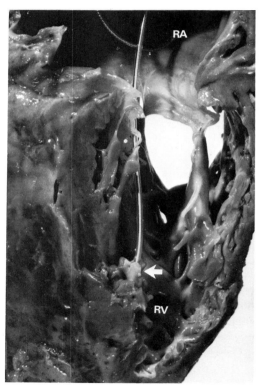

Fig. 44–70. Right ventricular (RV) view of standard ventricular pacemaker. Catheter tip (arrow) shows minimal fibrosis and was not associated with underlying myocardial scar. Compare catheter fibrosis with that in Fig. 44–66 to 44–68. RA, right atrium.

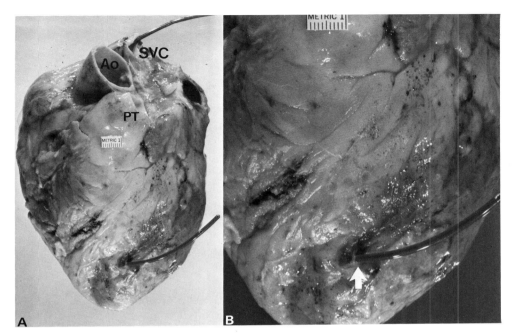

Fig. 44–71. (**A**) Perforation of left ventricle from temporary right ventricular pacing catheter. Catheter inserted via superior vena cava (SVC). Catheter perforated ventricular septum (internally), then left ventricular free wall (externally). (**B**) Closeup of perforation site. Ao, aorta; PT, pulmonary trunk.

cardiac assist (1) may be accomplished with a low complication rate; (2) should not be denied patients with existing myocardial necrosis, since necrosis does not preclude improvement or survival; and (3) frequently leads to functional myocardial recovery if patients survive early noncardiac complications, which often result from a long cardiopulmonary bypass.[214]

We examined the hearts of several patients who had left or right or combined ventricular assist devices for severe ventricular dysfunction following CABG or valve replacement (Fig. 43–72). In several cases, the atrial cannulas had thrombus on the tip. In addition, all had variable degrees of atrial wall hemorrhage at sites of atrial collapse surrounding the cannulas (Figs. 44–72 and 44–73). In one case, the hemorrhage encroached on the AV node. Cannulas in the aorta or pulmonary

trunk were generally free of thrombus, and the adjacent arterial walls showed no hemorrhage.

The pathogenesis of the myocardial abnormality accounting for reversibility of an early postoperative cardiac dysfunction remains unclear. Myocardial necrosis itself does not appear to preclude a favorable hemodynamic response. However, the extent of necrosis present on initial myocardial biopsy appeared to correlate with a poor prognosis.[213] Since repair of myocardial necrosis during left ventricular assist pump support is minimal, and because established areas of myocardial infarction are not affected by enhanced flows and pressures, the reversible abnormality must involve other factors (interstitial myocardial edema or hemorrhage) that causes decreased compliance of otherwise viable myocardium.[213]

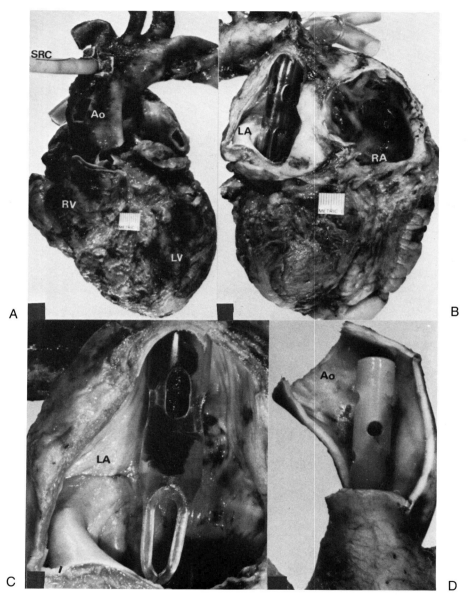

Fig. 44–72. Temporary left ventricular assist device in a patient who developed severe left ventricular (LV) dysfunction following aortocoronary bypass grafting. (**A**) External view showing systemic return cannula (SRC) in ascending aorta (Ao). RV, right ventricle. (**B**) Removal of posterior atrial walls to show exit cannula in left atrium (LA). Note hemorrhage in atrial septum as viewed from right atrium (RA). (**C**) Closeup of left atrial cannula showing tip thrombus and dimple of left atrial appendage, which has been sucked into cannula. (**D**) Closeup of systemic return cannula showing no thrombus or arterial wall damage. (From Waller,[245] with permission.)

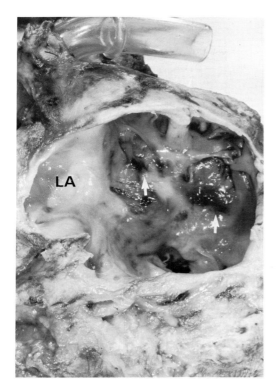

Fig. 44–73. Temporary left ventricular assist device. Closeup of left atrium (LA) seen in Fig. 44–72. Note atrial septal hemorrhage (arrows).

CATHETER BALLOON VALVULOPLASTY FOR TREATMENT OF NATIVE VALVE STENOSES

During the past several years, catheter balloon valvuloplasty has been used successfully as a nonsurgical treatment of stenosed cardiac valves in children and adults at all sites. Only pulmonic valve valvuloplasty has been approved by the Food and Drug Administration (FDA), while dilation of other stenotic cardiac valves is performed under investigational protocols. As more and more procedures are performed, pathologists will be called upon to review valves that have been dilated and are operatively excised or become autopsy specimens (Figs. 43–74 to 44–80).

Pulmonic Valve

History

In 1979, Semb and colleagues[216] reported the first successful use of a balloon catheter in a patient with pulmonic valve stenosis. The balloon was inflated with carbon dioxide and pulled back across the valve. The first pulmonic valvuloplasty in an adult was performed in 1982 by Pepine and colleagues.[184] They used a 20-mm balloon inflated to 5 atm in a patient with congenital pulmonary stenosis. Following successful reports of the procedure used in children and adults,[115,126,184,216,262] it has become the primary therapy for children and adults with pulmonic stenosis. Recent data from a 15-center valvuloplasty registry at the Mansfield Scientific Corporation (Mansfield, MA)[157] indicated that more than 800 pulmonic valve balloon valvuloplasty procedures have been performed with success in about 90 percent of patients.

Mechanisms and Morphologic Changes

The mechanism of balloon valvuloplasty depends in part on the etiology of the stenosis. In congenital pulmonic valve stenosis, the valve is dome shaped with undeveloped or primitive commissures. Catheter balloon valvuloplasty tears or avulses the valve cusps. In patients with congenital pulmonic stenosis of the dysplastic type, well-formed commissures are present but unfused, and the pulmonic valve cusps are severely thickened. Balloon valvuloplasty in these instances produces cuspal tearing and stretching of the pulmonary artery at sites of nonfused commissures. In the rare case of acquired pulmonic valve stenosis (rheumatic, carcinoid), fused commissures and thickened cusps are present. Balloon valvuloplasty results in cuspal tears and splitting of fused commissures.

Mitral Valve

History

In 1984, Inoue and colleagues[104] provided the first report of successful percutaneous catheter balloon valvuloplasty of a stenotic mitral valve. Six patients underwent single-balloon valvuloplasty. In 1985 Lock and colleagues[146] reported successful balloon dilation of eight patients with mitral stenosis; again, a single balloon was used. In 1986, Al Zaibag and associates[4] reported the successful use of a double-balloon technique. The first reports of successful single-balloon valvuloplasty for calcified stenotic mitral valves in the United States came from R. McKay and colleagues[159] and Palacios and associates[178] in 1986. C. McKay and co-workers[158] reported similar results in mitral stenosis using a double-balloon technique.

Mechanism and Morphologic Changes

The mechanism of successful balloon valvuloplasty of stenosed mitral valves relates in part to the cause of mitral stenosis. For practical purposes, rheumatic disease is responsible in most cases, inducing fusion of commissures and fibrous thickening of leaflets. Catheter balloon valvuloplasty improves the mitral valve orifice by "splitting" or "cracking" fused commissures[255] (Figs. 44–74 to 44–76). Minor leaflet cracking may occur as well (Fig. 44–75). Subvalvular fusion of chordae tendineae may cause additional valve stenosis but does not appear to be relieved by balloon dilation.[255] The mechanism of successful balloon valvuloplasty was first described by Inoue and colleagues,[104] who noted separation of fused commissures on direct vision in patients who had percutaneous mitral valve valvuloplasty and subsequent mitral valve replacement. These results have been confirmed by investigators studying postmortem or surgical specimens.[27,118,160,256] Additional benefits that may accrue from the use of two small, versus one large, or progres-

sively larger balloons are under investigation (Fig. 44–76).

Technical Aspects and Cardiac Anatomy

Most laboratories employ transseptal catheterization to enter the left atrium (Fig. 44–74). A dilating balloon then widens the atrial septal opening to permit passage of the dilating balloon(s). Under fluoroscopic control, the dilating balloon is inflated. Repeated inflations are made until the "waist" of the balloon (at the level of the mitral valve) disappears.

Complications

Complications associated with balloon valvuloplasty of the mitral valve include systemic emboli; acute, severe mitral regurgitation from tearing of leaflets and rupture of the mitral valve annulus[255,262] (Fig. 44–75).

Aortic Valve

History

Percutaneous balloon valvuloplasty was first performed in children and young adults in 1984.[127] Successful balloon valvuloplasty of stenotic aortic valves was first reported by Cribier and colleagues[49] and subsequently by others.[48,109,161,162,177,211]

Mechanisms and Morphologic Changes

The mechanism involves splitting of fused commissures, stretching of aortic wall, and fracture of calcific nodules[59,202,254] (Figs. 44–76 to 44–80). The major factor determining which of these mechanisms results in a successful valvuloplasty is the etiology of the aortic stenosis. Stenotic aortic valves of rheumatic etiology (fusion of commissures with or without calcific deposits) are dilated by the balloon splitting fused commissures (Figs. 44–76 and 44–79). Stenosed congenitally anom-

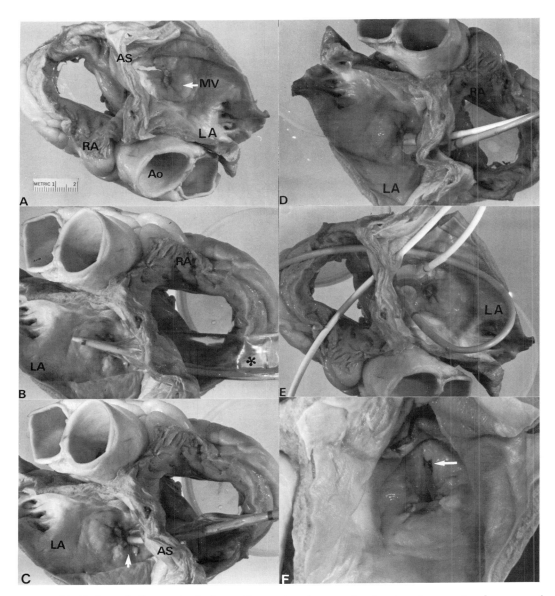

Fig. 44–74. Catheter balloon valvuloplasty. Composite photographs showing placement and passage of single- (Figs. B and C) and double- (Figs. D and E) catheter balloons. (**A**) Mitral valve (MV) stenosis. (**B**) Passage of single valvuloplasty balloon (asterisk) across fossa ovale area of atrial septum (AS). (**C**) Position of deflated balloon across stenotic MV (arrow). A portion of the dilated balloon still remains across AS. (**D**) Two dilating balloons are passed across the AS. (**E**) Dilating balloons across stenotic MV. (**F**) Fused commissural split achieved by dilating balloons (arrow). RA, right atrium; LA, left atrium; Ao, aorta.

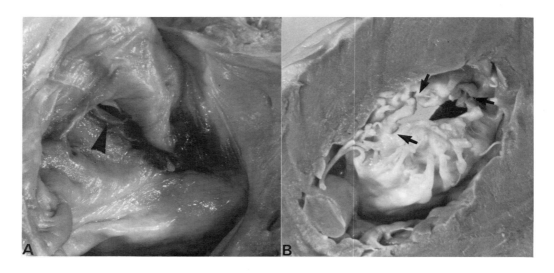

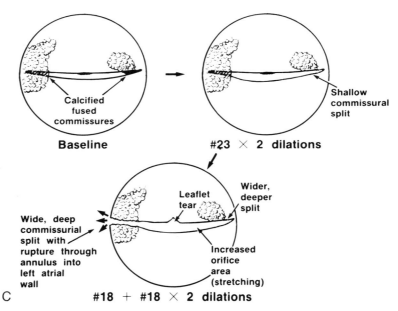

Fig. 44–75. Catheter balloon valvuloplasty of stenosed mitral valve during life studied at autopsy. **(A)** Residual atrial septal defect with surrounding hemorrhage following passage of dilating balloon. **(B)** Ventricular view of dilated mitral valve showing two commissural splits and cracked leaflet (arrows). **(C)** Diagram showing progressive changes of catheter balloon valvuloplasty of a stenosed mitral valve. A single #23 balloon causes a superficial commissural split, whereas two #18 balloons produce split commissures and a ruptured annulus.

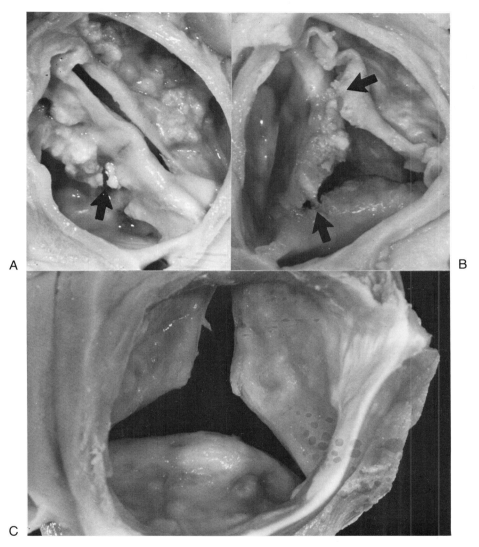

Fig. 44–76. Catheter balloon valvuloplasty of stenotic aortic valves. Depending on etiology of aortic stenosis, balloon valvuloplasty has varied effects. (**A**) Catheter balloon valvuloplasty of congenitally bicuspid aortic valve results in minimal cuspal cracking (arrow). (**B**) Valvuloplasty of rheumatic valve produces commissural splitting (arrows). (**C**) Catheter balloon valvuloplasty of degenerative valve results in stretching of aortic wall at nonfused commissural sites.

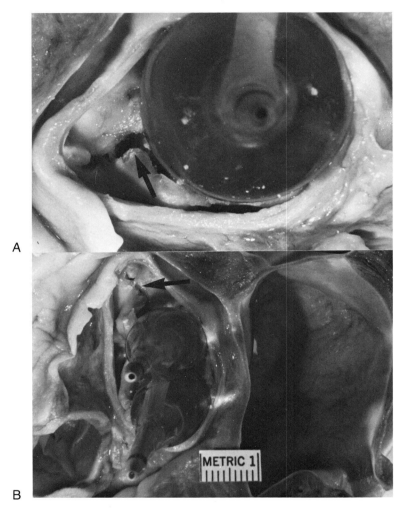

Fig. 44–77. Catheter balloon valvuloplasty of stenosed aortic valves at autopsy. **(A)** Inflated dilating balloon splits fused commissure (arrow). Note deformed aorta. **(B)** Double balloon valvuloplasty splits fused commissure (arrow).

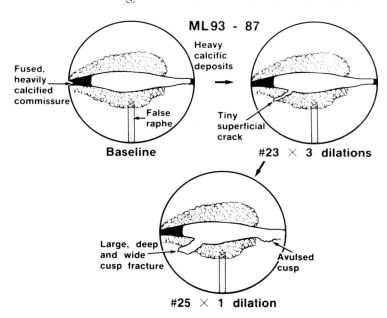

Fig. 44–78. Changes of catheter balloon valvuloplasty of a stenotic congenitally bicuspid aortic. Larger balloon causes progressive valve injury.

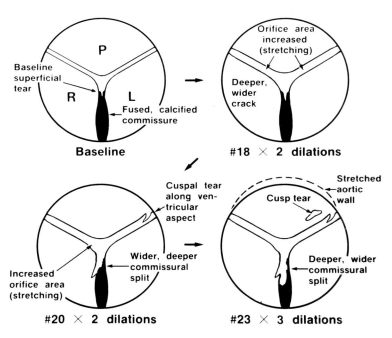

Fig. 44–79. Changes in stenosed aortic valve of rheumatic etiology, caused by catheter balloon valvuloplasty. Progressively larger balloons cause progressive commissural splitting and cuspal injury. Cusps: L, left; P, posterior; R, right.

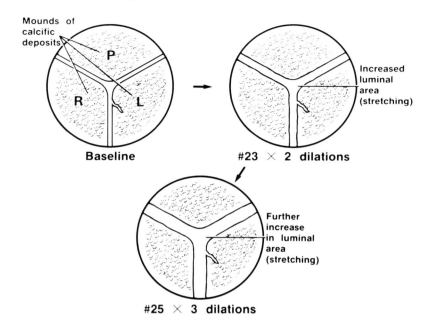

Fig. 44–80. Effects of catheter balloon valvuloplasty on stenotic aortic valve of degenerative etiology. Dilation with larger balloons progressively stretches aortic valve at unfused commissure sites, increasing central luminal area. Cusps: L, left; P, posterior; R, right.

alous valves (bicuspid valves usually unassociated with commissure fusion but heavily calcified) are dilated primarily by stretching the aortic wall at sites of unfused commissures (Figs. 44–76 and 44–78). Stenosed valves of degenerative etiology (absent commissural fusion and heavy calcific deposits in sinuses of Valsalva) are dilated by stretching the wall of the aorta and splitting of calcific nodules[202,254] (Figs. 44–76 to 44–80). Cuspal tears may occur in all three types.

Complications

As with mitral valvuloplasty, complications include systemic emboli, massive acute aortic regurgitation, aortic rupture, and aortic dissection.

Tricuspid Valve

History

Relative few stenosed tricuspid valves have received catheter balloon valvuloplasty. Zaibag and colleagues,[271] Shalilullah and asso-

ciates,[219] and Mullins and associates[171] all reported dilation of stenotic tricuspid valves in 1987. Bourdillon and colleagues[28] reported hemodynamic and pathologic findings in a patient receiving balloon dilation for tricuspid stenosis.

Mechanisms and Morphologic Changes

Double balloons have been used for tricuspid valve dilation. Mechanisms include splitting of fused commissures and minor leaflet injury.[28] Theoretically, dilation of stenotic tricuspid valves might be more successful clinically than dilation of stenotic mitral valves for several reasons: (1) heavily calcified commissures, which are more difficult to crack, are rare in tricuspid stenosis but common in mitral stenosis; (2) severely fused chordae tendineae, which produce a subvalvular element of stenosis not significantly affected by catheter balloon valvuloplasty, are less frequent with tricuspid stenosis than with mitral stenosis; and (3) the direct approach to the tricuspid valve through the right atrium avoids the potential complication of residual secundum atrial septal defects with the transseptal approach to the mitral valve.[28]

ARTIFICIAL HEART

Recently, scientific efforts have focused on the use of implantable artificial hearts as a mean of supporting or replacing a severely dysfunctioning heart.[40,41,53–56,79,94,125,132,186,191,194,257] The shortage of donor hearts for patients needing immediate cardiac transplantation gave rise to the use of the total artificial heart as a "bridge" to transplantation. The first total artificial heart was implanted in a dog by Akutsu and Kolff[2] in 1957. Human use occurred initially in April 1969. Between April 1969 and June 1988, there were at least 87 implants of biventricular pneumatic pulsable artificial hearts (Figs. 44–81 and 44–82). Five were "permanent implants" (Table 44–5). Of the 87 patients, 67 devices were implanted to keep the patient alive until a heart was available for transplantation. Several artificial heart devices have been used, such as the Liotta, Akutsu, Phenix, Jarvik 7 (7–70), Penn State, Berlin, and Ungar, but Jarvik devices have had the longest implant times (total of 4.1 years experience).[41] There has been only one mechanical device failure, a strut fracture of a Shiley disk valve in DeVries's first patient, Barney Clark.[55] Implant times for "bridge"

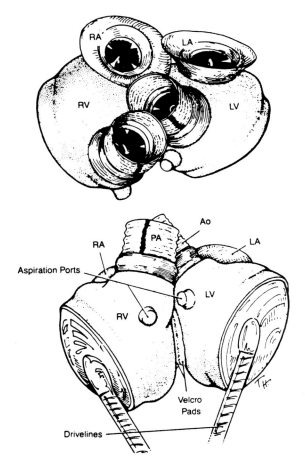

Fig. 44–81. Diagram of Jarvik 7–100 total artificial heart. RA, right atrium, LA, left atrium; RV, right ventricle; LV, left ventricle; Ao, aorta. (From DeVries,[55] with permission.)

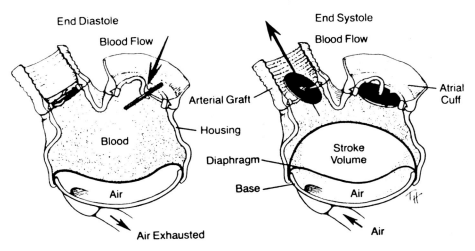

Fig. 44–82. Diagram showing diaphram function of pneumatic ventricle, demonstrating full-filling and complete ejection. (From Mayes et al.,[156] with permission.)

patients has averaged less than 2 weeks (range 0.5 to 244 days), while for "permanent" devices has averaged 292 days (range 10 to 622 days).[41] Only 4 patients survived after implant times of more than 21 days. Hemorrhage, hemolysis, emboli, and infections have been major complications.[2,40,41,53–56,79,94,125, 132,186,191,194] Pathologic findings in artificial hearts removed at transplantation or at autopsy disclosed macroscopic thrombus formation, fibrinous deposits in crevices at junctions of the valve housing and ventricle, and a fractured strut of a Shiley prosthesis.[40,54,55,132]

Dobbins and colleagues[56] reported in detail the postmortem microbiologic findings and

related gross pathology at autopsy in patients who had survived the longest after implantation of the Jarvik 7–100 total artificial heart. Extensive polymicrobial colonization at the site of the device and adjacent structures was observed. The internal drive lines were free of bacterial colonization despite evidence of infection at the skin junction. A mass of tissue that was adherent to the device and to portions of the drive lines contained inflammatory cells, fibrinous debris, and colonies of microorganisms.[56] Development of "partial" and "total" artificial heart devices will continue and will be used as effective bridges to cardiac transplantation.

Table 44–5.   Permanent Artificial Heart Implants

Implant Date	Patient	Age (years)	Surgeon/Site	Device	Days	Outcome
1. 12/02/82	Clark	61	DeVries/Utah	Jarvik 7	112	Death
2. 11/25/84	Schroeder	52	DeVries/Kentucky	Jarvik 7	622	Death
3. 02/17/85	Haydon	58	DeVries/Kentucky	Jarvik 7	488	Death
4. 04/07/85	Stenberg	53	Semb/Stockholm	Jarvik 7	227	Death
5. 04/14/85	Burcham	62	DeVries/Kentucky	Jarvik 7	10	Death

ACKNOWLEDGMENT

I wish to thank Marcy Culp for outstanding secretarial service in the preparation of this chapter.

REFERENCES

1. Abela GS, Seeger JM, Barbieri E, Conti CR: Laser angioplasty with angioscopic guidance in humans. J Am Coll Cardiol 8:184, 1986

2. Akutsu T, Kolff W: Permanent substitutes for valves and hearts. Trans Am Soc Artif Intern Organs 4:230, 1958

3. Althaus U, Gwitner HP, Bauer H, et al: Consequences of myocardial reperfusion following temporary coronary occlusion in pigs: Effects on morphologic, biochemical and hemodynamic findings. Eur J Clin Invest 7:437, 1977

4. Al Zaibag M, Kasab SA, Ribeiro PA, Fagih MR: Percutaneous double balloon mitral valvotomy for the rheumatic stenosis. Lancet 1:757, 1986

5. Anderson JL, Marshall HW, Askins JC, et al: A randomized trial of intravenous and intracoronary streptokinase in patients with acute myocardial infarction. Circulation 70:606, 1984

6. Angelini P, Leachman R, Heibig J: Distal coronary hemoperfusion during balloon angioplasty. Cardiology 5(3):31, 1988

7. Atkinson JB, Forman MB, Perry JM, Virmani R: Correlation of saphenous vein bypass graft angiograms with histologic changes at necropsy. Am J Cardiol 55:952, 1985

8. Aueron F, Gruentzig A: Distal embolization of a coronary artery bypass graft atheroma during percutaneous transluminal coronary angioplasty. Am J Cardiol 53:953, 1984

9. Austin GE, Norman NB, Hollman J, et al: Intimal proliferation of smooth muscle cells as an explanation for recurrent coronary artery stenosis after percutaneous transluminal coronary angioplasty. J Am Coll Cardiol 6:369, 1985

10. Baim DS (ed): A Symposium: Interventional Cardiology—1987. Am J Cardiol 61(14):1G, 1988

11. Baim DS: Interventional catheterization techniques: Percutaneous transluminal balloon angioplasty, valvuloplasty, and related procedures. p. 1379. In Braunwald E (ed): Heart Disease. A Textbook of Cardiovascular Medicine. 3rd Ed. WB Saunders, Philadelphia, 1988

12. Baim DS, Ignatius EJ: Use of percutaneous transluminal coronary angioplasty: Results of a current survey. Am J Cardiol 61(14):3G, 1988

13. Banka VS, Chadda KD, Helfant RH: Limitations of myocardial revascularization in restoration of regional contraction abnormalities produced by coronary occlusion. Am J Cardiol 34:164, 1974

14. Baroldi G: Diseases of the coronary arteries. p. 341. In Silver MD (ed): Cardiovascular Pathology. Churchill Livingstone, New York, 1983

15. Bashour TT, Hanna ES, Edgett J, Geiger J: Iatrogenic left main coronary artery stenosis following PTCA or valve replacement. Clin Cardiol 8:11, 1985

16. Batayias GE, Barboriak JJ, Korns ME, Pintar K: The spectrum of pathologic changes in aortocoronary saphenous vein grafts. Circulation 56(suppl II):11, 1977

17. Baughman KL, Pasternak RC, Fallon JT, Block PC: Transluminal coronary angioplasty of postmortem human hearts. Am J Cardiol 48:1044, 1981

18. Belhassen B, Miller HI, Landiado S: Catheter ablation of incessant ventricular tachycardia refractory to external cardioversions. Am J Cardiol 55:1637, 1985

19. Berry CL: Thrombolytic therapy and myocardial infarction. J Clin Pathol 28:352, 1975

20. Bertrand ME, LeBranche JM, Thieuleux FA, et al: Comparative results of percutaneous transluminal coronary angioplasty in patients with dynamic versus fixed coronary stenosis. J Am Coll Cardiol 8:504, 1986

21. Block PC: Histological and ultrastructural studies in animals. p. 155. In Proceedings of the Workshop on Percutaneous Transluminal Coronary Angioplasty. DHEW Publ. No. 80–2030. Department of Health and Human Services, Washington, DC, 1980

22. Block PC, Baughman KL, Pasternak RC, Fallon JT: Transluminal angioplasty: Correlation of morphologic and angiographic findings in

an experimental model. Circulation 61:778, 1980

23. Block PC, Cowley MJ, Kaltenbach M, et al: Percutaneous angioplasty of stenosis by bypass grafts or of bypass graft anastomatic sites. Am J Cardiol 53:666, 1984

24. Block PC, Elmer D, Fallon JT: Release of atherosclerotic debris after transluminal angioplasty. Circulation 65:950, 1982

25. Block PC, Fallon JT, Elmer D: Experimental angioplasty: Lessons from the laboratory. AJR 135:907, 1980

26. Block PC, Myler RK, Stertzer S, Fallon JT: Morphology after transluminal angioplasty in human beings. N Engl J Med 305:382, 1981

27. Block PC, Palacios IF, Jacobs ML, Fallon JT: Mechanism of percutaneous mitral valvuloplasty. Am J Cardiol 59:178, 1987

28. Bourdillon PDV, Hookman DK, Morris SN, Waller BF: Percutaneous balloon valvuloplasty for tricuspid stenosis: Hemodynamic and pathologic findings. Am Heart J, in press

29. Bredlau CE, Roubin GS, Leimgruber PP, et al: In hospital morbidity and mortality in patients undergoing elective coronary angioplasty. Circulation 72:1044, 1985

30. Breshnahan GF, Roberts R, Shell WE, et al: Deleterious effects due to hemorrhage after myocardial reperfusion. Am J Cardiol 33:82, 1974

31. Brown BG, Bolson E, Frimer M, Dodge HT: Quantitative coronary arteriography. Estimation of dimensions, hemodynamic resistance and atheroma mass of coronary artery lesions using the arteriogram and digital computation. Circulation 55:329, 1977

32. Bulkley BH, Hutchins G: Accelerated "atherosclerosis." A morphologic study of 97 saphenous vein coronary artery bypass grafts. Circulation 55:163, 1977

33. Campeau L, Lesperance J, Bourassa MG: Natural history of saphenous vein aortocoronary bypass grafts. Mod Concepts Cardiovasc Dis 53:59, 1984

34. Capone RJ, Most AS: Myocardial hemorrhage after coronary reperfusion in pigs. Am J Cardiol 41:259, 1978

35. Castaneda-Zuniga WR, Formarek A, Todavarthy M, Edwards JE: The mechanism of balloon angioplasty. Radiology 135:565, 1980

36. Castellot JJ, Favreau LV, Karnovsky MJ, Rosenberg RR: Inhibition of vascular smooth muscle cell growth by endothelial cell-derived heparin. J Biol Chem 257:11256, 1982

37. Cerra FB, Lajos TZ, Montes M, Siegel JH: Hemorrhagic infarction: A reperfusion injury following prolonged myocardial ischemia anoxia. Surgery 78:95, 1975

38. Chapman PD, Klopfenstein S, Troup PJ, et al: Evaluation of a percutaneous catheter technique for ablation of ventricular tachycardia in a canine model. Am Heart J 110:1, 1985

39. Colavita PG, Ideker RE, Reimer KA, et al: The spectrum of pathology associated with percutaneous transluminal coronary angioplasty during acute myocardial infarction. J Am Coll Cardiol 8:855, 1986

40. Copeland JG, Levinson MM, Smith R, et al: The total artificial heart as a bridge to transplantation. A report of two cases. JAMA 256:2991, 1986

41. Copeland JG, Smith RG, Icenogle TB, et al: Early experience with the total artificial heart as a bridge to cardiac transplantation. Surg Clin North Am 68:621, 1988

42. Corbelli J, Franco I, Hollman J, et al: Percutaneous transluminal coronary angioplasty after previous coronary artery bypass surgery. Am J Cardiol 56:398, 1985

43. Corcos T, David PR, Val PG, et al: Failure of dilitazem to prevent restenosis after percutaneous transluminal coronary angioplasty. Am Heart J 109:926, 1985

44. Cowley MJ, Dorros G, Kelsey SF, et al: Emergency coronary bypass surgery after coronary angioplasty: The National Heart Lung, and Blood Institute's Percutaneous Transluminal Coronary Angioplasty Registry experience. Am J Cardiol 53:22C, 1984

45. Cowley MJ, Dovros G, Kelsey SF, et al: Emergency coronary bypass surgery after coronary angioplasty: The National Heart, Lung and Blood Institute's Percutaneous Transluminal Coronary Angioplasty Registry experience. Am J Cardiol 53:22C, 1984

46. Cox JL: The status of surgery for cardiac arrhythmias. Circulation 71:413, 1985

47. Cragg A, Lund G, Rysavy J, et al: Nonsurgical placement of arterial endoprostheses: A new technique using nitinol wire. Radiology 147:261, 1983

48. Cribier A, Savin T, Berland J, et al: Percu-

taneous transluminal balloon valvuloplasty of adult aortic stenosis: Report of 92 cases. J Am Coll Cardiol 9:381, 1987

49. Cribier A, Savin T, Saoudi N, et al: Percutaneous transluminal valvuloplasty of acquired aortic stenosis in elderly patients. An alternative to valve replacement? Lancet 1:63, 1986

50. Cumberland DC, Sanborn TA, Taylor DI, et al: Percutaneous laser thermal angioplasty—Initial clinical results with a laser probe in a total peripheral artery occlusion. Lancet 1:1457, 1986

51. Deloche A, Fabiani JN, Camilleri JP, et al: The effect of coronary artery reperfusion on the extent of myocardial infarction. Am Heart J 93:358, 1977

52. de Morais CF, Lopez EA, Checchi H, et al: Percutaneous transluminal coronary angioplasty: Histopathological analysis of nine necropsy cases. Virchows Arch [A] 410:195, 1986

53. DeVries WC: Surgical technique for implantation of the Jarvik-7–100 total artificial heart. JAMA 259:875, 1988

54. DeVries WC: The permanent artificial heart. Four case reports. JAMA 259:849, 1988

55. DeVries WC, Anderson JL, Joyce LD, et al: Clinical use of the total artificial heart. N Engl J Med 310:273, 1988

56. Dobbins JJ, Johnson S, Kunin CM, DeVries WC: Postmortem microbiological findings of two total artificial heart recipients. JAMA 259:865, 1988

57. Dorros G, Cowley MJ, Simpson J, et al: Percutaneous transluminal coronary angioplasty: Report of complications from the National Heart, Lung and Blood Institute PTCA Registry. Circulation 67:723, 1983

58. Dorros G, Johnson WD, Tector AJ, et al: Percutaneous transluminal coronary angioplasty in patients with prior coronary artery bypass grafting. J Thorac Cardiovasc Surg 87:17, 1984

59. Dorros G, Lewin RF, King JF, Janke LM: Percutaneous transluminal valvuloplasty in calcific aortic stenosis: The double-balloon technique. Cath Cardiovasc Diagn 13:151, 1987

60. Dotter CT: Transluminally placed coil-spring endarterial tube grafts: Long-term patency in canine popliteal artery. Invest Radiol 4:329, 1969

61. Dotter CT, Judkins MP: Transluminal treatment of atherosclerotic obstructions: Description of new technic and a preliminary report of its application. Circulation 30:654, 1964

62. Dotter CT, Bushmann RW, McKinney MK, Rosch J: Transluminal expandable nitinol coil stent grafting: Preliminary report. Radiology 147:259, 1983

63. Douglas JS Jr, Gruentzig AR, King SB III, et al: Percutaneous transluminal coronary angioplasty in patients with prior coronary bypass surgery. J Am Coll Cardiol 2:745, 1983

64. Epstein AE, Kay GN, Plumb VJ, et al: Combined automatic implantable cardioverter-defibrillator and pacemaker systems: Implantation techniques and follow-up. J Am Coll Cardiol 13:121, 1989

65. Erbel R, Clas W, Busch U, et al: New balloon catheter for prolonged percutaneous transluminal coronary angioplasty and bypass flow in occluded vessels. Cathet Cardiovasc Diagn 12:116, 1986

66. Essed CD, Brand MVD, Becker AE: Transluminal coronary angioplasty and early restenosis. Br Heart J 49:393, 1983

67. Famularo M, Vasilomanolakis EC, Schrager B, et al: Percutaneous transluminal angioplasty of aortocoronary saphenous vein graft: Morphologic observations. JAMA 249:3347, 1983

68. Faxon DP, Weber VJ, Haudenschild C, et al: Acute effects of transluminal angioplasty in three experimental models of atherosclerosis. Arteriosclerosis 2:125, 1982

69. Fenoglio JJ Jr, Pham TD, Harken AH, et al: Recurrent sustained ventricular tachycardia: Structure and ultrastructure of subendocardial regions in which tachycardia originates. Circulation 68:518, 1983

70. Ferguson TB Jr, Hinohara T, Simpson J, et al: Catheter reperfusion to allow optimal coronary bypass grafting following failed transluminal coronary angioplasty. Ann Thorac Surg 42:399, 1986

71. Fishbein MC, Ganz W, Y-Rit J, et al: Relevance of hemorrhage after reperfusion in acute myocardial infarction. p. 284. In Kaltenback M (ed): Transluminal Coronary Angioplasty and Intracoronary Thrombolysis. Springer-Verlag, Berlin, 1982

72. Fishbein MC, Y-Rit J, Lando U, et al: The

relationship of vascular injury and myocardial hemorrhage to necrosis after reperfusion. Circulation 62:1274, 1980

73. Ford WB, Wholey MH, Zikria EA, et al: Percutaneous transluminal angioplasty in the management of occlusive disease involving the coronary arteries and saphenous vein bypass grafts: Preliminary results. J Thorac Cardiovasc Surg 79:11, 1980

74. Ford WB, Wholey MH, Zikria EA, et al: Percutaneous transluminal dilation of aortocoronary saphenous vein bypass grafts. Chest 79:529, 1981

75. Forrester JS, Litvack F, Grundfest W: Vaporization of atheroma in man: The role of lasers in the era of balloon angioplasty. Int J Cardiol 20:1, 1988

76. Fouvier JL, Marache P, Brunetand JM, et al: Laser recanalization of peripheral arteries by contact sapphire in man. Circulation 74(suppl II):231, 1986 (abst)

77. Fujiwara H, Onodera T, Tanaka M, et al: A clinicopathologic study of patients with hemorrhagic myocardial infarction treated with selective coronary thrombolysis with urokinase. Circulation 73:749, 1986

78. Fuster V, Adams PC, Badimon JJ, Chesebro JH: Platelet-inhibitor drugs role in coronary artery disease. Prog Cardiovasc Dis 29:325, 1987

79. Galletti PM: Replacement of the heart with a mechanical device. The case of Dr. Barney Clark. N Engl J Med 310:312, 1984

80. Ganz W, Buchbinder N, Marcus H, et al: Intracoronary thrombolysis in evolving myocardial infarction. Am Heart J 101:4, 1981

81. Gold HK, Cowley MJ, Palacios IF, et al: Combined intracoronary streptokinase infusion and coronary angioplasty during acute myocardial infarction. Am J Cardiol 53:122C, 1984

82. Gold HK, Cowley MJ, Palacios IF, et al: Combined intracoronary streptokinase infusion and coronary angioplasty during acute myocardial infarction. Am J Cardiol 53:122C, 1984

83. Graf RH, Vernai MS: Left main coronary artery stenosis: A possible complication of transluminal coronary angioplasty. Cathet Cardiovasc Diagn 10:163, 1984

84. Gruntzig AR: Transluminal dilatation of coronary artery stenosis. Lancet 1:263, 1978

85. Gruentzig AR, Myler RK, Hanna EH, Turina MI: Coronary transluminal angioplasty. Circulation 55–56:III–84, 1977 (abst)

86. Guiraudon GM, Fontaine G, Frank R, et al: Encircling endocardial ventriculotomy: A new surgical treatment for life-threatening ventricular tachycardias resistant to medial treatment following myocardial infarction. Ann Thorac Surg 26:438, 1978

87. Hall DP, Gruentzig AR: Percutaneous transluminal coronary angioplasty: An update on indications, techniques, and results. Cardiol Clin 3:37, 1985

88. Harrison DG, Ferguson DW, Collins SM, et al: Rethrombosis after reperfusion with streptokinase: Importance of geometry of residual lesions. Circulation 69:991, 1984

89. Hartzler GO: Electrode catheter ablation of refractory focal ventricular tachycardia. J Am Coll Cardiol 2:1107, 1983

90. Hartzler GO, Rutherford BD, McConahay DR: Percutaneous transluminal coronary angioplasty with and without thrombolytic therapy for treatment of acute myocardial infarction. Am Heart J 106:965, 1983

91. Hartzler GO, Rutherford BD, McConahay DR: Percutaneous transluminal coronary angioplasty: Application for acute myocardial infarction. Am J Cardiol 53:117C, 1984

92. Health and Public Policy Committee, American College of Physicians: Thrombolysis for evolving myocardial infarction. Ann Intern Med 103:463, 1985

93. Henson DE, Kajafi H, Callaghan R, et al: Myocardial lesions following open heart surgery. Arch Pathol 88:423, 1969

94. Hill JD, Farrar DJ, Hershon JJ, et al: Use of a prosthetic ventricle as a bridge to cardiac transplantation for postinfarction cardiogenic shock. N Engl J Med 314:626, 1986

95. Hill JA, Margolis JR, Feldman RL, et al: Coronary arterial aneurysm formation after balloon angioplasty. Am J Cardiol 52:261, 1983

96. Hofling B, Simpson JB, Rmeberger K, et al: Percutaneous atherectomy in iliac, femoral and popliteal arteries. Klin Wochenschr 65:528, 1987

97. Holems DR Jr, Vlietstra RE, Mock MB, et al: Angiographic changes produced by percutaneous transluminal coronary angioplasty. Am J Cardiol 51:676, 1983

98. Hollander G, Ozick H, Anselmo M, et al:

Myocardial rupture following intracoronary thrombolysis therapy. NY State J Med 84:129, 1984

99. Holmes DR Jr, Vlietstra RE, Mock MB: Angiographic changes produced by percutaneous transluminal coronary angioplasty. Am J Cardiol 51:676, 1983

100. Holmes DR Jr, Vlietstra RE, Smith HC, et al: Restenosis after percutaneous transluminal coronary angioplasty (PTCA): A report from the PTCA Registry of the National Heart, Lung, and Blood Institute. Am J Cardiol 53:77C, 1984

101. Horowitz LN, Harken AH, Kastor JA, et al: Ventricular resection guided by epicardial mapping for treatment of recurrent ventricular tachycardia. N Engl J Med 302:489, 1980

102. Hutchins GM, Bulkley BH: Correlation of myocardial contraction band necrosis and vascular patency. Lab Invest 36:642, 1977

103. Inoue H, Ealler BF, Zipes DP: Intracoronary ethyl alcohol or phenol injection ablates aconitine-induced ventricular tachycardia in dogs. J Am Coll Cardiol 10:1342, 1987

104. Inoue K, Owaki T, Nakamura T, et al: Clinical application of transvenous mitral commissurotomy by a new balloon catheter. J Thorac Cardiovasc Surg 87:394, 1984

105. Isner JM, Clarke RH: Laser angioplasty: Unraveling the Gordian knot. J Am Coll Cardiol 7:705, 1986

106. Isner JM, Donaldson RF, Deckelbaum LI, et al: The excimer laser: Gross, light microscopic and ultrastructural analysis of potential advantages for use in laser therapy of cardiovascular disease. J Am Coll Cardiol 6:1102, 1985

107. Isner JM, Fortin RV: Frequency in nonangioplasty patients of morphologic findings reported in coronary arteries treated with transluminal angioplasty. Am J Cardiol 51:689, 1983

108. Isner JM, Konstam MA, Fortin RV, et al: Delayed thrombolysis of streptokinase-resistant occlusive thrombus: Documentation by pre and postmortem coronary angiography. Am J Cardiol 52:210, 1982

109. Isner JM, Salem DN, Desnoyers MR, et al: Treatment of calcific aortic stenosis by balloon valvuloplasty. Am J Cardiol 59:313, 1987

110. Jenkins RD, Sinclair IN, Anand RK, et al: Laser balloon angioplasty: Effect of exposure duration on shear strength of welded layers of postmortem human aorta. Circulation 76(suppl IV):IV-46, 1987 (abst)

111. Jenkins RD, Sinclair IN, Leonard BM, et al: Laser balloon angioplasty vs balloon angioplasty in normal rabbit iliac arteries. Circulation 76(suppl IV):IV-47, 1987 (abst)

112. Jennings RB, Reimer KA: Factors involved in salvaging ischemic myocardium: Effect of reperfusion of arterial blood. Circulation 68(suppl I):I-25, 1983

113. Josephson ME, Horowitz LN, Harken AH: Endocardial excision: A new surgical technique for the treatment of ventricular tachycardia. Circulation 60:1430, 1979

114. Kaltenback M, Kober G, Scherer D, Vallbracht C: Recurrence rate after successful coronary angioplasty. Eur Heart J 6:276, 1985

115. Kan J, White RI, Mitchell SE, Gardner TJ: Percutaneous balloon valvuloplasty: A new method for treating congenital pulmonary valve stenosis. N Engl J Med 307:540, 1982

116. Kao K-J, Hackel DB, Kong Y: Hemorrhagic myocardial infarction after streptokinase treatment for acute coronary thrombosis. Arch Pathol Lab Med 108:121, 1984

117. Kaplan J, Barry KJ, Connolly RJ, et al: Thermal angioplasty with a radiofrequency balloon system. Circulation 78(suppl II):II-503, 1988 (abst)

118. Kaplan JD, Isner JM, Karas RH, et al: In-vitro analysis of mechanisms of balloon valvuloplasty of stenotic mitral valves. Am J Cardiol 59:318, 1987

119. Kennedy JW, Ritchie JL, Davis KB, Friz JK: Western Washington randomized trial of intracoronary streptokinase in acute myocardial infarction. N Engl J Med 309:1477, 1983

120. Keon WJ, Heggtveit HA, Leduc J: Perioperative myocardial infarction caused by atheroembolism. J Thorac Cardiovasc Surg 84:849, 1982

121. Khaja F, Walton JA, Brymer JF, et al: Intracoronary fibrinolytic therapy in acute myocardial infarction. Report of a prospective randomized trial. N Engl J Med 308:1305, 1983

122. Kloner RA, Alker KJ: The effect of streptokinase on intramyocardial hemorrhage, infarct size and the no-reflow phenomena during coronary reperfusion. Circulation 70:513, 1984

123. Kloner RA, Ellis SG, Lange R, Braunwald E: Studies of experimental coronary artery reperfusion. Effects on infarct size, myocardial function, biochemistry, ultrastructure, microvascular damage. Circulation 68(suppl I):I-8, 1983

124. Kloner RA, Rude RE, Carlson N, et al: Ultrastructural evidence of microvascular damage and myocardial injury after coronary artery occlusion: Which comes first? Circulation 62:945, 1980

125. Kunin CM, Dobbins JJ, Melo JC, et al: Infectious complications in four long-term recipients of the Jarvik-7 artificial heart. JAMA 259:860, 1988

126. Lababidi Z, Wu JR: Percutaneous balloon valvuloplasty. Am J Cardiol 52:560, 1983

127. Lababidi Z, Wu RJ, Walls JT: Percutaneous balloon aortic valvuloplasty: Results in 23 patients. Am J Cardiol 53:194, 1984

128. La Delia V, Rossi PA, Sommers S, Kreps E: Coronary histology after percutaneous transluminal coronary angioplasty. Tex Heart Inst J 15:113, 1988

129. Lang TW, Corday E, Gold H, et al: Consequences of reperfusion after coronary occlusion. Effects of hemodynamic and regional myocardial metabolic function. Am J Cardiol 33:69, 1974

130. Laurie GM, Pacifico A: Surgical treatment of ventricular tachycardia. Cardiology 1:99, 1989

131. Lawrence DD, Charnsangavej C, Wright KC, et al: Percutaneous endovascular graft: Experimental evaluation. Radiology 163:357, 1987

132. Lawrie GM: Permanent implantation of the Jarvik-7 total artificial heart: A clinical perspective. JAMA 259:892, 1988

133. Lee BI, Becker GJ, Waller BF, et al: Thermal compression and molding of atherosclerotic vascular tissue using radiofrequency energy: Implications for radiofrequency balloon angioplasty. J Am Coll Cardiol, in press

134. Lee G, Lee MH, Ikeda RM, et al: Effects of laser radiation on the morphology of human coronary atherosclerotic disease. p. 621. In Waller BF (ed): Cardiac Morphology. Vol. 2. WB Saunders, Philadelphia, 1984

135. Leiboff RH, Katz RJ, Wasserman AG, et al: A randomized angiographically controlled trial of intracoronary streptokinase in acute myocardial infarction. Am J Cardiol 53:404, 1984

136. Leimgruber PP, Roubin GS, Anderson HV, et al: Influence of intimal dissection on restenosis after successful coronary angioplasty. Circulation 72:530, 1985

137. Leimgruber PP, Roubin GS, Hollman J, et al: Restenosis after successful coronary angioplasty in patients with single vessel disease. Circulation 73:710, 1986

138. Levine S, Ewels CJ, Rosing DR, Kent KM: Coronary angioplasty: Clinical and angiographic followup. Am J Cardiol 55:673, 1985

139. Lie JT, Lawrie GM, Morris GC Jr: Aortocoronary bypass saphenous vein graft atherosclerosis: Anatomic study of 99 vein grafts from normal and hyperlipoproteinemic patients up to 74 months postoperatively. Am J Cardiol 40:906, 1977

140. Lie JT, Lawrie GM, Morris GC Jr, Winters VL: Hemorrhagic myocardial infarction associated with aortocoronary bypass revascularization. Am Heart J 96:295, 1978

141. Little WC: Thrombolytic therapy of acute myocardial infarction. Curr Probl Cardiol 8(9):7, 1983

142. Little WC, Rogers EW: Angiographic evidence of hemorrhagic myocardial infarction after intracoronary thrombolysis with streptokinase. Am J Cardiol 51:906, 1983

143. Litvack F, Grundfest W, Mohr F, et al: "Hot-tip" angioplasty by a novel radiofrequency catheter. Circulation 16(suppl IV):IV-47, 1987 (abst)

144. Lo YSA: Intravenous versus intracoronary streptokinase in acute myocardial infarction. Clin Cardiol 8:609, 1985

145. Lock JE, Khalilullah M, Shrivasta S, et al: Percutaneous catheter commissurotomy in rheumatic mitral stenosis. N Engl J Med 313:1515, 1985

146. Maass D, Kropf L, Egloff L, et al: Transluminal implantation of intravascular "double-helix" spiral prostheses: Technical and biological considerations. Proc Eur Soc Artif Organs 9:252, 1982

147. Maass D, Zollikofer CL, Largiader F, Senning A: Radiological follow-up of transluminally inserted vascular endoprostheses: An experimental study using expanding spirals. Radiology 152:659, 1984

148. Mabin TA, Holmes DR, Smith HC, et al:

Follow-up clinical results in patients undergoing percutaneous transluminal coronary angioplasty. Circulation 71:754, 1985

149. MacDonald RG, Feldman RL, Conti CR, Pepine CJ: Thromboembolic complications of coronary angioplasty. Am J Cardiol 54:916, 1984

150. Markis JE, Malagould M, Parker A, et al: Myocardial salvage after intracoronary thrombolysis with streptokinase in acute myocardial infarction. N Engl J Med 305:777, 1981

151. Marti M-C, Bouchardy B, Cox JN: Aortocoronary by-pass with autogenous saphenous vein grafts: Histopathological aspects. Virchows Arch [A] 352:255, 1971

152. Mathews BJ, Ewels CJ, Kent KM: Coronary dissection: A predictor of restenosis? Am Heart J 115:547, 1988

153. Mathey DG, Juch KH, Tilsner V, et al: Nonsurgical coronary artery recanalization in acute transmural myocardial infarction. Circulation 63:489, 1981

154. Mathey DG, Schofer J, Kuck K-H, et al: Transmural hemorrhagic myocardial infarction after intracoronary streptokinase. Clinical, angiographic and necropsy findings. Br Heart J 48:546, 1982

155. Mattfeldt T, Schwarz F, Schuler G, et al: Necropsy evaluation in seven patients with evolving acute myocardial infarction treated with thrombolytic therapy. Am J Cardiol 54:530, 1984

156. Mayes JB, Williams MA, Barker LE, et al: Clinical management of total artificial heart drive systems. JAMA 259:881, 1988

157. McKay RG, Grossman W: Balloon valvuloplasty for treating pulmonic, mitral, aortic and prosthetic valve stenoses. p. 1. In Braunwald E (ed): Heart Disease. 3rd Ed. Update 1. WB Saunders, Philadelphia, 1988

158. McKay CR, Kawanishi DT, Rahimtoola SH: Double catheter balloon valvuloplasty in patients with mitral stenosis. Initial experience and long-term improvement in rest and exercise hemodynamics. Clin Res 35:180A, 1987

159. McKay RG, Lock JE, Keane FJ, et al: Percutaneous mitral valvuloplasty in an adult patient with calcific rheumatic stenosis. J Am Coll Cardiol 77:1410, 1986

160. McKay RG, Lock JE, Safian RD, et al: Balloon dilation of mitral stenosis in adults: Post-mortem and percutaneous mitral valvuloplasty studies. J Am Coll Cardiol 9:773, 1987

161. McKay RG, Safian RD, Lock JE, et al: Assessment of left ventricular and aortic valve function after aortic balloon valvuloplasty in adult patients with critical aortic stenosis. Circulation 75:192, 1987

162. McKay RG, Safian RD, Lock JE, et al: Balloon dilatation of calcific aortic stenosis in elderly patients: Postmortem intraoperative, and percutaneous valvuloplasty studies. Circulation 74:119, 1986

163. Meier B, King SB, Gruentzig AR, et al: Repeat coronary angioplasty. J Am Coll Cardiol 4:463, 1984

164. Menke DM, Jordan MD, Aust CH, et al: Histologic evidence of distal coronary thromboembolism: A complication of acute proximal coronary artery thrombolysis therapy. Chest 9:614, 1986

165. Meyer J, Marks W, Effert S: Percutaneous transluminal coronary angioplasty immediately after intracoronary streptolysis of transluminal myocardial infarction. Circulation 66:905, 1982

166. Mirowski M, Mower MM, Staewen WS, et al: Standby automatic defibrillator. Arch Intern Med 126:158, 1970

167. Mirowski M, Reid PR, Mower MM, et al: Termination of malignant ventricular arrhythmias with an implanted automatic defibrillator in human beings. N Engl J Med 303:22, 1980

168. Mizuno K, Jurita A, Imazeki N: Pathologic findings after percutaneous transluminal coronary angioplasty. Br Heart J 52:588, 1984

169. Morady F, Scheinman MM, Hess DS, et al: Electrophysiology testing in the management of survivors of out-of-hospital cardiac arrest. Am J Cardiol 51:85, 1983

170. Morales AR, Fine G, Taber RE: Cardiac surgery and myocardial necrosis. Arch Pathol 83:71, 1967

171. Mullins CE, Nihill MR, Vick GW, et al: Double balloon techniques for dilation of valvular or vessel stenosis in congenital and acquired heart disease. J Am Coll Cardiol 10:107, 1987

172. Myler RK, Cumberland DA, Clark DA, et al: High and low power thermal laser angioplasty for total occlusions and restenosis in man. Circulation 76(suppl IV):IV-230, 1987 (abst)

173. Myler RM, Shaw RE, Stertzer SH, et al: Recurrence after coronary angioplasty. Cathet Cardiovasc Diagn 13:77, 1987

174. Nobuyoski M, Kimura T, Nosaka H, et al: Restenosis after successful percutaneous transluminal coronary angioplasty: Serial angiographic followup of 229 patients. J Am Coll Cardiol 12:616, 1988

175. Olson HG, Butman SM, Piters KM, et al: A randomized controlled trial of intravenous streptokinase in evolving acute myocardial infarction. Am Heart J 111:1021, 1986

176. O'Neill W, Timmis GC, Bourdillon PD, et al: A prospective randomized clinical trial of intracoronary streptokinase versus coronary angioplasty for acute myocardial infarction. N Engl J Med 314:812, 1986

177. Palacios I, Block PC: Antegrade balloon valvotomy for aortic stenosis. J Am Coll Cardiol 9:14A, 1987

178. Palacios I, Lock JE, Keane JF, Block PC: Percutaneous transvenous balloon valvotomy in a patient with severe calcific mitral stenosis. J Am Coll Cardiol 7:1416, 1986

179. Palmaz JC, Richter GM, Noeldge G, et al: Intraluminal stents in atherosclerotic iliac artery stenosis: Preliminary report of a multicenter study. Inter Radiol 168:727, 1988

180. Palmaz JC, Sibbitt RR, Reuter SR, et al: Expandable intraluminal graft: A preliminary study. Radiology 156:73, 1985

181. Palmaz JC, Sibbitt RR, Tio FO, et al: Expandable intraluminal vascular graft: A feasibility study. Surgery 99:199, 1986

182. Palmaz JC, Windeler SA, Garcia F, et al: Atherosclerotic rabbit aortas: Expandable intraluminal grafting. Radiology 160:723, 1986

183. Papaiotro SE, Machean WAH, Stanley AWH Jr, et al: Percutaneous transluminal coronary angioplasty in acute myocardial infarction. Am J Cardiol 55:48, 1985

184. Pepine CJ, Gessner JH, Feldman RL: Percutaneous balloon valvuloplasty for pulmonic valve stenosis in the adult. Am J Cardiol 51:1442, 1982

185. Peuch P, Gallay P, Grolleau R, et al: Traitement par electrofulguration endocavitaire d'une tachycardie ventriculaire par dysplasie ventriculaire droite. Arch Mal Coeur 77:826, 1984

186. Pierce WS: Permanent heart substitution: Better solutions lie ahead. JAMA 259:891, 1988

187. Reeder GS, Bresnahan JF, Holmes DR Jr, et al: Angioplasty for aortocoronary bypass graft stenosis. Mayo Clin Proc 61:14, 1986

188. Reduto LA, Smalling RW, Freund GC, et al: Intracoronary infusion of streptokinase in patients with acute myocardial infarction: Effects of reperfusion on left ventricular performance. Am J Cardiol 48:403, 1981

189. Reimer KA: Overview of potential mechanisms. p. 387. In Wagner GS (ed): Myocardial Infarction: Measurement and Intervention. Martinus Nijhoff, The Hague, 1982

190. Relman AS: Intravenous thrombolysis in acute myocardial infarction. A progress report. N Engl J Med 312:915, 1985

191. Relman AS: Artificial hearts—Permanent and temporary. N Engl J Med 314:644, 1986

192. Rentrop P, Blanke H, Karsch KR, et al: Selective intracoronary thrombolysis in acute myocardial infarction and unstable angina pectoris. Circulation 63:489, 1981

193. Rentrop P, DeVivie ER, Karsch KR, et al: Acute myocardial infarction: Intracoronary application of nitroglycerin and streptokinase in combination with transluminal recanalization. Clin Cardiol 5:354, 1979

194. Rice LB: Artificial heart implantation: What limitations are imposed by infectious complications? JAMA 259:894, 1988

195. Roberts WC: Coronary embolism: A review of causes, consequences and diagnostic considerations. Cardiovasc Med 3:699, 1978

196. Roberts WC, Morrow AG: Causes of early postoperative death following cardiac valve replacement. J Thorac Cardiovasc Surg 54:433, 1967

197. Roberts CS, Schoen FJ, Kloner RA: Effect of coronary reperfusion on myocardial infarct healing and hemorrhage. Am J Cardiol 52:610, 1983

198. Roubin G, Giaturco C, Brown J, et al: Intracoronary stenting of canine coronary arteries after percutaneous coronary angioplasty. Circulation 74:11, 1986 (abst)

199. Roubin GS, Robinson KA, King SB, et al: Acute and late results of intracoronary arterial stenting after coronary angioplasty in dogs. Circulation 76:891, 1987

200. Saber RS, Edwards WD, Holmes DR, et al: Balloon angioplasty of aortocoronary saphenous vein bypass grafts: A histopathologic study of six grafts from five patients with em-

phasis on restenosis and embolic complications. J Am Coll Cardiol 12:1501, 1988

201. Saffitz JE, Rose TE, Oaks JB, Roberts WC: Coronary arterial rupture during coronary angioplasty. Am J Cardiol 51:902, 1983

202. Safian RD, Mandell VS, Thurer RE, et al: Postmortem and intraoperative balloon valvuloplasty of calcific aortic stenosis in elderly patients: Mechanisms of successful dilation. J Am Coll Cardiol 9:655, 1987

203. Saner HE, Gobel FL, Salomonowitz E, et al: The disease-free wall in coronary atherosclerosis: Its relation to degree of obstruction. J Am Coll Cardiol 6:1096, 1985

204. Sanborn TA: Laser thermal angioplasty. p. 75. In White RA, Grundfest WS (eds): Lasers in Cardiovascular Disease. Year Book Medical Publishers, Chicago, 1987

205. Sanborn TA: Laser angioplasty. What has been learned from experimental studies and clinical trials? Circulation 78:769, 1988

206. Sanborn TA, Cumberland, Greenfield AJ, et al: Percutaneous laser thermal angioplasty: Initial results and 1-year followup in 129 femoropopliteal lesions. Radiology 168:121, 1988

207. Sanborn TA, Cumberland DC, Welsh CL, et al: Laser thermal angioplasty as an adjunct to peripheral balloon angioplasty: One year follow-up results. Circulation 16(suppl IV):IV-230, 1987 (abst)

208. Sanborn TA, Faxon DP, Haudenschild CC, Ryan TJ: Experimental angioplasty: Circumferential distribution of laser thermal energy with a laser probe. J Am Coll Cardiol 5:934, 1985

209. Sanborn TA, Haudenschild CC, Faxon DP, Ryan TJ: Angiographic and histologic followup of laser angioplasty with a laser probe. J Am Coll Cardiol 5:408, 1985 (abst)

210. Schachenmayr W, Haferkamp O: Der hamorrhagische Herzinfarkt. Dtsch Med Wochenschr 97:1172, 1972

211. Schneider JF, Wilson M, Gallant TE: Percutaneous balloon aortic valvuloplasty for aortic stenosis in elderly patients at high risk for surgery. Ann Intern Med 106:696, 1987

212. Schatz R, Palmaz J, Garcia F, et al: Balloon expandable intracoronary stents in dogs. Circulation 76:450, 1987

213. Schoen FJ, Bernhard WF, Khuri SF, et al: Pathologic findings in postcardiotomy patients managed with a temporary left ventricular assist pump. Am J Surg 143:508, 1982

214. Schoen FJ, Palmer DC, Bernhard WF, et al: Clinical temporary assist: Pathologic findings and their implications in a multi-institutional study of 41 patients. J Thorac Cardiovasc Surg, in press

215. Schwarz F, Schuler G, Katus H, et al: Intracoronary thrombolysis in acute myocardial infarction: Duration of ischemia is a major determinant of late results after recanalization. Am J Cardiol 50:933, 1982

216. Semb BKH, Tjonneland S, Stake G, Aabyholm G: Balloon valvotomy of congenital pulmonary valve stenosis with tricuspid insufficiency. Cardiovasc Radiol 2:239, 1979

217. Serruys DW, Juiliere Y, Bertrand ME, et al: Additional improvement of stenosis geometry in human coronary arteries by stenting after balloon dilatation. Am J Cardiol 61:71G, 1988

218. Serruys PW, Wijns W, Van den Brand M, et al: Is transluminal coronary angioplasty mandatory after successful thrombolysis? Quantitative coronary angiographic study. Br Heart J 50:257, 1983

219. Shalilullah M, Tyagi S, Yadau BS, et al: Double balloon valvuloplasty of tricuspid stenosis. Am Heart J 114:1232, 1987

220. Shaw RE, Myler RK, Stertzer SH, Clark DA: Restenosis after coronary angioplasty. Cardiology 4:42, 1987

221. Sigwart U, Puel J, Mirkowitch V, et al: Intravascular stents to prevent occlusion and restenosis after transluminal angioplasty. N Engl J Med 316:701, 1987

222. Silver MA, Cohen AI, Katz NM, et al: Cardiac morphologic findings late after partial left ventricular endomyocardial resection for recurrent ventricular tachycardia. Am J Cardiol 54:233, 1984

223. Simpfendorfer C, Belardi J, Bellamy G, et al: Frequency, management and followup of patients with acute coronary occlusions after percutaneous coronary angioplasty. Am J Cardiol 59:267, 1987

224. Simpson JB, Selmon MR, Robertson GC, et al: Transluminal atherectomy for occlusive peripheral vascular disease. Am J Cardiol 61:965, 1988

225. Simpson JB, Zimmerman JJ, Selmon MR, et al: Transluminal atherectomy: Initial clinical results in 27 patients. Circulation 74(suppl II):II-203, 1986 (abst)

226. Sinclair IN: Effect of laser balloon angioplasty on normal dog coronary arteries in vivo. J Am Coll Cardiol 11:108A, 1988 (abst)

227. Sinclair IN, McCabe CH, Sipperly ME, Baim DS: Predictors, therapeutic options and long-term outcome of abrupt reclosure. Am J Cardiol 61(14):615, 1988

228. Slack JD, Pinkerton CA: Subacute left main coronary stenosis: An unusual but serious complication of percutaneous transluminal angioplasty. Angiology 36:130, 1985

229. Smith SH, Geer JC: Morphology of saphenous vein-coronary artery bypass grafts: Seven to 116 months after surgery. Arch Pathol Lab Med 107:13, 1983

230. Sobel BE, Bergmann SR: Coronary thrombolysis: Some unresolved issues. Am J Med 72:1, 1982

231. Soward AL, Essed CE, Serruys PW: Coronary arterial findings after accidental death immediately after successful percutaneous transluminal coronary angioplasty. Am J Cardiol 56:794, 1985

232. Spears JR: Percutaneous transluminal coronary angioplasty restenosis: Potential prevention with laser balloon angioplasty. Am J Cardiol 60:61B, 1987

233. Stroh JA, Sanborn TA, Haudenschild CC: Experimental argon laser thermal angioplasty as an adjunct to balloon angioplasty. J Am Coll Cardiol 11(suppl A):108A, 1988 (abst)

234. Sugita Y, Shimomitsu T, Oku T, et al: Nonsurgical implantation of a vascular ring prosthesis using thermal shape memory Ti/Ni Alloy (nitinol wire). Trans Am Soc Artif Intern Organs 32:30, 1986

235. The TIMI Study Group: The thrombolysis in myocardial infarction (TIMI) Trial: Phase I findings. N Engl J Med 312:932, 1985

236. Turi ZG, Campbell CA, Gottimukkala MV, Kloner RA: Preservation of distal coronary perfusion during prolonged balloon inflation with an autoperfusion angioplasty catheter. Circulation 75:1273, 1987

237. Turi ZG, Rezkalla S, Campbell CA, Kloner RA: Amelioration of ischemia during angioplasty of the left anterior descending coronary artery with an autoperfusion catheter. Am J Cardiol 62:513, 1988

238. Unni KK, Kottke BA, Titus JL, et al: Pathologic changes in aortocoronary saphenous vein grafts. Am J Cardiol 34:526, 1974

239. Verstraete M, van de Loo J, Jesdinsky HJ: Streptokinase in acute myocardial infarction. Acta Med Scand 648(suppl):7, 1981

240. Vlodaver Z, Edwards JE: Pathology of coronary atherosclerosis. Prog Cardiovasc Dis 14:256, 1971

241. Vlodaver Z, Edwards JE: Pathologic analysis in fatal cases following saphenous vein coronary arterial bypass. Chest 64:555, 1973

242. Waldo AL, Arciniegas JG, Klein H: Surgical treatment of left-threatening ventricular arrhythmias: The role of intraoperative mapping and consideration of the presently available surgical techniques. Prog Cardiovasc Dis 23:247, 1981

243. Waller BF: Early and late morphologic changes in human coronary arteries after percutaneous transluminal coronary angioplasty. Clin Cardiol 6:363, 1983

244. Waller BF: Coronary luminal shape and the arc of disease-free wall: Morphologic observations and clinical relevance. J Am Coll Cardiol 6:1100, 1985

245. Waller BF: Pathology of new interventions used in the treatment of coronary heart disease. Curr Probl Cardiol 11:665, 1986

246. Waller BF: Pathology of transluminal balloon angioplasty used in the treatment of coronary heart disease. Hum Pathol 18:476, 1987

247. Waller BF: Morphologic correlates of coronary angiographic patterns at the site of percutaneous transluminal coronary angioplasty. Clin Cardiol 11:817, 1988

248. Waller BF: The eccentric coronary atherosclerotic plaque: Morphologic observations and clinical relevance. Clin Cardiol 12:14, 1989

249. Waller BF: "Crackers, breakers, stretchers, drillers, scrapers, shavers, burners, welders and melters"—The future treatment of atherosclerotic coronary artery disease? A clinical-morphologic assessment. J Am Coll Cardiol, in press

250. Waller BF, Dillon JC, Cowley MH: Plaque hematoma and coronary dissection with percutaneous transluminal angioplasty (PTCA) of severely stenotic lesions. Morphologic coronary observations in 5 men within 30 days of PTCA. Circulation 68(suppl III):III-144, 1983 (abst)

251. Waller BF, Dixon DS, Kim RW, et al: Em-

bolus to the left main coronary artery. Am J Cardiol 50:658, 1982

252. Waller BF, Roberts WC: Amount of luminal narrowing in bypassed and nonbypassed native coronary arteries in necropsy patients dying early and late after aortocoronary bypass operations. p. 503. In Mason DT, Collins JJ (eds): Myocardial Revascularization. Medical and Surgical Advances in Coronary Disease. York Medical Books, New York, 1981

253. Waller BF, Gorfinkel HJ, Rogers FJ, et al: Early and late morphologic changes in major epicardial coronary arteries after percutaneous transluminal coronary angioplasty. Am J Cardiol 53:42C, 1984

254. Waller BF, McKay CR, Hookman LD: Catheter balloon valvuloplasty of congenital and acquired types of aortic stenosis: Morphologic changes using single, double and oversized balloon dilation. Circulation 76(suppl IV):IV-189, 1987

255. Waller BF, McKay CR, Hookman LD, Rahimtoola SH: Incremental changes following single and double catheter balloon valvuloplasty of 12 stenotic mitral valves: Morphologic analysis of operatively-excised and intact necropsy mitral valves. J Am Coll Cardiol 11:220A, 1988

256. Waller BF, McKay CR, Lewin RF, et al: Morphologic analysis of 23 operatively-excised and intact necropsy stenotic cardiac valves from patients undergoing previous clinical catheter balloon valvuloplasty. Circulation 78(suppl II):II-593, 1988

257. Waller BF, McManus BM, Gorfinkel HJ, et al: Status of the major coronary arteries 80 to 150 days after percutaneous transluminal coronary angioplasty. Analysis of 5 necropsy patients. Am J Cardiol 5:403, 1983

258. Waller BF, Pinkerton CA, Foster LN: Morphologic evidence of accelerated left main coronary artery stenosis: A late complication of percutaneous transluminal balloon angioplasty of the proximal left anterior descending coronary artery. J Am Coll Cardiol 9:1019, 1987

259. Waller BF, Rothbaum DA, Gorfinkel HJ, et al: Morphologic observations after percutaneous transluminal balloon angioplasty of early and late aortocoronary saphenous vein bypass grafts. J Am Coll Cardiol 4:784, 1984

260. Waller BF, Rothbaum DA, Pinkerton CA, et al: Status of the myocardium and infarct-related coronary artery in 19 necropsy patients with acute recanalization using pharmacologic, mechanical or combined types of reperfusion therapy. J Am Coll Cardiol 9:785, 1987

261. Waller TJ, Kay HR, Spielman SR, et al: Reduction in sudden death and total mortality by antiarrhythmic therapy evaluated by electrophysiologic drug testing. J Am Coll Cardiol 10:83, 1987

262. Walls JT, Curtis JJ: Assessment of percutaneous balloon pulmonary and aortic valvuloplasty. J Thorac Cardiovasc Surg 88:352, 1984

263. Walts AE, Fishbein MC, Sustaita H, Matloff JM: Ruptures atheromatous plaques in saphenous vein coronary bypass grafts: A mechanism of acute, thrombotic, late graft occlusion. Circulation 65:197, 1982

264. White RA, Grundfest WS: Lasers in Cardiovascular Disease. Year Book Medical Publishers, Chicago, 1987, pp. 1–129

265. Whitworth HB, Roubin GS, Hollman J, et al: Effects of nifedipine on recurrent stenosis after percutaneous transluminal coronary angioplasty. J Am Coll Cardiol 8:1271, 1986

266. Wilson GJ: The pathology of cardiac pacing. p. 1297. In Silver MD (ed): Cardiovascular Pathology. Churchill Livingstone, New York, 1983

267. Winkle RA, Stinson EB, Echt AS, et al: Practical aspects of cardioverter/defibrillator implantation. Am Heart J 108:1335, 1984

268. Wright KC, Wallace S, Charnsangavej C, et al: Percutaneous endovascular stents: An experimental evaluation. Radiology 156:69, 1985

269. Yasuno M, Endo S, Takakashi M, et al: Angiographic and pathologic evidence of hemorrhage into the myocardium after coronary reperfusion. Angiology 35:797, 1984

270. Zacca NM, Raizner AE, Noon GP, et al: Treatment of symptomatic peripheral atherosclerotic disease with a rotational atherectomy device. Am J Cardiol 63:77, 1989

271. Zaibag MA, Ribeiro P, Kasah SA: Percutaneous balloon valvotomy in tricuspid stenosis. Br Heart J 57:51, 1987

272. Zarkins CK, Lu CT, Gewertz BL, et al: Arterial disruption and remodel following balloon dilation. Surgery 92:1086, 1982

45

Postoperative Congenital Cardiac Disease: Selected Topics with Emphasis on Morphologic Alterations and Correlative Angiocardiography

Robert M. Freedom
J. A. G. Culham
Meredith M. Silver

Although the natural history of many infants and children with congenitally malformed hearts has been positively influenced by surgical intervention, it is only with rare exception that such patients can be considered unequivocally cured, despite the restoration of a circulation that is functionally closer to normal than it was.

As summarized in a monograph[204] and in a legion of published papers,[5,56,85,138,150,200,267,268,307,384,400] the child with congenital heart disease is potentially liable to a variety of postsurgical sequelae. In addition, changes in the form and function of the malformed heart may further compromise the structure and func-tion of the myocardium before surgical intervention.[354,355] Yet, many patients with congenital heart disease having undergone extracardiac palliative and open heart surgery will survive to adulthood. In this chapter, we examine several types of congenital heart disease from the morphologic standpoint, to ascertain how changes in form and function alter the natural history of a patient with the given malformation. Finally, we discuss those alterations of structure and function that result from operative intervention and how such changes may be recognized in the adult with congenital heart disease.

VENTRICULAR SEPTAL DEFECT

Ventricular septal defect is the most common congenital cardiac defect, occurring in about 2 per 1,000 live births.[89] An extensive literature is devoted to the morphology, clinical features, angiocardiography, surgical results, and natural history of patients with ventricular septal defect. Most defects are small to moderate in size and occupy the membranous or perimembranous septum. Numerous analyses of natural history phenomena (summarized by Freedom[102]) show that these membranous or perimembranous ventricular septal defects tend to undergo a spontaneous diminution in size, or indeed complete anatomic closure. This had been surmised because ventricular septal defect occurs in 2 of 1,000 live births, yet its prevalence in school age children is about 1 in 1,000, and in adults 0.5 in 1,000.[89]

Although it is likely that most defects destined to close spontaneously do so early in childhood, instances of closure in adulthood have been reported.[89,341] Keith estimated that 25 to 30 percent of defects recognized at birth would close spontaneously,[202] and Hoffman, who was even more optimistic, suggested that at least 50 percent close in childhood, most frequently in the first year of life.[171] The Joint Natural History Study for congenital heart disease reported an overall incidence of complete spontaneous closure of 7 percent.[345] This low incidence can be explained, at least in part, by the fact that only 5 percent of the infants had trivial defects, that follow-up was relatively short, and that most patients were beyond five years of age and thus somewhat older than those in whom one might anticipate closure.[61,62,93,186,277,308,395,396]

The mechanisms by which ventricular septal defects undergo a spontaneous diminution in size or complete anatomic closure have been reviewed (summarized by Freedom,[102] and Mesko et al.[260]). One might anticipate that defects which occupy different positions in the ventricular septum might close by different processes and at different rates.[102] Yet, with rare exception, analyses of natural history data treat all ventricular septal defects as being membranous in position.[3,4]

There is convincing morphologic and clinical/angiocardiographic evidence that ventricular septal defects occupying the membranous or perimembranous septum become smaller and may possibly close by so-called aneurysmal transformation.[92,102,123,218,262,278,292,306,341,387] The so-called aneurysm of the membranous or perimembranous ventricular septum is a cup-shaped sac of fibrous tissue attached to the margins of a ventricular septal defect. This sac protrudes from left ventricle into the right ventricle under the septal leaflet of the tricuspid valve. In some instances, the aneurysm is intact, so that no interventricular communication is present. In others, one or more fenestrations in the fibrous sac allow left-to-right shunting of varying magnitude. Aneurysm of the membranous septum—described initially by Laennec in 1826 and thought by Mall to be congenital in origin.[99,102]—was first diagnosed during life by Steinberg in 1957.[362] Subsequently, numerous reports documented the association between these aneurysms and other congenital cardiac malformations; their angiocardiograhic appearance (Fig. 45–1) and their complications (summarized by Freedom et al.[123]). It soon became evident that most commonly associated cardiac anomaly was a small membranous ventricular septal defect.[102,123] During the same period, several authors suggested that these aneurysms might be related to anatomic closure of a ventricular septal defect.[123,218,262,292,306] And, in 1969, Varghese and Rowe presented angiocardiographic evidence of spontaneous closure of a small ventricular septal defect previously shown to have an associated aneurysm.[387] Subsequently, other studies[123,218,292] presented data on the association.

Such an aneurysm is common, usually but not invariably occuring after infancy, and is present in about 50 percent of patients with small ventricular septal defects before they reach 6 years of age. Coincident with aneurysm is a decrease in the magnitude of the left-to-right shunt, or complete cessation of the shunt. Although numerous complications have been attributed to aneurysms of the membranous septum, complications during childhood are rare.[123] These include right ventricular outflow tract obstruction, bundle branch block, aortic cusp prolapse, tricuspid insufficiency, and infective endocarditis.[123]

Finally, although the term "aneurysm of the membranous septum" has been used since the earliest reports to describe a circumferential deposition of tissue about the margins of a membranous or perimembranous ventricular septal defect, it is evident that some lesions that bear this name, including pouches of the septal leaflet of the tricuspid valve, are not truly aneurysms—nor did they, in many cases, derive their tissue from the membranous septum.[102,366]

Right ventricular outflow obstruction may complicate the natural history of a patient with a ventricular septal defect. It is thought to occur in from 1 to 7 percent of affected patients.[62,134,191,243,277,393,395] The acquisition of right ventricular outflow tract obstruction usually occurs in childhood and, if severe, may result in tetralogy physiology (right ventricular hypertension, normal pulmonary artery pressure, and bidirectional or right to left shunting at the ventricular level). The morphologic basis for the obstruction may be related to progressive hypertrophy of an anteriorly deviated infundibular septum or to hypertrophy of abnormally positioned right ventricular anomalous muscle bundles (proximal to the ostium of the infundibulum). Such obstructing right ventricular anomalous muscle bundles can cause the so-called double-chambered right ventricle[102,134,191,234,393] (see Fig. 45–1). It has been our experience that a ventricular septal defect associated with progressive right ventricular outflow tract obstruction usualy involves the membranous or perimembranous septum, or the infundibular septum.[102] However, a precise morphologic

characterization of the ventricular septal defect, in those patients in whom right ventricular outflow tract obstruction develops has not been presented.

A right-sided aortic arch may increase the propensity towards right ventricular outflow tract obstruction,[386] with this occurrence being reported as high as 40 to 50 percent among patients with ventricular septal defect and right-sided aortic arch.

Subaortic stenosis rarely complicates the natural history of isolated ventricular septal defect. Subaortic stenosis was not recorded in any patient in the U.S. Natural History Study, nor among those in the study of Corone.[277,395,396] The morphologic mechanisms responsible for subaortic obstruction include discrete fibrous or fibromuscular obstruction or subaortic obstruction secondary to a leftward deviation of the infundibular septum (see Ch. 26). When the latter mechanism is responsible, the ventricular septal defect results from a malalignment of the infundibular septum and the trabecular septum. Fibrous subaortic stenosis has been identified in patients with membranous ventricular septal defects.[281]

The malalignment type ventricular septal defect is similar to that seen in patients with obstructive anomalies of the aortic arch.[17,108,270,369] The leftward deviated infundibular septum may hypertrophy and cause muscular subaortic stenosis; or, if the patient had previously undergone palliative pulmonary artery banding, concentric hypertrophy of the infundibular septum in response to the banding may lead to subaortic obstruction.

The association of aortic regurgitation with ventricular septal defect is well recognized and is thought to occur in about 3 percent of patients with ventricular septal defect[17,48,60,62,89,102,369,381,395] (see Ch. 27). Among patients with both ventricular septal defect and aortic incompetence, a deficiency of anatomic structures supporting the aortic valve and sinus of Valsalva is highly correlated with the eventual prolapse of the valve through the ventricular septal defect.[17,102,199]

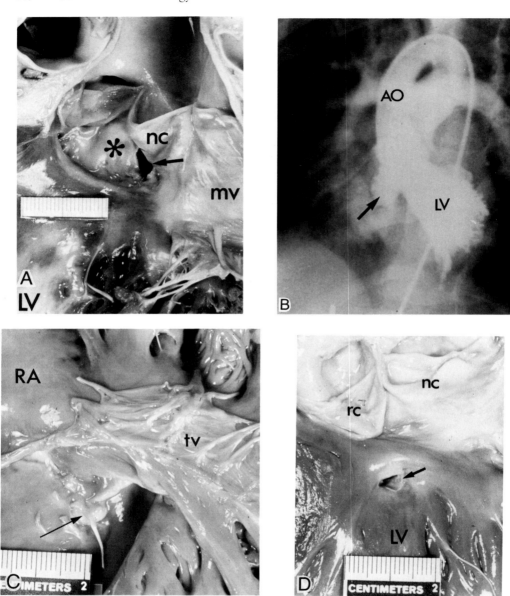

Fig. 45–1. (**A**) Ventricular septal defect with aneurysm formation viewed from left ventricle (LV). The ventricular septal defect is partially closed by fibrous tissue (asterisk) and the noncoronary aortic leaflet (nc) is partially prolapsing into it. There is a small, residual defect (arrow). Mitral valve (mv) to aortic valve fibrous continuity is evident. (**B**) Aneurysm of membranous ventricular septum in a patient with a small left-to-right shunt. Selective left ventriculogram was performed via a retrograde arterial catheter in an elongated axial view. With opacification of the left ventricle (LV) and aorta (AO), there is opacification of the so-called aneurysm of the membranous ventricular septum (arrow). (**C**) Small aneurysm of perimembranous septum (arrow) viewed from right side (RA, right atrium). The tricuspid valve (tv) is reflected to show the aneurysm. (**D**) When viewed from the left side, the small ventricular septal defect associated with the aneurysm illustrated in Fig. C (arrow) occupies the perimembranous muscular septum, proximal to commissure between the right coronary (rc) and the noncoronary (nc) aortic leaflets. (*Figure continues.*)

Fig. 45–1 (*continued*). (**E**) Child with perimembranous ventricular septal defect who developed right ventricular outflow tract obstruction. This aortopulmonary right ventriculogram demonstrates the relatively smooth inlet septum (is), the coarsely trabeculated trabecular septum (ts), and the smooth infundibular septum (inf), that supports the pulmonary artery (PA). The right ventricular outflow tract obstruction is related to a circumferential deposit of fibromuscular tissue (arrows) at the junction of the trabecular septum and infundibular septum. (Figs. A, C & D courtesy of M. D. Silver, M.D.)

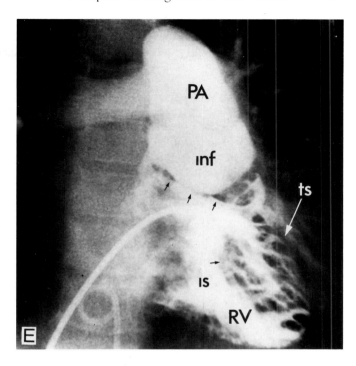

The patient with aortic regurgitation and a ventricular septal defect resulting from deficiency of the infundibular septum (so-called supracristal type) is a prime example. Among patients with membranous or perimembranous ventricular septal defects, the morphologic basis for aortic regurgitation is less clearly defined. A primary deficiency of the aortic commissure has been suggested as a mechanism by Van Praagh and McNamara,[199] but this viewpoint is not universally shared. Furthermore, hemodynamic influences present both in systole and diastole, contribute to progressive deformity of the prolapsing aortic valve. In accordance with the Bernouilli principle, the high velocity of blood jetting through the defect results in forces that tend to pull the cusp down into the defect. It is of interest that infundibular septal defects (so-called supracristal ventricular septal defect) seems more common among Orientals than among Occidentals.[17,89,102,199]

Infective endocarditis remains an important consideration in the medical and surgical history of patients with ventricular septal defects.[89,102,137,195,346] Among 266 patients with congenital heart disease and infective endocarditis reviewed by Kaplan,[195] ventricular septal defect accounted for 16 percent. From the studies of Shah and others, it would appear that the risk of endocarditis among patients with isolated ventricular septal defect is one episode in every 500 patient years, although the reported incidence has varied from 1:200 to 1:1,200 patient years.[137,346] Translated into a 70-year life span, any individual with ventricular septal defect has about a 10 to 15 percent chance of developing endocarditis. Endocarditis associated with ventricular septal defect is more common in patients older than 20 years of age and male. The incidence rate is greater in patients with smaller ventricular septal defects, and most infected lesions are frequently right-sided (valve and mural) at the site of impaction of the presumed jet of left-to-right shunted blood,[148] although infections of aortic, mitral, and left ventricular outflow tract have also been reported.

It is not clear whether patients with small ventricular septal defects and associated aneurysms of the membranous septum are more susceptible to endocarditis than are those with small defects but without aneurysms. Although a variety of pathogens have been isolated from patients with ventricular septal defect and bacterial endocarditis, *Streptococcus viridans* and *Staphylococcus aureus* were the most common causal agents identified in the report from the Joint Natural History Study for Congenital Heart Disease.[137]

Ventricular Septal Defect and Pulmonary Vascular Disease

Fortunately, today, most patients in North America come to medical attention before developing progressive and irrevocable pulmonary vascular obstructive disease. If not, death generally results from cyanotic heart disease or right-sided cardiac failure, or both.[405] The so-called Eisenmenger syndrome develops only in patients with a large ventricular septal defect and not in those with small ones.[34,48,60,89,102,171,202,277,395,396] Symptoms of exertional dyspnea and findings of shunt-reversal usually appear in the late teens or twenties, but in some patients symptoms develop much later. Once clinical deterioration begins, the prognosis for more than 5 to 10 years of life is poor.

The ventricular septal defect can occupy any portion of the ventricular septum. The cardiovascular findings at necropsy are well described.[34,102,277,395,396,405] Basically, the right heart chambers are dilated and hypertrophied, and the pulmonary artery is considerably dilated, often with conspicuous atheromatous changes of the pulmonary arterial intima. The pulmonary vascular tree will display the features of severe arteriopathy (see Ch. 15).

Postoperative Status

The postoperative status of the patient with ventricular septal defect has been exhaustively reviewed.[102] Briefly, among any group who survive open heart repair, a subset will be found to have a residual ventricular septal defect.[1,169,277,286,395,396] Among 105 patients from the joint study on the natural history of congenital heart disease and in whom the septal defect was found completely closed at postoperative catheterization, only four had a pulmonary arterial mean pressure at systemic levels; in 80 percent, the mean pulmonary arterial pressure had decreased to a value lower than 20 mmHg, and the postoperative pulmonary resistance was normal or only slightly elevated in all those operated on at less than 2 years of age.[325]

Rhythm disturbances, including heart block, among surgically treated patients with ventricular septal defect are fortunately uncommon, and the incidence of surgical heart block in most centers is less than 2 percent. Postoperative conduction disturbances have been well documented, and attention has been focused on the electrophysiologic-morphologic abnormality.[102,170,190,296,361,404,412] For instance, what does the postoperative development of a complete right bundle branch block (RBBB) signify? Although several centers have reported an incidence on the order of 40 percent, what this data does not provide is the site of origin of the block, that is, central or distal. Hobbins and colleagues have data suggesting that the atrial approach (as opposed to a right ventriculotomy) to the repair of ventricular septal defect significantly reduced the incidence of RBBB alone and that occurring with left axis deviation (so-called bifascicular block).[170]

Izukawa and his associates reviewed conduction disturbances after repair in 443 patients with ventricular septal defects and 506 patients, with tetralogy of Fallot.[190] Of 729 patients, 122 had immediate postoperative complete heart block, which was transient in

102 and persistent in 20. Of 607 patients who did not have complete heart block, 116 did not develop RBBB, 340 developed complete RBBB, and 127 developed RBBB with left anterior hemiblock. Although this latter conduction disturbance (bifascicular block) has been associated with a significant incidence of late complete heart block and sudden death at some centers, this has not been the experience at The Hospital for Sick Children in Toronto. The incidence of complete RBBB and left anterior hemiblock has ranged from 8 to 22 percent, and in our institution, the incidence is 16.7 percent, with a varying incidence of late complete heart block. A tragedy is for a patient to have complete anatomic closure of the ventricular septal defect, only to develop late-onset heart block, ventricular arrhythmias, or sudden death.[269] Damage to specialized cardiac conduction tissue certainly has a potential for initiating late-onset morbidity and mortality.

ATRIAL SEPTAL DEFECT

Considerable attention has been focused on the patient with secundum type atrial septal defect, and a clinical profile with physiologic correlates has emerged in children and adults with this defect.[66,75,165,305,309,391,413] In most cases, symptoms, atrial arrhythmias, right ventricular hypertrophy, right atrial and pulmonary arterial pressure, and systemic oxygen desaturation increased progressively with advancing age.

Survivors of a successful secundum atrial septal defect closure by means of open heart surgery are almost invariably asymptomatic and seldom have residual cardiomegaly, unless the operation was performed after the second decade of life. Most postoperative patients are in sinus rhythm, but there is no evidence that pre-existing arrhythmias have

been significantly ameliorated by surgery, nor is it known whether early surgery prevents the late appearance of atrial arrhythmias. Left ventricular performance before repair is mildly diminished.[66,305] This dysfunction is thought to be more related to volume overload of the right ventricle than to primary impairment of left ventricular myocardial contractility.[66,305] Echocardiographic studies document that right ventricular dilation and abnormal motion of the ventricular septum frequently persist after repair of an atrial septal defect.[66,305] Pearlman and colleagues found persistent right ventricular dilation in 35 percent of postoperative patients and abnormal septal motion in nearly 70 percent. These abnormalities, noted by echocardiography, could be correlated with age at operation and length of follow-up, but not with the preoperative right ventricular enlargement, shunt size, or right ventricular pressure. The long-term functional and morphologic sequelae of these findings are unclear.

Similar abnormalities of right ventricular dimension and ventricular septal motion have been found in patients with sinus venosus atrial septal defects.[214] This type, which accounts for about 10 percent of all atrial septal defects, is located high in the atrial septum, where the superior vena cava enters the right atrium and is commonly associated with partial anomalous pulmonary venous connections. Its repair may be technically difficult because of its location adjacent to the superior vena cava and sinus node. Postoperative problems including late-onset arrhythmias (including coronary sinus or low atrial rhythm, nodal or junctional rhythm. Atrioventricular dissociation, atrial flutter and fibrillation), obstruction of the superior vena cava, and incomplete repair have been reported.[214] At The Hospital for Sick Children, Toronto, we have analyzed, noninvasively, 29 children 2 to 14 years after surgical repair of sinus venosus atrial septal defect. Eighteen had also undergone cardiac catheterization and angiocardiograms. Four patients had mild symptoms. Trivial to slight superior caval narrowing was found in eight, and one child had a significant caval-right atrial gradient. Small left-to-right shunts were found in the superior vena cava of four children. Thirteen had minor electrocardiographic abnormalities at rest, during Holter monitering, or during exercise test, but sinus node recovery times were normal in all 12 children tested.

We will not consider postoperative follow-up studies of patients with ostium primum atrial septal defect,[227,233] or the complete form of atrioventricular defect. A comprehensive review of the genetic, morphologic, and hemodynamic factors influencing the natural history and postsurgical history of the patient with complete forms of atrioventricular defect has been published.[109]

TOTAL ANOMALOUS PULMONARY VENOUS CONNECTIONS

An extensive literature is devoted to the embryology, anatomy, diagnosis, and surgical management of patients with total anomalous pulmonary venous connections.[23,35,53,73,79,98,166,167,196,245,302,311,398,406] Although this group is somewhat heterogeneous, infants with obstructed pulmonary venous connections (to portal or gastric vein, or ductus venosus; to azygos vein; or supracardiac with obstruction) present early in infancy, usually with severe pulmonary edema, and require urgent surgical intervention. The patient with nonobstructed total anomalous pulmonary venous connections (cardiac level, coronary sinus, or right atrium) or to the left innominate vein usually comes to medical attention somewhat later in life. Indeed, some patients with nonobstructed total anomalous pulmonary venous connections present clinically like patients with a large atrial septal defect. Because of the heterogeneity of clinical presentations and the variable age at operation, it is difficult to summarize longitudinal follow-up data concisely.

Preoperatively, among most patients with total anomalous pulmonary venous connections, left atrial volume is diminished and its shape abnormal.[73] Left atrial contraction is normal, but excessive cephalad and posterior movement of the left atrium has been observed during atrial systole.[65] The right ventricular volume is increased, often markedly (especially in patients with nonobstructed total anomalous pulmonary venous connections), and ventricular septal motion is flattened or reversed. The study conducted by Mathew and colleagues demonstrated normal right ventricular ejection fraction preoperatively.[245] Left ventricular output was low, both in patients with either obstructed or nonobstructed total anomalous pulmonary venous connections. In this regard, Bove and associates found in an autopsy study of the left ventricle in anomalous pulmonary venous connections, that the mass of the left ventricle was normal, but that the ventricular cavity was compromised by significant leftward displacement of the interventricular septum.[35] Furthermore, severe septal displacement was associated with distorted myocardial architecture in the region of the septal attachment of the left ventricular free wall.

Cardiac performance has been evaluated during the immediate postoperative period in a small group of patients after repair of total anomalous pulmonary venous connections.[302] The stroke index was reduced, and abnormal phasic fluctuations in the left atrial pressure tracings suggested a restrictive left atrium. Our own data, and those of Mathew and colleagues,[245] suggest that cardiac function is often restored to normal after surgery.

Certain late complications have been reported following surgical repair of total anomalous pulmonary venous return below the diaphragm.[245] Scarring and progressive contraction at the junction of the pulmonary veins with the left atrium may cause pulmonary edema, necessitating reoperation. Kinking of one pulmonary vein at its juncture

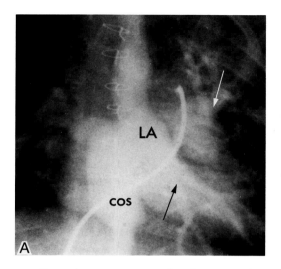 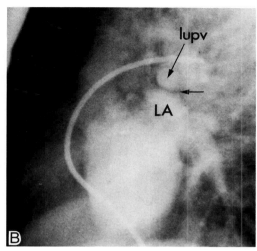

Fig. 45–2. This youngster was found at 1 year of age to have the mixed type of total anomalous pulmonary venous connections: all the right pulmonary veins and the left lower veins drained to the coronary sinus, and the left upper vein drained to the innominate vein. Total correction was performed. One year postoperatively, a cardiac catheterization demonstrated normal hemodynamics and no evidence of intracardiac shunting. (**A**) Selective left pulmonary arteriography demonstrated prompt venous return to left lower pulmonary vein to the coronary sinus (cos) and left atrium (LA) but delayed drainage from the left upper pulmonary vein (arrow). (**B**) In the lateral exposure the stenosis at the surgical anastomosis between left atrium (LA) and left upper pulmonary vein (lupv) is clearly seen (arrow).

with the left atrium may produce a picture of segmental pulmonary edema. Such complications usually occur in infancy or within a few months of operation, but it is conceivable that obstruction of one or two pulmonary veins may be clinically silent and be detected only at autopsy or clinically by ventilation-perfusion scans, or by postoperative cardiac catheterization with angiocardiograms (Fig. 45–2).

Whight and colleagues drew attention to late pulmonary venous obstruction after repair of total anomalous pulmonary venous connections to the coronary sinus.[398] In their study, for the most part, the anastomosis between the common pulmonary venous channel and left atrium increases in size as the infant grows.

Finally, some patients with repaired total anomalous pulmonary venous connections may have a residual atrial septal defect (incompletely repaired at the initial operation) or an atrial arrhythmia. It is our impression that most patients surviving early surgical intervention have excellent postoperative hemodynamics. This has been confirmed by other studies.[55,65,79,98,167,196,245,302,311,398,406]

PALLIATIVE EXTRACARDIAC OR INTRACARDIAC OPERATIONS

A number of operative procedures have been designed for palliation of potentially "correctable" and noncorrectable types of congenitally malformed hearts. Basically, these procedures may be divided into three generic groups: (1) procedures designed to augment pulmonary blood flow[33]; (2) procedures designed to reduce pulmonary blood flow and to ameliorate signs and symptoms of congestive heart failure (a direct corollary is a protection of the pulmonary vascular bed[271,301,321])—both procedures may set the stage for alterations of cardiac structure and function that may be reflected in unfavorable postoperative results; finally (3) some palliative procedures are designed primarily to afford mixing between the pulmonary and systemic circulations when the ventriculoarterial connections are discordant.[32]

Procedures Designed to Augment Pulmonary Blood Flow

Blalock-Taussig Shunt

A subclavian artery is surgically anastomosed to a pulmonary artery (usually end to side). Initially, the Blalock-Taussig shunt[32] was performed to the pulmonary artery opposite the aortic arch (because of the more favorable geometry of the subclavian artery originating from an innominate artery); the introduction of a proximal subclavian arterioplasty has allowed construction of this type of shunt on the same side as the aortic arch without excessive kinking of the down-turned subclavian artery. This type of shunt only rarely causes a significant elevation of pulmonary artery pressures and rarely severely distorts the geometry and distribution of the branch pulmonary arteries. "Tenting-up" or elevation of the shunted pulmonary artery is a not-infrequent angiocardiographic finding among patients who have had a Blalock-Taussig anastomosis. Prosthetic materials have also been used to construct systemic-to-pulmonary anastomoses (Fig. 45–3).

The use of Goretex in the construction of a modified Blalock-Taussig shunt may be accompanied by seroma formation. Such a seroma may produce a rather significant pleural effusion.[221] If there is a connection with the pericardial space, hemodynamics may be compromised by acute pericardial tamponade.

Waterston Shunt

An anastomosis between the right pulmonary artery and the ascending aorta, the Waterston shunt, is usually performed outside the pericardial reflection, but may be performed via an intrapericardial approach. Although the Waterston shunt[392] may provide acceptable short-term palliation, a number of studies have addressed themselves to the potential for excessive pulmonary blood flow and pulmonary vascular disease.[135,156,285,323,370,389] Of 54 Waterston anastomoses performed at The Hospital for Sick Children, Toronto, from 1966 to 1979, 61 percent had no narrowing or mild narrowing of the right pulmonary artery: 37 percent had mild-to-moderate narrowing; and 2 percent had moderate-to-severe narrowing as determined at subsequent angiocardiographic evaluations.[372]

Potts Shunt

This anastomosis between the left pulmonary artery and descending thoracic aorta, which is performed outside the pericardial reflection, is all too frequently characterized by distortion of the pulmonary artery (Fig. 45–4) and has the potential for growth of the anastomosis and excessive pulmonary blood flow.[279,282,312] In addition, this anastomosis is considered difficult to take down at subsequent surgical repair. Pulmonary vascular disease is a well-recognized sequel of this operation. Of 45 Potts shunts performed between 1968 and 1979, subsequent angiocardiographic investigations revealed no or very mild narrowing of the left pulmonary artery in 47 percent; mild to moderate narrowing in 51 percent and severe distortion of the left pulmonary artery in 2 percent. Sigifnicant elevation of pulmonary artery pressure was revealed in about 15 percent.[221]

Cavopulmonary Artery Anastomosis

The concept of anastomosing a large systemic vein to the right pulmonary artery to increase pulmonary blood flow in patients with cy-

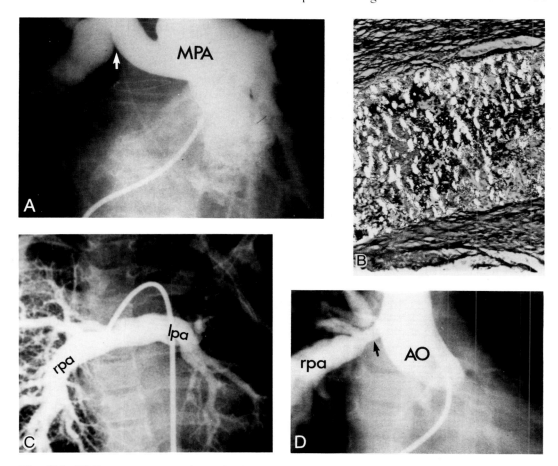

Fig. 45-3. (**A**) Postoperative tetralogy of Fallot in a patient with a previously constructed right Blalock-Taussig anastomosis. This selective injection into the main pulmonary artery (mpa) demonstrates superior elevation of the right pulmonary artery (arrow) by the previously constructed surgical anastomosis. (**B**) The doubly refractile meshwork of a Goretex prosthetic shunt is infiltrated by fibrin and calcium and lined by connective tissue. (Picro Mallory stain, partially polarized light, × 125.) (**C**) Waterston anastomosis: aortopulmonary projection with a retrograde aortic catheter in place. There is no significant stenosis of the right pulmonary artery (rpa). There is no main pulmonary artery. The left pulmonary artery (lpa) is slightly less well developed than the right pulmonary artery. (**D**) Narrowed right pulmonary artery (rpa) following a Waterston anastomosis. Both the ascending aorta (AO) and narrowed right pulmonary artery (rpa) (arrow) are clearly opacified.

anotic congenital heart disease was proposed by Carlon[49] in 1951. Glenn and Patino, in 1954, described a modification by anastomosing the superior vena cava directly to the right pulmonary artery.[145,147] A variety of complications may occur.[16,144,217,246,252] They have been summarized by McFaul and associates,[252] and include the superior vena cava syndrome, hemothorax, chylothorax, venous collateralization around the anastomotic site, pulmonary artery thrombosis, pulmonary infarction, abnormal perfusion patterns, and the late development of pulmonary arteriovenous fistula with significant intrapulmonary right-to-left shunting.[285,389] A very common finding is preferential blood flow to the right lower

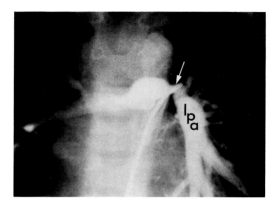

Fig. 45–4. Left Pott's anastomosis and narrowed (arrow) proximal left pulmonary artery (lpa).

lung field with decreased flow to the upper lobe (Fig. 45–5). This probably results from the nonpulsatile nature of superior vena cava flow and increases with time. Creation of an axillary arteriovenous fistula in patients with a cavopulmonary arterial shunt may supplement blood flow to the right lung when the patient has outgrown the cavopulmonary anastomosis.[146]

Because of the difficulty in reconstituting cavo-right atrial continuity at definitive intracardiac repair, it is not attempted frequently.

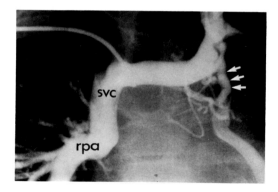

Fig. 45–5. Functioning Glenn anastomosis between superior vena cava (SVC) and right pulmonary artery (rpa). There is preferential flow to the right middle and lower lobe, as well as collateral venous connections to the oblique vein of Marshall and coronary sinus (arrows).

Procedure Designed to Reduce Pulmonary Blood Flow

Pulmonary artery banding, reported by Muller and Dammann[271] in 1952, was designed to decrease pulmonary blood flow, to alleviate features of congestive heart failure, and to protect the pulmonary artery bed from hypertensive arteriopathy. Complications of pulmonary arterial banding include pulmonary valve cusp thickening, secondary infundibular hypertrophy, local distortion of the pulmonary arterial trunk, rupture of the pulmonary artery with intraluminal or extraluminal migration of the band and distal migration of the pulmonary band, with narrowing of the right, left, or both branch pulmonary arteries.[102,188]

Procedures Designed to Augment Atrial Mixing in Transposition of the Great Arteries

Blalock and Hanlon, in 1950, devised an atrial septectomy procedure to augment atrial mixing and effective pulmonary blood flow in patients with transposition of the great arteries.[32] Basically, this is a closed procedure in which a curved vascular clamp is placed with one blade anterior to the right atrium and the other posterior to the left atrium. Parallel incisions are made in the right atrium and the anterior surface of the right pulmonary vein confluence; the atrial septum is grasped, withdrawn, and excised. Complications include atrial arrhythmias and stenosis of the right pulmonary veins. Balloon atrioseptostomy, as originally described by Rashkind and Miller,[321] opened the door for the medical treatment of the patient with complete transposition of the great arteries. One-year survival statistics markedly improved in these patients and thus can be linked directly to this development.[160,229] A number of reviews of such palliative therapy for the patient with complete transposition provide an interesting historical and current perspective.[20,374] Finally, Park and associates designed a blade-tipped catheter for medical septostomy in selected patients.[301]

TETRALOGY OF FALLOT

Tetralogy of Fallot accounts for about 5 percent of patients with congenital heart disease. Malalignment of the infundibular and trabecular septum causes subpulmonary obstruction and an infundibular septal defect that frequently extends into the perimembranous septum. These features—together with right ventricular hypertrophy and aortic override, both hemodynamic consequences of the subpulmonary obstruction and ventricular septal defect—are the pertinent morphologic features of Fallot's tetralogy. Frequent additional findings include a bicuspid pulmonary valve, varying degrees of pulmonary arterial hypoplasia, or discrete pulmonary artery branch stenoses. Rarely, anomalies of pulmonary venous connections, valvular or supravalvular pulmonary stenosis, or subaortic stenosis may complicate Fallot's tetralogy.

Surgical repair of Fallot's tetralogy, first accomplished in 1955, can currently be achieved in anatomically favorable cases, with a mortality of less than 10 percent, and has markedly altered the natural history of this disorder.[22] Surgical results are quite variable and reflect many factors.[29,37,45,52,59,95,96,133,153,183,205,239, 259,326,328,330,331,336,345] Closure of the ventricular septal defect is accomplished with a prosthetic patch of Dacron. Resection of the obstructing infundibular muscle and pulmonary valvotomy are frequently combined with an infundibular patch of pericardium. Not infrequently, the patch extends across the annulus and to the branch pulmonary arteries. This surgical approach requires a ventriculotomy, as it sacrifices infundibular coronary arteries of varying size, that originate from the right coronary artery.

Numerous studies have assessed the postoperative findings in patients with tetralogy of Fallot.[29,45,52,59,95,96,133,141,153,180,181,183,192, 259,317,326,328,331,336,345] A small but definite proportion have a residual ventricular septal defect, resulting either from detachment of the prosthetic patch or from failure to recognize a second ventricular septal defect (Fig. 45–6). Unrelieved infundibular or valvular pulmonary stenosis is fairly uncommon today. However, pulmonary incompetence of varying severity is common and is most exaggerated in those patients with too generous a transannular patch and unrelieved pulmonary artery branch stenoses. Although it has been suggested that mild pulmonary incompetence is well tolerated, clinical assessment of the severity of deleterious effects of pulmonary incompetence remains difficult (Fig. 45–6).

Postoperatively, dilation of the pulmonary infundibulum is not uncommon, and aneurysmal bulging of a pericardial outflow tract patch is occasionally encountered.[292,345] False or mycotic aneurysms are fortunately not common. Among those patients with severe pulmonary incompetence, the right ventricle may dilate progressively. This in concert with a paradoxically moving pericardial outflow tract patch may induce progressive right ventricular failure, secondary to fibrosis. Tricuspid incompetence may further exaggerate the pattern of diastolic overloading. Indeed, tricuspid regurgitation may result from right ventricular dilation and failure, or distortion of the septal leaflet of the tricuspid valve by the prosthetic patch used in the repair of the ventricular septal defect.

The proximity of the right aortic cusp to the ventricular septal defect in tetralogy of Fallot has been emphasized previously. Surgical incorporation of part of the right aortic leaflet in the ventricular septal defect may result in aortic incompetence of varying severity. Diastolic overload of the left ventricle may be

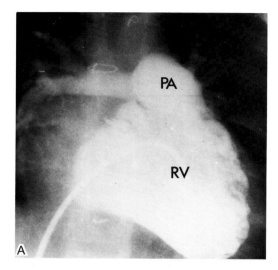

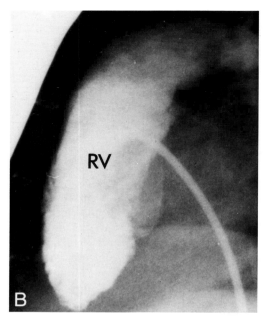

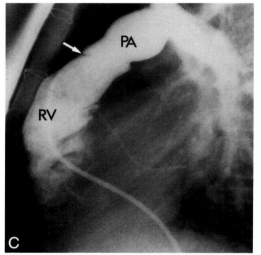

Fig. 45–6. Postoperative tetralogy of Fallot: aortopulmonary (**A**) and lateral (**B**) right ventriculogram in a patient with good surgical result. The right ventricle (RV) is mildly dilated, as is the main pulmonary artery (PA). (**C**) Lateral pulmonary arteriogram with catheter in proximal right pulmonary artery. There is regurgitation from the pulmonary artery (PA) to the right ventricle (RV). An anterior pulmonary valve leaflet (arrow) is just visible. (*Figure continues.*)

further aggravated by persistence of systemic to pulmonary artery collateral vessels (Table 45–1).

One hundred and eighteen patients with tetralogy of Fallot have undergone postoperative hemodynamic and angiocardiographic evaluation at The Hospital for Sick Children, Toronto (Dickinson D, unpublished data). Of these, 78 (66 percent) had some form of previous palliative surgery. The mean age at total correction was 6.75 years, with a range of 0.75 to 17.67 years. The mean interval from op-

eration to restudy was 48 months, ranging from 9 days to 10 years, 10 months. A residual left-to-right shunt was found in 30 patients (25 percent). A residual ventricular septal defect was identified in 18, atrial septal defect in 7, persistent Blalock-Taussig shunt in 7, and anomalous pulmonary venous drainage in one. Three of the 30 patients had shunting at more than one level. Only eight had a residual shunt with a pulmonary-to-systemic flow ratio of greater than 1.5. Five patients had aneurysmal bulging of a patched right ventricular

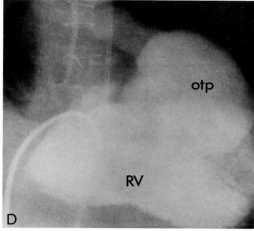

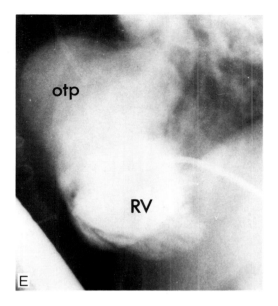

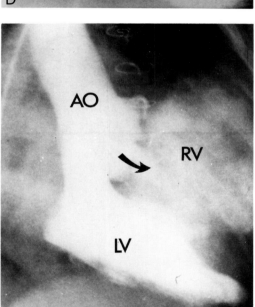

Fig. 45–6 (*continued*). (**D–F**) Postoperative tetralogy of Fallot with residual ventricular septal defect and aneurysmal dilation of right ventricular outflow tract. (**D**) Standard aortopulmonary right ventriculogram demonstrating dilation of morphologic right ventricle (RV) and akinetic, aneurysmal right ventricular outflow tract patch (otp). (**E**) Lateral right ventriculogram demonstrating same features. (**F**) Right anterior oblique left ventriculogram (LV) in systole. There is a residual ventricular septal defect (arrow) with left-to-right shunt into aneurysmally dilated right ventricular outflow (RV). AO, aorta. (*Figure continues.*)

outflow tract. Significant tricuspid or aortic incompetence occurred in about 1 percent. Significant residual right ventricular outflow tract obstruction was identified in 5 patients.

Garson and colleagues[133] from the Texas Children's Hospital summarized the status of the adult and adolescent after repair of tetralogy of Fallot. Of 233 patients born before January 1962, 120 underwent postoperative cardiac catheterization. Thirty-nine had an unsatisfactory hemodynamic result, but 30 of these were asymptomatic. A large left-to-right shunt was identified in eight patients, persistent significant right ventricular outflow tract obstruction in 25 patients, pulmonary vascular obstructive disease in five patients, and left ventricular cardiomyopathy in one patient. Complete right bundle branch block (RBBB) was found in 183 of 203 patients (88 percent). Seventeen of the 183 patients (9.2

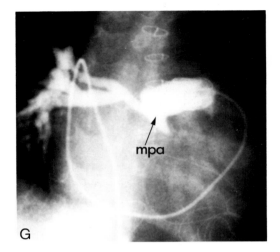

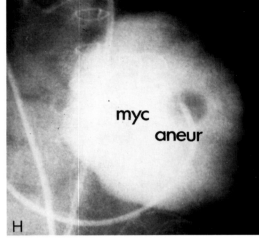

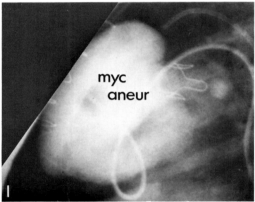

Fig. 45–6 (*continued*). (**G–I**) Formation of a mycotic aneurysm in a patient with ventricular septal defect and pulmonary atresia. (**G**) This injection in the left pulmonary artery demonstrates the blind main pulmonary artery (mpa) and the small right pulmonary artery. (**H,I**) Aortopulmonary and lateral of the mycotic aneurysm (myc aneur).

Table 45–1.   Potential Problems After Total Repair of Tetralogy of Fallot

Residual ventricular septal defect

Residual pulmonary outflow tract stenosis

Pulmonary regurgitation

Unrelieved pulmonary artery branch stenoses

Aneurysmal bulging of right ventricular outflow tract patch

Tricuspid valve incompetence

Disruption of large right ventricular infundibular coronary arterial supply

Right ventricular dysfunction

Aortic valve incompetence

Persistence of large systemic-pulmonary collateral vessels

Arrhythmias

percent) had additional left axis deviation. Twenty-one of the 203 patients (11.2 percent) had premature ventricular depolarization, and most had right ventricular hypertension with a systolic pressure greater than 60 mmHg and elevated right ventricular end-diastolic pressures. Multiple premature ventricular ectopic beats and ventricular tachycardia are ominous in postoperative patients, and sudden death has resulted.

Patients with the most severe form of tetralogy of Fallot, the so-called pulmonary atresia with ventricular septal defect, may have such prohibitively small pulmonary arteries that total correction is not possible.[140,207,256,297] Although a systemic-to-pulmonary artery anastomosis may promote growth of the pulmonary arteries in such cases,[207] not infrequently, hypoplasia of the branch pulmonary arteries, even after surgical shunt augmentation may still preclude complete correction. Reconstitution of continuity between right ventricle and main pulmonary artery with either pericardium or a valved external conduit (without closing the ventricular septal defect) has been advocated as one form of palliation.[140] Some patients, so palliated, may eventually become suitable candidates for closure of the ventricular septal defect, while in others, continued pulmonary arterial hypoplasia may never allow "total" correction. Such patients will subsequently die from the effects of chronic hypoxia.

COMPLETE TRANSPOSITION OF THE GREAT ARTERIES

Complete transposition of the great arteries is characterized by atrioventricular concordance (morphologic right atrium connected to morphologic right ventricle, and left atrium to left ventricle) and ventriculoarterial discordance (aorta originates above the morphologic right ventricle, and pulmonary artery above the morphologic left ventricle). This malformation accounts for about 9 percent of congenital cardiac malformations. The hemodynamic consequence is two parallel circulations—one systemic, and the other pulmonary. Survival for even a short time demands mixing between the two circulations, at either the atrial, ventricular, or great arterial level. Without surgical intervention, only about 5 percent of patients with complete transposition and intact ventricular septum survive to 1 year of age.[160,229] Closed atrial septectomy, as advocated by Blalock and Hanlon,[32] affords one surgical approach to enhance mixing at the atrial level. Balloon atrioseptostomy, originally introduced by Rashkind and Miller[321] in 1966, opened a new era in treatment.

Before the intraatrial baffle operation of Mustard, a variety of other operations had been designed to augment mixing between the pulmonary and systemic circulations (including Baffles's[15] and Senning's procedures[342]).

Intra-atrial Baffle Operation to Correct Transposition

The Mustard procedure required excision of the patient's atrial septum and construction of an intra-atrial baffle. The baffle diverted blood from the inferior and superior vena cavae through the mitral valve, and thus to the left ventricle and pulmonary artery, and the pulmonary venous blood through the tricuspid valve and into the morphologic right ventricle and aorta[273] (Fig. 45–7). The coronary sinus usually drains to the new pulmonary venous atrium. Although this inflow type of operation restores a circulation that is "functionally" closer to normal, postoperatively the morphologic right ventricle continues to pump blood into the aorta and systemic circulation, while the left ventricle supplies the pulmonary artery and the pulmonary circulation.

Different materials have been used to construct an atrial baffle. Currently, autologous pericardium is favored at most institutions. Experience with Dacron has been disappointing because its shrinkage causes obstruction to either caval or pulmonary venous connections. In this regard, superior or inferior vena caval obstruction (or rarely both) has been reported in about 2 to 4 percent of patients following Mustard's procedure using pericardium[58,87,250,274,324,359,360,388,407] (Fig. 45–7). Usually, even complete obstruction to the superior vena cava is well tolerated because an adequate runoff is provided by a rich venous collateral circulation via the azygos or hemiazygos vein or the paraspinal venous plexus. Rarely, an acute superior vena cava syndrome[250] or a protein-losing enteropathy[265] results from superior or in-

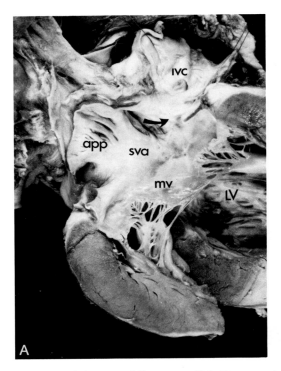
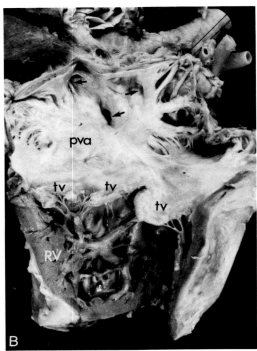

Fig. 45–7. (A) Mustard "intra-atrial" baffle operation: systemic venous atrium (sva) and left ventricle (LV). The inferior vena cava (IVC) and superior vena cava (arrow) are diverted through the mitral valve (mv) to the morphologic left ventricle (LV) and pulmonary artery (not shown) app, left atrial appendage. **(B)** Status post-Mustard procedure: internal view of pulmonary venous atrium (pva) and morphologic right ventricle. The endothelialized pericardium diverts the nonobstructed pulmonary veins (arrows) through the tricuspid valve into the morphologic right ventricle (RV) and aorta (not shown). The tricuspid valve (tv) is thickened, and at cardiac catheterization was severely regurgitant. The pulmonary venous atrium (pva) is dilated, reflecting the tricuspid regurgitation. (*Figure continues.*)

ferior vena caval obstruction, respectively. Massively dilated paraspinal venous collaterals resulting from caval obstruction may mimic paravertebral neoplasms[51] (Fig. 45–7). Severe inferior vena caval obstruction is usually symptomatic immediately.

Obstruction to right and left pulmonary venous return is, fortunately, uncommon when pericardium is used,[58,87,274,359,360] when present, clinical manifestations occur reasonably earlier, almost invariably dictating surgical intervention. Unilateral obstruction to pulmonary venous return may be clinically silent because of preferential pulmonary blood flow to the nonobstructed side.[231] However, some

patients with unilateral obstruction to pulmonary venous return may demonstrate clinical and radiologic evidence of severe pulmonary edema.

To avoid caval or pulmonary venous obstruction, variations in the shape of the baffle have been tried.[314] Following the Mustard procedure, a disconcertingly high number of patients present with atrial arrhythmias, including atrial flutter, junctional brady- or tachyarrhythmias, with features of *sick sinus syndrome.* Several investigators have discussed the pertinent electrophysiologic features and investigations of these patients.[56,83,88,161,203,228,254,258,337,373,375]   Al-

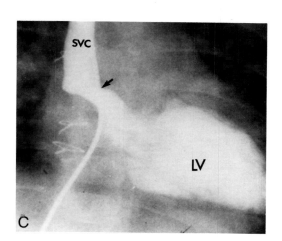

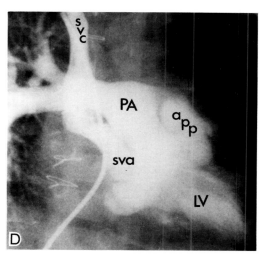

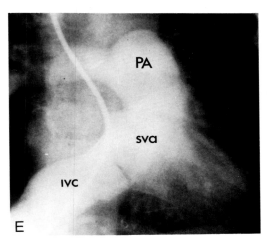

Fig. 45–7 *(continued).* **(C–E)** Postoperative Mustard's inflow "correction" for complete transposition of the great arteries. **(C)** Injection of contrast material into the superior vena cava (SVC) demonstrates the functional redirection of venous blood from the superior vena cava through the mitral valve into the morphologic left ventricle (LV). Mild dynamic narrowing of the superior vena caval channel is evident (arrow). **(D)** Slightly later in the injection, the new systemic venous atrium (sva), left atrial appendage (app), left ventricle and pulmonary artery (PA) are sequentially opacified. There is preferential flow into the right pulmonary artery. **(E)** Injection of contrast material into the inferior vena cava (IVC) demonstrates a widely patent inferior caval channel, the systemic venous atrium, and the pulmonary artery (this specific frame does not show the morphologic left ventricle). *(Figure continues.)*

though there is no unanimity as to the etiology of the arrhythmias, there is a consensus that interruption of the sinoatrial nodal artery, with subsequent ischemic damage or infarction of the sinus node, may be partially to blame[86,88] (Fig. 45–7). There is considerably less support for the idea that interruption of the various interatrial pathways has a role in the genesis of the rhythm disturbances.[187] Rarely, complete atrioventricular block may

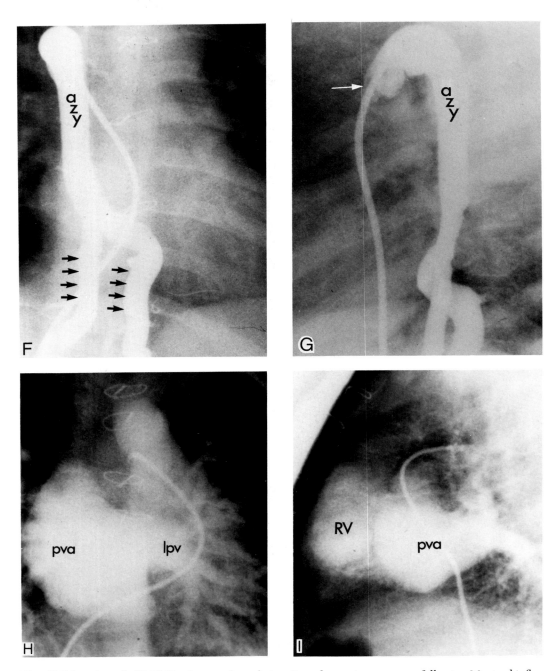

Fig. 45–7 *(continued).* **(F,G)** Nearly complete obstruction of superior vena cava following Mustard inflow correction for complete transposition of the great arteries. Catheter was advanced from femoral vein to new systemic venous atrium and through very narrowed channel to superior vena cava. **(F)** Injection of contrast in the proximal superior vena cava. The catheter virtually occludes the channel from the superior vena cava to the new systemic venous atrium. The superior vena cava decompresses through the azygos vein (azy) and an extensive paraspinal venous plexus (arrows). **(G)** The lateral of this injection demonstrates the very severe narrowing of the superior vena caval channel (arrow). **(H,I)** Following injection of contrast media in main pulmonary artery, the pulmonary veins (lpv) drain to the new pulmonary venous atrium (pva) and into the morphologic right ventricle (RV). *(Figure continues.)*

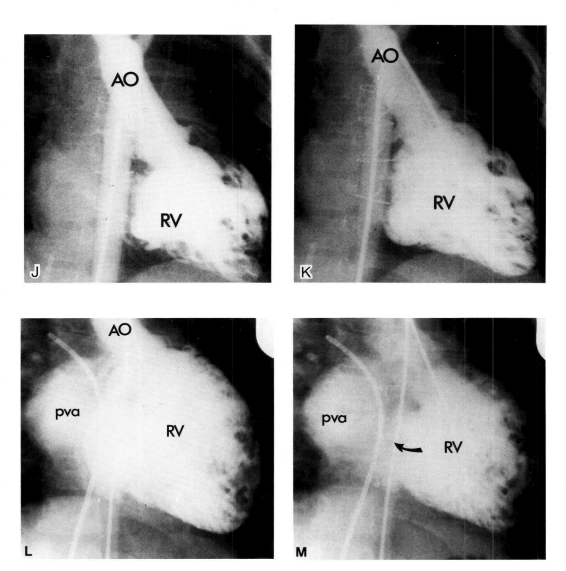

Fig. 45–7 *(continued).* Systolic (**J**) and diastolic (**K**) frames of aortopulmonary right ventriculogram 3 years after a Mustard inflow type of correction. The right ventricle is only mildly impaired in function. AO, aorta. (**L,M**) Postoperative inflow "correction" of Mustard for complete transposition of the great arteries and intact ventricular septum. The postoperative right ventriculogram (**L**, systole; **M**, diastole) demonstrates severe impairment of right ventricular function, with regurgitation of contrast from the poorly functioning right ventricle (RV) into the enlarged pulmonary venous atrium (pva). AO, aorta. (*Figure continues.*)

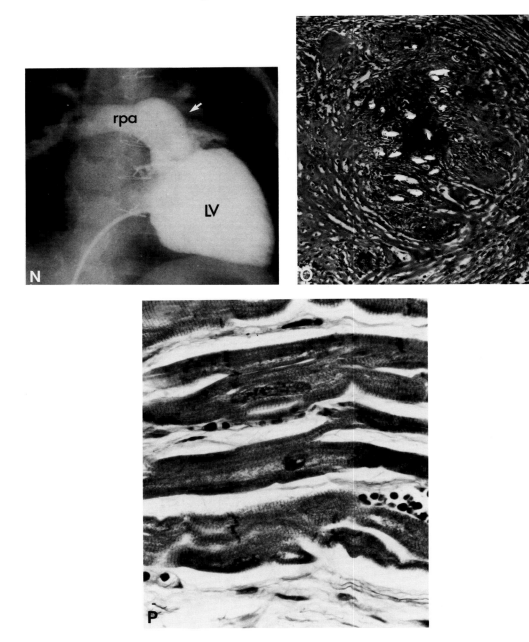

Fig. 45–7 *(continued)*. **(N,O)** Preferential flow into the right pulmonary artery. **(N)** Selective left ventriculogram **(LV)** in aortopulmonary projection demonstrating preferential flow into the right pulmonary artery because of the orientation of the left ventricular outflow tract. Arrow indicates poor filling of the left pulmonary artery. **(O)** Granulomatous inflammation in a scarred sinoatrial node region. Doubly refractile remnants of suture material appear white. Chronic inflammatory cells are plentiful in the scar. (H&E, partly polarized light, × 125.) **(P)** Right ventricular muscle fibers show marked hypertrophy, their nuclei are enlarged and collagenous tissue separates them. (H&E, × 680.)

occur as a result of damage to the specialized atrioventricular conduction tissue in the region of the coronary sinus. It is for this reason that the coronary sinus is usually left to drain into the new pulmonary venous atrium.

Although some rhythm disturbances are benign, patients with symptoms of the sick sinus syndrome are susceptible to sudden death, even when pacemakers are used. A variety of modifications of the atrial baffle have been introduced to avoid injury to the sinoatrial nodal artery and the node itself.[314] Sudden death some years subsequent to a Mustard operation usually results from a rhythm disturbance. There have been sporadic attempts to provide histopathologic correlation in such clinical events,[27] but unfortunately such reports are rare. A preference for the Senning procedure[342] to avoid arrhythmias and superior caval obstruction, is currently a vogue at some centers.[299,315]

Tricuspid regurgitation has been observed in some patients after the inflow type of "correction." The mechanism(s) responsible is/are uncertain (e.g., direct disruption of the valve or tensor apparatus, annular malorientation; or functional tricuspid regurgitation, resulting from impaired right ventricular function.) In our experience, significant tricuspid incompetence after an inflow operation occurs in less than 1 percent of patients and is usually related to severe impairment of right ventricular myocardial contractility.[80,376]

Finally, after the atrial baffle procedure, the morphologic right ventricle continues to support the aorta and the systemic circulation. There have been increasing numbers of reports describing progressive right ventricular dysfunction among these patients[2,151,152,162,193,283] and although the etiology of such myocardial depression is uncertain, long-term myocardial ischemia, chronic pressure overload, and perhaps differences in the pattern of contraction are possible. Certainly histologic examination of the right ventricular myocardium of patients who succumb with right ventricular failure demonstrates diffuse fibrosis in addition to

muscle fiber hypertrophy (Fig. 45–7P). It is of interest that an abnormal right ventricular morphology has been identified as a distinctive feature of transposition of the great arteries.[19] Furthermore, as Yacoub[409] summarized in an editorial, other problems exist with the inflow approach of Mustard or Senning. Abnormal function of the mitral valve and left ventricular outflow, as manifested by echocardiographic findings of systolic anterior movement and coarse diastolic fluttering of the mitral valve, probably result from the abnormal shape and bulge of the interventricular septum into the left ventricular outflow tract. Partial loss of the reservoir and contractile function of the atria may also impair cardiac performance. Abnormal distribution of pulmonary blood flow with preferential flow into the right lung, resulting from the orientation of the left ventricular outflow tract, leads to progressvie hypoplastic changes in the left pulmonary vascular bed. Also, the long-term effects of preferential flow into the right lung are unknown.[275,276,390,409]

A summary of results from this institution of the Mustard operation (inflow correction) for patients with complete transposition can be seen in Table 45–2.[371]

Surgical Procedures Producing Anatomic Correction of Transposition

Concern about atrial arrhythmias and right ventricular dysfunction following the Mustard atrial baffle operation for complete transposition of the great arteries[83] led to interest in an anatomic correction. This approach requires dividing, contraposing, and reanastomosing the great arteries as well as transferring the coronary arteries; the latter proves a major technical difficulty.

Subsequent to Jatene's[153] report of the successful anatomic correction many others have been published, with emphasis on anastomotic considerations and various technical

Table 45–2.   Potential Problems After an "Inflow Correction" for Complete Transposition of the Great Vessels

Complication	Incidence (%)
Superior or inferior vena caval obstruction[a]	<2
Obstruction of pulmonary venous channel (usually presents early)[a]	<3
Atrial arrhythmia	~30
Right ventricular dysfunction[a]	~40
Preferential flow to right pulmonary artery	~35
Dynamic left ventricular outflow (pulmonary) obstruction[a]	~10
Tricuspid valve incompetence[a]	<5

[a] Based on 140 postoperative cardiac catheterizations at The Hospital for Sick Children, Toronto. More than 300 Mustard operations had been performed as of January 1, 1980.

modifications.[7,13,179,213,240,248,332,335,348] There are relatively few long-term follow-up data and some have cautioned against a rapid swing to the arterial switch procedure.[97] Yacoub[409] summarized the potential problems with anatomic correction. One relates to the need to transpose the coronary arteries without tension, torsion, or kinking to the posterior vessel at a very young age. A second results from the need to bridge the gap between the proximal end of the transected aorta and the distal pulmonary artery. Although direct anastomosis has been accomplished, undue tension may result in pulmonary arterial stenosis or pressure on the coronary arteries. The gap may be bridged by a Dacron or homologous dura tube, but their long-term behavior is not known, and they may eventually require replacement. Will the coronary and aortic anastomoses grow? Unpublished data from Radley-Smith and Yacoub in a small series of patients who have undergone an arterial switch procedure with reimplantation of the coronary arteries demonstrated no signs of narrowing of either anastomosis, although the

longest follow-up was only 2.5 years. In older children with complete transposition, a marked discrepancy in size between the pulmonary arterial root and ascending aorta (after the arterial switch) causes an angiographic appearance similar to an aneurysm of the aortic root[113] (Fig. 45–8). This abnormality in geometry, combined with the thin arterial wall of the pulmonary artery, may lead to progressive dilatation and incompetence of the left aortic valve.

Of concern to all those who perform the arterial switch procedure is the fate of the coronary arterial anastomosis. Data collected over nearly a decade indicate that growth of the coronary arterial anastomosis does occur.[28,210,316] Instances of sudden death have been recorded, and at our institution two patients have died suddenly after the arterial switch procedure. In one of these cases, the ostium of the left coronary artery was severely narrowed, and the left ventricular myocardium demonstrated diffuse ischemic injury. Thus far, the arterial switch procedures have seemingly avoided significant atrial arrhythmias, and in those infants assessed after the arterial switch repair, both sinoatrial node and atrioventricular node function has been normal.[12] Finally, right ventricular outflow tract obstruction of varying severity has been assessed postoperatively in about 20 percent of patients evaluated after arterial repair despite implementation of the LeCompte maneuver.[222,244]

The morphologic left ventricle has to support the systemic circulation after a successful arterial switch procedure. This poses no difficulty in patients with additional lesions, such as a large ductus arteriosus or ventricular septal defect, that help maintain a high left ventricular pressure (and, possibly, mass). However, most patients with complete transposition have an intact ventricular septum, and a rapid diminution in left ventricular mass begins after birth because of the normal fall in left ventricular pressure associated with the normal regression of pulmonary vascular resistance. Thus, left ventricular

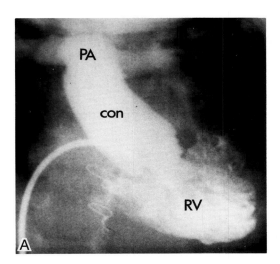

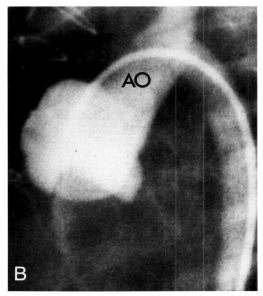

Fig. 45–8. Patient with complete transposition and large ventricular septal defect, status post-patch closure of ventricular septal defect, arterial switch, and retransposition and implantation of the coronary arteries. **(A)** Aortopulmonary right ventriculogram showing right ventricle (RV) and pulmonary artery (PA). A nonvalved Dacron conduit (con) is interposed between the right ventricular semilunar valve and pulmonary artery (PA). **(B)** Lateral of selective angiocardiogram performed proximal to left ventricular semilunar valve in aorta (AO). Note the discrepancy in size between the aorta and the bulbus left ventricular semilunar valve. (From Freedom et al.,[113] with permission.)

mass must be augmented in these patients. This is successfully accomplished by banding the pulmonary artery with or without an aortopulmonary shunt proximal to the band. Such patients require a banding procedure as an initial step, followed by an arterial switch at a later date. Whether the left ventricle can maintain long-term normal function after anatomic correction is uncertain (Table 45–3).

Almost simultaneously, Damus,[67] Stansel,[357] and Kaye[198] proposed a type of great vessel switch operation without coronary relocation for transposition of the great arteries. In this procedure, the aorta is left in anatomic continuity with the right ventricle but is functionally isolated from it because the aortic pressure remains greater than the right ventricular pressure throughout the cardiac cycle and keeps the aortic valve closed. This ne-

cessitates reconstruction of the right ventricular outflow tract with a conduit which will not grow with the patient. This procedure carries a high operative mortality, and a late morbidity will certainly result from the need to replace the ventricular conduit. Limited

Table 45–3. Potential Problems After "Anatomic Correction" for Complete Transposition of the Great Vessels

Fate of retransposed and reimplanted coronary arteries

Form and function of left ventricular semilunar valve (reconstituted aortic valve)

Growth of arterial anastomoses

Form and function of morphologic left ventricle

Fate of prosthetic conduit interposed between right ventricular semilunar valve (reconstituted pulmonary valve) and pulmonary artery initial surgical success has been reported by Danielson and colleagues from the Mayo Clinic.[71] Others have proposed, on theoretical grounds and with animal models, intra-aortic septation for anatomical correction of transposition of the great vessels.[81]

Surgical Treatment of Transposition, Ventricular Septal Defect, and Severe Valvular and Subvalvular Pulmonary Stenosis

Most youngsters with complete transposition of the great arteries, large ventricular septal defect, and subvalvular and valvular pulmonary stenosis require augmentation of pulmonary blood flow in infancy or during the first few years of life. Long-term palliation can be afforded by (1) diversion of left ventricle through the ventricular septal defect as advocated by Rastelli,[322] or (2) restoration of right ventricular to pulmonary artery continuity with a valved external conduit.[206,253,287,322] Left ventricular to pulmonary artery continuity must be disrupted, and is usually accomplished by oversewing the proximal end of the main pulmonary artery or by intracardiac closure of the pulmonary outflow tract. The advantages of this operation are that the procedure permits satisfactory relief of subvalvular and valvular pulmonary stenosis, which is frequently difficult to accomplish by direct means because of the proximity to the anterior leaflet of the mitral valve, ventricular septum, and coronary arteries.[7,189,338,347] In addition, the operation restores normal ventriculoarterial connections and allows the left ventricle to support the aorta and systemic circulation, with the right ventricle supporting the pulmonary artery (via a valved external conduit). Furthermore, the atrial anatomy is altered less by incisions and suture than it is with the inflow "correction" of Mustard, and troublesome atrial arrhythmias should be less frequent. Finally, late ob-

Table 45–4.   Potential Problems with Use of Valved External Conduit for Ventricular-Pulmonary Artery Continuity

Biologic life of conduit itself
Stenosis at cardiac or pulmonary artery anastomotic site
Stenosis of xenograft valve (or regurgitation)
Loss of function of ventricular free wall (site of proximal anastomosis)

struction of the systemic or pulmonary venous return will not be a problem.

As pointed out by Marcelletti and colleagues,[241] potential disadvantages of this procedure are related mainly to the xenograft valve in the conduit (see Ch. 42). This valve may become either regurgitant or stenotic. When pulmonary vascular resistance is normal, little difficulty should result from a regurgitant xenograft valve. Nonetheless, significant and progressive obstruction of the valve will eventually necessitate its replacement (Table 45–4). Furthermore, the dimensions of the patch used to construct the intracardiac tunnel from the left ventricle must be sufficient to permit a nonobstructed flow of blood. Most frequently, subaortic stenosis results when the ventricular septal defect is considerably smaller than the orifice of the aortic valve (Fig. 45–9). Indeed, the obstruction was localized to the proximal end of the left ventricle to aortic tunnel in five patients with subaortic obstruction after the Rastelli procedure reported by Rocchini.[327,329]

In some patients with complete transposition, ventricular septal defect, and severe subvalve pulmonary stenosis, the position of the ventricular septal defect may preclude the Rastelli procedure. Certainly, if the ventricular defects are small and multiple and are removed from the usual perimembranous and infundibular location, it would not be possible to divert the left ventricle to the aorta via the ventricular septal defect. Such patients, fortunately few, require an inflow correction of the Mustard or Senning type, closure of the

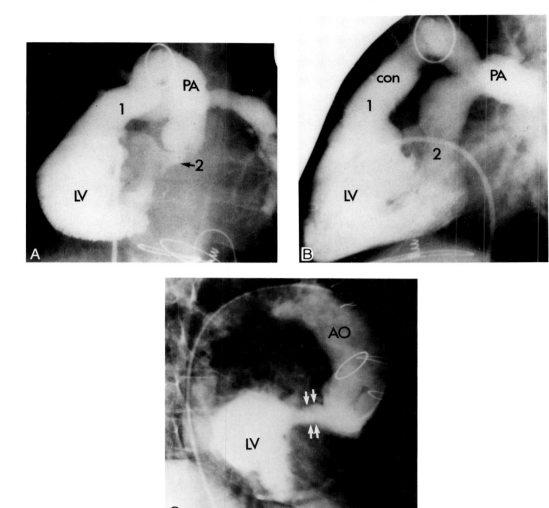

Fig. 45–9. (A,B) Total repair of corrected transposition, ventricular septal defect, and valvular and subvalvular pulmonary stenosis. Relief of the pulmonary outflow tract obstruction was afforded by a valved external conduit (con) interposed between the morphological left ventricle (LV) and the pulmonary artery (PA). Thus, there are two points of exit from left ventricle to pulmonary artery: (1) conduit, and (2) stenotic pulmonary outflow tract. **(C)** Postoperative complete repair of double-outlet right ventricle, ventricular septal defect, and pulmonary stenosis. The left ventricle (LV) is "connected" to the aorta (AO) via the ventricular septal defect. Postoperatively, this patient developed subaortic stenosis, which resulted from a restrictive ventricular septal defect (arrows). (From Rocchini et al.,[327] with permission.)

ventricular defect, and a left ventricular to pulmonary artery valved external conduit.[154,206,352] Similarly, patients with complete transposition of the great arteries, intact ventricular septum, and severe subvalvular left ventricular outflow tract obstruction require an inflow type of "correction" as well as a valved external conduit from left ventricle to pulmonary artery.

Surgical Correction of Transposition, Ventricular Septal Defect, and Pulmonary Vascular Obstructive Disease

The patient with markedly elevated pulmonary vascular resistance is not a candidate for either total "correction" by either an inflow operation or by an arterial switch with transposition of the coronary arteries. Nonetheless, these patients are often very cyanotic and limited in their activity.

Some experience supports the viewpoint that they may benefit by the so-called palliative Mustard operation.[21,44,230,236] The ventricular septal defect is not closed, but an inflow operation is performed. In suitable candidates, the systemic oxygen saturation improves with amelioration of symptoms resulting from hypoxia and polycythemia. Such patients may experience the complications of an inflow type of operation and, in the presence of pulmonary vascular obstructive disease, atrial tachyarrhythmias are poorly tolerated. Whether the palliative Mustard operation actually prolongs life is uncertain. There is no doubt, however, that the quality of life is improved.

In an occasional patient with transposition of the great arteries and intact ventricular septum, pulmonary vascular obstructive disease will develop. Creation of an apical ventricular septal defect combined with an inflow "correction" type of operation has successfully palliated some.[44] Whether patients so treated

actually live longer than nonoperated patients is uncertain, but clinical observations indicate that their quality of life is enhanced.

The application of the arterial switch operation to the patient with transposition of the great arteries and fixed, irrevocable pulmonary vascular disease would have merit theoretically, but, to our knowledge, this has not yet been reported.

Finally, bronchopulmonary circulation has been assessed by Aziz and his associates in patients with complete transposition of the great arteries, and was marked in 20 of 138 patients having cardiac catheterizations before two years of age.[14] Such collateral vessels were more frequently demonstrated in the patients with an intact ventricular septum than in those with ventricular septal defect or left ventricular outflow tract stenosis. It was suggested that the extensive bronchopulmonary circulation might be one factor predisposing an occasional patient with complete transposition to accelerated pulmonary vascular disease. The extent to which such extensive bronchopulmonary collaterals regress after either an inflow or anatomic correction is unknown.

TRUNCUS ARTERIOSUS

Truncus arteriosus is an uncommon cardiac malformation characterized by a single arterial vessel supplying systemic, coronary, and pulmonary arteries.[6,18,26,43,47,50,136,350,380,383] With the exception of only one or two published cases, a ventricular septal defect involving the infundibular septum is always present.[50] Abnormalities of the truncal valve are very frequent, with truncal valve regurgitation of varying severity occurring in about 20 percent.[126,471] Truncal valve stenosis, when severe, is usually fatal, often in the neonatal period.[14,18,21,26,43,44,47,50,230,236,303,352,380,383] Truncus arteriosus, if untreated, is usually fatal[242]; the median age of death in Van Praagh's autopsy series was 5 weeks,[383] although some patients develop pulmonary vas-

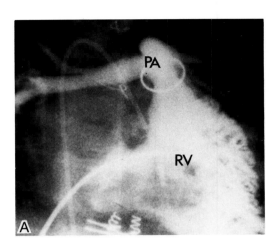
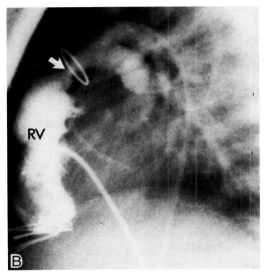

Fig. 45–10. Postoperative complete repair of type 1 truncus arteriosus in infancy. Several years later, this asymptomatic patient developed a loud murmur, and cardiac catheterization demonstrated severe right ventricular hypertension with a normal distal pulmonary artery pressure. (**A**) Aortopulmonary right ventriculogram shows a large right ventricle (RV) and relatively small pulmonary arteries (PA). (**B**) The lateral of this injection demonstrates severe stenosis at the level of the porcine valve (arrow).

cular obstructive disease and survive two decades or more. An occasional patient, despite a torrential pulmonary blood flow and high pulmonary artery pressures, will survive several years without developing irreversible pulmonary vascular changes.[237] Anomalies of the pulmonary arteries in truncus arteriosus are common (including unilateral absence), complicate the clinical course, and render more difficult assessment of the status of the pulmonary vascular bed.[26,38,237,334]

The symptomatic neonate is usually in profound and often intractable congestive heart failure. There is a torrential blood flow into the low-resistance pulmonary circuit. Truncal valve abnormalities often pose a further burden to a compromised left ventricular myocardium.[303] Finally, the truncal diastolic pressure is frequently very low, both because of a large aortopulmonary runoff and because of truncal valve regurgitation, and the coronary arterial perfusion pressure is low. For these reasons, the myocardium is particularly vul-

nerable to ischemic damage. Furthermore, the left coronary ostium is often directly posteroinferior to the ostium of the pulmonary artery(s).[6,350] This abnormal configuration may lessen coronary blood flow and further potentiate ischemic myocardial damage.[251,351]

Although pulmonary arterial banding or, more recently, the creation of pulmonary ostial stenosis, has been advocated for short-term palliation,[263] the early and late surgical mortality from these procedures have prompted a more aggressive surgical approach: total correction in infancy and childhood.[11,157,257,358,364] This involves separation of the pulmonary arteries from the truncus, closure of the truncal wall defect, patch closure of the ventricular septal defect, and reconstitution of right ventricular-pulmonary artery continuity with a valved external conduit (Fig. 45–10). Presently, with rare exception, the surgical mortality in infants remains unacceptably high. In large part, long-term follow-up and morbidity are predicated on the fate of the xenograft valve in the conduit and on the inevitable need to replace the conduit because of growth of the patient. Because the truncal valve is so often abnormal, some patients surviving "correction" in infancy suffer progressive insufficiency and/or stenosis of this valve, which may necessitate later surgical intervention. Indeed, some patients have required replacement of their truncal valve at the same time as total correction.

TRICUSPID ATRESIA WITH NORMAL VENTRICULOARTERIAL CONNECTIONS

Most patients with tricuspid atresia and normal ventriculoarterial connections become progressively cyanosed during the first year of life.[77,320,402] Since there is no direct connection between right atrium and ventricle, flow into the pulmonary artery is via either a communication from the left ventricular chamber to the small right ventricular outflow chamber, or via some form of aortopulmonary communication. The morphologic bases for restriction in pulmonary blood flow are frequently related to progressive narrowing of the ventricular communication, although infundibular or valve stenosis may also lead to a reduction in pulmonary blood flow.[9,25,159,319,320,367] Most patients require some form of systemic to pulmonary artery or cavopulmonary artery anastomosis in the first few years of life to palliate progressive hypoxia.[402]

In 1971, Fontan and Baudet[99] reported an operation that provided a better circulation for the patient with tricuspid atresia and reduced pulmonary blood flow. Basically, the atrial septal defect is closed, and right atrial to pulmonary artery continuity is provided by either an external conduit or a direct anastomosis between atrium and pulmonary artery. Early procedures with this right ven-

tricular bypass operation included caval valves, but more recent experience suggests that this is not necessary. A number of modifications of the initial Fontan and Baudet operation have been recorded, including Kreutzer's incorporation of the patient's own infundibulum and pulmonary artery (when both are normal) into the circuit.[30,36,100,130,168,177,212,272,333,368,408] In some centers, a cavopulmonary anastomosis has been performed at the same time to "underload" the right atrium, but this is not done consistently. In the patient with tricuspid atresia and a well-expanded outlet chamber, atrio- "right" ventricular continuity may be provided with a valved external conduit.

Success, for even a short time, in direct atriopulmonary artery anastomosis is determined by the status of the pulmonary vascular bed and the lack of significant stenoses in the pulmonary arterial tree.[261,343] Even with a low pulmonary pressure and normal pulmonary resistance, features of right heart failure with hepatomegaly, pleural effusion, and ascites may be conspicuous in the immediate postoperative period, although these features do eventually abate[261,343] (Fig. 45–11).

Of obvious concern is the ability of the right atrium to tolerate elevated pressures (as compared with normal atrial dynamics). One might anticipate that atrial fibrillation or other supraventricular tachyarrhythmias might seriously compromise the efficacy of this approach. Sharratt and colleagues[349] have shown that atrial systole is necessary for pulsatile pulmonary blood flow and a good hemodynamic result.

Although atrial systole (and a normal sinus mechanism) would seem important in any patients with atrial to pulmonary artery anastomoses, patients with tricuspid atresia, especially the older patient, may be susceptible to ventricular arrhythmias. Ventricular performance is impaired in older patients with tricuspid atresia who have had longstanding large aortopulmonary shunts and chronic left ventricular diastolic overload.[215] The histopathologic equivalent of this impaired left ventricular function is myocardial fibrosis resulting from ischemia (certainly these features have been observed in autopsied patients). While these comments have been directed to the patient with tricuspid atresia, normal ventriculoarterial connections, and naturally occurring pulmonary stenosis, a Fontan-like surgical approach is also applicable in the patient with tricuspid atresia, transposition of the great arteries, and naturally occurring pulmonary stenosis (Table 45–5).

For the patient with tricuspid atresia, transposition of the great arteries, and banded pulmonary artery, a Fontan-like approach may accomplish reconstitution of the circulation—provided that the pulmonary artery pressure distal to the band is normal. However, because the outlet foramen in this situation often becomes obstructed after pulmonary artery banding (thus causing subaortic obstruction), reconstitution of atriopulmonary continuity must be combined with some procedure

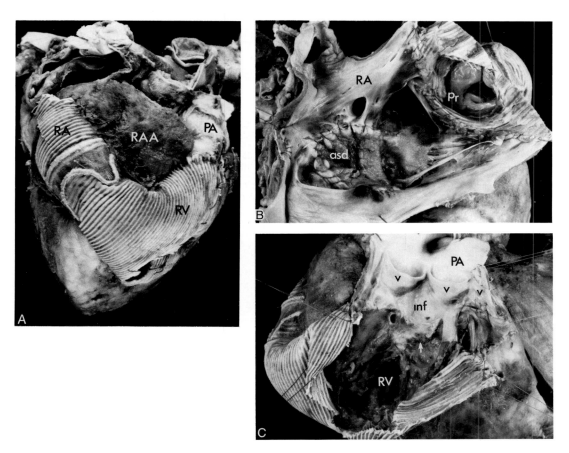

Fig. 45–11. Postoperative modified Fontan procedure. (**A**) External view of heart with tricuspid atresia. Right atrial (RA) to right ventricular continuity (RV) was obtained using a valved external conduit. The right atrial appendage (RAA) is enlarged, and the pulmonary artery (PA) is seen at the distal end of the conduit. (**B**) The right atrium (RA) is opened. The atrial septal defect (asd) has been closed with a prosthetic patch, and the proximal end of the valved external conduit (Pr) is seen. (**C**) The right ventricular (RV) outflow tract is opened to expose the pulmonary artery (PA) infundibulum (inf) and the tricuspid pulmonary valve (v). Subpulmonary infundibular obstructing muscle (arrow) has been surgically resected. (*Figure continues.*)

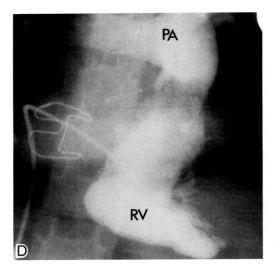

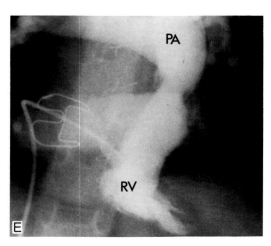

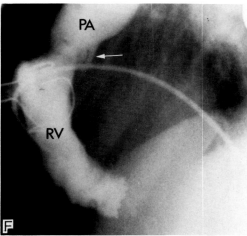

Fig. 45–11 *(continued)*. **(D,E)** Modified Fontan procedure for total correction of tricuspid atresia, normal ventriculoarterial connections, and pulmonary stenosis resulting from a narrowed outlet foramen. Total repair included (1) patch closure of atrial septal defect and ventricular septal defect, and (2) surgical anastomosis of a valved external conduit between right atrium and infundibular chamber. Figs. D&E show diastolic and systolic frames from selective injection of contrast material in new right ventricle (RV) with subsequent opacification of pulmonary artery (PA). The apical portion of the right ventricle contracts well. **(F)** Lateral projection of this injection demonstrates slightly thickened pulmonary valve (arrow). Postoperative right ventricular and pulmonary artery pressures were normal. The right atrial mean pressure was 10 mmHg.

Table 45-5. Potential Problems After Fontan or Fontan-like Operation for Tricuspid Atresia and Normal Ventriculoarterial Connections[a]

Form and function of right atrium (function related in part to atrial rhythm)

Form and function of external (valved or nonvalved) conduit (if used)

Form and function of left ventricle

Problems attendant to Glenn anastomosis (if used)

[a] See Figure 45–12. For other surgical approaches to outlet foramen stenosis and subaortic stenosis, see section on univentricular heart.

to ameliorate the subaortic stenosis.[114,115,118,122,280,403] One approach taken at our Institute is to combine an arterial switch procedure with coronary artery reimplantation plus constitution of right atrial- "right ventricular" continuity with a valved external conduit[124] (Fig. 45–12). (For other surgical approaches to outlet foramen stenosis and subaortic stenosis, see the section on univentricular heart.)

SINGLE VENTRICLE (UNIVENTRICULAR HEART)

The past decade has witnessed an exponential growth in the literature devoted to the morphology, nosology, and angiocardiographic and echocardiographic features of the univentricular heart. This interest was initially stimulated by some surgical success in the "repair" of this malformation by a combination of ventricular septation and correction of the associated cardiac malformations.[68–70,78,84,164,187,255,266,365]

It is impossible to discuss the postoperative features of patients with univentricular heart without discussing the morphology of the condition. For this, we will consider a univentricular heart as one with both atrioventricular valves connected to one ventricular chamber.

The univentricular heart may therefore be of left ventricular type, with or without an infundibular chamber; of right ventricular type; or of indeterminate type. The ventriculoarterial connections may be normal (concordant), discordant (transposition), or double outlet (from main chamber or outlet chamber in the left ventricular type). The arterial relationships may be normal, side by side, or leftward or rightward an anterior aorta. (An excellent review of the univentricular heart can be found in the April 1979 issue of Herz.)

Most patients with single ventricle present either in the neonatal period, infancy, or early childhood with one or a combination of the following features:

1. Hypoxia secondary to pulmonary outflow tract obstruction
2. Congestive heart failure with an unobstructed pulmonary outflow tract, frequently in combination with an obstructive anomaly of the aortic arch
3. Atrioventricular valve incompetence
4. Congenital heart block or other arrhythmias
5. Severe left atrioventricular valve stenosis with an inadequate interatrial communication and pulmonary edema

Although the symptomatic young infant with severe pulmonary outflow tract obstruction and single ventricle can be palliated by one or more systemic to pulmonary artery anastomoses or by a cavopulmonary artery anastomoses, restoration of a functionally normal circulation depends on (1) preservation of low or normal pulmonary vascular resistance, (2) a myocardium that is not irrevocably damaged by chronic volume overload and/or hypoxia, and (3) the surgical ability to deal with other complicating cardiac anomalies.

Although there was some success in septation of the univentricular heart with constitution of "right" ventricular to pulmonary continuity with a valved external conduit, most centers have abandoned this approach, except for the patient with single left ventricle, left-sided infundibular chamber support-

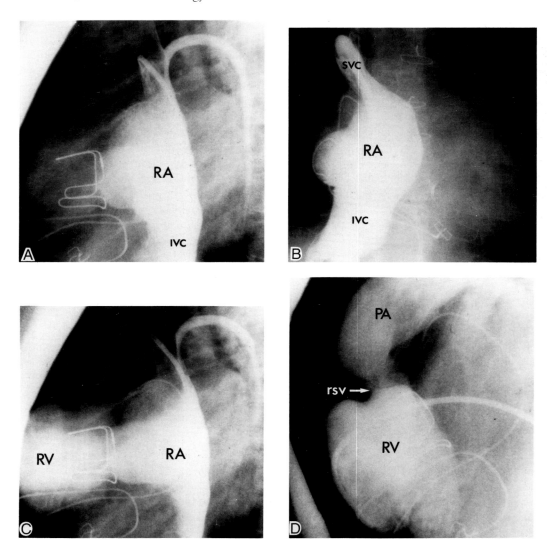

Fig. 45–12. Patient, aged 15 years, with tricuspid atresia, transposition of the great arteries, large ventricular septal defect, banded pulmonary artery, and atrial septal defect. Patient underwent an anatomic repair including arterial switch, coronary artery reimplantation, constitution of right atrial-right ventricular continuity with a valved external conduit, patch closure of ventricular septal defect, and patch closure of atrial septal defect. (**A**) Selective injection in right atrium (RA) with reflux into superior (SVC) and inferior vena cava (IVC). (**B**) Lateral of this injection. (**C**) Lateral of right atriogram with filling of right ventricle (RV) via a valved external conduit. (**D**) Selective injection in right ventricle (RV) in lateral projection. Note the discrepancy between the right ventricular semilunar valve (rsv; former aortic valve; new pulmonary valve) and pulmonary artery. (*Figure continues.*)

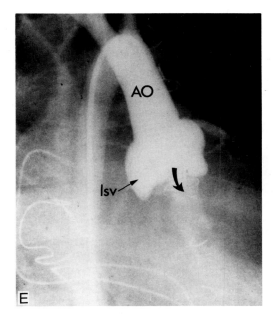
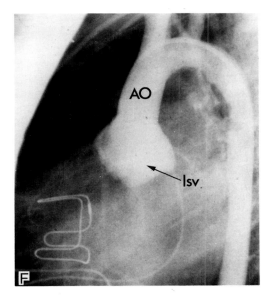

Fig. 45–12 (*continued*). (**E,F**) Aortopulmonary and lateral aortogram of same patient showing incompetence of left ventricular semilunar valve (lsv). Again, there is a significant discrepancy between the caliber of the ascending aorta and the left ventricular semilunar valve (former pulmonary valve; new aortic valve). The coronary arteries fill normally following reimplantation. AO, aorta. Curved arrow indicates presence of aortic regurgitation. (Operation performed by W. G. Williams, M.D., Hospital for Sick Children, Toronto.) (From Freedom et al.,[124] with permission.)

ing a discordantly connected and levopositioned aorta, naturally occurring pulmonary outflow tract obstruction, or two functionally normal atrioventricular valves.

Some of the mechanical reasons for both the high initial surgical mortality and the considerable ongoing morbidity include (1) the inability of septation to provide two ventricular chambers of adequate size and the likelihood of damage to, or the need to replace, abnormal atrioventricular valves, (2) a high incidence of surgical heart block, (3) damage to the coronary arteries, and (4) a paradoxically moving ventricular septation patch.[201] Certainly, a few patients have been palliated by ventricular septation. Even in these patients the long-term results will be affected by: the alteration of ventricular function by the large, ventricular septation patch: the long-term durability of any valved external conduit; any

distortion of atrioventricular valves, and remote disturbances of atrioventricular conduction. In this regard, LaCorte and colleagues drew attention to impaired left ventricular function among a large series of patients with tricuspid atresia and related this deterioration to the age of the patient and the presence of long-standing, large, surgically created aortopulmonary communications.[215] Perhaps even more disturbing are the findings of Gibson and colleagues[139] that architectural abnormalities in univentricular hearts lead to disturbances of myocardial function that particularly affect the apex, and that such changes are detectable from an early age and are independent of age, volume overload, or degree of cyanosis. It is uncertain just how these data will affect survival/morbidity curves in patients with univentricular heart who have survived septation.

Because of disappointingly high early and late surgical mortality and morbidity, ventricular septation procedures have been more or less abandoned in favor of a Fontan-like procedure combined with oversewing or closure of the right atrioventricular valve (thus converting the patient with univentricular heart and two atrioventricular valves into a patient with tricuspid atresia).[410,411] In this context, the abnormalities described by Gibson in patients with univentricular hearts were more common in those with univentricular hearts and an absent right atrioventricular connection (tricuspid atresia).[139] Thus, in patients with univentricular heart and two atrioventricular valves treated by a Fontan procedure, any of the problems associated with that operation may develop.

The patient with univentricular heart and two atrioventricular valves with unobstructed pulmonary outflow presents with features of severe congestive heart failure and pulmonary artery hypertension. Digoxin and diuretics rarely provide symptomatic relief, and survival of these patients, usually neonates or infants, requires pulmonary arterial banding, often associated with reconstruction of an obstructed anomaly of the aortic arch. Usually, a transposed aorta originates above the infundibular chamber, while the pulmonary artery originates above the main ventricular chamber, which receives both atrioventricular valves.[114,115,118,122,124,318,382,399] Since the chamber supporting the aorta does not receive any atrioventricular valve, flow into the aorta is through the outlet foramen (the communication between the main ventricular chamber receiving the atrioventricular valves and the outlet chamber). When there is no obstruction to pulmonary blood flow, the dimensions of the outlet foramen are frequently marginal and potentially obstructive (and if obstructive, would cause subaortic stenosis).[114,115,118,122] We and others have suggested that concentric muscular hypertrophy in response to pulmonary arterial banding may result in a progressive diminution in size of the outlet foramen and therefore in severe

suboartic   stenosis.[114,115,118,122,355,356,410,411] When this complication occurs, obstruction to both arterial outlets is present: (1) the pulmonary outlet because of previous pulmonary arterial banding, and (2) the aortic outlet because of restriction of the outlet foramen. Concentric ventricular muscular hypertrophy in this situation can nearly obliterate the ventricular cavity, and if unrecognized and untreated, is invariably fatal (Fig. 45–13). Yet any long-term hope for survival and restoration of a "normal" circulation requires protection of the pulmonary arterial bed from the ravages of pulmonary artery hypertension.[118]

Outlet foramen stenosis can be treated in several ways. Attempts at surgical ventricular septation, surgical enlargement of the outlet foramen and pulmonary arterial debanding and reconstruction have, with rare exception, proved fatal. Furthermore, the complication of outlet foramen stenosis frequently occurs in young infants, often within a few months of pulmonary artery banding; in this age group, ventricular septation (even in those with naturally occurring pulmonary stenosis) carries nearly a 100 percent operative mortality. Direct surgical enlargement of the outlet foramen has met with limited success. Often because of the disposition of the cardiac conduction tissue or because of the proximity of atrioventricular valve tissue to the circumference of the outlet foramen, this surgical approach has caused heart block, atrioventricular valve regurgitation, or both. However, using the approach advocated by Neches[280] for a patient with tricuspid atresia, transposition of the great arteries, banded pulmonary artery, and a restrictive outlet foramen, we have created an aorticopulmonary window proximal to the pulmonary artery band. In a small series of patients, this has effectively abolished the subaortic gradient, but none has yet gone on to a modified Fontan-approach, although Yacoub[410,411] reported a surgical success.

A modified Fontan procedure can be used effectively to palliate some patients with univentricular heart of left ventricular type,

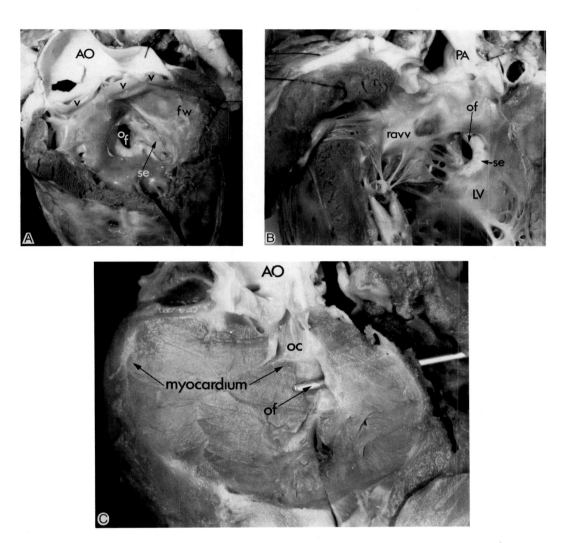

Fig. 45–13. Subaortic stenosis in single left ventricle, transposition of the great arteries, and banded pulmonary artery. (**A**) Internal view of small outlet chamber supporting the discordantly connected aorta (AO). The outlet foramen (of) is restrictive, with an area considerably less than the aortic valve (v). Sclerotic endocardium (se) about the margins of the outlet foramen extends to the free wall (fw) of the outlet foramen. (**B**) Internal view of the main left ventricular cavity (LV) demonstrates the transposed pulmonary artery (PA). The outlet foramen (of) is small, and sclerotic endocardium (se) is a testament to its restrictive nature. The proximity of the right atrioventricular valve (ravv) and its tensor apparatus to the outlet foramen is apparent. (**C**) Sagittal "transectional" view in a patient with single left ventricle, transposed great arteries, and banded pulmonary artery who developed severe subaortic stenosis. The outlet chamber (oc) is small, and the outlet foramen accommodates a 2.0-mm probe (of). The left ventricular free wall myocardium is severely hypertrophied, indicative of the severe subaortic stenosis. AO, aorta. (*Figure continues.*)

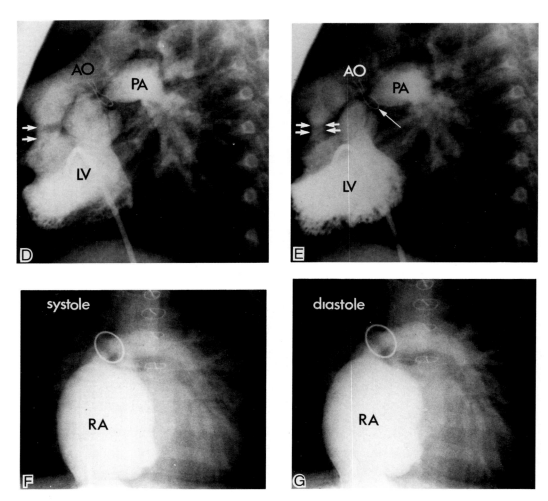

Fig. 45–13 *(continued).* **(D,E)** Patient with double inlet atrioventricular connection in whom subaortic stenosis developed after pulmonary artery banding. Selective diastolic **(D)** and systolic **(E)** frames of left ventricle (LV) show that the transposed aorta (AO) is anterior to the banded pulmonary artery (PA). The subaortic stenosis involves the subaortic infundibulum (arrows). Patient underwent a "functional" correction by construction of a Glenn anastomosis, closure of the right atrioventricular valve, division of proximal main from distal main pulmonary artery, establishment of right atrial-distal main pulmonary artery anastomosis with external conduit, and interposition of short Dacron graft between proximal main pulmonary artery and ascending aorta. Chronic right "heart" failure resulted from severe impairment of right atrial function. **(F,G)** Systolic and diastolic frames from right atrial injection. The right atrium (RA) is large, and its contractility is severely impaired. *(Figure continues.)*

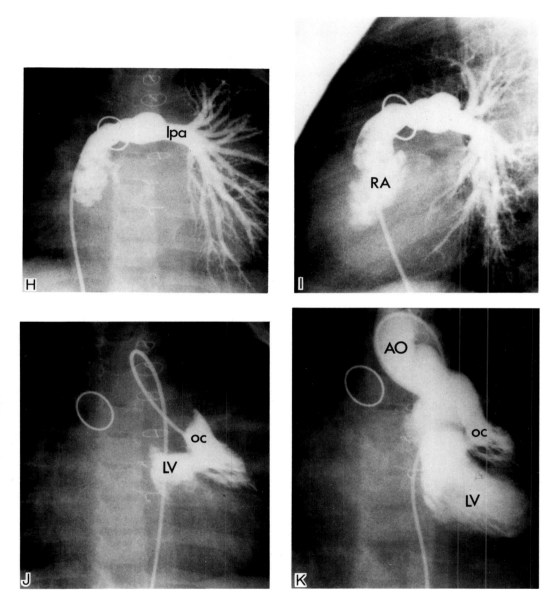

Fig. 45–13 *(continued).* **(H,I)** Selective injection in distal main pulmonary artery. Flow through the left pulmonary artery (lpa) is very slow. **(J)** Retrograde arterial injection in small outlet chamber (oc) with opacification of left ventricle (LV) via outlet foramen. **(K)** The anatomy of the single left ventricle (LV), outlet chamber (oc) and aorta are clearly visualized in this aortopulmonary projection. *(Figure continues.)*

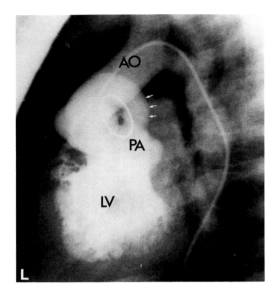
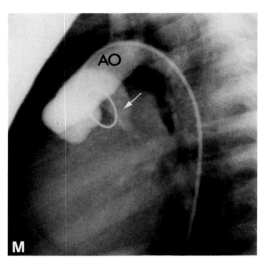

Fig. 45–13 *(continued)*. (**L**) In this lateral projection of the left ventriculogram, the Dacron conduit (arrows) connects the left ventricular semilunar valve to the aorta. (**M**) This retrograde aortogram opacifies the ascending aorta (AO) and the aortic end of the dacron conduit (arrow). (Performed by A. Dobell, M.D., Montreal Children's Hospital.)

transposition of the great arteries, with the aorta supported by an infundibular chamber, two atrioventricular valves connected to main left ventricular cavity, banded pulmonary artery, and acquired subaortic stenosis secondary to narrowing of the outlet foramen.[131,356] Oversewing of the right atrioventricular valve is combined with (1) a conduit to provide continuity between right atrium and distal pulmonary artery; (2) closure of any atrial septal defect, and (3) anastomosis of the proximal end of the divided pulmonary artery to the side of the ascending aorta.[410,411] This usually requires interposition of a woven Dacron graft. The procedure provides two outlets to the ascending aorta: (1) the natural outlet via the narrowed outlet foramen, and (2) the pulmonary outlet (i.e., main left ventricle to left ventricular semilunar valve to proximal main pulmonary artery to woven Dacron graft to ascending aorta) (Fig. 45–13). This surgical tour de force provides physiologic palliation, but the potential problems and their anatomic substrate include: (1) right atrial function and rhythm, (2) fate of atriopulmonary conduits, (3) fate of woven Dacron graft interposed between main pulmonary artery and side of ascending aorta, and (4) function of left ventricle. Finally, subaortic obstruction in univentricular hearts can rarely occur with normal ventriculoarterial connections, with or without an infundibular chamber. Nonetheless, the acquisition of subaortic obstruction in a univentricular heart causes such profound hemodynamic, anatomic, and myocardial disturbances that only a few such patients can be anticipated to survive to adulthood.

The patient with severely incompetent atrioventricular valve(s) will rarely survive infancy; however, in a rare patient operated on some years ago, ventricular septation has been combined with replacement of one atrioventricular valve. The combination of congenital heart block and univentricular heart is frequently fatal. It is not the disturbance of atrioventricular conduction so much as the associated cardiac defects that predestine early death. Finally, the condition of a patient with univentricular heart and severely obstructive left atrioventricular valve can be palliated by atrial decompression (balloon atrioseptostomy, Blalock-Hanlon atrial septectomy, or blade atrioseptostomy), in combination with pulmonary arterial banding to palliate torrential pulmonary blood flow or by creation of a systemic to pulmonary artery anastomosis to augment pulmonary blood flow. Whether such patients are afforded long-term palliation by closure of the left atrioventricular valve, diversion of pulmonary venous return through the right atrioventricular valve and into the aorta, with construction of a right atriopulmonary conduit, is at present conjectural.

The Fontan procedure or one of its variations has been performed for about two decades. It has been applied to a wide spectrum of congenitally abnormal hearts when a biventricular repair is not possible.[175,249,313] Currently at The Hospital for Sick Children, Toronto, the most common operation performed in patients older than 2 years of age is the Fontan or one of its modifications.

The criteria for a successful atriopulmonary connection with atrial partitioning have been published elsewhere; these criteria have been thoroughly scrutinized. It has become increasingly evident that myocardial hypertrophy may have an impact on both early and late Fontan results.[104,111,208] Such myocardial hypertrophy could result from banding of the pulmonary trunk in patients with increased pulmonary blood flow, pulmonary hypertension, and absence of pulmonary outflow tract obstruction.[104,111] This procedure also potentiates and accelerates the natural tendency of the potentially restrictive muscular ventricular septal defect to a further reduction in size. Thus, in the patient with a univentricular atrioventricular connection of left ventricular type and transposition of the great arteries, the result of a restrictive ventricular septal defect is subaortic stenosis and myocardial hypertrophy. One would assume that an increasing myocardial mass would impact on

Table 45–6. Results with the Fontan Procedure[a]

Type of Heart	Patients (N)	Operative Deaths (%)	Late Deaths (%)
TAT, I	74	9	4
TAT, II	21	2	2
TAT, III	2	0	0
Non-TAT	148	23	8
Totals	245	13.9	6.6

[a] Except in the totals, where operative deaths and late deaths are given as percentages, the remaining data are presented as numbers related to the entire Fontan experience of 245 patients.
TAT, tricuspid atresia.

ventricular compliance or stiffness, and thus diastolic function.[104,111,208] At this institution, the overall Fontan results through March 1989 are shown in Table 45–6. Thus, our institutional experience provides a nearly 14 percent operative or 30 day mortality, with 6.6 percent late deaths as well. These results are comparable to those of colleagues at the Mayo Clinic, who reported in 1985 an overall mortality of 12 percent for patients with tricuspid atresia, noting that in the previous 5 years the mortality had fallen to 7 percent.[235] A number of reports addressing follow-up have been published. Late functional problems relate to arrhythmias, atrioventricular valve regurgitation, subaortic stenosis, or ventricular dysfunction.[76,147,176,224,363] Those patients whose major ventricle is of right ventricular morphology seem to have a poorer outcome than do those with a major ventricle of left ventricular morphology.[247]

HYPOPLASTIC LEFT HEART SYNDROME

Hypoplastic left heart syndrome is an invariably lethal condition affecting the newborn.[105,107,284] Like a dinosaur surviving into the 1990s, an occasional patient with this anomaly will live to 4 to 5 years of age. This condition is characterized by varying degrees of aortic outflow tract, inflow tract, and left ventricular hypoplasia. In the most severe expression of hypoplastic left heart syndrome, aortic and mitral atresia are present. The left ventricle is represented only by an endothelium lined slit that may be recognizable by histologic examination.[24,105,107,225] A normal-sized left ventricle is found in 2 to 7 percent of patients with aortic atresia.[24,105,116] Aortic atresia has also been described in hearts exhibiting complete and corrected transposition of the great arteries, dominant right form of atrioventricular septal defect, double-outlet right ventricle, a univentricular heart of left ventricular morphology, and in patients with so-called right or left atrial isomerism.[105,107] Uncommon associations include interruption of the aortic arch, aorticopulmonary window, and aortico-left ventricular tunnel.[105,107]

The mode of death in those babies with the usual representation of this disorder is related to normal events of the transitional circulation, that is, functional and anatomic closure of the ductus arteriosus and closure of the interatrial communication.[105,107,129,284] Survival for even a short time depends on patency of the ductus arteriosus and an adequate-sized interatrial communication. In more than 75 percent of infants with hypoplastic left heart syndrome, the atrial septum is obstructive, and premature closure of the foramen ovale is not uncommon. The impact on the pulmonary circulation of a severely obstructive interatrial communication may be quite dramatic, and pulmonary lymphangiectasia may be very conspicuous, complicating pulmonary edema which may be hemorrhagic.[105,107,264] Progressive postnatal ductal closure will lead to a rapidly inadequate systemic and coronary circulation, and death.

The past decade has witnessed a dramatic evolution in the treatment of patients with hypoplastic left heart syndrome. This has been stimulated in large part by (1) data obtained from the New England Regional Infant Cardiac Program,[129] (2) the application and extension of Fontan's operation to patients with diverse forms of complex congenital heart malformations,[99] and (3) neonatal heart transplantation. Heart transplantation is not described here. (See Chapter 43.)

The New England Regional Infant Cardiac Program

Data obtained from the New England Regional Infant Cardiac Program indicate that most infants with hypoplastic left heart syndrome were full term, and only 21 percent of all patients identified with this syndrome had extracardiac anomalies.[129] Four percent were considered severe, 7 percent moderate, and 10 percent mild. Of infants with aortic atresia, severe extracardiac anomalies were identified in only 2 percent. Thus these babies seemed excellent candidates for palliative and later definitive reconstructive surgery.

The Fontan Principle

The concept of atrial partitioning with an atriopulmonary connection was initially conceived and applied by Fontan and Baudet to patients with tricuspid atresia.[99] When the atrial septal defect was closed in the patient with tricuspid atresia, this effectively partitioned the systemic venous from the pulmonary venous return. Connection of the surgically isolated systemic venous atrium receiving the superior and inferior caval veins to the pulmonary artery combined with ligation or division of the main pulmonary trunk as it left the heart provided separate systemic and pulmonary venous circulations. Thus, blood would be delivered to the lungs without an intervening pump (the right ventricle), and the patient would function with a 'single' left ventricle. A number of hemodynamic and anatomic criteria had to be satisfied before Fontan's operation could be applied to a patient. Subsequent to the benchmark report of Fontan and Baudet, the anatomic matrix was extended; this operation was performed on patients with a wide range of complex cardiac malformations, including some with a single right ventricle. When the anatomy of those infants with aortic atresia and hypoplastic left heart syndrome is surveyed, it is the morphologically right ventricle that supports the circulation. It was the vision and perseverance of Dr. William Norwood that led to the successful staged surgical palliation of patients with the hypoplastic left heart syndrome.[219,288–290]

This first stage includes atrial septectomy, reconstruction of the ascending aorta when it is diminutive with repair of the frequently associated coarctation of the aorta, and construction of a controlled systemic-to-pulmonary anastomosis to provide pulmonary blood flow.[184,219,288–290] In a series of papers, Norwood described those technical modifications used in the repair of the ascending aorta, coarctation of the aorta, and, as well, the modifications in the construction of the shunt.[219,288–290] The second stage is a Fontan operation.[99] The right and left atria are partitioned such that the pulmonary veins are diverted through the tricuspid valve to the right ventricle, the systemic-to-pulmonary artery connection is disrupted, and a connection is made between the systemic venous atrium and the pulmonary artery confluence.

In presenting the experience of Norwood and colleagues of the Children's Hospital of Philadelphia, Pigott reviewed the surgical results in 104 consecutive nonselected infants ranging in age from 1 to 30 days (median age, 6 days).[291,310] These infants weighed 1.7 to 4.2 kg. There were 30 early and 11 late deaths in this cohort subjected to the first stage of the surgical program. Thirty-three patients had undergone the second stage procedure (Fontan's operation) with 21 survivors.

We have suggested elsewhere in this review particular concern about the long-term well-being of patients undergoing Fontan's operation if the major or dominant ventricle is of right ventricular morphology.[105,107]

There are other reasons to show concern about the morphologic right ventricle in patients with the hypoplastic left heart syndrome. Some hearts with this disorder examined at postmortem by Lloyd and colleagues[231] exhibited extensive myocardial necrosis. Whether lesser degrees of myocardial necrosis will eventuate in ventricular dysfunction and failure in those survivors of staged palliative surgery is unclear. Wenink and colleagues[397] have studied the ventricular septum in patients with hypoplastic left heart syndrome, concluding that formation of the ventricular septum in these patients is abnormal, leading to pathology of the right ventricle. Thus, both acquired and developmental changes in the myocardium have the potential to affect the functional status of these patients after palliative surgery.

Ventriculocoronary connections have been described in hypoplastic left hearts.[105,107,293,340] Some years ago, we suggested that such ventriculocoronary connections may disadvantage the myocardium of patients with hypoplastic left heart syndrome, similar to the situation in patients with ventriculocoronary connections complicating pulmonary atresia and intact ventricular septum.[105–107] In hearts with hypoplastic left heart syndrome, ventriculocoronary connections have not been identified in those with absent or imperforate mitral valves (mitral atresia); thus, we suggested that such patients would be better candidates for staged palliative surgery than those with a perforate mitral valve.[105,107] Others have examined the coronary arteries in patients with the hypoplastic left heart syndrome, reaching a similar conclusion: in the presence of an open mitral valve, the coronary circulation may be so disadvantaged that a staged surgical approach is contraindicated.[293,340] Pigott addressed this particular theoretical concern and, at least for first-stage survivors, could not find a difference in survival between those with mitral hypoplasia and those with mitral atresia ($P = 0.4$).[291,310] Whether this concern will manifest itself at or beyond the second stage is unknown. Finally, we have addressed earlier concerns about the fate of the morphologically right ventricle as the systemic ventricle after Fontan's operation.

PULMONARY ATRESIA AND INTACT VENTRICULAR SEPTUM

In the first edition, we did not specifically address the postoperative pathology of pulmonary atresia and intact ventricular septum. The past several years have seen increased interest in the surgical management of this extremely complex and heterogeneous malformation. This is not the appropriate forum to address all the complexities of this malformation, (but a recently published monograph describes all aspects of this disorder[106]). Nevertheless, a few comments seem appropriate.

Pulmonary atresia and intact ventricular septum is an uncommon congenital anomaly, accounting for less than 1 percent of all congenitally malformed hearts.[119] Yet among cyanotic newborns, this disorder is third in frequency after transposition of the great arteries and tetralogy/pulmonary atresia and ventricular septal defect. Pulmonary atresia and intact ventricular septum is an extremely complex disorder with a wide morphologic substrate.[42,120,125–127,304] Only recently have we begun to understand the role of the disordered coronary circulation and the impact of abnormalities of the coronary circulation on surgical management and outcome.

The Endomyocardium: The Target Organ of a Disordered Coronary Circulation

The myocardium may be parchment thin and transilluminate in those patients with extreme tricuspid regurgitation complicating pulmonary atresia and intact ventricular septum.[64,112,378] As such patients are unlikely to have a disordered coronary circulation, they are not considered here. The endomyocardium of patients with pulmonary atresia, intact ventricular septum, and a small and hypertensive right ventricle exhibits a wide range of abnormalities, including evidence of myocardial ischemia, infarction, and even cardiac rupture; myocardial disarray; endocardial sclerosis; and so-called spongy myocardium.[39–41,74,82,90,91,94,101,111,174,211,298,344] Ischemic changes have been observed in the myocardium of newborns dying shortly after birth with pulmonary atresia and intact ventricular septum and in patients surviving for a number of years.[211] One can catalogue several reasons for an ischemic myocardium in these patients, including arterial hypoxemia, increased myocardial wall stress or tension from chronic isometric contraction, the chronic effects of a volume-loaded left ventricle secondary to one or more systemic-to-pulmonary artery connections, and the effects of a low coronary arterial driving pressure secondary to one or more systemic-to-pulmonary artery connections.[149,172] All these factors can and do affect the form and function of the myocardium of these patients.

The Nature of the Coronary Circulation

Peculiarities of the coronary arterial circulation have been recognized in these patients for more than half a century.[155,394] Such abnormalities have been designated myocardial or intramyocardial sinusoids, sinusoidal-coronary artery connections or fistulae, and more recently ventriculocoronary connections.[10,63,117,143,158,197] Other than patients with primary anomalies of the coronary circulation, abnormalities of the coronary circulation are intrinsic to many patients with pulmonary atresia and intact ventricular septum. Thus, the recognition of a disordered coronary arterial circulation in these patients is not new. The pathologist and the angiocardiographer have each shown communications between the cavity of the right ventricle and one or both coronary arteries mediated by ventriculocoronary connections. In addition, pathologists have defined the nature of the coronary arterial obstructive lesions.[10, 46,63,117,143,158,185,197,220,234,339,353,401] But it has taken many years for our understanding of the role of these coronary artery abnormalities to evolve from that of a pathologic curiosity to an appreciation of their dominant role in determining the prognosis for many patients afflicted with pulmonary atresia and intact ventricular septum.[103,294,295]

Factors Influencing Survival of Patients with Pulmonary Atresia and Intact Ventricular Septum

A disordered coronary circulation may affect in an important way the outcome of infants with pulmonary atresia and intact ventricular septum. We suggested 15 years ago that intramyocardial sinusoids in this disorder "predispose to ischemic myocardial dysfunction."[117] There is now no doubt that abnormalities in the coronary circulation compete with normal coronary artery dynamics and that the secondary changes in the involved coronary arteries will promote an ischemic myocardium and, in some, a right ventricular-dependent coronary circulation. Data recently published from this institution defined those morphologic variables that impacted negatively on survival: (1) profound Ebstein's anomaly of the tricuspid valve, and (2) ventriculocoronary connections, also designated as sinusoids.[106] It is well established that these two entities in the setting of pulmonary atresia and intact ventricular septum are mutually exclusive. Right ventricular hypertension at systemic levels or higher is required for right ventriculocoronary arterial flow. The right ventricle in such patients is thick walled, and the cavity of the right ventricle underdeveloped. By contrast, patients with a florid expression of Ebstein's anomaly rarely achieve systemic pressures in their right ventricle, and the right ventricular myocardium is profoundly thinned, occasionally dramatically so. Thus, there must be some relationship between the small hypertensive right ventricle and ventriculocoronary connections.

The Right Ventricle and Ventriculocoronary Artery Connections

In recent years, there has been a desire to catalogue the right ventricle in patients with pulmonary atresia and intact ventricular septum as (1) *tripartite*, with all three components (inlet, apical trabecular, and outlet) well-represented; (2) *bipartite*, with inlet and outlet components, both usually hypoplastic; or (3) *unipartite*, the most severely affected hearts, with profound attenuation of the apical trabecular and outlet components and with severe tricuspid valve and annular stenosis.[42,72] While this categorization has clinical relevance, Richard Van Praagh has cautioned that the approach is both simplistic and morphogically incorrect.[385] However, when those hearts with pulmonary atresia, intact ventricular septum, and ventriculocoronary artery connections are surveyed, hypoplasia of the right ventricle is a rather consistent feature. Moreover, there seems to be a predilection for ventriculocoronary artery connections in those hearts that one would categorize as either unipartite or bipartite. Ventriculocoronary artery connections can be observed in hearts with all three components well represented but are far less common than in those hearts in which the right ventricle is severely disadvantaged.

The Concept of a Right Ventricular-Dependent Coronary Circulation

In patients with pulmonary atresia, an intact ventricular septum, and a unipartite or bipartite, hypertensive right ventricle ventriculocoronary connections can be identified in about 50 percent.[106] Because of the intrinsic abnormalities of coronary circulation coronary artery blood flow in some patients will be driven not by aortic diastolic pressure, but by right ventricular systolic pressure. Thus, the coronary circulation in these specific situations will be considered right ventricular-dependent.[46,103,111,125,126,143,185,211,294,295,339]

The corollary to this statement is that reduction of right ventricular systolic pressure or right ventricular blood flow may impair myocardial perfusion, promoting myocardial ischemia and infarction. Those conditions requiring right ventricular blood flow and hypertension to maintain systolic coronary blood flow include (1) absence of connection of one or both coronary arteries from the aortic root,[31,132,163,223,377] (2) coronary artery stenosis or interruption,[46,103,111,125,126,128,143,185,211,294,295,339] and (3) substantial coronary artery–right ventricular flow.[72,111,125,126,143,339]

Absence of proximal connection between both coronary arteries and the aorta in a patient with pulmonary atresia and intact ventricular was first described by Lenox and Briner.[223] Subsequently, other patients with discontinuity between aorta and one or both coronary arteries have been recorded.[31,103,132,163,377] In patients with discontinuity between both proximal coronary arteries and the aorta, coronary blood flow is mediated entirely from retrograde systolic right ventricular flow through ventriculocoronary artery connections. Attempts to reduce the degree of right ventricular hypertension by any of a variety of means or to reduce right ventricular blood flow by thromboexclusion of the right ventricle would immediately jeopardize myocardial perfusion resulting in myocardial infarction.

Coronary artery stenosis or interruption can be found in the newborn with pulmonary atresia and intact ventricular septum. Such lesions have been noted to progress from an apparently normal coronary artery to stenosis or frank interruption. The impact of a major coronary artery stenosis or interruption that goes unappreciated is clear. We found a severe stenosis or interruption of the proximal anterior descending coronary artery to be a uniformly lethal risk factor for patients undergoing either right ventricular outflow tract reconstruction or thromboexclusion of the right ventricle ($P = 0.0003$).[106]

SUMMARY

Structure and function provides the foundation upon which much of the discipline of pediatric cardiology is based. Yet, the structure of the malformed heart, even in gross morphologic terms, is not static, and dynamic alterations of cardiac structure may either improve or worsen the quality of life. Superimposed on the changing form and function of congenitally malformed hearts are the primary and secondary effects of direct surgical intervention. We have briefly reviewed some of the postoperative features of patients with congenital heart disease but for many with more complex lesions, a Pandora's box of potential problems exists.

As the infant with complex congenital heart disease survives to adulthood, having been palliated by one or more closed or open cardiac procedures (thereby sustaining a scarred and fibrosed mediastinum and pericardium; with obliteration of the saphenofemoral venous system by one, or several cardiac catheter investigations), such patients will still, we think, be subject to the ravages of atherosclerotic cardiovascular disease. In such patients, aortocoronary bypass operations may be rendered impossible by mediastinal and pericardial scarring and obliteration sustained during childhood.

Will the patient with transposition of the great arteries, following an inflow type of correction, develop the same pattern of aortic or coronary atherosclerosis as the patient with normal ventriculoarterial connections? Follow-up evaluation of these patients with congenital heart disease will reveal many problems that need answers.

REFERENCES

1. Allen HD, Anderson RC, Noren GR, Moller JH: Post-operative follow-up of patients with ventricular septal defects. Circulation 50:465, 1974
2. Alpert BS, Bloom KR, Olley PM, et al: Echocardiographic evaluation of right ventricular function in complete transposition of the great arteries: Angiographic correlates. Am J Cardiol 44:270, 1979
3. Alpert BS, Cook DH, Varghese PJ, Rowe RD: Spontaneous closure of small ventricular septal defects. Ten year follow-up. Pediatrics 62:204, 1979
4. Alpert BS, Mellits ED, Rowe RD: Spontaneous closure of small ventricular septal defects. Probability rates in the first five years of life. Am J Dis Child 125:194, 1973
5. Amplatz K, Formanek A, Knight L, et al: Radiographic changes in the postoperative patient. Prog Cardiovasc Dis 17:403, 1975
6. Anderson KR, McGoon DC, Lie JT: Surgical significance of the coronary arterial anatomy in truncus arteriosus sommunis. Am J Cardiol 41:76, 1978
7. Anderson KR, McGoon DC, Lie JT: Vulnerability of coronary arteries in surgery for transposition of the great arteries. J Thorac Cardiovasc Surg 76:135, 1979
8. Anderson RH, Tynan M, Freedom RM, et al: Ventricular morphology in the univentricular heart. Herz 4:184, 1979
9. Anderson RH, Wilkinson JL, Gerlis LM, et al: Atresia of the right atrioventricular orifice. Br Heart J 39:44, 1977
10. Anselmi G, Munoz S, Blanco P, et al: Anomalous coronary artery connecting with the right ventricle associated with pulmonary stenosis and atrial septal defect. Am Heart J 62:406, 1961
11. Appelbaum A, Bargeron LM Jr, Pacifico AD, Kirklin JW: Surgical treatment of truncus arteriosus with emphasis on infants and small children. J Thorac Cardiovasc Surg 71:436, 1976
12. Arensman FW, Bostock J, Radley-Smith R, Yacoub MH: Cardiac rhythm and conduction before and after anatomic correction of transposition of the great arteries. Am J Cardiol 52:836, 1983
13. Aubert J, Pannetier A, Courelly JP, et al: Transposition of the great arteries. New technique for anatomic correction. Br Heart J 40:204, 1978
14. Aziz KU, Paul MH, Rowe RD: Bronchopulmonary circulation in D-transposition of the great arteries. Possible role in genesis of accelerated pulmonary vascular disease. Am J Cardiol 39:432, 1977
15. Baffes TG: A method for surgical correction of transposition of the great arteries. Surg Gynecol Obstet 102:227, 1956
16. Bargeron LM Jr, Karp RB, Barcia A, et al: Late deterioration of patients after superior vena cava to right pulmonary artery anastomosis. Am J Cardiol 30:211, 1972
17. Baumstark A, Fellows KE, Rosenthal A: Combined double chambered right ventricle and discrete subaortic stenosis. Circulation 57:299, 1978
18. Becker AE, Becker MJ, Edwards JE: Pathology of the semilunar valve in persistent truncus arteriosus. J Thorac Cardiovasc Surg 62:16, 1971
19. Becu L, Gallo A: Abnormal right ventricular morphology—A distinctive feature of transposition of the great arteries. p. 259. In Abstracts of the Thirteenth Annual General Meeting of the Association of European Pediatric Cardiologists, 1975
20. Behrendt DM, Kirsh MM, Orringer MB, et al: The Blalock-Hanlon procedure. A new look at an old operation. Ann Thorac Surg 20:424, 1975
21. Bernhard WF, Dick M, Sloss LJ, et al: The palliative Mustard operation for double outlet right ventricle or transposition of the great arteries associated with ventricular septal defect, pulmonary arterial hypertension and pulmonary vascular obstructive disease: A report of 8 patients. Circulation 5:810, 1976
22. Bertranou EG, Blackstone EH, Hazelrig JB,

et al: Life expectancy without surgery in tetralogy of Fallot. Am J Cardiol 42:458, 1978

23. Bharati S, Lev M: Congenital anomalies of the pulmonary veins. Cardiovasc Clin 5:23, 1973

24. Bharati S, Lev M: The surgical anatomy of hypoplasia of aortic tract complex. J Thorac Cardiovasc Surg 88:97, 1984

25. Bharati S, McAllister HA Jr, Tatooles CJ, et al: Anatomic variations in underdeveloped right ventricle related to tricuspid atresia and stenosis. J Thorac Cardiovasc Surg 72:383, 1976

26. Bharati S, McAllister HA Jr, Rosenquist GC, et al: The surgical anatomy of truncus arteriosus. J Thorac Cardiovasc Surg 67:501, 1974

27. Bharati S, Moltham ME, Veasy LG, Lev M: Conduction system in two cases of sudden death two years after the Mustard operation. J Thorac Cardiovasc Surg 77:101, 1979

28. Bical O, Hazan E, LeCompte Y, et al: Anatomic correction of transposition of the great arteries associated with ventricular septal defect: Midterm results in 50 patients. Circulation 70:891, 1984

29. Bjarke B: Functional studies in palliated and totally corrected adult patients with tetralogy of Fallot. Scand J Thorac Cardiovasc Surg 16(suppl):1, 1974

30. Bjork VO, Olin CL, Bjarke BB, Thoren CA: Right atrial-right ventricular anastomosis for correction of tricuspid atresia. J Thorac Cardiovasc Surg 77:452, 1979

31. Blackman MS, Schneider B, Sondheimer HM: Absent proximal left main coronary artery in association with pulmonary atresia. Br Heart J 46:449, 1981

32. Blalock A, Hanlon CR: The surgical treatment of complete transposition of the aorta and the pulmonary artery. Surg Gynecol Obstet 90:1, 1950

33. Blalock A, Taussig HB: Surgical treatment of malformations of the heart in which there is pulmonary stenosis or pulmonary atresia. JAMA 128:189, 1945

34. Bloomfield DK: Natural history of ventricular septal defect in patients surviving infancy. Circulation 29:194, 1964

35. Bove KE, Geiser EA, Mayer RA: The left ventricle in anomalous pulmonary venous return. Morphometric analysis of 36 fatal cases in infancy. Arch Pathol 99:522, 1975

36. Bowman FO Jr, Malm JR, Hayes CJ, Gersony WM: Physiological approach to surgery for tricuspid atresia. Circulation 58(suppl 1):83, 1978

37. Bregman D, Bush HL Jr, Bowman FO Jr, Malm JR: Longterm results of surgical correction of tetralogy of Fallot. p. 347. In Davila JC (ed): Second Henry Ford Hospital International Symposium on Cardiac Surgery. Appleton-Century-Crofts. East Norwalk, CT, 1971

38. Bricker DL, King SM, Edwards JE: Anomalous aortic origin of the right and left pulmonary arteries in a normally septated truncus arteriosus. Chest 68:591, 1975

39. Bryan C, Oppenheimer EH: Ventricular endocardial fibroelastosis. Basis for its presence or absence in cases of pulmonic and aortic atresia. Arch Pathol 87:82, 1969

40. Bulkley BH, Weisfeldt ML, Hutchins GM: Isometric contraction. A possible cause of the disorganised myocardial pattern of idiopathic hypertrophic subaortic stenosis. N Engl J Med 296:135, 1977

41. Bulkley BH, D'Amico B, Taylor AL: Extensive myocardial fiber disarray in aortic and pulmonary atresia. Relevance to hypertrophic cardiomyopathy. Circulation 67:191, 1983

42. Bull C, de Leval M, Mercanti C, et al: Pulmonary atresia and intact ventricular septum: A revised classification. Circulation 66:266, 1982

43. Burnell RM, McEnery G, Miller GAH: Truncal valve stenosis. Br Heart J 33:423, 1971

44. Byrne J, Clarke D, Taylor JFN, et al: Treatment of patients with transposition of the great arteries and pulmonary vascular obstructive disease. Br Heart J 40:221, 1978

45. Calder AL, Barratt-Boyes BG, Brandt PWT, Neutze JM: Postoperative evaluation of patients with tetralogy of Fallot repaired in infancy including criteria for use of outflow patching and radiologic assessment of pulmonary regurgitation. J Thorac Cardiovasc Surg 77:704, 1979

46. Calder AL, Co EE, Sage MD: Coronary arterial abnormalities in pulmonary atresia with intact ventricular septum. Am J Cardiol 59:437, 1987

47. Calder AL, Van Praagh R, Van Praagh S, et al: Truncus arteriosus communis. Clinical, angiocardiographic and pathologic findings in 100 patients. Am Heart J 92:23, 1976

48. Campbell M: The natural history of ventricular septal defect. Br Heart J 33:246, 1971

49. Carlon CA, Mondini PG, de Marchi R: Surgical treatment of some cardiovascular diseases (new vascular anastomosis). J Int Coll Surg 16:1, 1951

50. Carr I, Bharati S, Kusnoor VS, Lev M: Truncus arteriosus with intact ventricular septum. Br Heart J 42:97, 1979

51. Castellino RA, Blank N, Adams DF: Dilated azygos and hemiazygos veins presenting as paravertebral intrathoracic masses. N Engl J Med 278:1087, 1968

52. Castaneda AR, Freed MD, Williams RG, Norwood WI: Repair of tetralogy of Fallot in infancy. Early and late results. J Thorac Cardiovasc Surg 74:372, 1977

53. Choussat A, Fontan F, Besse P, et al: Selection criteria for Fontan's procedure. p. 559. In Anderson RH, Shinebourne EA (eds): Paediatric Cardiology, 1977. Churchill Livingstone, Edinburgh, 1978

54. Ciaravella JM Jr, McGoon DC, Danielson GK, et al: Experience with the extracardiac conduit. J Thorac Cardiovasc Surg 78:920, 1979

55. Clarke DR, Stark J, De Leval M, et al: Total anomalous pulmonary venous drainage in infancy. Br Heart J 39:436, 1977

56. Clark DS, Hirsh HD, Tawer DM, Gelband H: Electrocardiographic changes following surgical treatment of congenital cardiac malformations. Prog Cardiovasc Dis 17:451, 1975

57. Clarkson PM, Barratt-Boyes BG, Neutze JM: Late dysrhythmias and disturbances of conduction following Mustard operation of the great arteries. Circulation 53:519, 1976

58. Clarkson PM, Neutze JM, Barratt-Boyes BG, Brandt PWT: Late post-operative hemodynamic results and cineangiocardiographic findings after Mustard atrial baffle repair for transposition of the great arteries. Circulation 53:525, 1976

59. Clayman JA, Ankeney JL, Liebman J: Results of complete repair of tetralogy of Fallot in 156 consecutive patients. Am J Surg 130:601, 1975

60. Collins G, Calder L, Rose V, et al: Ventricular septal defect: Clinical and hemodynamic changes in the first five years of life. Am Heart J 84:695, 1972

61. Cook DH, Alpert BS, Rowe RD, Varghese PJ: Sex difference in rates of spontaneous closure of ventricular septal defect. (Letter.) J Pediatr 95:371, 1979

62. Corone P, Doyon F, Gaudeau S, et al: Natural history of ventricular septal defect. A study involving 790 cases. Circulation 55:908, 1977

63. Cornell SH: Myocardial sinusoids in pulmonary valvular atresia. Radiology 86:421, 1966

64. Cote M, Davignon A, Fouron J-C: Congenital hypoplasia of right ventricular myocardium (Uhl's anomaly) associated with pulmonary atresia in a newborn. Am J Cardiol 31:658, 1973

65. Coussement AM, Gooding CA, Carlson E: Left atrial volume, shape, and movement in total anomalous pulmonary venous return. Radiology 107:139, 1973

66. Covitz W, Meyer RA, Korfhagen J, Kaplan S: Late post-operative changes following closure of secundum atrial septal defect. Am J Cardiol 39:294, 1977 (abstr)

67. Damus P: Letter to the Editor. Ann Thorac Surg 20:724, 1975

68. Danielson GK, Giuliani ER, Ritter DG: Successful repair of common ventricle associated with complete atrioventricular canal. J Thorac Cardiovasc Surg 67:152, 1974

69. Danielson GK, McGoon DC, Maloney JD, Ritter DG: Surgery of primitive ventricle with outlet chamber. p. 381. In Anderson RH, Shinebourne EA (eds): Paediatric Cardiology, 1977. Churchill Livingstone, London, 1978

70. Danielson GK, McGoon DC, Maloney JD, Ritter DG: Surgical septation of univentricular heart with outlet chamber. Herz 4:262, 1979

71. Danielson GK, Tabry IM, Mair DD, Fulton RE: Great vessel switch operation without coronary relocation for transposition of great arteries. Mayo Clin Proc 53:675, 1978

72. De Leval M, Bull C, Stark J, et al: Pulmonary atresia and intact ventricular septum: Surgical management based on a revised classification. Circulation 66:272, 1982

73. Delisle G, Ando M, Calder AL, et al: Total anomalous pulmonary venous connection: Report of 93 autopsied cases with emphasis on diagnostic and surgical considerations. Am Heart J 91:99, 1976

74. De Morais CF, Fiorelli AI, Marcial MB, et al: Infarto do miocardio e lesao coronaria em paciente portador de atresia pulmonar. Rev Lat Cardiol Infect 1:201, 1985

75. Desnick SJ, Neal WA, Nicoloff DM, Moller JH: Residual right to left shunt following repair of atrial septal defect. Ann Thorac Surg 21:291, 1976

76. de Vivie E-R, Rupprath G: Long-term results after Fontan procedure and its modifications. J Thorac Cardiovasc Surg 91:690, 1986

77. Dick M, Fyler DC, Nadas AS: Tricuspid atresia: Clinical cause in 101 patients. Am J Cardiol 36:327, 1975

78. Doty DB, Schieken RM, Lauer RM: Septation of the univentricular heart. Transatrial approach. J Thorac Cardiovasc Surg 78:423, 1979

79. Duff DF, Nihill MR, McNamara DG: Infradiaphragmatic total anomalous pulmonary venous return. Review of clinical and pathological findings and results of operation in 28 cases. Br Heart J 39:619, 1977

80. Dunn J, Perry B, Kirsh MM: The treatment of tricuspid insufficiency after the Mustard procedure with a Carpentier annuloplasty ring. J Thorac Cardiovasc Surg 74:784, 1977

81. Dureau G, Kepenekian G, Paul J, et al: Intra-aortic septation: Experimental model for "anatomical" correction of transposition of the great vessels. J Thorac Surg 19:251, 1978

82. Dusek J, Ostadal B, Duskova M: Postnatal persistence of spongy myocardium with embryonic blood supply. Arch Pathol 99:312, 1975

83. Ebert PA, Gay WA Jr, Engle MA: Correction of transposition of the great arteries. Relationship of the coronary sinus and post-operative arrhythmias. Ann Surg 180:433, 1974

84. Edie RN, Ellis K, Gersony WM, et al: Surgical repair of single ventricle. J Thorac Cardiovasc Surg 66:350, 1973

85. Edwards JE: Survey of operative congenital heart disease. Am J Pathol 82:408, 1976

86. Edwards WD, Edwards JE: Pathology of the sinus node in D-transposition following the Mustard operation. J Thorac Cardiovasc Surg 75:213, 1978

87. Egloff LP, Freed MD, Dick M, et al: Early and late results with the Mustard operation in infancy. Ann Thorac Surg 26:474, 1978

88. El-Said GM, Gillette PC, Cooley DA, et al: Protection of the sinus node in Mustard's operation. Circulation 53:788, 1976

89. Engle MA, Kline SA: Ventricular septal defect in the adult. p. 279. In Roberts WL (ed): Congenital Heart Disease in Adults. FA Davis, Philadelphia, 1979

90. Essed CE, Klein HW, Krediet P, Vorst EJ: Coronary and endocardial fibroelastosis of the ventricles in the hypoplastic left and right heart syndromes. Virchows Arch [A] 368:87, 1975

91. Esterly JR, Oppenheimer EH: Some aspects of cardiac pathology in infancy and childhood. I. Neonatal myocardial necrosis. Johns Hopkins Bull 119:191, 1966

92. Evan JR, Rowe RD, Keith JD: Spontaneous closure of ventricular septal defect. Circulation 22:1044, 1960

93. Farina MA, Hook ED: Apparent sex differences in spontaneous closure of ventricular septal defect. J Pediatr 93:1065, 1978

94. Finegold MJ, Klein KM: Anastomotic coronary vessels in hypoplasia if the right ventricle. Am Heart J 82:678, 1971

95. Finley KH, Buse ST, Popper MP, Collart DS, Riggs N: Intellectual functioning of children with tetralogy of Fallot: Influence of open heart surgery and earlier palliative operations. J Pediatr 85:318, 1974

96. Finnegan P, Harder R, Patel RG, et al: Results of total correction of the tetralogy of Fallot. Longerm hemodynamic evaluation at rest and during exercise. Br Heart J 38:934, 1976

97. Fleming WH: Why switch? J Thorac Cardiovasc Surg 78:1, 1979

98. Fleming WH, Clark EB, Dooley KJ, et al: Late complications following surgical repair of total anomalous pulmonary venous return below the diaphragm. Ann Thorac Cardiovasc Surg 27:435, 1978

99. Fontan F, Baudet E: Surgical repair of tricuspid atresia. Thorax 26:240, 1971

100. Fontan F, Choussat A, Brom AG, et al: Repair of tricuspid atresia—surgical considerations and results. p. 567. In Anderson RH, Shinebourne EA (eds): Paediatric Cardiology 1977. Churchill Livingstone, Edinburgh, 1978

101. Franciosi RA, Blanc WA: Myocardial infarcts in infants and children. 1. A necropsy study in congenital heart disease. J Pediatr 73:309, 1968

102. Freedom RM: The natural history of ventricular septal defect; with morphologic considerations. p. 251. In Moss AJ (ed): Pediatrics Update. Elsevier Science Publishing, New York, 1979

103. Freedom RM: The morphological variations of pulmonary atresia with intact ventricular septum: Guidelines for surgical intervention. Pediatr Cardiol 183, 1983

104. Freedom RM: The dinosaur and banding of the main pulmonary trunk in the heart with functionally one ventricle and transposition of the great arteries: A saga of evolution and caution. J Am Coll Cardiol 10:427, 1987

105. Freedom RM: Atresia or hypoplasia of the left atrio-ventricular and/or ventriculoarterial junction. p. 739. In Anderson RH, Macartney FJ, Shinebourne EA, Tynan M (eds): Paediatric Cardiology. Churchill Livingstone, Edinburgh, 1987

106. Freedom RM: Pulmonary Atresia and Intact Ventricular Septum. Futura, Mt. Kisco, NY, 1989

107. Freedom RM: Hypoplastic left heart syndrome. p. 515. In Adams FH, Emmanoulides GC, Riemenschneider TA (eds): Moss' Heart Disease in Infants, Children, and Adolescents. Williams & Wilkins, Baltimore, 1989

108. Freedom RM, Bain HH, Esplugas E, et al: Ventricular septal defect in interruption of the aortic arch. Am J Cardiol 39:572, 1977

109. Freedom RM, Benson LN, Olley PM, Rowe RD: The natural history of the complete atrioventricular canal defect: An analysis of selected genetic, hemodynamic and morphological variables. p. 45. In Gallucci V, Bini RM, Thiene G (eds): Selected Topics in Cardiac Surgery. Patron Editors, Bologna, 1980

110. Freedom RM, Benson LN, Smallhorn JF, et al: Subaortic stenosis, the univentricular heart, and banding of the pulmonary artery: An analysis of the courses of 43 patients with univentricular heart palliated by pulmonary artery banding. Circulation 73:758, 1986

111. Freedom RM, Benson L, Wilson GJ: The coronary circulation and myocardium in pulmonary and aortic atresia with an intact ventricular septum. p. 78. In Marcelletti C, Anderson RH, Becker AE, et al (eds): Paediatric Cardiology, Vol. 6. Churchill Livingstone, Edinburgh, 1986

112. Freedom RM, Culham G, Moes F, et al: Differentiation of functional and structural pulmonary atresia: Role of aortography. Am J Cardiol 41:914, 1978

113. Freedom RM, Culham JAG, Olley PM, et al: Anatomic correction of transposition of the great arteries: Pre- and postoperative catheterization, with angiography in five patients. Circulation 63:905, 1981

114. Freedom RM, Culham JAG, Rowe RD: Angiocardiography of subaortic obstruction in infancy. AJR 129:813, 1977

115. Freedom RM, Dische MR, Rowe RD: Pathologic anatomy of subaortic stenosis and atresia in the first year of life. Am J Cardiol 39:1035, 1977

116. Freedom RM, Dische MR, Rowe RD: Conal anatomy in aortic atresia, ventricular septal defect, and normally developed left ventricle. Am Heart J 94:689, 1977

117. Freedom RM, Harrington DP: Contribution of intramyocardial sinusoids in pulmonary atresia and intact ventricular septum to a right-sided circular shunt. Br Heart J 36:1061, 1974

118. Freedom RM, Hirose M, Patel RG, et al: The morphologic basis of subaortic stenosis in single ventricle, with angiocardiographic and therapeutic considerations. Unpublished observations

119. Freedom RM, Keith JD: Pulmonary atresia with normal aortic root. p. 506. In Keith JD, Rowe RD, Vlad P (eds): Heart Disease in Infancy and Childhood. Macmillan, New York, 1978

120. Freedom RM, Moes CAF: The hypoplastic right heart complex. Semin Roentgenol 20:169, 1985

121. Freedom RM, Rowe RD: Morphological and topographical variations of the outlet chamber in complex congenital heart disease. An angiocardiographic study. Cath Cardiovasc Diagn 4:345, 1978

122. Freedom RM, Sondheimer H, Dische MR, Rowe RD: Development of "subaortic stenosis" after pulmonary arterial banding for common ventricle. Am J Cardiol 39:778, 1977

123. Freedom RM, White RD, Pieroni DR, et al: The natural history of the so-called aneurysm of the membranous septum in childhood. Circulation 49:375, 1974

124. Freedom RM, Williams WG, Fowler RS, et al: Tricuspid atresia, transposition of the great arteries and banded pulmonary artery: Repair by arterial switch, coronary artery reimplantation and right atrial ventricular valved conduit. J Thorac Cardiovasc Surg 80:621, 1980

125. Freedom RM, Wilson GJ: The anatomic substrate of pulmonary atresia and intact

ventricular septum. p. 217. In Tucker BL, Lindesmith GC, Takahashi M (eds): Third Clinical Conference on Congenital Heart Disease. Obstructive Lesions of the Right Heart. University Park Press, Baltimore, 1984

126. Freedom RM, Wilson G, Trusler GA, et al: Pulmonary atresia and intact ventricular septum. A review of the anatomy, myocardium, and factors influencing right ventricular growth and guidelines for surgical intervention. Scand J Thorac Cardiovasc Surg 17:1, 1983

127. Fricker FJ, Zuberbuhler JR: Pulmonary atresia with intact ventricular septum. p. 711. In Anderson RH, Macartney FJ, Shinebourne EA, Tynan M (eds): Paediatric Cardiology. Vol. 2. Churchill Livingstone, London, 1987

128. Fyfe DA, Edwards WD, Driscoll DJ: Myocardial ischaemia in patients with pulmonary atresia and intact ventricular septum. J Am Coll Cardiol 8:402, 1986

129. Fyler DC: Report of the New England Regional Infant Cardiac Program. Pediatrics 65(suppl 2):436, 1980

130. Gago O, Salles CA, Stern AM, et al: A different approach for the total correction of tricuspid atresia. J Thorac Cardiovasc Surg 72:209, 1976

131. Gale AW, Danielson GK, McGoon DC, Mair DD: Modified Fontan operation for univentricular heart and complicated congenital lesions. J Thorac Cardiovasc Surg 78:831, 1979

132. Garcia OL, Gelband H, Tamer DF, Fojaco RM: Exclusive origin of both coronary arteries from a hypoplastic right ventricle complicating an extreme tetralogy of Fallot: Lethal myocardial infarction following a palliative shunt. Am Heart J 115:198, 1988

133. Garson A Jr, Nihill MR, McNamara DG, Cooley DA: Status of the adult and adolescent after repair of tetralogy of Fallot. Circulation 59:1232, 1979

134. Gasul B, Dillon R, Urla V: The natural transformation of ventricular septal defect into ventricular septal defects with pulmonary stenosis and/or tetralogy of Fallot: Clinical and physiologic findings. Am J Dis Child 94:424, 1957

135. Gay WA Jr, Ebert PA: Aorta to right pulmonary artery anastomosis causing obstruction of the right pulmonary artery. Ann Thorac Surg 16:402, 1973

136. Gelband H, Van Meter S, Gersony WM: Truncal valve abnormalities in infants with persistent truncus arteriosus. A clinicopathologic study. Circulation 45:397, 1972

137. Gersony WM, Hayes CJ: Bacterial endocarditis in patients with pulmonary stenosis, aortic stenosis, or ventricular septal defect. Circulation 56(suppl I):84, 1977

138. Gersony WM, Krongrad E: Evaluation and management of patients after surgical repair of congenital heart diseases. Prog Cardiovasc Dis 18:39, 1975

139. Gibson DG, Traill TA, Brown DJ: Abnormal ventricular function in patients with univentricular heart. Herz 4:226, 1979

140. Gill CC, Moodie DS, McGoon DC: Staged surgical management of pulmonary atresia with diminutive pulmonary arteries. J Thorac Cardiovasc Surg 73:436, 1972

141. Gillette PC, Yeoman MA, Mullins CE, McNamara DG: Sudden death after repair of tetralogy of Fallot. Electrocardiographic and electrophysiologic abnormalities. Circulation 56:566, 1977

142. Girod DA, Fontan F, Deville C, et al: Long-term results after the Fontan operation. Circulation 75:605, 1987

143. Gittenberger-De Groot AC, Sauer U, et al: Competition of coronary arteries and ventriculo-coronary arterial communications in pulmonary atresia with intact ventricular septum. Int J Cardiol 18:243, 1988

144. Gleason WA, Roodman ST, Laks H: Protein-losing enteropathy and intestinal lymphangiectasis after superior vena cava to right pulmonary artery (Glenn) shunt. J Thorac Cardiovasc Surg 77:843, 1979

145. Glenn WWL: Circulatory bypass of the right side of the heart. IV. Shunt between superior vena cava and distal right pulmonary artery: Report of clinical application. N Engl J Med 259:117, 1958

146. Glenn WWL, Fenn JE: Axillary arteriovenous fistula. A means of supplementary blood flow through a cavo-pulmonary artery shunt. Circulation 46:1013, 1972

147. Glenn WWL, Patino JF: Circulatory by-pass of the right heart. Yale J Biol Med 27:147, 1954

148. Goor DA, Edwards JE: Friction lesions of the right ventricular endocardium. Arch Pathol 87:100, 1969

149. Gorlin R: Dynamic vascular factors in the genesis of myocardial ischemia. J Am Coll Cardiol 1:897, 1983

150. Graham TP Jr: Myocardial performance after anatomic or physiologic corrective surgery. Prog Cardiovasc Dis 17:439, 1975

151. Graham TP Jr, Atwood GF, Boucek RJ Jr, Boerth RC: Transposition of the great arteries—Right and left ventricular function problems. p. 207. In Kidd BSL, Rowe RD (eds): The Child with Congenital Heart Disease after Surgery. Futura, Mt. Kisco, NY, 1976

152. Graham TP Jr, Atwood GF, Boucek RJ Jr: Abnormalities of right ventricular function following Mustard's operation for transposition of the great arteries. Circulation 52:678, 1975

153. Graham TP Jr, Cordell D, Atwood GF, et al: Right ventricular volume characteristics before and after palliative and reparative operation in tetralogy of Fallot. Circulation 54:417, 1976

154. Graham TP Jr, Friesinger GC: Complex cyanotic congenital heart disease in adults. p. 383. In Roberts WL (ed): Congenital Heart Disease in Adults. FA Davis, Philadelphia, 1979

155. Grant RT: An unusual anomaly of the coronary vessels in the malformed heart of a child. Heart 13:273, 1926

156. Greenwood RD, Nadas AS, Rosenthal A, et al: Ascending aorta to pulmonary artery anastomosis for cyanotic congenital heart disease. Am Heart J 94:14, 1977

157. Griepp RB, Stinson EB, Shumway NE: Surgical correction of types II and III truncus arteriosus. J Thorac Cardiovasc Surg 73:345, 1977

158. Guidici C, Becu L: Cardio-aortic fistula through anomalous coronary arteries. Br Heart J 22:729, 1960

159. Guller B, Titus JL: Morphological studies in tricuspid atresia. Circulation 38:977, 1968

160. Gutgesell HP, Garson A, McNamara DG: Prognosis for the newborn with transposition of the great arteries. Am J Cardiol 44:96, 1979

161. Hagler DJ, Ritter DG, Mair DD, et al: Clinical angiocardiographic and hemodynamic assessment of late results after Mustard's operation. Circulation 57:1214, 1978

162. Hagler DJ, Ritter DG, Main DD, et al: Right and left ventricular function after the Mustard operation in transposition of the great arteries. Am J Cardiol 44:276, 1979

163. Hamazaki M: Congenital coronary arterioventricular fistulae, associated with absence of proximal coronary artery from aorta. Jpn Heart J 23:271, 1982

164. Hamilton DI, Arnold R, Wilkinson JL: Surgery of univentricular heart without outlet chamber. p. 388. From Anderson RH, Shinebourne EA (eds): Paediatric Cardiology, 1977. Churchill Livingstone, London, 1978

165. Hamilton WT, Haffajee CI, Dalen JE, et al: Atrial septal defect secundum: Clinical profile with physiologic correlates in children and adults. p. 2617. In Roberts WC (ed): Congenital Heart Disease in Adults. FA Davis, Philadelphia, 1979

166. Haworth SG, Reid L: Structural study of pulmonary circulation and of heart in total anomalous pulmonary venous return in early infancy. Br Heart J 39:80, 1977

167. Hayes CJ, Gersony WM, Griffiths SP, et al: Results of total anomalous pulmonary venous connections in infancy. Adv Cardiol 11:36, 1974

168. Henry JN, Danielson GK: Successful "correction" of tricuspid atresia: Results of a detailed anatomical study. Surg Forum 15:163, 1974

169. Ho CS, Krovetz LJ, Strife JL, et al: Postoperative assessment of residual defects following cardiac surgery in infants and children. II. Ventricular septal defects. Johns Hopkins Med J 133:278, 1973

170. Hobbins SM, Izukawa T, Radford DJ, et al: Conduction disturbances after surgical correction of ventricular septal defect by the atrial approach. Br Heart J 41:289, 1979

171. Hoffman JIE: Natural history of congenital heart disease. Problems in its assessment with special reference to ventricular septal defects. Circulation 37:97, 1968

172. Hoffman JIE: Determinants and prediction of transmural myocardial perfusion. Circulation 58:381, 1978

173. Hofschire PJ, Rosenquist GC, Ruckerman RN, et al: Pulmonary vascular disease complications in Blalock-Taussig anastomosis. Circulation 56:124, 1977

174. Hubbard JF, Girod DA, Caldwell RL, et al: Right ventricular infarction with cardiac rupture in an infant with pulmonary atresia with

intact ventricular septum. J Am Coll Cardiol 2:363, 1983

175. Humes RA, Feldt RH, Porter CJ, et al: The modified Fontan operation for asplenia and polysplenia syndromes. J Thorac Cardiovasc Surg 96:212, 1988

176. Humes RA, Porter CJ, Mair DD, et al: Intermediate follow-up and predicted survival after the modified Fontan procedure for tricuspid atresia and double-inlet ventricle. Circulation 76(suppl 3):76, 1987

177. Hunt CE, Formanek G, Leving MA, et al: Banding of the pulmonary artery: Results in ill children. Circulation 43:395, 1971

178. Hurwitt ES, Young D, Escher DJUS: The rationale of anastomosis of the right auricular appendage of the pulmonary artery in the treatment of tricuspid atresia. J Thorac Cardiovasc Surg 30:503, 1955

179. Hvass U: Coronary arteries in D-transposition. A necropsy study of reimplantation. Br Heart J 39:1234, 1977

180. Idriss FS, Deleon SY, Nikaidoh H, et al: Resection of left ventricular outflow obstruction in D-transposition of the great arteries. J Thorac Casrdiovasc Surg 74:343, 1977

181. Isaacson R, Titus JL, Merideth J, et al: Apparent interruption of atrial conduction pathways after surgical repair of transposition of the great arteries. Am J Cardiol 30:533, 1972

182. Izukawa T, Sondheimer HM, Trusler GA, Mustard WT: Conduction disturbances after repair of ventricular septal defect and tetralogy of Fallot. p. 241. In Kidd BSL, Rowe RD (eds): The Child with Congenital Heart Disease After Surgery. Futura, Mt. Kisco, NY, 1977

183. Jain V, Subramanian S, Lambert EC: Concomitant development of infundibular pulmonary stenosis and spontaneous closure of ventricular septal defect. Am J Cardiol 24:247, 1969

184. James FW, Kaplan S: Sudden unexpected cardiac arrests in patients after surgical correction for tetralogy of Fallot. Am J Cardiol 35:146, 1975 (abst)

185. James FW, Kaplan S, Chou TC: Unexpected cardiac arrest in patients after surgical correction of tetralogy of Fallot. Circulation 52:691, 1975

186. James FW, Kaplan S, Schwartz DC: Response to exercise in patients following total

surgical correction of tetralogy of Fallot. Circulation 54:671, 1976

187. Janse MJ, Anderson RH: Specialized internodal atrial pathways—Fact of fiction? Eur J Cardiol 2:117, 1974

188. Jarmakani JMM, Canent RV Jr: Pre-operative and Post-operative right ventricular function in children with transposition of the great vessels. Circulation 49/50(suppl II):39, 1974

189. Jarmakani JMM, Graham TP Jr, Canent RV Jr, Jewett PH: Left heart function in children with tetralogy of Fallot before and after palliative or corrective surgery. Circulation 46:478, 1972

190. Jatene AD, Fontes VF, Paulista PP, et al: Anatomic correction of transposition of the great vessels. J Thorac Cardiovasc Surg 72:364, 1976

191. Jonas RA, Lang P, Hansen D, et al: First-stage palliation of hypoplastic left heart syndrome. The importance of coarctation and shunt size. J Thorac Cardiovasc Surg 92:6, 1986

192. Kaplan EL: Infective Endocarditis in the Pediatric Age Group. An Overview. American Heart Association Monograph No. 52, 1975

193. Kasznica J, Ursell PC, Blanc WA, Gersony WM: Abnormalities of the coronary circulation in pulmonary atresia and intact ventricular septum. Am Heart J 114:1415, 1987

194. Kato H, Hirose M, Fukuda H, Nagayama T: Natural history of ventricular septal defect. Jpn Circ J 36:814, 1972

195. Katz NM, Kirklin JW, Pacifico AD: Concepts and practices in surgery for total anomalous pulmonary venous connection. Ann Thorac Surg 25:479, 1978

196. Kauffman SL, Andersen DH: Persistent venous valves, maldevelopment of the right heart, and coronary artery-ventricular communications. Am Heart J 66:664–669 1963

197. Kawashima Y, Mori T, Matsuda H, et al: Intraventricular repair of single ventricle associated with transposition of the great arteries. J Thorac Cardiovasc Surg 72:21, 1976

198. Kaye MP: Anatomic correction of transposition of the great arteries. Mayo Clin Proc 59:638, 1975

199. Keane JF, Plauth WH Jr, Nadas AS: Ventricular septal defect with aortic regurgitation. Circulation 56(2)(suppl I):72, 1977

200. Keane JF, Williams R, Treves S, Rosenthal

A: Assessment of the postoperative patient by non-invasive means. Prog Cardiovasc Dis 18:57, 1975

201. Keeton BR, Lie JT, McGoon DC, et al: Anatomy of coronary arteries in univentricular hearts and its surgical implications. Am J Cardiol 43:569, 1979

202. Keith JD, Rose V, Collins G, Kidd BSL: Ventricular septal defect. Incidence, morbidity and mortality in various age groups. Br Heart J 33:81, 1971

203. Kidd BSL, Humphries JO: Transposition of the great arteries in the adult. p. 365. In Roberts WL (ed): Congenital Heart Disease in Adults. FA Davis, Philadelphia, 1979

204. Kidd BSL, Rowe RD (eds): The Child with Congenital Heart Disease After Surgery. Futura, New York, 1976

205. Kinsley RH, McGoon DC, Danielson GK, et al: Pulmonary arterial hypertension after repair of tetralogy of Fallot. J Thorac Cardiovasc Surg 67:110, 1974

206. Kirklin JW, Bailey WW: Valved external conduits to pulmonary arteries. Ann Thorac Surg 24:202, 1977

207. Kirklin JW, Bargeron LM Jr, Pacifico AD: The enlargement of small pulmonary arteries by preliminary palliative operations. Circulation 56:612, 1977

208. Kirklin JK, Blackstone EH, Kirklin JW, et al: The Fontan operation. Ventricular hypertrophy, age, and date of operation as risk factors. J Thorac Cardiovasc Surg 92:1049, 1986

209. Kitamura S, Kawashima Y, Shimazak Y, et al: Characteristics of ventricular function in single ventricle. Circulation 60:849, 1979

210. Klautz RJM, Ottenkamp J, Quaegebeur JM, et al: Anatomic correction for tranposition of the great arteries: First follow-up (38 patients). Pediatr Cardiol 10:1, 1989

211. Koike K, Wilson GJ, Perrin DG, Freedom RM: Coronary artery involvement and myocardial ischemia in newborn babies with pulmonary atresia and intact ventricular septum. Circulation 78(suppl II-356, 1988 (abst)

212. Kreutzer G, Galindez E, Bono H, et al: An operation for the correction of tricuspid atresia. J Thorac Cardiovasc Surg 66:613, 1973

213. Kreutzer G, Neirott R, Galindez E, et al: Anatomic correction of transposition of the great arteries. J Thorac Cardiovasc Surg 73:538, 1977

214. Kyger ER III, Frazler OH, Cooley DA, et al: Sinus venosus atrial septal defects: Early and late results following closure in 109 patients. Ann Thorac Surg 25:44, 1978

215. LaCorte MA, Dick M, Scheir G, et al: Left ventricular function in tricuspid atresia. Angiographic analysis in 28 patients. Circulation 52:996, 1975

216. Laks H, Castaneda AR: Subclavian arterioplasty for the ipsilateral Blalock-Taussig shunt. Ann Thorac Surg 19:319, 1975

217. Laks H, Mudd JG, Standeven JW, et al: Longterm effect of the superior vena cava to pulmonary artery anastomosis in pulmonary blood flow. J Thorac Cardiovasc Surg 74:253, 1977

218. Lambert ME, Widlansky S, Franken EA, et al: Natural history of ventricular septal defects with ventricular septal aneurysms. Am Heart J 88:566, 1974

219. Lang P, Norwood WI: Hemodynamic assessment after palliative surgery for hypoplastic left heart syndrome. Circulation 68:104, 1983

220. Lauer RM, Fink HP, Petry EL, et al: Angiographic demonstration of intramyocardial sinusoids in pulmonary-valve atresia with intact ventricular septum and hypoplastic right ventricle. N Engl J Med 271:68, 1964

221. Leblanc J, Albus R, Williams WG, et al: Serous fluid leakage: A complication following the modified Blalock-Taussig shunt. J Thorac Cardiovasc 88:259, 1984

222. LeCompte Y, Zannini L, Hazan E: Anatomic correction of transposition of the great arteries. J Thorac Cardiovasc Surg 82:629, 1981

223. Lenox CC, Briner J: Absent proximal coronary arteries associated with pulmonic atresia. Am J Cardiol 30:666, 1972

224. Leung MP, Benson LN, Smallhorn JF, et al: Abnormal cardiac signs after Fontan type of operation: Indicators of residua and sequelae. Br Heart J 61:52, 1989

225. Lev M: Pathologic anatomy and interrerlationship of hypoplasia of the aortic tract complexes. Lab Invest 1:61, 1952

226. Lev M, Liberthson RR, Kirkpatrick JR, et al: Single (primitive) ventricle. Circulation 39:577, 1969

227. Levy S, Blondeau P, Dubost C: Longterm follow-up after surgical correction of the partial form of common atrioventricular canal

(ostium primum). J Thorac Cardiovasc Surg 67:353, 1974

228. Lewis AB, Lindesmith GG, Takahashi M, et al: Cardiac rhythm following the Mustard procedure for transposition of the great vessels. J Thorac Cardiovasc Surg 73:919, 1977

229. Liebman J, Cullan L, Beloc NB: Natural history of transposition of the great arteries. Anatomy and birth and death characteristics. Circulation 40:237, 1969

230. Lindesmith GG, Stanton RE, Lurie PR, et al: An assessment of Mustard's operation as a palliative procedure for transposition of the great vessels. Ann Thorac Surg 19:514, 1975

231. Lloyd TR, Evans TC, Marvin WJ Jr: Morphologic determinants of coronary blood flow in the hypoplastic left heart syndrome. Am Heart J 112:666, 1986

232. Lock JE, Lucas RV Jr, Amplatz K, Bessinger FB: Silent unilateral pulmonary venous obstruction. Occurrence after surgical correction of transposition of the great arteries. Chest 73:224, 1978

233. Losay J, Rosenthal A, Nadas AS, Castaneda A: Prognosis after repair of primum atrial septal defect. Am J Cardiol 39:294, 1977 (abst)

234. MacMahon HE, Dickinson PCT: Occlusive fibroelastosis of coronary arteries in the newborn. Circulation 35:3, 1967

235. Mair DD, Rice MJ, Hagler DJ, et al: Outcome of the Fontan procedure in patients with tricuspid atresia. Circulation 72(suppl II):88, 1985

236. Mair DD, Ritter DG, Danielson GK, et al: The palliative Mustard operation: Rationale and results. Am J Cardiol 37:762, 1976

237. Mair DD, Ritter DG, Danielson GK, et al: Truncus arteriosus with unilateral absence of a pulmonary artery. Criteria for operability and surgical results. Circulation 55:641, 1977

238. Mair DD, Ritter DG, Davis GD, et al: Selection of patients with truncus arteriosus for surgical correction. Anatomic and hemodynamic considerations. Circulation 49:144, 1974

239. Malm JR, Bregman D, Bush HL Jr: Complications following correction of tetralogy of Fallot. p. 127. In Cordell AR, Ellison RG (eds): Complications of Intrathoracic Surgery. Little, Brown, Boston, 1979

240. Mamiya RT, Moreno-Cabral RJ, Nakamura FT, Sprague AY: Retransposition of the great vessels for transposition with ventricular septal defect and pulmonary hypertension. J Thorac Cardiovasc Surg 73:340, 1977

241. Marcelletti C, McGoon DC, Danielson GK, et al: Early and late results of surgical repair of truncus arteriosus. Circulation 55:636, 1977

242. Marcelletti C, McGoon DC, Mair DD: The natural history of truncus arteriosus. Circulation 54:108, 1976

243. Maron BJ, Ferrans VJ, White RI Jr: Unusual evolution of acquired infundibular stenosis in patients with ventricular septal defect. Clinical and morphological implications. Circulation 48:1092, 1973

244. Martin MM, Snider AR, Bove EL, et al: Two-dimensional and Doppler echocardiographic evaluation after arterial switch repair in infancy for complete transposition of the great arteries. Am J Cardiol 63:332, 1989

245. Mathew R, Thilenius OG, Replogle RL, Arcilla RA: Cardiac function in total anomalous pulmonary venous return before and after surgery. Circulation 55:361, 1977

246. Mathur M, Glenn WWL: Long-term evaluation of cava-pulmonary artery anastomoses. Surgery 74:899, 1973

247. Matsuda H, Kawashima Y, Kishimoto H, et al: Problems in the modified Fontan operation for univentricular heart of right ventricular type. Circulation 76(suppl 3):45, 1987

248. Mauck HP Jr, Robertson LW, Parr EL, Lower RR: Anatomic correction of transposition of the great arteries without significant ventricular septal defect or patent ductus arteriosus. J Thorac Cardiovasc Surg 74:631, 1977

249. Mayer JE Jr Helgason H, Jonas RA, et al: Extending the limits for modified Fontan procedures. J Thorac Cardiovasc Surg 92:1021, 1986

250. Mazzei EA, Mulder DG: Superior vena cava syndrome following complete correction (Mustard repair) of transposition of the great vessels. Ann Thorac Surg 11:243, 1971

251. McFaul RC, Mair DD, Feldt RH, et al: Truncus arteriosus and previous pulmonary arterial banding: Clinical and hemodynamic assessment. Am J Cardiol 38:626, 1976

252. McFaul RC, Tajik AJ, Mair DD, et al: Development of pulmonary arteriovenous shunt

after superior vena cava or right pulmonary artery (Glenn) anastomosis. Report of four cases. Circulation 55:212, 1977

253. McGoon DC: Left ventricular and biventricular extracardiac conduits. J Thorac Cardiovasc Surg 72:7, 1976

254. McGoon DC: The baffle baffle. Ann Thorac Surg 23:202, 1977

255. McGoon DC, Danielson GK, Ritter DG, et al: Correction of the univentricular heart having two atrioventricular valves. J Thorac Cardiovasc Surg 74:218, 1977

256. McGoon MD, Fulton RE, Davis GD, et al: Systemic collateral and pulmonary artery stenosis in patients with congenital pulmonary valve atresia and ventricular septal defect. Circulation 56:473, 1977

257. McGoon DC, Rastelli GC, Ongley PA: An operation for the correction of truncus arteriosus. JAMA 205:59, 1968

258. McNamara DG, El-Said GM, Gillette PC, Mullins CE: The problem of arrhythmias following the Mustard operation. p. 201. In Kidd BSL, Rowe RD (eds): The Child with Congenital Heart Disease after Surgery. Futura, Mt. Kisco, NY, 1976

259. McNamara DG, Nihill MR, Ruzyllo W, Mullins CE: Cardiac catheterization in 221 patients after tetralogy of Fallot repair. p. 55. In Kidd BSL, Rowe RD (eds): The Child with Congenital Heart Disease after Surgery. Futura, Mt. Kisco, NY, 1976

260. Mesko ZG, Jones JE, Nadas AS: Diminution and closure of large ventricular septal defects after pulmonary artery banding. Circulation 48:847, 1973

261. Miller RA, Pahlajani D, Serratto M, Tatooles CJ: Clinical studies after Fontan's operation for tricuspid atresia. Am J Cardiol 33:157, 1974

262. Misra WP, Kildner FJ, Cohen LS, et al: Aneurysms of the membranous ventricular septum. A mechanism for spontaneous closure of ventricular septal defect. N Engl J Med 283:58, 1970

263. Mistrott JJ, Varco RL, Nicoloff DM: Palliation of infants with truncus arteriosus through creation of a pulmonary artery ostial stenosis. Ann Thorac Surg 22:495, 1976

264. Moerman PL, van Dijck H, Lawweryns JM, et al: Premature closure of the foramen ovale and congenital pulmonary cystic lymphangiectasis in aortic valve atresia or in severe aortic valve stenosis. Am J Cardiol 57:703, 1986

265. Moodie DS, Feldt RH, Wallace RB: Transient protein-losing enteropathy secondary to elevated caval pressures and caval obstruction after the Mustard procedure. J Thorac Cardiovasc Surg 72:379, 1976

266. Moodie DS, Tajik AJ, Ritter DG: The natural history of common (single) ventricle. Am J Cardiol 39:311, 1977

267. Morriss JH, McNamara DG: Residual, sequelae, and complications of surgery for congenital heart disease. Prog Cardiovasc Dis 18:1, 1975

268. Moss AJ: What every primary physician should know about the post-operative cardiac patient. Pediatrics 63:320, 1979

269. Moss AJ, Klyman G, Emmanouilides GC: Late onset complete heart block—A newly recognized sequelae of cardiac surgery. Am J Cardiol 30:659, 1972

270. Moulaert AJ, Bruins CC, Oppenheimer-Dekker A: Anomalies of the aortic arch and ventricular septal defects. Circulation 53:1011, 1976

271. Muller WH Jr, Dammann JF Jr: Treatment of certain congenital malformations by the creation of pulmonic stenosis to reduce pulmonary hypertension and excessive pulmonary blood flow. Preliminary report. Surg Gynecol Obstet 95:213, 1952

272. Murray GF, Herrington RT, Delany DJ: Tricuspid atresia: Corrective operation without a bioprosthetic valve. Ann Thorac Surg 23:209, 1977

273. Mustard WT: Successful two-stage correction of transportation of the great vessels. Surgery 55:469, 1964

274. Mustard WT: Baffle problems in transposition of the great arteries. p. 195. In Kidd BSL, Rowe RD (eds): The Child with Congenital Heart Disease after Surgery. Futura, Mt. Kisco, NY, 1976

275. Muster AJ, Paul MH, Van Grondelle A, Conway JJ: Abnormal distribution of the pulmonary blood flow between the two lungs in transposition of the great arteries. p. 165. In Kidd BSL, Rowe RD (eds): The Child with Congenital Heart Disease after Surgery. Futura, Mt. Kisco, NY, 1976

276. Muster AJ, Paul MH, Van Grondelle A, Con-

way JJ: Asymmetrical distribution of pulmonary blood flow between the right and left lungs in D-transposition of the great arteries. Am J Cardiol 38:352, 1976

277. Nadas AS: Clinical course. Summary and conclusions. Circulation 56(suppl I):70, 1977

278. Nadas AS, Scott LP, Hauck AJ, Rudolph AM: Spontaneous functional closing of ventricular septal defects. N Engl J Med 264:309, 1961

279. Neches WH, Naifeh JG, Park SC, et al: Systemic to pulmonary artery anastomoses in infancy. J Thorac Cardiovasc Surg 70:921, 1975

280. Neches WH, Park SC, Lenox CC, et al: Tricuspid atresia with transposition of the great arteries and closing ventricular septal defect: Sucessful surgical palliation by banding of the pulmonary artery and creation of an aorticopulmonary window. J Thorac Cardiovasc Surg 65:538, 1973

281. Newfeld EA, Muster AJ, Paul MH: Discrete subvalvular aortic stenosis in childhood. Study of 51 patients. Am J Cardiol 38:53, 1976

282. Newfeld EA, Waldman JD, Paul MH, et al: Pulmonary vascular disease after systemic to pulmonary arterial shunt operations. Am J Cardiol 39:715, 1977

283. Nixon JV, Atkins JM, Curry GC, et al: Late right ventricular failure after Mustard operation for transposition of the great arteries. Cath Cardiovasc Diagn 4:175, 1978

284. Noonan JA, Nadas AS: The hypoplastic left heart syndrome. An analysis of 101 cases. Pediatr Clin North Am 5:1029, 1958

285. Norberg WJ, Tadavarthy M, Knight L, et al: Late hemodynamic and angiographic findings after ascending aorta to pulmonary artery anastomoses. J Thorac Cardiovasc Surg 76:345, 1978

286. Norwood WI, Castaneda AR: Complications of the surgical repair of defects in the ventricular septum. p. 127. In Cordell AR, Ellison RG (eds): Complications of Intrathoracic Surgery. Little, Brown, Boston, 1979

287. Norwood WI, Freed MD, Rocchini AP, et al: Experience with valved conduits for repair of congenital cardiac lesions. Ann Thorac Surg 24:223, 1977

288. Norwood WI, Kirklin JK, Sanders SP: Hypoplastic left heart syndrome: Experience with palliative surgery. Am J Cardiol 45:87, 1980

289. Norwood WI, Lang P, Castaneda AR, Campbell DN: Experience with operations for hypoplastic left heart syndrome. J Thorac Cardiovasc Surg 82:511, 1981

290. Norwood WI, Lang P, Hansen DD: Physiologic repair of aortic atresia-hypoplastic left heart syndrome. New Engl J Med 308:23, 1983

291. Norwood WI, Pigott JD: Recent advances in congenital cardiac surgery. Clin Perinatol 15:713, 1988

292. Nugent EW, Freedom RM, Rowe RD, et al: Aneurysm of the membranous septum in ventricular septal defect. Circulation 56(suppl 1):82, 1977

293. O'Connor WN, Cash JB, Cottrill CM, et al: Ventriculocoronary connections in the hypoplastic left hearts: An autopsy microscopic study. Circulation 66:1078, 1982

294. O'Connor WN, Cottrill CM, Johnson GL, et al: Pulmonary atresia with intact ventricular septum and ventriculocoronary communications: Surgical significance. Circulation 65:805, 1982

295. O'Connor WN, Stahr BJ, Cottrill CM, et al: Ventriculocoronary connections in hypoplastic right heart syndrome: Autopsy serial section study of six cases. J Am Coll Cardiol 11:1961, 1988

296. Okoroma ED, Guller B, Maloney JD, Weidman WH: Etiology of right bundle branch block pattern after surgical closure of ventricular septal defects. Am Heart J 90:14, 1975

297. Olin CL, Ritter DG, McGoon DC, et al: Pulmonary atresia: Surgical considerations and results in 103 patients undergoing definitive repair. Circulation 56(suppl 3):35, 1976

298. Oppenheimer EH, Esterly JR: Some aspects of cardiac pathology in infancy and childhood. II. Unusual coronary endarteritis with congenital cardiac malformations. Johns Hopkins Bull 119:343, 1966

299. Parenzan L, Locatelli G, Alfieri O, Villani M, Invernizzi G: The Senning operation for transposition of the great arteries. J Thorac Cardiovasc Surg 76:305, 1978

300. Park SC, Neches WH, Lenox CC, Zuberbuhler JR, Bahnson HT: Massive calcification and obstruction in a Homograft after the Rastelli procedure for transposition of the great arteries. Am J Cardiol 32:860, 1973

301. Park SC, Neches WH, Zuberbuhler JR, Lenox CC, Mathews RA, Fricker FJ, Zoltan

RA: Clinical use of blade atrial septostomy. Circulation 58:600, 1978

302. Parr GVS, Kirklin JW, Pacifico AD, Blackstone EH, Lauridsen P: Cardiac performance in infants after repair of total anomalous pulmonary venous connections. Ann Thorac Surg 17:561, 1974

303. Patel RG, Freedom RM, Bloom KR, Rowe RD: Truncal or aortic valve stenosis in functionally single arterial trunk. A clinical, hemodynamic and pathologic study of six cases. Am J Cardiol 43:800, 1978

304. Patel R, Freedom RM, Moes CAF, et al: Right ventricular volume determinations in 18 patients with pulmonary atresia and intact ventricular septum. Analysis of factors influencing right ventricular growth. Circulation 61:428, 1980

305. Pearlman AS, Borer JS, Clark CE, et al: Abnormal right ventricular size and ventricular motion after atrial septal defect closure. Am J Cardiol 41:295, 1978

306. Perloff JK: Therapeutics of nature. The invisible suture of "spontaneous closure." Am Heart J 82:581, 1971

307. Perloff JK: Pediatric congenital cardiac becomes a post-operative adult. The changing population of congenital heart disease. Circulation 47:606, 1973

308. Perloff JK, Lindgren KM: Adult survival in congenital heart disease. Part I. Common defects with expected adult survival. Geriatrics 29:54, 1974

309. Pieroni DR, Strife JL, Donahoo JS, Korvetz LJ: Post-operative assessment of residual defects following cardiac surgery in infants and children. III. Atrial septal defects. Johns Hopkins BULL 133:287, 1973

310. Pigott JD, Murphy JD, Barber G, Norwood WI: Palliative reconstructive surgery for hypoplastic left heart syndrome. Ann Thorac Surg 45:122, 1988

311. Porter CJ, Vargo TA, McNamara DG, Cooley DA: Successful surgical correction of infradiaphragmatic total anomalous pulmonary venous return into the inferior vena cava. A fourteen year follow-up. J Thorac Cardiovasc Surg 75:68, 1978

312. Potts WJ, Smith S, Gibson S: Anastomosis of the aorta to a pulmonary artery. Certain types in congenital heart disease. JAMA 132:627, 1946

313. Puga FJ, Chiavarelli M, Hagler DJ: Modifications of the Fontan operation applicable to patients with left atrioventricular valve atresia or single atrioventricular valve. Circulation 76(suppl 3):53, 1987

314. Quaegebeur JM, Brom AG: The trousers-shaped baffle for use in the Mustard operation. Ann Thorac Surg 25:240, 1978

315. Quaegebeur JM, Rohmer J, Brom AG, Tinkelenberg J: Revival of the Senning operation in the treatment of transposition of the great arteries. Thorax 32:517, 1977

316. Quaegebeur JM, Rohmer J, Ottenkamp J, et al: The arterial switch operation. An eight year experience. J Thorac Cardiovasc Surg 92:361, 1986

317. Quattlebaum TG, Varghese PJ, Neill CA, Donahoo JS: Sudden death among post-operative patients with tetralogy of Fallot. Circulation 54:289, 1976

318. Quero-Jiminiz M, Cameron AH, Acerete F, Quero-Jiminiz C: Univentricular hearts: pathology of the atrioventricular valves. Herz 4:161, 1979

319. Quero-Jiminez M, Maitre Azcarate MJ, Alvarez Bejarno H, Vazquez Martul E: Tricuspid atresia. An anatomical study of 17 cases. Eur J Cardiol 3:337, 1975

320. Rao PS: Natural history of the ventricular septal defect in tricuspid atresia and its surgical implications. Br Heart J 39:276, 1977

321. Rashkind WJ, Miller WW: Creation of an atrial septal defect without thoracotomy: A palliative approach to complete transposition of the great arteries. JAMA 196:991, 1966

322. Rastelli GC: A new approach to "anatomic" repair of transposition of the great arteries. Mayo Clin Proc 44:1, 1969

323. Reitman MJ, Galioto FM Jr, El-Said GM, et al: Ascending aorta to right pulmonary artery anastomosis. Immediate results in 123 patients and one month to six year follow-up in 74 patients. Circulation 49:952, 1974

324. Reul GJ Jr, Coolley DA, Sandiford FM, Hallman GL: Complications following the contoured Dacron baffle in correction of transposition of the great arteries. Surgery 76:946, 1974

325. Ritter DG, Dushane JW: Long-term follow-up of operated patients with ventricular septal defect and pulmonary hypertension. p. 243. In Davila JC (ed): Second Henry Ford Hos-

pital International Symposium on Cardiac Surgery. Appleton-Century-Crofts, East Norwalk, CT, 1977

326. Rocchini AP, Keane JF, Freed MD, et al: Left ventricular function following attempted surgical repair of tetralogy of Fallot. Circulation 57:798, 1978

327. Rocchini AP, Rosenthal A, Castaneda AR, et al: Subaortic obstruction after the use of an intracardiac baffle to tunnel the left ventricle to the aorta. Circulation 54:957, 1976

328. Rocchini AP, Rosenthal A, Freed M, et al: Chronic congestive heart failure after repair of tetralogy of Fallot. Circulation 56:305, 1977

329. Rocchini AP, Rosenthal A, Keane JF, et al: Hemodynamics after surgical repair with right ventricle to pulmonary artery conduit. Circulation 54:951, 1976

330. Rosenthal AR, Gross RE, Pasternac A: Aneurysms of right ventricular outflow patches. J Thorac Cardiovasc Surg 63:735, 1972

331. Rosing DR, Borer JS, Kent KM, et al: Long-term hemodynamic and electrocardiographic assessment following operative repair of tetralogy of Fallot. Circulation 58(suppl I):209, 1978

332. Ross D, Rickards A, Somerville J: Transposition of the great arteries: logical anatomical arterial correction. Br Med J 1:1109, 1976

333. Ross DN, Somerville J: Surgical correction of tricuspid atresia. Lancet 1:845, 1973

334. Rossiter SJ, Silverman JF, Shumway NE: Patterns of pulmonary arterial supply in patients with truncus arteriosus. J Thorac Cardiovasc Surg 75:73, 1978

335. Rowlatt UF: Coronary artery distribution in complete transposition. JAMA 179:269, 1962

336. Ruzyllo W, Nihill MR, Mullins CE, McNamara DG: Hemodynamic evaluation of 221 patients after intracardiac repair of tetralogy of Fallot. Am J Cardiol 34:565, 1974

337. Saalouke MG, Rios J, Perry LW, et al: Electrophysiologic studies after Mustard's operation for D-transposition of the great vessels. Am J Cardiol 41:1104, 1978

338. Sansa M, Tonkin IL, Bargeron LM Jr, Elliott LD: Left ventricular outflow tract obstruction in transposition of the great arteries: An angiocardiographic study of 74 cases. Am J Cardiol 44:88, 1979

339. Sauer U, Bindl L, Pilossoff V, et al: Pulmonary atresia with intact ventricular septum

and right ventricle-coronary artery fistulae: Selection of patients for surgery. p. 566. In Doyle EF, Engle MA, Gersony WM, Rashkind WJ, Talner NS (eds): Pediatric Cardiology. Springer-Verlag, New York, 1986

340. Sauer U, Gittenberger-de Groot AC, et al: Coronary arteries in hypoplastic left heart syndrome: Histopathological and histometrical study, implications for surgery. Circulation 78(II):II-87, 1988 (abst)

341. Schott GD: Documentation of spontaneous functional closure of a ventricular septal defect during adult life. Br Heart J 35:1214, 1973

342. Senning A: Surgical correction of transposition of the great vessels. Surgery 45:966, 1959

343. Serratto M, Miller RA, Tatooles C, Ardekani R: Hemodynamic evaluation of Fontan operation in tricuspid atresia. Circulation 54(suppl 3):99, 1976

344. Setzer E, Ermocilla R, Tonkin I, et al: Papillary muscle necrosis in a neonatal autopsy population: Incidence and associated clinical manifestations. J Pediatr 96:289, 1980

345. Seybold-Epting W, Chiariello L, Hallman GL, Cooley DA: Aneurysm of pericardial right ventricular outflow tract patches. Ann Thorac Surg 24:237, 1977

346. Shah P, Singh WSA, Rose V, Keith JD: Incidence of bacterial endocarditis in ventricular septal defects. Circulation 32:127, 1966

347. Shaher RM: Complete Transposition of the Great Arteries. Academic Press, San Diego, 1973

348. Shaher RM, Pudou GC: Coronary arterial anatomy in complete transposition of the great vessels. Am J Cardiol 17:355, 1966

349. Sharatt GP, Johnson AM, Monro JL: Persistence and effects of sinus rhythm after Fontan procedure for tricuspid atresia. Br Heart J 42:74, 1979

350. Shrivastava S, Edwards JE: Coronary arterial origin in persistent truncus arteriosus. Am J Cardiol 55:551, 1977

351. Singh AK, de Leval MR, Pincott JR, Stark J: Pulmonary artery banding for truncus arteriosus in the first year of life. Circulation 54(suppl 3):17, 1976

352. Singh AK, Stark J, Taylor JFN: Left ventricle to pulmonary artery conduit in treatment of transposition of great arteries, restrictive ventricular septal defect, and acquired pulmonary atresia. Br Heart J 38: 1213, 1976

353. Sissman NJ, Abrams HL: Bidirectional shunting in a coronary artery—Right ventricular fistula associated with pulmonary atresia and an intact ventricular septum. Circulation 32:582, 1965

354. Somerville J: Congenital heart disease. Changes in form and function. Br Heart J 41:1, 1979

355. Somerville J: Changing form and function in one ventricle hearts. Herz 4:206, 1979

356. Somerville J, Beer L, Ross D: Common ventricle with acquired subaortic obstruction. Am J Cardiol 34:206, 1974

357. Stansel HC: A new operation for D-loop transposition of the great vessels. Ann Thorac Surg 19:565, 1975

358. Stark J, Gandhi D, de Leval M, et al: Surgical treatment of persistent truncus arteriosus in the first year of life. Br Heart J 40:1280, 1978

359. Stark J, Silove ED, Taylor JFN, Graham GR: Obstruction to systemic venous return following the Mustard operation for transposition of the great arteries. J Thorac Cardiovasc Surg 68:742, 1974

360. Stark J, Singh A, de Leval M, Taylor JFN: Early versus late Mustard operation for "simple" transposition of the great arteries. p. 195. In Kidd BSL, Rowe RD (eds): The Child With Congenital Heart Disease after Surgery. Futura, Mt. Kisco, NY, 1976

361. Steeg CN, Krongrad E, Davachi F, et al: Postoperative left anterior hemiblock and right bundle branch block following repair of tetralogy of Fallot. Clinical and etiologic considerations. Circulation 51:1026, 1979

362. Steinberg I: Diagnosis of congenital aneurysm of the ventricular septum during life. Br Heart J 19:8, 1957

363. Stellin G, Mazzucco A, Bortolotti U, et al: Tricuspid atresia versus other complex lesions. Comparison of results with a modified Fontan procedure. J Thorac Cardiovasc Surg 96:204, 1988

364. Sullivan H, Sulaman R, Replogle R, Arcilla RA: Surgical correction of truncus arteriosus in infancy. Am J Cardiol 38:113, 1976

365. Tabry IF, McGoon DC, Danielson GK, et al: Surgical management of straddling atrioventricular valve. J Thorac Cardiovasc Surg 77:191, 1979

366. Tandon R, Edwards JE: Aneurysm-like formation in relation to membranous ventricular septum. Circulation 47:1089, 1973

367. Tandon R, Edwards JE: Tricuspid atresia. A re-evaluation and classification. J Thorac Cardiovasc Surg 67:530, 1974

368. Tatooles CJ, Ardekani RG, Miller RA, Serratto M: Operative repair for tricuspid atresia. Ann Thorac Surg 21:499, 1976

369. Tatsuno K, Ronno S, Sakakibara S: Ventricular septal defect with aortic regurgitation. Angiocardiographic aspects and a new classification. Am Heart J 85:13, 1973

370. Tay DJ, Engle MA, Enhlers KH, Levin AR: Early results and late developments of the Waterston anastomosis. Circulation 50:220, 1974

371. Trusler GA: Complications of atrial partitioning for transposition of the great arteries. p. 153. In Cordell AR, Ellison RG (eds): Complications of Intrathoracic Surgery. Little, Brown, Boston, 1979

372. Trusler GA, Miyamura H, Culham JAG, et al: Pulmonary artery stenosis following aortopulmonary anastomoses. J Thorac Cardiovasc Surg 82:398, 1981

373. Trusler GA, Mulholland HC, Takeuchi Y, et al: Longterm results of intra-atrial repair of transposition of the great arteries. p. 368. In Davila JC (ed): Second Henry Ford Hospital International Symposium on Cardiac Surgery. Appleton-Century-Crofts, East Norwalk, CT, 1977

374. Trusler G, Mustard WT: Palliative and reparative procedures for transposition of the great arteries. Ann Thorac Surg 17:410, 1974

375. Turley K, Ebert PA: Total correction of transposition of the great arteries. Conduction disturbances in infants younger than three months of age. J Thorac Cardiovasc Surg 76:312, 1978

376. Tynan M, Aberdeen E, Stark J: Tricuspid incompetence after the Mustard operation for transposition of the great arteries. Circulation 51, 52(suppl I):111, 1972

377. Ueda K, Saito A, Nakano H, Hamazaki Y: Absence of proximal coronary arteries associated with pulmonary atresia. Am Heart J 106:596, 1983

378. Uhl HMS: Previously undescribed congenital malformation of the heart: Almost total absence of the myocardium of the right ventricle. Johns Hopkins Bull 91:197, 1953

379. Van Den Bogaert-Van Heesvelde AM, Derom F, Kunnen M, et al: Surgery for arteriovenous fistulas and dilated vessels in the right lung after the Glenn procedure. J Thorac Cardiovasc Surg 76:195, 1978

380. Van Praagh R: Classification of truncus arteriosus communis (TAC). Am Heart J 92:129, 1976

381. Van Praagh R, McNamara JJ: Anatomic type of ventricular septal defect with aortic insufficiency. Am Heart J 75:604, 1968

382. Van Praagh R, Plett JA, Van Praagh S: Single ventricle. Pathology, embryology, terminology and classification. Herz 4:113, 1979

383. Van Praagh R, Van Praagh S: The anatomy of common aorticopulmonary trunk (truncus arteriosus communis) and its embryologic implications. A study of 57 necropsy cases. Am J Cardiol 16:406, 1965

384. Van Praagh R, Visner MS: Postoperative pathology of congenital heart disease. Am J Cardiol 38:225, 1976

385. Van Praagh R: Discussion. In First World Congress of Pediatric Cardiac Surgery, Bergamo, June 1989

386. Varghese PJ, Allen JR, Rosenquist GC, Rowe RD: Natural history of ventricular septal defect with right sided aortic arch. Br Heart J 32:537, 1970

387. Varghese PJ, Rowe RD: Spontaneous closure of ventricular septal defects by aneurysmal formation of the membranous septum. J Pediatr 75:700, 1969

388. Venables AW, Edis B, Clarke CP: Vena caval obstruction complicating the Mustard operation for complete transposition of the great arteries. Eur J Cardiol 1:401, 1974

389. Vetter VL, Rashkind WJ, Waldhausen JA: Ascending aorta to right pulmonary artery anastomoses in 137 patients with cyanotic congenital heart disease. J Thorac Cardiovasc Surg 76:115, 1978

390. Vidne BA, Duxzynski D, Subramanian S: Pulmonary flow distribution in transposition of the great arteries. Am J Cardiol 37:178, 1976

391. Wanderman KL, Ovsyshcher I, Gueron M: Left ventricular performance in patients with atrial septal defect: Evaluation with non-invasive methods. Am J Cardiol 41:487, 1978

392. Waterston DJ: Treatment of Fallot's tetralogy in children under one year of age. Rozhl Chir 41:181, 1962

393. Watson H, McArthur P, Somerville J, Ross

D: Spontaneous evaluation of ventricular septal defect into isolated pulmonary stenosis. Lancet 2:1225, 1969

394. Wearn JT, Mettier SR, Klumpp TG, Zschiesche LJ: The nature of the vascular communications between the coronary arteries and the chambers of the heart. Am Heart J 9:143, 1933

395. Weidman WH, Blount SG Jr, Dushane JW, et al: Clinical course in ventricular septal defect. Circulation 56(suppl I):56, 1977

396. Weidman WH, Dushane JW, Ellison RC: Clinical course in adults with ventricular septal defect. Circulation 56(suppl I):178, 1977

397. Wenink ACG, Sauer U, Gittenberger-de Groot AC: The ventricular septum in the hypoplastic left heart syndrome. Pediatr Cardiol 4:82, 1983 (abst)

398. Whight CM, Barratt-Boyes BG, Calder AL, et al: Total anomalous pulmonary venous connection. Longterm results following repair in infancy. J Thorac Cardiovasc Surg 75:52, 1978

399. Whilkinson JL, Becker AE, Tynan M, et al: Nomenclature of univentricular heart. Herz 4:107, 1979

400. Whitman V, Ellis NG: Pulmonary hemodynamics after repair of left to right shunt lesions associated with pulmonary artery hypertension. Prog Cardiovasc Dis 17:467, 1975

401. Williams RR, Kent GB Jr, Edwards JE: Anomalous cardiac blood vessel communicating with the right ventricle. Arch Pathol 52:480, 1951

402. Williams WG, Rubis L, Fowler RS, et al: Tricuspid atresia: Results in 160 children. Am J Cardiol 38:235, 1976

403. Williams WG, Rubis L, Trusler GA, Mustard WT: Palliation of tricuspid atresia. Arch Surg 110:1383, 1975

404. Wolff GS, Rowland TW, Ellison RC: Surgically induced right bundle branch block with left anterior hemiblock. Circulation 46:587, 1972

405. Wood P: The Eisenmenger syndrome or pulmonary artery hypertension with reversed central shunt. Br Med J 2:701, 1958

406. Wukash DC, Deutsch M, Reul GJ, et al: Total anomalous pulmonary venous return: Review of 125 patients treated surgically. Ann Thorac Surg 19:622, 1975

407. Wyse RKH, Haworth SG, Taylor JFN, Macartney FJ: Obstruction of superior vena caval pathway after Mustard's repair. Reliable di-

agnosis by transcutaneous Doppler ultrasound. Br Heart J 42:167, 1979

408. Yacoub MH: Fontan's operation—Are caval valves necessary? p. 581. In Anderson RH, Shinebourne EA (eds): Paediatric Cardiology, 1977. Churchill Livingstone, Edinburgh, 1978

409. Yacoub MH: The case for anatomic correction of transposition of the great arteries. J Thorac Cardiovasc Surg 78:5, 1979

410. Yacoub MH, Radley-Smith R: The use of a valved conduit from right atrium to pulmonary artery for "creation" of single ventricle. Circulation 54 (suppl III):63, 1976

411. Yacoub M, Radley-Smith R: The use of the Fontan procedure for treatment of single ventricle. p. 396. In Anderson RH, Shinebourne EA (eds): Paediatric Cardiology, 1977. Churchill Livingstone, Edinburgh, 1978

412. Yasui H, Takeda Y, Yamauchi S, et al: The deterious effects of surgically induced complete right bundle branch block on longterm follow-up results of closure of ventricular septal defect. J Thorac Cardiovasc Surg 74:210, 1977

413. Young D: Later results of closure of secundum atrial septal defect in children. Am J Cardiol 31:14, 1973

Index

Page numbers followed by f indicate figures; those followed by t indicate tables.

A

Abdominal angina, due to atherosclerosis, 409

Abdominal apoplexy, 369–370

Abetalipoproteinemia
  cardiovascular findings in, 1108
  dilated cardiomyopathy in, 756

Abscess
  annular, in infective endocarditis, 910, 913f–914f
    natural valve and, 913
    prosthetic valve and, 910, 913f, 1514f, 1514–1515
  of brain
    in congenital heart disease, 1052
    in infective endocarditis, 1039
  of mitral valve, 913, 914f
  of myocardium
    complicating myocardial infarction, 701
    in infective endocarditis, 914, 915f

Absent spleen syndrome, cardiovascular anomalies in, 1130t

Acid maltase deficiency, 1073

Aciduria
  L-glyceric, 1084
  glycolic, 1084

Acquired immune deficiency syndrome. *See* AIDS.

Acrocyanosis, 366

Acromegaly, 1181–1183
  cardiomegaly in, 1181–1182, 1182f
  cardiomyopathy in, 1181–1183, 1182f–1183f
    coronary arteriole intimal and medial fibromuscular hyperplasia in, 1182, 1183f
    interstitial fibrous tissue increase in, 1182, 1182f
    left ventricular hypertrophy in, 1182
    sudden death in, 1182
  diagnosis of, 1182–1183

Actin filament(s)
  of endothelial cells, 106
    in atherogenesis, 236, 249
    in vascular repair processes, 248, 248f
    shear stress effects on, 142f, 143
  of smooth muscle cells, 110f–112f, 111, 239
    in atherogenesis, 252

Acyl-Co-A-dehydrogenase deficiency, dilated cardiomyopathy in, 757

Addison's disease, 1190–1191
  causes of, 1190–1191
  heart size in, 1191
  hypotension in, 1191
  metabolic abnormalities in, 1191

in vasculitis
  with cryoglobulinemia, 460
  hypersensitivity, 458–462
  radiation, 462
  with systemic disease, 460
in Whipple's disease, 467
in *Yersinia pestis* infection, 467
Smith-Lemli-Opitz syndrome, 1130t
Smoking. *See* Cigarette smoking.
Smooth muscle cell(s), 108–113. *See also*
        Myocyte(s).
  actin (thin, micro-) filaments of, 110f–112f,
        111, 239
    in atherogenesis, 252
  in aortic media, 271
  in arterial intima, 126
  in arterial media, 126
  in atherogenesis, 238t, 238–239, 249–252,
        250f–251f
  in atherosclerotic plaque, 233, 234f
  cell membrane and external lamina of, 112
  collagen bridge artifact of, 112f, 112–113
  endocytotic structures of, 111, 111f–112f
  filaments of, 110f–112f, 111–112
  gap junctions of, 112f, 112–113
  general features of, 108–111, 109f–111f
  glycogen in, 108
  lipid droplets in, 108
    in fatty streaks, 274–275
  lipofuscin granules of, 108
  micropinocytotic vesicles in, 108, 111f–112f
  myosin (thick) filaments of, 111–112
  subplasmalemmal densities of, 111, 111f
  transformation into foam cells of, 233
  ultrastructure of, 74–76, 75f
  vascular
    contractile-state, 239
    injury response of, 239
    normal function of, 238t, 238–239
    synthetic-state, 239
  vimentin (intermediate, desmin) filaments of,
        112
    in atherogenesis, 252
Socioeconomic group, ischemic heart disease and,
        674
Sodium azide, dilated cardiomyopathy due to,
        755t, 763
Soldier's (milk) patch
  in chronic pericarditis, 882
  epicardial, 7
  pericardial, 854f
SPARC, endothelial cell secretion of, 240

Spasm
  arterial, 414–415
  coronary artery, 414–415
    in angina pectoris, 678–679
    in floppy mitral valve syndrome, 415
    ischemic heart disease and, 551
    in myocardial infarction, 676–677
    in nitrate withdrawal, 414
    in small arteries, 589
Spermatic cord, varicocele of, 203
Spherical microparticles, 120, 121f–122f
  in arteries, 120
  in heart, 121
Sphingolipidoses, 1109–1112
Spider cells, in rhabdomyoma, 1314, 1315f
Spinal cord
  arteriovenous fistula of, congenital, 344
  ischemia of
    due to abdominal aortic aneurysm surgery,
        294
    cardiovascular causes of, 1059
Spinal muscular atrophy, juvenile
  cardiovascular findings in, 1127
  dilated cardiomyopathy in, 757
Spirinolactone, hypersensitivity vasculitis due to,
        1223t
Spleen
  absent, cardiovascular anomalies in, 1130t
  arteriosclerosis of, hyaline, 406–407,
        407f
Splenic artery, aneurysms of, 357
Spondylitis, ankylosing
  aortic incompetence in, 1014, 1018, 1159,
        1162f, 1162–1163
  etiology of, 1153
  HLA-B27 in, 1153
  mitral incompetence in, 1162
  valvular stretch lesions of, 182
St. Jude Medical prosthesis, 1491f
Stab wound trauma, 1335, 1336f
Stains, histologic, 33
Staphylococcal endocarditis, 920
Staphylococcal pericarditis, 869
Starr-Edwards 1200 ball valve prosthesis, 1492f
Starvation
  severe, 1120–1121
  therapeutic, 1121
Steatosis, dilated cardiomyopathy and, 757
Steinert's disease, 1122
Stenosis. *See under individual anatomic types.*
Stent(s), arterial, 1745–1746, 1746f–1747f
Stenting, biologic, 1749–1751, 1750f–1751f